WR 544

D0717612

Contemporary Targeted Therapies in Rheumatology

Contemporary Targeted Therapies in Rheumatology

Edited by

Josef S Smolen MD
Medical University of Vienna and
Hietzing Hospital
Vienna, Austria

Peter E Lipsky MD
Bethesda, MD
USA

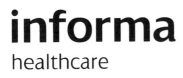

informa
healthcare

© 2007 Informa UK Ltd

First published in the United Kingdom in 2007 by Informa Healthcare,
Telephone House, 69-77 Paul Street, London EC2A 4LQ.
Informa Healthcare is a trading division of Informa UK Ltd.
Registered Office: 37/41 Mortimer Street, London W1T 3JH.
Registered in England and Wales number 1072954.

Tel: +44 (0)20 7017 5000
Fax: +44 (0)20 7017 6699
Website: www.informahealthcare.com

Second printing 2007

Although every effort has been made to ensure that all owners of copyright material have been acknowledged in this publication, we would be glad to acknowledge in subsequent reprints or editions any omissions brought to our attention.

Although every effort has been made to ensure that drug doses and other information are presented accurately in this publication, the ultimate responsibility rests with the prescribing physician. Neither the publishers nor the authors can be held responsible for errors or for any consequences arising from the use of information contained herein. For detailed prescribing information or instructions on the use of any product or procedure discussed herein, please consult the prescribing information or instructional material issued by the manufacturer.

A CIP record for this book is available from the British Library.
Library of Congress Cataloging-in-Publication Data

Data available on application

ISBN-10: 1 84184 484 5
ISBN-13: 978 1 84184 484 8

Distributed in North and South America by
Taylor & Francis
6000 Broken Sound Parkway, NW, (Suite 300)
Boca Raton, FL 33487, USA

Within Continental USA
Tel: 1 (800) 272 7737; Fax: 1 (800) 374 3401
Outside Continental USA
Tel: (561) 994 0555; Fax: (561) 361 6018
Email: orders@crcpress.com

Distributed in the rest of the world by
Thomson Publishing Services
Cheriton House
North Way
Andover, Hampshire SP10 5BE, UK
Tel: +44 (0)1264 332424
Email: tps.tandfsalesorder@thomson.com

Composition by Cepha Imaging Pvt. Ltd, Bangalore, India.
Printed and bound in India by Replika Press Pvt Ltd

Contents

Section III - Transcription factors and signaling molecules

Section IV - Inflammatory mediators and matrix molecules

Section V - Targeted therapies in human and experimental rheumatic diseases

Contributors

Daniel Aletaha MD
Medical University of Vienna
Vienna, Austria

Gunnar Alm MD PhD
Department of Biomedical Sciences and
Veterinary Public Health
Swedish University of Agricultural Sciences
Uppsala, Sweden

William P Arend MD
Division of Rheumatology
University of Colorado Health Sciences Center
Denver CO, USA

Dolores Baksh PhD
National Institute of Arthritis, and
Musculoskeletal and Skin Diseases
Bethesda, MD, USA

Bradley J Bloom MD
Clinical Research and Development
Pfizer Global Research and Development
New London, CT, USA

Jürgen Braun MD
Rheumazentrum Ruhrgebiet
Herne, Germany

Ferdinand C Breedveld MD PhD
Leiden University Medical Center Department
of Rheumatology
C1-R
RC, Leiden
The Netherlands

Michael B Brenner MD PhD
Harvard Medical School
Division of Rheumatology
Immunology and Allergy
Boston, MA, USA

Damien Bresson PhD
La Jolla Institute for Allergy and Immunology
Developmental Immunology
La Jolla, CA, USA

Constantinos Brikos MD
Trinity College Dublin
School of Biochemistry and Immunology
Dublin, Ireland

Keith Brown PhD
National Institute of Allergy and Infectious
Diseases
Laboratory of Immunoregulation
Bethesda, MD, USA

Danielle Burger MD
University Hospital
Clinical Immunology Unit
Division of Immunology and Allergy
Geneva, Switzerland

Leonard H Calabrese DO
Cleveland Clinic Foundation
Department of Rheumatic and Immunologic
Diseases
Cleveland, OH, USA

John C Cambier PhD
University of Colorado Health Sciences Center
and National Jewish Medical Research Center
Integrated Department of Immunology
Denver, CO, USA

Paul Changelian PhD
Pfizer Global Research and Development
New London, CT, USA

Brenda J Classon PhD
Bristol-Myers Squibb
Pharmaceutical Research Institute
Princeton, NJ, USA

Estefania Claudio PhD
National Institute of Allergy and Infectious
Diseases
Laboratory of Immunoregulation
National Institutes of Health
Bethesda, MD, USA

Mary Collins PhD
Wyeth Research
Immunology/RA/MS Inflammation
Cambridge, MA, USA

Sally Cox MD
Chapel Allerton Hospital
Academic Unit of Musculoskeletal Disease
Chapel Allerton
Leeds, UK

Leslie J Crofford MD
Kentucky Clinic
Department of Internal Medicine
Rheumatology Division University of Kentucky
Lexington, KY, USA

John J Cush MD PhD
Southwestern Medical School
Division of Rheumatology
University of Texas
Dallas, Tx, USA

Jean-Michel Dayer MD
University Hospital
Faculty of Medicine
Division of Immunology and Allergy
Department of Internal Medicine
Geneva, Switzerland

Charles A Dinarello MD
University of Colorado Health Sciences Center
Department of Medicine
Division of Infectious Diseases
Denver, CO, USA

Stefan K Drexler PhD
Kennedy Institute of Rheumatology Division
Faculty of Medicine
Imperial College of Science
London, UK

Paul John Egan MSc PhD
Walter and Eliza Hall Institute of Medical
Research
Parkville
Victoria, Australia

Maija-Leena Eloranta PhD
Department of Medical Sciences
Uppsala University
Uppsala, Sweden

Paul Emery MA MD FRCP
Chapel Allerton Hospital
Academic Unit of Musculoskeletal Disease
Leeds, UK

Gary S Firestein MD
University of California San Diego School of
Medicine
Division of Rheumatology
Allergy and Immunology
La Jolla, CA, USA

Marc Feldmann FMEDSCI FAA FRS
Head Kennedy Institute of Rheumatology
Division
Imperial College London
London, UK

Brian M Foxwell BSc PhD DSc FRCPATH
Kennedy Institute of Rheumatology Division
Faculty of Medicine
Imperial College London
London, UK

Cem Gabay MD PhD
University Hospital of Geneva
Division of Rheumatology
Geneva, Switzerland

Stephen Gauld
University of Colorado Health Sciences Center
and National Jewish Medical Research Center
Integrated Department of Immunology
Denver, CO, USA

Steffen Gay MD PhD
University Hospital Zürich
Department of Rheumatology
Zurich, Switzerland

J Alastair Gracie BSc PhD
Centre for Rheumatic Diseases and Department
of Immunology
Infection and Inflammation Faculty of Medicine
University of Glasgow, UK
Glasgow, UK

Amrie Grammer PhD
National Institute of Arthritis, and
Musculoskeletal and Skin Diseases
Intramural Research Program
Bethesda, MD, USA

Ellen M Gravallese MD PhD
Harvard Medical School
Beth Israel Deaconess Medical Center
Harvard Institutes of Medicine
Boston, MA, USA

Bevra Hannahs Hahn MD
UCLA David Geffen School of Medicine
Division of Rheumatology
Los Angeles, CA, USA

Gary S Hoffman MD MS
Cleveland Clinic Foundation
Cleveland Clinic Lerner College of Medicine
Lerner College of Medicine, Department of
Rheumatic and Immunologic Diseases
Cleveland, OH, USA

Michael Holers MD
University of Colorado at Denver and Health
Sciences Center
Division of Rheumatology
Aurora, CO, USA

David A Isenberg MD FRCP
Arthritis Research Campaign
University College London
London, UK

Joachim R Kalden MD
University of Erlangen-Nuremberg
Institute of Clinical Immunology
Department of Internal Medicine
Erlangen, Germany

Mohit Kapoor MD
Kentucky Clinic, Department of Internal Medicine
Rheumatology Division
University of Kentucky
Lexington, KY, USA

Marion T Kasaian PhD
Wyether Research
Respiratory Diseases Wyeth
Cambridge, MA, USA

Arthur Kavanaugh MD
Professor of Medicine
Center for Innovative Therapy
Division of Rheumatology
Allergy and Immunology
La Jolla, CA, USA

Soo-Hyun Kim
Division of Infectious Diseases
University of Colorado Health Sciences Center
Denver, Co, USA

Tadamitsu Kishimoto MD
Osaka University
Graduate School of Frontier Biosciences
Osaka, Japan

Alisa Erika Koch MD
University of Michigan Health System
Department of Internal Medicine
Division of Rheumatology
Ann Arbor, MI, USA

Fumiaki Kojima MD
Institute of Medical Science
St Marianna University School of Medicine
Kawasaki, Japan

Carol A Langford MD MHS FACP
Cleveland Clinic Foundation
Department of Rheumatic and Immunologic
Diseases Cleveland, OH, USA

Sonwoo Lee MD
UCLA
David Geffen School of Medicine
Division of Rheumatology
Los Angeles, CA, USA

Warren J Leonard MD
National Heart, Lung, and Blood Institute
Laboratory of Molecular Immunology
Bethesda, MD, USA

Foo Y Liew MD
Centre for Rheumatic Diseases and Department
of Immunology
Infection and Inflammation Faculty of Medicine
University of Glasgow
Glasgow, UK

Peter E Lipsky MD
Bethesda, MD
USA

Thomas A Luger MD PhD
University of Münster
Department of Dermatology
Münster, Germany

Viviana Lutzky BSc PhD
Diamantina Institute
University of Queensland
Princess Alexandra Hospital
Brisbane, Queensland
Australia

Sir Ravinder N Maini FRCP FMedSci FRS
Emeritus Professor of Rheumatology
Kennedy Institute of Rheumatology Division
Imperial College London
London, UK

Iain B McInnes FRCP PhD
Glasgow Royal Infirmary
Centre for Rheumatic Diseases and Department
of Immunology Infection and Inflammation
Faculty of Medicine
Glasgow, UK

Philip J Mease MD
Swedish Rheumatology Research
Seattle, WA, USA

Kevin Merrell MD
University of Colorado Health Sciences Center
and National Jewish Medical Research Center
Integrated Department of Immunology
Denver, CO, USA

Pierre Miossec MD PhD
University Claude Bernard of Lyon
Department of Immunology and Rheumatology
Hospital Edouard Herriot
Lyon, France

Anthony Milici MD
Pfizer Global Research and Development
New London, CT, USA

Frederick W Miller MD PhD
National Institute of Environmental Health
Sciences
National Institutes of Health HHS
Bethesda, MD, USA

Nicolas Molnarfi MD
University Hospital
Division of Immunology and Allergy
Clinical Immunology Unit
Department of Internal Medicine
Geneva, Switzerland

Haralampos M Moutsopoulos MD FACP
FRCP(Edin)
National University of Athens
School of Medicine
Department of Pathophysiology
Athens, Greece

Gillian Murphy PhD
University of Cambridge
Cambridge Institute for Medical Research
Department of Oncology
Cambridge, UK

Steven G Nadler PhD
Bristol-Myers Squibb
Pharmaceutical Research Institute
Princeton, NJ, USA

Hideaki Nagase MD
Kennedy Institute of Rheumatology Division
Imperial College London
London, UK

Norihiro Nishimoto MD
Osaka University
Graduate School of Frontier Biosciences
Osaka, Japan

Kristine P Ng MBBS BSc (MED) FRACP
University College London
Centre for Rheumatology
University College Hospital
London, UK

Erika H Noss MD PhD
Harvard Medical School
Division of Rheumatology
Immunology and Allergy Brigham and
Women's Hospital
Boston, MA, USA

Esra Nutku-Bilir MD
University of Colorado Health Sciences Center
and National Jewish Medical Research Center
Integrated Department of Immunology
Denver, CO, USA

Luke AJ O'Neill PhD
Trinity College School of Biochemistry and
Immunology
Dublin, Ireland

Andrew Parker MD
AstraZeneca, Respiratory and Inflammation
Research, Macclesfield
Cheshire, UK

Thomas Pap MD PhD
University Hospital Munster
Division of Molecular Medicine of
Musculoskeletal Tissue
Munster, Germany

Allison Robyn Pettit PhD
Institute for Molecular Bioscience
QBP University of Queensland
Brisbane, Australia

Aimee E Pugh-Bernard MD
University of Colorado Health Sciences Center
and National Jewish Medical Research Center
Integrated Department of Immunology
Denver, CO, USA

Kurt Redlich MD
Medical University of Vienna, Division of
Rheumatology
Vienna, Austria

Lars Edvard Rönnblom MD PhD
Uppsala University Hospital
Section of Rheumatology
Uppsala University
Uppsala, Sweden

Kathleen T Rousche PhD
National Institute of Arthritis
Musculoskeletal and Skin Diseases
Cartilage Biology and Orthopaedics Branch
National Institutes of Health
Bethesda, MD, USA

Jane E Salmon MD
Weill Medical College of Cornell University
Hospital for Special Surgery
New York, NY, USA

Georg Schett MD PhD
University of Erlangen-Nuremberg
Institute for Clinical Immunology
Erlangen, Germany

Hendrik Schulze-Koops MD PhD
University of Munich
Division of Rheumatology
Munich, Germany

Edgar Serfling MD
Institute of Pathology
Department of Molecular Pathology
Würzburg, Germany

Ulrich K Siebenlist PhD
National Institute of Allergy and Infectious
Diseases
Laboratory of Immunoregulation
National Institutes of Health
Bethesda, MD, USA

Joachim Sieper MD
Universit Medicine Charité
Berlin
Medical Department I
Rheumatology
Berlin, Germany

Josef S Smolen MD
Medical University of Vienna and Hietzing
Hospital
Vienna, Austria

Rosanne Spolski PhD
National Institute of Allergy and Infectious
Diseases
Laboratory of Molecular Immunology
National Institutes of Health
Bethesda, MD, USA

William Stohl MD PhD
University of Southern California
Division of Rheumatology
Los Angeles, CA, USA

Suzanne J Suchard PhD
Bristol-Myers Squibb
Pharmaceutical Research Institute
Princeton, NJ, USA

Susan E Sweeney MD PhD
University of California
San Diego School of Medicine
Rheumatology
Allergy, and Immunology
La Jolla, CA, USA

Zoltán Szekanecz MD PhD
University of Debrecen Medical and Health
Sciences Center
Division of Rheumatology
Debrecen, Hungary

Ranjeny Thomas MBBS MD FRACP
Diamantina Institute
University of Queensland
Princess Alexandra Hospital
Brisbane, Australia

Myew-Ling Toh MD PhD
Hôpital Edouard Herriot
Department of Immunology and Rheumatology
Lyon, France

Rocky S Tuan MD PhD
National Institute of Arthritis
Musculoskeletal and Skin Diseases Cartilage
Biology and Orthopaedics Branch
National Institutes of Health Bethesda MD,
USA

Jeremy JO Turner MBBS BSc DPHIL MRCP
Imperial College London
Faculty of Medicine
Division of Investigative Science
London, UK

Wim B Van Den Berg PhD
Radboud University Nijmegen Medical Centre
Rheumatology Research Laboratory
Nijmegen, The Netherlands

Peter van Lent PhD
Radboud University Nijmegen Medical Centre
Rheumatology Research Laboratory
Nijmegen, The Netherlands

Harald von Boehmer MD PhD
Harvard Medical School
Dana-Farber Cancer Institute
Boston, MA, USA

Matthias von Herrath MD PhD
La Jolla Institute for Allergy and Immunology
Developmental Immunology
La Jolla, CA, USA

Michael Voulgarelis MD
National University of Athens
Department of Pathophysiology
School of Medicine
Athens, Greece

Ian Peter Wicks MBBS FRACP PhD
Walter and Eliza Hall Institute of Medical
Research
Reid Rheumatology Laboratory
Parkville, Australia

PKK Wong MBBS FRACP PhD
Royal Melbourne Hospital
Department of Rheumatology
Victoria, Australia

Patricia Woo PhD
Windeyer Institute of Medical Sciences
Centre for Paediatric and Adolescent
Rheumatology
London, UK

Sam Zwillich MD
Pfizer Global Research and Development
New London, CT, USA

Saloua Zrioual
Hôpital Edouard Herriot
Department of Immunology and Rheumatology
Lyon, France

1

T cells – overview – update

Hendrik Schulze-Koops and Joachim R Kalden

Introduction • Lymphopenia and autoimmunity • T-cell-directed therapy by immunosuppressive drugs • T-cell-directed therapy with biologicals • T-cell-directed therapy by blocking T-cell costimulation • T-cell-directed therapy by blocking T-cell migration • T-cell-directed therapy with statins • T-Cell-directed therapy in non-rheumatic diseases • Conclusion • Acknowledgment • References

INTRODUCTION

Because of the central role that CD4[+] T cells play in the pathogenesis of autoimmune diseases, different T-cell-directed therapies were introduced for the treatment of autoimmune rheumatic diseases. The initial approaches that aimed to ameliorate inflammatory activity by reducing T-cell numbers, however, provided only modest and inconsistent clinical benefit. Compounds that specifically interfere with T-cell activation – such as some of the disease-modifying anti-rheumatic drugs currently used as standard therapy in rheumatic inflammation – are clinically effective in a majority of patients, but are still associated with a number of side effects related to toxicity and general immunosuppression. Owing to the substantially increased knowledge of cellular and molecular mechanisms of the pathogenesis of rheumatic diseases and the increased understanding of molecular and cellular biology, molecules (biologicals) can now be specifically designed to exclusively target only those cells perpetuating the chronic inflammation, with minimal effects on other aspects of the immune or inflammatory systems. Various T-cell-directed biologicals have been employed in rheumatic diseases with different clinical successes. This chapter updates the currently available clinical data on T-cell-directed interventions in rheumatic diseases.

T cells are central for both the induction and the effector phases of specific immune responses in autoimmune diseases. Of particular importance for initiating, controlling, and driving inflammatory autoimmune responses are CD4[+] T cells that, once activated, determine to a large extent the outcome of immune reactions by activating different effector functions of the immune system. Thus, T cells and in particular CD4[+] T cells represent an ideal target for immunotherapy in diseases driven by specific immunity to autologous antigens.

LYMPHOPENIA AND AUTOIMMUNITY

However, initial T-cell-directed therapies that were designed to control disease progression by means of reducing the number of T cells, for example, by total lymphoid irradiation or thoracic duct drainage,[1–3] have provided only modest and inconsistent clinical benefit and have been associated with a number of side effects. It became obvious from these approaches that the generation of T-cell lymphopenia is insufficient to combat established autoimmune responses. Moreover, numerous studies have subsequently shown that manipulations that generate functional T-cell lymphopenia in animals result in the development of a variety of organ-specific autoimmune disease in these models.[4] Impressive examples of such manipulations include the interleukin (IL)-2 knockout (KO) mouse, that develops prominent autoimmune colitis,[5] the T-cell receptor (TCR) α-chain deficient mice which develop inflammatory bowel disease associated with an array of autoantibodies,[6,7] TCR-α chain transgenic mice,[8] neonatal application of cytotoxic intervention protocols, such as cyclosporin A,[9] total lymphoid irradiation[10] or thymectomy,[11] and lymphotoxic treatment of adult animals.[12] Further studies revealed that the development of autoimmunity was critically dependent on α/β CD4+ T cells, indicating that lymphopenia promotes the induction of autoimmune inflammation by self-reactive peripheral blood CD4 T cells in these animals. In fact, it could be demonstrated that the peripheral T-cell population that emerged in mice in which lymphopenia was induced by cytotoxic treatment with cyclophosphamide or streptozotocin, preferentially consisted of interferon (IFN)-γ secreting pro-inflammatory Th1-like cells.[13] Although lymphopenia is not sufficient for the development of autoimmune diseases in humans,[14] it is conceivable that lymphopenia in patients with existing autoimmune diseases permits the homeostatic expansion of autoreactive T cells, thereby resulting in the reappearance of autoimmune inflammation and, thus, the reoccurrence of clinically overt autoimmune phenomena.

T-CELL-DIRECTED THERAPY BY IMMUNOSUPPRESSIVE DRUGS

Owing to the significant advances in the understanding of T-cell biology, compounds were designed in recent years that specifically interfere with T-cell activation without reducing T-cell numbers. Cyclosporin A and FK506 (tacrolimus), for example, inhibit T-cell activation by interfering with calcineurin-mediated transcriptional activation of a number of cytokine genes, such as IL-2, IL-3, IL-4, IL-8, and IFN-γ. Leflunomide, a potent non-cytotoxic inhibitor of the key enzyme of the *de novo* synthesis of uridine monophosphate,[15] dihydro-orotate dehydrogenase, blocks clonal expansion and terminal differentiation of T cells as activated T cells critically depend on the *de novo* pyrimidine synthesis to fulfill their metabolic needs. These compounds are clinically

effective in ameliorating autoimmune inflammation and are important components of the current therapeutic repertoire in autoimmune diseases. It is of interest to note that besides the established ability of some of these so-called disease-modifying anti-rheumatic drugs (DMARDs), such as cyclosporine, FK506, or leflunomide, to directly inhibit T-cell activation, many DMARDs have been associated with a shift in the balance of proinflammatory Th1 cells to immunomodulatory Th2 cells.[1,16] This immunomodulatory effect might contribute to the beneficial therapeutic potential of DMARDs in inflammatory autoimmune diseases that reflect ongoing inflammation largely mediated by activated proinflammatory Th1 cells without the sufficient differentiation of immunoregulatory Th2 cells to down-modulate inflammation, such as rheumatoid arthritis (RA).[17–20]

T-CELL-DIRECTED THERAPY WITH BIOLOGICALS

Despite the progress that has been made in the treatment of rheumatic diseases, standard immunosuppressive therapy (even if T-cell-directed) is still clinically ineffective in many patients and is associated with a number of side effects related to toxicity and general immunosuppression. Moreover, as yet standard therapy with DMARDs and corticosteroids has failed to interrupt and permanently halt autoimmune inflammation. The substantial progress in our understanding of molecular and cellular biology in recent years has permitted the design of therapeutic tools with defined targets and effector functions ('biologicals') that might fulfill these hopes of an optimal therapy. Based on the increased knowledge of molecular mechanisms involved in the pathogenesis of rheumatic diseases, biologicals have been developed to selectively target only those cells and/or pathways driving the disease, while maintaining the integrity of the remainder of the immune system. Based on the concept that activated T cells are the key mediators of chronic autoimmune inflammation, a number of approaches have been designed in autoimmune diseases to specifically target mature circulating T cells. However, although the concept of T-cell-directed immunotherapy with biologicals is evidence-based and has been successfully employed in animal models of autoimmune diseases, T-cell-directed biologicals have generally failed to induce sustained clinical improvement in patients with RA.[1, 21]

A number of reasons, such as the selection of the targeted molecules, the design of the biologicals, and the selection of patients at advanced stages of their disease, might have contributed to the unfavorable results of some T-cell-directed therapies with biologicals in man. A further problem in targeting specifically the disease-promoting T cells in human autoimmune rheumatic diseases is the fact that neither the eliciting (auto)antigens nor the specific disease initiating or perpetuating T cells are known. Therefore, the most rational approach to treat human autoimmune diseases has been interference with the activation of CD4+ T cells in a rather non-antigen-specific manner.

T-cell-directed therapies have been performed with biologicals that target T-cell surface receptors or disrupt the cell/cell interactions that are important for the recruitment of T cells to sites of inflammation and/or for T-cell costimulation. The T-cell surface receptors that have been targeted in clinical trials include CD2, CD3, CD4, CD5, CD7, CD25, and CD52. These molecules are more or less specific for T cells or T-cell subsets and were thus considered promising targets in attempts to down-modulate sustained inflammation by virtue of interfering with T-cell activation. A detailed review of experiences with the *in vivo* use of monoclonal antibodies (mAbs) to these individual surface receptors and the outcome of clinical trials with such mAbs was presented in our earlier review.[1] Although some of the mAbs employed were clearly associated with convincing and prolonged clinical benefit, the conception arose from these trials that targeting surface receptors of CD4 T cells by mAbs was generally not sufficient to ameliorate established autoimmune inflammation.[1,21] Of importance, the induction of permanent unresponsiveness of autoreactive T cells that would have resulted in sustained clinical improvement without the need for continuous immunosuppressive therapy was never achieved in any of the studies. With the exception of a limited number of trials with biologicals blocking CD2,[22] CD3,[23] or CD4,[24] clinical studies with mAbs to

T-cell surface receptors in rheumatic diseases have largely been discontinued for the past few years.

T-CELL-DIRECTED THERAPY BY BLOCKING T-CELL COSTIMULATION

An alternative approach to inhibit T-cell activation in inflammatory diseases is to interrupt the interaction between T-cells and neighboring cells by blocking the ligand for a T-cell surface molecule on the surface of the cells interacting with T cells, thereby preventing receptor/counter receptor interaction. This approach has been successfully employed in an attempt to block CD28-mediated costimulation in T cells.[25–28] Costimulation is an absolute requirement for the activation of naive T cells. Therefore, costimulation controls the initiation of specific immunity. In fact, activation of a naive T-cell through its TCR without providing appropriate costimulation renders the T cell anergic, which essentially restricts the initiation of specific immune responses to professional antigen-presenting cells (APCs), such as dendritic cells, that are able to engage costimulatory molecules on naive T cells. CD28-mediated costimulation can be blocked by coating the binding partners of CD28 on APCs, CD80, and CD86, with a soluble immunoglobulin fusion protein of the extracellular domain of CD152 (cytotoxic T-lymphocyte antigen 4, CTLA-4). CTLA-4 is a homolog to CD28 and is expressed by activated T cells. It can bind both CD80 and CD86 with higher affinity than CD28. Because CD152 has a high affinity for CD80 and CD86, soluble forms of CTLA-4 inhibit the interaction of CD28 with its ligands. The various clinical trials in which signaling through CD28 was inhibited will be discussed in detail elsewhere in this book.

An alternative costimulatory pathway involved in T-cell activation is the CD2/CD58 pathway. Following the promising results from an open-label study with alefacept, a soluble fully human recombinant fusion protein comprising the first extracellular domain of CD58 and the hinge, CH2 and CH3 sequences of human IgG1, in patients with psoriatic arthritis,[29] a phase II study of alefacept in combination with methotrexate for psoriatic arthritis has recently been presented.[22] Three months after a 12-week period of weekly intramuscular application of 15 mg alefacept, 54% of the verum-treated patients (compared with 23% of the placebo-treated control) achieved an ACR20 response. The data suggest that prevention of T-cell activation by targeting CD2/CD58 interactions is feasible and might result in reduction of autoimmune joint inflammation. Further studies are required to substantiate these observations.

Together, the successful therapy of clinically active rheumatic diseases with biologicals interrupting T-cell costimulatory pathways clearly emphasize the important role of T cells in the pathogenesis even at advanced stages of these diseases. Importantly, as in contrast to naive T cells, memory and effector T cells are independent of costimulation, the data also strongly suggest that inflammatory joint activity in RA and psoriasis depends on the continuous activation and recruitment of naive T cells.

T-CELL-DIRECTED THERAPY BY BLOCKING T-CELL MIGRATION

T-cell recruitment to sites of inflammation was successfully prevented with a murine mAb to CD54 (ICAM-1), which is critical for transendothelial migration of T cells and their subsequent activation.[30] Because of the immunogenicity of this mAb, however, retreatment with this agent was associated with immune complex-mediated side effects, including urticaria, angioedema, and serum complement protein consumption[31] and therefore further studies were not conducted. The concept of modulating autoimmune inflammation by selectively interfering with T-cell migration, however, was tested again in a more recent randomized placebo-controlled trial of an antisense oligodeoxynucleotide to ICAM-1 in patients with severe RA.[32] In this study, clinical efficacy was not noted, presumably because of insufficient dosage, as suggested by a subsequent study in Crohn's disease, in which the dose required for therapeutic efficacy was higher than the dose employed in the RA trial.[33] Thus the clinical value of an antisense oligodeoxynucleotide approach to CD54 in RA remains to be shown.

T-CELL-DIRECTED THERAPY WITH STATINS

Apart from the treatment principles described herein in more detail, other innovative T-cell-directed therapeutic strategies have been defined, some of which have already entered preliminary clinical trials. For example, the anti-inflammatory role of 3-hydroxy-3-methylglutaryl-CoA reductase inhibitors (statins) has been documented in a murine model of inflammatory arthritis. Simvastatin not only markedly inhibited developing but also clinically established collagen-induced arthritis in doses that were unable to significantly alter cholesterol concentrations *in vivo*.[34] Importantly, simvastatin reduced anti-CD3/anti-CD28-induced T-cell proliferation and IFN-γ production and, moreover, demonstrated a significant suppression of collagen-specific Th1 humoral and cellular immune responses. Studies in humans, though, have not been reported to date.

T-CELL-DIRECTED THERAPY IN NON-RHEUMATIC DISEASES

In non-rheumatic autoimmune diseases, several interesting T-cell-directed approaches have been performed. For example, altered peptide ligands (APLs) of myasthenogenic peptides that are single amino acid-substituted analogons of the pathogenic peptides were able to inhibit the proliferative responses of the pathogenic peptide-specific T-cell lines *in vitro* and to prevent *in vivo* priming to the myastenogenic peptides.[35] A dual APL composed of two tandemly arranged single altered peptide analogs was also able to inhibit those responses *in vitro* and *in vivo*. Interestingly, the dual APL activated CD4+CD25+-expressing regulatory T cells in the lymph nodes of injected mice, suggesting that the active suppression exerted by the dual APL is mediated by the recently identified CD4+CD25+ regulatory T-cell population. The potency of these cells in ameliorating autoimmune inflammation has been documented in non-obese diabetic mice, in which small numbers of antigen-specific CD25+ regulatory T cells were able to reverse diabetes after disease onset.[36] As it was possible to expand these antigen-specific regulatory T cells *in vitro*, the vaccination with CD4+CD25+ regulatory

T cells might open novel avenues for T-cell-mediated cellular immunotherapy in autoimmune diseases. Whether the obstacle of unknown antigens in most human autoimmune diseases can be overcome and whether the numbers of regulatory T cells required for down-modulating systemic autoimmune inflammation in humans can be generated *in vitro* remain to be shown.

CONCLUSION

Based on the concept that activated T cells are the key mediators of chronic autoimmune inflammation, different T-cell-directed approaches have been introduced for the treatment of inflammatory rheumatic disease. Whereas attempts to down-modulate rheumatic inflammation by reducing T cell numbers have largely failed, novel treatment approaches with biologicals that specifically inhibit T-cell activation by preventing costimulation are associated with considerable clinical efficiency. These compounds have clearly established the feasibility of targeted T-cell-directed interventions and the clinical benefit induced by inhibiting T-cell activation supports the dominant role of T cells in rheumatic inflammation even at advanced stages of the diseases. Some interesting novel treatment approaches have been tested in animal models of autoimmune disease, but their value for clinical use in humans needs to be established.

ACKNOWLEDGMENT

The work of HSK was supported in part by the Deutsche Forschungsgemeinschaft (Schu 786/2-4) and the Interdisciplinary Center for Clinical Research in Erlangen (Projects B3 and A18).

REFERENCES

1. Schulze-Koops H, Kalden JR. Targeting T cells in rheumatic diseases. In: Smolen JS, Lipsky PE, eds. Biological Therapy in Rheumatology. London: Martin Dunitz, 2003: 3.

2. Schulze-Koops H, Lipsky PE. T cells in the pathogenesis of rheumatoid arthritis. In: St Clair EW, Pisetsky DS, and Haynes BF, eds. Rheumatoid Arthritis. Philadelphia: Lippincott Williams & Wilkins, 2004: 184.

3. Emmrich F, Schulze-Koops H, Burmester G. Anti-CD4 and other antibodies to cell surface antigens for therapy. In: Immunopharmacology of Joints and Connective Tissue. Davies EM, Dingle JT, eds. London: Academic Press, 1994: 87.

4. Gleeson PA, Toh BH, van Driel IR. Organ-specific autoimmunity induced by lymphopenia. Immunol Rev 1996; 149: 97–125.

5. Sadlack B, Merz H, Schorle H et al. Ulcerative colitis-like disease in mice with a disrupted interleukin-2 gene. Cell 1993; 75: 253–61.

6. Mombaerts P, Mizoguchi E, Grusby MJ et al. Spontaneous development of inflammatory bowel disease in T cell receptor mutant mice. Cell 1993; 75: 274–82.

7. Mizoguchi A, Mizoguchi E, Smith RN, Preffer FI, Bhan AK. Suppressive role of B cells in chronic colitis of T cell receptor alpha mutant mice. J Exp Med 1997; 186: 1749–56.

8. Sakaguchi S, Ermak TH, Toda M et al. Induction of autoimmune disease in mice by germline alteration of the T cell receptor gene expression. J Immunol 1994; 152: 1471–84.

9. Sakaguchi S, Sakaguchi N. Organ-specific autoimmune disease induced in mice by elimination of T cell subsets. V. Neonatal administration of cyclosporin A causes autoimmune disease. J Immunol 1989; 142: 471–80.

10. Sakaguchi N, Miyai K, Sakaguchi S. Ionizing radiation and autoimmunity. Induction of autoimmune disease in mice by high dose fractionated total lymphoid irradiation and its prevention by inoculating normal T cells. J Immunol 1994; 152: 2586–95.

11. Kojima A, Prehn RT. Genetic susceptibility to post-thymectomy autoimmune diseases in mice. Immunogenetics 1981; 14: 15–27.

12. Barrett SP, Toh BH, Alderuccio F, van Driel IR, Gleeson PA. Organ-specific autoimmunity induced by adult thymectomy and cyclophosphamide-induced lymphopenia. Eur J Immunol 1995; 25: 238–44.

13. Ablamunits V, Quintana F, Reshef T, Elias D, Cohen IR. Acceleration of autoimmune diabetes by cyclophosphamide is associated with an enhanced IFN-gamma secretion pathway. J Autoimmun 1999; 13: 383–92.

14. Schulze-Koops H. Lymphopenia and autoimmune diseases. Arthritis Res Ther 2004; 6: 178–80.

15. Bruneau JM, Yea CM, Spinella-Jaegle S et al. Purification of human dihydro-orotate dehydrogenase and its inhibition by A77 1726, the active metabolite of leflunomide. Biochem J 1998; 336: 299–303.

16. Dimitrova P, Skapenko A, Herrmann ML et al. Restriction of de novo pyrimidine biosynthesis inhibits Th1 cell activation and promotes Th2 cell differentiation. J Immunol 2002; 169: 3392–9.

17. Simon AK, Seipelt E, Sieper J. Divergent T-cell cytokine patterns in inflammatory arthritis. Proc Natl Acad Sci USA 1994; 91: 8562–6.

18. Miltenburg AM, van Laar JM, de Kuiper R, Daha MR, Breedveld FC. T cells cloned from human rheumatoid synovial membrane functionally represent the Th1 subset. Scand J Immunol 1992; 35: 603–10.

19. Schulze-Koops H, Lipsky PE, Kavanaugh AF, Davis LS. Elevated Th1- or Th0-like cytokine mRNA in peripheral circulation of patients with rheumatoid arthritis: Modulation by treatment with anti-ICAM-1 correlates with clinical benefit. J Immunol 1995; 155: 5029–37.

20. Skapenko A, Wendler J, Lipsky PE, Kalden JR, Schulze-Koops H. Altered memory T cell differentiation in patients with early rheumatoid arthritis. J Immunol 1999; 163: 491–9.

21. Schulze-Koops H, and Lipsky PE. Anti-CD4 monoclonal antibody therapy in human autoimmune diseases. Curr Dir Autoimmun 2000; 2: 24–49.

22. Gottlieb AB. Alefacept for psoriasis and psoriatic arthritis. Ann Rheum Dis 2005; 64(Suppl 4): iv58–60.

23. Utset TO, Auger JA, Peace D et al. Modified anti-CD3 therapy in psoriatic arthritis: a phase I/II clinical trial. J Rheumatol 2002; 29: 1907–13.

24. Hepburn TW, Totoritis MC, Davis CB. Antibody-mediated stripping of CD4 from lymphocyte cell surface in patients with rheumatoid arthritis. Rheumatology 2003; 42: 54–61.

25. Moreland LW, Alten R, Van den Bosch F et al. Costimulatory blockade in patients with rheumatoid arthritis: a pilot, dose-finding, double-blind, placebo-controlled clinical trial evaluating CTLA-4Ig and LEA29Y eighty-five days after the first infusion. Arthritis Rheum 2002; 46: 1470–9.

26. Kremer JM, Westhovens R, Leon M et al. Treatment of rheumatoid arthritis by selective inhibition of T-cell activation with fusion protein CTLA4Ig. N Engl J Med 2003; 349: 1907–15.

27. Kremer JM, Dougados M, Emery P et al. Treatment of rheumatoid arthritis with the selective costimulation modulator abatacept: twelve-month results of a phase iib, double-blind, randomized, placebo-controlled trial. Arthritis Rheum 2005; 52: 2263–71.

28. Genovese MC, Becker JC, Schiff M et al. Abatacept for rheumatoid arthritis refractory to tumor necrosis factor alpha inhibition. N Engl J Med 2005; 353: 1114–23.

29. Patel S, Veale D, FitzGerald O, McHugh NJ. Psoriatic arthritis – emerging concepts. Rheumatology 2001; 40: 243–6.

30. Kavanaugh AF, Davis LS, Nichols LA et al. Treatment of refractory rheumatoid arthritis with a monoclonal antibody to intercellular adhesion molecule 1. Arthritis Rheum 1994; 37: 992–9.

31. Kavanaugh AF, Schulze-Koops H, Davis LS, Lipsky PE. Repeat treatment of rheumatoid arthritis patients with a murine anti-intercellular adhesion molecule 1 monoclonal antibody. Arthritis Rheum 1997; 40: 849–53.

32. Maksymowych WP, Blackburn WD, Jr., Tami JA, Shanahan WR, Jr. A randomized, placebo controlled trial of an antisense oligodeoxynucleotide to intercellular adhesion molecule-1 in the treatment of severe rheumatoid arthritis. J Rheumatol 2002; 29: 447–53.

33. Yacyshyn BW, Chey W, Salzberg GB et al. Double-blinded, randomized, placebo-controlled trial of the remission inducing and steroid sparing properties of two schedules of ISIS 2302 (ICAM-1 antisense) in active, steroid-dependent Crohn's disease. Gastroenterology 2000; 118: S2: 2977.

34. Leung BP, Sattar N, Crilly A et al. A novel anti-inflammatory role for simvastatin in inflammatory arthritis. J Immunol 2003; 170: 1524–30.

35. Paas-Rozner M, Sela M, Mozes E. A dual altered peptide ligand down-regulates myasthenogenic T cell responses by up-regulating CD25- and CTLA-4-expressing CD4+ T cells. Proc Natl Acad Sci U S A 2003; 100: 6676–81.

36. Tang Q, Henriksen KJ, Bi M et al. In vitro-expanded antigen-specific regulatory T cells suppress autoimmune diabetes. J Exp Med 2004; 199: 1455–65.

2

Pathways of T-cell costimulation

Brendan J Classon, Steven G Nadler and Suzanne J Suchard

Introduction • Costimulatory pathways • Coinhibitory pathways • Conclusion and summary • References

INTRODUCTION

It has been recognized since the 1970s that T cells require at least two signals for full activation leading to maximum proliferation and cytokine production.[1–3] The first signal is provided by the clonotypic cell surface T-cell receptor (TCR) when it engages a specific major histocompatibility complex (MHC) molecule–peptide complex on an antigen-presenting cell (APC). The second activating signal(s) is provided by costimulatory ligands expressed on the T-cell surface that engage cognate receptors on the surface of APCs. The initiation and progression of the immune response is controlled by spatial and temporal regulation of the expression of costimulatory and coinhibitory ligands and their receptors. In general, T cells that receive only the first signal through the TCR in the absence of a second costimulatory signal become anergic and non-responsive. However, in certain circumstances, T cells may become activated after receiving a potent agonist signal via the TCR. In addition to receiving costimulatory signals, T cells may also receive coinhibitory signals, which results in the attenuation of costimulatory signals and interruption of T-cell activation and cytokine secretion. The expression pattern of costimulatory and coinhibitory ligands and their receptors is regulated over the course of the immune response, ensuring an optimal balance of stimulatory and inhibitory signals to enable effective clearance of antigen or pathogen and a diminution of the response once the antigen or pathogen is cleared. Thus, T-cell costimulation and coinhibitory pathways have evolved to facilitate initiation of appropriate immune responses, which are subsequently regulated to avoid uncontrolled T-cell activation and the attendant potential risk of autoimmunity.

There are two major families of cell surface costimulatory molecules that can be classified according to their structural characteristics (Figure 2.1). Firstly, there is the CD28:B7 family, whose ligands and receptors comprise immunoglobulin (Ig)-like domains. The second family of costimulatory molecules is the CD40/CD40L family, whose ligands are homologous to tumor necrosis factor (TNF), and whose receptors are homologous to the TNF-receptor. In contrast to costimulatory molecules, the cell surface coinhibitory ligands and their receptors are predominantly composed of Ig-like domains. This chapter reviews the important costimulatory and coinhibitory ligands and receptors, with an emphasis on their function in normal immune responses, and how these functions may contribute to the pathogenesis of autoimmune disease, particularly, rheumatoid arthritis.

COSTIMULATORY PATHWAYS

CD28 AND CD80/CD86

The most well characterized T-cell costimulatory ligand is CD28, which interacts with the costimulatory receptors CD80 and CD86. CD28 is a transmembrane protein comprising a single

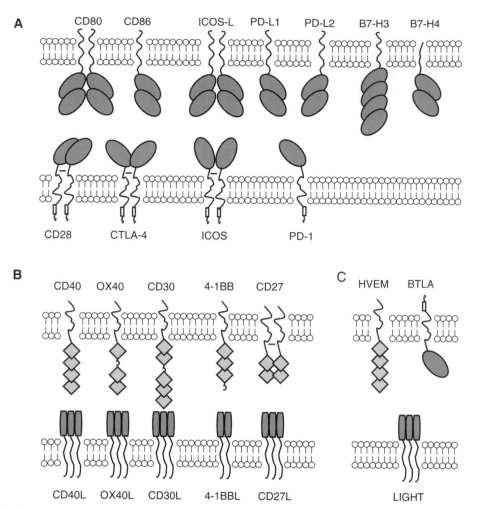

Figure 2.1 (A) Molecular interactions between costimulatory and coinhibitory receptor/ligand pairs of the immunoglobulin super-family. Putative cognate ligands for the B7-H3 and B7-H4 receptors remain unidentified. (B) Molecular interactions between co-stimulatory receptor/ligand pairs of the TNF/TNFR superfamily. (C) Receptor/ligand interactions that mediate costimulatory (LIGHT/HVEM) and coinhibitory response (BTLA/LIGHT) that involve members of both the Ig and TNF/TNFR superfamilies.

extracellular Ig variable-like (IgV) domain.[4] In humans and in mice, CD28 is constitutively expressed on the majority of CD4+ T cells and a subset of CD8+ T cells.[5,6] Costimulation through CD28 in T cells leads to initiation of the cell cycle, enhanced metabolic activity, up-regulation of anti-apoptotic genes, and enhanced cytokine production, particularly IL-2.[7–9] CD28 plays a key role in activation of naive T cells; however, recent data suggest that CD28 also plays a role in the activation of memory T cells.[10]

The first receptor to be identified for CD28 was CD80 (also termed B7-1).[11] The second

receptor, CD86 (also termed B7-2), was identified subsequently.[12,13] CTLA-4 is a second ligand that binds CD80 and CD86, but CTLA-4 function differs from CD28 because it plays an important role in coinhibitory signaling (see below). The CD80 receptor is expressed constitutively at very low levels on APCs including dendritic cells (DCs), B cells, and Langerhans cells, but its expression is markedly up-regulated on APCs and T cells following activation, which may occur during infection and exposure to proin-flammatory cytokines.[14] In contrast, CD86 is expressed constitutively and increased only moderately after APC stimulation.[12] CD80 and CD86 are structurally similar and they have overlapping but distinct functions.[15] Considering their tissue distribution and timing of expression, it is generally believed that CD86 is critical for the initiation of immune responses, whereas CD80 plays a more prominent role in maintenance and subsequent attenuation of the immune response.[16]

Extensive *in vitro* analysis of CD28 and CD80/CD86 function has been performed using monoclonal antibodies (mAbs) and fusion proteins, including CTLA-4-Ig, in blocking experiments. Antibody blockade of CD28 was shown to inhibit T-cell proliferation in a mixed lymphocyte reaction (MLR).[17,18] Similarly, antibody blockade of either CD80 or CD86 also inhibited T-cell proliferation, although dual blockade of both CD80 and CD86 was required for maximum inhibition.[19] A soluble derivative of the alternative CD80/CD86 ligand, CTLA-4, expressed as an Ig-fusion protein (CTLA-4-Ig) was also shown to inhibit T-cell proliferation.[19] In this study, the degree of inhibition observed with CTLA-4-Ig was similar to that observed with CD80 plus CD86 mAbs, a result that is consistent with the notion that CTLA-4-Ig is an effective dual antagonist of CD80 and CD86. Several studies have demonstrated that CTLA-4-Ig is also an effective inhibitor of the CD80/CD86 interaction with CD28 *in vivo*,[20,21] and the functional effect of this reagent has been studied in a significant number of experimental animal models of autoimmune disease.[22] CTLA-4-Ig inhibits T-cell-dependent antibody responses, ameliorates autoimmune disease progression and severity, and prolongs allograft survival.[23,24] In the collagen-induced arthritis model, CTLA-4-Ig inhibits anti-collagen antibody production, paw swelling, serum cytokine production, and bone erosion.[25]

Analysis of CD28-deficient mice has confirmed a key role for CD28 in the activation of naive T cells, differentiation of T-helper cells, Ig isotype class switching, and T-cell survival.[26] Furthermore, the impaired T-cell responses observed in these mice have established that CD28 is the single major CD80/CD86 binding costimulatory ligand on T cells.[27] Similarly, it has been shown that mice deficient for either CD80 or CD86 also exhibit impaired T-cell responses. CD80-deficient mice exhibited reduced T-cell proliferative responses in MLRs[28] and CD86-deficient mice are defective in Ig isotype switching and have impaired splenic germinal center formation.[29] CD80/CD86-double deficient mice exhibited a similar phenotype to CD86-deficient mice, although the deficiency in Ig isotype switching was more pronounced.[29]

To date, CTLA-4-Ig (abatacept) is the only clinically approved drug that selectively targets CD28-mediated costimulation. A phase I clinical trial was conducted in patients with psoriasis, where approximately half the abatacept-treated patients exhibited a sustained improvement in disease symptoms.[30] In this study, it was established that abatacept effectively inhibited Ig production in response to a neoantigen as well as measures of inflammation in the psoriatic lesion. Abatacept was also shown to be effective in reducing the signs and symptoms of rheumatoid arthritis in phase III clinical trials.[31–33] In December 2005, abatacept was approved for the treatment of moderate to severe rheumatoid arthritis in the United States and Canada.[22] Other biologics that target the CD28 pathway and have been in development for autoimmune disease but are now discontinued include anti-CD80 (Galiximab) and anti-CD86. A small molecule inhibitor of CD80[34] is currently entering a phase II clinical trial in rheumatoid arthritis patients.[35]

ICOS and ICOS-L

Inducible costimulatory molecule (ICOS) is a CD28-related molecule whose expression is induced on differentiated T cells following activation.[36] Costimulation of T cells through ICOS initiates secretion of cytokines other than IL-2.[37] The lack of IL-2 production following ICOS costimulation limits the long-term expansion potential of ICOS-costimulated T cells.[38] Because ICOS seems to play a more prominent role in driving T-cell effector function, rather than expansion, it has been suggested that ICOS facilitates rapid activation of T-cell memory responses.[9] Thus, while CD28 costimulation is required for initiation of the response, ICOS appears to play a more prominent role in the ongoing response through maintenance of T-cell effector function.[39]

ICOS binds B7h (also called B7RP-1, B7H2, LICOS, and GL50), which is expressed on activated myeloid cells. ICOS does not bind CD80 or CD86, and B7h does not bind CD28 or CTLA-4. Both ICOS- and B7h-deficient mice display similar phenotypes, suggesting that they function as a monogamous receptor/ligand pair. Analysis of mice deficient for ICOS or B7h suggests that the ICOS/B7h interaction is not an obligate requirement for T-cell expansion, but rather ICOS acts co-operatively with CD28 in T-cell costimulation.[40–42] The major functional role of ICOS/ICOS-L appears to be in the induction of T-cell effector function during T-cell differentiation. The phenotype of ICOS-deficient mice and analysis of mice treated with soluble ICOS-Ig fusion protein to block ICOS/B7h interactions reveal that ICOS is required for Ig isotype switching and germinal center formation.[40,41,43] ICOS seems to play little if any role in the generation of CD8+ T-cell effector function, since viral CTL and antibody responses in mice treated with soluble ICOS-Ig fusion protein were relatively unaffected.[44] The importance of ICOS in late B-cell differentiation and Ig class switching was confirmed following the identification of a homozygous loss of ICOS in a subset of patients suffering from adult-onset common variable immunodeficiency.[45,46]

CD40 and CD40L

CD40 is a member of the TNFR superfamily, which was first identified as a B-cell surface receptor capable of inducing polyclonal activation and differentiation into antibody-producing cells.[47] CD40 is constitutively expressed on B cells, monocytes, macrophages, DCs, epithelial cells, endothelial cells, fibroblasts, and platelets.[48] The ligand for CD40 is CD40L (CD154), which was reported to induce contact-dependent differentiation of B cells.[49,50] CD40L is a type II transmembrane protein expressed predominantly by activated CD4+ T cells and activated platelets.[51] CD40L expression on T cells is induced shortly after T-cell activation, and thus represents an early activation marker of T lymphocytes. The expression of CD40L on activated platelets is thought to

mediate recruitment of inflammatory cells to the damaged endothelium. In a manner similar to membrane-bound TNF-α, CD40L is cleaved from the cell surface of activated T cells by a matrix metalloproteinase, releasing a homotrimeric form of sCD40L into the circulation.[52] Like membrane-bound CD40L, sCD40L can also promote B-cell activation and differentiation.

Engagement of CD40 by CD40L induces up-regulation of CD80 and CD86 on B cells, and up-regulation of CD54 and CD86 on DCs.[53,54] Ligation of CD40 on DCs induces the secretion of cytokines such as IL-8, TNF-α, MIP-1α, and IL-12. Functional interactions between CD40L and CD40 are bidirectional, and engagement of CD40L on T cells by CD40+ APCs can induce apoptosis in CD4+ T cells and leads to the generation of CD8+ memory T cells.[55,56] Ligation of CD40 on endothelial cells triggers production of chemokines and cytokines such as IL-8, MCP-1, MIP-1α, RANTES, IL-1, IL-6, IL-12, and TNF-α, and leads to the up-regulation of adhesion molecules and matrix metalloproteinases.[57–60]

Cognate interactions between CD40 and CD40L are crucial for the switch in recombination and synthesis of immunoglobulins by B cells.[61] In addition to its role in Ig isotype switching, binding of CD40L to CD40 is crucial for activation, proliferation, and maturation of B cells. A critical role for CD40L in B-cell function was confirmed when genetic mutations in CD40L were reported in patients suffering from hyper-IgM syndrome.[62] These individuals exhibit defective antibody production manifest by a lack of circulating IgG and IgA due to the inability of the B cell to switch the IgM isotype. Similar defects were recapitulated in mice following genetic disruption of the CD40/CD40L pathway.[63,64]

Antibody blockade of CD40L has been a relatively successful immunosuppressive strategy in animal transplantation models. In combination with CTLA-4-Ig, CD40L blockade has both additive and synergistic effects in the context of prolonging kidney allograft survival in primates and skin graft survival in mice.[65,66] Preclinical animal models also demonstrate the potential for antagonizing the CD40L/CD40 pathway for the treatment of autoimmune diseases. Treatment with an anti-CD40L mAb suppresses the development of collagen-induced arthritis, ameliorating disease symptoms including joint inflammation, cartilage erosion, and infiltration by inflammatory cells of the subsynovial tissue.[67] In a transgenic mouse model of Ig-mediated arthritis, anti-CD40L mAb significantly diminished the development of arthritis in a prophylactic treatment regimen.[68] In a mouse model of lupus, animals treated with continuous anti-CD40L mAb infusion exhibited a delay in disease onset, with increased efficacy in combination with CTLA-4-Ig. In both cases, there was a decrease in anti-dsDNA autoantibodies and the spleens from these animals had reduced numbers of B cells.

Monotherapeutic applications of anti-CD40L mAbs in human lupus have been published. In a phase II trial, a humanized anti-CD40L antibody (IDEC-131) was shown to be safe and well tolerated but failed to demonstrate significant efficacy over placebo.[69] In another study, another humanized anti-CD40L antibody (BG9588) appeared to have a beneficial impact on the course of disease[70] but the study was terminated early due to adverse thromboembolytic complications.[71]

OX40 and OX40L

OX40 (CD134) is a member of the TNFR superfamily originally identified by an antibody generated against activated rat T cells.[72,73] Subsequently, the human OX40 homolog was identified.[74] OX40 is absent from resting T cells but is expressed on CD4+ and some CD8+ T cells following activation.[75] Costimulation through OX40 has been implicated in the generation of T-helper responses as well as in the maintenance of memory T-cell populations.[76] OX40L (gp34) was first identified as a type II transmembrane protein induced by HTLV-1 infection of T cells.[77] OX40L is expressed on activated T cells, B cells, DCs, macrophages, epithelial cells, and endothelial cells, and similar to OX40, OX40L expression is prolonged for several days following cell activation.[78]

Studies using OX40L or anti-OX40 antibody to mediate T-cell activation demonstrated that OX40 signaling on T cells enhances cytokine production and proliferation of CD4+ T cells,

an effect that can occur in the absence of CD28 signaling.[79,80] OX40/OX40L interactions appear to be important in sustaining T-cell function at later stages of the primary immune response and during the memory response.[75,81] T cells from OX40-deficient mice produce IL-2 and proliferate normally, but as the response proceeds, T-cell expansion and cytokine production are not sustained.

Agonistic anti-OX40 antibody can elicit CD4+ and CD8+ T-cell expansion *in vivo*, with transient splenomegaly and lymphadenopathy observed in non-human primates.[82] CD40L transgenic mice demonstrate an accumulation of activated CD4+ OX40+ T cells in the B-cell follicles of secondary lymphoid organs following antigenic stimulation, suggesting that OX40 regulates T-cell homing within secondary lymphoid organs.[83] OX40+ T cells have been demonstrated at the site of inflammation in a number of animal models of autoimmunity, including experimental allergic encephalomyelitis (EAE), rheumatoid arthritis (RA), and graft versus host disease (GVHD).[84-86] Consistent with these observations, transgenic expression of OX40L by DCs increases the number of antigen-responding CD4+ and autoimmune events in rodents.[83] Administration of soluble OX40-Ig fusion protein to colitic mice ameliorates disease, with a concomitant reduction in T-cell infiltrates and TNF-α, IL-1, IL-12, and IFN-γ production.[87] In mice, a neutralizing anti-OX40L antibody administered before, but not after a second immunization with a model autoantigen (type II collagen), inhibits the development of collagen-induced arthritis,[88] suggesting that the OX40/OX40L interaction is involved in the early stages of disease induction. Treatment with anti-OX40L antibody or depletion of OX40+ T cells has been shown to ameliorate EAE symptoms in both an induced disease model and an adoptive transfer model.[85,89] OX40L antibody treatment does not inhibit the development of pathogenic T cells but rather their accumulation in the spinal cord.[90] The opposite effect is observed with an activating OX40 antibody which can exacerbate disease.[91] Similarly, agonistic anti-OX40 can break peripheral T-cell tolerance induced in mice by administering antigen-specific peptides. In general, these data support a role for

OX40/OX40L in maintaining the ongoing immune response following antigen-specific T-cell activation, and as such, manipulation of the OX40/OX40L pathway has significant clinical potential for treatment of autoimmune disease.

4-1BB and 4-1BBL pathway

4-1BB (CD137) was first discovered as a TNFR-related cDNA whose expression was induced in activated mouse T-cell clones.[92] 4-1BB is absent from resting T cells, but is expressed on activated CD4[+] and CD8[+] T cells, some DCs, and on activated natural killer (NK) cells, with expression peaking at 42–72 hours after activation.[93,94] The ligand for 4-1BB (4-1BB-L) was first identified in a human B-cell line, using a 4-1BB-Ig fusion protein as a probe for the counter structure.[95] Although a member of the TNF superfamily, 4-1BBL is unusual in that it exists at the cell surface as a disulfide-linked homodimer, rather than the more typical homotrimer. 4-1BB-L is expressed on mature DCs, activated T cells and B cells and macrophages.[96,97]

Antibody-induced cross-linking of 4-1BB on anti-CD3 activated mouse T cells was shown to enhance T-cell proliferation.[93] Likewise, engagement of 4-1BB by 4-1BBL was shown to elicit a similar response.[95] Engagement of 4-1BB on activated T cells by its ligand leads to a preferential expansion of CD8[+] T cells, rather than CD4[+] T cells.[98] Thus, signaling through 4-1BB appears to be important for CD8[+] T-cell survival, enhancing cytokine production and differentiation of CTL effector function.[98,99] In addition to 4-1BB signaling on T cells, 4-1BBL is capable of inducing a 'reverse' signal to APCs. For example, engagement of 4-1BBL induces B-cell proliferation and inflammatory cytokine production by monocytes.[97,100,101] In T cells, proliferation induced by anti-CD3 antibody is inhibited by cross-linking of 4-1BBL, which ultimately leads to apoptosis.[102]

Although 4-1BB mAbs have been shown to effectively costimulate CD4[+] and CD8[+] T cells, they can also block the development of humoral immunity when administered early during immunization.[103] Consistent with this finding, an anti-CD137 mAb can effectively block the onset of SLE in young mice and block its progression in

animals with advanced disease.[104] Administration of the 4-1BB agonist antibody at the time of collagen immunization blocks development of disease in a model of collagen-induced arthritis,[105,106] but it has only a modest effect on progression of established disease. [106]

HVEM and LIGHT

LIGHT is a TNF-related cell surface ligand that was originally identified from a human activated T-cell library. It is expressed on the surface of activated T cells, NK cells, and immature DCs.[107–109] LIGHT is a homotrimeric cell surface protein, which exists in three distinct forms. Full-length LIGHT is expressed on the cell surface, an alternatively spliced isoform lacking the transmembrane domain is retained in the cytoplasm, and there is a soluble form which is released from the cell surface by a metalloprotease activity.[110,111]

There are two cell surface receptors that interact with LIGHT. The first, HVEM (herpesvirus-entry mediator), is expressed on T cells, B cells, monocytes, and immature DCs[112,113] and the second, lymphotoxin-β receptor (LTβR), is expressed on epithelial cells and stromal cells but not on lymphocytes.[107] HVEM expression decreases following T-cell activation and it has been suggested that LIGHT may be responsible for this phenomenon.[111] This reciprocal regulation of LIGHT and HVEM expression may be important for limiting the duration of LIGHT-HVEM-mediated T-cell activation. HVEM also interacts with the BTLA (B- and T-lymphocyte attenuator) ligand. BTLA is a coinhibitory ligand which down-regulates B- and T-cell responses and will be discussed further below. LIGHT can also costimulate T-cell proliferation in a manner that is CD28-independent.[108,114,115] This response can be inhibited with either an anti-HVEM antibody or an HVEM/Fc fusion protein, indicating that LIGHT-mediated T-cell immune responses are mediated through its interaction with HVEM. Splenocytes from HVEM-deficient mice fail to proliferate in response to triggering with an anti-TCR antibody plus recombinant soluble LIGHT, demonstrating that HVEM signaling is essential for LIGHT-mediated costimulation.[116] CD8[+] T cells from LIGHT-deficient mice exhibit reduced *in vitro* proliferative responses,[115,117] although LIGHT deficiency does not appear to impact their cytolytic effector function.

Transgenic mice with enhanced LIGHT expression on T cells exhibit a lymphoproliferative phenotype, with expanded populations of both CD4+ and CD8+ T cells.[118] In transplantation models, antibody blockade of LIGHT or targeted disruption of the LIGHT gene has been shown to ameliorate graft rejection and GVHD, further supporting a role for LIGHT in regulation of T-cell effector function.[114,119] Blockade of the LTβR/LIGHT interaction by a soluble LTβR-Ig fusion protein has been shown to ameliorate disease severity in a colitis model.[118,120] Consistent with these findings, transfer of transgenic T cells overexpressing LIGHT into RAG−/− recipient mice induces a rapid disease onset with a pathology similar to Crohn's disease.[116] Up-regulation of LIGHT is also associated with active disease in Crohn's patients, suggesting that LIGHT may contribute to pathogenesis of Crohn's disease.[116]

CD27 and CD70

The CD27 receptor is a member of the TNFR superfamily originally identified as a novel T-cell differentiation antigen.[121] CD27 is a disulfide-linked homodimer expressed on CD4+ and CD8+ T, NK cells, and antigen-primed B cells. The CD27 counter structure, CD70, is expressed on activated T and B cells, activated DCs, NK cells, and Hodgkin's lymphoma cells.[121,122] CD70 expression on T cells is up-regulated following antigen activation and it is further modulated by cytokines.[123] On DCs, CD70 expression is induced by CD40 ligation.[124] Interestingly, anomalous expression of CD27 in B cells has proved a useful marker for assessing disease activity in lupus patients.[125]

Costimulation mediated by CD27/CD70 induces expansion and differentiation of effector T-cell and memory T-cell populations.[126] Engagement of CD27 on B cells promotes cell expansion, germinal center formation, plasma cell differentiation, and Ig production.[126,127] CD27-deficient mice have reduced numbers of antigen-specific T cells in lymphoid organs and recruitment of CD4+ and CD8+ effector T cells to sites of viral challenge in these animals

is also impaired.[128] CD27 signaling in T cells is thought to enhance cell survival rather than directly affecting proliferation. CD70 transgenic mice exhibit an accumulation of CD4+ and CD8+ effector T cells, which leads to progressive depletion of naïve T cells in secondary lymphoid tissue.[129] In a vascularized cardiac transplant model, CD70 blockade has little effect on CD4+ T-cell function but prevents CD8+ T-cell-mediated graft rejection.[130]

CD30 and CD30L

CD30 (Ki-1) is a TNFR-related cell surface receptor originally discovered as a marker of Reed-Sternberg cells in Hodgkin's lymphoma, where it was discovered that CD30 overexpression led to malignancy.[131] CD30 is expressed on activated T cells and B cells, and some NK cells, and is inducible on T cells by signaling through the TCR in combination with CD28 or IL-4 signaling. CD30+ cells are also present at inflammatory sites in several human diseases, including atopic dermatitis, RA, chronic GVHD, and systemic sclerosis.[132] CD30L (CD153) is primarily expressed by CD4+ T cells, B cells, and some tumors. [133]

Signaling through CD30 can induce proliferation, differentiation or apoptosis depending upon the cell type, stage of development, and other stimuli.[133–136] CD30-deficient mice have an impaired capacity to sustain follicular germinal center responses and have reduced recall responses to T-dependent antigens.[137] Memory T-cell responses are reduced in these mice because the T cells fail to receive adequate survival signals from CD30+ OX40L+ accessory cells in B-cell follicles. Consistent with this finding, a non-depleting anti-CD30L mAb inhibits class switching in antibody responses to T-dependent antigens, but it does not affect primary antibody responses.[132] As expected, the phenotype of CD30L-transgenic mice is generally the opposite of that observed with the CD30-deficient mice. It has been suggested that CD30 is a candidate for a diabetes-susceptible gene (*Idd 9*) in NOD mice,[138] and an anti-CD30L antibody has been used to implicate the CD30/CD30L pathway in autoimmune diabetes.[139] The CD30/CD30L pathway has also been implicated in CD4[+] T-cell-mediated GVHD disease.[139,140] Currently, there are anti-CD30 antibodies in the clinic for the treatment of hematopoietic malignancies but none for autoimmune disease.

COINHIBITORY PATHWAYS

CTLA-4 AND CD80/CD86

The coinhibitory ligand counterpart to CD28 is CTLA-4, which was first identified as an activation-induced gene in mouse T cells.[141,142] In contrast to CD28, CTLA-4 delivers a negative signal to T cells, and even low levels of constitutively expressed cell surface CTLA-4 are capable of inhibiting early events in T-cell activation and IL-2 secretion.[143] CTLA-4 binds both CD80 and CD86, although the apparent affinity of CTLA-4 interaction with CD80 is significantly higher than the corresponding interaction with CD86, as a consequence of multivalent avidity enhancement.[144] The mechanism of CTLA-4 function involves inhibition of TCR signal transduction through binding of CTLA-4 to the zeta chain of the TCR, with concomitant inhibition of tyrosine phosphorylation via phosphatases associated with the cytoplasmic tail of CTLA-4.[145] More recently, CTLA-4 was shown to effect the immune synapse and length of time of interaction between T cells and APCs.[146,147] An alternatively sliced variant of CTLA-4 which lacks the CD80/CD86 binding domain has been identified and shown to induce potent inhibition of T-cell proliferation and cytokine secretion,[148] suggesting that CTLA-4 can function as a negative regulator of T cell responses in a CD80/CD86-independent fashion. Thus, the mechanism of CTLA-4-mediated down-regulation of T-cell activation is complex, because it involves ligand competition, perturbation of the immune synapse, and recruitment of intracellular phosphatase activity, which may occur in a ligand-dependent or a ligand-independent fashion.[149]

The crucial role of CTLA-4 in down-regulating T-cell responses was most clearly evident in the phenotype of CTLA-4-deficient mice. These animals develop a pronounced lymphoproliferative disorder and die at around 3 weeks of age as a consequence of multiorgan lymphocytic infiltration and tissue destruction.[150] In humans, susceptibility to the cluster of autoimmune disorders including Graves' disease, autoimmune hypothyroidism, and type I diabetes is correlated with lower levels of an alternatively spliced transcript which encodes a soluble form of CTLA-4.[151]

PD-1 and PDL-1/PD-L2

Programmed death-1 (PD-1) was initially described as an abundant transcript in a mouse T-cell hybridoma undergoing programmed cell death. Subsequently, it was shown that PD-1 is also expressed on activated T cells, B cells, and myeloid cells in humans and mice. PD-1 is a single IgV-like domain, but unlike CD28 and CTLA-4, it exists as a monomer at the cell surface. Like CTLA-4, even low levels of PD-1 at the cell surface are sufficient to mediate inhibition of T-cell activation. PD-1 has two counter-receptors, PD-L1 (B7h1) and PD-L2 (B7-DC), which share 38% sequence identity. PD-L1 mRNA is widely expressed in parenchymal tissue, including heart, placenta, skeletal muscle, and lung, but PD-L1 protein appears to be restricted to cancer cells, activated myeloid cells, and a subset of activated T cells. PD-L2 expression is restricted to activated macrophages and DCs.

Genetically modified mice deleted for expression of PD-1, PD-L1, or PD-L2 exhibit immune phenotypes consistent with an inhibitory role for this receptor ligand/pair in T-cell activation. PD-1-deficient mice spontaneously develop a lupus-like disease or autoimmune dilated cardiomyopathy, depending on the genetic background. PD-1-deficient mice crossed with H-2L[d]-specific TCR transgenic mice on an H-2[b/d] background develop splenomegaly and a lethal GVHD. In NOD mice, PD-1 deficiency or blockade accelerates progression of autoimmune diabetogenic disease. In humans, PD-1 has been identified as a candidate gene within a disease-susceptibility locus for systemic lupus erythematosus (SLE). In PD-L1-deficient mice, CD8[+] T cells exhibited enhanced clonal expansion and were capable of secreting higher levels of IFN-γ. Likewise, PD-L2-deficient mice exhibit enhanced *in vivo* T-cell activation and augmented APC function. A second study of PD-L2-deficient mice reported contradictory findings of diminished CD4[+] T-cell-dependent humoral responses and impaired CD8[+] T-cell anti-tumor responses, suggesting a costimulatory function for PD-L2. These studies suggest that mouse PD-L2 possesses dual stimulatory and inhibitory functions, invoking the presence of an additional costimulatory ligand analogous to PD-1. Nevertheless, it appears that the primary role of PD-L2 in humans is inhibitory.

Consistent with its function as a coinhibitory ligand, it has been shown that PD-1 attenuates immune responses to both viruses and tumors. In humans and mice, it has been shown that during chronic viral infection, T cells that have become non-responsive as a consequence of PD-1 overexpression, can be functionally reactivated following PD-1 blockade. It has been demonstrated that overexpression of PD-L1 in human cancer cells confers resistance to cytolysis by T cells, thought to be mediated by PD-L1-induced apoptosis in the T cell. Similarly, enhanced anti-tumor responses were observed in mice treated with T cells activated by APCs under conditions where PD-L1 function was blocked. Taken together, these results show that the primary function of the PD-1-PD-L1/PD-L2 pathway is to mediate downregulation of the immune response.

B7-H3 (B7RP-2)

B7 homolog 3 (B7-H3) was first identified in humans as a truncated sequence derived from a more abundant, full-length sequence ubiquitously expressed in many tissues including, heart, liver, lung, kidney, pancreas, and colon. Human B7-H3 protein is expressed on immature and mature DCs, activated monocytes, subsets of activated T cells, B cells, and NK cells, and also neuroblastomas and many other cancer cell lines. Mouse B7-H3 is similarly expressed in a wide variety of tissues, including osteoblasts. In mice, the abundant form of B7-H3 corresponds to the truncated form of human B7-H3, a consequence of selective exon loss that occurred in rodents, but not in humans. The putative counter structure for B7-H3 has not been identified.

Blocking experiments conducted with soluble B7-H3-Ig fusion proteins and antibodies have yielded conflicting functional results, although in mice, B7-H3 appears to function predominantly

as an attenuator of immune responses. For example, it has been shown that immobilized soluble B7-H3-Ig fusion protein induces a dose-dependent inhibition of mouse T-cell proliferation and reduced IL-2 and IFN-γ production. Furthermore, blockade of B7-H3 with an antagonist antibody was shown to enhance T-cell proliferation and enhance EAE. However, it has been shown that B7-H3 was capable of delivering a positive costimulation signal leading to expansion of antigen-specific CD8[+] cytolytic cells.

Genetically modified mice lacking B7-H3 developed more severe disease symptoms in both an airway inflammation model and an EAE model. An inhibitory role for B7-H3 was further supported by the finding that mouse APCs lacking B7-H3 expression exhibit enhanced stimulatory capacity. B7-H3-deficient mice developed a spontaneous autoimmune phenotype and develop anti-DNA autoantibodies with age. The relatively broad tissue distribution of B7-H3 suggests pleiotropic effects outside the immune system and a recent report describing reduced bone mineral density in B7-H3-deficient mice suggests a role for B7-H3 in osteoblast differentiation and bone mineralization. In humans, there is less evidence to support the role of B7-H3 as an inhibitory receptor, although it has been reported that B7-H3 expressed ectopically on APCs can attenuate T-cell proliferative responses. Interestingly, a recent report has shown that B7-H3 expression affords tumor cells protection from NK cell-mediated lysis. Taken together, it appears that B7-H3 functions predominantly as a coinhibitory receptor. The lack of structural conservation between human and mouse B7-H3 may further reflect species-specific differences in B7-H3 function in mice and humans.

B7-H4 (B7x, B7s1)

B7-H4 was identified by sequence database mining based on similarities to other known members of the gene family. Like B7-H3, B7-H4 mRNA is also expressed in many tissues, including lung, kidney, stomach, and small intestine, but the relatively broad distribution of the mRNA contrasts with the more restricted expression pattern of B7-H4 protein. In mice,

B7-H4 protein is expressed on splenic B cells and peritoneal macrophages, but not on T cells. In humans, B7-H4 is absent from resting T cells, B cells, monocytes, and DCs, but its expression is up-regulated on activated T cells and B cells. Aside from its expression on lymphoid cells, B7-H4 is highly expressed in human cancers, including breast, ovarian, renal, and kidney cancers. Moreover, B7-H4 is abundantly expressed on tumor-infiltrating macrophages in ovarian cancer. Initially, B7-H4 was thought to interact with the coinhibitory ligand BTLA (see below), but this has since been disproved. Binding studies with soluble B7-H4 have demonstrated a putative ligand on activated human T cells, although it remains unidentified.

There are relatively few data on the functional outcome of B7-H4 blockade on T-cell responses. However, one study reported that antisense oligo-mediated down-regulation of B7-H4 expression on tumor-infiltrating macrophages enhanced their ability to prime T cells when coinjected into ovarian tumors in a xenogeneic model. Recently, analysis of B7-H4-deficient mice revealed a mild enhancement in the magnitude of Th1-type responses, but the overall impact of B7-H4 deficiency on immune responses is subtle, possibly indicative of overlapping function between the ubiquitously expressed coinhibitory receptors such as B7-H3 and B7-H4.

BTLA

B- and T-lymphocyte attenuator (BTLA) was initially discovered in a mouse Th2 T-cell clone[183] and was subsequently shown to be also expressed at high levels on mouse B cells. In humans, BTLA is constitutively expressed on B and T cells and expression is diminished following activation.[184] The receptor for BTLA has been identified as HVEM,[185,186] a TNFR-related molecule which is relatively widely expressed on T cells, B cells, NK cells, DCs, and myeloid cells (see above). BTLA and HVEM are structurally unrelated and, as such, this interaction represents an unusual example of cross-talk between the two major structural classes of costimulatory and coinhibitory ligands and their receptors.[187]

In humans, cross-linking BTLA with an agonistic mAb inhibited T-cell proliferation and cytokine production in primary CD4$^+$ T-cell responses and secondary CD4$^+$ and CD8$^+$ responses.[184,188] At present, the function of BTLA on other cells is less clear. Unlike other costimulatory and coinhibitory ligands, BTLA is polymorphic and several alleles have been identified in various inbred mouse strains.[158] In humans, a BTLA gene polymorphism has been associated with an increased risk of RA.[190]

CONCLUSION AND SUMMARY

A regulated balance of activating and inhibitory signals is required to ensure an effective immune response while preserving self-tolerance. After its initiation, the magnitude and progression of the immune response are governed by an array of costimulatory and coinhibitory receptor ligand pairs whose expression is modulated both spatially and temporally. At the outset of the response, T-cell activation is directed largely by a combination of an antigen-specific signal via the TCR and a costimulatory signal delivered by CD28 ligation. As the response progresses, costimulation through other costimulatory ligands, such as ICOS, regulates the differentiation of T-cell effector function. At the height of the response, expression of coinhibitory molecules such as CTLA-4, BTLA, and PD-1 is up-regulated, which serves to dampen the response as the pathogen or antigen is cleared. While CTLA-4 is the predominant coinhibitory ligand, additional inhibitory signals are provided by BTLA, B7-H3, and B7-H4. The relatively broad distribution of some of the more recently discovered coinhibitory receptors suggests a key role for these molecules in the maintenance of tolerance and the regulation of immune responses in peripheral tissues. The molecules that direct costimulatory and coinhibitory signaling pathways represent tractable targets for therapeutic intervention in inflammatory autoimmune disease.

REFERENCES

1. Bretscher P, Cohn M. A theory of self-nonself discrimination. Science 1970; 169(950): 1042–9.
2. Cunningham AJ, Lafferty KJ. A simple conservative explanation of the H-2 restriction of interactions between lymphocytes. Scand J Immunol 1977; 6(1–2): 1–6.

3. Bretscher PA. A two-step, two-signal model for the primary activation of precursor helper T cells. Proc Natl Acad Sci U S A 1999; 96(1): 185–90.

4. Aruffo A, Seed B. Molecular cloning of a CD28 cDNA by a high-efficiency COS cell expression system. Proc Natl Acad Sci U S A 1987; 84(23): 8573–7.

5. Martin PJ, Ledbetter JA, Morishita et al. A 44 kilodalton cell surface homodimer regulates interleukin 2 production by activated human T lymphocytes. J Immunol 1986; 136(9): 3282–7.

6. Gross JA, Callas E, Allison JP. Identification and distribution of the costimulatory receptor CD28 in the mouse. J Immunol, 1992; 149(2): 380–8.

7. Harding FA, McArthur JG, Gross JA, Raulet DH, Allison JP. CD28-mediated signalling co-stimulates murine T cells and prevents induction of anergy in T-cell clones. Nature 1992; 356(6370): 607–9.

8. Ledbetter JA, Imbaten JB, Schieven GL et al. CD28 ligation in T-cell activation: evidence for two signal transduction pathways. Blood, 1990; 75(7): 1531–9.

9. Riley JL, June CH. The CD28 family: a T-cell rheostat for therapeutic control of T-cell activation. Blood, 2005; 105(1): 13–21.

10. Ndejembi MP, Teijaro JR, Patke DS et al. Control of memory CD4 T cell recall by the CD28/B7 costimulatory pathway. J Immunol, 2006; 177(11): 7698–706.

11. Freeman GJ, Freedman AS, Segil JM et al. B7, a new member of the Ig superfamily with unique expression on activated and neoplastic B cells. J Immunol, 1989; 143(8): 2714–22.

12. Azuma M, Ito D, Yagita H et al. B70 antigen is a second ligand for CTLA-4 and CD28. Nature, 1993; 366(6450): 76–9.

13. Freeman GJ, Gribben JG, Boussiotis VA et al. Cloning of B7-2: a CTLA-4 counter-receptor that costimulates human T cell proliferation. Science, 1993; 262(5135): 909–11.

14. Freedman AS, Freeman GJ, Rhynhart K, Nadler LM. Selective induction of B7/BB-1 on interferon-gamma stimulated monocytes: a potential mechanism for amplification of T cell activation through the CD28 pathway. Cell Immunol, 1991; 137(2): 429–37.

15. Lanier LL, O'Fallon S, Somoza C et al. CD80 (B7) and CD86 (B70) provide similar costimulatory signals for T cell proliferation, cytokine production, and generation of CTL. J Immunol, 1995; 154(1): 97–105.

16. Bhatia S, Edidin M, Almo SC, Nathensen SG. B7-1 and B7-2: similar costimulatory ligands with different biochemical, oligomeric and signaling properties. Immunol Lett, 2006; 104(1–2): 70–5.

17. Damle NK, Hansen JA, Good RA, Gupta S. Monoclonal antibody analysis of human T lymphocyte subpopulations exhibiting autologous mixed lymphocyte reaction. Proc Natl Acad Sci U S A, 1981; 78(8): 5096–8.

18. Damle NK, Doyle LV, Grosmaire LS, Ledbetter JA. Differential regulatory signals delivered by antibody binding to the CD28 (Tp44) molecule during the activation of human T lymphocytes. J Immunol, 1988; 140(6): 1753–61.

19. Gribben JG, Guinan EC, Boussiotis VA et al. Complete blockade of B7 family-mediated costimulation is necessary to induce human alloantigen-specific anergy: a method to ameliorate graft-versus-host disease and extend the donor pool. Blood, 1996; 87(11): 4887–93.

20. Linsley PS, Wallace PH, Johnson J et al. Immunosuppression in vivo by a soluble form of the CTLA-4 T cell activation molecule. Science, 1992; 257(5071): 792–5.

21. Judge TA, Tang A, Spain LM. The in vivo mechanism of action of CTLA4Ig. J Immunol, 1996; 156(6): 2294–9.

22. Bluestone JA. CTLA-4Ig is finally making it: a personal perspective. Am J Transplant, 2005; 5(3): 423–4.

23. Racke MK, Scott DE, Quigley L et al. Distinct roles for B7-1 (CD-80) and B7-2 (CD-86) in the initiation of experimental allergic encephalomyelitis. J Clin Invest, 1995; 96(5): 2195–203.

24. Lenschow DJ, Zeng Y, Thistlethwaite JR et al. Long-term survival of xenogeneic pancreatic islet grafts induced by CTLA4Ig. Science, 1992; 257(5071): 789–92.

25. Webb LM, Walmsley MJ and Feldmann M. Prevention and amelioration of collagen-induced arthritis by blockade of the CD28 co-stimulatory pathway: requirement for both B7-1 and B7-2. Eur J Immunol, 1996; 26(10): 2320–8.

26. Shahinian A, Pfeffer K, Lee KP et al. Differential T cell costimulatory requirements in CD28-deficient mice. Science, 1993; 261(5121): 609–12.

27. Green JM, Noel PJ, Sperling AI et al. Absence of B7-dependent responses in CD28-deficient mice. Immunity, 1994; 1(6): 501–8.

28. Freeman GJ, Borriello F, Hodes RJ et al. Uncovering of functional alternative CTLA-4 counter-receptor in B7-deficient mice. Science, 1993; 262(5135): 907–9.

29. Borriello F, Sethna MP, Boyd SD et al. B7-1 and B7-2 have overlapping, critical roles in immunoglobulin class switching and germinal center formation. Immunity, 1997; 6(3): 303–13.

30. Abrams JR, Lebwohl MG, Guzzo CA et al. CTLA4Ig-mediated blockade of T-cell costimulation in patients with psoriasis vulgaris. J Clin Invest, 1999; 103(9): 1243–52.

31. Kremer JM, Westhovens R, Leon M et al. Treatment of rheumatoid arthritis by selective inhibition of T-cell activation with fusion protein CTLA4Ig. N Engl J Med, 2003; 349(20): 1907–15.

32. Kremer JM, Dougados M, Emery P et al. Treatment of rheumatoid arthritis with the selective costimulation modulator abatacept: twelve-month results of a phase iib, double-blind, randomized, placebo-controlled trial. Arthritis Rheum, 2005; 52(8): 2263–71.

33. Kremer JM, Genant HK, Moreland LW et al. Effects of abatacept in patients with methotrexate-resistant active rheumatoid arthritis: a randomized trial. Ann Intern Med, 2006; 144(12): 865–76.

34. Huxley P, Sutton DH, Debnam P et al. High-affinity small molecule inhibitors of T cell costimulation: compounds for immunotherapy. Chem Biol, 2004; 11(12): 1651–8.

35. MacKenzie NM. New therapeutics that treat rheumatoid arthritis by blocking T-cell activation. Drug Discov Today, 2006; 11(19–20): 952–6.

36. Hutloff A, Dittrich AM, Beier KC et al. ICOS is an inducible T-cell co-stimulator structurally and functionally related to CD28. Nature, 1999; 397(6716): 263–6.

37. Riley JL, Mao M, Kobayashi S et al. Modulation of TCR-induced transcriptional profiles by ligation of CD28, ICOS, and CTLA-4 receptors. Proc Natl Acad Sci U S A, 2002; 99(18): 11790–5.

38. Riley JL, Blair PJ, Musser JT et al. ICOS costimulation requires IL-2 and can be prevented by CTLA-4 engagement. J Immunol, 2001; 166(8): 4943–8.

39. Coyle AJ, Lehar S, Lloyd C et al. The CD28-related molecule ICOS is required for effective T cell-dependent immune responses. Immunity, 2000; 13(1): 95–105.

40. Dong C, Juedes AE, Temann UA et al. ICOS co-stimulatory receptor is essential for T-cell activation and function. Nature, 2001; 409(6816): 97–101.

41. Tafuri A, Shahinian A, Bladt F et al. ICOS is essential for effective T-helper-cell responses. Nature, 2001; 409(6816): 105–9.

42. Nurieva R, Thomas S, Nguyen T et al. T-cell tolerance or function is determined by combinatorial costimulatory signals. EMBO J, 2006; 25(11): 2623–33.

43. Aicher A, Hayden-Ledbetter M, Brady WA et al. Characterization of human inducible costimulator ligand expression and function. J Immunol, 2000; 164(9): 4689–96.

44. Kopf M, Coyle AJ, Schmitz N et al. Inducible costimulator protein (ICOS) controls T helper cell subset polarization after virus and parasite infection. J Exp Med, 2000; 192(1): 53–61.

45. Grimbacher B, Hutloff A, Schlesier M et al. Homozygous loss of ICOS is associated with adult-onset common variable immunodeficiency. Nat Immunol, 2003; 4(3): 261–8.

46. Warnatz K, Bassaller L, Salzer U et al. Human ICOS deficiency abrogates the germinal center reaction and provides a monogenic model for common variable immunodeficiency. Blood, 2006; 107(8): 3045–52.

47. Clark EA. CD40: a cytokine receptor in search of a ligand. Tissue Antigens, 1990; 36(1): 33–6.

48. Danese S, Sans M and Fiocchi C. The CD40/CD40L costimulatory pathway in inflammatory bowel disease. Gut, 2004; 53(7): 1035–43.

49. Hollenbaugh D, Grosmaire LS, Kullas CD et al. The human T cell antigen gp39, a member of the TNF gene family, is a ligand for the CD40 receptor: expression of a soluble form of gp39 with B cell co-stimulatory activity. EMBO J, 1992; 11(12): 4313–21.

50. Noelle RJ, Roy M, Shepherd DM et al. A 39-kDa protein on activated helper T cells binds CD40 and transduces the signal for cognate activation of B cells. Proc Natl Acad Sci U S A, 1992; 89(14): 6550–4.

51. Buchner K, Henn V, Grafe M et al. CD40 ligand is selectively expressed on CD4+ T cells and platelets: implications for CD40-CD40L signalling in atherosclerosis. J Pathol, 2003; 201(2): 288–95.

52. Daoussis D, Andonopoulos AP, and Liossis SN. Targeting CD40L: a promising therapeutic approach. Clin Diagn Lab Immunol, 2004; 11(4): 635–41.

53. Caux C, Massacrier C, Vanbervliet B et al. Activation of human dendritic cells through CD40 cross-linking. J Exp Med, 1994; 180(4): 1263–72.

54. Roy M, Aruffo A, Ledbetter J et al. Studies on the interdependence of gp39 and B7 expression and function during antigen-specific immune responses. Eur J Immunol, 1995; 25(2): 596–603.

55. Blair PJ, Riley JL, Harlan DM et al. CD40 ligand (CD154) triggers a short-term CD4(+) T cell activation response that results in secretion of immunomodulatory cytokines and apoptosis. J Exp Med, 2000; 191(4): 651–60.

56. Bourgeois C, Rocha B, and Tanchot C. A role for CD40 expression on CD8+ T cells in the generation of CD8+ T cell memory. Science, 2002; 297(5589): 2060–3.

57. Mach F, Schonbeck U, Fabunmi RP et al. T lymphocytes induce endothelial cell matrix metalloproteinase expression by a CD40L-dependent mechanism: implications for tubule formation. Am J Pathol, 1999; 154(1): 229–38.

58. Thienel U, Loike J, and Yellin MJ. CD154 (CD40L) induces human endothelial cell chemokine production and migration of leukocyte subsets. Cell Immunol, 1999; 198(2): 87–95.

59. Dechanet J, Grasset C, Taupin JL et al. CD40 ligand stimulates proinflammatory cytokine production by human endothelial cells. J Immunol, 1997; 159(11): 5640–7.

60. Karmann K, Hughes CC, Schechner J, Fanslow WC, Pober JS. CD40 on human endothelial cells: inducibility by cytokines and functional regulation of adhesion molecule expression. Proc Natl Acad Sci U S A, 1995; 92(10): 4342–6.

61. Zan H, Cerutti A, Dramitinos P, Schaffer A, Casali P. CD40 engagement triggers switching to IgA1 and IgA2 in human B cells through induction of endogenous TGF-beta: evidence for TGF-beta but not IL-10-dependent direct S mu—>S alpha and sequential S mu—>S gamma,

S gamma—>S alpha DNA recombination. J Immunol, 1998; 161(10): 5217–25.

62. Callard RE, Armitage RJ, Fanslow WC, Spriggs MK. CD40 ligand and its role in X-linked hyper-IgM syndrome. Immunol Today, 1993; 14(11): 559–64.

63. Xu J, Foy TM, Laman JD et al. Mice deficient for the CD40 ligand. Immunity, 1994; 1(5): 423–31.

64. Grewal IS, Xu J and Flavell RA. Impairment of antigen-specific T-cell priming in mice lacking CD40 ligand. Nature, 1995; 378(6557): 617–20.

65. Kirk AD, Harlan DM, Armstrong NN et al. CTLA4-Ig and anti-CD40 ligand prevent renal allograft rejection in primates. Proc Natl Acad Sci U S A, 1997; 94(16): 8789–94.

66. Yu X, Carpenter P and Anasetti C. Advances in transplantation tolerance. Lancet, 2001; 357(9272): 1959–63.

67. Durie FH, Fava RA, Foy TM et al. Prevention of collagen-induced arthritis with an antibody to gp39, the ligand for CD40. Science, 1993; 261(5126): 1328–30.

68. Kyburz D, Carson DA and Corr M. The role of CD40 ligand and tumor necrosis factor alpha signaling in the transgenic K/BxN mouse model of rheumatoid arthritis. Arthritis Rheum, 2000; 43(11): 2571–7.

69. Kalunian KC, Davis JC Jr, Merrill JT et al. Treatment of systemic lupus erythematosus by inhibition of T cell costimulation with anti-CD154: a randomized, double-blind, placebo-controlled trial. Arthritis Rheum, 2002; 46(12): 3251–8.

70. Boumpas DT, Furie R, Manzis et al. A short course of BG9588 (anti-CD40 ligand antibody) improves serologic activity and decreases hematuria in patients with proliferative lupus glomerulonephritis. Arthritis Rheum, 2003; 48(3): 719–27.

71. Kawai T, Andrews D, Colvin RB, Sachs DH, Cosimi AB. Thromboembolic complications after treatment with monoclonal antibody against CD40 ligand. Nat Med, 2000; 6(2): 114.

72. Paterson DJ, Jefferies WA, Green JR et al. Antigens of activated rat T lymphocytes including a molecule of 50,000 Mr detected only on CD4 positive T blasts. Mol Immunol, 1987; 24(12): 1281–90.

73. Mallett S, Fossum S and Barclay AN. Characterization of the MRC OX40 antigen of activated CD4 positive T lymphocytes – a molecule related to nerve growth factor receptor. EMBO J, 1990; 9(4): 1063–8.

74. Latza U, Durkop H, Schnittger S et al. The human OX40 homolog: cDNA structure, expression and chromosomal assignment of the ACT35 antigen. Eur J Immunol, 1994; 24(3): 677–83.

75. Gramaglia I, Weinberg AD, Lemon M, Croft M. Ox-40 ligand: a potent costimulatory molecule for sustaining primary CD4 T cell responses. J Immunol, 1998; 161(12): 6510–17.

76. Weinberg AD, Evans DE, Thalhofer C, Shi T, Prell RA. The generation of T cell memory: a review describing the molecular and cellular events following OX40 (CD134) engagement. J Leukoc Biol, 2004; 75(6): 962–72.

77. Baum PR, Gayle RB 3rd, Ramsdell F et al. Molecular characterization of murine and human OX40/OX40 ligand systems: identification of a human OX40 ligand as the HTLV-1-regulated protein gp34. EMBO J, 1994; 13(17): 3992–4001.

78. Watts TH. TNF/TNFR family members in costimulation of T cell responses. Annu Rev Immunol, 2005; 23: 23–68.

79. Weinberg AD, Vella AT and Croft M. OX-40: life beyond the effector T cell stage. Semin Immunol, 1998; 10(6): 471–80.

80. Godfrey WR, Fagnoni FF, Harava MA, Buck D, Engleman EG. Identification of a human OX-40 ligand, a costimulator of CD4+ T cells with homology to tumor necrosis factor. J Exp Med, 1994; 180(2): 757–62.

81. Gramaglia I, Jember A, Pippig SD et al. The OX40 costimulatory receptor determines the development of CD4 memory by regulating primary clonal expansion. J Immunol, 2000; 165(6): 3043–50.

82. Weinberg AD, Thalhofer C, Morris N et al. Anti-OX40 (CD134) administration to nonhuman primates: immunostimulatory effects and toxicokinetic study. J Immunother, 2006; 29(6): 575–85.

83. Brocker T, Gulbranson-Judge A, Flynn S et al. CD4 T cell traffic control: in vivo evidence that ligation of OX40 on CD4 T cells by OX40-ligand expressed on dendritic cells leads to the accumulation of CD4 T cells in B follicles. Eur J Immunol, 1999; 29(5): 1610–16.

84. Weinberg AD, Wallin JJ, Jones RE et al. Target organ-specific up-regulation of the MRC OX-40 marker and selective production of Th1 lymphokine mRNA by encephalitogenic T helper cells isolated from the spinal cord of rats with experimental autoimmune encephalomyelitis. J Immunol, 1994; 152(9): 4712–21.

85. Weinberg AD, Bourdette EN, Sullivan TJ et al. Selective depletion of myelin-reactive T cells with the anti-OX-40 antibody ameliorates autoimmune encephalomyelitis. Nat Med, 1996; 2(2): 183–9.

86. Tittle TV, Weinberg AD, Steinketer CN, Maziarz RT. Expression of the T-cell activation antigen, OX-40, identifies alloreactive T cells in acute graft-versus-host disease. Blood, 1997; 89(12): 4652–8.

87. Higgins LM, McDonald SA, Whittle N et al. Regulation of T cell activation in vitro and in vivo by targeting the OX40-OX40 ligand interaction: amelioration of ongoing inflammatory bowel disease with an OX40-IgG fusion protein, but not with an OX40 ligand-IgG fusion protein. J Immunol, 1999; 162(1): 486–93.

88. Yoshioka T, Nakajima A, Akiba H et al. Contribution of OX40/OX40 ligand interaction to the pathogenesis of

rheumatoid arthritis. Eur J Immunol, 2000; 30(10): 2815–23.

89. Weinberg AD, Wegmann KW, Fanatake C, Whitham RH et al. Blocking OX-40/OX-40 ligand interaction in vitro and in vivo leads to decreased T cell function and amelioration of experimental allergic encephalomyelitis. J Immunol, 1999; 162(3): 1818–26.

90. Nohara C, Akiba H, Nakajima A et al. Amelioration of experimental autoimmune encephalomyelitis with anti-OX40 ligand monoclonal antibody: a critical role for OX40 ligand in migration, but not development of pathogenic T cells. J Immunol, 2001; 166(3): 2108–15.

91. Weinberg AD, Lemon M, Jones AJ et al. OX-40 antibody enhances for autoantigen specific V beta 8.2+ T cells within the spinal cord of Lewis rats with autoimmune encephalomyelitis. J Neurosci Res, 1996; 43(1): 42–9.

92. Kwon BS and Weissman SM. cDNA sequences of two inducible T-cell genes. Proc Natl Acad Sci U S A, 1989; 86(6): 1963–7.

93. Pollok KE, Kim YJ, Zhou Z et al. Inducible T cell antigen 4-1BB. Analysis of expression and function. J Immunol, 1993; 150(3): 771–81.

94. Melero I, Johnston JV, Shufford WW, Mittler RS, Chen L et al. NK1.1 cells express 4-1BB (CDw137) costimulatory molecule and are required for tumor immunity elicited by anti-4-1BB monoclonal antibodies. Cell Immunol, 1998; 190(2): 167–72.

95. Goodwin RG, Din WS, Davis-Smith T et al. Molecular cloning of a ligand for the inducible T cell gene 4-1BB: a member of an emerging family of cytokines with homology to tumor necrosis factor. Eur J Immunol, 1993; 23(10): 2631–41.

96. DeBenedette MA, Shahinian A, Mak TW, Watts TH et al. Costimulation of CD28- T lymphocytes by 4-1BB ligand. J Immunol, 1997; 158(2): 551–9.

97. Pollok KE, Kim YJ, Hurtado J et al. 4-1BB T-cell antigen binds to mature B cells and macrophages, and costimulates anti-mu-primed splenic B cells. Eur J Immunol, 1994; 24(2): 367–74.

98. Shuford WW, Klussman K, Tritchler DD et al. 4-1BB costimulatory signals preferentially induce CD8+ T cell proliferation and lead to the amplification in vivo of cytotoxic T cell responses. J Exp Med, 1997; 186(1): 47–55.

99. Takahashi C, Mittler RS and Vella AT. Cutting edge: 4-1BB is a bonafide CD8 T cell survival signal. J Immunol, 1999; 162(9): 5037–40.

100. Langstein J, Michel J, Fritsche J et al. CD137 (ILA/4-1BB), a member of the TNF receptor family, induces monocyte activation via bidirectional signaling. J Immunol, 1998; 160(5): 2488–94.

101. Langstein J and Schwarz H. Identification of CD137 as a potent monocyte survival factor. J Leukoc Biol, 1999; 65(6): 829–33.

102. Michel J, Pauly S, Langstein J, Krammer PH, Schwarz H et al. CD137-induced apoptosis is independent of CD95. Immunology, 1999; 98(1): 42–6.

103. Mittler RS, Baily TS, Klussman K, Trailsmith MD, Hoffmann MK. Anti-4-1BB monoclonal antibodies abrogate T cell-dependent humoral immune responses in vivo through the induction of helper T cell anergy. J Exp Med, 1999; 190(10): 1535–40.

104. Foell J, McCausland M, Burch J et al. CD137-mediated T cell co-stimulation terminates existing autoimmune disease in SLE-prone NZB/NZW F1 mice. Ann NY Acad Sci, 2003; 987: 230–5.

105. Foell JL, Diez-Mendiondo BI, Deiz OH et al. Engagement of the CD137 (4-1BB) costimulatory molecule inhibits and reverses the autoimmune process in collagen-induced arthritis and establishes lasting disease resistance. Immunology, 2004; 113(1): 89–98.

106. Seo SK, Choi JH, Kim YH et al. 4-1BB-mediated immunotherapy of rheumatoid arthritis. Nat Med, 2004; 10(10): 1088–94.

107. Mauri DN, Ebner R, Montgomery RI et al. LIGHT, a new member of the TNF superfamily, and lymphotoxin alpha are ligands for herpesvirus entry mediator. Immunity, 1998; 8(1): 21–30.

108. Tamada K, Shimozaki K, Chapoval AI et al. LIGHT, a TNF-like molecule, costimulates T cell proliferation and is required for dendritic cell-mediated allogeneic T cell response. J Immunol, 2000; 164(8): 4105–10.

109. Zhai Y, Guo R, Hsu TL et al. LIGHT, a novel ligand for lymphotoxin beta receptor and TR2/HVEM induces apoptosis and suppresses in vivo tumor formation via gene transfer. J Clin Invest, 1998; 102(6): 1142–51.

110. Granger SW, Butrovich KD, Houshmand P, Edwards WR, Ware CF. Genomic characterization of LIGHT reveals linkage to an immune response locus on chromosome 19p13.3 and distinct isoforms generated by alternate splicing or proteolysis. J Immunol, 2001; 167(9): 5122–8.

111. Morel Y, Schiano de colelta JM, Harrop J et al. Reciprocal expression of the TNF family receptor herpes virus entry mediator and its ligand LIGHT on activated T cells: LIGHT down-regulates its own receptor. J Immunol, 2000; 165(8): 4397–404.

112. Kwon BS, Tan KB, Ni J et al. A newly identified member of the tumor necrosis factor receptor superfamily with a wide tissue distribution and involvement in lymphocyte activation. J Biol Chem, 1997; 272(22): 14272–6.

113. Morel Y, Truneh A, Sweet RW, Olive D, Costello RT. The TNF superfamily members LIGHT and CD154 (CD40 ligand) costimulate induction of dendritic cell maturation and elicit specific CTL activity. J Immunol, 2001; 167(5): 2479–86.

114. Tamada K, Shimozaki K, Chapoval AI et al. Modulation of T-cell-mediated immunity in tumor

and graft-versus-host disease models through the LIGHT co-stimulatory pathway. Nat Med, 2000; 6(3): 283–9.

115. Liu J, Schmidt CS, Zhao F et al. LIGHT-deficiency impairs CD8+ T cell expansion, but not effector function. Int Immunol, 2003; 15(7): 861–70.

116. Wang J, Anders RA, Wang Y et al. The critical role of LIGHT in promoting intestinal inflammation and Crohn's disease. J Immunol, 2005; 174(12): 8173–82.

117. Tamada K, Ni J, Zhu G et al. Cutting edge: selective impairment of CD8+ T cell function in mice lacking the TNF superfamily member LIGHT. J Immunol, 2002; 168(10): 4832–5.

118. Shaikh RB, Santee S, Granjer SW et al. Constitutive expression of LIGHT on T cells leads to lymphocyte activation, inflammation, and tissue destruction. J Immunol, 2001; 167(11): 6330–7.

119. Ye Q, Fraser CC, Gao W et al. Modulation of LIGHT-HVEM costimulation prolongs cardiac allograft survival. J Exp Med, 2002; 195(6): 795–800.

120. Mackay F, Browning JL, Lawton P et al. Both the lymphotoxin and tumor necrosis factor pathways are involved in experimental murine models of colitis. Gastroenterology, 1998; 115(6): 1464–75.

121. van Lier RA, Borst J, Vroom TM et al. Tissue distribution and biochemical and functional properties of Tp55 (CD27), a novel T cell differentiation antigen. J Immunol, 1987; 139(5): 1589–96.

122. Gravestein LA, Blom B, Nolten LA et al. Cloning and expression of murine CD27: comparison with 4-1BB, another lymphocyte-specific member of the nerve growth factor receptor family. Eur J Immunol, 1993; 23(4): 943–50.

123. Lens SM, Tesselaar K, Van Oers MH, van Lier RA. Control of lymphocyte function through CD27-CD70 interactions. Semin Immunol, 1998; 10(6): 491–9.

124. Tesselaar K, Xiao Y, Arens R et al. Expression of the murine CD27 ligand CD70 in vitro and in vivo. J Immunol, 2003; 170(1): 33–40.

125. Dorner T and Lipsky PE. Correlation of circulating CD27high plasma cells and disease activity in systemic lupus erythematosus. Lupus, 2004; 13(5): 283–9.

126. Borst J, Hendriks J and Xiao Y. CD27 and CD70 in T cell and B cell activation. Curr Opin Immunol, 2005; 17(3): 275–81.

127. Agematsu K, Nagumo H, Oguchi Y et al. Generation of plasma cells from peripheral blood memory B cells: synergistic effect of interleukin-10 and CD27/CD70 interaction. Blood, 1998; 91(1): 173–80.

128. Hendriks J, Xiao Y and Borst J. CD27 promotes survival of activated T cells and complements CD28 in generation and establishment of the effector T cell pool. J Exp Med, 2003; 198(9): 1369–80.

129. Tesselaar K, Arens R, Van Schijndel GM et al. Lethal T cell immunodeficiency induced by chronic costimulation via CD27-CD70 interactions. Nat Immunol, 2003; 4(1): 49–54.

130. Yamada A, Salama AD, Sho M et al. CD70 signaling is critical for CD28-independent CD8+ T cell-mediated alloimmune responses in vivo. J Immunol, 2005; 174(3): 1357–64.

131. Horie R, Higashihara M and Watanabe T. Hodgkin's lymphoma and CD30 signal transduction. Int J Hematol, 2003; 77(1): 37–47.

132. Kennedy MK, Willis CR and Armitage RJ. Deciphering CD30 ligand biology and its role in humoral immunity. Immunology, 2006; 118(2): 143–52.

133. Gruss HJ, Boiani N, Williams DE et al. Pleiotropic effects of the CD30 ligand on CD30-expressing cells and lymphoma cell lines. Blood, 1994; 83(8): 2045–56.

134. Smith CA, Grass HJ, Davis T et al. CD30 antigen, a marker for Hodgkin's lymphoma, is a receptor whose ligand defines an emerging family of cytokines with homology to TNF. Cell, 1993; 73(7): 1349–60.

135. Shanebeck KD, Maliszewski CR, Kennedy MK et al. Regulation of murine B cell growth and differentiation by CD30 ligand. Eur J Immunol, 1995; 25(8): 2147–53.

136. Bowen MA, Olsen KJ, Cheng L, Avila D, Podack ER et al. Functional effects of CD30 on a large granular lymphoma cell line, YT. Inhibition of cytotoxicity, regulation of CD28 and IL-2R, and induction of homotypic aggregation. J Immunol, 1993; 151(11): 5896–906.

137. Gaspal FM, Kim MY, McConnell FM et al. Mice deficient in OX40 and CD30 signals lack memory antibody responses because of deficient CD4 T cell memory. J Immunol, 2005; 174(7): 3891–6.

138. Siegmund T, Armitage N, Wicker LS et al. Analysis of the mouse CD30 gene: a candidate for the NOD mouse type 1 diabetes locus Idd9.2. Diabetes, 2000; 49(9): 1612–16.

139. Chakrabarty S, Nagata M, Yasuda H et al. Critical roles of CD30/CD30L interactions in murine autoimmune diabetes. Clin Exp Immunol, 2003; 133(3): 318–25.

140. Blazar BR, Levy RB, Mak TW et al. CD30/CD30 ligand (CD153) interaction regulates CD4+ T cell-mediated graft-versus-host disease. J Immunol, 2004; 173(5): 2933–41.

141. Brunet JF, Denizot F, Luciani MF et al. A new member of the immunoglobulin superfamily – CTLA-4. Nature, 1987; 328(6127): 267–70.

142. Dariavach P, Mattei MG, Golstein P, Lefranc MP. Human Ig superfamily CTLA-4 gene: chromosomal localization and identity of protein sequence between murine and human CTLA-4 cytoplasmic domains. Eur J Immunol, 1988; 18(12): 1901–5.

143. Blair PJ, Riley JL, Levine BL et al. CTLA-4 ligation delivers a unique signal to resting human CD4 T cells that inhibits interleukin-2 secretion but allows Bcl-X(L) induction. J Immunol, 1998; 160(1): 12–15.

144. Stamper CC, Zhang Y, Tobin JF et al. Crystal structure of the B7-1/CTLA-4 complex that inhibits human immune responses. Nature, 2001; 410(6828): 608–11.

145. Lee KM, Chaung E, Griffin M et al. Molecular basis of T cell inactivation by CTLA-4. Science, 1998; 282(5397): 2263–6.

146. Egen JG and Allison JP. Cytotoxic T lymphocyte antigen-4 accumulation in the immunological synapse is regulated by TCR signal strength. Immunity, 2002; 16(1): 23–35.

147. Chikuma S, Imboden JB and Bluestone JA. Negative regulation of T cell receptor-lipid raft interaction by cytotoxic T lymphocyte-associated antigen 4. J Exp Med, 2003; 197(1): 129–35.

148. Vijayakrishnan L, Salvik JM, Illes Z et al. An autoimmune disease-associated CTLA-4 splice variant lacking the B7 binding domain signals negatively in T cells. Immunity, 2004; 20(5): 563–75.

149. Teft WA, Kirchhof MG and Madrenas J. A molecular perspective of CTLA-4 function. Annu Rev Immunol, 2006; 24: 65–97.

150. Tivol EA, Borriello F, Schweitzer AN et al. Loss of CTLA-4 leads to massive lymphoproliferation and fatal multiorgan tissue destruction, revealing a critical negative regulatory role of CTLA-4. Immunity, 1995; 3(5): 541–7.

151. Ueda H, Howson JM, Esposito L et al. Association of the T-cell regulatory gene CTLA4 with susceptibility to autoimmune disease. Nature, 2003; 423(6939): 506–11.

183. Watanabe N, Gavrieli M, Sedy JR et al. BTLA is a lymphocyte inhibitory receptor with similarities to CTLA-4 and PD-1. Nat Immunol, 2003; 4(7): 670–9.

184. Otsuki N, Kamimura Y, Hashiguchi M, Azuma M. Expression and function of the B and T lymphocyte attenuator (BTLA/CD272) on human T cells. Biochem Biophys Res Commun, 2006; 344(4): 1121–7.

185. Sedy JR, Gavrieli M, Potter KG et al. B and T lymphocyte attenuator regulates T cell activation through interaction with herpesvirus entry mediator. Nat Immunol, 2005; 6(1): 90–8.

186. Gonzalez LC, Loyet KM, Calemine-Fenaux J et al. A coreceptor interaction between the CD28 and TNF receptor family members B and T lymphocyte attenuator and herpesvirus entry mediator. Proc Natl Acad Sci U S A, 2005; 102(4): 1116–21.

187. Murphy KM, Nelson CA and Sedy JR. Balancing co-stimulation and inhibition with BTLA and HVEM. Nat Rev Immunol, 2006; 6(9): 671–81.

188. Krieg C, Han P, Stone R, Goularte OD, Kaye J et al. Functional analysis of B and T lymphocyte attenuator engagement on CD4+ and CD8+ T cells. J Immunol, 2005; 175(10): 6420–7.

189. Hurchla MA, Sedy JR, Gavrieli M et al. B and T lymphocyte attenuator exhibits structural and expression polymorphisms and is highly induced in anergic CD4+ T cells. J Immunol, 2005; 174(6): 3377–85.

190. Lin SC, Kuo CC and Chan CH. Association of a BTLA gene polymorphism with the risk of rheumatoid arthritis. J Biomed Sci 2006; 13(6): 853–60.

3

Regulatory T cells

Harald von Boehmer

INTRODUCTION

Cellular therapy employing Foxp3-expressing regulatory T cells (Tregs) holds the promise to replace and/or supplement indiscriminatory immunosuppression by drugs. In order to achieve this goal in the clinic we need to learn more about the generation, lifestyle, and function of Tregs. One way to generate Tregs of any desired antigen specificity is the retroviral introduction of the Foxp3 gene into activated CD4 T cells. Foxp3 is mostly but not exclusively a transcriptional repressor that interferes with T-cell receptor (TCR)-dependent activation of genes and may exert its effect, at least in part, by compromising NF-AT-dependent gene activation. Another way of generating Tregs extrathymically *in vivo* is the introduction of low amounts of peptides under subimmunogenic conditions. Such artificially induced Tregs have a long lifespan in the absence of the inducing antigen and can thus mediate antigen-specific tolerance. Antigen specificity of Tregs-mediated immunosuppression is due to effective co-recruitment and expression of Tregs and T effector cells to antigen-draining lymph nodes and sites of inflammation such that Tregs effectively suppress neighboring effector T cells at early or late stages of their differentiation. The latter allows for interference with already established unwanted immunity and may thus be employed to treat rather than prevent unwanted immune reactions.

The notion that the immune system employs different mechanisms to prevent autoimmune disease or maintain self-tolerance has been around for decades, but definitive evidence emphasizing the essential role of negative selection as well as that of suppressor or regulatory T cells is of more recent origin. Today we distinguish negative selection in the form of deletion[1] of certain antigen-specific cells as well as in the form of 'anergy'[2] by cell-autonomous mechanisms, also referred to as 'recessive' tolerance, from tolerance that relies on the silencing of immune cells by regulatory or suppressor T cells by non-cell-autonomous mechanisms,[3] also referred to as 'dominant' tolerance. Both forms of tolerance can achieve antigen-specific non-responsiveness of the immune system in contrast to pharmacological interventions that usually result in undesirable general immunosuppression with potentially deadly side effects. In many clinical situations antigen-specific non-responsiveness represents the desired goal but in general present day treatment does not achieve that goal. For that reason it remains a great challenge for immunologists to design strategies and protocols that achieve antigen-specific non-responsiveness, since there is little hope that the pharmaceutical industry will come up with suitable procedures to effectively and specifically interfere with unwanted immunity in the near future. Given this goal, it appears a reasonable strategy to exploit evolutionarily selected mechanisms effective in self-tolerance for clinical purposes. This requires a thorough understanding of how the immune system manages to avoid self-aggression. It is now appreciated that so-called negative selection of potentially self-reactive T cells by antigens inside and probably also outside the thymus essentially contributes to self-tolerance.[4] Likewise it has become clear that the generation of Foxp3-expressing regulatory T cells is mandatory to achieve self-tolerance.[5] The progress in understanding the contribution of such reasonably well-defined mechanisms to tolerance has thus established the somewhat limited usefulness of models that solely consider the absence of 'danger' signals as an essential feature of self-tolerance.

While we have some basic ideas about mechanisms that can be exploited to induce antigen-specific non-responsiveness, much needs to be learned in detail before this will become clinically applicable. Experiments have shown that overexpression of certain crucial self-antigens (such as insulin) that results in more profound tolerance by negative selection,[6] can be helpful in preventing autoimmune disease, perhaps because certain autoimmune diseases, such as type 1 diabetes, begin with a rather limited autoimmune response to antigens such as insulin,[6,7] while later on a variety of other antigens in pancreatic β cells are recognized. However, clinically, such maneuvers would be limited to introducing such antigens prior to disease outbreak or when the immune system is 'reset' after elimination of mature lymphocytes by x-irradiation and/or cytotoxic drugs.

In contrast, the manipulation of regulatory T cells appears to represent a more widely applicable approach not only to prevent but potentially also to interfere with already ongoing unwanted immunity. With such a clinical goal in mind it is clear that we need to have a much better understanding of how antigen-specific regulatory T cells are and can be generated and/or amplified and how they can achieve antigen-specific non-responsiveness. It is the purpose of this chapter to review recent progress in the understanding of several aspects of regulatory T cells with the hope that some of this information may find its way into the clinic, with the challenge that ensuing procedures will eventually replace or at least supplement the present day practice of indiscriminate immunosuppression.

CHARACTERISTICS OF REGULATORY T CELLS

Recent years have seen rapid progress in the characterization of regulatory T cells (Tregs). There is not one particular cell surface marker that defines Tregs but the CD25 surface molecule is at least expressed on the vast majority of cells that express the Foxp3 transcription factor, which has become a signature gene expressed in Tregs. The recognition that CD25+ cells are enriched in Tregs has thus contributed considerably to establishing their role in suppressing the activation and function of other lymphocytes.[8] In the meantime other molecules such as neuropilin 1,[9] CD103,[10] GPR83,[11] GITR,[12] and CTLA-4[13] have been shown to have a characteristic expression profile in Tregs and thus can be helpful in achieving optimal purification in combination with the CD25 marker. Recent evidence shows that CD4+25+ Tregs are IL-7R-negative, in contrast to CD4+25+ cells that just represent activated T cells without obvious regulatory function.[14] Intracellular staining by Foxp3 antibodies represents a useful means to identify Tregs in various tissues[15] and in the meantime various Foxp3 reporter mice[16,17] have become available, which allow purification of functional Foxp3-expressing cells. While Foxp3 expression represents a good signature for Tregs it can have its drawbacks, because Foxp3 can be transiently expressed in activated T cells that do not qualify as stable Tregs.[15]

A variety of studies indicate that stable Foxp3 expression is sufficient to confer a regulatory T-cell phenotype to CD4 T cells.[18–20] Thus retroviral Foxp3 transduction is a valuable means to endow antigen-specific T cells with a regulatory phenotype. This represents an important tool because, unlike the *in vitro* expansion[21,22] of Tregs that have been preformed *in vivo*, it allows production of Tregs of any desired specificity.

Recent data suggest that Foxp3 can interact with NF-AT in a DNA binding complex to regulate gene expression such as down-regulation of the IL-2 gene and up-regulation of CTLA-4 and CD25 molecules.[23] It is presently not clear whether all Foxp3-dependent gene regulation involves NF-AT and whether NF-AT plays a crucial role in the generation of Tregs. It has become clear from the combined analysis of Foxp3 binding and genome-wide gene expression, however, that Foxp3 is predominantly but not exclusively a repressor that silences genes that are normally activated after T-cell stimulation, especially genes associated with T-cell receptor (TCR) signaling.[43] This fact may contribute to the relatively poor response of Tregs in response to antigenic stimulation *in vitro*, while exogenous growth factors may permit effective clonal expansion *in vivo*. The latter feature is likely essential for effective *in vivo* suppression.

Among the genes that fail to be up-regulated in Foxp3-expressing cells is the PTPN22 phosphatase that has a role in dephosphorylating p56[lck] and Zap-70. Interestingly, a gain of function mutation of this gene is associated with several autoimmune diseases and it is presently not clear whether this mutant affects Tregs that control autoimmune disease or effector T cells that cause autoimmune disease.[24]

Another important characteristic of Tregs is that they do express an αβ,TCR that confers antigen specificity. This is worthwhile pointing out, since many studies on Tregs ignore this fact. It is our belief that antigen specificity of Tregs is absolutely crucial for antigen-specific suppression of immune responses and hence considerable attention has to be paid to the role of TCR specificity in the generation, homing, and effector function of Tregs.[25] As all T cells with αβ, TCRs, Tregs also undergo stringent TCR-dependent selection in primary and secondary lymphoid organs,[26] which eventually may be exploited to generate Tregs of any desired specificity and to interfere specifically with unwanted immune responses in the clinic.

INTRA- AND EXTRA-THYMIC GENERATION OF TREGS

Experiments in TCR transgenic mice, in which the transgenic TCR was the only TCR expressed, by developing T cells have clearly shown that ligation of the αβ,TCR by strong agonist ligands plays an essential role in the intrathymic generation of Tregs.[27,28] These results are compatible with analysis of the Tregs TCR repertoire in normal mice, suggesting a focus on self-antigens.[29] It became especially obvious that expression of TCR ligands by thymic epithelial cells represented a powerful means to commit developing CD4+ T cells to the Treg lineage.[28] In this context it is of considerable interest to note that thymic epithelial cells, and especially thymic medullary epithelial cells, can express 'ectopically' a variety of proteins that otherwise would be considered 'organ-specific' such as preproinsulin2 that is expressed in pancreatic β cells but also in thymic medullary epithelial cells.[30,31] Such ectopic expression can be regulated, at least in part, by the AIRE (autoimmuneimmune regulator) transcription factor[32] and it is thus conceivable that the ectopic expression of 'organ-specific' antigen by thymic epithelium plays a decisive role in the generation of Tregs specific for such antigens, even though experiments addressing that question have so far yielded negative results.[33,34] However, negative results by no means rule out the possibility that AIRE-regulated antigens contribute to the generation of Tregs under more favorable experimental conditions.

The intrathymic generation of Tregs by strong agonist ligands appears to require costimulation of developing cells by B7-1 (CD80)[35] ligands that are expressed on thymic epithelial cells as well as on antigen-presenting cells (APCs) of hemopoietic origin, at least under certain experimental conditions. This is a somewhat astonishing observation in the light of findings that Treg generation in peripheral lymphoid tissue is most effective under conditions that avoid costimulation (see below). Conceivably this could be due to the different stages of development of thymic and extrathymic T cells, which may require different signaling inputs for Treg commitment. From thymus transplantation experiments it is clear that Tregs generated by ligands expressed on thymic epithelium only can migrate into peripheral lymphoid tissue and patrol the body for long periods of time without being confronted with the same ligand that was involved in their generation.[28,36] This does not exclude the possibility that lower affinity ligands in peripheral lymphoid tissue may contribute to survival, much as they can contribute to survival of CD4 and CD8 conventional T cells.[37]

Considering the intrathymic generation of Tregs it is of interest to note that generation of Tregs from cells with one particular αβ,TCR is not mutually exclusive to deletion of some of these cells.[28] Thus both processes depend on recognition of agonist ligands by developing CD4+ T cells but under some conditions such recognition results in deletion and under other conditions in Treg generation, even within the same thymus, perhaps because some of these cells encounter their TCR ligands on different cells, i.e. either on cross-presenting dendritic cells (DCs) or directly on thymic epithelial cells.[38]

Whereas the intrathymic generation of Tregs would mostly depend on instruction of lineage commitment by self-antigens, the peripheral generation of Tregs may also include instruction by foreign antigens. It is therefore of considerable interest to define conditions permissible for extrathymic Treg generation. To this end we have exploited protocols of subimmunogenic antigen presentation, because circumstantial and historic evidence suggested that one might be able to induce 'dominant' tolerance in this way. Indeed it was found that either constant delivery of peptides by osmotic mini-pumps[39] or by targeting DCs with peptide-containing fusion antibodies directed against the DEC205 endocytic receptor on DCs allowed the conversion of naïve T cells into Foxp3 regulatory T cells.[15] The conversion process depended on an intact TGF-βRII receptor on naïve T cells a similiar and conditions that avoided activation of DCs as well as IL-2 production by naïve T cells. It was clear that Tregs were generated by conversion rather than expansion of already committed Tregs, since the experiments were performed in mice expressing only one particular transgenic TCR in the absence of coexpression of a TCR agonist ligand, resulting in the unique constellation that none of the generated CD4+ T cells initially exhibited a Treg phenotype and only a certain percentage (15–20%) assumed it after the artificial introduction of the respective TCR agonist ligand.[15] Importantly, the Tregs generated in this way exhibited i.e. was TGF-β-dependent the same global gene expression pattern as intrathymically generated Tregs[38] and much like intrathymically generated Tregs exhibited a long lifespan that was independent of further supply

of the TCR agonist ligand. Thus by these maneuvers a Treg 'memory' to external TCR ligands could be induced, resulting in the subsequent suppression of immune responses elicited by the same agonist ligand, i.e. this protocol succeeded in generating specific immunological tolerance to one particular antigen ("by stander" supression, see below). Hopefully this protocol can be extended to many other antigens and thus help the prevention of unwanted immune responses. Of note, this particular protocol only works with naïve T cells and not with T cells that have already been activated *in vivo* and thus can presumably not be used to suppress already established autoimmunity in which most antigen-specific T cells are already activated. In such cases the *in vitro* generation of Tregs by Foxp3 transduction would likely be more appropriate (see below).[38]

LIFESTYLE OF TREGS

As pointed out above, Tregs can survive for relatively long periods of time as resting cells at an intermitotic stage but as soon as they encounter their TCR agonist ligand they will express activation markers and begin to home to antigen-draining lymph nodes and undergo considerable expansion.[21,22,36] This is usually accompanied by loss of CD62L and acquisition of CD44 expression and followed by expression of the α_E integrin (CD103) receptor (at least in the mouse). Such activated cells to extravasate and accumulate together with other T effector cells in inflamed tissue.[10] It is in fact the co-recruitment of CD4 and/or CD8 effector cells with activated Tregs in draining lymph nodes and/or inflamed tissue that determines the specificity of immunosuppression:[36] since Tregs suppress neighboring T cells in a 'bystander' fashion it can only be effective when most antigen-specific effector cells are co-recruited to the same anatomical location, which depends on presentation of TCR ligands in these places, such as antigen-draining lymph nodes.[20] Thus while Tregs may suppress 'innocent' bystanders that happen to be in their vicinity, this will not result in general immunosuppression, because the majority of such 'innocent' cells will be distributed throughout the body and not recruited by antigen such that they will not be subject to suppression. It is for this reason that injection of Tregs specific for a pancreas-derived antigen are far more effective in suppressing diabetes than polyclonal Tregs that will not all accumulate and be activated in pancreatic lymph nodes.[20]

'Bystander suppression' is well documented by the fact that, for instance, CD4+ Tregs recognizing a class II major histocompatibility complex (MHC)-presented epitope from one particular protein can suppress CD8 T cells recognizing a different class I MHC-presented epitope from the same protein.[40] Thus the antigen specificity of Tregs and effector T cells does not need to match for effective immunosuppression to occur: it is sufficient that the different T cells are co-recruited to the same tissue. This of course is good news since this will permit a Treg of one particular specificity to suppress a variety of effector cells with different specificity, as long as all these different epitopes are present within the same draining lymph node or anatomical site.

Since many intrathymically generated Tregs are specific for self-antigen it is perhaps not surprising that normally there are always 'activated' Tregs present in the organism[41] and some of these Tregs may be engaged in locally preventing autoimmunity. In fact neonatal removal of Tregs will result in the 'scurfy' phenotype associated with multiorgan-specific autoimmunity.[42] Other Tregs are apparently not 'in action' and patrol the body by exhibiting a phenotype of naïve T cells that do not divide.[30,41]

FUNCTION OF TREGS

One of the questions that has remained rather elusive concerns the molecular mechanisms by which Tregs control other T cells. There are probably several not mutually exclusive mechanisms that may dominate in certain situations.[25] *In vitro* data have emphasized the role of close cell-to-cell contact and a nonessential role of cytokines such as IL-10 or TGF-β. All *in vivo* data published so far have emphasized the crucial role of the TGF-βRII on suppressed cells, since a dominant negative form of that receptor is usually associated with ineffective Treg suppression and with generalized autoimmunity. It is still not clear whether this results from the fact that Tregs produce TGF-β (which they do but only in

moderate amounts) or whether in general TGF-β-induced signaling 'conditions' effector cells for more stringent suppression by a mechanism that does not involve increased TGF-β production but depends on specific Treg activation.[25] A good example for such a scenario is the suppression of tumor-specific CD8 T cells by CD4 Tregs that crucially depends on an intact TGF-βRII receptor on the CD8 T cells. In this particular model the suppression affects the function of fully differentiated cytotoxic T lymphocytes (CTLs), notably the secretion of cytolytic granules. However, *in vitro* experiments with fully differentiated CTLs have shown that TGF-β does not have any negative impact on cytolysis when added during the effector phase. This is consistent with the hypothesis that TGF-β-dependent signaling 'conditions' the CD8 T cells for Treg suppression rather than representing the sole suppressor mechanism.[40]

These experiments also make another important point, namely that it is apparently never too late to interfere with an immune response by Treg suppression, since the experiments show that suppression can affect fully differentiated effector cells. This is good news in the sense that the obviously effective suppression late during an immune response can revert rather than prevent unwanted immunity, a concept that may become extremely useful in the clinic.

Different experiments attempting to reverse rather than prevent diabetes are fully consistent with that view: CD4 T cells specific for an islet-derived antigen of unknown nature could be activated *in vitro* and retrovirally transduced with Foxp3 such that within 24 hours they assumed a phenotype of Tregs. When 10^5 of such converted cells were injected into NOD mice that had become just diabetic because of beginning destruction of their islet cells, these islet-specific Tregs cured the mice of diabetes and they remained diabetes-free for at least 3 months when the experiment was terminated. Again this experiment suggests that Tregs can silence already fully developed effector cells.[20]

Additional controls make important points with regard to the role of Treg antigen receptors in this process and hence the specificity of immunosuppression: while the injection of 10^5 cells with islet-antigen specificity was sufficient to abolish disease, the injection of even 10^6 Tregs with specificity for a large variety of different antigens or the injection of Tregs with specificity for an antigen not present in the pancreatic lymph node did not have any effect and the animals died several days later from complete destruction of β cells and resulting diabetes that obviously at this point could no longer be reversed by Tregs.[20] These results and similar results by others employing *in vitro* expanded Tregs[21,22] are very encouraging, since they suggest that by adoptive Treg therapy early-diagnosed diabetes may be cured, in spite of the fact that the generation of sufficient numbers of islet-antigen-specific Tregs still represents a staggering logistic problem.

Thus in spite of our ignorance concerning molecular mechanisms of Treg-mediated suppression (even though a variety has been proposed)[25] we have promising evidence from murine models of disease that Tregs have the capacity to interfere with unwanted immunity early and/or late during the immune response in an antigen-specific way, since they interfere with such immunity in a local milieu only while leaving the rest of the immune system intact.

There is also no compelling reason why the findings made in the somewhat popular models of type 1 diabetes should not be extended to other autoimmune diseases such as rheumatic diseases, provided that there are clues about relevant antigens that are presented in local lymphoid tissue.

CONCLUDING REMARKS

The described properties of Tregs, i.e. the possibility of generating them extrathymically *in vivo* or *in vitro* with any desired antigen specificity, their ability to co-home with T effector cells into antigen-draining lymph nodes and/or sites of inflammation, their potential to suppress effector cells at early and late stages of differentiation, and last but not least the ability to suppress neighboring T effector cells of any antigenic specificity, make these cells an ideal tool with which to intervene in unwanted immunity in an antigen-specific way. Thus one would hope that eventually the exploitation of evolutionarily selected mechanisms to deal with unwanted immune responses against self will replace indiscriminate immunosuppression by drugs with potentially deadly side effects. This is not to say that such drugs may be completely useless: their transient application may help to set the immune system to a stage where Tregs can be more effective in dealing specifically with unwanted immunity. What should be avoided, however, is the long-term indiscriminate use of the drugs that eventually will ruin the protection against infections and malignant disease afforded by the immune system.

ACKNOWLEDGMENT

This work was supported by NIH grant R37A1053102

REFERENCES

1. von Boehmer H, Kisielow P. Negative selection of the T-cell repertoire: where and when does it occur? Immunol Rev 2006; 209: 284–9.
2. Rocha B, von Boehmer H. Peripheral selection of the T cell repertoire. Science 1991; 251: 1225–8.
3. Sakaguchi S, Ono M, Setoguchi R et al. Foxp3CD25CD4 natural regulatory T cells in dominant self-tolerance and autoimmune disease. Immunol Rev 2006; 212: 8–27.
4. von Boehmer H, Aifantis I, Gounari F et al. Thymic selection revisited: how essential is it? Immunol Rev 2003; 191: 62–78.
5. Khattri R, Cox T, Yasayko SA, Ramsdell F. An essential role for Scurfin in CD4+CD25+ T regulatory cells. Nat Immunol 2003; 4: 337–42.
6. Jaeckel E, Lipes MA, von Boehmer H. Recessive tolerance to preproinsulin 2 reduces but does not abolish type 1 diabetes. Nat Immunol 2004; 5: 1028–35.
7. Nakayama M, Abiru N, Moriyama H et al. Prime role for an insulin epitope in the development of type 1 diabetes in NOD mice. Nature 2005; 435: 220–3.
8. Itoh M, Takahashi T, Sakaguchi N et al. Thymus and autoimmunity: production of CD25+CD4+ naturally anergic and suppressive T cells as a key function of the thymus in maintaining immunologic self-tolerance. J Immunol 1999; 162: 5317–26.
9. Bruder D, Probst-Kepper M, Westendorf AM et al. Neuropilin-1: a surface marker of regulatory T cells. Eur J Immunol 2004; 34: 623–30.
10. Huehn J, Siegmund K, Lehmann JC et al. Developmental stage, phenotype, and migration distinguish naive- and effector/memory-like CD4+ regulatory T cells. J Exp Med 2004; 199: 303–13.
11. Hansen W, Loser K, Westendorf AM et al. G protein-coupled receptor 83 overexpression in naive

CD4+CD25- T cells leads to the induction of Foxp3+ regulatory T cells in vivo. J Immunol 2006; 177: 209–15.

12. Stephens GL, McHugh RS, Whitters MJ et al. Engagement of glucocorticoid-induced TNFR family-related receptor on effector T cells by its ligand mediates resistance to suppression by CD4+CD25+ T cells. J Immunol 2004; 173: 5008–20.

13. Bachmann MF, Kohler G, Ecabert B, Mak TW, Kopf M. Cutting edge: lymphoproliferative disease in the absence of CTLA-4 is not T cell autonomous. J Immunol 1999; 163: 1128–31.

14. Liu W, Putnam AL, Xu-Yu Z et al. CD127 expression inversely correlates with FoxP3 and suppressive function of human CD4+ T reg cells. J Exp Med 2006; 203: 1701–11.

15. Kretschmer K, Apostolou I, Hawiger D et al. Inducing and expanding regulatory T cell populations by foreign antigen. Nat Immunol 2005; 6: 1219–27.

16. Fontenot JD, Rasmussen JP, Williams LM et al. Regulatory T cell lineage specification by the forkhead transcription factor foxp3. Immunity 2005; 22: 329–41.

17. Wan YY, Flavell RA. Identifying Foxp3-expressing suppressor T cells with a bicistronic reporter. Proc Natl Acad Sci U S A 2005; 102: 5126–31.

18. Hori S, Nomura T, Sakaguchi S. Control of regulatory T cell development by the transcription factor Foxp3. Science 2003; 299: 1057–61.

19. Fontenot JD, Gavin MA, Rudensky AY. Foxp3 programs the development and function of CD4+CD25+ regulatory T cells. Nat Immunol 2003; 4: 330–6.

20. Jaeckel E, von Boehmer H, Manns MP. Antigen-specific FoxP3-transduced T-cells can control established type 1 diabetes. Diabetes 2005; 54: 306–10.

21. Tang Q, Henriksen KJ, Bi M et al. In vitro-expanded antigen-specific regulatory T cells suppress autoimmune diabetes. J Exp Med 2004; 199: 1455–65.

22. Tarbell KV, Yamazaki S, Olson K, Toy P, Steinman RM. CD25+ CD4+ T cells, expanded with dendritic cells presenting a single autoantigenic peptide, suppress autoimmune diabetes. J Exp Med 2004; 199: 1467–77.

23. Wu Y, Borde M, Heissmeyer V et al. FOXP3 controls regulatory T cell function through cooperation with NFAT. Cell 2006; 126: 375–87.

24. Bottini N, Vang T, Cucca F, Mustelin T. Role of PTPN22 in type 1 diabetes and other autoimmune diseases. Semin Immunol 2006; 18: 207–13.

25. von Boehmer H. Mechanisms of suppression by suppressor T cells. Nat Immunol 2005; 6: 338–44.

26. von Boehmer H. Selection of the T-cell repertoire: receptor-controlled checkpoints in T-cell development. Adv Immunol 2004; 84: 201–38.

27. Jordan MS, Boesteanu A, Reed AJ et al. Thymic selection of CD4+CD25+ regulatory T cells induced by an agonist self-peptide. Nat Immunol 2001; 2: 301–6.

28. Apostolou I, Sarukhan A, Klein L, von Boehmer H. Origin of regulatory T cells with known specificity for antigen. Nat Immunol 2002; 3: 756–63.

29. Hsieh CS, Liang Y, Tyznik AJ et al. Recognition of the peripheral self by naturally arising CD25+ CD4+ T cell receptors. Immunity 2004; 21: 267–77.

30. Derbinski J, Schulte A, Kyewski B, Klein L. Promiscuous gene expression in medullary thymic epithelial cells mirrors the peripheral self. Nat Immunol 2001; 2: 1032–9.

31. Vafiadis P, Bennett ST, Todd JA et al. Insulin expression in human thymus is modulated by INS VNTR alleles at the IDDM2 locus. Nat Genet 1997; 15: 289–92.

32. Anderson MS, Venanzi ES, Klein L et al. Projection of an immunological self shadow within the thymus by the aire protein. Science 2002; 298: 1395–401.

33. Liston A, Gray DH, Lesage S et al. Gene dosage – limiting role of Aire in thymic expression, clonal deletion, and organ-specific autoimmunity. J Exp Med 2004; 200: 1015–26.

34. Anderson MS, Venanzi ES, Chen Z et al. The cellular mechanism of Aire control of T cell tolerance. Immunity 2005; 23: 227–39.

35. Tai X, Cowan M, Feigenbaum L, Singer A. CD28 costimulation of developing thymocytes induces Foxp3 expression and regulatory T cell differentiation independently of interleukin 2. Nat Immunol 2005; 6: 152–62.

36. Klein L, Khazaie K, von Boehmer H. In vivo dynamics of antigen-specific regulatory T cells not predicted from behavior in vitro. Proc Natl Acad Sci U S A 2003; 100: 8886–91.

37. Hao Y, Legrand N, Freitas AA. The clone size of peripheral CD8 T cells is regulated by TCR promiscuity. J Exp Med 2006; 203: 1643–9.

38. Kretschmer K, Apostolou I, Jaeckel E, Khazaie K, von Boehmer H. Making regulatory T cells with defined antigen specificity: role in autoimmunity and cancer. Immunol Rev 2006; 212: 163–9.

39. Apostolou I, Von Boehmer H. In vivo instruction of suppressor commitment in naive T cells. J Exp Med 2004; 199: 1401–8.

40. Mempel TR, Pittet MJ, Khazaie K et al. Regulatory T cells reversibly suppress cytotoxic T cell function independent of effector differentiation. Immunity 2006; 25: 129–41.

41. Fisson S, Darrasse-Jeze G, Litvinova E et al. Continuous activation of autoreactive CD4+ CD25+ regulatory T cells in the steady state. J Exp Med 2003; 198: 737–46.

42. Lin W, Truong N, Grossman WJ et al. Allergic dysregulation and hyperimmunoglobulinemia E in Foxp3 mutant mice. J Allergy Clin Immunol 2005; 116: 1106–15.

43. Marson A, Kretschmer K, Frompton GM, et al. Foxp3 occupancy and regulation of key target genes during T-cell stimulation. Nature 2007; 445: 931–5.

4

B-cell antigen receptor signaling and autoimmunity

Esra Nutku-Bilir, Aimee E Pugh-Bernard, Stephen Gauld, Kevin Merrell and John C Cambier

Introduction • BCR signaling pathway • Anergy as a mechanism for silencing self-reactive B cells: differential B-cell signaling • References

INTRODUCTION

A number of illnesses affecting joints or muscles are associated with antibodies to 'self' molecules and are classified as autoimmune rheumatic diseases. They include rheumatoid arthritis (RA), systemic lupus erythematosus (SLE), anti-phospholipid syndrome, polymyalgia rheumatica, systemic sclerosis, Sjögren's syndrome, polymyositis and dermatomyositis, myasthenia gravis, and a spectrum of related syndromes. Altered development and function of B cells may play a prominent role in the development and progression of autoimmune rheumatic disorders, with RA and SLE being the classic and most widely studied.

Loss of self-tolerance leading to production of self-reactive antibodies is integral to the development and progression of RA and SLE. By largely stochastic processes, immunoglobulin (Ig) gene arrangement gives rise to B cells with an enormous range of antigen specificity. Although optimally protective, a disadvantage of such diversity is the potential to generate self-reactive antibodies. Indeed, B cells contribute to the pathophysiology of autoimmune rheumatic diseases in part by production of germ-line encoded and/or somatically mutated self-reactive antibodies.[1–3] The successful treatment of RA, SLE, multiple sclerosis, and Sjögren's syndrome with anti-CD20 monoclonal antibodies that eliminate B cells further supports the key role of B cells in the development of autoimmune rheumatic diseases.[4–8] In animal models, the absence of B cells prevents the spontaneous development of SLE.[9] Interestingly, this does not merely reflect a role for self-reactive antibody production. SLE-associated T-cell accumulation in lymphoid organs does not occur in the absence of B cells, suggesting a role for B cells apart from secretion of self-reactive antibodies in the development of SLE. These findings and those of several other studies suggest that B cells may also be involved in presentation of self-antigen to T cells, or some novel form of regulation of T-cell activation and recruitment.[10,11]

The critical role of B cells in rheumatological diseases has become increasingly evident as a consequence of insights gained from studies of B-cell antigen receptor (BCR) signaling pathways. The BCR plays a key role in B-cell development and function, and has a central role in regulation of self-tolerance. To ensure self-tolerance, self-reactive B cells are efficiently silenced by one of three distinct mechanisms: receptor editing, clonal deletion, or anergy.[12] Studies suggest that a key determinant of the mode of silencing is the strength of BCR signaling and developmental stage.[13] Antigen avidity, i.e valency, affinity, and concentration, as well as involvement of co-receptors and adaptor molecules, play a role in determining signal quality and strength. At extremes, high avidity antigen interactions with immature B cells lead to receptor editing in an anthropomorphic effort to eliminate autoantigen binding activity. Failing this, these cells are eliminated by apoptotic death, referred to as clonal deletion. Lower avidity interactions with self, particularly in the periphery, lead to anergy wherein cells remain viable for some time and bind antigen yet are unresponsive to immunogenic stimulation.

In this chapter, we have incorporated the most recent and salient findings regarding BCR signaling, its role in the maintenance of self-tolerance and its impact on the development and progression of autoimmune rheumatic diseases, particularly focusing on SLE and RA. We discuss the primary signaling pathways emanating from the BCRs and their downstream effectors (Figure 4.1). Our review is divided into sections addressing (i) signal initiation, (ii) signal propagation and integration focusing on the role of inositol lipids, and (iii) signal modulation with an emphasis on

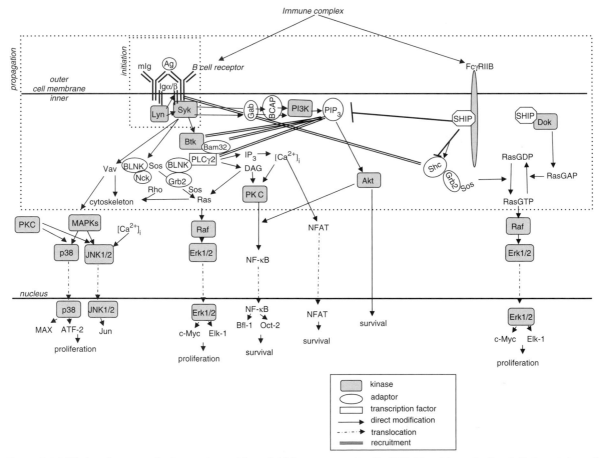

Figure 4.1 BCR signaling cascade: interactions with an inhibitory co-receptor, FcγRIIB. Signal transduction initiates at the cell membrane following ligand-induced aggregation of the membrane immunoglobulin (mIg) and associated Igα/β. Signals are propagated by means of protein phosphorylation, modification, and integration. BCR signaling strength is modulated by activatory and inhibitory co-receptors and their effectors. Finally, activation of transcription factors and gene expression determines B-cell fate. For example, BCR-FcγRIIB co-aggregation leads to inhibition of certain BCR-coupled signaling pathways, terminating cell proliferation, survival and antibody production. Down-regulation of PIP3 levels by FcγRIIB-recruited SHIP is most probably the mechanism underlying the reported inhibition of BCR-mediated activation of Akt, Btk, and PLCγ2, and consequently, the calcium mobilization response. An alternative mechanism of FcγRIIB-SHIP-mediated inhibition involves RasGAP. BCR-FcγRIIB co-aggregation on B cells leads to association of SHIP with the RasGAP-binding protein Dok. Co-aggregation of this complex results in complete inhibition of BCR-induced Erk activation. Please refer to the text for the definitions of abbreviations.

the role of inhibitory receptors and their effectors in prevention of autoimmunity. Our discussion is further refined as we discuss anergy as a mechanism for silencing self-reactive B cells.

BCR SIGNALING PATHWAY

Signal initiation

The B-cell antigen receptor or BCR is a multiprotein structure that is composed of membrane Ig, which serves as the antigen binding subunit, and a non-covalent associated heterodimer composed of Ig-α (CD79a) and Ig-β (CD79b). This complex serves as the signaling subunit. The Ig-α and Ig-β signaling proteins are disulfide-linked heterodimers that contain an _i_mmunoreceptor _t_yrosine-based _a_ctivation _m_otif (ITAM) within each cytoplasmic tail.[14,15] The ITAM is a conserved 18 amino acid motif containing six conserved residues including two tyrosines. The N-terminal of ITAM tyrosine in Ig-α, YEGL, is most strongly phosphorylated upon receptor aggregation and binds to the _src_ family protein tyrosine kinases (PTKs) (i.e. Lyn, Fyn, Blk, Lck).[16,17] BCR aggregation results in the phosphorylation of one or more ITAM tyrosines within the Ig-α and Ig-β cytoplasmic tails and this initiates downstream signaling events. Ig-α and Ig-β ITAMs are not equivalent in their contribution to BCR signaling. Several proteins have been shown to associate differentially with Ig-α and Ig-β, which suggests that they may activate distinct downstream pathways.[18] Both Ig-α and Ig-β are essential for BCR chaperone functions, transporting BCRs to the cell surface.[19] Ig-α plays a prominent role in activating PTKs, contains a BLNK docking site, and apparently also contains a negative signaling function.[20–23] Thus, Ig-α and Ig-β are only partially redundant in function and have distinct biological activities.

BCR aggregation activates downstream signaling pathways through the _src_ family PTKs and SYK. Following receptor aggregation, initial ITAM phosphorylation of Ig-α/β primarily occurs asymmetrically, with most phosphorylation occurring on the N-terminal or membrane proximal ITAM tyrosines.[23] This phosphorylation is mediated by _src_ family PTKs.[17] In part by virtue of their lipid acylation _src_ family PTKs interact with the non-phosphorylated ITAMs of the resting BCR.[18,24] Maximal receptor signaling requires the binding of phosphorylated ITAMs to _src_ family kinase SH2 domains, which amplifies ITAM phosphorylation and the subsequent recruitment and activation of downstream cytosolic tyrosine kinases, such as Syk. Association of BCRs with _src_ family PTKs may further be enhanced by the propensity of ligand aggregated molecules, but not monomeric BCRs, to partition into glycosphingolipid-rich microdomains or lipid rafts of the plasma membrane that have been shown to contain increased concentrations of PTKs.[25] Binding and activation of Syk requires recognition of two ITAM phosphotyrosines via its tandem domains.[26,27] The spacing of ITAM phosphotyrosines by ~12 residues is critical for binding Syk's SH2 domains, which are in fixed orientation to one another. Syk activation, and thus Ig-α or Ig-β biphosphorylation, is critical for all downstream signaling.

The ordered dual phosphorylation of ITAMs and activation of Lyn, Syk, and Bruton's tyrosine kinase (Btk, a Tec family PTK) are essential for proper initiation of BCR signal transduction. Deficiencies in any of these result in defective and aberrant B-cell development and function.[28–32] The protein tyrosine kinase Lyn is believed to be primarily responsible for phosphorylating Ig-α/β ITAM tyrosines. Lyn plays a unique role in BCR signaling as it activates both positive and negative signaling circuitry.[33] While the positive role of Lyn is redundant, as demonstrated by normal B-cell development in the bone marrow of Lyn-deficient mice,[34] its inhibitory role in BCR signaling is not. Lyn's inhibitory signaling function depends on its ability to phosphorylate receptors such as FcγRIIB, PIR-B, LMIR, and CD22, as well as the adaptors such as Dok. These inhibitory co-receptors contain _i_mmunoreceptor _t_yrosine-based _i_nhibitory _m_otifs (ITIMs) that recruit phosphatases, such as src homology 2 (SH2) domain-containing inositol 5′-phosphatase (SHIP)-1 and SH2 domain-containing tyrosine phosphatase (SHP)-1.[35–37] Recruited phosphatases suppress BCR signaling by dephosphorylating and deactivating signal transducers.

The outcome of BCR signaling is determined by the balance between kinase and phosphatase activity. Thus, Lyn plays a central role in the equilibrium between activation and inhibition of B-cell signaling pathways, determining, at extremes, B-cell tolerance versus autoimmunity. This latter hypothesis is further supported by studies in which mice overexpressing or deficient in Lyn demonstrated breakdown of self-tolerance, and developed circulating autoantibodies, and lupus-like nephritis.[38–40]

The recruitment and activation of Syk is essential to couple the BCR to downstream signaling events.[41] Studies in Syk-deficient B cells showed a profound defect in BCR-mediated activation of downstream signaling pathways while *src* family PTK activation and Ig-α/β phosphorylation remained intact. Singly phosphorylated ITAMs, or chimeric Ig-α or Ig-β in which one of the tyrosines is absent, do not bind and consequently fail to activate Syk kinase.[26] Thus recruitment of Syk to doubly phosphorylated Ig-α and/or Ig-β ITAMs results in activation of the kinase and initiation of multiple distinct downstream signaling pathways.[42] For example, the activation and recruitment of Lyn and Syk to the BCR complex both precede and influence the activity of Btk, a cytoplasmic tyrosine kinase that is required for the sustained calcium influx that follows B-cell activation.[43]

Loss of function mutations in Btk affects B-cell development and B-cell activation in response to antigen.[44] In humans this type of mutation results in the disease X-linked agammaglobulinemia (XLA).[45,46] This disorder is characterized by the absence of mature B cells in the periphery and a serious deficiency of serum antibodies.[45] In mice, Btk inactivation results in a disorder called X-linked immunodeficiency (*xid*).[47,48] Studies using *xid* mice suggest that disrupting the kinase function of Btk could result in desensitization of B-cell signaling and possibly provide a therapeutic effect in autoimmune disorders, including RA.[49] However, several lines of recent evidence challenge the positive role of Btk in regulation of BCR signaling and suggest that Btk may be required for tolerance. Patients with XLA had increased numbers of self-reactive B cells in the periphery and failed to establish proper B-cell tolerance.[50] Btk-deficient B cells obtained from these patients display unusual Ig light chain repertoires showing impaired secondary recombination regulation,

which indicates that receptor editing, one of the mechanisms that normally ensures B-cell tolerance, may be defective. Interestingly, in a recent study conducted by the same group, similar self-reactive B cells were detected in RA patients, suggesting that Btk may be essential for regulation of B-cell tolerance in humans.[51] It is not clear from this study whether occurrence of self-reactive B cells from RA patients was associated with defects in Btk, or other B-cell intrinsic defects, or whether the association between B-cell self-reactivity and Btk deficiency observed in XLA patients was just an outcome of genetic co-segregation with unknown mechanisms. These findings, however, suggest that Btk deficiency may allow the release of self-reactive B cells into the periphery. Studies are ongoing in an effort to delineate the role of Btk as a therapeutic target for treatment of B-cell-mediated diseases.[52]

The propagation of downstream BCR signals requires that a number of effector molecules become activated via tyrosine phosphorylation after the proximal signaling molecules (i.e. Lyn, Syk, Btk) are activated. A second mechanism by which Syk couples the BCR to downstream signal transduction molecules is by its interaction with and subsequent phosphorylation of the adaptor molecule B-cell linker protein (BLNK, also known as SLP-65 or BASH). BLNK acts as a platform for effector molecule assembly and transduces initial BCR-proximal events into several divergent signaling pathways (Figure 4.1).[53–56] Particularly important events are the recruitment and activation of PLCγ2, and elevation in intracellular calcium ($[Ca^{2+}]_i$).

The adaptor molecule BLNK is essential for PLCγ2 recruitment from the cytosol to the plasma membrane and for coupling BCR aggregation to calcium influx.[53,56,57] Syk rapidly phosphorylates BLNK following BCR aggregation and provides a primary docking site for the SH2 domain of PLCγ2, as well as other effector and adaptor molecules involved in BCR signaling.[53–55] For example, phospho-BLNK has been shown to associate with the SH2 domain of Btk, which is significant since dual phosphorylation of PLCγ2 by Syk and Btk is required for optimal activation of PLCγ2. In the absence of BLNK, B cells fail to recruit PLCγ2 to the plasma membrane and have severely impaired distal BCR signaling.[54] Furthermore, the guanine exchange factor, Vav, and adaptor complex of Grb2/SOS also associate with phosphorylated BLNK and can activate Rac and Ras. BLNK recruits other adaptors, such as Nck, which associates with cytoskeletal elements and has been proposed to connect BCR signaling to morphological reorganization and cellular migration.[58,59] BLNK$^{-/-}$ mice exhibit attenuated but not abolished BCR-mediated calcium mobilization, suggesting that partially redundant mechanisms must exist for BCR-mediated PLCγ2 activation.[60] A potential candidate mediator of this function is cytosolic adaptor Bam32, which contains single pleckstrin homology (PH) and SH2 domains, the latter shown to associate with PLCγ2.[61] Ablation of Bam32 in B cells results in a decreased BCR-mediated calcium influx and proliferation.[62,63] These findings suggest that alternative and often redundant pathways are activated following BCR ligation.

Signal propagation and integration: role of inositol lipids

BCR signal transduction involves a complex network of interactions. For example, BCR-mediated activation of calcium mobilization does not depend solely on the linear activation of Lyn, Syk, Btk, BLNK, and PLCγ2. Inner leaflet membrane phospholipids are of paramount importance to B-cell signaling. Ligation of the BCR leads to the activation of PI-3K, which phosphorylates plasma membrane phosphatidylinositol 4,5-biphosphate [PI(4,5)P2] yielding phosphatidylinositol 3,4,5-triphosphate [PI(3,4,5)P3]. PI(3,4,5)P3 is critical to retain multiple PH domain-containing cytosolic proteins at the membrane and also to co-localize PH domain containing proteins that may function in same signaling pathway, e.g. Akt (PKB) and phosphoinositide-dependent kinase-1 (PDK-1).[64,65] Although the activation/recruitment of Lyn and Syk to the BCR complex both precedes and influences the activity of Btk, PI(3,4,5)P3 production is a rate-limiting step in Btk function. PI(3,4,5)P3 production is critical for the translocation and activation of Btk, and the subsequent Btk-mediated phosphorylation of PLCγ2.

Moreover, the subcellular localization and activity of Btk are regulated by PH domain binding. In mice with X-linked immunodeficiency (Xid) there is a point mutation in the PH domain of Btk which prohibits recruitment to PI(3,4,5)P3 and results in defective BCR signaling and impaired B-cell maturation and responsiveness.[47,66]

PI-3K-dependent activation of PLCγ2 causes the mobilization of calcium from both intracellular and extracellular stores through cleavage of the ubiquitous plasma membrane lipid phosphoinositide PI(4,5)P2 into the second messengers I(1,4,5)P3 and DAG. Pharmacological inhibitors of PI-3K completely abolish BCR-mediated calcium mobilization.[67–69] B cells deficient in effectors involved in PI-3K recruitment, such as CD19, exhibit diminished PI(3,4,5)P3 production, PLCγ2 activation, and calcium mobilization.[69–73]

Elevated [Ca^{2+}]$_i$ levels are required for the activation of certain transcription factors that are necessary for B-cell activation and survival, such as NF-κB and NF-AT.[74–78] DAG activates conventional protein kinase C (PKC) isoforms that regulate the MAPK family (i.e. ERKs, JNKs, SAPKs, p38).[79,80] Following activation of these kinases, different sets of transcription factors are phosphorylated, e.g. Elk-1 and c-Myc by Erk, c-Jun and ATF-2 by JNK, and ATF-2 and MAX by p38 MAPK (Figure 4.1). It is the profile of these activated transcription factors that determines B-cell fate.

Signal modulation: role of ITIM-containing proteins and their effectors in prevention of autoimmunity

The strength of the BCR signal is determined in part by co-receptors and accessory molecules that either augment or attenuate the potency of the signal. The temporal and spatial regulation of these processes ultimately defines signal quality and quantity.

It is important to note that several studies have demonstrated genetic alterations in BCR co-receptors in patients with autoimmune diseases. For example, in SLE, polymorphisms were identified in the genes that encode FcγRIIB,[81–84] programmed cell death 1 (PD-1),[85] and CD22.[86] Similarly, alterations in the levels of CD19,[87] functional CD45,[88] and SHP-1[88,89] have been observed in patients with B-cell-mediated autoimmune diseases.

In a simplistic model of BCR signaling, co-receptors can be classified according to whether they increase or decrease the threshold for B-cell activation and survival after co-aggregation. Those that increase the threshold, dampen the immune response, while those that decrease the BCR signaling threshold increase immune responses. Thus, an increase in BCR signaling threshold may result in immunodeficiency, while a decreased BCR threshold may result in autoimmunity. For example, CD45 and CD19/CD21 co-receptor complex decrease BCR signaling threshold and act as positive regulators. Negative regulators include FcγRIIB, CD22, CD72, the paired immunoglobulin-like receptor (PIR-B), and the myeloid-associated immunoglobulin-like receptors (MAIRs or LMIRs), which are characterized by content of ITIM signaling domains.

Most inhibitory receptors recruit SH2 containing phosphatases and function through one of two pathways. ITIMs in FcγRIIB, and MAIR recruit the inositol phosphatase SHIP-1, while those in CD22, CD72, and PIR-B recruit the protein tyrosine phosphatase SHP-1. SHP-1 dephosphorylates proteins in the signalsome thus dampening signaling and SHIP-1 converts PI (3,4,5)P3 to PI(3,4)P2. The inhibitory effects of SHIP-1 can be more global, modulating signaling by distantly stimulated PI3 kinase-dependent receptors, while the inhibitory effect of SHP-1 is localized to the signalsome in which it is engaged. The importance of these inhibitory pathways to autoimmunity is demonstrated by the autoimmune diseases seen in SHP-1 deficient (*moth eaten*) mice.[90] We have observed production of self-reactive antibodies in SHIP-1-deficient mice (K Merrell and JC Cambier, unpublished observations).

A detailed description of co-receptors and cell surface molecules that modulate the BCR signal was reviewed in several recent articles.[33,91,92] Here we will present an overview of the ITIM-containing inhibitory co-receptors including: FcγRIIB, CD22, PIR-B, and MAIRs/LMIRs. We will also discuss the recent findings regarding CD45 and autoimmunity.

IgG-containing immune complexes can co-ligate BCR and the low affinity IgG receptor, FcγRIIB,

leading to inhibition of BCR-induced phosphatidylinositol 3,4,5-triphosphate [PI(3,4,5)P3] accumulation, proliferation, and calcium mobilization.[93] Inhibition through FcγRIIB is primarily mediated by its ITIM region, which recruits SHIP-1.[36,94,95] SHIP-1 degrades PIP3 to PI(3,4)P2 and recruits the adaptor molecule downstream of kinase (DOK), which acts to inhibit other downstream signaling pathways (i.e. Ras/Erk activation) (Figure 4.1).[96] Thus, co-ligation of FcγRIIB with BCR provides a mechanism that may promote deletion of low-affinity self-reactive B cells during high affinity maturation and controls autoantibody production.[96] Conversely, ablation of FcγRIIB renders mice susceptible to experimental autoimmune diseases upon immunization with autoantigens and they spontaneously develop SLE-like syndrome on the C57BL/6 background.[97,98] This spontaneous autoimmunity is strain-specific, e.g. BALB/c/FcγRIIB deficient mice do not show any autoimmunity, suggesting the presence of other genetic factors that influence disease susceptibility. These findings may also imply the existence of other inhibitory mechanisms that play a compensatory role in the regulation of autoimmune diseases in different strains of mice.[98] Indeed, a locus in chromosome 1, which contains the FcγRIIB gene, is associated with autoimmunity in multiple mouse models (i.e. NZB, BXSB).[99,100] Polymorphisms in the transmembrane region of the FcγRIIB gene were identified in a study done in 193 Japanese patients and 303 healthy controls, where homozygosity for I232T polymorphism was significantly increased in SLE patients compared with controls.[82] FcγRIIB-I232T polymorphism was associated with reduced FcγRIIB-mediated inhibition of B-cell proliferation.[83]

Recent work by Okazaki et al., reported that co-deficiency of two inhibitory receptors, FcγRIIB and PD-1, induced an autoimmune disease state, hydronephrosis, accompanied by self-reactive antibody production in BALB/c mice, which was not observed in either FcγRIIB- or PD-1-deficient mice.[101] PD-1 is a type 1 transmembrane protein that belongs to the Ig superfamily and contains cytoplasmic tyrosine residues within a consensus ITIM. Studies have shown that PD-1 provides a signal that limits response to antigen by recruiting SHP-2.[102] PD-1[−/−] mice develop lupus-like glomerulonephritis and arthritis on the C57BL/6 background.[103] In humans, gene mapping studies suggested that there was an association between 7 and 12% of SLE patients and a SNP in PD-1.[85] Although the mechanism of FcγRIIB and PD-1 complementarity is not clear, in their study, Okazaki et al. clearly demonstrated that FcγRIIB and PD-1 cooperatively regulate autoimmunity in the mouse, suggesting that some human autoimmune diseases may also be regulated by the combination of dysfunction of human FcγRIIB and PD-1 genes. These findings may suggest that polymorphisms affecting the strength and quality of Ig signaling are important in determining the genetic susceptibility or resistance to autoimmune disease. Predisposition to human autoimmunity occurs when different combinations of susceptibility alleles combine to reach some threshold.

Consistent with these observations, it has been shown that CD72 polymorphisms, which are associated with the relative quantity of an alternative splicing product, and also with the presence of nephritis among the patients with SLE, may modify susceptibility to human SLE through interacting with FcγRIIB.[104] CD72 functions as a negative regulator of BCR signaling.[105] Interactions were also identified between FcγRIIB and CD19, where FcγRIIB-mediated inhibition can be mediated through selective dephosphorylation of CD19 leading to abrogated PI-3K recruitment.[95]

Finally, a recent study by McGaha et al. demonstrated that the partial restoration of FcγRIIB levels on B cells in lupus-prone mouse restored tolerance and prevented autoimmunity.[106] The physiologic consequences of cell-bound IgG and immune complexes are modulated by a balance between activating (i.e. FcγRIA, FcγRIIA, FcγRIII, and FcγRIV) and inhibitory Fcγ receptors and include immune regulatory and inflammatory responses.[98,107–109] B cells express FcγRIIB but not other Fc receptors. Thus, findings from McGaha et al. illustrate an important role for FcγRIIB in regulation of a common B-cell check-point, and suggest that relative changes in its expression can result in either tolerance or autoimmunity.[106] Similar observations were also made for CD22.[87]

CD22 is a B-cell-specific inhibitory co-receptor that belongs to the Ig superfamily, and contains seven Ig-like domains and three cytoplasmic ITIMs. CD22 regulates BCR signaling through recruitment of SHP-1 to its ITIM motifs.[110] Activation of SHP-1 regulates the strength of the BCR-induced calcium signal.[111] In this manner, CD22 is thought to control signaling threshold of B cells, preventing overstimulation. CD22[−/−] mice show higher BCR-mediated calcium signaling, and their B cells show evidence of basal activation, such as expression of activation markers, and increased sensitivity to apoptosis.[112,113] CD22[−/−] mice may develop high affinity autoantibodies.[112] Also, CD22[−/−] mice show characteristic changes in B-cell maturation, such as a higher proportion of mature, follicular cells,[114] and a reduced number of marginal zone B cells in the spleen,[115] thought to be direct consequences of increased signaling. However, the effect of CD22 deficiency on BCR signaling is sensitive to the strain of the mice used,[116,117] suggesting a role of other genetic factors in CD22-mediated modulation of BCR signaling.

Recent studies suggested that one of these regulatory factors for CD22 may be its own ligand, namely, sialic acid α2-6 linked to galactose (Siaα2-6Gal). Siaα2-6Gal is a glycan that specifically binds to CD22 *in vivo*.[118,119] The interaction of CD22 with its ligand modulates its activity as a negative regulator of BCR signaling.[120] For example, lupus-prone mice, whose B cells have lower expression of CD22 ligand than those of wild-type mice, have reduced production of autoimmune antiboby.[121] Inhibition of CD22–ligand interactions or the absence of ligands decrease SHP-1 recruitment and increase calcium influx, enhancing BCR signaling.[120,122,123] These studies suggest that CD22 regulates B-cell function *in vivo* in a ligand-dependent manner, with mechanisms still under investigation.[124,125] Interestingly, Siaα2-6Gal is typically found on N-linked glycans of glycoproteins, including those involved in BCR signaling, such as CD45, and IgM.[126–128] Both IgM and CD45 were shown to be CD22 binding partners.[129] Recently, an open-label pilot study of anti-CD22 (epratuzumab) in the treatment of active SLE showed some B-cell depletion but no consistent changes in autoantibody levels.[130] The role of CD22 ligands in regulation of BCR signaling and utility for therapeutic applications are yet to be determined.

CD45 is a receptor-like protein tyrosine phosphatase that establishes the sensitivity of the BCR to stimulation. Both CD45-deficient mice and humans develop severe combined immunodeficiency (SCID) with defects in B-cell development and function. B cells from CD45-deficient mice are hyporesponsive to BCR stimulation and display reduced calcium responses, demonstrating a positive regulatory role for CD45 in BCR signaling.[131,132] In part, this is accomplished by maintaining an adequate supply of BCR-associated *src* family kinases.[133] CD45 can also negatively regulate signals emanating from BCR. Acting in opposition to CD45 is Csk, which functions to phosphorylate the C-terminal inhibitory tyrosine of the *src* family PTKs, keeping them in a 'repressed' state.[134] Whether CD45 positively and negatively regulates protein kinase phosphorylation depends upon its subcellular localization relative to its substrate and the phosphorylation state of the protein kinases.[135] Recent studies showed that introducing a point mutation into the CD45 juxtamembrane wedge (CD45 E613R) abolished the inhibitory effect of CD45.[136] The analogous point mutation introduced into the germ-line of mice leads to lymphoproliferative disorder and a lupus-like autoimmune disease and autoantibody production.[137] CD45 E613R-mediated negative regulation was also suggested by a recent study, where CD45 E613R B cells were hyperproliferative and have augmented calcium responses.[138] Thus, CD45-deficient and CD45 E613R mice reflect the positive and negative regulatory role of CD45 on B-cell function, with mechanisms still under investigation.

The paired Ig-like receptors (PIRs) and the myeloid-associated immunoglobulin-like receptors (MAIRs or LMIRs) are transmembrane glycoproteins that play a role in BCR regulation. They exist in activating and inhibitory isoforms and are often expressed in pair-like fashion on the same cell.[139,140] The expression of the inhibitory isoform, PIR-B, can have an attenuating effect on BCR signaling, while the activating form, PIR-A, appears to function independently of the BCR.[141,142] PIR-B contains multiple ITIMs, which are constitutively phosphorylated and

associated with SHP-1 in B cells.[143,144] The inhibitory form of MAIR, MAIR-I, contains ITIM sequences in its cytoplasmic tail that can recruit SH2-domain containing inhibitory effectors, like SHIP, although much more needs to be worked out regarding MAIR signaling and regulation of the BCR signal.[145]

ANERGY AS A MECHANISM FOR SILENCING SELF-REACTIVE B CELLS: DIFFERENTIAL B-CELL SIGNALING

It was recently estimated that 50–75% of newly produced B cells are self-reactive and must be silenced by tolerance mechanisms.[13,146] Evidence of receptor editing is seen in ~25% of peripheral B cells,[147] and 10% of B cells appear to be silenced by deletion.[148] The remaining self-reactive cells are presumably silenced by other mechanisms, e.g. deletion or anergy. It is also clear that self-reactive B cells develop by somatic mutation during the germinal center response. These are likely silenced by anergy or clonal deletion.

Anergy is a reversible state of unresponsiveness determined by the binding of cognate self-antigen.[149] It is the consequence of reception of signal one (antigen) without signal two (cognate T-cell help, Toll-like receptor agonists). Thus, anergy can be prevented by provision of T-cell help immediately following exposure to antigen.[150,151] The reversibility of anergy suggests that continuous presence of the antigen in the microenvironment is essential to maintain unresponsiveness. Based on the assumption that some self-antigens are tissue-specific, it is reasonable to suggest that loss of anergy *in vivo* could result from the lodging of self-reactive B cells to anatomical sites free of self-antigen. Such a situation could lead to restoration of responsiveness and activation by cross-reactive immunogens, leading to autoimmunity. Understanding molecular mechanisms involved in anergy may provide insights to target autoimmune diseases.

Anergic B cells provide a particularly interesting example of differential BCR signaling leading to altered physiologic responses. Anergic cells persist in the periphery without deletion and receptor editing. Instead, they become refractory to further BCR stimulation.[152] This refractoriness is multifactorial, which begins with a decrease in the strength of association between mIgM and Ig-α/β.[153] This may result in decreased Ig-α/β, and Syk phosphorylation upon BCR aggregation.[152,154] Anergic cells also exhibit chronic low level increases in intracellular free calcium but are unable to further elevate intracellular calcium upon BCR aggregation.[155] Normally, stimulation of B cells leads to the calcium-dependent activation of NF-AT and NF-κB, both necessary for B-cell activation and survival.[74-76] However, in anergic cells, altered calcium levels result in constitutive NF-AT activation but impaired NF-κB activation.[77,156] Alteration in transcription factor activation in anergic cells may cause their shortened lifespan.

REFERENCES

1. Anolik J, Sanz I. B cells in human and murine systemic lupus erythematosus. Curr Opin Rheumatol 2004; 16(5): 505–12.
2. Lipsky PE. Systemic lupus erythematosus: an autoimmune disease of B cell hyperactivity. Nat Immunol 2001; 2(9): 764–6.
3. Leslie D, Lipsky P, Notkins AL. Autoantibodies as predictors of disease. J Clin Invest 2001; 108(10): 1417–22.
4. Silverman GJ, Weisman S. Rituximab therapy and autoimmune disorders: prospects for anti-B cell therapy. Arthritis Rheum 2003; 48(6): 1484–92.
5. Edwards JC, Leandro MJ, Cambridge G. B lymphocyte depletion in rheumatoid arthritis: targeting of CD20. Curr Dir Autoimmun 2005; 8: 175–92.
6. Anolik JH, Barnard J, Cappione A et al. Rituximab improves peripheral B cell abnormalities in human systemic lupus erythematosus. Arthritis Rheum 2004; 50(11): 3580–90.
7. Press OW, Howell-Clark J, Anderson S, Bernstein I. Retention of B-cell-specific monoclonal antibodies by human lymphoma cells. Blood 1994; 83(5): 1390–7.
8. Reff ME, Carner K, Chambers KS et al. Depletion of B cells in vivo by a chimeric mouse human monoclonal antibody to CD20. Blood 1994; 83(2): 435–45.
9. Chan OT, Madaio MP, Shlomchik MJ. The central and multiple roles of B cells in lupus pathogenesis. Immunol Rev 1999; 169: 107–21.
10. Tian J, Zekzer D, Lu Y, Dang H, Kaufman DL. B cells are crucial for determinant spreading of T cell autoimmunity among beta cell antigens in diabetes-prone nonobese diabetic mice. J Immunol 2006; 176(4): 2654–61.
11. Looney RJ, Anolik J, Sanz I. B cells as therapeutic targets for rheumatic diseases. Curr Opin Rheumatol 2004; 16(3): 180–5.
12. Ferry H, Leung JC, Lewis G et al. B-cell tolerance. Transplantation 2006; 81(3): 308–15.
13. Wardemann H, Yurasov S, Schaefer A et al. Predominant autoantibody production by early human B cell precursors. Science 2003; 301(5638): 1374–7.
14. Teh YM, Neuberger MS. The immunoglobulin (Ig)alpha and Igbeta cytoplasmic domains are independently sufficient to signal B cell maturation and activation in transgenic mice. J Exp Med 1997; 185(10): 1753–8.
15. Pike KA, Ratcliffe MJ. Dual requirement for the Ig alpha immunoreceptor tyrosine-based activation motif (ITAM) and a conserved non-Ig alpha ITAM tyrosine in supporting Ig alpha beta-mediated B cell development. J Immunol 2005; 174(4): 2012–20.
16. Cambier JC. Antigen and Fc receptor signaling. The awesome power of the immunoreceptor tyrosine-based activation motif (ITAM). J Immunol 1995; 155(7): 3281–5.
17. Kurosaki T. [B cell signaling]. Nihon Rinsho Meneki Gakkai Kaishi 1999; 22(6): 378–81.[in Japanese]
18. Clark MR, Campbell KS, Kazlauskas A et al. The B cell antigen receptor complex: association of Ig-alpha and Ig-beta with distinct cytoplasmic effectors. Science 1992; 258(5079): 123–6.
19. Reichlin A, Hu Y, Meffre E et al. B cell development is arrested at the immature B cell stage in mice carrying a mutation in the cytoplasmic domain of immunoglobulin beta. J Exp Med 2001; 193(1): 13–23.
20. Torres RM, Hafen K. A negative regulatory role for Ig-alpha during B cell development. Immunity 1999; 11(5): 527–36.
21. Flaswinkel H, Reth M. Dual role of the tyrosine activation motif of the Ig-alpha protein during signal transduction via the B cell antigen receptor. EMBO J 1994; 13(1): 83–9.
22. Kraus M, Saijo K, Torres RM, Rajewsky K. Ig-alpha cytoplasmic truncation renders immature B cells more sensitive to antigen contact. Immunity 1999; 11(5): 537–45.
23. Kraus M, Pao LI, Reichlin A et al. Interference with immunoglobulin (Ig)alpha immunoreceptor tyrosine-based activation motif (ITAM) phosphorylation modulates or blocks B cell development, depending on the availability of an Igbeta cytoplasmic tail. J Exp Med 2001; 194(4): 455–69.
24. Pleiman CM, Abrams C, Gauen LT et al. Distinct p53/56lyn and p59fyn domains associate with nonphosphorylated and phosphorylated Ig-alpha. Proc Natl Acad Sci U S A 1994; 91(10): 4268–72.
25. Cheng PC, Brown BK, Song W, Pierce SK. Translocation of the B cell antigen receptor into lipid rafts reveals a novel step in signaling. J Immunol 2001; 166(6): 3693–701.
26. Kurosaki T, Johnson SA, Pao L et al. Role of the Syk autophosphorylation site and SH2 domains in B cell

antigen receptor signaling. J Exp Med 1995; 182(6): 1815–23.

27. Rowley RB, Burkhardt AL, Chao HG, Matsueda GR, Bolen JB. Syk protein-tyrosine kinase is regulated by tyrosine-phosphorylated Ig alpha/Ig beta immunoreceptor tyrosine activation motif binding and autophosphorylation. J Biol Chem 1995; 270(19): 11590–4.

28. Allman D, Lindsley RC, DeMuth W et al. Resolution of three nonproliferative immature splenic B cell subsets reveals multiple selection points during peripheral B cell maturation. J Immunol 2001; 167(12): 6834–40.

29. Khan WN, Sideras P, Rosen FS, Alt FW. The role of Bruton's tyrosine kinase in B-cell development and function in mice and man. Ann N Y Acad Sci 1995; 764: 27–38.

30. Chan VW, Meng F, Soriano P, DeFranco AL, Lowell CA. Characterization of the B lymphocyte populations in Lyn-deficient mice and the role of Lyn in signal initiation and down-regulation. Immunity 1997; 7(1): 69–81.

31. Nishizumi H, Taniuchi I, Yamanashi Y et al. Impaired proliferation of peripheral B cells and indication of autoimmune disease in lyn-deficient mice. Immunity 1995; 3(5): 549–60.

32. Turner M, Mee PJ, Costello PS et al. Perinatal lethality and blocked B-cell development in mice lacking the tyrosine kinase Syk. Nature 1995; 378(6554): 298–302.

33. Xu Y, Harder KW, Huntington ND, Hibbs ML, Tarlinton DM. Lyn tyrosine kinase: accentuating the positive and the negative. Immunity 2005; 22(1): 9–18.

34. Law DA, Chan VW, Datta SK, DeFranco AL. B-cell antigen receptor motifs have redundant signalling capabilities and bind the tyrosine kinases PTK72, Lyn and Fyn. Curr Biol 1993; 3(10): 645–57.

35. D'Ambrosio D, Hippen KL, Minskoff SA et al. Recruitment and activation of PTP1C in negative regulation of antigen receptor signaling by Fc gamma RIIB1. Science 1995; 268(5208): 293–7.

36. D'Ambrosio D, Fong DC, Cambier JC. The SHIP phosphatase becomes associated with Fc gammaRIIB1 and is tyrosine phosphorylated during 'negative' signaling. Immunol Lett 1996; 54(2–3): 77–82.

37. Nishizumi H, Horikawa K, Mlinaric-Rascan I, Yamamoto T. A double-edged kinase Lyn: a positive and negative regulator for antigen receptor-mediated signals. J Exp Med 1998; 187(8): 1343–8.

38. Hibbs ML, Tarlinton DM, Armes J et al. Multiple defects in the immune system of Lyn-deficient mice, culminating in autoimmune disease. Cell 1995; 83(2): 301–11.

39. Du C, Sriram S. Increased severity of experimental allergic encephalomyelitis in lyn−/− mice in the absence of elevated proinflammatory cytokine response in the central nervous system. J Immunol 2002; 168(6): 3105–12.

40. Hibbs ML, Harder KW, Armes J et al. Sustained activation of Lyn tyrosine kinase in vivo leads to autoimmunity. J Exp Med 2002; 196(12): 1593–604.

41. Takata M, Sabe H, Hata A et al. Tyrosine kinases Lyn and Syk regulate B cell receptor-coupled Ca2+ mobilization through distinct pathways. EMBO J 1994; 13(6): 1341–9.

42. Pao LI, Famiglietti SJ, Cambier JC. Asymmetrical phosphorylation and function of immunoreceptor tyrosine-based activation motif tyrosines in B cell antigen receptor signal transduction. J Immunol 1998; 160(7): 3305–14.

43. de Weers M, Brouns GS, Hinshelwood S et al. B-cell antigen receptor stimulation activates the human Bruton's tyrosine kinase, which is deficient in X-linked agammaglobulinemia. J Biol Chem 1994; 269(39): 23857–60.

44. Tsukada S, Saffran DC, Rawlings DJ et al. Deficient expression of a B cell cytoplasmic tyrosine kinase in human X-linked agammaglobulinemia. Cell 1993; 72(2): 279–90.

45. Conley ME. B cells in patients with X-linked agammaglobulinemia. J Immunol 1985; 134(5): 3070–4.

46. Rosen FS, Cooper MD, Wedgwood RJ. The primary immunodeficiencies. N Engl J Med 1995; 333(7): 431–40.

47. Rawlings DJ, Saffran DC, Tsukada S et al. Mutation of unique region of Bruton's tyrosine kinase in immunodeficient XID mice. Science 1993; 261(5119): 358–61.

48. Thomas JD, Sideras P, Smith CI et al. Colocalization of X-linked agammaglobulinemia and X-linked immunodeficiency genes. Science 1993; 261(5119): 355–8.

49. Satterthwaite AB, Cheroutre H, Khan WN, Sideras P, Witte ON. Btk dosage determines sensitivity to B cell antigen receptor cross-linking. Proc Natl Acad Sci U S A 1997; 94(24): 13152–7.

50. Ng YS, Wardemann H, Chelnis J, Cunningham-Rundles C, Meffre E. Bruton's tyrosine kinase is essential for human B cell tolerance. J Exp Med 2004; 200(7): 927–34.

51. Samuels J, Ng YS, Coupillaud C, Paget D, Meffre E. Human B cell tolerance and its failure in rheumatoid arthritis. Ann N Y Acad Sci 2005; 1062: 116–26.

52. Mahajan S, Ghosh S, Sudbeck EA et al. Rational design and synthesis of a novel anti-leukemic agent targeting Bruton's tyrosine kinase (BTK), LFM-A13 [alpha-cyano-beta-hydroxy-beta-methyl-N-(2,5-dibromophenyl) propenamide]. J Biol Chem 1999; 274(14): 9587–99.

53. Fu C, Turck CW, Kurosaki T, Chan AC. BLNK: a central linker protein in B cell activation. Immunity 1998; 9(1): 93–103.

54. Ishiai M, Kurosaki M, Pappu R et al. BLNK required for coupling Syk to PLC gamma 2 and Rac1-JNK in B cells. Immunity 1999; 10(1): 117–25.

55. Kurosaki T, Tsukada S. BLNK: connecting Syk and Btk to calcium signals. Immunity 2000; 12(1): 1–5.

56. Wienands J, Schweikert J, Wollscheid B et al. SLP-65: a new signaling component in B lymphocytes which requires expression of the antigen receptor for phosphorylation. J Exp Med 1998; 188(4): 791–5.

57. Goitsuka R, Fujimura Y, Mamada H et al. BASH, a novel signaling molecule preferentially expressed in B cells of the bursa of Fabricius. J Immunol 1998; 161(11): 5804–8.

58. Chiu CW, Dalton M, Ishiai M, Kurosaki T, Chan AC. BLNK: molecular scaffolding through 'cis'-mediated organization of signaling proteins. EMBO J 2002; 21(23): 6461–72.

59. Mizuno K, Tagawa Y, Mitomo K et al. Src homology region 2 (SH2) domain-containing phosphatase-1 dephosphorylates B cell linker protein/SH2 domain leukocyte protein of 65 kDa and selectively regulates c-Jun NH2-terminal kinase activation in B cells. J Immunol 2000, 165(3): 1344–51.

60. Jumaa H, Wollscheid B, Mitterer M et al. Abnormal development and function of B lymphocytes in mice deficient for the signaling adaptor protein SLP-65. Immunity 1999; 11(5): 547–54.

61. Niiro H, Maeda A, Kurosaki T, Clark EA. The B lymphocyte adaptor molecule of 32 kD (Bam32) regulates B cell antigen receptor signaling and cell survival. J Exp Med 2002; 195(1): 143–9.

62. Fournier E, Isakoff SJ, Ko K et al. The B cell SH2/PH domain-containing adaptor Bam32/DAPP1 is required for T cell-independent II antigen responses. Curr Biol 2003; 13(21): 1858–66.

63. Han A, Saijo K, Mecklenbrauker I, Tarakhovsky A, Nussenzweig MC. Bam32 links the B cell receptor to ERK and JNK and mediates B cell proliferation but not survival. Immunity 2003; 19(4): 621–32.

64. Alessi DR, Downes CP. The role of PI 3-kinase in insulin action. Biochim Biophys Acta 1998; 1436(1–2): 151–64.

65. Andjelkovic M, Alessi DR, Meier R et al. Role of translocation in the activation and function of protein kinase B. J Biol Chem 1997; 272(50): 31515–24.

66. Takata M, Kurosaki T. A role for Bruton's tyrosine kinase in B cell antigen receptor-mediated activation of phospholipase C-gamma 2. J Exp Med 1996; 184(1): 31–40.

67. Brennan P, Mehl AM, Jones M, Rowe M. Phosphatidylinositol 3-kinase is essential for the proliferation of lymphoblastoid cells. Oncogene 2002; 21(8): 1263–71.

68. Beckwith M, Fenton RG, Katona IM, Longo DL. Phosphatidylinositol-3-kinase activity is required for the anti-Ig-mediated growth inhibition of a human B-lymphoma cell line. Blood 1996; 87(1): 202–10.

69. Aagaard-Tillery KM, Jelinek DF. Phosphatidylinositol 3-kinase activation in normal human B lymphocytes. J Immunol 1996; 156(12): 4543–54.

70. Buhl AM, Cambier JC. Phosphorylation of CD19 Y484 and Y515, and linked activation of phosphatidylinositol 3-kinase, are required for B cell antigen receptor-mediated activation of Bruton's tyrosine kinase. J Immunol 1999; 162(8): 4438–46.

71. Fruman DA, Snapper SB, Yballe CM et al. Impaired B cell development and proliferation in absence of phosphoinositide 3-kinase p85alpha. Science 1999; 283(5400): 393–7.

72. Ingham RJ, Holgado-Madruga M, Siu C, Wong AJ, Gold MR. The Gab1 protein is a docking site for multiple proteins involved in signaling by the B cell antigen receptor. J Biol Chem 1998; 273(46): 30630–7.

73. Suzuki H, Terauchi Y, Fujiwara M, et al. Xid-like immunodeficiency in mice with disruption of the p85alpha subunit of phosphoinositide 3-kinase. Science 1999; 283(5400): 390–2.

74. Antony P, Petro JB, Carlesso G et al. B-cell antigen receptor activates transcription factors NFAT (nuclear factor of activated T-cells) and NF-kappaB (nuclear factor kappaB) via a mechanism that involves diacylglycerol. Biochem Soc Trans 2004; 32(Pt 1): 113–15.

75. Pham LV, Tamayo AT, Yoshimura LC, Lin-Lee YC, Ford RJ. Constitutive NF-κB and NFAT activation in aggressive B-cell lymphomas synergistically activates the CD154 gene and maintains lymphoma cell survival. Blood 2005; 106(12): 3940–7.

76. Fu L, Lin-Lee YC, Pham LV et al. Constitutive NF-κB and NFAT activation leads to stimulation of the BLyS survival pathway in aggressive B-cell lymphomas. Blood 2006; 107(11): 4540–8.

77. Dolmetsch RE, Lewis RS, Goodnow CC, Healy JI. Differential activation of transcription factors induced by Ca2+ response amplitude and duration. Nature 1997; 386(6627): 855–8.

78. Saijo K, Mecklenbrauker I, Santana A et al. Protein kinase C beta controls nuclear factor kappaB activation in B cells through selective regulation of the IkappaB kinase alpha. J Exp Med 2002; 195(12): 1647–52.

79. Dong C, Davis RJ, Flavell RA. MAP kinases in the immune response. Annu Rev Immunol 2002; 20: 55–72.

80. Johnson GL, Lapadat R. Mitogen-activated protein kinase pathways mediated by ERK, JNK, and p38 protein kinases. Science 2002; 298(5600): 1911–12.

81. Hatta Y, Tsuchiya N, Ohashi J et al. Association of Fc gamma receptor IIIB, but not of Fc gamma receptor IIA and IIIA polymorphisms with systemic lupus erythematosus in Japanese. Genes Immun 1999; 1(1): 53–60.

82. Kyogoku C, Dijstelbloem HM, Tsuchiya N et al. Fcgamma receptor gene polymorphisms in Japanese patients with systemic lupus erythematosus: contribution of FCGR2B to genetic susceptibility. Arthritis Rheum 2002; 46(5): 1242–54.

83. Floto RA, Clatworthy MR, Heilbronn KR et al. Loss of function of a lupus-associated FcgammaRIIb polymorphism through exclusion from lipid rafts. Nat Med 2005; 11(10): 1056–8.

84. Blank MC, Stefanescu RN, Masuda E et al. Decreased transcription of the human FCGR2B gene mediated by the -343 G/C promoter polymorphism and association with systemic lupus erythematosus. Hum Genet 2005; 117(2–3): 220–7.

85. Prokunina L, Castillejo-Lopez C, Oberg F et al. A regulatory polymorphism in PDCD1 is associated with susceptibility to systemic lupus erythematosus in humans. Nat Genet 2002; 32(4): 666–9.

86. Hatta Y, Tsuchiya N, Matsushita M et al. Identification of the gene variations in human CD22. Immunogenetics 1999; 49(4): 280–6.

87. Sato S, Hasegawa M, Fujimoto M, Tedder TF, Takehara K. Quantitative genetic variation in CD19 expression correlates with autoimmunity. J Immunol 2000; 165(11): 6635–43.

88. Huck S, Le Corre R, Youinou P, Zouali M. Expression of B cell receptor-associated signaling molecules in human lupus. Autoimmunity 2001; 33(3): 213–24.

89. Cyster JG, Goodnow CC. Protein tyrosine phosphatase 1C negatively regulates antigen receptor signaling in B lymphocytes and determines thresholds for negative selection. Immunity 1995; 2(1): 13–24.

90. Shultz LD, Rajan TV, Greiner DL. Severe defects in immunity and hematopoiesis caused by SHP-1 protein-tyrosine-phosphatase deficiency. Trends Biotechnol 1997; 15(8): 302–7.

91. Nitschke L. The role of CD22 and other inhibitory co-receptors in B-cell activation. Curr Opin Immunol 2005; 17(3): 290–7.

92. Dal Porto JM, Gauld SB, Merrell KT et al. B cell antigen receptor signaling 101. Mol Immunol 2004; 41(6–7): 599–613.

93. Muta T, Kurosaki T, Misulovin Z et al. A 13-amino-acid motif in the cytoplasmic domain of Fc gamma RIIB modulates B-cell receptor signalling. Nature 1994; 368(6466): 70–3.

94. Famiglietti SJ, Nakamura K, Cambier JC. Unique features of SHIP, SHP-1 and SHP-2 binding to FcgammaRIIb revealed by surface plasmon resonance analysis. Immunol Lett 1999; 68(1): 35–40.

95. Hippen KL, Buhl AM, D'Ambrosio D et al. Fc gammaRIIB1 inhibition of BCR-mediated phosphoinositide hydrolysis and Ca2+ mobilization is integrated by CD19 dephosphorylation. Immunity 1997; 7(1): 49–58.

96. Tamir I, Stolpa JC, Helgason CD et al. The RasGAP-binding protein p62dok is a mediator of inhibitory FcgammaRIIB signals in B cells. Immunity 2000; 12(3): 347–58.

97. Takai T, Nakamura A, Akiyama K. Fc receptors as potential targets for the treatment of allergy, autoimmune disease and cancer. Curr Drug Targets Immune Endocr Metabol Disord 2003; 3(3): 187–97.

98. Bolland S, Ravetch JV. Spontaneous autoimmune disease in Fc(gamma)RIIB-deficient mice results from strain-specific epistasis. Immunity 2000; 13(2): 277–85.

99. Davis RS, Dennis G Jr, Odom MR et al. Fc receptor homologs: newest members of a remarkably diverse Fc receptor gene family. Immunol Rev 2002; 190: 123-36.

100. Mechetina LV, Najakshin AM, Alabyev BY, Chikaev NA, Taranin AV. Identification of CD16-2, a novel mouse receptor homologous to CD16/Fc gamma RIII. Immunogenetics 2002; 54(7): 463–8.

101. Okazaki T, Otaka Y, Wang J et al. Hydronephrosis associated with antiurothelial and antinuclear autoantibodies in BALB/c-Fcgr2b–/–Pdcd1–/– mice. J Exp Med 2005; 202(12): 1643–8.

102. Okazaki T, Maeda A, Nishimura H, Kurosaki T, Honjo T. PD-1 immunoreceptor inhibits B cell receptor-mediated signaling by recruiting src homology 2-domain-containing tyrosine phosphatase 2 to phosphotyrosine. Proc Natl Acad Sci U S A 2001; 98(24): 13866–71.

103. Nishimura H, Nose M, Hiai H, Minato N, Honjo T. Development of lupus-like autoimmune diseases by disruption of the PD-1 gene encoding an ITIM motif-carrying immunoreceptor. Immunity 1999; 11(2): 141–51.

104. Hitomi Y, Tsuchiya N, Kawasaki A et al. CD72 polymorphisms associated with alternative splicing modify susceptibility to human systemic lupus erythematosus through epistatic interaction with FCGR2B. Hum Mol Genet 2004; 13(23): 2907–17.

105. Adachi T, Wakabayashi C, Nakayama T, Yakura H, Tsubata T. CD72 negatively regulates signaling through the antigen receptor of B cells. J Immunol 2000; 164(3): 1223–9.

106. McGaha TL, Sorrentino B, Ravetch JV. Restoration of tolerance in lupus by targeted inhibitory receptor expression. Science 2005; 307(5709): 590–3.

107. Bolland S, Yim YS, Tus K, Wakeland EK, Ravetch JV. Genetic modifiers of systemic lupus erythematosus in FcgammaRIIB(–/–) mice. J Exp Med 2002; 195(9): 1167–74.

108. Ravetch JV, Bolland S. IgG Fc receptors. Annu Rev Immunol 2001; 19: 275–90.

109. Clynes RA, Towers TL, Presta LG, Ravetch JV. Inhibitory Fc receptors modulate in vivo cytoxicity against tumor targets. Nat Med 2000; 6(4): 443–6.

110. Doody GM, Justement LB, Delibrias CC et al. A role in B cell activation for CD22 and the protein tyrosine phosphatase SHP. Science 1995; 269(5221): 242–4.

111. Chen J, McLean PA, Neel BG et al. CD22 attenuates calcium signaling by potentiating plasma membrane calcium-ATPase activity. Nat Immunol 2004; 5(6): 651–7.

112. O'Keefe TL, Williams GT, Davies SL, Neuberger MS. Hyperresponsive B cells in CD22-deficient mice. Science 1996; 274(5288): 798–801.

113. Nitschke L, Carsetti R, Ocker B, Kohler G, Lamers MC. CD22 is a negative regulator of B-cell receptor signalling. Curr Biol 1997; 7(2): 133–43.

114. Gerlach J, Ghosh S, Jumaa H et al. B cell defects in SLP65/BLNK-deficient mice can be partially corrected by the absence of CD22, an inhibitory coreceptor for BCR signaling. Eur J Immunol 2003; 33(12): 3418–26.

115. Samardzic T, Marinkovic D, Danzer CP et al. Reduction of marginal zone B cells in CD22-deficient mice. Eur J Immunol 2002; 32(2): 561–7.

116. Morel L, Mohan C, Yu Y et al. Functional dissection of systemic lupus erythematosus using congenic mouse strains. J Immunol 1997; 158(12): 6019–28.

117. Mohan C, Morel L, Yang P, Wakeland EK. Genetic dissection of systemic lupus erythematosus pathogenesis: Slc2 on murine chromosome 4 leads to B cell hyperactivity. J Immunol 1997; 159(1): 454–65.

118. Kelm S, Schauer R, Manuguerra JC, Gross HJ, Crocker PR. Modifications of cell surface sialic acids modulate cell adhesion mediated by sialoadhesin and CD22. Glycoconj J 1994; 11(6): 576–85.

119. Powell LD, Jain RK, Matta KL, Sabesan S, Varki A. Characterization of sialyloligosaccharide binding by recombinant soluble and native cell-associated CD22. Evidence for a minimal structural recognition motif and the potential importance of multisite binding. J Biol Chem 1995; 270(13): 7523–32.

120. Poe JC, Fujimoto Y, Hasegawa M et al. CD22 regulates B lymphocyte function in vivo through both ligand-dependent and ligand-independent mechanisms. Nat Immunol 2004; 5(10): 1078–87.

121. Lajaunias F, Ida A, Kikuchi S et al. Differential control of CD22 ligand expression on B and T lymphocytes, and enhanced expression in murine systemic lupus. Arthritis Rheum 2003; 48(6): 1612–21.

122. Jin L, McLean PA, Neel BG, Wortis HH. Sialic acid binding domains of CD22 are required for negative regulation of B cell receptor signaling. J Exp Med 2002; 195(9): 1199–205.

123. Kelm S, Gerlach J, Brossmer R, Danzer CP, Nitschke L. The ligand-binding domain of CD22 is needed for inhibition of the B cell receptor signal, as demonstrated by a novel human CD22-specific inhibitor compound. J Exp Med 2002; 195(9): 1207–13.

124. Collins BE, Smith BA, Bengtson P, Paulson JC. Ablation of CD22 in ligand-deficient mice restores B cell receptor signaling. Nat Immunol 2006; 7(2): 199–206.

125. Ghosh S, Bandulet C, Nitschke L. Regulation of B cell development and B cell signalling by CD22 and its ligands α2,6-linked sialic acids. Int Immunol 2006; 18(4): 603–11.

126. Sgroi D, Varki A, Braesch-Andersen S, Stamenkovic I. CD22, a B cell-specific immunoglobulin superfamily member, is a sialic acid-binding lectin. J Biol Chem 1993; 268(10): 7011–18.

127. Law CL, Aruffo A, Chandran KA, Doty RT, Clark EA. Ig domains 1 and 2 of murine CD22 constitute the ligand-binding domain and bind multiple sialylated ligands expressed on B and T cells. J Immunol 1995; 155(7): 3368–76.

128. Han S, Collins BE, Bengtson P, Paulson JC. Homomultimeric complexes of CD22 in B cells revealed by protein-glycan cross-linking. Nat Chem Biol 2005; 1(2): 93–7.

129. Zhang M, Varki A. Cell surface sialic acids do not affect primary CD22 interactions with CD45 and surface IgM nor the rate of constitutive CD22 endocytosis. Glycobiology 2004; 14(11): 939–49.

130. Domer T, Kaufmann J, Wegener WA, Teoh N, Goldenberg DM, Burmester GR. Initial clinical study of epratuzumab (humanized anti-CD22 antibody). Arthritis Res. Ther. 2006; 8(3): R74.

131. Kung C, Pingel JT, Heikinheimo M et al. Mutations in the tyrosine phosphatase CD45 gene in a child with severe combined immunodeficiency disease. Nat Med 2000; 6(3): 343–5.

132. Justement LB, Campbell KS, Chien NC, Cambier JC. Regulation of B cell antigen receptor signal transduction and phosphorylation by CD45. Science 1991; 252(5014): 1839–42.

133. Hermiston ML, Xu Z, Weiss A. CD45: a critical regulator of signaling thresholds in immune cells. Annu Rev Immunol 2003; 21: 107–37.

134. Hata A, Sabe H, Kurosaki T, Takata M, Hanafusa H. Functional analysis of Csk in signal transduction through the B-cell antigen receptor. Mol Cell Biol 1994; 14(11): 7306–13.

135. Gupta N, DeFranco AL. Visualizing lipid raft dynamics and early signaling events during antigen receptor-mediated B-lymphocyte activation. Mol Biol Cell 2003; 14(2): 432–44.

136. Majeti R, Bilwes AM, Noel JP, Hunter T, Weiss A. Dimerization-induced inhibition of receptor protein tyrosine phosphatase function through an inhibitory wedge. Science 1998; 279(5347): 88–91.

137. Majeti R, Xu Z, Parslow TG et al. An inactivating point mutation in the inhibitory wedge of CD45 causes lymphoproliferation and autoimmunity. Cell 2000; 103(7): 1059–70.

138. Hermiston ML, Tan AL, Gupta VA, Majeti R, Weiss A. The juxtamembrane wedge negatively regulates CD45 function in B cells. Immunity 2005; 23(6): 635–47.

139. Hayami K, Fukuta D, Nishikawa Y et al. Molecular cloning of a novel murine cell-surface glycoprotein homologous to killer cell inhibitory receptors. J Biol Chem 1997; 272(11): 7320–7.

140. Kubagawa H, Burrows PD, Cooper MD. A novel pair of immunoglobulin-like receptors expressed by B cells and myeloid cells. Proc Natl Acad Sci U S A 1997; 94(10): 5261–6.

141. Maeda A, Scharenberg AM, Tsukada S et al. Paired immunoglobulin-like receptor B (PIR-B) inhibits BCR-induced activation of Syk and Btk by SHP-1. Oncogene 1999; 18(14): 2291–7.

142. Maeda A, Kurosaki M, Kurosaki T. Paired immunoglobulin-like receptor (PIR)-A is involved in activating mast cells through its association with Fc receptor gamma chain. J Exp Med 1998; 188(5): 991–5.

143. Blery M, Kubagawa H, Chen CC et al. The paired Ig-like receptor PIR-B is an inhibitory receptor that recruits the protein-tyrosine phosphatase SHP-1. Proc Natl Acad Sci U S A 1998; 95(5): 2446–51.

144. Ho LH, Uehara T, Chen CC, Kubagawa H, Cooper MD. Constitutive tyrosine phosphorylation of the inhibitory paired Ig-like receptor PIR-B. Proc Natl Acad Sci U S A 1999; 96(26): 15086–90.

145. Yotsumoto K, Okoshi Y, Shibuya K et al. Paired activating and inhibitory immunoglobulin-like receptors, MAIR-I and MAIR-II, regulate mast cell and macrophage activation. J Exp Med 2003; 198(2): 223–33.

146. Nemazee D. Antigen receptor 'capacity' and the sensitivity of self-tolerance. Immunol Today 1996; 17(1): 25–9.

147. Casellas R, Shih TA, Kleinewietfeld M et al. Contribution of receptor editing to the antibody repertoire. Science 2001; 291(5508): 1541–4.

148. Pelanda R, Schwers S, Sonoda E et al. Receptor editing in a transgenic mouse model: site, efficiency, and role in B cell tolerance and antibody diversification. Immunity 1997; 7(6): 765–75.

149. Gauld SB, Benschop RJ, Merrell KT, Cambier JC. Maintenance of B cell anergy requires constant antigen receptor occupancy and signaling. Nat Immunol 2005; 6(11): 1160–7.

150. Cooke MP, Heath AW, Shokat KM et al. Immunoglobulin signal transduction guides the specificity of B cell-T cell interactions and is blocked in tolerant self-reactive B cells. J Exp Med 1994; 179(2): 425–38.

151. Rathmell JC, Goodnow CC. The in vivo balance between B cell clonal expansion and elimination is regulated by CD95 both on B cells and in their microenvironment. Immunol Cell Biol 1998; 76(5): 387–94.

152. Vilen BJ, Burke KM, Sleater M, Cambier JC. Transmodulation of BCR signaling by transduction-incompetent antigen receptors: implications for impaired signaling in anergic B cells. J Immunol 2002; 168(9): 4344–51.

153. Vilen BJ, Nakamura T, Cambier JC. Antigen-stimulated dissociation of BCR mIg from Ig-alpha/Ig-beta: implications for receptor desensitization. Immunity 1999; 10(2): 239–48.

154. Parent BA, Wang X, Song W. Stability of the B cell antigen receptor modulates its signaling and antigen-targeting functions. Eur J Immunol 2002; 32(7): 1839–46.

155. Benschop RJ, Brandl E, Chan AC, Cambier JC. Unique signaling properties of B cell antigen receptor in mature and immature B cells: implications for tolerance and activation. J Immunol 2001; 167(8): 4172–9.

156. Healy JI, Dolmetsch RE, Timmerman LA et al. Different nuclear signals are activated by the B cell receptor during positive versus negative signaling. Immunity 1997; 6(4): 419–28.

5

Macrophages in rheumatoid arthritis

Peter LEM van Lent and Wim B van den Berg

Introduction • Resident intima macrophages in rheumatoid arthritis • Differentiation and function of macrophages in RA synovium • Activation of synovial macrophages • Macrophages and joint destruction • Depletion of type A intima cells inhibits onset of arthritis • Final remarks • References

INTRODUCTION

Rheumatoid arthritis (RA) is characterized by chronic inflammation in multiple joints and concomitant destruction of cartilage and bone. Macrophages play a crucial role in both the inflammatory process and tissue destruction.[1-3] Macrophages become activated by the RA process in the synovial tissue, either directly through stimulation with bacterial or viral triggers, or indirectly through T- and B-cell-mediated events. The latter responses can be directed to joint-specific autoantigens, but may also include reactions to persistent viral and bacterial elements. Although RA has been considered an autoimmune process, a crucial autoantigen has not been defined and it seems more likely that multiple candidate triggers are involved. This argues for general therapeutic approaches at a downstream level, making activated macrophages an obvious target.

RA is a systemic disease, with its main expression in body compartments that are surrounded by a synovial lining layer, containing large amounts of macrophages. Such compartments include diarthrodial joints and precipitation of the RA process in such areas underlines the crucial role of tissue macrophages in disease onset. During active arthritis monocytes infiltrate from the blood into the synovium, differentiate into mature macrophages, and form the dominant cell type in the inflamed synovium. However, synovial lining macrophages remain a crucial

source of inflammatory mediators and contribute significantly to local cytokine and chemokine production. Of great interest, RA synovial macrophages appear to express deranged levels of Fcγ receptors, and proof is accumulating that an aberrant reaction of macrophages to immune complexes, leading to prolonged activation, contributes to increased and prolonged release of proinflammatory and cartilage destructive cytokines. Therapeutic approaches targeting the macrophage itself or its dominant proinflammatory mediators have already been shown to be efficient in the treatment of RA. Inhibition of the macrophage-derived master cytokines tumor necrosis factor (TNF)-α and interleukin (IL)-1 created a major breakthrough in the treatment of this crippling disease. Insight into mechanisms of macrophage activation and mediators involved in that process may provide novel targets for further optimization of therapy.

RESIDENT INTIMA MACROPHAGES IN RHEUMATOID ARTHRITIS

The inside of diarthrodial joints, the preferential site for development of RA, is lined by a layer of cells, usually one to three cells in thickness, which is called the intima. This layer contains two types of cells, the fibroblast-like type B cell and the macrophage-like type A cell, which interdigitate using cytoplasmic processes.[4] These cells are enclosed within a matrix, probably produced by the lining cell itself, containing collagen type IV, forming a covalently stabilized polygonal framework and a second interlocking polymer network of laminin. Immunohistologic investigations have shown that three of the four constituents forming a basement membrane (collagen type IV, heparan sulfate, proteoglycan, and laminin) are present but that entactin, a sulfated glycoprotein that connects laminin and type IV collagen, is absent. The intima lining sits on compact loose connective tissue bearing a vascular plexus that gives a close contact with the blood vessels. The origin of the type A cell is probably a monocyte, as shown in elegant studies using mice with the Chediak Higashi syndrome. Monocytes of these mice that contain crystals were transferred to control mice and kinetic studies showed accumulation of crystal-containing type A cells in the lining layer.[5] These cells are constantly replaced via the circulation, although the turnover is slow. After selective removal of type A cells in the intima of mice, it takes more than 30 days before the lining cell layer returns to normal levels.[6]

As a first sign of onset of arthritis, intima cells become activated. Intima cells form a strategic barrier within the joint. Substances leaking from the joint, bacterial infections, or immune complexes formed within the synovial fluid first meet this layer and the abundance of receptors expressed by type A cells leads to phagocytosis and activation of these cells. Moreover, this layer lies just above the vascular plexus in the synovium, which also makes these cells very accessible for substances arriving via the bloodstream. Immunolocalization studies have shown that phagocytic intima cells express many proinflammatory factors like cytokines IL-1α, TNF-α, IL-6, IL-15, IL-18, IL-32,[7,8] and chemokines like IL-8 or MCP-1, but also growth factors like GM-CSF and TGF-β.[9] As type A cells produce various chemokines, these cells are involved in attraction of inflammatory cells during the onset of arthritis and probably also in arresting of inflammatory cells within the synovium during the chronic phase.

DIFFERENTIATION AND FUNCTION OF MACROPHAGES IN RA SYNOVIUM

Activation of the lining layer directs the influx of inflammatory cells, such as polymorphonuclear leukocytes (PMNs), lymphocytes (T and B cells), and large amounts of monocytes (Figure 5.1).

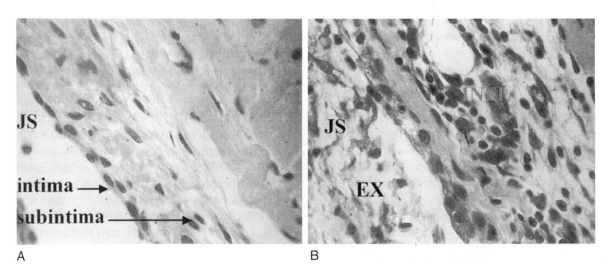

A   B

Figure 5.1 Synovial lining layer in knee joints of normal (A) and arthritic (B) mice. JS, joint space; Ex, exudate; Infl, infiltrate. Original magnification ×400. Hematoxylin/eosin staining.

During RA, a number of alterations in the synovial membrane are observed. Synovial lining cells increase many-fold. Type A macrophages still form the predominant population in the hypertrophied intima, approaching 50–70% of cells.[4] Superimposed on this is a highly vascular subintima filled with mononuclear cells, including T and B cells and large numbers of macrophages, often forming aggregates around the blood vessels. Most of the macrophages are thought to stem from monocytes which have infiltrated into the joint, where they diffentiate into macrophages.[10] A small proportion may be derived from locally dividing mononuclear phagocytes. Chemokine receptor expression is different on RA monocytes in peripheral blood and synovial fluid (significantly higher CCR3, 4, and 5 levels in synovial fluid). CCR1 and CCR2 seem to be crucial for monocyte recruitment. CCR3 and CCR5 may play a role in monocyte/macrophage tissue migration or retention. Therapeutic application of chemokine inhibitors seems hampered by redundancy.[11] *In vivo*, generation of monocytes is controlled by various growth factors including IL-3, GM-CSF, and M-CSF. These factors are abundantly present in the RA joint, and are potent stimulators of CD34[+] stem cells, which have been found to infiltrate the joints. As such, local production and maturation may contribute to the total macrophage cell mass.

Monocyte differentiation into macrophages in the RA synovium is highly versatile. Many differentiation stadia are found, reflecting various subpopulations of cells that are probably involved in different aspects of immune and effector mechanisms. Some of the maturation stages are now identified by CD markers, as listed in Table 5.1. It is a recent finding that an unexpectedly large subpopulation of CD68[+] macrophages express DC-SIGN, a receptor which normally is expressed only on dendritic cells (DCs).[12] DC-SIGN is a crucial receptor involved in the initial interaction with ICAM-3-containing naive T cells, which are abundantly present in RA synovia, and blockade of DC-SIGN prevents binding and subsequent antigen presentation. It may suggest that these DC-SIGN-positive macrophages contribute to

Table 5.1 CD markers on human tissue macrophages

Functional aspects	CD markers
Adhesion and migration	CD33, CD169, CCR2, CCR5
Cytokine receptors	CD25, CD119, CDw121b, EMR-1
Fcγ and complement receptor (CR)	CD16, CD32, CD64, CD23
Microbial pattern recognition receptors	CD11b, CD204, CD68, CD14, CD206
T-cell activation	MHC class II

Differences between type 1 and type 2 cytokine polarized macrophages

	Type 1	Type 2
Adhesion/migration	CCR-5	CCR-2
Microbial pattern recognition receptor	CD206 Mannose R	CD206++ Mannose R

local immune activation, apart from the scant numbers of fully matured DCs.

Expression of different surface markers probably has consequences for macrophage effector function, ranging from more proinflammatory to anti-inflammatory activity. Such a mixture of cell types was found earlier in the chronically inflamed lung, where proinflammatory and suppressor macrophage populations were identified.[13] This diversity is in line with findings in RA synovia. Only a limited number of CD68[+] cells produce TNF and IL-1, whereas others produce none or even anti-inflammatory cytokines like IL-10 and TGF-β. Further research into the identification of cell surface markers akin to various subgroups of macrophages is warranted, as it may provide targets for more selective anti-inflammatory therapy.

Normal tissue macrophages and young monocytes that have recently immigrated into normal tissues are quiescent. In an activated state, as found in the synovium of RA patients, macrophages acquire multiple functions. Under conditions of cell stress, macrophages produce alarmins, or damage-associated molecular pattern proteins (DAMPS).

Important members of DAMPS are S100 proteins, characterized by calcium binding motifs, and to date more than 20 members have been described. S100A8 and A9, formerly called MRP 8 and 14, are not only markers of activation, but also display prominent proinflammatory activity when released.[14,15] S100 A8/9 induced marked TNF and IL-1 production and expression of S100A8/9 is seen at sites of joint erosion.

Activated macrophages also elaborate chemokines involved in PMN, monocyte, and T-cell migration. Integrins and vascular cell adhesion molecules (VCAMs) are up-regulated under the influence of IL-1,TNF-α, and interferon (IFN)-γ release. Moreover, reactive oxygen and nitrogen intermediates are produced, eliciting local tissue damage. Production of cytokines like platelet-derived growth factor (PDGF), fibroblast growth factor (FGF), and TNF-α enhance the growth and proliferation of lining macrophages through paracrine interaction with the fibroblast-like lining cells. Activated macrophages also release angiogenesis-promoting factors like TGF-β, angiotropin, and vascular endothelial growth factor (VEGF), responsible for neovascularization and further increase of the subintimal layer.

Apart from a role in synovial activation and growth, matured macrophages may function as antigen-presenting cells (APCs), initiating local antigen-specific T- and B-cell responses, and herein amplifying immune-mediated macrophage activation. Moreover, macrophages producing TNF, IL-1, and destructive enzymes will contribute to cartilage erosion. The ultimate fate of macrophages in the RA synovium is not known but a large proportion of the CD68+ lining cells show signs of apoptosis.[4] A minority may traffic to other sites like remote secondary lymphoid organs.

ACTIVATION OF SYNOVIAL MACROPHAGES

The pathogenic mechanisms involved in synovial macrophage activation are as yet unknown. Theoretically, there is either direct activation by phlogistic stimuli such as bacteria or viruses, or the system is turned on indirectly, as an effector

mechanism of immune-mediated events. In principle, the latter can be caused by T- and B-cell-mediated recognition of exogenous antigens reaching the joints, including bacteria and viruses, or by immune responses to joint-specific autoantigens (Figure 5.2). Chronicity of the process of macrophage activation may be due to persistence of stimuli, which is obvious in the case of autoantigens, and/or deranged responsiveness of the cells, acquiring tumor-like properties. In particular, viral stimuli have been suggested to be involved in the latter process, although a viral contribution to chronicity of RA is still to be proven.

Endogenous bacterial fragments enter the joint as a continuous process and, when poorly degraded by the macrophages, do form an obvious persistent stimulus for macrophage activation. It was identified that bacterial DNA fragments bearing a CpG motif are powerful stimulants of macrophages.[16] More recent developments provided further insight into receptors involved in cell activation by environmental stimuli. At present up to 10 TLRs (Toll-like receptors) are described. Bacterial cell wall fragments stimulate TLR2,[17,18] lipopolysaccharide (LPS) interacts with TLR4, and viruses mainly trigger TLR3 and 7. CPG motifs trigger TLR9. Additional diversity in response patterns is created by receptor crosstalk and differential use of adapter molecules. The TLR4 receptor is intriguing since it is not only stimulated by LPS but also by breakdown fragments of connective tissue components. This pathway stimulates TNF and IL-1 production and links tissue damage as a sustaining factor of chronic joint inflammation. Regulation of tolerance to these persistent triggers is a delicate

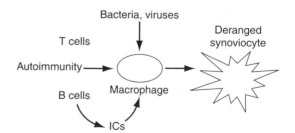

Figure 5.2 Stimuli involved in synovial macrophage activation.

process and disturbances in receptor activation may underlie autoimmune responses.[19] In fact, deranged TLR4 signaling and excessive cytokine production have been demonstrated in RA patients.[20]

When T-cell tolerance against bacterial fragments is lost, T cells are turned on locally and their products activate the macrophage. As a further element of local immune events, antibodies can be generated, forming immune complexes at the site and stimulating macrophages through their Fc receptors. In principle, any protein antigen reaching the joint in sufficient quantities and retained in avascular joint structures, either due to charge-mediated binding or antibody-mediated trapping, may function as a persistent trigger. As such, the difference between autoantigens of joint structures or endogenous and exogenous proteins sticking to joint structures is mainly semantic, although it may be argued that regulation of tolerance is different.

Animal model studies have identified a number of potential autoantigens, including cartilage-derived collagen type II, proteoglycan, GP-39, citrullinated proteins, and even the ubiquitously expressed enzyme GPI (glucose phosphate isomerase), showing cartilage-adhering potential.[21-23] There is reason to believe that the antigen causing RA might be associated with cartilage, since removal of cartilage at joint replacement is sufficient to silence such a joint, without the need of synovectomy. Nevertheless, it seems unlikely that one particular autoantigen is at the base of RA pathology and a multiple trigger concept is more obvious. This leaves us with therapeutic options that interfere with general elements of immune functions, such as suppressive T-cell cytokines. Attempts to use joint-specific antigens to induce tolerance and to generate bystander suppression of nonrelated T-cell responses were successful in animal models, but convincing effects and therapeutic applicability in RA patients have yet to be shown.

Efforts to treat RA by depleting CD4 T cells, using monoclonal antibodies or immunotoxins, have been disappointing and questioned the relevance of T cells. However, it is now clear that different subsets of T cells exist, ranging from IFN-γ- and IL-17-producing effector cells to regulatory T cells, and more selective targeting of subsets seems warranted. The recent development of therapeutic targeting of the T-cell activation marker CTLA-4 looks promising and underlines the importance of T cells in RA.

T cell macrophage activation and regulating cytokines

The belief in T-cell activation of macrophages was reduced by the difficulty of finding significant amounts of IL-2 or IFN-γ in inflamed RA synovia. However, the recent identification of IL-17 as a pathogenic mediator of a distinct subset of Th17 cells[24,25] and its clear presence in many RA patients[26,27] boosted renewed interest. This revival in thinking is strengthened by the old finding of virtual absence of the counteracting cytokine IL-4. IL-17 itself stimulated the production of IL-1 and TNF-α by human macrophages and synovial fibroblasts and amplified the effect of IL-1 and TNF-α on synoviocytes. Furthermore, data from animal models support the arthritogenic potential of this cytokine. When IL-17 is overexpressed in the joints of mice with experimental collagen type II arthritis (CIA), it strongly aggravates joint inflammation and cartilage destruction, independent of IL-1.[28,29] In addition, it enhances immune complex-mediated arthritis and renders the arthritis independent of TNF. Blockade of IL-17 in classic CIA significantly ameliorated the disease and combined TNF/IL-17 neutralization was superior.

A further argument for IL-17 and T-cell involvement is the abundance of IL-15 in RA synovia. This cytokine is produced by macrophages and is a major stimulus of T-cell activation. Such IL-15-exposed T cells become TNF-producing cells and are potent activators of macrophage TNF production, in an IL-17- and cell–cell contact-dependent fashion.[30-32] Intriguingly, apolipoprotein A-I blocks contact activation and seems a natural regulator.[33]

Additional cytokines involved in boosting T-cell responses are IL-12 and IL-18.[34,35] IL-12 and IL-18, in particular, are found in significant quantities in RA synovia and are products of activated macrophages. Although IL-18 alone is not a potent maturation factor, it markedly synergizes with IL-12 in Th1 maturation. Both mediators are induced in macrophages by bacterial activation and this provides the intriguing possibility that bacteria are not only phlogistic triggers but also amplify autoimmune responses in the joint through release of IL-12 and IL-18 (Figure 5.3). It may fit with the often suggested relationship between bacterial infections and arthritis. Apart from septic arthritis, arthritis occurs in patients with Lyme disease and infections of the throat and the gastrointestinal tract. In animal models IL-12 was shown to promote an acute, nondestructive joint inflammation to a chronic, destructive process. Early neutralization of IL-12 as well as IL-18 markedly reduced autoimmune collagen type II arthritis, but also nonimmune Zymosan arthritis, underlining that these cytokines are both immune-potentiating as well as directly proinflammatory.[36–38] However, when neutralization is done in established stages of arthritis, opposite effects are noted. With the identification of IL-23 further insight is now provided. IL-23 knockout (KO) mice are

protected from disease, whereas selective IL-12 KO mice exhibit more severe disease.[39] It is becoming clear that not IL-12, but IL-23, is the main driving force of Th17 cells. In fact, IL-12/IFN-γ could mediate regulatory functions in a ying-yang relationship with IL-23/IL-17. IL-6, formerly seen as a driver of the Th2 pathway and responsible for inhibiting excessive development of the Th1 population, is now considered a major driver of Th17 differentiation, with IL-23 as a maturation factor. This would fit well with the marked therapeutic effect of IL-6 neutralization in RA trials.

Macrophage activation induced by immune complexes

One of the characteristic features of RA is the presence of high titers of autoantibodies. Impaired B-cell responses have been found within RA synovium and may be caused by impaired antigen presentation or clonal deletion. Autoantibodies are released in large amounts and target many antigens, forming immune

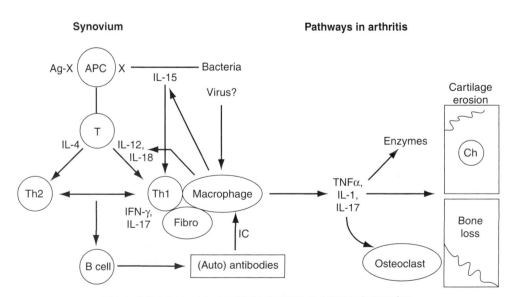

Figure 5.3 Cytokines in synovial activation and tissue destruction.

complexes residing in the inflamed joint, which contribute to macrophage activation. Immune complexes are found abundantly in the synovial fluid, synovial layer, and even in the superficial layer of the cartilage. Many potential autoantigens have been defined, including citrullin and IgG. In the latter case, immune complexes include IgG isotype antibodies directed against the constant part of the IgG isotype. These often large immune complexes are recognized by Fcγ receptors (FcγR) expressed on the membrane of macrophages.

In the mouse four FcγR classes have been described. FcγRI is a high affinity receptor, whereas FcγRII and III are low affinity receptors. FcγRIV was recently identified[40,41] and binds IgGs with intermediate affinity. FcγRI, III, and IV are activating receptors. Upon binding intracellular signaling is mediated by an ITAM motif present in the intracytoplasmic part of the receptor leading to production of syk kinases, resulting in selective activation of genes. In contrast, FcγRII is an inhibiting receptor. Co-ligation of FcγRII with FcγRI, III, or IV leads to inactivation mediated by the ITIM motif present in the intracytoplasmic receptor. All four FcγR classes are expressed on macrophages and a balance between activating versus inhibiting receptors determines the net reaction of the cell if exposed to immune complexes.

In humans, three classes of FcγR receptors are described and all are elevated on RA synovial macrophages (Figure 5.4). Two types of FcγRII are identified, with IIa being an activating receptor, whereas IIb probably is the equivalent of the mouse type II inhibitory receptor. To identify which activating FcγRs are important in onset and prolongation of arthritis, experimental models were studied in various FcγR KO mice. When experimental arthritis was induced passively by immune complexes, FcγRIII appeared the dominant FcγR in joint inflammation. In FcγRIII−/− mice onset of arthritis was completely prevented, whereas in FcγRI−/−, joint inflammation continued and was not different from controls. In contrast, using a

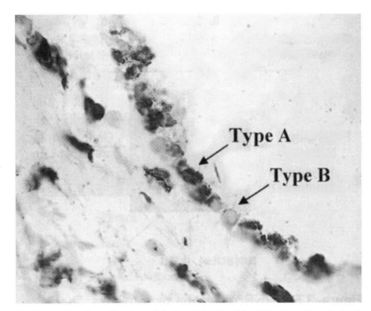

Figure 5.4 FcγRIII expression by macrophage-like type A but not by fibroblast-like type B cells in the intima of knee joints of normal mice.

mixture of T-cell and immune complex-mediated arthritis (antigen-induced arthritis model), we found that not FcγRIII but FcγRI was crucial.[42–44] Antigen-induced arthritis was not reduced in FcγRIII KO mice, but profoundly suppressed in FcγRI- deficient mice. As collagen type II arthritis is also FcγRIII-dependent,[45] this may suggest that the onset of this model is driven more by anti-collagen type II antibodies than by anti-CII T cells.

The contribution of FcγRI, III, and IV with respect to inflammation and cartilage pathology may differ and suggestive evidence is accumulating that FcγRI is crucial in destruction, even in FcγRIII-dependent immune complex arthritis. FcγRIV is mainly expressed during the late phase of collagen arthritis and then contributes to destruction. Cytokines released during arthritis may influence the expression of activating FcγR. IFN-γ, a cytokine produced mainly by activated Th1 cells but also in lower amounts by activated macrophages, up-regulates FcγRI and may explain why FcγRI becomes the dominant FcγR in the T-cell-mediated arthritis model. Other cytokines found in RA patients may also contribute to skewing of FcγR expression patterns.[46] IL-4 and IL-13 down-regulate activating FcR. IL-10 up-regulates FcγRI, whereas TGF-β up-regulates FcγRIII (Figure 5.5). So far, a direct effect of IL-17 on up-regulation in macrophages has not been identified, although IL17 does have this capacity *in vivo*, herein enhancing erosive progression of arthritis.[47]

Apart from the type of FcγR, the degree of FcγR expression and the relative balance between activating and inhibitory receptor may be of utmost importance in regulating inflammation. Certain mouse strains appear to be hyperreactive to immune complexes. Immune complex-mediated arthritis passively induced within knee joints of DBA/1 mice caused a severe phenotype, which became chronic, whereas the same amount of immune complexes brought into the knee joints of C57BL6 mice only induced a mild arthritis, which was already extinguished after 3 days.[48] As synovial macrophages are crucial for development of arthritis in both strains, peritoneal macrophages were screened for FcR expression. It appeared that normal macrophages from DBA/1 mice expressed higher FcγRIII and lower FcγRI levels if compared with peritoneal macrophages derived from C57BL6 mice. Upon activation by immune complexes a prolonged

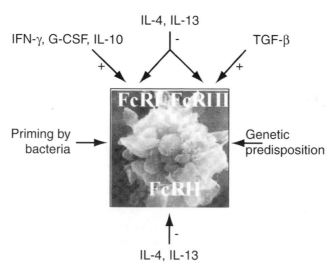

Figure 5.5 FcγR regulation by cytokines.

rise in FcγRI and FcγRIII expression was found, whereas in C57BL6 mice the rise in FcγR was normalized within 1 day.[49] Up-regulation of activatory FcγR showed physiological consequences, since a high prolonged release of IL-1 was found in immune complex-activated DBA/1 macrophages, whereas release of IL-1 was much lower and only short-lasting in immune complex-activated BL/6 macrophages. This suggests that genetic differences in macrophages may be responsible for a different regulation of FcγR expression, resulting in prolonged higher expression of activatory receptors, and lower expression of the inhibiting FcγRII receptor, leading to an aberrant response upon contacting immune complexes. A significant correlation was found between genes on the chromosome also containing FcγR and susceptibility of mice to develop arthritis.[50,51] In line with this, mice that are not prone to develop arthritis become highly vulnerable after deletion of the FcγRII gene.[52] Moreover, the ameliorating effect of intravenous IgG treatment is probably mediated by binding to the inhibiting FcγRII, leading to abrogation of intracellular signaling caused by immune complexes and regulated by the activatory FcR.[53]

MACROPHAGES AND JOINT DESTRUCTION

Destruction of bone and cartilage is a characteristic feature of RA. The number of lining layer macrophages has been found to correlate with both clinical disease activity and radiographic progression in chronic RA.[54] Macrophages may be involved in cartilage destruction by direct release of enzymes, by activation of fibroblasts, and indirectly by activation of catabolic pathways in chondrocytes.

The production of proteolytic enzymes by the inflamed synovium may contribute to the pathogenesis of articular damage,[55] in particular at sites of pannus overgrowth, where there is direct access of activated synovial cells to the cartilage matrix and more limited inhibition by enzyme inhibitors, abundantly present in the synovial fluid. Four families of proteases (metallo, aspartic, cysteine, and serine) have been implicated and probably act synergistically to destroy the connective tissue components of the joint. Proteoglycan loss is an early feature and a crucial role of ADAMTS5 (aggrecanase-2) has been demonstrated.[56] Although this level of proteoglycan loss is reversible, its absence in ADAMTS5 KO mice prevents progression of erosions in experimental arthritis, thereby confirming the old dogma that proteoglycans cover and therefore protect the collagen network. Further cleavage of aggrecan, the largest proteoglycan in the cartilage, occurs with metalloproteinases (MMPs). Amino acid sequence analysis of proteoglycan breakdown products in RA synovial fluid has defined a major site of proteolytic cleavage in aggrecan within the first interglobular domain of the aggrecan core protein.[57] Cleavage of this site results in the neoepitope VDIPEN, which remains in the cartilage whereas the other part ending on FFGVG is found within the synovial fluid. Among the many MMP members, collagenase is thought to be of particular importance since it forms the rate-limiting step in collagen breakdown and eventually leads to cartilage erosions. MMP-1 is strongly elevated in synovial fluid but also in the synovial membrane of patients with RA. More recently, MMP-13 has been identified and implicated in cartilage pathology.[58] Neoepitopes identifying collagenase-mediated collagen breakdown in RA cartilage are abundant, and also present in deep cartilage layers, which may suggest involvement of bone marrow-derived mediators in the destructive process. Proteolytic enzymes are already up-regulated in the synovial layer at a very early stage in the course of inflammatory arthritis. The number of MMP-1 and MMP-13 mRNA-positive cells in the synovial lining layer was significantly correlated with the development of new joint erosions. Apart from macrophage-derived proteolytic enzymes, fibroblasts stimulated by macrophage interaction are a major source of proteases and believed to contribute to direct matrix attack at the pannus invasive front.[59]

In addition to direct enzyme release, macrophages contribute to cartilage destruction by the production of TNF-α and IL-1. Both IL-1 and TNF-α activate surrounding macrophages or fibroblasts to produce MMPs, but these cytokines also modulate the metabolism of chondrocytes. IL-1 is the dominant cytokine involved in inhibition of cartilage proteoglycan and collagen synthesis (Figure 5.6). Moreover, IL-1 stimulates chondrocytes to produce MMPs. MMPs are released in a latent form, are stored in the cartilage matrix, and additionally are activated by as yet unknown factors. Members of other enzyme groups might be involved in this activation step. Cysteine proteases (e.g. cathepsins) or serine proteases (e.g. elastases) can activate pro-MMPs. These enzymes may derive from granulocytes or connective tissue cells but also from the macrophages. In animal models a crucial role of MMP-3 (stromelysin) is evident in activating pro-MMP1 inside the cartilage.[60,61] Immune complexes are potent inducers of MMP-3 and crucial in activation of pro-MMPs. Comparing various experimental arthritis models, MMP-mediated cartilage erosion was only found in those models in which immune complexes were present. Furthermore, in the absence of functional activating FcγR, immune complex-mediated arthritis did not show cartilage erosion, although latent pro-MMPs were present in the cartilage in large amounts. FcγRI appeared to be the dominant activating FcγR in

cartilage destruction. Intriguingly, in mice deficient for FcγI, II, and III, inflammation was enhanced after induction of antigen-induced arthritis, yet cartilage destruction was completely absent. In strong contrast, bone erosion was markedly enhanced, roughly following the degree of inflammation. This illustrates that cartilage and bone erosion are distinct processes and suggests that FcγR activation by immune complexes is not essential in osteoclast activation.[62] In line with this, FcγR expression is high on macrophages, but diminishes dramatically upon differentiation and full maturation of osteoclasts.

Osteoclasts are the principal effector cells involved in bone resorption. Both maturation of precursor cells and activation of mature cells is highly stimulated by the macrophage-derived cytokines TNF and IL-1, whereas an amplifying role is attributed to T-cell-derived IL-17. Recent studies identified RANKL (receptor activator of nuclear factor kappaB ligand) as a crucial stimulus of osteoclast activation, and the interplay between RANKL, its receptor RANK and OPG (osteoprotegerin), which is the natural inhibitor of RANKL, determines the

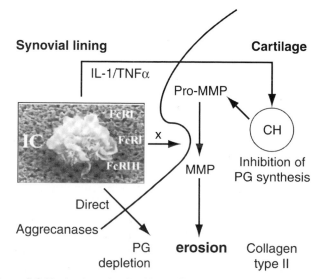

Figure 5.6 Mechanisms involved in cartilage destruction during arthritis.

erosive nature of an arthritic process.[63–65] Bone erosion is completely blocked in arthritis in RANKL-deficient mice, whereas progression of cartilage destruction is evident, illustrating the lack of a role of RANKL in cartilage destruction. Of note, RANK is clearly expressed on chondrocytes, but apparently its activation does not drive cartilage erosion.

DEPLETION OF TYPE A INTIMA CELLS INHIBITS ONSET OF ARTHRITIS

The above studies have identified macrophages as crucial cells in inflammation and joint erosion, herein providing a rationale for therapeutic macrophage targeting. As intima type A cells become activated before arthritis development and are dominant producers of proinflammatory cytokines, these cells seem very important in regulating the early onset of arthritis. Transfer studies, using macrophage-like synovial cells from preinflammatory synovia from rats with developing experimental adjuvant arthritis were able to transfer arthritis to control rats.[66] The ultimate proof that these cells are crucial in regulating arthritis was provided by selective removal of these cells from the intima.

Several methods to eliminate synovial intima cells have been described. Local deposition of osmium tetroxide or radioisotopes[67] in knee joints indeed showed down-regulation of the lining function. However, the disadvantages of these methods are that they are non-selective and often cause side effects in other joint tissues. Another more selective approach is the use of liposomes encapsulating the drug clodronate (dichloromethylene bisphosphonate: Cl_2MDP). This drug belongs to a class of synthetic compounds structurally related to pyrophosphate, an endogenous regulator of calcium metabolism. Macrophages preferentially phagocytose relatively large (1 μm) multilamellar liposomes. Once inside the cell, the lipid bilayer is degraded by enzymes, clodronate is set free and induces cell death by apoptosis. The exact mechanism by which clodronate induces apoptosis is not known but

most likely it is due to intracellular arrestment of Fe^{2+}.[68] A single injection of 6 μl of liposomes containing 75 μg clodronate into murine knee joints resulted in selective depletion of type A cells. Optimal depletion was found within 6–11 days after liposome injection, but even after 30 days no full recovery of the lining was found. No side effects were found on cartilage metabolism.[69] The free drug, ^{14}C-labeled clodronate, is not taken up by cells and had no effect on macrophages.

The role of type A intima cells in onset of arthritis was demonstrated in murine experimental arthritis models. Selective depletion of type A intima cells, starting 7 days before arthritis induction, completely prevented cell influx.[69,70] Washouts of the joints showed significantly reduced chemotactic activity and reduced levels of IL-1. The most important reduction was noted in complement factor C5a and IL-1-induced chemokines such as MCP-1. In addition it was found that elimination of type A lining cells also suppressed the onset of autoimmune collagen arthritis, herein identifying that processes initiated by antibodies directed against cartilage epitopes are also dependent on lining cells. Moreover, it markedly reduced joint damage. Intriguingly, elimination of macrophages also prevented cartilage destruction in murine osteoarthritis.[71]

As type A cells and macrophages can remain in an activated state in RA for prolonged periods, selective removal might be very beneficial for bringing the inflamed synovium to rest. A serious caveat as regards targeting lining macrophages selectively during active arthritis is that many PMNs and monocytes are present in the synovial fluid. The abundance of these cells largely prevents proper access of the locally injected liposomes to the intima, and much is destroyed by lipases produced by, for example, PMNs. In line with this, injection of an adenoviral vector expressing the reporter gene luciferase only identified infection of exudate cells of the inflamed joint and the virus failed to reach the synovium. Moreover, injection of an adenoviral IL-1ra vector, which largely prevents the onset of arthritis when given before onset, was less effective in arthritis when given during the acute phase.[72] To make it more applicable to the human situation, either synovial fluid aspiration has to be performed before liposome injection, or the joint has to be pretreated with a potent anti-inflammatory drug, e.g. steroid.

It is re-assuring to note that clodronate-containing liposomes injected locally in chronically inflamed murine knee joints, in which only few exudate cells are present, easily targeted the lining cells. Fluorescent liposomes accumulated in the superficial intima layer when injected in joints of mice with antigen-induced arthritis, induced 2 weeks before. The sustained inflammation in the synovium was largely resolved 1 week later (Figure 5.7). Of great interest, exacerbation of the inflammation by oral or intra-articular rechallenge with antigen was largely prevented in these lining-depleted joints, suggesting that apart from sustaining chronic arthritis, these cells are also crucial players in the flare-up reaction.

Promising results were found when clodronate liposomes were injected locally into the human RA joint. Seven days after injection the intima layer was eliminated whereas the inflammation in the subintima was significantly reduced.

The treatment was well tolerated and no side effects were found.[73] A recent improvement focused on silencing rather than elimination of activated macrophages. A single i.v. treatment with glucocorticoids encapsulated in long-circulating liposomes suppressed murine collagen arthritis.[74] These PEG liposomes were primarily taken up by activated macrophages, showed good safety, and are now tested in RA patients.

Other macrophage targeted therapies

Apart from liposome targeting of macrophages, more recent approaches are those using gene therapy. Local injection of adenoviral vectors harboring the herpes simplex virus thymidine kinase (Tk) gene in the knees of rhesus monkeys with developing collagen type II arthritis followed by treatment of gangciclovir for 14 days resulted in increased apoptotic cell death in the synovium. Although the procedure showed no toxic side effects, the Tk gene therapy approach is not selective for macrophages. An interesting clinical application is the killing of interface cells in prosthesis loosening.[75]

AIA day 21   AIA day 21: liop treatment

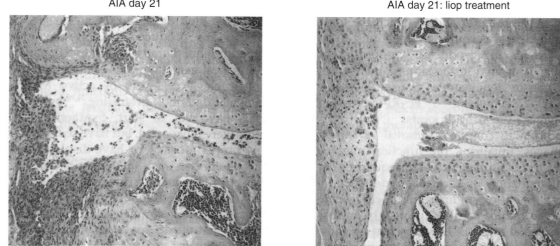

Figure 5.7 Intra-articular injection of clodronate liposomes in mouse arthritic knee joints ameliorates synovitis. Original magnification ×250. Hematoxylin/eosin staining.

In addition, direct intra-articular injection of adenoviral vectors harboring FasL resulted in extensive apoptosis in the synovium without affecting chondrocyte viability. As both type A and type B cells express Fas, this approach might also not be selective for type A cells. A further option to target particular cell types more specifically is to use modified viruses or liposomes, for instance carrying RGD motifs and preferentially touching cells which heavily express adhesion molecules.[76] It is expected that those cells are primarily the ones actively involved in inflammatory mediator release.

Another promising approach to eliminate macrophages is the use of FcγRI as a targeting element. As FcγRs and FcγRI in particular are present on macrophages and play an important role in joint inflammation and severe cartilage destruction, this receptor may be used to deplete these cells from the synovium. Since FcγRI is a high affinity IgG receptor, which is saturated with serum IgG *in vivo*, conventional antibodies are ineffective in targeting FcγRI. Anti-FcγRI antibodies directed against non-antigen binding epitopes of the receptor, and to which the toxic compound ricin was coupled, were found to be very efficient in producing apoptosis of macrophages *in vivo* in the skin and studies are ongoing to prove that it might be an effective tool to selectively remove FcγRI-expressing macrophages from arthritic joints.[77]

Therapeutic scavengers of macrophage mediators

Among the most successful therapeutic approaches to combat RA is blockade of macrophage mediators, such as cytokines. As RA is a versatile disease, it is important to emphasize that therapies directed at one target mediator may be only partially effective.

The most obvious way to block severe cartilage destruction is blockade of MMPs. The use of naturally occurring inhibitors has apparent disadvantages. Broad-spectrum inhibitors such as α2-macroglobulin have a large size, which prevents these inhibitors from penetrating the cartilage matrix. Other inhibitors like TIMPs,

which bind tightly to the active sites of all MMPs, are produced in low amounts. This makes additional therapy, in particular using local gene therapy, obvious an way to combat elevated levels of active MMPs. Experimental data with synthetic inhibitors looked promising,[78] but clinical trials still suffer from safety concerns, in particular enhanced tumor spreading or ligament stiffening. It is still unclear whether selective targeting of MMP-13 is beneficial and may eliminate most side effects. It argues that we do not know enough about the homeostatic functions of most MMPs.

The most successful treatment of RA to date is blocking the macrophage cytokine TNF-α.[79] Given the vast abundance of a whole range of inflammatory mediators in RA synovial tissue it is encouraging to note that there seems to be substantial hierarchy. TNF-α and IL-1, mainly produced by macrophages, are probably master cytokines regulating inflammation and cartilage destruction. Using culture studies of RA synovial membranes it was claimed that TNF-α drives most of the IL-1 production. However, in experimental arthritis IL-1 rather than TNF-α regulated cartilage destruction and erosions were absent in a range of arthritis models in IL-1-deficient mice, but not in TNF-deficient mice.[80,81] IL-1Ra trials show benefit in RA, including reduction of erosions.[82,83] Trials with high quality neutralizing antibodies have just started and hopefully will provide further insight. It remains an option that IL-1 produced locally in the cartilage is not optimally targeted. On the other hand, IL-1ra-deficient mice, displaying uncontrolled IL-1 effects, develop a T-cell-dependent arthritis.[84]

FINAL REMARKS

RA is probably a macrophage-driven disease. Resident synovial macrophages present in the intima become activated, which may be a consequence of an aberrant response to various triggers such as bacterial products or immune complexes released within the joint. Inflammation starting in the intimal layer attracts blood monocytes which differentiate into mature macrophages, potentially with deranged function. Genetic preponderance or inadequate feedback mechanisms may be the cause for the aberrant responses to triggers that are normally cleared without many side effects. Activated macrophages produce a myriad of mediators, many of which are involved in inflammation and cartilage destruction. As therapies directed at only one target mediator may not be fully effective, selective removal of activated synovial macrophages or combination treatments leading to general inactivation of these cells, such as methotrexate or steroids, remain of interest.

REFERENCES

1. Kinne RW, Brauer R, Stuhlmuller B et al. Macrophages in rheumatoid arthritis. Arthritis Res 2000; 2: 189–202.

2. Van den Berg WB, van Lent PL. The role of macro-phages in chronic arthritis. Immunobiology 1996; 195: 614–23.

3. Burmester GR, Stuhlmuller B, Rittig M. The monocyte/macrophage system in arthritis – leopard tank or Trojan horse? Scand J Rheumatol Suppl 1995; 101: 77–82.

4. Zvaifler NJ. Macrophages and the synovial lining. Scand J Rheumatol Suppl 1995; 101: 67–75.

5. Dreher R. Origin of synovial type A cells during inflammation. An experimental approach. Immunobiology 1982; 161: 232–45.

6. van Lent PL, van den Bersselaar L, van den Hoek AE et al. Reversible depletion of synovial lining cells after intra-articular treatment with liposome-encapsulated dichloromethylene diphosphonate. Rheumatol Int 1993; 13: 21–30.

7. Joosten LAB, Radstake TRD, Lubberts E et al. Association of IL-18 expression with enhanced levels of both IL-1β and TNFα in synovial knee tissue of patients with RA, Arthritis Rheum 2003; 48: 339–47.

8. Joosten LAB, Netea MG, Kim SH et al. IL-32, a new pro-inflammatory cytokine in rheumatoid arthritis, Proc Natl Acad Sci U S A 2006; 103: 3298–303.

9. Smolen JS, Tohidast-Akrad M, Gal A et al. The role of T-lymphocytes and cytokines in rheumatoid arthritis, Scand J Rheumatol 1996; 25: 1–4.

10. Gordon S, Macrophage-restricted molecules: role in differentiation and activation, Immunol Lett 1999; 65: 5–8.

11. Tak PP, Chemokine inhibition in inflammatory arthritis, Best Pract Res Clin Rheumatol 2006; 20: 929–39.

12. Geijtenbeek TB, Torensma R, van Vliet SJ et al. Identification of DC-SIGN, a novel dendritic cell-specific ICAM-3 receptor that supports primary immune responses, Cell 2000; 100: 575–85.

13. Zeibecoglou K, Ying S, Meng Q et al. Macrophage subpopulations and macrophage-derived cytokines in sputum of atopic and nonatopic asthmatic subjects and atopic and normal control subjects, J Allergy Clin Immunol 2000; 106: 697–704.

14. Foell D, Roth J, Proinflammatory S100 proteins in arthritis and autoimmune disease, Arthritis Rheum 2004; 50: 3762–71.

15. Youssef P, Roth J, Frosch M et al. Expression of myeloid related proteins (MRP) 8 and 14 and the MRP8/14 heterodimer in rheumatoid arthritis synovial membrane, J Rheumatol 1999; 26: 2523–8.

16. Deng GM, Tarkowski A, The role of bacterial DNA in septic arthritis, Int J Mol Med 2000; 6: 29–33.

17. Joosten LAB, Koenders MI, Smeets RL et al. Toll-like receptor 2 pathway drives streptococcal cell wall induced joint inflammation: critical role of MYD88. J Immunol 2003; 171: 6145–53.

18. Radstake TRDJ, Roelofs M, Jenniskens YM et al. Expression of Toll-like receptors 2 and 4 in rheumatoid synovial tissue and regulation by proinflammatory cytokines IL-12 and IL-18 via interferon-gamma, Arthritis Rheum 2004; 50: 3856–65.

19. Ehlers M, Ravetch JV, Opposing effects of TLR stimulation induce autoimmunity or tolerance. Trends Immunol, 2006 Epub ahead of print.

20. Roelofs MF, Joosten LAB, Abdollahi-Roodsaz S et al. The expression of Toll-like receptor 3 and 7 in RA synovium is increased and costimulation of TLR3, 4, 7/8 results in synergistic cytokine production by dendritic cells, Arthritis Rheum 2005; 52: 2313–22.

21. Kraetsch HG, Unger C, Wernhoff P et al. Cartilage-specific autoimmunity in rheumatoid arthritis: characterization of a triple helical B cell epitope in the integrin-binding-domain of collagen type II, Eur J Immunol 2001; 31: 1666–73.

22. Li NL, Zhang DQ, Zhou KY et al. Isolation and characteristics of autoreactive T cells specific to aggrecan G1 domain from rheumatoid arthritis patients, Cell Res 2000; 10: 39–49.

23. Monach PA, Benoist C, Mathis D, The role of antibodies in mouse models of arthritis, and relevance to human disease, Adv Immunol, 2004; 82: 217–48.

24. Harrington LE, Hatton RD, Mangan PR et al. IL-17 producing CD4+ effector T cells develop via a lineage distinct from the T helper type 1 and 2 lineages, Nat Immunol 2005; 6: 1123–32.

25. Hirota K, Hashimoto M, Yoshitomi H et al. T cell self-reactivity forms a cytokine milieu for spontaneous development of IL-17+ Th cells that cause autoimmune arthritis, J Exp Med 2007; 204: 41–7.

26. Miossec P, van den Berg WB, Th1/Th2 cytokine balance in arthritis, Arthritis Rheum 1997; 40: 2105–15.

27. Chabaud M, Durand JM, Buchs N et al. Human IL-17: a T cell derived proinflammatory cytokine produced by the RA synovium, Arthritis Rheum 1999; 42: 962–71.

28. Lubberts E, Joosten LA, Oppers B et al. IL-1-independent role of IL-17 in synovial inflammation and joint destruction during collagen-induced arthritis, J Immunol 2001; 167: 1004–13.

29. Lubberts E, Koenders MI, van den Berg WB, The role of T cell IL-17 in conducting destructive arthritis: lessons from animal models, Arthritis Res Ther 2005; 7: 29–37.

30. McInnes IB, Liew FY, IL-15: a proinflammatory role in rheumatoid arthritis synovitis, Immunol Today 1998; 19: 75–9.

31. Connell L, McInnes IB, New cytokine targets in inflammatory rheumatic diseases, Best Pract Res Clin Rheumatol 2006; 20: 865–78.

32. Dayer JM, Burger D, Cytokines and direct cell contact in synovitis: relevance to therapeutic intervention, Arthritis Res 1999; 1: 17–20.

33. Bresnihan B, Gogarty M, Fitzgerald O et al. Apolipoprotein A-I infiltration in RA synovial tissue: a control mechanism of cytokine production?, Arthritis Res Ther, 2004; 6: R563–566.

34. Dinarello CA, Interleukin-18, a proinflammatory cytokine, Eur Cytokine Netw 2000; 11: 483–6.

35. Gracie JA, Forsey RJ, Chan WL et al. A proinflammatory role for IL-18 in rheumatoid arthritis, J Clin Invest 1999; 104: 1393–401.

36. Joosten LA, Lubberts E, Helsen MM et al. Dual role of IL-12 in early and late stages of murine collagen type II arthritis, J Immunol 1997; 159: 4094–102.

37. Joosten LAB, van de Loo FAJ, Lubberts E et al. An IFN-gamma-independent proinflammatory role of IL-18 in murine streptococcal cell wall arthritis, J Immunol 2000; 165: 6553–8.

38. Plater Zyberk C, Joosten LAB, Helsen MMA et al. Therapeutic effect of neutralizing endogenous IL-18 activity in the collagen-induced model of arthritis, J Clin Invest 2001; 108: 1825–32.

39. Murphy CA, Langrish CL, Chen Y et al. Divergent pro- and antiinflammatory roles for IL-23 and IL-12 in joint autoimmune inflammation, J Exp Med 2003; 198: 1951–7.

40. Nimmerjahn F, Bruhns P, Horiuchi K, Ravetch JV, FcgammaRIV; a novel FcR with distinct IgG subclass specificity, Immunity 2005; 23: 41–51.

41. Nimmerjahn F, Ravetch JV, Fcgamma receptors: old friends and new family members, Immunity 2006; 24; 19–28.

42. Ioan-Facsinay A, de Kimpe SJ, Hellwig SM et al. FcgammaRI (CD64) contributes substantially to severity of arthritis, hypersensitivity responses, and protection from bacterial infection, Immunity 2002; 16: 391–402.

43. Van Lent PL, Nabbe K, Blom AB et al. Role of activatory Fc gamma RI and Fc gamma RIII and inhibitory Fc gamma RII in inflammation and cartilage destruction during experimental antigen-induced arthritis, Am J Pathol 2001; 159: 2309–20.

44. Van Lent PLEM, Nabbe K, Boross P et al. The inhibitory receptor FcγRII reduces joint inflammation and destruction in experimental immune complex mediated arthritides not only by inhibition of FcγRI/III but also by efficient clearance of immune complexes by endocytosis of immune complexes, Am J Pathol 2003; 163: 1839–48.

45. Kleinau S, Martinsson P, Heyman B, Induction and suppression of collagen-induced arthritis is dependent on distinct fcgamma receptors, J Exp Med 2000; 191: 1611–16.

46. Gerber JS, Mosser DM, Stimulatory and inhibitory signals originating from the macrophage Fcgamma receptors, Microbes Infect 2001; 3: 131–9.

47. Koenders MI, Lubberts E, van de Loo FAJ et al. Interleukin-17 acts independently of TNF-α under arthritic conditions, J Immunol 2006; 176: 6262–9.

48. Blom AB, van Lent PL, Holthuysen AE et al. Immune complexes, but not streptococcal cell walls or zymosan, cause chronic arthritis in mouse strains susceptible for collagen type II auto-immune arthritis, Cytokine 1999; 11: 1046–56.

49. Blom AB, van Lent PL, van Vuuren H et al. Fc gamma R expression on macrophages is related to severity and chronicity of synovial inflammation and cartilage destruction during experimental immune-complex-mediated arthritis (ICA), Arthritis Res 2000; 2: 489–503.

50. Johansson ACM, Hansson AS, Nandakumar KS et al. IL-10-deficient B10.Q mice develop more severe collagen-induced arthritis, but are protected from arthritis induced with anti-type II collagen antibodies, J Immunol 2001; 167: 3505–12.

51. Ortmann RA, Shevach EM, Susceptibility to collagen-induced arthritis: cytokine-mediated regulation, Clin Immunol 2001; 98: 109–18.

52. Yuasa T, Kubo S, Yoshino T et al. Deletion of fcgamma receptor IIB renders H-2(b) mice susceptible to collagen-induced arthritis, J Exp Med 1999; 189: 187–94.

53. Samuelsson A, Towers TL, Ravetch JV, Anti-inflammatory activity of IVIG mediated through the inhibitory Fc receptor, Science 2001; 291: 484–6.

54. Mulherin D, Fitzgerald O, Bresnihan B, Synovial tissue macrophage populations and articular damage in rheumatoid arthritis, Arthritis Rheum 1996; 39: 115–24.

55. Cawston T, Matrix metalloproteinases and TIMPs: properties and implications for the rheumatic diseases, Mol Med Today 1998; 4:130–7.

56. Stanton H, Rogerson FM, East CJ et al. ADAMTS5 is the major aggrecanase in mouse in vivo and in vitro. Nature, 2005, 434:648–52.

57. Fosang AJ, Last K, Maciewicz RA et al. Aggrecan is degraded by matrix metalloproteinases in human arthritis. Evidence that matrix metalloproteinase and aggrecanase activities can be independent, J Clin Invest 1996; 98: 2292–9.

58. Ishiguro N, Ito T, Oguchi T et al. Relationships of MMPs and their inhibitors to cartilage proteoglycan and collagen turnover and inflammation as revealed by analysis of synovial fluids from patients with RA, Arthritis Rheum 2001; 44: 2503–11.

59. Pap T, Muller-Ladner U, Gay RE et al. Fibroblast biology. Role of synovial fibroblasts in the pathogenesis of RA, Arthritis Res 2000; 2: 361–7.

60. Van Meurs J, van Lent P, Stoop R et al. Cleavage of aggrecan at the Asn341-Phe342 site coincides with the initiation of collagen damage in murine antigen-induced arthritis: a pivotal role for stromelysin 1 in matrix metalloproteinase activity, Arthritis Rheum 1999; 42: 2074–84.

61. Van Meurs J, van Lent PL, Holthuysen A et al. Active MMPs are present in cartilage during immune complex mediated arthritis: a pivotal role for stromelysin-1 in cartilage destruction, J Immunol 1999; 163: 5633–9.

62. Van Lent PLEM, Grevers L, Lubberts E et al. Fcγ receptors directly mediate cartilage, but not bone, destruction in murine antigen-induced arthritis, Arthritis Rheum 2006; 54: 3868–77.

63. Pettit AR, Ji H, von Stechow D et al. TRANCE/RANKL knockout mice are protected from bone erosion in a serum transfer model of arthritis, Am J Pathol 2001; 159: 1689–99.

64. Lubberts E, Schwarzenberger P, Huang W et al. Requirement of IL-17 receptor signaling in resident synoviocytes for development of full blown destructive arthritis, J Immunol 2005; 175: 3360–68.

65. Schett G, Hayer S, Zwerina J et al. Mechanisms of disease: the link between RANKL and arthritic bone disease, Nat Clin Pract Rheumatol 2005; 1: 47–54.

66. Ramos-Ruiz R, Bernabeu C, Ariza A et al. Arthritis transferred by cells derived from pre-inflammatory rat synovium, J Autoimmun 1992; 5: 93–106.

67. Boerbooms AM, Buijs WC, Danen M et al. Radio-synovectomy in chronic synovitis of the knee joint in patients with rheumatoid arthritis, Eur J Nucl Med 1985; 10: 446–9.

68. Van Rooijen N, Bakker J, Sanders A, Transient suppression of macrophage functions by liposome-encapsulated drugs, Trends Biotechnol 1997; 15: 178–85.

69. Van Lent PL, van den Hoek AE, van den Bersselaar LA et al. In vivo role of phagocytic synovial lining cells in onset of experimental arthritis, Am J Pathol 1993; 143:1226–37.

70. Van Lent PL, Holthuysen AE, van den Bersselaar LA et al. Phagocytic lining cells determine local expression of inflammation in type II collagen-induced arthritis, Arthritis Rheum 1996; 39: 1545–55.

71. Blom AB, van Lent PLEM, Libregts S et al. Crucial role of macrophages in MMP mediated cartilage destruction during experimental OA; involvement of MMP-3. Arthritis Rheum, 2007; 56: 147–57.

72. van de Loo FA, Geurts J, van den Berg WB, Gene therapy works in animal models of RA, .. so what, Curr Rheumatol Rep, 2006; 8: 386–93.

73. Barrera P, Blom A, van Lent PL et al. Synovial macrophage depletion with clodronate-containing liposomes in rheumatoid arthritis, Arthritis Rheum 2000; 43: 1951–9.

74. Metselaar JM, van den Berg WB, Holthuysen AE et al. Liposomal targeting of glucocorticoids to synovial lining cells strongly increases therapeutic benefit in collagen type II arthritis, Ann Rheum Dis 2004; 63: 348–53.

75. de Poorter JJ, Tolboom TC, Rabelink MJ et al. Towards gene therapy in prosthesis loosening. J Gene Med 2005; 7: 1421–8.

76. Bakker AC, van de Loo FA, Joosten LA et al. A tropism-modified adenoviral vector increased the effectiveness of gene therapy for arthritis, Gene Ther 2001; 8: 1785–93.

77. van Roon JA, Bijlsma JW, van de Winkel JG et al. Depletion of synovial macrophages in RA, Ann Rheum Dis 2005; 64: 865–70.

78. Milner JM, Cawston TE, MMP knockout studies and the potential use of MMP inhibitors in RA, Curr Drug Targets Inflamm Allergy 2005; 4: 363–75.

79. Feldmann M, Brennan FM, Williams RO et al. The transfer of a laboratory based hypothesis to a clinically useful therapy: the development of anti-TNF therapy of RA, Best Pract Res Clin Rheumatol 2004, 18; 59–80.

80. Van den Berg WB, Arguments for interleukin 1 as a target in chronic arthritis, Ann Rheum Dis 2000; 59 (Suppl) 1: i81–84.

81. Van den Berg WB, Joosten LAB, van de Loo FAJ, TNFα and IL-1β are separate targets in chronic arthritis, Clin Exp Rheumatol 1999; 17 (Suppl 18): S105–S114.

82. Dayer JM, Bresnihan B, Targeting interleukin-1 in the treatment of rheumatoid arthritis, Arthritis Rheum 2002; 46: 574–8.

83. Furst DE, Anakinra: review of recombinant IL-1ra in the treatment of RA, Clin Ther 2004; 26: 1960–75.

84. Nakae S, Saijo S, Horai R et al. IL-17 production from activated T cells is required for the spontaneous development of destructive arthritis in mice deficient in IL-1 receptor antagonist. Proc Natl Acad Sci U S A 2003; 100: 5986–90.

6

Dendritic cells

Viviana Lutzky and Ranjeny Thomas

Introduction • Dendritic cells • Vaccination to reduce autoantigen-specific immune responses in rheumatic diseases • Role of dendritic cells in induction and maintenance of autoimmune disease • Generation of dendritic cells for tolerance • Use of dendritic cells for tolerance • Therapeutic applications of regulatory dendritic cells • Blocking dendritic cell function in rheumatic disease • Conclusion • References

INTRODUCTION

Autoimmune rheumatic diseases result from a process involving three distinct but related components – a break in self-tolerance, development of chronic inflammation in one or several organs, and if ongoing, tissue destruction and its resultant detrimental effects. It has been proposed that dendritic cells (DCs) are the critical decision-making cells in the immune system.[1] Through their role in the generation of central and peripheral tolerance, as well as in priming immune responses and stimulation of memory and effector T cells, DCs are likely to play essential roles in both the initiation and perpetuation of autoimmunity and autoimmune diseases. However, the understanding of the means by which DCs contribute to peripheral tolerance has opened the exciting possibility of harnessing them for antigen-specific immunotherapy of autoimmune diseases and transplantation. This chapter will consider the use of DCs as a biological therapy for the induction of tolerance in rheumatic autoimmune diseases. After consideration of the known mechanisms of peripheral tolerance, we will focus on the various means by which effector function is regulated in the periphery. Means and pathways by which DCs have induced peripheral tolerance in autoimmune models will be discussed, followed by consideration of the potential and relative merits of

this approach for future therapy of autoimmune rheumatic diseases. Finally, other strategies for the blockade of DC function will be examined.

DENDRITIC CELLS

DCs are now recognized as essential regulators of both innate and acquired arms of the immune system.[2] They are responsible for the stimulation of naive T lymphocytes, a property that distinguishes them from all other antigen-presenting cells (APCs). DCs are also essential accessory cells in the generation of primary antibody responses[3] and are powerful enhancers of natural killer (NK) cell cytotoxicity.[4] DCs are crucial for the initiation of primary immune responses of both helper and cytotoxic T lymphocytes, and thus act as 'nature's adjuvant'.[5] Conversely, DCs are also involved in the maintenance of tolerance to antigens. DCs contribute to thymic central tolerance and shaping of the T-cell repertoire by presenting antigens to T cells and deleting those T cells that exhibit strong autoreactivity.[6] However, DCs also play a role in peripheral tolerance. Here, DCs contribute by deletion of autoreactive lymphocytes and expansion of the population of regulatory T cells (Tregs). Therefore, DCs offer potential utility in protective and therapeutic strategies for tolerance restoration in autoimmune diseases.

DC precursors from the bone marrow migrate via the bloodstream to peripheral tissues where they reside as immature DCs. Immature DCs efficiently capture invading pathogens and other particulate and soluble antigens. After antigen uptake, DCs rapidly cross the endothelium of lymphatic vessels and migrate to the draining secondary lymphoid organs. Following the uptake of immunogenic antigens and lymphatic migration, DCs undergo a process of maturation, which is characterized by down-regulation of the capacity to capture antigens and up-regulation of antigen processing and presentation, expression of costimulatory molecules and altered dendritic morphology.[7–9] After presentation of antigen to naïve T cells in the T-cell area of secondary lymphoid organs, most DCs disappear, probably by apoptosis. Thus, under optimal conditions, the same DC sequentially carries out distinct functions such as capture and processing of antigens, antigen presentation to rare, naïve antigen-specific T cells, and induction of antigen-specific T-cell clonal expansion.

Dendritic cells and immune tolerance

Considering the crucial role of DCs in antigen processing and presentation and thus in the regulation of immune reactivity, DCs are important directors of immune responsiveness, through the interactions with responding lymphocytes and other accessory cells. Broadly, evidence suggests that under steady-state conditions, recruitment of DC precursors into tissues and migration/maturation into secondary lymphoid organs occurs at low rates and may favor tolerance induction. On the other hand, stimulation of immature DCs leading to DC maturation and activation may induce a productive immune response.[10]

The process of DC maturation can be stimulated by various mechanisms, including pathogen-derived molecules (LPS, DNA, RNA), proinflammatory cytokines (TNF-α, IL-1, IL-6), tissue factors such as hyaluronan fragments, migration of DCs across endothelial barriers between inflamed tissues and lymphatics, and T-cell-derived signals (CD154).[11–13] In contrast, anti-inflammatory signals, such as IL-10, TGF-β, prostaglandins, and corticosteroids tend to inhibit maturation.[14–16] Thus, DCs represent an attractive therapeutic target, either to enhance or to attenuate immunity for modulation of disease. To date, *ex vivo* modulation of DCs and exposure to antigen before transfer into an animal or human recipient has been the major approach to achieve protective and therapeutic immunity. This relates in part to complexity of the DC system in the context of a whole person with an immune system disorder, and in part to the difficulty of delivery of specific antigens and immunomodulators to DCs *in vivo*.

NF-κB and DC function

The ability of a myeloid DC to induce immunity or tolerance is linked to its maturation state and thus to NF-κB activity.[17–20] Immature DCs generated from murine bone marrow induce T-cell unresponsiveness *in vitro* and prolonged cardiac allograft survival.[21] Various drugs and cytokines, and inhibitors of NF-κB inhibit myeloid DC maturation,[16,22–26] including corticosteroids, salicylates, mycophenolate mofetil, transforming growth factor (TGF)-β, and IL-10. DCs generated in the presence of these agents alter T-cell function *in vitro* and *in vivo*, including promotion of allograft survival.[27–30] NF-κB activity leads to transcription of a number of genes involved in the immune response. RelB activity is required for myeloid DC differentiation.[31–33] RelB regulates DC- and B-cell APC function through regulation of CD40 and MHC molecule expression.[34–36] We have shown that antigen-exposed DCs in which RelB function is inhibited lack cell surface CD40, prevent priming of immunity, and suppress previously primed immune responses. While immature DCs, which maintain the potential for subsequent activation, were only moderately suppressive of primed immune responses, RelB-deficient DCs lacking this potential were much more suppressive.[36]

VACCINATION TO REDUCE AUTOANTIGEN-SPECIFIC IMMUNE RESPONSES IN RHEUMATIC DISEASES

Loss of tolerance to self-antigens is a critical component in the pathogenesis of autoimmunity. Active mechanisms of peripheral tolerance include deletion of self-reactive cells or survival of antigen-specific cells long term after antigen recognition while the animal remains tolerant. The regulation of self-reactive effector responses by specialized populations of regulatory T cells constitutes a major mechanism whereby the tolerant state is maintained and autoimmune disease is avoided long term. Several T-cell and NKT-cell populations with the ability to inhibit the response of other (effector) T cells have been described. Understanding and harnessing these mechanisms therapeutically using DCs has great potential for therapy of autoimmune diseases, including rheumatoid arthritis (RA).

Regulatory T cells as targets for vaccination approaches

CD4+CD25+ regulatory T cells

Mice thymectomized on day 3 after birth develop a syndrome of organ-specific autoimmune disease, including oophoritis, gastritis, and/or thyroiditis. The mice can be rescued from illness by transfer of CD4+CD25+ T cells from a syngeneic adult spleen, and depletion of this population from non-thymectomized mice leads to a similar spectrum of autoimmune disease.[37–40] Transfer of CD4+CD25- T-cells into syngeneic nude recipients leads to similar autoimmune disease, as well as a wasting syndrome and immune complex-mediated glomerulonephritis in some animals. Since these discoveries were made in the 1960s and 1970s, the CD4+CD25+ T-cell subset has been well characterized as a thymic-derived suppressor or regulatory population with the capacity to reduce the strength of effector responses.[41,42] By this means, the T cells down-regulate immune responses to self and foreign antigens, and prevent autoimmune disease. These T cells constitute about 5% of murine and human spleen or blood T cells and characteristically express the transcription factor FoxP3. They proliferate in response to mitogen or APC and IL-2 *in vitro*, and inhibit CD4+CD25- T-cell proliferative responses after T-cell receptor (TCR) ligation.[43] Autoantigen-specific CD25+ Tregs are also inducible in the periphery *in vivo*, and can be expanded *in vitro* by antigen-exposed DCs.[44,45]

Expanded Tregs have been shown to suppress pancreatic inflammation and disease after adoptive transfer to mice prone to autoimmune diabetes.[46,47]

Other CD4+ regulatory T cells

TR1 cells

This population of T cells was first shown to emerge after several rounds of stimulation of human blood T cells by allogeneic monocytes in the presence of IL-10. The clones themselves secrete high levels of IL-10 and moderate levels of TGF-β but little IL-4 and varying levels of IFN-γ.[48] An early phase clinical trial of adoptive immunotherapy with donor T lymphocytes tolerized *in vitro* by IL-10, in patients transplanted with T-cell-depleted haploidentical allogeneic stem cells, is in progress in Italy.

Th3 cells

The Th3 regulatory subpopulation refers to a specific subset induced following antigen delivery via the oral (or other mucosal) route. They produce predominantly TGF-β, and only low levels of IL-10, IL-4, or IFN-γ, and provide specific help for IgA production.[49] They are able to suppress both Th1- and Th2-type effector T cells.

Th2 cells

This subpopulation produces high levels of IL-4, IL-5, and IL-10 but low levels of IFN-γ and TGF-β. Th2 cells are generated in response to a relative abundance of IL-4 and lack of IL-12 in the environment at the time of presentation of their cognate peptide ligands.[50] T-cell signaling by CD86 may also be important for generation of Th2 cells.[51,52] Prostaglandin E_2 (PGE$_2$) inhibits the ability of DCs to produce IL-12 but promotes T-cell stimulatory capacity, thereby resulting in Th2 cell differentiation.[53] The precise definition of the costimulatory molecules involved in Th2 as opposed to regulatory T-cell induction are not entirely clear, but it appears that the effects of PGE$_2$ are cAMP-dependent and NF-κB-independent. Novel candidate genes that have potential for the production of DCs capable of Th2 immune deviation include galectin1, an endogenous lectin that promotes T-cell apoptosis and Th2 skewing, and OX2, a DC surface antigen that suppresses Th1 responses OX40 ligand and Notch ligands.[54,55] The importance of Th2 cells as a regulatory subset is unclear. However, suppressive effects may result from deviation away from a Th1-type immune response, or as a result of DC factors which commonly stimulate Th2 cells and Tregs simultaneously.

CD8+ regulatory T cells

A distinct CD8+CD28− regulatory or 'suppressor' subset of T cells can be induced by repetitive antigenic stimulation *in vitro*. These cells are also found *in vivo* in patients with chronic inflammation, transplantation, or tumors such as melanoma.[56–59] They are major histocompatibility complex (MHC) class I-restricted, and suppress CD4+ T-cell responses. A related CD4+CD28− subset is found in patients with RA, particularly in patients with vascular complications. Like CD8+CD28− T cells, this subset expresses killer cell immunoglobulin-like receptors (KIRs), including the stimulatory KIR2DS2, which is potentially involved in endothelial damage.[60]

NK T cells

This T-cell population that expresses the NK cell marker, CD161, and whose TCRs are Vα24JαQ in human and Vα14Jα281 in mouse, is activated specifically by the non-polymorphic CD1d molecule through presentation of various glycolipid antigens.[61] They have been shown to be immunoregulatory in a number of experimental systems. Administration of the glycolipid, α-galactosyl ceramide (α-gal cer), presented by CD1d, results in accumulation of NKT cells and amelioration of diabetes in non-obese diabetic mice.[62]

γδ T cells

γδ T cells have been implicated in the suppression of immune responses in various inflammatory diseases and reduction of inflammation associated with induction of mucosal tolerance. However, γδ T cells with a contra-suppressive effect have also been described.[63]

ROLE OF DENDRITIC CELLS IN INDUCTION AND MAINTENANCE OF AUTOIMMUNE DISEASE

In autoimmune diseases, when tolerance against self-determinants is impaired, activated autoreactive lymphocytes participate in the process of tissue damage. As translocation of antigens from the periphery to secondary lymphoid organs and their presentation to naive T cells are primarily mediated by DCs, these cells play an essential role in the priming of lymphocytes in autoimmunity.[64,65] DCs are also important cells at the inflammatory site. For example, in the NOD mouse model of type 1 diabetes, DCs are among the first cells to infiltrate the islets.[66] Moreover, DCs are critical APCs for the activation of CD25+ Tregs.[45] Therefore, abnormalities of DCs have implications not only for immune priming but for immune regulation.

Self-Antigen Presentation

Presentation of viral or modified self-antigens, of which the immune system has been ignorant, represents a common theme in the initiation of autoimmunity. For example, in a transgenic animal model, chronic stimulation of organ-specific immune responses by DCs was shown to initiate severe cardiovascular immunopathology.[65] In a transgenic rat insulin promoter-glycoprotein model of autoimmune diabetes, DC-mediated antigen transport primed an autoimmune response against a pancreatic neo-self antigen. Continued antigenic stimulation by DCs and repeated stimulation of T cells induced local inflammation, resulting in the formation of ectopic lymphoid structures in the pancreas.[67,68]

A number of modified self-antigens have been described in human autoimmune diseases. In patients with type 1 diabetes, a recent paper elegantly demonstrated the immunogenicity of a post-translationally modified region of the insulin A-chain, presented in the context of HLA-DR4.[69] In RA, a variety of citrullinated autoantigens are described. Citrullination is a physiological process in which protein is altered during apoptosis and inflammation. Citrulline-specific autoantibodies are known as anti-CCP (citrullinated cyclic peptide). In RA, anti-CCPs are present in approximately 70% of patients.[70]

Anti-CCPs are highly specific for RA and are associated with more severe joint damage and radiographic outcome.[70] Recent data implicate immune system reactivity towards citrullinated antigens in patients with RA-associated HLA genotype as a fundamental element in the pathogenesis of RA.[71,72]

In many different populations it has been observed that specific HLA-DR gene variants in the MHC region are highly associated with RA. The association has been mapped to the third hypervariable region of DRβ-chains, especially amino acids 70–74, encoding a conserved amino acid sequence that forms the fourth anchoring pocket (P4) in the HLA groove (Figure 6.1). This susceptibility epitope, known as the 'shared epitope', is found in multiple RA-associated DR molecules, including DRB1*0401, DRB1*0404, DRB*0101, and DRB1*1402. The shared epitope is positively charged and would bind proteins or peptides containing a negatively charged or nonpolar amino acid. The shared epitope-encoding

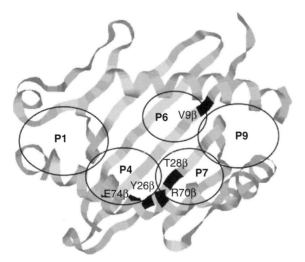

Figure 6.1 A ribbon diagram depicting the structure of the peptide binding groove of HLA-DRB1*01, a susceptibility allele for RA. Residues in pockets 4, 6, and 7 as outlined on the DRB1*01 structure. E74β is predicted to interact with arginine/citrulline. The regions that compose pockets 1, 4, 6, 7, and 9 have been circled and labeled accordingly. Reproduced with permission from Pearson CI, Gautam AM, Rulifson IC, Liblau RS, McDevitt HO. Proc Natl Acad Sci USA 1999; 96: 197–202. Copyright (1999) National Academy of Sciences, USA.

HLA alleles are particularly associated with anti-CCP-positive RA.[71–73] Citrullination replaces charged imino side chain groups with an uncharged carbonyl group, dramatically increasing the affinity of citrullinated proteins with the shared epitope. Fibrin and vimentin are two citrullinated proteins identified thus far in synovial extracts from inflamed joints and are prominent synovial candidate antigens in anti-CCP-positive RA.[74,75] Collagen type II is a further protein candidate.[76] Recent data suggest that smoking may trigger citrulline-specific autoimmunity in individuals with shared epitope-encoding HLA alleles, which may or may not subsequently develop into clinical inflammatory joint disease.[72,77] The definition of this group of autoantigens in RA and their contribution to disease pathogenesis has been a major recent advance. As discussed later, this advance should aid the development of antigen-specific therapies for RA. Given their specificity for RA, and strong evidence for their role in disease severity, our strategy has been to develop citrullinated antigen-specific DCs as a therapeutic, with the aim of altering the immune response to citrullinated antigens in anti-CCP⁺ patients with the HLA shared-epitope and established RA. In the future, one could also conceive that such a strategy might also be used preventatively in anti-CCP⁺ HLA shared-epitope⁺ first degree relatives of RA patients.

Dendritic cells at sites of autoimmune disease

DCs have been studied in a number of common autoimmune conditions. In autoimmune diseased sites, DCs share some common characteristics. These include enrichment of activated DCs in inflamed tissues, particularly in a perivascular distribution. Moreover, DCs infiltrate tissues at very early stages of disease. At inflammatory sites in general, early DC infiltration contributes to the recruitment of other immune cells. Indeed the same process occurs during the development of lymphoid organs, such that if lymphotoxin-β is not produced by DCs, the organ cannot develop. Similarly, DC infiltration is an early feature of islet cell autoimmunity in diabetes mellitus[78] and contributes to local lymphoid tissue formation in the pancreas.[79] Organization of tissue into lymph node-like structures, including lymphoid follicles, is a common feature of tissues affected by autoimmune inflammation.[80]

Increased numbers of the myeloid and plasmacytoid subsets of DCs have been shown in synovial fluid and perivascular regions of synovial tissues in patients with RA and other autoimmune rheumatic diseases.[81–86] The sustained immunomodulatory effect of TNF blockade in RA relates in part to the traffic of DCs and other immunocytes to the inflammatory site.[87,88]

GENERATION OF DENDRITIC CELLS FOR TOLERANCE

Anti-rheumatic disease-modifying drugs act systemically, and as a result of non-specific immune suppressive effects, opportunistic infections may occur. Thus, it is desirable to develop a therapeutic means to modulate immune responses in an antigenic-specific manner. DCs are an attractive target for a therapeutic strategy that attenuates autoimmune responses.

During the last decade, the development of techniques to generate large numbers of DCs *in vitro*, together with advances in gene transfer technology and understanding of the role of DCs in peripheral tolerance, have opened up the possibility of generating DCs with regulatory properties in the laboratory. Strategies used to generate DCs with such potential include modification of tissue culture conditions, pharmacological modification, and genetic engineering.[22,89,90] Regulatory DCs have potential utility as a platform for prevention or therapy of a range autoimmune diseases, including type 1 diabetes, RA, and multiple sclerosis (MS), as well as allergies, transplantation, and graft-versus-host disease (GVHD). The theoretical principles employed to generate regulatory DCs *in vitro* are based mainly on the mechanisms elucidated experimentally which DCs use to maintain self-tolerance in the healthy steady state. Thus, *in vivo* administration of regulatory DCs may promote T-cell tolerance through induction of antigen-specific T-cell apoptosis, anergy, or the generation of Tregs.[18]

In vitro, human DCs can be isolated directly from peripheral blood, or generated in larger numbers from peripheral blood monocytes or bone marrow $CD34^+$ hematopoietic precursor cells.[91–93] Alternatively, regulatory DCs can be directly differentiated from embryonic stem cells.[94] This approach generates stable, long-term DC cultures, which can be manipulated subsequently by viral or non-viral gene transfer. Recently, Hirata et al. reported that treatment of mice with embryonic stem cell DCs (ES-DCs) presenting antigenic peptide in the context of MHC class II and simultaneously expressing immunosuppressive genes significantly reduced the severity of central nervous system (CNS) autoimmunity.[95]

USE OF DENDRITIC CELLS FOR TOLERANCE

Increasing evidence in humans and rodents strongly suggests that immature or NF-κB-deficient DCs may control peripheral tolerance by inducing the differentiation of regulatory T cells.[17,18,36,96] Thus, repetitive *in vitro* stimulation of allogeneic human T cells with immature, monocyte-derived DCs leads to the generation of nonproliferating, suppressive, IL-10-producing Tregs.[18] Dhodapkar et al. injected autologous, monocyte-derived immature DCs, pulsed with influenza matrix peptide and keyhole limpet hemocyanin, subcutaneously in two human volunteers. They reported an antigen-specific inhibition of $CD8^+$ T-cell killing activity and the appearance of peptide-specific IL-10-producing T cells, accompanied by a decrease in the number of interferon (IFN)-γ-producing T cells.[17]

CD40 is a key determinant of DC immunogenicity. Inhibition of the RelB transcription factor or of CD40 itself produces regulatory DCs that are able to generate IL-10-producing T-regulatory cells *in vivo*.[36] Conversely, tumor antigen-specific immunity can be markedly heightened by engineering DCs which are able to express CD40 for prolonged periods *in vivo*.[97] IL-10 and TGF-β produced by T-regulatory cells may contribute to tolerance by limiting expression of MHC class II and costimulatory molecules by DCs.[18,96]

In conjunction with decreased expression of costimulatory molecules, expression of ILT3 and ILT4 may be increased by regulatory DCs.[98]

These Ig-like inhibitory receptors, related to NK cell killer inhibitory receptors (KIRs), are up-regulated by the APCs as a result of interaction with CD8+CD28− regulatory T cells. These receptors negatively signal monocytes and DCs through immunoreceptor tyrosine-based inhibitory motifs (ITIMs).[99–101] CD4+ T-cell-induced NF-κB activation of APCs is reduced in the presence of CD8+CD28− T cells, potentially through this signaling pathway.[56]

IL-10 is an important cytokine involved in the generation of regulatory T cells by DCs. Treatment of DCs with IL-10 can convert immature DCs into regulatory DCs by suppressing NF-κB and therefore arresting maturation. This drives the differentiation of IL-10 producing T regulatory type 1-producing cells *in vitro* and *in vivo*.[25,102,103] Human DCs exposed to IL-10 induce a state of antigen-specific anergy in CD4+ T cells and CD8+ T cells by similarly converting DCs into an immuoregulatory state.[104] IL-10 inhibits IL-12 production and costimulatory molecule expression by DCs, giving rise to regulatory DCs.[53]

DCs could also be manipulated *in situ* to induce peripheral tolerance. For example Flt3L, a growth factor that expands DCs, enhanced the induction of oral tolerance *in vivo*.[105] In contrast, treatment with Flt-3L increased the severity of experimental autoimmune thyroiditis due to enhanced Th1 responses, while GM-CSF either prevented or significantly suppressed disease development even at a late stage, due to enhanced Th2 responses.[106]

THERAPEUTIC APPLICATIONS OF REGULATORY DENDRITIC CELLS

Animal models

Several procedures to induce tolerance have been developed using either DCs modified as just described, or different routes of DC administration. For example, subcutaneous (s.c.) injection of antigen-pulsed splenic DCs or epidermal Langerhans cells induces antigen-specific immunity, whereas intravenous (i.v.) injections of the same preparation result in tolerance.[107,108] Specific strategies for autoimmune diseases might include the promotion of regulatory T-cell

development using regulatory DCs, or genetic engineering of DCs to introduce molecules that have immunosuppressive functions, such as IL-10, TGF-β, Fas-ligand, ILT3, and ILT4. Evidence for the ability of DCs to suppress autoimmune inflammatory disease so far comes from the application of DCs to models of autoimmune disease, as detailed below. Syngeneic DCs, with or without exposure to autoantigens, have been shown to inhibit the development of autoimmune diseases of the neuromuscular system, such as experimental allergic encephalomyelitis (EAE), autoimmune endocrinopathies, such as type 1 diabetes, and models of autoimmune arthritis, such as collagen-induced arthritis.

Neuromuscular diseases

After exposure to TGF-β *in vitro*, splenic DCs from healthy syngeneic donor rats could transfer suppression to recipients with EAE. In contrast, TGF-β-exposed DCs from donor rats with EAE had no effect when transferred. DCs were administered 5 days after immunization of Lewis rats with encephalitogenic myelin basic protein peptide 68–86 (MBP68–86) and complete Freund's adjuvant (CFA), during the incipient phase of EAE.[109] S.C. injection of immature, but not lipopolysaccharide (LPS)-treated, bone marrow-derived DCs prior to immunization also prevented EAE.[110] TGF-β-modified DCs similarly inhibited the development of clinical signs of experimental autoimmune myasthenia gravis (EAMG) in Lewis rats when given during the incipient phase of EAMG.[111]

In autoimmune disease of the eye, peptide-loaded immature DCs inhibited the production of IFN-γ by uveitogenic T cells and therefore the induction of experimental autoimmune uveoretinitis (EAU) *in vivo*.[112] Draining lymph node T cells secreted high levels of IL-10 and IL-15. In another model, transfer of inter-photoreceptor retinoid binding protein-pulsed TGF-β$_2$-treated APCs to inter-photoreceptor retinoid binding protein-immunized mice successfully suppressed the induction of experimental uveoretinitis in mice.[113]

Myelin antigen-pulsed splenocytes were shown to suppress EAE by selective induction of anergy in encephalitogenic T cells.[114] Regulatory APCs, generated by exposure to TGF-β_2 and MBP antigen, promoted development of CD8[+] Tregs that suppressed EAE.[115] These results provide evidence that DCs can induce tolerance in experimental autoimmune diseases through effects on responding T cells. In an alternative approach, EAE could be prevented by i.v. injection of splenic DCs exposed *ex vivo* to MBP and CTLA-4-Ig fusion protein, presumably through *ex vivo* blockade of CD28–CD80 interactions.[116]

In a number of models, repetitive intravenous administration of so-called 'semimature' DCs, prepared *in vitro* by exposure to TNF-α, induced antigen-specific protection. TNF-α-DCs have been shown to express high levels of MHC and T-cell costimulatory molecules, but unlike mature DCs, they produce low levels of proinflammatory cytokines and are unable to secrete IL-12p70. These DCs suppress EAE through generation of autoantigen-specific IL-10-secreting CD4[+] T cells,[117] possibly as a result of the lack of expression of costimulatory 'signal 3'.[118] Finally, DCs exposed to TGF-β_1 or IFN-γ suppressed the onset and relapses of EAE, in comparison with animals receiving untreated DC or saline injections.[119]

Type 1 diabetes and diseases of the endocrine glands

In the NOD mouse model of diabetes, transfer of DCs treated with IFN-γ also induced long-lasting protection against type 1 diabetes mellitus.[120] Transfer of pancreatic lymph node DCs also suppressed the development of diabetes by the induction of regulatory cells in NOD mice.[121] In other experiments, a single i.v. injection of syngeneic splenic DCs from euglycemic NOD mice exposed to human IgG protected mice from diabetes. Supernatants of islets from these mice contained increased levels of IL-4 and IL-10 and diminished levels of IFN-γ compared with diabetic controls, suggesting a favorable effect of type 2 cytokines on disease.[122]

Mature bone marrow-derived DCs could also prevent diabetes development in NOD, an effect ascribed to the generation of CD25[+]CD4[+] regulatory T cells, secreting Th2 cytokines.[123] Bone marrow-derived DCs generated in the presence of NF-κB inhibitory oligo-dinucleotides or the soluble NF-κB inhibitor Bay11-7082 could also prevent diabetes.[124] (unpublished data).

However, no studies have demonstrated that transferred DCs can ameliorate established type 1 diabetes in NOD mice.

Experimental autoimmune thyroiditis (EAT), a murine model of Hashimoto's thyroiditis in humans, can be induced upon challenge of susceptible animals with thyroglobulin and adjuvant.[125] This disease is mediated by CD4[+] T cells and is characterized by lymphocytic infiltration of the thyroid gland.[126] DCs exposed to TNF-α and antigen induced antigen-specific CD4[+]CD25[+] T cells with the ability to inhibit development of EAT, confirming results previously published for a model of EAE.[127]

Arthritis

Several studies in experimental arthritis have evaluated the therapeutic effect of DCs transduced with various immunomodulatory genes. Transduction of DCs with TNF-related apoptosis-induced ligand (TRAIL) was evaluated in mice with collagen-induced arthritis (CIA). TRAIL expression was controlled by a doxycycline-inducible tetracycline response element. Transfected DCs were capable of inducing apoptosis of arthritogenic T cells.[128] Genetic modification of primary DCs to express Fas-L, eliminated or reduced the number of antigen-specific T cells responsible for the progression of CIA.[129] Moreover, DCs transfected with Fas-L could induce antigen-specific tolerance after exposure to a peptide to which they had previously been sensitized. This observation provides evidence that it may also be possible to delete autoreactive T cells from the repertoire using modified DCs.[130]

Adoptive transfer of immature DCs expressing IL-4 after adenoviral infection, into mice with established CIA suppressed disease for up to 4 weeks.[131] Similarly, IL-4-transduced bone marrow-derived DCs adoptively transferred before disease onset reduced the incidence and severity of murine CIA, whereas IL-4 delivery by retrovirally transduced T cells and NIH 3T3 cells had no effect.[132] Whereas each of these approaches suppressed Th1-mediated T-cell and antibody responses, they typically did not deviate the immune response towards a Th2-type or regulatory response. In contrast, DCs generated in the presence of vasoactive intestinal peptide (VIP) were able to suppress CIA in an IL-10-dependent fashion.[133] TNF-DCs also suppressed CIA, when delivered i.v. in high doses, in a partially IL-10-dependent manner.[127] Both TNF-DCs and VIP-DCs stimulate peripheral conversion of CD4[+]CD25[+] regulatory T cells and Tr1-type Tregs. VIP has been shown to reduce DC NF-κB activation and CD40 expression.[133]

Human studies

DC immunotherapy has been introduced in the clinical trials, and has proven to be feasible, non-toxic and effective in some patients with cancer, particularly if the DCs have been appropriately activated.[134–136] In vivo activation and targeting of DCs, as well as exploitation of DCs to suppress autoimmunity, will expand the application of DCs to a wide variety of immune-mediated diseases. However, a number of technical questions also need to be addressed in autoimmune immunotherapy, including the frequency and route of administration, the subset and number of DCs to be used, and the concentration and duration of cytokine treatment. For example, while a single i.v. or s.c. dose of 0.5×10^6 DCs treated with an NF-κB inhibitor was sufficient to suppress priming or antigen-induced arthritis, TNF-treated DCs must be given repeatedly i.v. in high doses.

Data relating to human DCs are scarce, but certain studies have reported encouraging results. Using a human in vitro model system, immature DCs exposed to allospecific CD8[+]CD28[−] T-suppressor cells or CD4[+]CD25[+] Tregs exhibited increased surface expression of the inhibitory molecules ILT3 and 4.[98] These human regulatory DCs induced reversible anergy in unprimed or primed T-helper cells, promoting the conversion of alloreactive CD4[+] T-cells to Tregs. Human blood CD4[+]CD123[+]CD11c[−] precursor DCs can be generated when cultured in the presence of IL-3.[137–139] After in vitro activation by TNF-α, these DCs promoted production of IL-4 and IL-10 by T cells.[138] Such DCs have potential for the treatment of autoimmune diseases and acute GVHD.[140]

Peripheral blood monocyte-derived DCs, exposed to IFN-β, secrete high levels of IL-10 but low levels of IL-12, and suppress IFN-γ production by mononuclear cells.[141] DCs from MS patients treated with IFN-β in vivo produced less IFN-γ and TNF-α than DCs from control patients.[142] These findings suggest that exposure of DCs to IFN-β and IL-10 may curtail the production of proinflammatory cytokines, and after re-infusion, such DCs may represent a promising direction for therapy of MS. Signaling through NF-κB was also shown to determine the capacity of DCs to stimulate T-cell proliferation in vitro, in that CD40[−] human monocyte-derived DCs generated in the presence of an NF-κB inhibitor, signal little T-cell proliferation or IFN-γ production.[143]

In a human study of two healthy volunteers, in vivo responses to recall antigens were suppressed when normal volunteers were injected with antigen-exposed immature DCs.[17] This effect was linked to the generation of regulatory type CD4[+] and CD8[+] T cells and the production of IL-10, and is in marked contrast to the active immunity that can be achieved with mature DCs. This small study is the only clinical evidence to date illustrating the potential of immature DCs as a tool for immunosuppression. However, it is not yet clear whether this potential will translate into patients with immune system defects that have led to the development of spontaneous autoimmune disease. DC modified by differentiation in the presence of an NF-κB inhibitor, Bay 11-7082 suppressed antigen-induced arthritis is an antigen-specific fashion, even after disease was fully clinically expressed.[155]

Route of injection

Studies analysing in vivo biodistribution of labeled DCs demonstrated that DCs injected i.v. localize to the lungs, followed by redistribution to the liver, spleen, and bone marrow, but not lymph nodes. After s.c. administration, DCs preferentially accumulate in the T-cell areas of the draining lymph nodes.[44] To a lesser extent, DCs are also found in the abdominal draining lymph nodes after i.p. administration.

BLOCKING DENDRITIC CELL FUNCTION IN RHEUMATIC DISEASE

Patients with SLE have been shown to display major alterations in DC homeostasis in that plasmacytoid DCs are reduced in blood and IFN-α-activated monocytes from these patients are effective APCs *in vitro*.[145] It was speculated that monocyte-derived DCs might efficiently capture apoptotic cells and nucleosomes, present in SLE patients' blood and tissues.[146] In view of the high levels of IFN-α in serum, and its detrimental effects in SLE, IFN-α is being developed as a potential target for therapeutic intervention in SLE.[147] IFN-α activates not only myeloid cells, including monocytes and myeloid DCs, but also plasmacytoid DCs themselves, which are enriched in the inflammatory site in SLE skin lesions.[148] Of interest, the RNA components of the Ro 60 and Sm/RNP small ribonucleoprotein autoantigens have recently been shown to act as endogenous adjuvants which stimulate plasmacytoid DC (PDC) maturation and type I IFN production.[149–151] Type I IFN production by PDCs can also be triggered in cutaneous LE by UV light, which stimulates local production of chemokines for T cells and PDCs.

Other investigators have suggested the blockade of chemokines or chemokine receptors for inhibition of the ectopic lymphoid development characteristic of the chronic inflammatory response in RA and other autoimmune rheumatic diseases. Thus, DCs in perivascular, T-cell enriched areas of synovial tissue are associated with CCL19 and 21 expression and are characterized by CCR7 expression, and immature DCs in the lining and sublining layers are characterized by CCR6 expression and are associated with CCL20 expression.[152] It remains to be seen whether such treatments might be effective in animal models. However, ectopic expression of CCL19 is sufficient for formation of lymphoid tissue.[153] Similarly, BCA-1/CXCL13 is found, predominantly in follicular DCs, in germinal centers in RA synovium. B cells aggregate in these regions, likely attracted by the FDCs.[154] The data suggest that blockade of these chemokines would have a marked but potentially toxic effect on the process of lymphoid tissue development in synovial tissue.

CONCLUSION

Restoration of tolerance to self-antigens is currently an exciting field. After many years in the doldrums, progress in our understanding of how T-cell regulation occurs, how to control the

APCs for generation of regulation, and the nature of the autoantigens driving rheumatic diseases has recently surged ahead. DCs are an attractive target to attenuate immune responses in autoimmune diseases. The plasticity of DCs provides a wide platform, enabling expansion of DCs, modification of DC function, and promotion of immunity towards a predicted direction. Further detailed understanding of the phenotype and function of DCs may aid the development of therapeutic strategies in future clinical application. There are still challenges, not least of which is the commercial development of DCs or regulatory T-cell therapy for widespread use in patients with autoimmune disease, including issues of product quality control, cost, broad distribution, and business modelling. In this regard, a significant challenge remains to develop cell-free antigen-specific therapy to target APCs with appropriate autoantigens and immunomodulators *in vivo*. However, convincing clinical trial evidence that the principles of antigen-specific therapy using DCs that are already demonstrated in animal models can actually work in practice in patients with spontaneous autoimmunity would be a very good starting point.

REFERENCES

1. Fazekas de St Groth B. The evolution of self-tolerance: a new cell arises to meet the challenge of self-reactivity. Immunol Today 1998; 19: 448–54.
2. Bancherau J, Steinman RM. Dendritic cells and the control of immunity. Nature 1998; 392(6673): 245–52.
3. Inaba K, Steinman RM, Van Voorhis WC, Muramatsu S. Dendritic cells are critical accessory cells for thymus-dependent antibody responses in mouse and in man. Proc Natl Acad Sci U S A 1983; 80(19): 6041–5.
4. Kitamura H, Iwakabe K, Yahata T et al. The natural killer T (NKT) cell ligand alpha-galactosylceramide demonstrates its immunopotentiating effect by inducing interleukin (IL)-12 production by dendritic cells and IL-12 receptor expression on NKT cells. J Exp Med 1999; 89(7): 1121–8.
5. Schuler G, Steinman RM. Dendritic cells as adjuvants for immune-mediated resistance to tumors. J Exp Med 1997; 186(8): 1183–7.
6. Brocker T. Survival of mature CD4 T lymphocytes is dependent on major histocompatibility complex class II-expressing dendritic cells. J Exp Med 1997; 186(8): 1223–32.

7. Steinman RM. The dendritic cell system and its role in immunogenicity. Annu Rev Immunol 1991; 9: 271–96.

8. Cella M, Sallusto F, Lanzavecchia A. Origin, maturation and antigen presenting function of dendritic cells. Curr Opin Immunol 1997; 9(1): 10–16.

9. Cella M, Scheidegger D, Palmer-Lehmann K et al. Ligation of CD40 on dendritic cells triggers production of high levels of interleukin-12 and enhances T cell stimulatory capacity: T-T help via APC activation. J Exp Med 1996; 184(2): 747–52.

10. Sallusto F, Lanzavecchia A. Mobilizing dendritic cells for tolerance, priming, and chronic inflammation. J Exp Med 1999; 189(4): 611–14.

11. Sparwasser T, Koch ES, Vabulas RM et al. Bacterial DNA and immunostimulatory CpG oligonucleotides trigger maturation and activation of murine dendritic cells. Eur J Immunol 1998; 28(6): 2045–54.

12. Cella M, Salio M, Sakakibara Y et al. Maturation, activation, and protection of dendritic cells induced by double-stranded RNA. J Exp Med 1999; 189(5): 821–9.

13. De Smedt T, Pajak B, Muraille E et al. Regulation of dendritic cell numbers and maturation by lipopolysaccharide in vivo. J Exp Med 1996; 184(4): 1413–24.

14. De Smedt T, Van Mechelen M, De Becker G et al. Effect of interleukin-10 on dendritic cell maturation and function. Eur J Immunol 1997; 27(5): 1229–35.

15. Geissmann F, Revy P, Regnault A et al. TGF-beta 1 prevents the noncognate maturation of human dendritic Langerhans cells. J Immunol 1999; 162(8): 4567–75.

16. de Jong EC, Vieira PL, Kalinski P, Kapsenberg ML. Corticosteroids inhibit the production of inflammatory mediators in immature monocyte-derived DC and induce the development of tolerogenic DC3. J Leukoc Biol 1999; 66(2): 201–4.

17. Dhodapkar MV, Steinman RM, Krasovsky J, Munz C, Bhardwaj N. Antigen-specific inhibition of effector T cell function in humans after injection of immature dendritic cells. J Exp Med 2001; 193(2): 233–8.

18. Jonuleit H, Schmitt E, Schuler G, Knop J, Enk AH. Induction of interleukin 10-producing, nonproliferating CD4(+) T cells with regulatory properties by repetitive stimulation with allogeneic immature human dendritic cells. J Exp Med 2000; 192(9): 1213–22.

19. Lutz MB, Kukutsch NA, Menges M, Rossner S, Schuler G. Culture of bone marrow cells in GM-CSF plus high doses of lipopolysaccharide generates exclusively immature dendritic cells which induce alloantigen-specific CD4 T cell anergy in vitro. Eur J Immunol 2000; 30(4): 1048–52.

20. Mehling A, Grabbe S, Voskort M et al. Mycophenolate mofetil impairs the maturation and function of murine dendritic cells. J Immunol 2000; 165(5): 2374–81.

21. Lutz MB, Suri RM, Niimi M et al. Immature dendritic cells generated with low doses of GM-CSF in the absence of IL-4 are maturation resistant and prolong allograft survival in vivo. Eur J Immunol 2000; 30(7): 1813–22.

22. Griffin MD, Lutz W, Phan VA et al. Dendritic cell modulation by 1alpha,25 dihydroxyvitamin D3 and its analogs: a vitamin D receptor-dependent pathway that promotes a persistent state of immaturity in vitro and in vivo. Proc Natl Acad Sci U S A 2001; 98(12): 6800–5.

23. Hackstein H, Morelli AE, Larregina AT et al. Aspirin inhibits in vitro maturation and in vivo immunostimulatory function of murine myeloid dendritic cells. J Immunol 2001; 166(12): 7053–62.

24. Lee JI, Ganster RW, Geller DA et al. Cyclosporine A inhibits the expression of costimulatory molecules on in vitro-generated dendritic cells: association with reduced nuclear translocation of nuclear factor kappa B. Transplantation 1999; 68(9): 1255–63.

25. Steinbrink K, Wolfl M, Jonuleit H, Knop J, Enk AH. Induction of tolerance by IL-10-treated dendritic cells. J Immunol 1997; 159(10): 4772–80.

26. Yoshimura S, Bondeson J, Foxwell BM, Brennan FM, Feldmann M. Effective antigen presentation by dendritic cells is NF-kappaB dependent: coordinate regulation of MHC, co-stimulatory molecules and cytokines. Int Immunol 2001; 13(5): 675–83.

27. Giannoukakis N, Bonham CA, Qian S et al. Prolongation of cardiac allograft survival using dendritic cells treated with NF-kB decoy oligodeoxyribonucleotides. Mol Ther 2000; 1(5 Pt 1): 430–7.

28. Griffin MD, Lutz W, Phan VA et al. Dendritic cell modulation by 1alpha,25 dihydroxyvitamin D3 and its analogs: a vitamin D receptor-dependent pathway that promotes a persistent state of immaturity in vitro and in vivo. Proc Natl Acad Sci U S A 2001; 98(12): 6800–5.

29. Rea D, van Kooten C, van Meijgaarden KE et al. Glucocorticoids transform CD40-triggering of dendritic cells into an alternative activation pathway resulting in antigen-presenting cells that secrete IL-10. Blood 2000; 95(10): 3162–7.

30. Adorini L, Penna G, Giarratana N, Uskokovic M. Tolerogenic dendritic cells induced by vitamin D receptor ligands enhance regulatory T cells inhibiting allograft rejection and autoimmune diseases. J Cell Biochem 2003; 88(2): 227–33.

31. Burkly L, Hession C, Ogata L et al. Expression of relB is required for the development of thymic medulla and dendritic cells. Nature 1995; 373(6514): 531–6.

32. Weih F, Carrasco D, Durham SK et al. Multiorgan inflammation and hematopoietic abnormalities in mice with a targeted disruption of RelB, a member of the NF-kappa B/Rel family. Cell 1995; 80(2): 331–40.

33. Wu L, D'Amico A, Winkel KD et al. RelB is essential for the development of myeloid-related CD8alpha-dendritic cells but not of lymphoid-related CD8alpha+ dendritic cells. Immunity 1998; 9(6): 839–47.

34. O'Sullivan BJ, MacDonald KP, Pettit AR, Thomas R. RelB nuclear translocation regulates B cell MHC molecule, CD40 expression, and antigen-presenting cell function. Proc Natl Acad Sci U S A 2000; 97(21): 11421–6.

35. O'Sullivan BJ, Thomas R. CD40 Ligation conditions dendritic cell antigen-presenting function through sustained activation of NF-kappaB. J Immunol 2002; 168(11): 5491–8.

36. Martin E, O'Sullivan B, Low P, Thomas R. Antigen-specific suppression of a primed immune response by dendritic cells mediated by regulatory T cells secreting interleukin-10. Immunity 2003; 18(1): 155–67.

37. Nishizuka Y, Sakakura T. Thymus and reproduction: sex-linked dysgenesia of the gonad after neonatal thymectomy in mice. Science 1969; 166(906): 753–5.

38. Kojima A, Tanaka-Kojima Y, Sakakura T, Nishizuka Y. Prevention of postthymectomy autoimmune thyroiditis in mice. Lab Invest 1976; 34(6): 601–5.

39. Sakaguchi S, Sakaguchi N, Shimizu J et al. Immunologic tolerance maintained by CD25+ CD4+ regulatory T cells: their common role in controlling autoimmunity, tumor immunity, and transplantation tolerance. Immunol Rev 2001; 182: 18–32.

40. Itoh M, Takahashi T, Sakaguchi N et al. Thymus and autoimmunity: production of CD25+CD4+ naturally anergic and suppressive T cells as a key function of the thymus in maintaining immunologic self-tolerance. J Immunol 1999; 162(9): 5317–26.

41. Sakaguchi S, Sakaguchi N, Shimizu J et al. Immunologic tolerance maintained by CD25+ CD4+ regulatory T cells: their common role in controlling autoimmunity, tumor immunity, and transplantation tolerance. Immunol Rev 2001; 182: 18–32.

42. McHugh RS, Shevach EM, Thornton AM. Control of organ-specific autoimmunity by immunoregulatory CD4(+)CD25(+) T cells. Microbes Infect 2001; 3(11): 919–27.

43. Thornton AM, Shevach EM. Suppressor effector function of CD4+CD25+ immunoregulatory T cells is antigen nonspecific. J Immunol 2000; 164(1): 183–90.

44. Zheng Z, Narita M, Takahashi M et al. Induction of T cell anergy by the treatment with IL-10-treated dendritic cells. Comp Immunol Microbiol Infect Dis 2004; 27(2): 93–103.

45. Yamazaki S, Iyoda T, Tarbell K, Olson K et al. Direct expansion of functional CD25+ CD4+ regulatory T cells by antigen-processing dendritic cells. J Exp Med 2003; 198(2): 235–47.

46. Tarbell KV, Yamazaki S, Olson K, Toy P, Steinman RM. CD25+ CD4+ T cells, expanded with dendritic cells presenting a single autoantigenic peptide, suppress autoimmune diabetes. J Exp Med 2004; 199(11): 1467–77.

47. Tang Q, Henriksen KJ, Bi M et al. In vitro-expanded antigen-specific regulatory T cells suppress autoimmune diabetes. J Exp Med 2004; 199(11): 1455–65.

48. Groux H, O'Garra A, Bigler M et al. A CD4+ T-cell subset inhibits antigen-specific T-cell responses and prevents colitis. Nature 1997; 389(6652): 737–42.

49. Weiner HL. Oral tolerance: immune mechanisms and the generation of Th3-type TGF-beta-secreting regulatory cells. Microbes Infect 2001; 3(11): 947–54.

50. O'Garra A, Arai N. The molecular basis of T helper 1 and T helper 2 cell differentiation. Trends Cell Biol 2000; 10(12): 542–50.

51. Lenschow DJ, Herold KC, Rhee L et al. CD28/B7 regulation of Th1 and Th2 subsets in the development of autoimmune diabetes. Immunity 1996; 5(3): 285–93.

52. Xu H, Heeger PS, Fairchild RL. Distinct roles for B7-1 and B7-2 determinants during priming of effector CD8+ Tc1 and regulatory CD4+ Th2 cells for contact hypersensitivity. J Immunol 1997; 159(9): 4217–26.

53. Kalinski P, Hilkens CM, Wierenga EA, Kapsenberg ML. T-cell priming by type-1 and type-2 polarized dendritic cells: the concept of a third signal. Immunol Today 1999; 20(12): 561–7.

54. Rabinovich GA, Daly G, Dreja H et al. Recombinant galectin-1 and its genetic delivery suppress collagen-induced arthritis via T cell apoptosis. J Exp Med 1999; 190(3): 385–98.

55. Gorczynski L, Chen Z, Hu J et al. Evidence that an OX-2-positive cell can inhibit the stimulation of type 1 cytokine production by bone marrow-derived B7-1 (and B7-2)-positive dendritic cells. J Immunol 1999; 162(2): 774–81.

56. Chang CC, Ciubotariu R, Manavalan JS et al. Tolerization of dendritic cells by T(S) cells: the crucial role of inhibitory receptors ILT3 and ILT4. Nat Immunol 2002; 3(3): 237–43.

57. Becker JC, Vetter CS, Schrama D, Brocker EB, thor Straten P. Differential expression of CD28 and CD94/NKG2 on T cells with identical TCR beta variable regions in primary melanoma and sentinel lymph node. Eur J Immunol 2000; 30(12): 3699–706.

58. Speiser DE, Valmori D, Rimoldi D et al. CD28-negative cytolytic effector T cells frequently express NK receptors and are present at variable proportions in circulating lymphocytes from healthy donors and melanoma patients. Eur J Immunol 1999; 29(6): 1990–9.

59. Vallejo AN, Brandes JC, Weyand CM, Goronzy JJ. Modulation of CD28 expression: distinct regulatory pathways during activation and replicative senescence. J Immunol 1999; 162(11): 6572–9.

60. Yen JH, Moore BE, Nakajima T et al. Major histocompatibility complex class I-recognizing receptors are disease risk genes in rheumatoid arthritis. J Exp Med 2001; 193(10): 1159–67.

61. Kawano T, Cui J, Koezuka Y et al. CD1d-restricted and TCR-mediated activation of valpha14 NKT cells by glycosylceramides. Science 1997; 278(5343): 1626–9.

62. Naumov YN, Bahjat KS, Gausling R et al. Activation of CD1d-restricted T cells protects NOD mice from developing diabetes by regulating dendritic cell subsets. Proc Natl Acad Sci U S A 2001; 98(24): 13838–43.

63. Fujihashi K, Taguchi T, Aicher WK et al. Immuno-regulatory functions for murine intraepithelial lymphocytes: gamma/delta T cell receptor-positive (TCR+) T cells abrogate oral tolerance, while alpha/beta TCR+ T cells provide B cell help. J Exp Med 1992; 175(3): 695–707.

64. Drakesmith H, Chain B, Beverley P. How can dendritic cells cause autoimmune disease? Immunol Today 2000; 21(5): 214–7.

65. Ludewig B, Zinkernagel RM, Hengartner H. Transgenic animal models for virus-induced autoimmune diseases. Exp Physiol 2000; 85(6): 653–9.

66. Morel PA, Vasquez AC, Feili-Hariri M. Immunobiology of DC in NOD mice. J Leukoc Biol 1999; 66(2): 276–80.

67. Ludewig B, Odermatt B, Ochsenbein AF, Zinkernagel RM, Hengartner H. Role of dendritic cells in the induction and maintenance of autoimmune diseases. Immunol Rev 1999; 169: 45–54.

68. Rosmalen JG, Homo-Delarche F, Durant S et al. Islet abnormalities associated with an early influx of dendritic cells and macrophages in NOD and NODscid mice. Lab Invest 2000; 80(5): 769–77.

69. Mannering SI, Harrison LC, Williamson NA et al. The insulin A-chain epitope recognized by human T cells is posttranslationally modified. J Exp Med 2005; 202(9): 1191–7.

70. Meyer O, Nicaise-Roland P, Santos MD et al. Serial determination of cyclic citrullinated peptide autoantibodies predicted five-year radiological outcomes in a prospective cohort of patients with early rheumatoid arthritis. Arthritis Res Ther 2006; 8(2): R40.

71. van Gaalen F, Ioan-Facsinay A, Huizinga TW, Toes RE. The devil in the details: the emerging role of anti-citrulline autoimmunity in rheumatoid arthritis. J Immunol 2005; 175(9): 5575–80.

72. Klareskog L, Stolt P, Lundberg K et al. A new model for an etiology of rheumatoid arthritis: smoking may trigger HLA-DR (shared epitope)-restricted immune reactions to autoantigens modified by citrullination. Arthritis Rheum 2006; 54(1): 38–46.

73. van Gaalen FA, van Aken J, Huizinga TW et al. Association between HLA class II genes and autoantibodies to cyclic citrullinated peptides (CCPs) influences the severity of rheumatoid arthritis. Arthritis Rheum 2004; 50(7): 2113–21.

74. Hida S, Miura NN, Adachi Y, Ohno N. Influence of arginine deimination on antigenicity of fibrinogen. J Autoimmun 2004; 23(2): 141–50.

75. Hill JA, Southwood S, Sette A et al. Cutting edge: the conversion of arginine to citrulline allows for a high-affinity peptide interaction with the rheumatoid arthritis-associated HLA-DRB1*0401 MHC class II molecule. J Immunol 2003; 171(2): 538–41.

76. Dessen A, Lawrence CM, Cupo S, Zaller DM, Wiley DC. X-ray crystal structure of HLA-DR4 (DRA*0101, DRB1*0401) complexed with a peptide from human collagen II. Immunity 1997; 7(4): 473–81.

77. Linn-Rasker SP, van der Helm-van Mil AH, van Gaalen FA et al. Smoking is a risk factor for anti-CCP antibodies only in rheumatoid arthritis patients who carry HLA-DRB1 shared epitope alleles. Ann Rheum Dis 2006; 65(3): 366–71.

78. Dahlen E, Dawe K, Ohlsson L, Hedlund G. Dendritic cells and macrophages are the first and major producers of TNF-alpha in pancreatic islets in the nonobese diabetic mouse. J Immunol 1998; 160(7): 3585–93.

79. Ludewig B, Odermatt B, Landmann S, Hengartner H, Zinkernagel RM. Dendritic cells induce autoimmune diabetes and maintain disease via de novo formation of local lymphoid tissue. J Exp Med 1998; 188(8): 1493–501.

80. Thompson AG, Thomas R. Induction of immune tolerance by dendritic cells: implications for preventative and therapeutic immunotherapy of autoimmune disease. Immunol Cell Biol 2002; 80(6): 509–19.

81. Harding B, Knight SC. The distribution of dendritic cells in the synovial fluids of patients with arthritis. Clin Exp Immunol 1986; 63(3): 594–600.

82. Thomas R, Lipsky PE. Presentation of self peptides by dendritic cells: possible implications for the pathogenesis of rheumatoid arthritis. Arthritis Rheum 1996 39(2): 183–90.

83. Pettit AR, MacDonald KPA, O'Sullivan B, Thomas R. Differentiated dendritic cells expressing nuclear RelB are predominantly located in rheumatoid synovial tissue perivascular mononuclear cell aggregates. Arthritis Rheum 2000; 43(4): 791–800.

84. Pettit AR, Ahern M, Zehntner S, Smith MD, Thomas R. Comparison of differentiated dendritic cell infiltration of autoimmune and osteoarthritic synovial tissue. Arthritis Rheum 2001; 44: 105–10.

85. Cavanagh LL, Boyce A, Smith L et al. Rheumatoid arthritis synovium contains plasmacytoid dendritic cells. Arthritis Res Ther 2005; 7(2): R230–40.

86. Van Krinks CH, Matyszak MK, Gaston JS. Characterization of plasmacytoid dendritic cells in inflammatory arthritis synovial fluid. Rheumatology (Oxford) 2004; 43(4): 453–60.

87. Camussi G, Lupia E. The future role of anti-tumour necrosis factor (TNF) products in the treatment of rheumatoid arthritis. Drugs 1998; 55(5): 613–20.

88. Paleolog EM, Hunt M, Elliott MJ et al. Deactivation of vascular endothelium by monoclonal anti-tumor necrosis factor alpha antibody in rheumatoid arthritis. Arthritis Rheum 1996; 39(7): 1082–91.

89. Niimi M, Shirasugi N, Ikeda Y et al. Operational tolerance induced by pretreatment with donor dendritic cells under blockade of CD40 pathway. Transplantation 2001; 72(9): 1556–62.

90. Min WP, Gorczynski R, Huang XY, et al. Dendritic cells genetically engineered to express Fas ligand induce donor-specific hyporesponsiveness and prolong allograft survival. J Immunol 2000; 164(1): 161–7.

91. Romani N, Gruner S, Brang D et al. Proliferating dendritic cell progenitors in human blood. J Exp Med 1994; 180(1): 83–93.

92. Sallusto F, Lanzavecchia A. Efficient presentation of soluble antigen by cultured human dendritic cells is maintained by granulocyte/macrophage colony-stimulating factor plus interleukin 4 and downregulated by tumor necrosis factor alpha. J Exp Med 1994; 179(4): 1109–18.

93. Caux C, Dezutter-Dambuyant C, Schmitt D, Banchereau J. GM-CSF and TNF-alpha cooperate in the generation of dendritic Langerhans cells. Nature 1992; 360(6401): 258–61.

94. Fairchild PJ, Brook FA, Gardner RL et al. Directed differentiation of dendritic cells from mouse embryonic stem cells. Curr Biol 2000; 10(23): 1515–18.

95. Hirata S, Senju S, Matsuyoshi H et al. Prevention of experimental autoimmune encephalomyelitis by transfer of embryonic stem cell-derived dendritic cells expressing myelin oligodendrocyte glycoprotein peptide along with TRAIL or programmed death-1 ligand. J Immunol 2005; 174(4): 1888–97.

96. Roncarolo MG, Levings MK, Traversari C. Differentiation of T regulatory cells by immature dendritic cells. J Exp Med 2001; 193(2): F5–9.

97. Hanks BA, Jiang J, Singh RA et al. Re-engineered CD40 receptor enables potent pharmacological activation of dendritic-cell cancer vaccines in vivo. Nat Med 2005; 11(2): 130–7.

98. Chang CC, Ciubotariu R, Manavalan JS et al. Tolerization of dendritic cells by T(S) cells: the crucial role of inhibitory receptors ILT3 and ILT4. Nat Immunol 2002; 3(3): 237–43.

99. Colonna M, Nakajima H, Cella M. A family of inhibitory and activating Ig-like receptors that modulate function of lymphoid and myeloid cells. Semin Immunol 2000; 12(2): 121–7.

100. Colonna M, Navarro F, Bellon T et al. A common inhibitory receptor for major histocompatibility complex class I molecules on human lymphoid and myelomonocytic cells. J Exp Med 1997; 186(11): 1809–18.

101. Colonna M, Samaridis J, Cella M et al. Human myelomonocytic cells express an inhibitory receptor for classical and nonclassical MHC class I molecules. J Immunol 1998; 160(7): 3096–100.

102. Steinbrink K, Jonuleit H, Muller G et al. Interleukin-10-treated human dendritic cells induce a melanoma-antigen-specific anergy in CD8(+) T cells resulting in a failure to lyse tumor cells. Blood 1999; 93(5): 1634–42.

103. Liu L, Rich BE, Inobe J, Chen W, Weiner HL. Induction of Th2 cell differentiation in the primary immune response: dendritic cells isolated from adherent cell culture treated with IL-10 prime naive CD4+ T cells to secrete IL-4. Int Immunol 1998; 10(8): 1017–26.

104. Steinbrink K, Graulich E, Kubsch S, Knop J, Enk AH. CD4(+) and CD8(+) anergic T cells induced by interleukin-10-treated human dendritic cells display antigen-specific suppressor activity. Blood 2002; 99(7): 2468–76.

105. Viney JL, Mowat AM, O'Malley JM, Williamson E, Fanger NA. Expanding dendritic cells in vivo enhances the induction of oral tolerance. J Immunol 1998; 160(12): 5815–25.

106. Vasu C, Dogan RN, Holterman MJ, Prabhakar BS. Selective induction of dendritic cells using granulocyte macrophage-colony stimulating factor, but not fms-like tyrosine kinase receptor 3-ligand, activates thyroglobulin-specific CD4+/CD25+ T cells and suppresses experimental autoimmune thyroiditis. J Immunol 2003; 170(11): 5511–22.

107. Morikawa Y, Furotani M, Kuribayashi K, Matsuura N, Kakudo K. The role of antigen-presenting cells in the regulation of delayed-type hypersensitivity. I. Spleen dendritic cells. Immunology 1992; 77(1): 81–7.

108. Morikawa Y, Furotani M, Matsuura N, Kakudo K. The role of antigen-presenting cells in the regulation of delayed-type hypersensitivity. II. Epidermal Langerhans' cells and peritoneal exudate macrophages. Cell Immunol 1993; 152(1): 200–10.

109. Huang YM, Yang JS, Xu LY, Link H, Xiao BG. Autoantigen-pulsed dendritic cells induce tolerance to experimental allergic encephalomyelitis (EAE) in Lewis rats. Clin Exp Immunol 2000; 122(3): 437–44.

110. Xiao BG, Huang YM, Yang JS, Xu LY, Link H. Bone marrow-derived dendritic cells from experimental allergic encephalomyelitis induce immune tolerance to EAE in Lewis rats. Clin Exp Immunol 2001; 125(2): 300–9.

111. Yarilin D, Duan R, Huang YM, Xiao BG. Dendritic cells exposed in vitro to TGF-beta1 ameliorate experimental autoimmune myasthenia gravis. Clin Exp Immunol 2002; 127(2): 214–19.

112. Jiang HR, Muckersie E, Robertson M, Forrester JV. Antigen-specific inhibition of experimental autoimmune uveoretinitis by bone marrow-derived immature dendritic cells. Invest Ophthalmol Vis Sci 2003; 44(4): 1598–607.

113. Okamoto S, Kosiewicz M, Caspi R, Streilein J. ACAID as a potential therapy for established experimental autoimmune uveitis. In: Nussenblatt RB, Whitcup SH, Cospi RR, Geri I, eds. Advances in Ocular Immunology. Proceedings of the 6th International Symposium on the Immunology and Immunopathology of the Eye, Bethesda, MD, 1994. Amsterdam: Elsevier, 1994: 195–8.

114. Vandenbark AA, Celnik B, Vainiene M, Miller SD, Offner H. Myelin antigen-coupled splenocytes suppress experimental autoimmune encephalomyelitis in Lewis rats through a partially reversible anergy mechanism. J Immunol 1995; 155(12): 5861–7.

115. Faunce DE, Terajewicz A, Stein-Streilein J. Cutting edge: in vitro-generated tolerogenic APC induce CD8+ T regulatory cells that can suppress ongoing experimental autoimmune encephalomyelitis. J Immunol 2004; 172(4): 1991–5.

116. Khoury SJ, Gallon L, Verburg RR et al. Ex vivo treatment of antigen-presenting cells with CTLA4Ig and encephalitogenic peptide prevents experimental autoimmune encephalomyelitis in the Lewis rat. J Immunol 1996; 157(8): 3700–5.

117. Menges M, Rossner S, Voigtlander C et al. Repetitive injections of dendritic cells matured with tumor necrosis factor alpha induce antigen-specific protection of mice from autoimmunity. J Exp Med 2002; 195(1): 15–21.

118. Thomas R. Signal 3 and its role in autoimmunity. Arthritis Res Ther 2004; 6: 26–7.

119. Xiao BG, Wu XC, Yang JS et al. Therapeutic potential of IFN-gamma-modified dendritic cells in acute and chronic experimental allergic encephalomyelitis. Int Immunol 2004; 16(1): 13–22.

120. Shinomiya M, Fazle Akbar SM, Shinomiya H, Onji M. Transfer of dendritic cells (DC) ex vivo stimulated with interferon-gamma (IFN-gamma) down-modulates autoimmune diabetes in non-obese diabetic (NOD) mice. Clin Exp Immunol 1999; 117(1): 38–43.

121. Clare-Salzler MJ, Brooks J, Chai A, Van Herle K, Anderson C. Prevention of diabetes in nonobese diabetic mice by dendritic cell transfer. J Clin Invest 1992; 90(3): 741–8.

122. Papaccio G, Nicoletti F, Pisanti FA, Bendtzen K, Galdieri M. Prevention of spontaneous autoimmune diabetes in NOD mice by transferring in vitro antigen-pulsed syngeneic dendritic cells. Endocrinology 2000; 141(4): 1500–5.

123. Feili-Hariri M, Dong X, Alber SM et al. Immunotherapy of NOD mice with bone marrow-derived dendritic cells. Diabetes 1999; 48(12): 2300–8.

124. Ma L, Qian S, Liang X et al. Prevention of diabetes in NOD mice by administration of dendritic cells deficient in nuclear transcription factor-kappaB activity. Diabetes 2003; 52(8): 1976–85.

125. Charreire J. Immune mechanisms in autoimmune thyroiditis. Adv Immunol 1989; 46: 263–334.

126. Weetman AP, McGregor AM. Autoimmune thyroid disease: further developments in our understanding. Endocr Rev 1994; 15(6): 788–830.

127. Verginis P, Li HS, Carayanniotis G. Tolerogenic semimature dendritic cells suppress experimental autoimmune thyroiditis by activation of thyroglobulin-specific CD4+CD25+ T cells. J Immunol 2005; 174(11): 7433–9.

128. Liu Z, Xu X, Hsu HC et al. CII-DC-AdTRAIL cell gene therapy inhibits infiltration of CII-reactive T cells and CII-induced arthritis. J Clin Invest 2003; 112(9): 1332–41.

129. Kim SH, Kim S, Oligino TJ, Robbins PD. Effective treatment of established mouse collagen-induced arthritis by systemic administration of dendritic cells genetically modified to express FasL. Mol Ther. 2002; 6(5): 584–90.

130. Matsue H, Matsue K, Walters M et al. Induction of antigen-specific immunosuppression by CD95L cDNA-transfected 'killer' dendritic cells. Nat Med 1999; 5(8): 930–7.

131. Kim SH, Kim S, Evans CH et al. Effective treatment of established murine collagen-induced arthritis by systemic administration of dendritic cells genetically modified to express IL-4. J Immunol 2001; 166(5): 3499–505.

132. Morita Y, Yang J, Gupta R et al. Dendritic cells genetically engineered to express IL-4 inhibit murine collagen-induced arthritis. J Clin Invest 2001; 107(10): 1275–84.

133. Chorny A, Gonzalez-Rey E, Fernandez-Martin A, Ganea D, Delgado M. Vasoactive intestinal peptide induces regulatory dendritic cells that can prevent acute graft-versus-host disease while maintain graft-versus-tumor. Blood 2006; 107: 3787–94.

134. Banchereau J, Palucka AK, Dhodapkar M et al. Immune and clinical responses in patients with metastatic melanoma to CD34(+) progenitor-derived dendritic cell vaccine. Cancer Res 2001; 61(17): 6451–8.

135. Nestle FO, Banchereau J, Hart D. Dendritic cells: on the move from bench to bedside. Nat Med 2001; 7(7): 761–5.

136. Dhodapkar MV, Krasovsky J, Steinman RM, Bhardwaj N. Mature dendritic cells boost functionally superior CD8(+) T-cell in humans without foreign helper epitopes. J Clin Invest 2000; 105(6): R9–R14.

137. Grouard G, Rissoan MC, Filgueira L et al. The enigmatic plasmacytoid T cells develop into dendritic cells

with interleukin (IL)-3 and CD40-ligand. J Exp Med 1997; 185(6): 1101–11.

138. Rissoan MC, Soumelis V, Kadowaki N et al. Reciprocal control of T helper cell and dendritic cell differentiation. Science 1999; 283(5405): 1183–6.

139. Arpinati M, Green CL, Heimfeld S, Heuser JE, Anasetti C. Granulocyte-colony stimulating factor mobilizes T helper 2-inducing dendritic cells. Blood 2000; 95(8): 2484–90.

140. Liu YJ, Blom B. Introduction: TH2-inducing DC2 for immunotherapy. Blood 2000; 95(8): 2482–3.

141. Huang YM, Hussien Y, Yarilin D et al. Interferon-beta induces the development of type 2 dendritic cells. Cytokine 2001; 13(5): 264–71.

142. Huang YM, Xiao BG, Ozenci V et al. Multiple sclerosis is associated with high levels of circulating dendritic cells secreting pro-inflammatory cytokines. J Neuroimmunol 1999; 99(1): 82–90.

143. Thompson AG, O'Sullivan BJ, Beamish H, Thomas R. T cells signaled by NF-kappa B- dendritic cells are sensitized not anergic to subsequent activation. J Immunol 2004; 173(3): 1671–80.

144. Morse MA, Deng Y, Coleman D et al. A Phase I study of active immunotherapy with carcinoembryonic antigen peptide (CAP-1)-pulsed, autologous human cultured dendritic cells in patients with metastatic malignancies expressing carcinoembryonic antigen. Clin Cancer Res 1999; 5(6): 1331–8.

145. Blanco P, Palucka AK, Gill M, Pascual V, Banchereau J. Induction of dendritic cell differentiation by IFN-alpha in systemic lupus erythematosus. Science 2001; 294(5546): 1540–3.

146. Amoura Z, Piette JC, Chabre H et al. Circulating plasma levels of nucleosomes in patients with systemic lupus erythematosus: correlation with serum antinucleosome antibody titers and absence of clear association with disease activity. Arthritis Rheum 1997; 40(12): 2217–25.

147. Vallin H, Blomberg S, Alm GV, Cederblad B, Ronnblom L. Patients with systemic lupus erythematosus (SLE) have a circulating inducer of interferon-alpha (IFN-alpha) production acting on leucocytes resembling immature dendritic cells. Clin Exp Immunol 1999; 115(1): 196–202.

148. Farkas L, Beiske K, Lund-Johansen F, Brandtzaeg P, Jahnsen FL. Plasmacytoid dendritic cells (natural interferon- alpha/beta-producing cells) accumulate in cutaneous lupus erythematosus lesions. Am J Pathol 2001; 159(1): 237–43.

149. Kelly KM, Zhuang H, Nacionales DC et al. 'Endogenous adjuvant' activity of the RNA components of lupus autoantigens Sm/RNP and Ro 60. Arthritis Rheum 2006; 54(5): 1557–67.

150. Savarese E, Chae OW, Trowitzsch S et al. U1 small nuclear ribonucleoprotein immune complexes induce type I interferon in plasmacytoid dendritic cells through TLR7. Blood 2006; 107(8): 3229–34.

151. Vollmer J, Tluk S, Schmitz C et al. Immune stimulation mediated by autoantigen binding sites within small nuclear RNAs involves Toll-like receptors 7 and 8. J Exp Med 2005; 202(11): 1575–85.

152. Page G, Lebecque S, Miossec P. Anatomic localization of immature and mature dendritic cells in an ectopic lymphoid organ: correlation with selective chemokine expression in rheumatoid synovium. J Immunol 2002; 168: 5333–41.

153. Fan L, Reilly CR, Luo Y, Dorf ME, Lo D. Cutting edge: ectopic expression of the chemokine TCA4/SLC is sufficient to trigger lymphoid neogenesis. J Immunol 2000; 164(8): 3955–9.

154. Shi K, Hayashida K, Kaneko M et al. Lymphoid chemokine B cell-attracting chemokine-1 (CXCL13) is expressed in germinal center of ectopic lymphoid follicles within the synovium of chronic arthritis patients. J Immunol 2001; 166(1): 650–5.

155. Martin E, Capini C, Duggan E, et al. Antigen-specific suppression of established arthritis by dendritic cells deficient in NF-kappa B. Arthritis Rhem 2007; 56: 2255-2266.

7

Osteoclasts

Georg Schett and Kurt Redlich

Introduction • Bone loss in rheumatic diseases • Joint destruction • Targeted therapies for the osteoclast • Summary • References

INTRODUCTION

Osteoclasts are the primary bone resorbing cells, which are essential for the remodelling of bone throughout life.[1] These composite structures are the product of up to 20 single cells having fused to form a syncytium. Osteoclasts enable the shaping of bone architecture in early life, remodel the skeleton during adulthood, and pave the way to bone loss in the senium. Osteoclasts have two pivotal molecular characteristics, which enable them to resorb bone. First, a proton/protein pump, which is molecularly characterized as a vacuolar ATPase. This pump creates an acidic milieu between the osteoclast surface (termed ruffled border) and the bone surface, which allows the cell to solubilize calcium from the bone matrix. Second, matrix enzymes like matrix metalloproteinases (MMPs) as well as cathepsins, cleave matrix molecules such as collagen type-1 and thus remove the non-mineralized substances from bone. These two specificities of the osteoclasts allow them to invade bone and create a resorption pit, which can later be filled up by osteoblasts synthesizing new bone matrix.

Osteoclasts are highly specified cells, which are particularly designed to degrade bone, a job that cannot be done by other cell types in a similar manner. Importantly, generation of osteoclasts is linked to the presence of bone, since these cells are not found at places where no mineralized tissue is present, meaning that bone provides key differentiation signals for these cells to develop. Osteoclasts are hematopoietic cells stemming from the monocytic lineage and undergo a series of differentiation steps until they ultimately end up as activated osteoclasts, which stick to bone and start resorbing it (Figure 7.1).

BONE LOSS IN RHEUMATIC DISEASES

Local bone destruction and systemic bone loss are frequently observed conditions in rheumatic diseases.[2] Patients with arthritis usually suffer from several risk factors for accelerated bone loss such as physical disability and long-term use of glucocorticoids, which can speed up bone loss.[3] As a consequence, the prevalence of osteoporosis in patients with rheumatic diseases is high and fracture risk is significantly increased at axial as well as peripheral skeletal sites.[4,5] Importantly, inflammation *per se* is a strong risk factor for increased skeletal breakdown in rheumatic diseases. This is based on the fact that inflammation is associated with the production of proinflammatory cytokines, which not only fuel the inflammatory process but also trigger the generation of osteoclasts. Cytokines such as tumor necrosis factor (TNF)-α and interleukin (IL)-1 are important triggers for osteoclast formation and can explain the link between inflammation and osteoporosis.[6] Parameters of bone resorption are increased in conditions such as rheumatoid arthritis (RA), indicating a

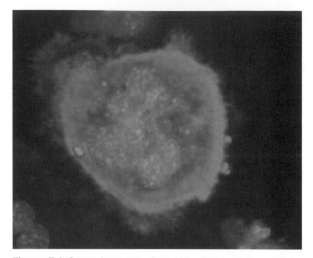

Figure 7.1 Osteoclasts are giant cells that contain multiple nuclei (blue) and attach tightly to bone by forming a ring-shaped structure containing actin (red).

systemically elevated level of bone resorption as a consequence of inflammation. Bisphosphonates, which are the most well known drugs to interfere with the function of osteoclasts, can indeed maintain bone density in patients with RA.[7] The deteriorative effect of systemic inflammation on bone is best illustrated by the finding that even differences in the lower range of the serum level of C-reactive protein are decisive for fracture risk (G. Schett, unpublished observation). This suggests that even a small increase in systemic inflammation leads to production of proinflammatory cytokines, which suffice to create a negative effect on bone balance.

JOINT DESTRUCTION

Apart from this systemic bone loss, chronic arthritis is complicated by the destruction of the joint architecture, composed of resorption of juxta-articular bone as well as destruction of the articular cartilage. This destructive phenotype of inflammatory rheumatic diseases such as RA and psoriatic arthritis contributes to a high burden, which leads to an inability to accomplish activities of daily life.[8] This clinical aspect is based on the ability of inflammatory tissue to build up osteoclasts.[9,10] Cells within the synovial tissue express factors such as macrophage colony stimulating factor (MCSF) as well as

receptor activator of NF-κB ligand (RANKL), which are critical for osteoclast development.[11,12] These factors are regulated by proinflammatory cytokines such as TNF-α as well as IL-1, IL-6, and IL-17, which can up-regulate the expression of RANKL in the synovial tissue. In fact, RANKL is up-regulated in experimental models of arthritis as well as human RA and psoriatic arthritis.[11,13,14] In addition, MCSF, the second essential factor for osteoclast formation, is also inducibly expressed in inflamed joints.[12]

In human disease, osteoclasts and their precursors are found within the synovial tissue close to the bone surface and also within the resorption pits of cortical bone.[9] There is a clear gradient in differentiation steps of the osteoclast within the synovial inflammatory tissue, showing a more differentiated phenotype the closer to the bone surface they are found. Osteoclast precursors within the synovium are mononuclear cells but are already committed to the osteoclast lineage. The high number of monocytic cells in the inflamed tissue facilitates accumulation of osteoclast precursors, which are typically CD68[+] and express tartrate-resistant acid phosphatase (TRAP), a key enzyme of the osteoclast. After further differentiation steps osteoclasts also express the calcitonin receptor, which is a highly specific molecule for the osteoclast lineage. Enzymes such as cathepsin K are also expressed by mononuclear cells within the synovial tissue; however, they are not completely confined to the osteoclast lineage, since synovial fibroblasts have the capacity to express cathepsin K.[15] From sections of samples of joint replacement surgery it is evident that osteoclasts invade the mineralized cartilage as well as the cortical bone, both of which are localized underneath the unmineralized surface cartilage. These holes are then filled by inflammatory tissue also called the pannus (Figure 7.2). Similar observations have been made in all the relevant animal models for RA such as collagen-induced arthritis, adjuvant-induced arthritis, and the serum transfer model of arthritis, as well as mice transgenic for human TNF. From these models it is evident that osteoclast formation is an early and rapidly occurring process, which starts right at the onset of arthritis and leads to a fast resorption of the juxta-articular bone.[16] Experiments that have induced

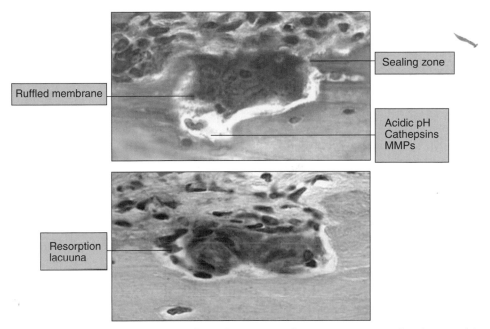

Figure 7.2 Inflammatory tissue can form osteoclasts. Osteoclasts emerge from monocytes, attach to bone, and form resorption pits. Characteristic features are the expression of tartrate-resistant acid phosphatase (TRAP) visualized in the upper panel as well as the calcitonin receptor depicted in the lower panel.

arthritis in osteoclast-free models such as the *c-fos* knockout mice,[17] or mice deficient in either *rankl* or *rank* have shown that osteoclasts are essential for joint destruction.[18,19] In these models no osteoclasts can be built up, which not only results in osteopetrosis but also in a complete protection of the joint from bone damage. Inflammatory signs of arthritis are not affected by the removal of osteoclasts, suggesting that osteoclasts are strictly linked to bone damage but not to the inflammatory features of arthritis.

TARGETED THERAPIES FOR THE OSTEOCLAST

Considering the fact that increased bone resorption and formation of osteoclasts not only contribute to an increased systemic bone loss but also to structural damage of joints, pharmacologic inhibition of the osteoclast is an attractive tool to preserve the skeleton from inflammatory damage. In fact, anti-inflammatory drugs such as TNF-blockers are potent inhibitors of inflammatory joint destruction.[20,21] Thus, clinical trials with TNF-blockers have shown an arrest of progression of radiological bone damage and this effect even extends to the population of patients

who did not achieve a significant clinical response according to the ACR (American College of Rheumatology) criteria. This suggests that TNF-blockers have a potential to preserve bone, which goes beyond their anti-inflammatory properties. In fact, TNF is a potent stimulator of RANKL as well, as it directly interacts with the osteoclast through TNF-RI.[22] Thus, blockade of TNF may not only decrease the burden of inflammation in the joint but also directly interfere with osteoclast formation. This has been shown in animal models of arthritis;[23] however, direct proof in human disease is difficult since there is only limited accessibility to the invasion front. How targeted therapies in RA such as IL-1, IL-6, or costimulation blockade, as well as the depletion of B-cells, affect osteoclast formation in the joint is far less clear. IL-1 and IL-6 can induce osteoclastogenesis, suggesting that effective blockade of these cytokines could also lead to additive structural benefits.

Bisphosphonates in inflammatory joint disease

The best studied drugs to inhibit osteoclast-mediated bone resorption are bisphosphonates.

Due to modifications by insertion of nitrogen moieties bisphosphonates have increased in their potency to inhibit bone resorption.[24] The exact mechanism by which bisphosphonates hamper resorption of bone by the osteoclast is not fully elucidated, but it is commonly accepted that they accumulate in bone and are taken up by osteoclasts and subsequently prevent osteoclast function, possibly due to interference with the mevalonate pathway. Bisphosphonates are very effective in increasing systemic bone mass and reduce the incidence of osteoporotic fracture. Interestingly, when bisphosphonates such as zolendronic acid are administered to arthritic mice, they protect them from inflammatory bone erosions.[25] This suggests that bisphosphonate therapy might also serve as a tool to interfere with structural damage in the joint, which exceeds their known role in maintaining systemic bone mass during inflammatory joint disease. However, the doses of bisphosphonates that have to be used to inhibit structural damage are rather high as compared with those needed to protect from systemic bone loss. This suggests that such an approach might not be easy to accomplish in human disease, which could explain the inconclusive picture of the value of bisphosphonates to protect from inflammatory joint damage, as reviewed by Goldring and Gravallese.[26] It is conceivable that the dose of bisphosphonates used to block inflammatory bone erosion could be similar to the dose that

protects from bone metastasis and which is higher than the dose used to treat osteoporosis. These differences may be based on a higher differentiation rate of osteoclasts during inflammatory disease or differences in the variations of susceptibility of different skeletal sites to take up bisphosphonates.

RANKL blockade

Other potential targets to inhibit synovial osteoclast formation are the ligand–receptor pair RANKL and RANK. RANKL is not only critical for the formation of osteoclasts but also for their activity.[27,28] Due to an imbalance of RANKL as compared with its natural antagonist osteoprotegenin (OPG) in the inflamed joint, inhibition of RANKL could be an effective tool to preserve joints from an inflammatory attack. There is extensive experience in using OPG as a blocker of RANKL in animal models of arthritis. In all relevant animal models of arthritis administration of OPG results in an almost complete protection of the articular bone and disappearance of osteoclasts from the inflamed synovium (Figure 7.3).[29–31] In contrast, inflammation is not affected by the inhibition of RANKL. Thus, inhibition of RANKL appears to selectively inhibit structural damage in the joint by sparing inflammatory disease activity. As a consequence, blockade of RANKL needs to be done in combination with a potent anti-inflammatory approach

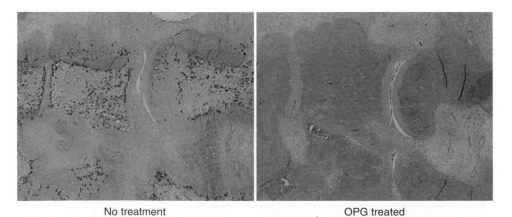

No treatment   OPG treated

Figure 7.3 Adjuvant-induced arthritis leads to rapid resorption of bone (left) by recruiting numerous osteoclasts (brown cells), as depicted by the expression of cathepsin K. Blockade of receptor agonist of NF-κB ligand (RANKL) by osteoprotegerin (OPG) completely blocks osteoclast formation and bone resorption (right).

to control synovitis. Whether RANKL inhibition is also effective to protect human joints from inflammatory damage remains to be elucidated. Currently, the best studied drug interfering with RANKL is a neutralizing human antibody termed denosumab (formerly AMG162), which is highly effective in suppressing bone resorption within days of administration.[32] Currently a phase II trial is testing the efficacy of denosumab to inhibit inflammatory bone erosions in arthritis. Inhibition of RANKL may thus provide an effective tool to preserve joints from inflammatory damage. Other molecular targets that can be targeted by drug therapy are enzymes which solubilize the bone matrix, such as cathepsin K.[33] Inhibitors of cathepsin K are currently being tested for the feasibility to increase bone mass in human in phase II trials; however, no data are available on their role in inflammatory arthritis so far.

Other targets

Other potential targets are the attachment of the osteoclast to bone, which is based on matrix-binding molecules such as the $\alpha v \beta 3$ integrin. Neutralizing antibodies have been developed which block $\alpha v \beta 3$ integrin; however, as with cathepsin K inhibitors, the role in inflammatory bone loss is still elusive.[34] Another interesting target is the vacuolar ATPase that is responsible for creating an acidic milieu necessary to remove calcium from bone.[35] This ATPase cannot be blocked by classical proton pump inhibitors used for interefering with acid production in the stomach, but selective inhibitors of this structurally different proton pump of the osteoclast are in development.

SUMMARY

During the past 10 years osteoclasts have been rediscovered as an important cell type in the inflammatory tissue of chronic arthritis. As hematopoietic cells, osteoclasts are part of the armada of cells trafficking from the bone marrow to the inflamed joint. Upon terminal differentiation they fulfil a very selective job, which is the degradation of mineralized tissue next to the joint. Whereas self-limiting arthritis

cannot produce osteoclasts in a proper way, chronic arthritis leads to a stable accumulation of cells in the synovial space, which are exposed to signals such RANKL long enough to differentiate into osteoclasts. Osteoclasts are essential for bone degradation in arthritis, although they depend on the help of activated T cells or synovial fibroblasts, which provide the essential signals to grow them.[30,36] Based on the highly specialized phenotype of the osteoclasts these cells are thus an objective and feasible target for future drug therapies in arthritis.

REFERENCES

1. Teitelbaum SL. Bone resorption by osteoclasts. Science 2000; 289: 1504–8.
2. Goldring SR, Gravallese EM. Pathogenesis of bone erosions in rheumatoid arthritis. Curr Opin Rheumatol 2000; 12: 195–9.
3. Kirwan JR. The effect of glucocorticoids on joint destruction in rheumatoid arthritis. The Arthritis and Rheumatism Council Low-Dose Glucocorticoid Study Group. N Engl J Med 1995; 333: 142–6.
4. Woolf AD. Osteoporosis in rheumatoid arthritis – the clinical viewpoint. Br J Rheumatol 1991; 30: 82–4.
5. Spector TD, Hall GM, McCloskey EV, Kanis JA. Risk of vertebral fracture in women with rheumatoid arthritis. BMJ 1993; 306: 558.
6. Azuma Y, Kaji K, Katogi R, Takeshita S, Kudo A. Tumor necrosis factor-alpha induces differentiation of and bone resorption by osteoclasts. J Biol Chem 2000; 275: 4858–64.
7. Eggelmeijer F, Papapoulos SE, van Paassen HC et al. Increased bone mass with pamidronate treatment in rheumatoid arthritis. Results of a three-year randomized, double-blind trial. Arthritis Rheum 1996; 39: 396–402.
8. Scott DL, Pugner K, Kaarela K et al. The links between joint damage and disability in rheumatoid arthritis. Rheumatology (Oxford) 2000; 39: 122–32.
9. Gravallese EM, Harada Y, Wang JT et al. Identification of cell types responsible for bone resorption in rheumatoid arthritis and juvenile rheumatoid arthritis. Am J Pathol 1998; 152: 943–51.
10. Bromley M, Woolley DE. Chondroclasts and osteoclasts at subchondral sites of erosion in the rheumatoid joint. Arthritis Rheum 1984; 27: 968–75.
11. Gravallese EM, Manning C, Tsay A et al. Synovial tissue in rheumatoid arthritis is a source of osteoclast differentiation factor. Arthritis Rheum 2000; 43: 250–8.
12. Seitz M, Loetscher P, Fey MF, Tobler A. Constitutive mRNA and protein production of macrophage colony-stimulating factor but not of other cytokines by

synovial fibroblasts from rheumatoid arthritis and osteoarthritis patients. Br J Rheumatol 1994; 33: 613–19.

13. Stolina M, Adamu S, Ominsky M et al. RANKL is a marker and mediator of local and systemic bone loss in two rat models of inflammatory arthritis. J Bone Miner Res 2005; 20: 1756–65.

14. Ritchlin CT, Haas-Smith SA, Li P, Hicks DG, Schwartz EM. Mechanisms of TNF-alpha- and RANKL-mediated osteoclastogenesis and bone resorption in psoriatic arthritis. J Clin Invest 2003; 111: 821–31.

15. Hummel KM, Petrow PK, Franz JK et al. Cystein proteinase cathepsin K mRNA is expressed in synovium of patients with rheumatoid arthritis and is detected at sites of synovial bone destruction. J Rheum 1998; 25: 1887–94.

16. Schett G, Stolina M, Bolon B et al. Analysis of the kinetics of osteoclastogenesis in arthritic rats. Arthritis Rheum 2005; 52: 3192–201.

17. Redlich K, Hayer S, Ricci R et al. Osteoclasts are essential for TNF-alpha-mediated joint destruction. J Clin Invest 2002; 110: 1419–27.

18. Pettit AR, Ji H, von Stechow D et al. TRANCE/RANKL knockout mice are protected from bone erosion in a serum transfer model of arthritis. Am J Pathol 2001; 159: 1689–99.

19. Li P, Schwarz EM, O'Keefe et al. RANK signaling is not required for TNF-mediated increase in CD11(hi) osteoclast precursors but is essential for mature osteoclast formation in TNF-alpha-mediated inflammatory arthritis. J Bone Miner Res 2004; 19: 207–13.

20. Elliott MJ, Maini RN, Feldmann M et al. Randomised double-blind comparison of chimeric monoclonal antibody to tumour necrosis factor alpha (cA2) versus placebo in rheumatoid arthritis. Lancet 1994; 344: 1105–10.

21. Lipsky PE, van der Heijde DM, St Clair EW et al. Infliximab and methotrexate in the treatment of rheumatoid arthritis. Anti-Tumor Necrosis Factor Trial in Rheumatoid Arthritis with Concomitant Therapy Study Group. N Engl J Med 2000; 343: 1594–602.

22. Lam J, Takeshita S, Barker JE et al. TNF-alpha induces osteoclastogenesis by direct stimulation of macrophages exposed to permissive levels of RANK ligand. J Clin Invest 2000; 106: 1481–8.

23. Zwerina J, Hayer S, Tohidast-Akrad M et al. Single and combined inhibition of tumor necrosis factor, interleukin-1, and RANKL pathways in tumor necrosis factor-induced arthritis: effects on synovial inflammation, bone erosion, and cartilage destruction. Arthritis Rheum 2004; 50: 277–90.

24. Watts NB. Pharmacology of agents to treat osteoporosis. In: Favus MJ, ed. Primer on the Metabolic Bone Diseases and Disorders of Mineral Metabolism, 4th ed. Philadephia: Lippincott Williams & Wilkins, 1999: 52, 278–83.

25. Herrak P, Gortz B, Hayer S et al. Zoledronic acid protects against local and systemic bone loss in tumor necrosis factor-mediated arthritis. Arthritis Rheum 2004; 50: 2327–37.

26. Goldring SR, Gravallese EM. Bisphosphonates: environmental protection for the joint? Arthritis Rheum 2004; 50: 2044–7.

27. Lacey DL, Timms E, Tan HL et al. Osteoprotegerin ligand is a cytokine that regulates osteoclast differentiation and activation. Cell 1998; 93: 165–76.

28. Kong YY, Yoshida H, Sarosi I et al. OPGL is a key regulator of osteoclastogenesis, lymphocyte development and lymph-node organogenesis. Nature 1999; 397: 315–23.

29. Redlich K, Hayer S, Maier A et al. Tumor necrosis factor α-mediated joint destruction is inhibited by targeting osteoclasts with osteoprotegerin. Arthritis Rheum 2002; 46: 785–92.

30. Kong YY, Feige U, Sarosi I et al. Activated T cells regulate bone loss and joint destruction in adjuvant arthritis through osteoprotegerin ligand. Nature 1999; 402: 304–9.

31. Romas E, Gillespie MT, Martin TJ. Involvement of receptor activator of NFκB ligand and tumor necrosis factor-α in bone destruction in rheumatoid arthritis. Bone 2002; 30: 340–6.

32. McClung MR, Lewiecki EM, Cohen SB et al. AMG 162 Bone Loss Study Group. Denosumab in postmenopausal women with low bone mineral density. N Engl J Med 2006; 354: 821–31.

33. Yasuda Y, Kaleta J, Bromme D. The role of cathepsins in osteoporosis and arthritis: rationale for the design of new therapeutics. Adv Drug Deliv Rev 200; 57: 973–93.

34. Wilder RL. Integrin alpha V beta 3 as a target for treatment of rheumatoid arthritis and related rheumatic diseases. Ann Rheum Dis 2002; 61: 96–9.

35. Farina C, Gagliardi S. Selective inhibition of osteoclast vacuolar H(+)-ATPase. Curr Pharm 2002; 8: 2033–48.

36. Shigeyama Y, Pap T, Kunzler P et al. Expression of osteoclast differentiation factor in rheumatoid arthritis. Arthritis Rheum 2000; 43: 2523–30.

8

Cell contact dependence of inflammatory events

Danielle Burger, Jean-Michel Dayer and Nicolas Molnarfi

Introduction • Monocytes/macrophages • Different ways of activating monocytes/macrophages • Monocytes/macrophages in chronic/sterile inflammation • T-cell signaling of monocytes/macrophages by direct cell–cell contact • Cell surface molecules involved in contact-mediated monocyte activation • Intracellular pathways involved in cytokine production by monocytes/macrophages • Stimulated T-cell contact-mediated activation of monocytes/macrophages as a potential therapeutic target in autoimmune chronic inflammatory diseases • Impact of gender on contact-mediated activation of monocytes/macrophages • T-cell contact-mediated activation of other cell types involved in RA • Conclusions • Acknowledgments • References

INTRODUCTION

Inflammation is a normal response of living tissues to mechanical injury, invasion by microorganisms, and chemical toxins. The main goal of the inflammatory response is to protect the organism by getting rid of the initial cause of cell injury (e.g. microorganisms or toxins) and the consequences of such injury (e.g. necrotic cells and tissues), and in turn to initiate mechanisms aimed at repairing surrounding tissues that were damaged by injury. Inflammation has to be tightly controlled in time and space to avoid detrimental developments such as those seen in sepsis and chronic inflammatory diseases including rheumatoid arthritis (RA). Indeed, in chronic inflammation, which is an inflammation of prolonged duration, tissue destruction and attempts at repair occur simultaneously. In RA, the outcome is joint cartilage and bone destruction together with accumulation of fibrotic tissue due to synovial cell proliferation and infiltration, angiogenesis, and fibrosis. It has been assumed for a long time that the proinflammatory cytokines tumor necrosis factor (TNF) and interleukin-1β (IL-1β) play an important part in

RA progression. This was confirmed since inhibitors of these cytokines are now successfully used for clinical treatment. Indeed, to restrain inflammation, proinflammatory reactions are closely interconnected with counter-regulatory anti-inflammatory pathways. In the extracellular space this function is fulfilled by specific inhibitors generated by the shedding of cell surface receptors, e.g. soluble TNF receptors, soluble IL-1 receptor II and IL-1 receptor accessory protein, and the release of secreted IL-1 receptor antagonist (sIL-1Ra). All these effectors are mainly produced by monocytes/macrophages, which together with T lymphocytes, are an important part of cellular infiltrate of joints in RA. This chapter reviews the state of the art of the mechanisms underlying the production of proinflammatory cytokines and cytokine inhibitors in chronic inflammation.

In many chronic inflammatory diseases, inflammation is characterized by the influx into the target tissue of immune cells such as T and B lymphocytes, granulocytes, and mononuclear phagocytes. The influx of inflammatory cells is associated with the proliferation of invading and resident cells and frequently with destruction and remodeling of the extracellular matrix. Tissue destruction is mainly achieved by proteases, including matrix metalloproteinases (MMPs). The expression of these proteases and their inhibitors is ruled by many factors including soluble factors (i.e. cytokines, hormones), contact with extracellular matrix components, and direct cell–cell contact. In pathological conditions, the production of cytokines and proteases by infiltrating and resident tissue cells escapes regulatory mechanisms. The activity of pro-inflammatory cytokines is counterbalanced by numerous mechanisms of which specific cytokine inhibitors, e.g. sIL-1Ra, IL-1 soluble receptor II (IL-1-sRII), soluble IL-1 receptor accessory protein (sIL-1RAcP), and TNF soluble receptors (TNFsR). It is generally acknowledged that the imbalance between cytokines and their respective inhibitors is responsible for the persistence of chronic inflammatory conditions and maybe even necessary for their initiation.[1,2] There is now considerable evidence that cytokines such as TNF and IL-1β are involved in many diseases resulting in tissue destruction. This has been demonstrated conclusively by human clinical trials in RA in which the blockade of TNF but also of IL-1 resulted in clinical improvement.[3–5] Cytokine blockade in the clinic has also proved useful in many other diseases including juvenile idiopathic arthritis, Crohn's disease, spondyloarthropathy, vasculitis, and psoriasis.[6–13]

MONOCYTES/MACROPHAGES

Proinflammatory cytokines such as IL-1β and TNF are mainly produced by cells of the monocyte/macrophage lineage. Monocytes/ macrophages play different parts in T-cell-mediated inflammatory diseases. Indeed, they function as proinflammatory cells, as accessory cells for T-cell activation, as effector cells that mediate tissue damage, and as anti-inflammatory cells that promote tissue repair. In general, monocytes display marked functional plasticity.[14] Blood monocytes are young cells that already possess migratory, chemotactic, pinocytic, and phagocytic activities, as well as receptors for IgG Fc-domains (FcγR) and iC3b complement. During migration into tissues, monocytes undergo further differentiation into multifunctional tissue macrophages. Although monocytes are currently considered to be immature macrophages, they tend to represent the circulating macrophage population and should be considered fully competent in their location, able to change phenotype in response to factors encountered in specific tissue after migration. Macrophages can be classified into normal/resident and inflammatory/infiltrating macrophages. Resident macrophages are found in connective tissue (histiocytes), liver (Kupffer's cells), lung (alveolar macrophages), lymph nodes (free and fixed macrophages), spleen (free and fixed macrophages), bone marrow (fixed macrophages), serous fluids (pleural and peritoneal macrophages), skin (histiocytes, Langerhans cells), central nervous system (microglial cells), and in other organs of the reticuloendothelial system.[15] The macrophage population of a given tissue is maintained due to influx of monocytes from the circulating blood, local proliferation, and biological turnover. Under normal steady-state conditions, the renewal of tissue macrophages occurs through local proliferation of progenitor cells and not via monocyte influx.[16–18] Monocytes selectively home to different tissues, presumably under the influence of chemokines or other tissue-specific homing factors.[19] Upon entry into a tissue, maturing monocyte/macrophages migrate into the parenchyma, the environment of which significantly influences the function of macrophages – so macrophages localized in different tissues display different patterns of function.[20,21] Upon inflammatory insult to the tissue, resident macrophages contribute to the innate immune response by expressing a wide variety of inflammatory and effector activities, the pattern of which is differentially regulated by the microenvironment of the various tissues. Moreover, priming of macrophages is a very effective first step towards full-scale activation. Upon priming, cells are educated by an initial insult,[22] and thus prepared for subsequent second insults, in such a manner that the priming alters or modulates cell response to the secondary stimulation. Both monocytes and macrophages are renowned for their apparent phenotypic heterogeneity and for the diversity of their activities.[23,24]

The classical immunophenotypic marker for monocytes is CD14, the receptor for complexes of lipopolysaccharides (LPS) and LPS-binding protein.[25] Human peripheral blood monocytes differ in phenotype and function in that they could be divided into two major populations that express or do not express CD16, the low affinity Fc-γ receptor III.[26] The CD14+/CD16+ subpopulation of monocytes represents approximately 10% of total blood monocytes. Compared with the major subpopulation of CD14++ monocytes, this subpopulation is characterized by the enhanced expression of MHC class II determinants, and an increased ability to produce proinflammatory cytokines (TNF, IL-1β, IL-6) following stimulation by TLRs agonists.[27,28] The CD14+CD16+ subset of peripheral blood monocytes is also thought to be a transitional stage in the development of monocytes to either macrophages or dendritic cells (DCs).[29–31] Consistent with this notion, an expansion of the CD14+CD16+ population has been found in septicemia[32] and other infectious or inflammatory disorders.[29] However, the latter phenotypic switch is still controversial in RA[33,34] and has so far not been observed in multiple sclerosis (MS).[35,36]

As stated above, cells of the monocyte/macrophage lineage are heterogeneous and as such are engaged in a variety of activities that may appear conflicting: proinflammatory versus anti-inflammatory activities, immunogenic versus tolerogenic activities, and tissue-destructive versus tissue-restorative activities.[23,24,37,38] To date, monocyte/macrophage heterogeneity is considered to reflect the plasticity and versatility of these cells in response to exposure to microenvironmental signals.

DIFFERENT WAYS OF ACTIVATING MONOCYTES/MACROPHAGES

Consistent with the premise that monocytes/macrophages can display opposite activities, the activation pathways leading to such activities vary according to tissue distribution and responsiveness to endogenous and exogenous stimuli. As recently reviewed,[37] activation of macrophages can be classified into five categories as follows. (a) *Innate activation* in which macrophages are activated by microbial stimuli, giving rise to the production of low molecular weight metabolites and proinflammatory and/or anti-inflammatory cytokines. (b) *Humoral activation* in which macrophages are activated via occupancy of FcR and complement receptors, giving rise to cytolytic activity and the production of proinflammatory and/or anti-inflammatory cytokines. (c) *Classical activation* consisting of interferon (IFN)-γ-dependent priming/activation of macrophages which after exposure to microbes/LPS produce proinflammatory cytokines (IL-1, TNF, IL-6), nitric oxide (NO), and respiratory burst that in turn lead to major histocompatibility complex (MHC) class II expression, microbicidal activity, tissue damage, cellular immunity, and delayed-type hypersensitivity (DTH). (d) *Alternative activation* mediated by the recruitment of IL-4 receptor-α by IL-4 and IL-13 that, upon antigen endocytosis, triggers the expression of MHC class II and mannose receptor and in turn leads to the involvement of macrophages in humoral immunity, allergic and anti-parasite response, and repair (arginase). (e) *Innate/acquired deactivation* occurring through the uptake of apoptotic cells or lyzosomal storage of host molecules which induce an anti-inflammatory response by down-regulating MHC class II expression and inducing the production of anti-inflammatory cytokines (transforming growth factor (TGF)-β, IL-10) and prostaglandin E_2 (PGE$_2$). In addition to these well-established activation mechanisms, those inducing proinflammatory cytokines (IL-1 and TNF) in chronic (i.e. sterile) inflammation remain elusive. However, research over the past few years has demonstrated that cell contact-dependent signaling occurring during stimulated T-cell–macrophage interaction is a crucial triggering event in the activation of monocyte/macrophage functions.

MONOCYTES/MACROPHAGES IN CHRONIC/STERILE INFLAMMATION

Based on animal models, it is currently thought that in chronic immuno-inflammatory diseases, infiltration of target tissue by T lymphocytes precedes tissue damage, suggesting a pathogenic effect. In RA, T lymphocytes displaying a mature helper phenotype (i.e. CD3+CD4+CD45RO+)

are the main infiltrating cells in the pannus, at percentages ranging from 16% of total cells in 'transitional areas' and 75% in 'lymphocyte-rich perivascular areas'.[39,40] T-lymphocyte extravasation occurs at the level of vessels presenting the characteristics of high endothelial venules.[41] Angiogenesis and proliferation of resident cells accompany this infiltration. Like other chronic destructive inflammatory diseases, RA is thought to be a T-helper 1 (Th1)-mediated disease,[42–45] although current evidence suggests that the role played by CD4+ T cells in the development of rheumatoid inflammation exceeds that of activated proinflammatory Th1 effector cells that drive the chronic autoimmune response.[46] However, the mechanisms by which T cells exert their pathogenic role in RA remain elusive. The infiltration by T lymphocytes is followed by that of monocytes/macrophages, which are rapidly found in the lesion, and cellular interactions occur between T lymphocytes and monocytes/macrophages mainly in the perivascular region.[47] Studies performed by our group and others strongly argue that direct cellular contact with stimulated T cells is a major pathway for the production of IL-1β and TNF in monocytes/macrophages.[23,48–57] Indeed, the contact-mediated activation of monocytes/macrophages by stimulated T lymphocytes is as potent as optimal doses of LPS in inducing IL-1β and TNF production in monocytes and cells of monocytic lineage such as THP-1 cells.[58,59] We therefore postulate that this mechanism is highly relevant to the pathogenesis and persistence of chronic inflammation in diseases such as RA.

T-CELL SIGNALING OF MONOCYTES/ MACROPHAGES BY DIRECT CELL–CELL CONTACT

The importance of T-cell contact-mediated activation of monocytes was first recognized in the mid-1980s when the expression of membrane-associated IL-1 (IL-1α) in mouse macrophages was found to be triggered by both soluble factors and direct contact with T cells.[60] Further studies in human monocytes confirmed the importance of cellular contact with stimulated T cells in the induction of IL-1.[61] Subsequently, direct contact

with stimulated T cells proved to be a potent stimulus of human monocytic cells and monocytes that not only induced IL-1 but other cytokines as well, including TNF, IL-6, IL-8, and MMP.[48–50] Furthermore, in vitro, cell–cell contact with stimulated T cells induces cytokine production by monocytes/macrophages of the inflammatory site of chronic inflammatory diseases such as synovial macrophages[62] and microglial cells.[63,64]

A clue to the actual importance of T-cell contact-mediated activation of monocytes/macrophages in the induction of cytokine production at the inflammatory site was recently brought forward. Indeed, T cells isolated from RA synovial tissue, without further in vitro activation, induce TNF synthesis in normal resting monocytes through direct cellular contact.[65] Besides, RA synovial cultures in which the CD3+ T cells had been depleted contained significantly reduced TNF levels.[65] These results strongly indicate that contact between T cells and monocytes/macrophages is required for TNF production in RA pannus. In vitro, upon unspecific and drastic stimulation by phytohemagglutinin and phorbol myristate acetate (PHA/PMA), most T cell types including T-cell clones, synovial T-cell clones, freshly isolated T lymphocytes and T-cell lines such as HUT-78 and Jurkat cells induce IL-1 and TNF in monocytes.[48,49,66–68] As depicted in Figure 8.1, various stimuli other than PHA/PMA induce T lymphocytes to activate monocytes by direct cellular contact: (i) cross-linking of CD3 by immobilized anti-CD3 monoclonal antibody (mAb) with or without cross-linking of the costimulatory molecule CD28,[52,56,64,65,69,70] (ii) antigen stimulation of antigen-specific T-cell clones,[63,69,71] and (iii) cytokines.[51,53,54,65,72] Noteworthy, synovial T cells isolated from RA joints per se are able to induce IL-1β and TNF production upon contact with syngeneic monocytes.[65,73] Interestingly, RA synovial T cells are similar to cytokine-activated T cells based on their ability to induce TNF but not IL-10 production in monocytes/macrophages; this does not apply to T-cell receptor-activated T lymphocytes.[65] Thus, depending on type and stimulus of T cells, direct cell–cell contact can induce different patterns of products in

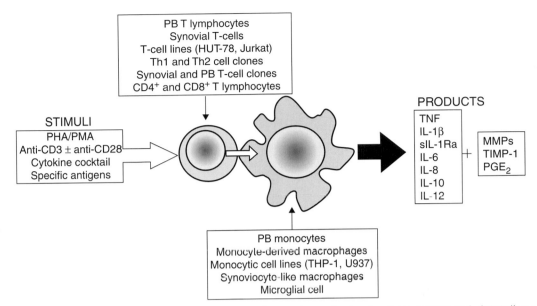

Figure 8.1 Most T-cell types are able to activate monocytes/macrophages by direct cellular contact and, depending on T-cell stimulus, different products are induced in cells of the monocytic lineage. PB, peripheral blood.

monocytes (Figure 8.1) (for review see Burger et al.).[57] In some cases, an imbalance in production between proinflammatory and anti-inflammatory cytokines has been observed, where Th1 cell clones preferentially induce the production of IL-1β rather than sIL-1Ra, and cytokine-stimulated T lymphocytes induce TNF production while failing to induce that of IL-10.[53,69] This suggests that multiple ligands and counter-ligands contribute to the contact-mediated activation of monocytes, which are differentially induced in T cells depending on the stimulus. In addition to variations due to T-cell type and stimulus, contact-mediated activation of monocytes/macrophages depends on the route of monocyte differentiation. Indeed, in monocyte-derived macrophages obtained by treatment with either IFN-γ or M-CSF, contact with cells transfected with CD40L induced diverse patterns of cytokines due to different usage of transduction pathways.[74,75] We also demonstrated that monocytes were more responsive to stimulated T-cell contact-mediated activation than macrophages, the latter requiring a stimulus concentration that was 10-fold higher to induce comparable production of cytokines.[76]

CELL SURFACE MOLECULES INVOLVED IN CONTACT-MEDIATED MONOCYTE ACTIVATION

A crucial issue arising from these observations is the identity of the molecules on the stimulated T-cell surface that are involved in contact-mediated signaling of monocyte activation as well as their counter-ligands. Although several T-cell surface molecules (CD69, CD23, LAG-3, CD45, LFA-1, intercellular adhesion molecule-1 (ICAM-1), and membrane-associated cytokines) have been proved to take part in the contact-mediated activation of monocytes/macrophages (for review see Burger),[58] the identity of the crucial molecule is still elusive.

Controversial results were obtained concerning the involvement of CD40 ligand (CD40L, CD154) in monocyte activation by T cells,[72,77,78] but recently we demonstrated that IL-1β and TNF were induced differentially by CD40L and cell–cell contact depending on the maturation stage of human monocytes, CD40L inducing the production of TNF but not that of IL-1β in IFN-γ-differentiated macrophages but not in monocytes.[76] These results ruled out a primary role for CD40L in contact-mediated activation on monocytes by stimulated T cells. Anti-inflammatory treatments with agents such as leflunomide, minocycline, IFN-β, and glatiramer that have been shown to diminish monocyte/macrophage activation induced by cell–cell contact display contrasting effects on the expression of CD40L at the surface of T cells. Indeed, the expression of CD40L on T cells is decreased by minocycline[79] but not affected by leflunomide, IFN-β, and glatiramer,[64,80–82] suggesting that this ligand may be co-activator but does not elicit a primary signal. Thus, CD40L as well as the above-mentioned surface molecules (i.e. CD69, CD23, LAG-3, CD45, LFA-1, ICAM-1, and membrane-associated cytokines) might be co-factors/activators, although this might depend on the type, differentiation stage, and differentiation route of the target cells (i.e. monocytes/macrophages). This might explain the discrepancies between different studies.

To date, attempts to identify the surface factor primarily involved in the induction of cytokine production in monocytes/macrophages have failed to reach a clear-cut answer, and although inhibitors (e.g. antibodies) of surface molecules display some inhibitory effects, they fail to abolish monocyte activation. This suggests that the factor(s) essential for T-cell signaling of human monocytes by direct contact remain(s) to be identified. Furthermore, hierarchy and sequence of events, and involvement of the different surface molecules during this cross-talk still need to be established.

A clue to the identity of the activating factor was provided by the identification of a specific inhibitor of T-cell contact-mediated activation of monocytes. Indeed, the inhibition of T-cell signaling of monocytes might be important in that it would maintain a low level of monocyte activation within the blood stream. We identified apolipoprotein A-I (apo A-I) as a specific inhibitor of contact-mediated activation of monocytes.[83] Apo A-I is a 'negative acute-phase protein' and the principal protein of high-density lipoproteins (HDL). Variations in apo A-I concentration were observed in several inflammatory diseases and low levels of apo A-I in patients with chronic inflammatory diseases might be a link between infection and chronic inflammation.[84] Results obtained by using either recombinant

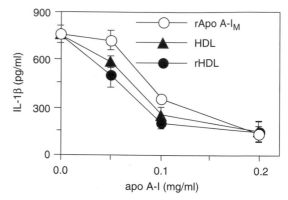

Figure 8.2 The production of IL-1β induced by contact with stimulated HUT-78 cells in human monocytes is inhibited to similar extents by isolated human HDL, reconstituted HDL (rHDL), and recombinant apo A-I$_{MILANO}$ (rApo A-I$_M$). Monocytes (50 × 10³ cells/200 µl/well; 96-well plates) were cultured for 24 hours with membranes isolated from PHA/PMA-stimulated HUT-78 cells (3 µg/ml proteins) in the presence of the indicated dose of HDL isolated from human blood (triangles), rHDL (closed circles), or rApo A-I$_M$ (open circles). IL-1β was measured in cultured supernatant as described previously.[83]

apo A-I$_{MILANO}$,[85] a natural mutant of apo A-I, or reconstituted HDL containing apo A-I as a single protein component[86] strengthened the importance of apo A-I in the inhibitory activity of HDL. Indeed, both forms of apo A-I displayed similar inhibitory activity to isolated human HDL in contact-mediated activation of monocytes (Figure 8.2). Recently, it was demonstrated that the T-cell contact-mediated induction of TNF in peripheral blood monocytes was inhibited by autologous sera from RA patients and that the production of TNF correlated inversely with apo A-I concentration in the latter sera.[87] This further confirms the anti-inflammatory effect of HDL-associated apo A-I. Besides, we observed that apo A-I was retained in the perivascular region of synovium of patients with active RA, i.e. in regions where infiltrating T cells were abundant.[88] We thus hypothesize that when the permeability of the vascular endothelium is increased due to inflammation, HDL-associated apo A-I diffuses into the pannus where it interacts with stimulating factors expressed on stimulated T cells, thus inhibiting cell–cell contact-induced cytokine production by monocytes/macrophages, as depicted in Figure 8.3.

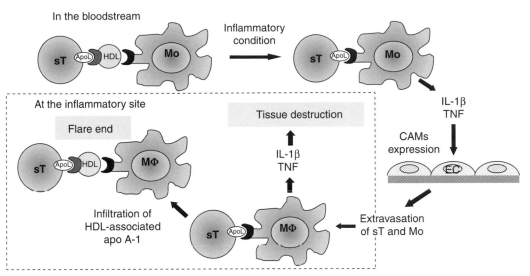

Figure 8.3 Hypothetical anti-inflammatory functions of HDL-associated apo A I in RA. In the bloodstream, upon remission or in health, HDL hamper the interaction between stimulated T cells (sT) and monocytes (Mo). Under inflammatory conditions, circulating HDL concentrations are lowered allowing the contact-mediated activation of monocytes and cytokine production; the latter in turn activate endothelial cells (EC) inducing cell adhesion molecules involved in the extravasation of T lymphocytes (sT) and monocytes (mo) into the inflammatory site. At the inflammatory site contact-mediated activation of macrophages (MΦ) occurs, leading to tissue destruction. At the same time, endothelial cells (EC) adopt an inflammatory phenotype allowing infiltration of HDL, which in turn inhibit contact-mediated activation of macrophages and thus temper inflammation, putting an end to the flare.

INTRACELLULAR PATHWAYS INVOLVED IN CYTOKINE PRODUCTION BY MONOCYTES/MACROPHAGES

LPS are the stimulus used most frequently *in vitro* in studies aiming to identify transduction pathways underlying cytokine production in monocytes/macrophages. However, other Toll-like receptor (TLR) ligands and cellular contact were also studied, although to a lesser extent. The induction of cytokine gene expression induced by the LPS receptor TLR4 involves components of transduction pathways that lead to the translocation of nuclear factor-κB (NF-κB) and activator protein-1 (AP-1).[89–91] Depending on the type of stimulus, different intracellular pathways in monocytes/macrophages lead to the production of a given cytokine. LPS and cellular contact with stimulated T cells can induce the production of both pro- and anti-inflammatory cytokines in human monocytes/macrophages (e.g. TNF, IL-1β, IL-12, sIL-1Ra, and IL-10). The tight control of proinflammatory cytokine production and activity is indeed a prerequisite

to avoiding a cascade of events that could lead to unbridled inflammation. For instance, in some cases sIL-1Ra is induced in the absence of IL-1, but from what is known at present, all stimuli eliciting IL-1β production also trigger sIL-1Ra production, at any rate in monocytes/macrophages. It is also well known that the production of both IL-1β and TNF is tightly regulated at several levels, including the dissociation between transcription, translation, and secretion.[92]

Some components of transcription pathways leading to cytokine synthesis have been identified after signaling by the engagement of specific cell surface molecules. For example, monocyte TNF production induced upon CD45 ligation (mimicking a cellular contact) or LPS activation was differentially modulated by phosphatidylinositide 3-kinases (PI3KS) and NF-κB but similarly regulated by p38 mitogen-activated protein kinase (MAPK). This suggests that both common and unique signaling pathways are utilized by different stimuli for the induction of TNF.[93] The differences in signaling pathway usage to induce identical cytokines were confirmed by data demonstrating the opposite effect of IFN-β on cytokine production by monocytes activated by LPS and contact with stimulated T cells.[59]

Macrophage colony-stimulating factor (M-CSF)-primed monocytes/macrophages produced IL-10 and TNF upon cellular contact with CD40L-transfected cells.[75] IL-10 production was dependent on PI3KS and their downstream substrates, protein kinase B (PKB, Akt) and p70 S6 kinase K (p70S6K), whereas TNF production was negatively regulated by PI3KS but dependent on p70S6K activity, bifurcating from the IL-10 pathway by utilizing p42/44 MAPK.[75] Thus, activation of macrophages by CD40L triggers two different pathways for the induction of IL-10 and TNF. In M-CSF-primed monocytes/macrophages activated by cellular contact with either cytokine-stimulated T cells or T cells isolated from RA synovial tissue, IL-10 was also triggered through a PI3K/p70S6K-dependent pathway.[94] Interestingly, the production of TNF by monocytes/macrophages upon contact with cytokine- but not anti-CD3-activated T lymphocytes is repressed by PI3KS.[65] Thus the production of pro- and anti-inflammatory cytokines upon monocytes/macrophages activation by cellular contact with T cells is utilizing different pathways, PI3KS being mainly involved in IL-10 induction, whereas NF-κB is involved in TNF production.[94,95] This strongly suggests that PI3KS are preferentially involved in pathways controlling the production of anti-inflammatory factors. We confirmed the involvement of PI3KS in the induction of anti-inflammatory cytokines in monocytes/macrophages by demonstrating that sIL-1Ra transcription required PI3K activation in human monocytes activated by IFN-β.[96] Furthermore, the balance between sIL-1Ra and IL-1β was controlled by PI3KS in both acute and chronic inflammatory conditions as exemplified by LPS and stimulated T-cell contact.[97] This was reminiscent of the control exerted by PI3KS in acute inflammatory conditions. Indeed, sIL-1Ra but not IL-1β translation is selectively triggerred via PI3K pathway, in 'septic' THP-1 cells.[97] Similarly, LPS from *Porphyromonas gingivalis* which bind TLR2 differentially induce IL-10 and IL-12 through PI3K activation.[99] Beside kinases

and NF-κB, upon contact with stimulated T cells, IL-1β and sIL-1Ra production in monocytic THP-1 cells is ruled by Ser/Thr phosphatase(s).[68] The latter cells express membrane-associated protease(s) neutralizing TNF activity both by degrading the cytokine and by cleaving its receptors at the cell surface.[67] Thus the triggering of these intra- and extracellular processes by direct contact with stimulated T lymphocytes may regulate the proinflammatory cytokines and their inhibitors, and the balance of their production in monocytes dictates in part the outcome of the chronic inflammatory process.[100]

STIMULATED T-CELL CONTACT-MEDIATED ACTIVATION OF MONOCYTES/MACROPHAGES AS A POTENTIAL THERAPEUTIC TARGET IN AUTOIMMUNE CHRONIC INFLAMMATORY DISEASES

Since the contact-mediated activation of monocytes/macrophages is a major pathway of cytokine production, the modulation of this mechanism, i.e. the blockade of IL-1 and TNF production at the triggering level, could be of therapeutic interest. We established that therapeutic agents administered to RA and MS patients, i.e. leflunomide, an inhibitor of dihydro-orotate dehydrogenase involved in pyrimidine synthesis[101–103] and IFN-β,[104,105] respectively, affected the contact-mediated activation of monocytes. Indeed, leflunomide inhibits the ability of stimulated T lymphocytes to trigger IL-1β production in monocytes, resulting in an enhancement of the sIL-1Ra/IL-1β molar ratio.[80] In addition to its effect on T-cell activating capacity, leflunomide also decreases the production of IL-1β and TNF, but not that of IL-1Ra in contact-activated monocytes, by directly acting on monocytes, as shown in Figure 8.4. Besides, the combination of methotrexate and leflunomide shows additive inhibitory effects on the production of inflammatory mediators (TNF, IL-1β, IL-6, ICAM-1, cyclooxygenase-1 and -2, and NF-κB) from synovial macrophages co-cultured with pre-activated Jurkat T cells.[62] This is consistent with clinical improvement observed in RA patients treated with leflunomide in combination therapy,

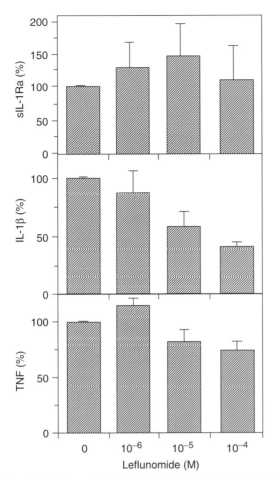

Figure 8.4 Leflunomide directly affects monocyte activation by cellular contact, inhibiting the production of both IL-1β and TNF but not that of sIL-1Ra. Monocytes were incubated for 2 hours in the presence or absence of the indicated dose of leflunomide before the addition of 3 μg/ml protein of membranes isolated from PHA/PMA-stimulated HUT-78 cells. Cells were activated for 24 hours and cytokines were measured in culture supernatants. Results are presented as the mean of three different experiments, 100% being defined as the production of the indicated cytokine in the absence of inhibitor.

although other synovial cells are affected by this drug including fibroblasts and articular chondrocytes.[106,107] In contact-mediated activation of monocytes, IFN-β not only inhibits IL-1β and TNF but it also stimulates sIL-1Ra production[108] in that it interferes with the activation of both T lymphocytes and monocytes.[81] More recently, we demonstrated that IFN-β displays opposite effects on cytokine homeostasis in

LPS- and T-cell contact-activated human monocytes.[59] Indeed, in monocytes activated by LPS, IFN-β enhanced the expression and production of IL-1β, TNF, and sIL-1Ra, suggesting that it does not display anti-inflammatory properties in this condition reflecting acute/infectious inflammation. In contrast, in monocytes activated by contact with stimulated T cells, i.e. in conditions mimicking chronic/ sterile inflammation, IFN-β inhibited the expression (mRNA) and production (protein) of IL-1β and TNF, while enhancing those of sIL-1Ra.[59] The premise that IFN-β displays opposite effects depending on the type of activation of human monocytes implies that it may affect different inflammatory mechanisms in opposite ways. Thus the induction of cytokines in acute and chronic inflammatory conditions occurs through different intracellular pathways. This might represent a clue to specific anti-inflammatory therapy. Another drug with anti-inflammatory properties, minocycline, that displays some efficacy in RA treatment,[109–111] was proved to affect contact-mediated activation of monocytes/macrophages. Indeed, minocycline attenuates T-cell and microglia activity thus affecting cytokine production in T-cell–microglia interaction, diminishing TNF production and simultaneously up-regulating IL-10 production.[79]

IMPACT OF GENDER ON CONTACT-MEDIATED ACTIVATION OF MONOCYTES/MACROPHAGES

RA and many other diseases associated with self-injury by the immune system are more common in women than in men.[112,113] As the distinct female preponderance in autoimmune diseases exists mainly during the reproductive age, sex hormone concentrations and metabolism have been evaluated in RA patients and have often been found to be changed.[114] Synovial fluid levels of proinflammatory estrogens relative to androgens are significantly elevated in both male and female RA patients, as compared with controls, which is most probably due to an increase in local enzymatic aromatase activity. Serum levels of estrogens have been found to be altered in RA patients, particularly estradiol in man. Thus, in the presence of inflammatory cytokines (i.e. TNF, IL-1, IL-6) available steroid prehormones are rapidly converted to proinflammatory estrogens in the synovial tissue.[115] *In vitro*, sex hormones influence cell proliferation and apoptosis of monocytic/ macrophage cells insofar as androgens increase the apoptosis, whilst estrogens tend to protect cells from death, both hormones acting as modulators of the NF-κB complex.[116] The influence of gender on contact-mediated activation of monocytes/macrophages was recently studied *in vitro* in a system related to MS, which like RA presents a gender bias, about 66% of all patients being female. In this study, myelin basic protein-primed T cells of female and castrated male but not normal male mice induced NO synthase and proinflammatory cytokine (IL-1β, IL-1α, IL-6, and TNF) production in microglial cells by cell–cell contact.[117] The mechanism underlying these differences was the activation of C/EBPβ by contact with neuroantigen-primed T cells from female but not from male mice. Thus contact-mediated activation of monocytes/macrophages by stimulated T cells could be one of the mechanisms behind the gender bias observed in chronic inflammatory diseases of autoimmune etiology like RA and MS.

T-CELL CONTACT-MEDIATED ACTIVATION OF OTHER CELL TYPES INVOLVED IN RA

A tremendous amount of information was generated identifying a variety of cell types involved in RA. Endothelial cells are present with an activated phenotype resembling high endothelial venule cells.[118] Infiltrating cells include T lymphocytes mainly in the perivascular region, monocytes/macrophages located together with fibroblast-like synoviocytes mainly in the pannus lining layer, and also B lymphocytes, mast cells, and DCs.[118–123] In contrast, neutrophils are mainly found in synovial fluid. Cytokines and contact with neighboring cells may affect the stage of activation of the above cell types. Although it is obvious that infiltrating cells (monocytes/macrophages, neutrophils) have to cross the perivascular layer of T cells or stay in T-cell-rich region (B cells), cell–cell contact with T cells is rarely seen in the pannus lining layer, i.e. the contact between fibroblast-like synoviocytes and T cells is hardly possible. However, cells can diffuse cell surface

molecules and thus ensure cellular contact by generating microparticles or microvesicles (MPs). MPs are fragments shed from the plasma membrane of stimulated or apoptotic cells. Having long been considered inert debris reflecting cellular activation or damage, MPs are now acknowledged as cellular effectors involved in cell–cell cross-talk.[124] Indeed, they harbor membrane proteins as well as bioactive lipids implicated in a variety of fundamental processes and are thus considered a disseminated storage pool of bioactive effectors.[125] MPs are found in the circulation of healthy subjects,[126–128] but their numbers can be increased in various pathological conditions such as thrombotic or infectious diseases.[127,129–133] Elevated MPs have also been reported in chronic inflammatory diseases[134–136] including RA.[137] In the latter disease, MPs are also abundant in the synovium,[138] where they may modulate fibroblast-like synoviocytes activity.[139,140] Since most cell types of which T cells can generate MPs,[139,141] this might represent a way for effector cells (e.g. T cells) to ship cellular contact from a distance. In this context preliminary data demonstrated that MPs generated by PHA/PMA-stimulated T cells induced IL-1β production in human monocytes that was inhibited in the presence of HDL (D. Burger, unpublished data). This suggests that similar activating molecules were present at the surface of stimulated T cells and MPs they released. Thus through the release of MPs, stimulated T cells might contact various cells other than mononuclear phagocytes that are involved in the pathogenic mechanisms. Such target cell types include interstitial fibroblast-like cells (synoviocytes), endothelial cells, and maybe migrating neutrophils. We observed that the latter cells were markedly affected by contact with stimulated T lymphocytes.[67,142–145] Indeed, cellular contact with stimulated T cells or MPs from the latter cells induces an imbalance between MMPs (MMP-1, MMP-3, MMP-9, and MMP-13) and tissue inhibitor of MMP (TIMP-1, TIMP-2, and TIMP-3) production by fibroblasts.[139,142] This was due to the length of the stimulation time of T lymphocytes. Indeed, T lymphocytes stimulated by PHA/PMA for 2–4 hours enhanced both TIMP-1 and MMP-1 production by synoviocytes, whereas T lymphocytes stimulated for 12–48 hours increased only the production of MMP-1 without affecting the expression of TIMP-1.[145] Since direct cell–cell contact with stimulated T lymphocytes induced an imbalance between the production *in vitro* of MMP and TIMP-1 by both monocytes and fibroblasts, it may, in analogy, favor tissue destruction *in vivo*. In addition to MMP-1 and TIMP-1, direct cell–cell contact with stimulated T lymphocytes induces PGE₂ production on human fibroblast-like synoviocytes[145] that also contributes to tissue destruction by favoring bone resorption. The T-cell surface molecules involved in MMP induction in fibroblasts are mainly membrane-associated IL-1 and TNF. Similarly, membrane-associated cytokines are involved in the inhibition of deposition of the major extracellular matrix components such as collagen types I and III. Indeed, direct contact with stimulated T cells markedly inhibited the synthesis of collagen types I and III in dermal fibroblasts and synoviocytes, whether untreated or treated with TGF-β. This inhibition was associated with a marked decrease in steady-state levels of pro-α I and pro-α III collagen mRNAs, which was due to a diminished transcription rate but not to a

significant alteration of the alpha 1(I) and alpha 1(III) transcript stability. This inhibition of extra-cellular matrix production mediated by T-cell contact was partially due to additive effects of T-cell membrane-associated IFN-γ, TNF, and IL-1α.[144] Thus, direct contact with stimulated T cells favors extracellular matrix catabolism by enhancing MMP production while diminishing collagen synthesis in fibroblasts and synoviocytes. Interestingly, similar membrane-associated cytokines were involved in both these processes. Cell-associated cytokines are not involved in contact-mediated activation of monocytes/ macrophages by T cells. By comparing the ability of T-cell clones to activate fibroblasts and monocytic cells, we found that there was no correlation (Figure 8.5). This confirms that different molecules at the surface of T cells are involved in the activation of these two target cell types.

It appears that the expression of ICAM-1, vascular cell adhesion molecule-1 (VCAM-1), and E-selectin is increased in the synovium of RA patients.[146-148] A similar phenomenon was observed in brain microvessels of MS patients.[149] In this regard, we demonstrated that membranes

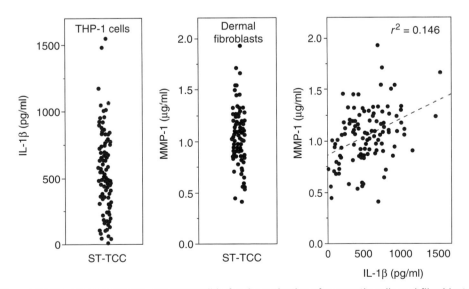

Figure 8.5 Different T-cell surface molecules are responsible for the activation of monocytic cells and fibroblasts. Eighty-eight T-cell clones generated from isolated T cells of RA synovium (ST-TCC) were stimulated for 48 hours with PHA/PMA and fixed[66] before coculture with THP-1 cells (50 × 10³ cells/200 µl/well; 96-well plate) and dermal fibroblasts (2 × 10⁴ cells/200 µl/well; 96-well plate) at 8:1 cellular ratio, respectively, for 48 hours. IL-1β and MMP-1 were measured in culture supernatants as described pereviously.[66,145]

of stimulated T lymphocytes induce the expression of ICAM-1, VCAM-1, and E-selectin on microvascular endothelial cells from human brain (HB-MVEC).[143] Beside cell adhesion molecules, contact-mediated activation of HB-MVEC induced the production of IL-6 and IL-8. The cell contact-induced expression of cell-adhesion molecules and the production of IL-6 and IL-8 were inhibited by TNF inhibitors, demonstrating that membrane-associated TNF was largely responsible for the activation of endothelial cells.[143] This suggests that both soluble and membrane-associated TNF can activate microvascular endothelium and that these two types of activation might be relevant to RA.[150] More recently, contact with T cells stimulated by either anti-CD3 or cytokines (TNF, IL-6, and IL-2) was shown to induce the expression and activation of tissue factor and the production of MCP-1, IL-8, and IL-6 in human umbilical vein endothelial cells (HUVEC) via CD40L–CD40 interaction.[151] Also in this case, different surface molecules are likely to play a part in the activation of endothelial cells upon direct cell–cell contact with stimulated T lymphocytes depending on the target cell type (i.e. microvascular or large vessel endothelial cells). These studies demonstrate that stimulated T lymphocytes could activate endothelial cells by direct contact, implying that this mechanism may be crucial to the extravasation of stimulated T lymphocytes into the target tissue. Furthermore, the induction of cytokine and chemokine production by endothelial cells upon contact with stimulated T lymphocytes might facilitate the invasion of the target tissue by other mononuclear cells.[143,151] TNF inhibitors decrease both endothelial cell and synoviocyte activation upon direct contact with stimulated T lymphocytes.[143–145] This may partly account for the beneficial effects of TNF blockade in RA.[152,153]

At an early stage of inflammation T lymphocytes could also be present in the tissue simultaneously with polymorphonuclear leukocytes (PMN), since the latter cells are recruited to sites of inflammation where they are in close vicinity to other immune cell types. This was recently confirmed by the premise that contact-mediated activation of human PMN respiratory burst was inhibited by HDLs.[154] Thus HDLs inhibit both T-cell contact-induced cytokine production in monocytes/macrophages and radical oxygen species (ROS) production induced in PMN upon contact with stimulated T cells. This confirms that similar molecules at the surface of T cells are involved in the activation of PMNs and monocytes/macrophages, as suggested by the premise that the activating capability of T-cell clones on PMNs correlates with that on THP-1 cells ($r^2 = 0.84$, $p < 0.001$).[66] This supports the emerging role of HDL as immunomodulators in inflammatory diseases. Furthermore, activated PMNs can in turn release potent anti-inflammatory MPs, in the form of ectosomes, which inhibit macrophage activation.[155]

Thus, the contact with stimulated T cells may activate several cell types involved in RA. While cytokine blockade prevents the activation of fibroblast-like synoviocytes and endothelial cells, HDL inhibit the activation of neutrophils and monocytes. This suggests that contact-mediated activation of neighboring cells is a fundamental process used by T cells to affect the activation status of other cells, even though the surface molecules involved in these processes are different. Furthermore, through the release of MPs, this T-cell activity might spread out and reach cells that are not directly in contact with the effector T cell.

CONCLUSIONS

As depicted in Figure 8.6, cell contact with stimulated T cells may affect the activity of several cell types involved in RA pathology either directly or by releasing MPs. To date, direct cell–cell contact with stimulated T cells is considered the main pathway triggering activation of monocytes/macrophages in the absence of infectious agents. The potency of this mechanism suggests that it is a major pathway by which T lymphocytes exert their pathogenic effect in chronic destructive immuno-inflammatory diseases. Additional investigations are needed to identify the surface molecules – ligands and counter-ligands – involved in this process. However, the control of contact-mediated signaling of monocytes and neutrophils by HDL-associated apo A-I might represent an interesting step toward developing a novel

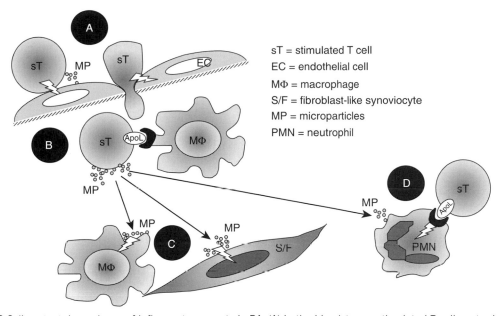

Figure 8.6 Cell contact dependence of inflammatory events in RA. (A) In the bloodstream stimulated T cells enter into contact with capillary endothelial cells in which they induce the expression of cell-adhesion molecules (ICAM-1, VCAM-1, E-selectin), cytokines (IL-6), and chemokines (IL-8)[143] leading to infiltrating cell extravasation. (B) In the perivascular region, stimulated T cells are in close contact with monocytes/macrophages, inducing cytokine and MMP production. (C) In the synovial lining layer, MPs produced by stimulated T cells might activate macrophage- and fibroblast-like synoviocytes. (D) In the synovial fluid, where both PMNs and T cells are present, stimulated T cells may activate PMNs through both direct cellular contact and MP projection. sT, stimulated T cell; EC, endothelial cell; MΦ, macrophage; S/F, fibroblast-like synoviocyte; MP, microparticles; PMN, neutrophil.

approach for dampening down the inflammatory response induced by cell–cell contact and leading to tissue destruction in chronic inflammatory diseases. It also extends the concept of inflammation in connection with lipid metabolism and other diseases such as arteriosclerosis. Stimulated T lymphocytes, which might establish cellular contact with fibroblasts or synoviocytes via the release of MPs, might also be responsible for the decrease in collagen synthesis and the increase in MMP production and may therefore play a part in the lack of repair process.

ACKNOWLEDGMENTS

The authors are indebted to Mrs Roswitha Rehm for skilful reading of the manuscript. We are grateful to Drs G. Franceschini and L. Calabresi (Center E. Grossi Paoletti, Milano, Italy) and to Dr P.G. Lerch (ZLB Central Laboratory, Bern, Switzerland) for the gifts of recombinant apo A-I$_{MILANO}$ and reconstituted HDL, respectively. Credit for experiments presented in Figures 8.2, 8.4, and 8.5 is due to Dr N. Hyka-Nouspickel, Dr J.M. Li, Mrs N. Begue-Pastor, and Mrs L. Gruaz. Unpublished results reported above were part of projects supported by grant #3200.068286.02 from the Swiss National Science Foundation as well as a grant from the Swiss Society for Multiple Sclerosis.

REFERENCES

1. Burger D, Dayer JM. Inhibitory cytokines and cytokine inhibitors. Neurology 1995; 45: S39–S43.
2. Burger D, Dayer JM. The balance between pro- and anti-inflammatory cytokines. In: Smolen JS, Lipsky PE, eds. Targeted Therapies in Rheumatology. London: Martin Dunitz, 2003: 329–43.
3. Dinarello CA. The many worlds of reducing interleukin-1. Arthritis Rheum 2005; 52(7): 1960–7.
4. Sacre SM, Andreakos E, Taylor P, Feldmann M, Foxwell BM. Molecular therapeutic targets in rheumatoid arthritis. Expert Rev Mol Med 2005; 7(16): 1–20.

5. Bresnihan B, Newmark R, Robbins S, Genant HK. Effects of anakinra monotherapy on joint damage in patients with rheumatoid arthritis. Extension of a 24-week randomized, placebo-controlled trial. J Rheumatol 2004; 31(6): 1103–11.

6. Bartolucci P, Ramanoelina J, Cohen P et al. Efficacy of the anti-TNF-alpha antibody infliximab against refractory systemic vasculitides: an open pilot study on 10 patients. Rheumatology (Oxford) 2002; 41(10): 1126–32.

7. Lorenz HM, Kalden JR. Perspectives for TNF-alpha-targeting therapies. Arthritis Res 2002; 4(Suppl 3): S17–S24.

8. Kalden JR. Emerging role of anti-tumor necrosis factor therapy in rheumatic diseases. Arthritis Res 2002; 4(Suppl 2): S34–S40.

9. Brandt J, Haibel H, Reddig J, Sieper J, Braun J. Successful short term treatment of severe undifferentiated spondyloarthropathy with the anti-tumor necrosis factor-alpha monoclonal antibody infliximab. J Rheumatol 2002; 29(1): 118–22.

10. Wollina U, Konrad H. Treatment of recalcitrant psoriatic arthritis with anti-tumor necrosis factor-alpha antibody. J Eur Acad Dermatol Venereol 2002; 16(2): 127–9.

11. Sfikakis PP. Behçet's disease: a new target for anti-tumour necrosis factor treatment. Ann Rheum Dis 2002; 61(Suppl 2): ii51–ii53.

12. Lee RZ, Veale DJ. Management of spondyloarthropathy: new pharmacological treatment options. Drugs 2002; 62(16): 2349–59.

13. Murray KJ, Lovell DJ. Advanced therapy for juvenile arthritis. Best Pract Res Clin Rheumatol 2002; 16(3): 361–78.

14. Stout RD, Suttles J. Functional plasticity of macrophages: reversible adaptation to changing microenvironments. J Leukoc Biol 2004; 76(3): 509–13.

15. Tracey KJ. The inflammatory reflex. Nature 2002; 420(6917): 853–9.

16. Daems WT, de Bakker JM. Do resident macrophages proliferate? Immunobiology 1982; 161(3–4): 204–11.

17. Metcalf D, Elliott MJ, Nicola NA. The excess numbers of peritoneal macrophages in granulocyte-macrophage colony-stimulating factor transgenic mice are generated by local proliferation. J Exp Med 1992; 175(4): 877–84.

18. Chen BD, Mueller M, Chou TH. Role of granulocyte/macrophage colony-stimulating factor in the regulation of murine alveolar macrophage proliferation and differentiation. J Immunol 1988; 141(1): 139–44.

19. Kennedy DW, Abkowitz JL. Kinetics of central nervous system microglial and macrophage engraftment: analysis using a transgenic bone marrow transplantation model. Blood 1997; 90(3): 986–93.

20. Laskin DL, Weinberger B, Laskin JD. Functional heterogeneity in liver and lung macrophages. J Leukoc Biol 2001; 70(2): 163–70.

21. Guillemin GJ, Brew BJ. Microglia, macrophages, perivascular macrophages, and pericytes: a review of function and identification. J Leukoc Biol 2004; 75(3): 388–97.

22. Meldrum DR, Cleveland JC Jr, Moore EE et al. Adaptive and maladaptive mechanisms of cellular priming. Ann Surg 1997; 226(5): 587–98.

23. Stout RD, Suttles J. T-cell signaling of macrophage activation: cell contact-dependent and cytokine signals. New York: Springer, 1995.

24. Gordon S, Fraser I, Nath D, Hughes D, Clarke S. Macrophages in tissues and in vitro. Curr Opin Immunol 1992; 4(1): 25–32.

25. Ziegler-Heitbrock HWL, Ulevitch RJ. CD14: cell surface receptor and differentiation marker. Immunol Today 1993; 14: 121–5.

26. Passlick B, Flieger D, Ziegler-Heitbrock HWL. Identification and characterization of a novel monocyte subpopulation in human peripheral blood. Blood 1989; 74: 2527–34.

27. Ziegler-Heitbrock HW, Fingerle G, Strobel M et al. The novel subset of CD14+/CD16+ blood monocytes exhibits features of tissue macrophages. Eur J Immunol 1993; 23(9): 2053–8.

28. Frankenberger M, Sternsdorf T, Pechumer H, Pforte A, Ziegler-Heitbrock HW. Differential cytokine expression in human blood monocyte subpopulations: a polymerase chain reaction analysis. Blood 1996; 87(1): 373–7.

29. Ziegler-Heitbrock HW. Heterogeneity of human blood monocytes: the CD14+ CD16+ subpopulation. Immunol Today 1996; 17(9): 424–8.

30. Siedlar M, Frankenberger M, Ziegler-Heitbrock LH, Belge KU. The M-DC8-positive leukocytes are a subpopulation of the CD14+ CD16+ monocytes. Immunobiology 2000; 202(1): 11–17.

31. de Baey A, Mende I, Riethmueller G, Baeuerle PA. Phenotype and function of human dendritic cells derived from M-DC8(+) monocytes. Eur J Immunol 2001; 31(6): 1646–55.

32. Fingerle G, Pforte A, Passlick B et al. The novel subset of CD14+/CD16+ blood monocytes is expanded in sepsis patients. Blood 1993; 82(10): 3170–6.

33. Kawanaka N, Yamamura M, Aita T et al. CD14+,CD16+ blood monocytes and joint inflammation in rheumatoid arthritis. Arthritis Rheum 2002; 46(10): 2578–86.

34. Cairns AP, Crockard AD, Bell AL. The CD14+ CD16+ monocyte subset in rheumatoid arthritis and systemic lupus erythematosus. Rheumatol Int 2002; 21(5): 189–92.

35. Then BF, Dayyani F, Ziegler-Heitbrock L. Impact of type-I-interferon on monocyte subsets and their differentiation to dendritic cells. An in vivo and ex vivo study in multiple sclerosis patients treated with interferon-beta. J Neuroimmunol 2004; 146(1–2): 176–88.

36. Kouwenhoven M, Teleshova N, Ozenci V, Press R, Link H. Monocytes in multiple sclerosis: phenotype and

cytokine profile. J Neuroimmunol 2001; 112(1–2): 197–205.

37. Gordon S. Alternative activation of macrophages. Nat Rev Immunol 2003; 3(1): 23–35.

38. Stout RD, Suttles J. T cell signaling of macrophage function in inflammatory disease. Front Biosci 1997; 2: 197–206.

39. Tak PP, Smeets TJM, Daha MR et al. Analysis of the synovial cell infiltrate in early rheumatoid synovial tissue in relation to local disease activity. Arthritis Rheum 1997; 40: 217–25.

40. Smeets TJ, Kraan MC, Galjaard S et al. Analysis of the cell infiltrate and expression of matrix metalloproteinases and granzyme B in paired synovial biopsy specimens from the cartilage-pannus junction in patients with RA. Ann Rheum Dis 2001; 60(6): 561–5.

41. Davis LS, Geppert TD, Meek K, Oppenheimer-Marks N, Lipsky PE. Immune and inflammatory responses. In: Kelley WN, Harris ED Jr, Ruddy S, Sledge CS, eds. Textbook of Rheumatology. Philadelphia: WB Saunders, 1997: 95–127.

42. Schulze-Koops H, Kalden JR. The balance of Th1/Th2 cytokines in rheumatoid arthritis. Best Pract Res Clin Rheumatol 2001; 15(5): 677–91.

43. Elliott CL, El Touny SY, Filipi ML, Healey KM, Leuschen MP. Interferon beta1a treatment modulates TH1 expression in gammadelta + T cells from relapsing-remitting multiple sclerosis patients. J Clin Immunol 2001; 21(3): 200–9.

44. Laman JD, Thompson EJ, Kappos L. Balancing the Th1/Th2 concept in multiple sclerosis. Immunol Today 1998; 19(11): 489–90.

45. Wong WM, Vakis SA, Ayre KR et al. Rheumatoid arthritis T cells produce Th1 cytokines in response to stimulation with a novel trispecific antibody directed against CD2, CD3, and CD28. Scand J Rheumatol 2000; 29(5): 282–7.

46. Skapenko A, Leipe J, Lipsky PE, Schulze-Koops H. The role of the T cell in autoimmune inflammation. Arthritis Res Ther 2005; 7(Suppl 2): S4–S14.

47. Harris ED. Rheumatoid Arthritis. Philadelphia: WB Saunders, 1997.

48. Vey E, Zhang JH, Dayer J-M. IFN-gamma and 1,25(OH)2D3 induce on THP-1 cells distinct patterns of cell surface antigen expression, cytokine production, and responsiveness to contact with activated T cells. J Immunol 1992; 149: 2040–6.

49. Isler P, Vey E, Zhang JH, Dayer JM. Cell surface glycoproteins expressed on activated human T-cells induce production of interleukin-1 beta by monocytic cells: a possible role of CD69. Eur Cytokine Netw 1993; 4: 15–23.

50. Lacraz S, Isler P, Vey E, Welgus HG, Dayer JM. Direct contact between T lymphocytes and monocytes is a major pathway for induction of metalloproteinase expression. J Biol Chem 1994; 269: 22027–33.

51. McInnes IB, Leung BP, Sturrock RD, Field M, Liew FY. Interleukin-15 mediates T cell-dependent regulation of tumor necrosis factor-alpha production in rheumatoid arthritis. Nat Med 1997; 3: 189–95.

52. Parry SL, Sebbag M, Feldmann M, Brennan FM. Contact with T cells modulates monocyte IL-10 production. Role of T cell membrane TNF-alpha. J Immunol 1997; 158: 3673–81.

53. Sebbag M, Parry SL, Brennan FM, Feldmann M. Cytokine stimulation of T lymphocytes regulates their capacity to induce monocyte production of tumor necrosis factor-alpha, but not interleukin-10: possible relevance to pathophysiology of rheumatoid arthritis. Eur J Immunol 1997; 27: 624–32.

54. Avice MN, Demeure CE, Delespesse G et al. IL-15 promotes IL-12 production by human monocytes via T cell-dependent contact and may contribute to IL-12-mediated IFN-gamma secretion by CD4+ T cells in the absence of TCR ligation. J Immunol 1998; 161(7): 3408–15.

55. Avice MN, Sarfati M, Triebel F, Delespesse G, Demeure CE. Lymphocyte activation gene-3, a MHC class II ligand expressed on activated T cells, stimulates TNF-alpha and IL-alpha production by monocytes and dendritic cells. J Immunol 1999; 162(5): 2748–53.

56. Chabot S, Charlet D, Wilson TL, Yong VW. Cytokine production consequent to T cell–microglia interaction: the PMA/IFN gamma-treated U937 cells display similarities to human microglia. J Neurosci Methods 2001; 105(2): 111–20.

57. Burger D, Roux-Lombard P, Chizzolini C, Dayer JM. Cell-cell contact in chronic inflammation: the importance to cytokine regulation in tissue destruction and repair. In: van den Berg WB, Miossec P, eds. Cytokines and Joint Injury. Basel: Birkhäuser Verlag, 2004: 165–88.

58. Burger D. Cell contact-mediated signaling of monocytes by stimulated T cells: a major pathway for cytokine induction. Eur Cytokine Netw 2000; 11(3): 346–53.

59. Molnarfi N, Gruaz L, Dayer JM, Burger D. Opposite effects of IFNbeta on cytokine homeostasis in LPS- and T cell contact-activated human monocytes. J Neuroimmunol 2004; 146(1–2): 76–83.

60. Weaver CT, Unanue ER. T cell induction of membrane IL-1 on macrophages. J Immunol 1986; 137: 3868–73.

61. Landis CB, Friedman ML, Fisher RI, Ellis TM. Induction of human monocyte IL-1 mRNA and secretion during anti-CD3 mitogenesis requires two distinct T cell-derived signals. J Immunol 1991; 146: 128–35.

62. Cutolo M, Capellino S, Montagna P et al. Antiinflammatory effects of leflunomide in combination with methotrexate

on co-culture of T lymphocytes and synovial macrophages from rheumatoid arthritis patients. Ann Rheum Dis 2006; 65: 728–35.

63. Dasgupta S, Jana M, Liu X, Pahan K. Role of very-late antigen-4 (VLA-4) in myelin basic protein-primed T cell contact-induced expression of proinflammatory cytokines in microglial cells. J Biol Chem 2003; 278(25): 22424–31.

64. Chabot S, Williams G, Yong VW. Microglial production of TNF-alpha is induced by activated T lymphocytes. Involvement of VLA-4 and inhibition by interferon beta-1b. J Clin Invest 1997; 100: 604–12.

65. Brennan FM, Hayes AL, Ciesielski CJ et al. Evidence that rheumatoid arthritis synovial T cells are similar to cytokine-activated T cells: involvement of phosphatidylinositol 3-kinase and nuclear factor kappaB pathways in tumor necrosis factor alpha production in rheumatoid arthritis. Arthritis Rheum 2002; 46(1): 31–41.

66. Li JM, Isler P, Dayer JM, Burger D. Contact-dependent stimulation of monocytic cells and neutrophils by stimulated human T-cell clones. Immunology 1995; 84: 571–6.

67. Vey E, Burger D, Dayer JM. Expression and cleavage of tumor necrosis factor-alpha and tumor necrosis factor receptors by human monocytic cell lines upon direct contact with stimulated T cells. Eur J Immunol 1996; 26: 2404–9.

68. Vey E, Dayer JM, Burger D. Direct contact with stimulated T cells induces the expression of IL-1 beta and IL-1 receptor antagonist in human monocytes. Involvement of serine/threonine phosphatases in differential regulation. Cytokine 1997; 9: 480–7.

69. Chizzolini C, Chicheportiche R, Burger D, Dayer JM. Human Th1 cells preferentially induce interleukin (IL)-1beta while Th2 cells induce IL-1 receptor antagonist production upon cell/cell contact with monocytes. Eur J Immunol 1997; 27(1): 171–7.

70. Chabot S, Williams G, Hamilton M, Sutherland G, Yong VW. Mechanisms of IL-10 production in human microglia-T cell interaction. J Immunol 1999; 162(11): 6819–28.

71. Dunlap NE, Tilden AB. T helper/inducer (CD4+) cells prestimulated with PPD induce monocytes to produce interleukin-1β. J Leukoc Biol 1991; 49: 542–7.

72. Ribbens C, Dayer JM, Chizzolini C. CD40-CD40 ligand (CD154) engagement is required but may not be sufficient for human T helper 1 cell induction of interleukin-2- or interleukin-15-driven, contact-dependent, interleukin-1beta production by monocytes. Immunology 2000; 99(2): 279–86.

73. Dai SM, Matsuno H, Nakamura H, Nishioka K, Yudoh K. Interleukin-18 enhances monocyte tumor necrosis factor alpha and interleukin-1beta production induced by direct contact with T lymphocytes: implications in

74. Foey AD, Feldmann M, Brennan FM. Route of monocyte differentiation determines their cytokine production profile: CD40 ligation induces interleukin 10 expression. Cytokine 2000; 12(10): 1496–505.

75. Foey AD, Feldmann M, Brennan FM. CD40 ligation induces macrophage IL-10 and TNF-alpha production: differential use of the PI3K and p42/44 MAPK-pathways. Cytokine 2001; 16(4): 131–42.

76. Burger D, Molnarfi N, Gruaz L, Dayer JM. Differential induction of IL-1beta and TNF by CD40 ligand or cellular contact with stimulated T cells depends on the maturation stage of human monocytes. J Immunol 2004; 173(2): 1292–7.

77. Stout RD, Suttles J, Xu J, Grewal IS, Flavell RA. Impaired T cell-mediated macrophage activation in CD40 ligand-deficient mice. J Immunol 1996; 156(1): 8–11.

78. Suttles J, Milhorn DM, Miller RW et al. CD40 signaling of monocyte inflammatory cytokine synthesis through an ERK1/2-dependent pathway. A target of interleukin (IL)- 4 and IL-10 anti-inflammatory action. J Biol Chem 1999; 274(9): 5835–42.

79. Giuliani F, Hader W, Yong VW. Minocycline attenuates T cell and microglia activity to impair cytokine production in T cell-microglia interaction. J Leukoc Biol 2005; 78(1): 135–43.

80. Déage V, Burger D, Dayer JM. Exposure of T lymphocytes to leflunomide but not to dexamethasone favors the production by monocytic cells of interleukin-1 receptor antagonist and the tissue-inhibitor of metalloproteinases-1 over that of interleukin-1beta and metalloproteinases. Eur Cytokine Netw 1998; 9(4): 663–8.

81. Jungo F, Dayer JM, Modoux C, Hyka N, Burger D. IFN-beta inhibits the ability of T lymphocytes to induce TNF-alpha and IL-1beta production in monocytes upon direct cell-cell contact. Cytokine 2001; 14(5): 272–82.

82. Chabot S, Yong FP, Le DM et al. Cytokine production in T lymphocyte-microglia interaction is attenuated by glatiramer acetate: a mechanism for therapeutic efficacy in multiple sclerosis. Mult Scler 2002; 8(4): 299–306.

83. Hyka N, Dayer JM, Modoux C et al. Apolipoprotein A-I inhibits the production of interleukin-1beta and tumor necrosis factor-alpha by blocking contact-mediated activation of monocytes by T lymphocytes. Blood 2001; 97(8): 2381–9.

84. Burger D, Dayer JM. High-density lipoprotein-associated apolipoprotein A-I: the missing link between infection and chronic inflammation? Autoimmun Rev 2002; 1: 111–17.

85. Soma MR, Donetti E, Parolini C et al. Recombinant apolipoprotein A-IMilano dimer inhibits carotid intimal thickening induced by perivascular manipulation in rabbits. Circ Res 1995; 76(3): 405–11.

86. Lerch PG, Fortsch V, Hodler G, Bolli R. Production and characterization of a reconstituted high density lipoprotein for therapeutic applications. Vox Sang 1996; 71(3): 155–64.

87. Rossol M, Kaltenhauser S, Scholz R et al. The contact-mediated response of peripheral-blood monocytes to preactivated T cells is suppressed by serum factors in rheumatoid arthritis. Arthritis Res Ther 2005; 7(6): R1189–R1199.

88. Bresnihan B, Gogarty M, Fitzgerald O, Dayer J-M, Burger D. Apolipoprotein A-I infiltration in rheumatoid arthritis synovial tissue: a control mechanism of cytokine production? Arthritis Res Ther 2004; 6: R563–R566.

89. Beutler B. Toll-like receptors: how they work and what they do. Curr Opin Hematol 2002; 9(1): 2–10.

90. Aderem A, Ulevitch RJ. Toll-like receptors in the induction of the innate immune response. Nature 2000; 406(6797): 782–7.

91. Beutler B. Inferences, questions and possibilities in Toll-like receptor signalling. Nature 2004; 430(6996): 257–63.

92. Schindler R, Gelfand JA, Dinarello CA. Recombinant C5a stimulates transcription rather than translation of interleukin-1 (IL-1) and tumor necrosis factor: translational signal provided by lipopolysaccharide or IL-1 itself. Blood 1990; 76(8): 1631–8.

93. Hayes AL, Smith C, Foxwell BM, Brennan FM. CD45-induced tumor necrosis factor alpha production in monocytes is phosphatidylinositol 3-kinase-dependent and nuclear factor- kappaB-independent. J Biol Chem 1999; 274(47): 33455–61.

94. Foey AD, Green P, Foxwell B, Feldmann M, Brennan F. Cytokine-stimulated T cells induce macrophage IL-10 production dependent on phosphatidylinositol 3-kinase and p70S6K: implications for rheumatoid arthritis. Arthritis Res 2002; 4: 64–70.

95. Foxwell BM, Browne K, Bondeson J et al. Efficient adenoviral infection with IkappaB alpha reveals that macrophage tumor necrosis factor alpha production in rheumatoid arthritis is NF-kappaB dependent. Proc Natl Acad Sci U S A 1998; 95(14): 8211–15.

96. Molnarfi N, Hyka-Nouspikel N, Gruaz L, Dayer JM, Burger D. The production of IL-1 receptor antagonist in IFN-{beta}-stimulated human monocytes depends on the activation of phosphatidylinositol 3-kinase but not of STAT1. J Immunol 2005; 174(5): 2974–80.

97. Molnarfi N, Gruaz L, Dayer JM, et al. Opposite regualtion of IL-1beta and secreted IL-1 receptor antagonist production by phosphatidylinositide-3 kinases in human monocytes activated by lipopolysaccharides or contact with T cells J Immunol 2007; 178(1):446-454.

98. Learn CA, Boger MS, Li L, McCall CE. The phosphatidylinositol 3-kinase pathway selectively controls sIL-1RA not interleukin-1beta production in the septic leukocytes. J Biol Chem 2001; 276(23): 20234–9.

99. Martin M, Schifferle RE, Cuesta N et al. Role of the phosphatidylinositol 3 kinase-Akt pathway in the regulation of IL-10 and IL-12 by *Porphyromonas gingivalis* lipopolysaccharide. J Immunol 2003; 171(2): 717–25.

100. Burger D, Dayer JM. Cell-cell interactions in chronic inflammation: modulation of surrounding cells by direct contact with stimulated T lymphocytes. In: Schneider CH, ed. Peptides in Immunology. Chichester: John Wiley and Sons, 1996: 159–64.

101. Williamson RA, Yea CM, Robson PA et al. Dihydroorotate dehydrogenase is a target for the biological effects of leflunomide. Transplant Proc 1996; 28(6): 3088–91.

102. Tugwell P, Wells G, Strand V et al. Clinical improvement as reflected in measures of function and health-related quality of life following treatment with leflunomide compared with methotrexate in patients with rheumatoid arthritis: sensitivity and relative efficiency to detect a treatment effect in a twelve-month, placebo-controlled trial. Leflunomide Rheumatoid Arthritis Investigators Group. Arthritis Rheum 2000; 43(3): 506–14.

103. Sharp JT, Strand V, Leung H, Hurley F, Loew-Friedrich I. Treatment with leflunomide slows radiographic progression of rheumatoid arthritis: results from three randomized controlled trials of leflunomide in patients with active rheumatoid arthritis. Leflunomide Rheumatoid Arthritis Investigators Group. Arthritis Rheum 2000; 43(3): 495–505.

104. Arnason BG. Treatment of multiple sclerosis with interferon beta. Biomed Pharmacother 1999; 53(8): 344–50.

105. Tak PP. IFN-beta in rheumatoid arthritis. Front Biosci 2004; 9: 3242–7.

106. Burger D, Begue-Pastor N, Benavent S et al. The active metabolite of leflunomide, A77 1726, inhibits the production of prostaglandin E(2), matrix metalloproteinase 1 and interleukin 6 in human fibroblast-like synoviocytes. Rheumatology (Oxford) 2003; 42(1): 89–96.

107. Palmer G, Burger D, Mezin F et al. The active metabolite of leflunomide, A77 1726, increases the production of IL-1 receptor antagonist in human synovial fibroblasts and articular chondrocytes. Arthritis Res Ther 2004; 6(3): R181–R189.

108. Coclet-Ninin J, Dayer JM, Burger D. Interferon-beta not only inhibits interleukin-1 beta and tumor necrosis factor-alpha but stimulates interleukin-1 receptor antagonist production in human peripheral blood mononuclear cells. Eur Cytokine Netw 1997; 8: 345–9.

109. Suresh E, Morris IM, Mattingly PC. Use of minocycline in rheumatoid arthritis: a district general hospital experience. Ann Rheum Dis 2004; 63(10): 1354–5.

110. O'Dell JR, Blakely KW, Mallek JA et al. Treatment of early seropositive rheumatoid arthritis: a two-year, double-blind comparison of minocycline and hydroxychloroquine. Arthritis Rheum 2001; 44(10): 2235–41.

111. O'Dell JR, Paulsen G, Haire CE et al. Treatment of early seropositive rheumatoid arthritis with minocycline: four-year followup of a double-blind, placebo-controlled trial. Arthritis Rheum 1999; 42(8): 1691–5.

112. Beeson PB. Age and sex associations of 40 autoimmune diseases. Am J Med 1994; 96(5): 457–62.

113. Fox HS. Sex steroids and the immune system. Ciba Found Symp 1995; 191: 203–11.

114. Cutolo M. Do sex hormones modulate the synovial macrophages in rheumatoid arthritis? Ann Rheum Dis 1997; 56(5): 281–84.

115. Cutolo M, Sulli A, Capellino S et al. Sex hormones influence on the immune system: basic and clinical aspects in autoimmunity. Lupus 2004; 13(9): 635–8.

116. Cutolo M, Capellino S, Montagna P et al. Sex hormone modulation of cell growth and apoptosis of the human monocytic/macrophage cell line. Arthritis Res Ther 2005; 7(5): R1124–R1132.

117. Dasgupta S, Jana M, Liu X, Pahan K. Myelin basic protein-primed T cells of female but not male mice induce nitric-oxide synthase and proinflammatory cytokines in microglia: implications for gender bias in multiple sclerosis. J Biol Chem 2005; 280: 32609–17.

118. Dinther-Janssen AC, Pals ST, Scheper R, Breedveld F, Meijer CJ. Dendritic cells and high endothelial venules in the rheumatoid synovial membrane. J Rheumatol 1990; 17(1): 11–17.

119. Kang YM, Zhang X, Wagner UG et al. CD8 T cells are required for the formation of ectopic germinal centers in rheumatoid synovitis. J Exp Med 2002; 195(10): 1325–36.

120. De Vita S, Zaja F, Sacco S et al. Efficacy of selective B cell blockade in the treatment of rheumatoid arthritis: evidence for a pathogenetic role of B cells. Arthritis Rheum 2002; 46(8): 2029–33.

121. Kim HJ, Berek C. B cells in rheumatoid arthritis. Arthritis Res 2000; 2(2): 126–31.

122. Tetlow LC, Woolley DE. Mast cells, cytokines, and metalloproteinases at the rheumatoid lesion: dual immunolocalisation studies. Ann Rheum Dis 1995; 54(11): 896–903.

123. Tetlow LC, Woolley DE. Distribution, activation and tryptase/chymase phenotype of mast cells in the rheumatoid lesion. Ann Rheum Dis 1995; 54(7): 549–55.

124. Morel O, Toti F, Hugel B, Freyssinet JM. Cellular microparticles: a disseminated storage pool of bioactive vascular effectors. Curr Opin Hematol 2004; 11(3): 156–64.

125. Hugel B, Martinez MC, Kunzelmann C, Freyssinet JM. Membrane microparticles: two sides of the coin. Physiology 2005; 20: 22–7.

126. Berckmans RJ, Neiuwland R, Boing AN et al. Cell-derived microparticles circulate in healthy humans and support low grade thrombin generation. Thromb Haemost 2001; 85(4): 639–46.

127. Joop K, Berckmans RJ, Nieuwland R et al. Microparticles from patients with multiple organ dysfunction syndrome and sepsis support coagulation through multiple mechanisms. Thromb Haemost 2001; 85(5): 810–20.

128. Nieuwland R, Berckmans RJ, Rotteveel-Eijkman RC et al. Cell-derived microparticles generated in patients during cardiopulmonary bypass are highly procoagulant. Circulation 1997; 96(10): 3534–41.

129. Nieuwland R, Berckmans RJ, McGregor S et al. Cellular origin and procoagulant properties of microparticles in meningococcal sepsis. Blood 2000; 95(3): 930–5.

130. Osmanovic N, Romijn FP, Joop K, Sturk A, Nieuwland R. Soluble selectins in sepsis: microparticle-associated, but only to a minor degree. Thromb Haemost 2000; 84(4): 731–2.

131. Fujimi S, Ogura H, Tanaka H et al. Activated polymorphonuclear leukocytes enhance production of leukocyte microparticles with increased adhesion molecules in patients with sepsis. J Trauma 2002; 52(3): 443–8.

132. Ogura H, Kawasaki T, Tanaka H et al. Activated platelets enhance microparticle formation and platelet-leukocyte interaction in severe trauma and sepsis. J Trauma 2001; 50(5): 801–9.

133. Geisbert TW, Young HA, Jahrling PB et al. Mechanisms underlying coagulation abnormalities in ebola hemorrhagic fever: overexpression of tissue factor in primate monocytes/macrophages is a key event. J Infect Dis 2003; 188(11): 1618–29.

134. Combes V, Simon AC, Grau GE et al. In vitro generation of endothelial microparticles and possible prothrombotic activity in patients with lupus anticoagulant. J Clin Invest 1999; 104(1): 93–102.

135. Brogan PA, Shah V, Brachet C et al. Endothelial and platelet microparticles in vasculitis of the young. Arthritis Rheum 2004; 50(3): 927–36.

136. Minagar A, Jy W, Jimenez JJ et al. Elevated plasma endothelial microparticles in multiple sclerosis. Neurology 2001; 56(10): 1319–24.

137. Knijff-Dutmer EA, Koerts J, Nieuwland R, Kalsbeek-Batenburg EM, van de Laar MA. Elevated levels of platelet microparticles are associated with disease activity in rheumatoid arthritis. Arthritis Rheum 2002; 46(6): 1498–503.

138. Berckmans RJ, Nieuwland R, Tak PP et al. Cell-derived microparticles in synovial fluid from inflamed arthritic joints support coagulation exclusively via a factor VII-dependent mechanism. Arthritis Rheum 2002; 46(11): 2857–66.

139. Distler JH, Jungel A, Huber LC et al. The induction of matrix metalloproteinase and cytokine expression in synovial fibroblasts stimulated with immune cell

microparticles. Proc Natl Acad Sci U S A 2005; 102(8): 2892–7.

140. Berckmans RJ, Nieuwland R, Kraan MC et al. Synovial microparticles from arthritic patients modulate chemokine and cytokine release by synoviocytes. Arthritis Res Ther 2005; 7(3): R536–R544.

141. Distler JH, Pisetsky DS, Huber LC et al. Microparticles as regulators of inflammation: novel players of cellular crosstalk in the rheumatic diseases. Arthritis Rheum 2005; 52(11): 3337–48.

142. Miltenburg AMM, Lacraz S, Welgus HG, Dayer JM. Immobilized anti-CD3 antibody activates T cell clones to induce the production of interstitial collagenase, but not tissue inhibitor of metalloproteinases, in monocytic THP-1 cells and dermal fibroblasts. J Immunol 1995; 154: 2655–67.

143. Lou J, Dayer JM, Grau GE, Burger D. Direct cell/cell contact with stimulated T lymphocytes induces the expression of cell adhesion molecules and cytokines by human brain microvascular endothelial cells. Eur J Immunol 1996; 26: 3107–13.

144. Rezzonico R, Burger D, Dayer JM. Direct contact between T lymphocytes and human dermal fibroblasts or synoviocytes down-regulates types I and III collagen production via cell-associated cytokines. J Biol Chem 1998; 273(30): 18720–8.

145. Burger D, Rezzonico R, Li JM et al. Imbalance between interstitial collagenase and tissue inhibitor of metalloproteinases 1 in synoviocytes and fibroblasts upon direct contact with stimulated T lymphocytes: involvement of membrane-associated cytokines. Arthritis Rheum 1998; 41(10): 1748–59.

146. Dinther-Janssen AC, Horst E, Koopman G et al. The VLA-4/VCAM-1 pathway is involved in lymphocyte adhesion to endothelium in rheumatoid synovium. J Immunol 1991; 147(12): 4207–10.

147. Matsuyama T, Kitani A. The role of VCAM-1 molecule in the pathogenesis of rheumatoid synovitis. Hum Cell 1996; 9(3): 187–92.

148. Postigo AA, Garcia-Vicuna R, Diaz-Gonzalez F et al. Increased binding of synovial T lymphocytes from rheumatoid arthritis to endothelial-leukocyte adhesion molecule-1 (ELAM-1) and vascular cell adhesion molecule-1 (VCAM-1). J Clin Invest 1992; 89(5): 1445–52.

149. Washington R, Burton J, Todd RF et al. Expression of immunologically relevant endothelial cell activation antigens on isolated central nervous system microvessels from patients with multiple sclerosis. Ann Neurol 1994; 35: 89–97.

150. Burger D, Lou J, Dayer JM, Grau GE. Both soluble and membrane-associated TNF activate brain microvascular endothelium: relevance to multiple sclerosis. Mol Psychiatry 1997; 2(2): 113–16.

151. Monaco C, Andreakos E, Young S, Feldmann M, Paleolog E. T cell-mediated signaling to vascular endothelium: induction of cytokines, chemokines, and tissue factor. J Leukoc Biol 2002; 71(4): 659–68.

152. Feldmann M, Maini RN. Anti TNF-alpha therapy of rheumatoid arthritis: what have we learned? Annu Rev Immunol 2001; 19: 163–96.

153. Maini RN, Feldmann M. How does infliximab work in rheumatoid arthritis? Arthritis Res 2002; 4(Suppl 2): S22–S28.

154. Cettour-Rose P, Nguyen TX, Serrander L et al. T cell contact-mediated activation of respiratory burst in human polymorphonuclear leukocytes is inhibited by high-density lipoproteins and involves CD18. J Leukoc Biol 2005; 77(1): 52–8.

155. Gasser O, Schifferli JA. Activated polymorphonuclear neutrophils disseminate anti-inflammatory microparticles by ectocytosis. Blood 2004; 104(8): 2543–8.

9

Toll-like receptors: possible targets for novel treatments for rheumatoid arthritis

Constantinos Brikos and Luke AJ O'Neill

Introduction • The family of Toll-like receptors • TLR signaling and arthritis • Final perspective • Acknowledgments • References

INTRODUCTION

At the time of writing, it is 15 years since the discovery of the similarity between the first Toll receptor in the fruit fly *Drosophila melanogaster* and the receptor for the proinflammatory cytokine interleukin-1 (IL-1RI).[1] Since then, at least 13 mammalian Toll-like receptors (TLRs) have been identified and the importance of their role in innate and adaptive immunity is now clear. When an organism is invaded by microbes such as bacteria, viruses, fungi and parasites, they are immediately detected by the TLRs. They exist in cell types involved in innate immunity such as macrophages and dendritic cells (DCs). They are also present in cells of the adaptive immune response, such as B and certain types of T cells. In addition, TLRs can be found in non-immune cells, such as fibroblasts and endothelial cells. TLRs are able to sense the invading microbes by recognizing a variety of molecules associated with them. The pathways that are induced by the majority of TLRs are very similar to those activated by the proinflammatory cytokine IL-1. TLRs as well as the IL-1RI induce a common set of genes via the activation of the transcription factor nuclear factor-κB (NF-κB) and the mitogen-activated protein kinases, p38 and c-Jun N-terminal kinase (JNK), leading to production of cytokines, chemokines, and

co-stimulatory molecules that play a central role in the activation and regulation of both innate and adaptive immunity. However, recent discoveries of the molecular basis of TLR-induced signal transduction, started to elucidate the differences among them. In contrast to IL-1, certain TLRs activate the interferon (IFN) regulatory factors (IRFs). These are a family of transcription factors that are responsible for the induction of type I IFNs and IFN-induced genes. In general, although all of the TLR signal transduction pathways have not been completely uncovered yet, it is clear that there is specificity in the genes which are expressed, depending on which TLRs are activated. This occurs to ensure that the host will respond efficiently to a certain invasion.

Apart from ligands of microbial origin, TLRs are also activated by endogenous stimuli, such as molecules from cells damaged because of infection, or as a result of chronic inflammation due to autoimmune diseases such as rheumatoid arthritis (RA). Consequently, as TLRs are key activators and regulators of innate and adaptive immunity and they have been observed to be activated in autoimmune diseases, it is very likely that they could be good targets for the development of new therapeutics.

In this chapter, we summarize the current knowledge on TLRs and discuss their possible involvement in the pathogenesis of chronic inflammatory and autoimmune diseases, with a focus on RA. We also review how some therapeutics, already used for the treatment of RA, inhibit components of the TLR signal transduction pathways, and discuss other possible approaches that could be used to target these pathways.

THE FAMILY OF TOLL-LIKE RECEPTORS

Historical overview

The first member of the family to be discovered was a transmembrane protein in *Drosophila melanogaster* which was essential for the formation of the dorsoventral axis of the fly embryo.[2] The finding that Toll had a cytosolic portion highly similar to that of IL-1RI was intriguing.[1,3–5] A lot of research had been focused on IL-1 because its local and systemic effects (reviewed by Dinarello)[6,7] placed it as a link between innate and adaptive immunity, playing a prominent role in the pathogenesis of certain chronic inflammatory autoimmune diseases such as RA. It was hoped that understanding of the signal transduction induced by IL-1 could lead to the discovery of new therapeutic targets – a notion that has since been proven true. Toll was subsequently shown to be important for the defence of the adult fly against fungi.[8] Later, the first human Toll was identified because of its similarity with the *Drosophila* Toll at both their intracellular and extracellular regions.[9] Soon afterwards, four more Tolls were reported.[10] One of them was TLR4, which is responsible for the recognition of lipopolysaccharide (LPS), also known as endotoxin. LPS is a main component of the cell wall of Gram-negative bacteria. TLR4 was discovered as the receptor that recognizes LPS, because mice that contain a mutation or are deficient in the *Tlr-4* gene, are defective in LPS signaling.[11–13] Comparably, TLR4 is the LPS receptor in humans, as a missense mutation (Asp299Gly) in the extracellular region of human TLR4 caused hyporesponsiveness to LPS.[14–16] In addition, it was shown that TLR4 mediates the response to the respiratory syncytial virus (RSV).[17] That was the first key evidence that TLRs detect molecules from invading microbial agents. In total, at least 12 more mammalian TLRs have been discovered and the list of the various pathogen-associated molecular patterns (PAMPs) and endogenous ligands they detect is continually growing.

Ligands

TLRs can be divided into two main groups, according to their ligands. One group of TLRs mainly recognize PAMPS from lipids and the other group detect PAMPS from nucleic acids. The first group consists of TLRs 1, 2, 4, and 6 and the other group consists of TLR3, 7, 8, and 9.

More specifically, TLR2 is responsible for the response to lipopeptides from the cell wall of Gram-positive bacteria, mycobacterial cell wall components, such as lipomannans, phospholipomannan from fungi, and glycosylphosphatidylinositolmucin from protozoan parasites. It was also believed to recognize peptidoglycan (PGN), although a more recent study[18] contradicts the earlier observations. TLR2 can also interact with proteins, such as porins from the outer membrane of the cell wall of Gram-negative bacteria and viral proteins such as the measles virus hemagglutinin protein. TLR2 actually heterodimerizes with TLR1 and TLR6, sensing even more microbial ligands in that way. For example, the TLR1/TLR2 complex can recognize bacterial and mycobacterial diacyl lipopeptides and bacterial triacylated lipoproteins, such as the synthetic compound Pam3Cys. The TLR6/TLR2 complex can recognize diacylated lipoproteins from mycoplasma, such as the mycoplasma lipoprotein-2 (MALP-2) and the bacterial glycolipid lipoteichoic acid (LTA).

TLR4, as mentioned, detects LPS from the cell wall of Gram-negative bacteria, lipid A (a lipid portion of LPS) and lipid A analogs, mannan from fungi, glycoinositolphospholipids from protozoan parasites, and several viral proteins, such as the fusion protein of the RSV.

TLR3 initiates signalling for double-stranded RNA.[19] As many viruses have double-stranded RNA during their replicative cycle, TLR3 is a key receptor for antiviral responses. In addition, it recognizes the synthetic analog of dsRNA polyriboinosinic:polyribocytidylic acid [poly(I:C)].

TLR7 is activated by viral single-stranded RNA but also by synthetic compounds such as guanosine analogs (e.g. Loxoribin) and various imidazoquinolines such as R-848 and imiquimod. R-848 also activates the human TLR8[20–23] but not the mouse TLR8 which is apparently inactive.

TLR9 recognizes unmethylated CpG motifs in bacterial and mycobacterial DNA and genomic DNA from parasites.[24,25]

Of the remaining TLRs, 5 and 11, do not belong to the above two groups. They recognize proteins. The ligand for TLR5 is bacterial flagellin,[26] whereas TLR11 recognizes a profilin-like molecule.[27] The human TLR11 is non-functional. Lastly, a ligand for TLR10, 12 and 13 have not been found. TLR10 is expressed in humans but not in mice and TLR12 and 13 are expressed in mice but not in humans.

As mentioned, TLRs also recognize endogenous ligands. TLR4 recognizes several proteins of its host, such as the heat-shock proteins (HSPs) 60, 70, Gp96, the high mobility group box 1 protein,[28–31] the extra domain A of fibronectin,[32] β-defensin 2,[33] fibrinogen,[34] and other ligands including heparan sulphate[35] and soluble hyaluronan.[36] TLR2 has also been reported to be activated by HSPs.[29–31] There is some evidence that TLR activation from HSPs is due to contaminations of the protein preparations with endotoxin.[37] Therefore, further investigation is required to clarify which of the endogenous proteins are actually ligands for TLR4. Among the other TLRs, TLR3 has been shown to recognize mRNA from the host[38] and TLR9 recognizes self-DNA.[39] A model has therefore emerged where the role of TLRs may not in fact be to recognize pathogen-derived molecules, but rather molecules out of context. For example, both host- and pathogen-derived nucleic acids will be sensed by TLRs if they are endocytosed into specialized endosomes. Fragmentation of host factors such as hyaluronan will be sensed by TLR2 and/or TLR4. It is in this context that TLRs might participate in inflammatory diseases, as may occur in RA and systemic lupus erythromatosus (SLE).[40,41]

The molecular interactions between the TLRs and their ligands, and the conformational changes that TLRs undergo in order to initiate signal transduction, have not been clarified yet. The reason is that only a limited number of structures of TLR domains have been solved.

Signaling

Structure of TLRs

In general, TLRs are type 1 transmembrane receptors with an extracellular domain consisting of 19–25 leucine-rich repeat (LRR) motifs which are 24–29 amino acids long. These LRR motifs are believed to recognize the ligands. Recently the crystal structure of the LRR domain of TLR3 was described at 2.3 Å.[42,43] There are 23 LRR motifs which form a structure like a horseshoe-shaped solenoid. Each of the LRRs contains asparagines that stabilize the structure by forming hydrogen bonding networks. TLR3 is highly glycosylated but it contains a surface which is free of glycosylation and hypothesized to be the site where dsRNA binds. Binding of dsRNA to one TLR3 molecule causes conformational changes that result in bringing the intracellular parts of TLR3 to close proximity, leading to signal transduction. Currently this is the model of how signal transduction is initiated by all TLRs. When the TLRs are liganded, they induce signal transduction either as homodimers (e.g. Drosophila Toll)[44,45] or heterodimers (i.e. TLR2 with TLR1 or TLR6).

In particular, all TLRs contain a highly homologous domain in their intracellular region. As already stated, this domain is also conserved in IL-1RI and the drosophila Toll and was named the Toll/IL-1 receptor (TIR) domain. The TIR domain is between 135 and 160 amino acids long. The molecular structures of the TIR domains of TLR1 and TLR2 have been resolved and show that they contain a central five-stranded parallel β-sheet which is surrounded by a total of five α-helices on both sides.[46] The hypothesized model is that upon the dimerization of the TLRs when liganded, a TIR–TIR interaction takes place intracellularly. The same TIR–TIR interaction also occurs in the case of IL-1RI, but instead of forming a homodimer, it associates with its accessory protein (IL-1RAcP), which also contains a TIR domain. The TIR–TIR structure provides the place of association with TIR domain-containing intracellular proteins.

These proteins are called adapters, because they link the receptors to other downstream proteins in the signalling cascade.

The first adapter to be identified was the myeloid differentiation primary response protein 88 (MyD88). MyD88 mediates the signaling of all TLRs, apart from TLR3 (Figure 9.1). It is also an adapter for IL-1RI. All TLRs that employ MyD88 signal in a MyD88-dependent way to activate NF-κB and the MAPKs, which is similar to the IL-1RI signaling.

MyD88-dependent pathways

Apart from a TIR domain at its C-terminus, MyD88 also contains a death domain which is a part of its N-terminus. FAS/Apo1/CD95 and tumor necrosis factor (TNF) receptors contain a death domain that is important for their cytotoxic function. However, in TLR signaling, the death domain of MyD88 does not induce apoptosis[47] but it is required for protein–protein interactions. Recruitment of MyD88 to liganded IL-1RI or TLRs, leads in it's turn to the recruitment of the IL-1 receptor-associated kinases (IRAKs) (Figure 9.1 – see downstream of TLR4). These kinases also have a death domain which is important for that interaction to occur. Recruited IRAK-4 phosphorylates IRAK-1, which is subsequently autophosphorylated to become fully activated.[48,49] Then, IRAK-1 leaves the receptor complex and binds to TNF-receptor-associated factor 6 (TRAF6). TRAF6[50] interacts with the E2 ubiquitin ligase complex of Ubc13 and Uev1A

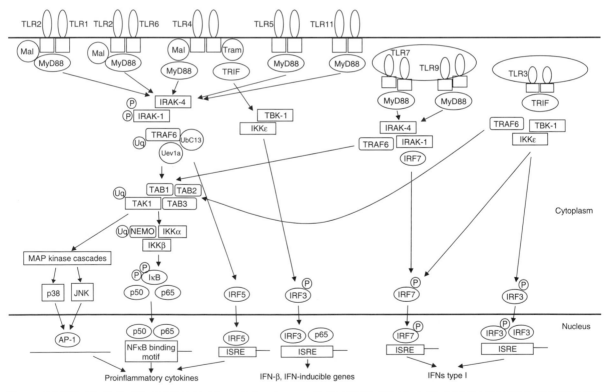

Figure 9.1 TLR signaling pathways (see text for details; please note that TLR3, 7,9 are expressed in endosomal compartments instead of the cell surface. The same applies for TLR8 which is not shown for simplicity reasons). Toll-like receptors, TLRs; myeloid differentiation primary response protein 88, MyD88; MyD88 adapter-like, Mal; TIR domain-containing adapter inducing IFN-β, TRIF; TRIF-related adapter molecule, TRAM; interleukin-1 receptor-associated kinase, IRAK; TNF-receptor-associated factor 6, TRAF6; interferon regulatory factor, IRF; TGF-β-activated kinase 1, TAK1; TAK1 binding protein, TAB; inhibitor of NF-κB kinases, IKKs; NF-κB essential modulator, NEMO; inhibitor of NF-κB, IκB; interferon regulatory factor, IRF; nuclear factor-κB, NF-κB; c-Jun N-terminal kinase, JNK; activator protein-1, AP-1; interferon-stimulated response element, ISRE; interferon, IFN; Uq, ubiquitination; P, phosphorylation.

and becomes polyubiquitinated. The same complex also polyubiquitinates the complex of the inhibitor of NF-κB (IκB) kinases (IKKs), on IKKγ-also known as NF-κB essential modulator (NEMO).[51] TRAF6 also forms a complex with the transforming growth factor (TGF)-β-activated kinase 1 (TAK1) and the TAK1 binding proteins, TAB1, TAB2, and TAB3.[52] TAK1 also undergoes ubiquitination and phosphorylates the IKK complex and MAP kinase kinase 6 (MKK6). The IKK complex phosphorylates the IκB proteins, which exist as a complex with the p50 and p65 subunits of the transcription factor NF-κB. This phosphorylation results in the degradation of IκB by the proteosome and the release of the NF-κB subunits, p50 and p65, that subsequently translocate to the nucleus and induce genes involved in inflammatory responses.

Phosphorylation of MKK6 leads to the activation of the MAPK cascades which activate the transcription factor, activator protein-1, which also plays a crucial role in the induction of inflammatory response genes.

Apart from IRAK-1 and IRAK-4 there are two additional members in the family of IRAKs, IRAK-2 and IRAK-M. They are both inactive kinases. IRAK-M is a negative regulator of IL-1RI and TLRs. It inhibits the dissociation of IRAK-1 from MyD88 and the formation of IRAK-TRAF6 complexes.[53] The role of IRAK-2 in signaling remains to be resolved. Overexpression of human IRAK-2, in cells that lack IRAK-1, seems to restore their responsiveness to IL-1 and LPS.[54] In mice there are four IRAK-2 splice isoforms, two of which induce signaling that leads to activation of NF-κB and two of which seem to inhibit such signaling.[55]

Other proteins that may be involved in the pathway, but their role is not totally clear, are the Toll-interacting protein (Tollip), Pellinos, MAPK kinase kinase-1(MEKK1) and MEKK3.

Apart from the MyD88-dependent pathway that leads to activation of NF-κB and the MAPKs, recent studies show that TLR7 and TLR9 signaling in plasmacytoid DCs (pDCs) but not conventional DCs (cDCs), also induce type I IFNs, in a MyD88-dependent manner (Figure 9.1 – see the pathway below TLR7 and TLR9). After these interactions, IRF7 translocates into the nucleus and binds to IFN-stimulated response element (ISRE) motifs that exist in the promoter

regions of several cytokine genes, inducing in that way, the production of type 1 IFNs. In particular, MyD88 associates directly with the transcription factor IRF7,[56–58] which can also interact with IRAK-1, IRAK-4, and TRAF6. In IRAK-1-deficient mice, IFN-α production is abolished, indicating that IRAK-1 plays an essential role in that pathway, perhaps by phosphorylating IRF7.

Lastly, another transcription factor, which also belongs to the family of IRFs and is activated in a MyD88-dependent way, is IRF5 (Figure 9.1). Several ligands for TLRs (such as LPS and unmethylated DNA) can induce IRF5. As in the case of IRF7, IRF5 has also been found in a complex with MyD88 and TRAF6[59] and to move into the nucleus where it binds ISRE motifs. IRF5 is a major inducer of IL-6, IL-12, and TNF-α but not of IFN-α.

MyD88 is essential for the signaling of IL-1RI, TLR2, TLR5, TLR7, TLR8, and TLR9, but not for the signaling of TLR4. In MyD88-deficient mice, NF-κB and MAPK activation is abolished in response to IL-1 and the ligands for TLR5, TLR7, TLR8, and TLR9, but is only delayed in response to TLR4. This observation led to the discovery of more adapter molecules homologous to MyD88. In total, four more adapters have been identified, the MyD88 adapter-like or TIR domain-containing adapter protein (Mal/TIRAP)[60,61] the TIR domain-containing adapter inducing IFN-β or TIR-containing adapter molecule-1 (TRIF/TICAM-1),[62,63] the TRIF-related adapter molecule (TRAM) TICAM-2[64] and sterile α and HEAT-Armadillo motifs (SARM).[65]

Mal was initially shown to have an important role in TLR4, but not in IL-1 signaling.[60] Later, Mal-deficient mice confirmed this original observation.[66,67] Their phenotype was very similar to that of the MyD88 knockout (KO) mice in terms of TLR2 and TLR4 signaling. The activation of NF-κB and MAPKs was delayed in response to TLR4, but was not affected by ligands for the other TLRs tested (TLR3, 5, 7 and 9) or by IL-1 and IL-18. Mal was the first proof that different TLRs recruit different adapter molecules. Very recently, the specific role of Mal in TLR4 signaling has been revealed. Mal contains a binding domain for phosphatidylinositol-4,5-bisphosphate (PIP2), one of the main structural components of the plasma membrane.[68,69] Upon activation of TLR4 (Figure 9.1), Mal binds to

PIP2 and facilitates the recruitment of MyD88 to the plasma membrane. In that way, Mal and MyD88 are in close proximity to liganded TLR4 and therefore, are able to interact with it. Thus, Mal is acting as a bridging adapter, bringing MyD88 to TLR4, and subsequently, MyD88, signals downstream. Thus, MyD88 can be termed as a signalling adapter .

The Mal-MyD88 double KO mice present a delayed instead of an abolished response, following TLR4 activation.[66] In addition, the MyD88 KO mice showed that TLR4 and TLR3 could initiate signal transduction that was independent of MyD88.[70,71] That MyD88-independent pathway leads to activation of the transcription factors IRF3 and IRF7, and consequently induction of IFN-α/β and IFN-inducible genes.

MyD88-independent pathways

The adapter responsible for the MyD88-independent pathway is TRIF.[63,72,73] It is recruited by both TLR3 and TLR4 (Figure 9.1) and signals via an IKK-like kinase named the TRAF-family-member-associated NF-κB activator (TANK)-binding kinase-1 (TBK-1)[70] and the IKK homolog, IKKε, in order to activate IRF3. In particular, TRIF forms a complex with TBK-1, IKKε, and IRF3. IRF3 becomes phosphorylated by TBK-1 and IKKε and thus activated. Then IRF3 binds to the ISRE on target genes inducing production of IFN α/β.[74] IRF7 also becomes phosphorylated and activated by TBK-1 and IKKε and binds to the ISRE of genes, thereby inducing their expression.[56–58]

In TLR3 signaling, TRIF has also been shown to activate NF-κB. TRIF associates with the TRAF6–TAK1–TAB2 complex that activates IKK (see the section on the MyD88-dependent pathway).[75] In addition, TRIF binds the receptor interacting protein-1 (RIP-1), an important mediator of both TLR3- and TLR4-induced NF-κB activation.[76,77] Following stimulation of TLR4, the TRIF-dependent signaling also leads to NF-κB activation indirectly. As mentioned, TRIF activates IRF3. IRF3 in its turn, binds to ISRE and induces TNF-α production. TNF-α is then secreted inducing its receptor (TNFR).[78] TNFR signaling also culminates in NF-κB activation.

It is believed that TLR3 associates with TRIF directly. On the contrary, TLR4 requires TRAM to engage TRIF.[64,71,79–81] Thus, in TLR4 signaling TRAM acts as a bridging adapter to bind TRIF and facilitate its recruitment to the receptor complex. Similar to Mal, TRAM associates with the plasma membrane, but unlike Mal, this depends on a myristic acid group in the N-terminus of TRAM. Activation of TRAM requires its phosphorylation on serine 16 by protein kinase Cε. This is required for TRAM to signal, but the exact mechanism is unknown. Another difference between TLR3 and TLR4 in the TRIF-dependent pathway, is that although TRIF is used by both TLR3 and TLR4 to drive IRF3, only TLR3 activates IRF3 homodimers that bind ISRE (Figure 9.1). When TLR4 initiates IRF3 activation, IRF3 forms a heterocomplex with the p65 subunit of NF-κB, which then binds ISRE.[82]

The fifth and final adapter with a TIR domain is SARM. Its role is however, inhibiting and very recent evidence indicates that it interacts specifically with TRIF.[83]

TLR SIGNALING AND ARTHRITIS

Our understanding of TLRs represents a remarkable achievement in basic research into the molecular functioning of the innate immune system. These findings are now being translated into disease relevance, and the study of TLRs in the context of autoimmune and inflammatory diseases is revealing important new insights into disease pathogenesis and potentially new treatments.

Evidence of the involvement of TLRs in autoimmune and inflammatory diseases

In tissue specimens from patients with autoimmune and/or inflammatory diseases, the expression of certain TLRs is altered.

In particular, in atherosclerosis, in areas of plaques where inflammatory cells are concentrated, the expression of TLR1, TLR2, and TLR4 is induced.[84] Some cells from atherotic plaques, showed expression of TLR5 of TLR3, and as well as that of.

In multiple sclerosis patients, in brain and spinal cord specimens, TLR3 and TLR4 expression is upregulated.[85]

In Crohn's disease (CD), TLR3 expression was downregulated in intestinal epithelial cells whereas TLR5 expression was unchanged, as in the case of ulcerative colitis (UC).[86] The way that the TLR2 expression levels are affected is not clear. Whereas in one report TLR2 was upregulated on submucosal cells during intestinal inflammation,[87] according to another study the levels of TLR2 were unchanged in the intestinal epithelium of patients with UC and CD.[86] Lastly, the TLR4 levels seem to be higher in these two diseases.[86,88]

The expression of TLRs is also altered in RA. TLR2, 3, 4 and 7 are expressed at higher levels in synovial tissue of RA patients.[88,89] In particular, TLR2 and TLR4 are expressed at higher levels in moderate but not severe inflammation.

The fact that TLRs are expressed in rheumatoid joints is crucial, because in these areas there is also availability of TLR ligands. Several exogenous ligands of bacterial origin such as bacterial DNA and PGNs have been detected.[92] In addition, a lot of endogenous ligands that are able to activate several TLRs have been identified, such as HSPs,[91] as well as hyaluronan fragments.[92,93] Moreover, in inflamed arthritic joints, where tissue destruction is taking place to a high extent, there are plenty of necrotic cells. These cells have been shown to activate TLR2[94] and TLR3.[95]

The significance of the TLR signaling pathways in RA, is also indicated by the fact that TLR ligands exhibit arthritogenic properties. There are mouse models in which arthritis is induced by the injection of TLR ligands. In particular, bacterial CpG DNA, staphylococcal PGNs and viral double-stranded RNA, when injected into mice, are able to induce arthritis.[96–98] The streptococcal cell wall can cause arthritis too. The role of TLR2, through the MyD88-dependent pathway,[99] is very important for this type of arthritis, as it cannot be induced in MyD88-deficient mice. Furthermore, in TLR2-deficient mice the symptoms of the disease are less severe.

The effect of TLRs on the severity of arthritis is also demonstrated by using the serum transferred arthritis model. In this model the injection of arthritogenic sera, intraperitoneally in mice, induces arthritis. This type of induction of arthritis is IL-1-dependent, because IL-1RI-deficient mice do not develop the disease.[100] When TLR4-deficient mice were used, the severity of arthritis was reduced. In addition, when LPS was administered together with arthritogenic sera to the IL-1RI-deficient mice, they developed arthritis. As a conclusion, LPS can substitute IL-1 in that model. This study shows that even when arthritis has started to develop and the adaptive immune system is activated against the host, TLRs might still play an important role in the progress of the disease.

Apart from activating the innate immune response in RA and other autoimmune and/or inflammatory diseases, TLRs have been reported to contribute in the induction of the adaptive immune system in such diseases.

A murine model of SLE and RA, has shown that TLR9 is likely to play a role in the production of autoantibodies. Immune complexes that contained host DNA, activated self IgG-specific B cells, by costimulating TLR9 and the B-cell antigen receptor (BCR).[39] In a similar way, RNA-associated autoantigens can also activate B cells, by the co-engagement of TLR7 and the BCR.[101] Moreover, two recent studies correlated the expression levels of TLR7, with an increase in B-cell responses to RNA-containing self-antigens.[102,103] It was found that male mice that contain the Y-linked autoimmune accelerator (*Yaa*) locus, develop SLE with a higher incidence. The disease is also more severe. The reason is that the *Yaa*-bearing mice express higher levels of TLR7.

Lastly, further evidence that might indicate the importance of TLRs in autoimmune diseases comes from TLR polymorphisms (Table 9.1). There is a rare nucleotide polymorphism in the *tlr4* gene that results in the expression of the Asp299Gly TLR4 variant. This amino acid substitution, reduces the ability of TLR4 to initiate signaling. Thus, as expected, this polymorphism increases susceptibility to Gram-negative bacterial infections. There are studies that show that this polymorphism might be associated with susceptibility in developing inflammatory diseases. In RA, there is a report that shows that individuals with the Asp299Gly TLR4 variant, are less susceptible to the disease.[104] However, this disagrees with two other studies, in which no association between this polymorphism with RA or SLE was observed.[106,107] In atherosclerosis, it was reported that this polymorphism was linked

Table 9.1 TLR polymorphisms and the diseases or infections in which they may be implicated in (see text for details).

Receptor	Polymorphism	Disease
TLR2	Arg677Trp	Lepromatous leprosy
	Arg753Gln	Staphylococcal infection in septic patients
	smaller number of guanine-thymine repeats in intron II of its gene	RA
TLR4	Asp299Gly	RA, atherosclerosis, CD, UC, type 2 diabetes, asthma
	Thr399Ile	UC, type 2 diabetes
TLR5	Truncated	SLE, Legionnaire's disease

TLR, Toll-like receptor; RA, rheumatoid arthritis; CD, Crohn's disease; UC, ulcerative colitis; SLE, systemic lupus erythromatosus.

to decreased susceptibility.[108] Another study associated this polymorphism with acute coronary syndromes.[109] However, in other studies, the polymorphism was not associated with coronary artery stenosis[110] and did not affect the progression of atherosclerosis.[111] In addition, the polymorphism was shown to play an important role in CD and UC,[112] whereas another study did not associate this it with UC.[113] A different polymorphism of TLR4 (Thr399Ile) was found to be important in this study. Both these polymorphisms are associated with reduced frequency of diabetic neuropathy in type 2 diabetes patients.[113] Lastly, the Asp299Gly variant does not seem to be associated with disease susceptibility in asthma, but the variant may increase atopy severity.[115]

Another polymorphism that was found in human TLR genes, leads to a substitution of Arg[677] with Trp in TLR2. This polymorphism is correlated with lepromatous leprosy.[116] It was also shown, that this polymorphism disables TLR2 from inducing NF-κB activation in response to *Mycobacterium leprae*.[116] Similarly, in the TLR2 gene there is a polymorphism that causes the Arg753Gln substitution. This substitution is associated with hyporesponsiveness to the bacteria *Borrelia burgdorferi* and *Treponema pallidum*, that cause the lyme and syphilis diseases respectively.[117] In addition, 2 out of 91 septic patients

had this polymorphism and both experienced staphylococcal infections. Polymorphisms in the TLR2 gene have not been linked with RA or SLE.[107]

On the contrary, in a recent study, a microsatellite polymorphism of the human TLR2 gene was associated with RA.[119] It has been suggested that a genotype which contains a smaller number of guanine-thymine repeats in intron II of the TLR2 gene may result in susceptibility to RA.

Lastly, a polymorphism in the TLR5 gene that results in the expression of a truncated (TLR5 392STOP) non-functional receptor, reduces susceptibility to SLE, but has the opposite effect for Legionnaire's disease.[119,120]

The contradictions in the studies mentioned above, show that it is not yet clear if certain TLR polymorphisms are definitely linked to inflammatory autoimmune diseases.

In general, there is not enough evidence that the initiation of certain inflammatory diseases is due to the overactivation or deficiency of TLRs. It is however clear, that TLR signaling is activated and involved in the pathogenesis of inflammatory diseases, including RA, or could even play a protective role against them. Thus, even in the case that induction of TLR signaling is a secondary phenomenon in these diseases, its inhibition or activation could be beneficial in reducing their severity.

Targeting TLR signaling for the discovery of new therapeutic agents

Several ways could be employed to inhibit TLR signaling. One method is to prevent the association of TLRs with their ligands. An approach to accomplish this is the development of molecules that would be able to occupy the ligand's binding site of the TLR, without initiating signal transduction (antagonists).

Another way, is to 'neutralize' TLRs by creating recombinant antibodies that could bind to them and hide their ligand-binding site. This technology has been successful in blocking the action of certain cytokines such as TNF-α.

Moreover, TLRs could be prevented from initiating a signal, by producing their extracellular domain as a recombinant protein, and using it as an antagonist for binding their ligands. In the case of the cytokine TNF-α, this method has also been successful.

Apart from developing medications that aim to inhibit the initiation of TLR signaling, a method, that has already been used, is to target important molecules in their signaling cascades.

As previously mentioned, a central molecule in NF-κB activation is IKK2. Several small molecules have been designed which can inhibit IKK2 and have anti-inflammatory effects. These molecules could be proven to be good agents for the treatment of RA.[122] Such compounds are SPC0023579, NVOIKK004[123] and SPC-839.[124] Moreover, several existing synthetic anti-inflammatory drugs, such as aspirin and salicylate,[125] or natural products such as parthenolide,[126] appear to target IKK2. Other molecules that inhibit NF-κB activation are sulfasalazine, leflunomide, and PS-1145.[126–128] In particular, sulfasalazine directly inhibits IKK1 and 2, and PS-1145 is an inhibitor of the proteosome that mediates the degradation of IκB. Other inhibitors of the proteosome are PR171[130] and Bortezomib.[131] Both might inhibit NF-κB activation. The first one is in clinical trials for multiple myeloma and the second one has already been approved for that disease (Velcade; Millennium Pharmaceuticals).

Pharmaceutical companies are also targeting several other protein kinases in the pathways. Two of these kinases are p38 and JNK.[132–134] As previously mentioned, both these proteins belong to the MAPK pathways. Several existing medications that are used to treat RA, inhibit these molecules. A molecule that targets JNK and has anti-inflammatory effects in animal models is SP-600125.[130] Additional compounds that inhibit both JNK and p38 signaling, are the glucocorticoids. A possible mechanism by which one glucocorticoid (dexamethasone) may inhibit proinflammatory gene expression, is via the induction of the MAPK phosphatase-1 (MKP-1), which is a potent inhibitor of p38 function.[135]

Recently, an important role of glucocorticoids was specifically highlighted in TLR signaling. As previously stated, both TLR3 and TLR4 activate IRF3-dependent gene expression (Figure 9.1). Glucocorticoids block the induction of these genes that contain ISRE, only in response to TLR4.[136] Thus, glucocorticoids may be able to inhibit the formation of the IRF3/p65 complex in TLR4 signaling, but cannot target the IRF3 homodimers that are formed in the TLR3 pathway.

Another group of compounds that inhibit p38 are the pyridinyl imidazoles.[136] In animal models of arthritis, they significantly reduced the severity of the disease.[137–139] Three other compounds that are currently used for clinical trials are BIRB-796 (RA, CD, and psoriasis), SCIO469 (RA, dental pain, and multiple myeloma), and VX-702 (RA).[129,140]

Apart from the proteins mentioned above, there are several other components in the TLR signaling cascades that could be good targets. Two of them are the protein kinases IRAK-4 and TAK1. IRAK-4 is essential for the phosphorylation and activation of IRAK-1. Designing specific inhibitors for them, could be a good approach to block the MyD88-dependent pathways. TAK1 plays a central role in linking the TLRs to the activation of NF-κB and the MAPKs. Thus, its inhibition could potentially inhibit all these signaling cascades.

Other proteins, that if inactivated, could have beneficial results in chronic inflammatory and autoimmune diseases, are the adapters MyD88 and TRAF-6. Designing peptides to prevent the association of MyD88 to TLRs or its downstream proteins, such as the IRAKs, could be a very successful approach to prevent inflammation. TRAF-6 participates in signaling induced by all TLRs including TLR3. TRAF-6 contains a binding motif for IRAK-1 and links it with downstream proteins. Most likely, peptides that block these interactions could block signaling. Nature offers examples of preventing such protein interactions in order to inhibit TLR signaling. The Vaccinia virus contains two proteins, A46R and A52R, that inhibit TLR signaling to limit the host defense against the virus.[141,142] A46R is a TIR containing protein that disrupts MyD88-dependent signaling. A52R blocus signaling downstream of MyD88, at the IRAK-2 and TRAF-6 level, and it is a strong inhibitor of TLR3 signaling, which is important for the defense of the host against viruses. It is therefore possible to use these proteins to design inhibitory peptides of the TLR signaling cascades. In a recent study, a peptide derived from the A52R protein, successfully blocked TLR activation *in vitro*. In particular, the peptide dramatically reduced middle ear inflammation, when used to treat mice that had been injected with heat-inactivated *Streptococcus pneumoniae* through their tympanic membrane (a murine model of otitis).[143]

Lastly, another method, which could potentially lead to the discovery of new therapeutic agents, is to try and inhibit the ubiquitination of certain proteins that play important roles in TLR signaling, such as TRAF6 and TAK1.

FINAL PERSPECTIVE

The importance of the function of TLRs in the activation of innate and adaptive immunity is clear. Extensive research into the function of TLRs continually increases the number of their discovered ligands. These ligands are deriving from invading microbial agents, but also from dead or damaged cells of the host, due to infection or autoimmune diseases.

Clarification of the differences among the TLR signaling cascades has started. Some of the dissimilarities are due to the fact that not all TLRs recruit the same adapter molecule(s). In addition, some TLRs, apart from proinflammatory cytokines, are able to induce IFNs or IFN-inducible genes. However, further research is required to identify all the protein interactions that take place in the TLR pathways and all the sets of genes that are activated by them.

The exact ways in which TLR signaling is associated with inflammatory and/or autoimmune diseases need clarification as well. Certain TLRs are expressed at higher levels in chronic inflammation sites of several diseases including RA. In these sites, there is a variety of exogenous and endogenous molecules that can associate with TLRs, thus activating innate as well as adaptive immunity. However, there is inconsistency between studies on polymorphisms that attempted to link the lack of function of certain TLRs with an alteration of the level of susceptibility to certain inflammatory or autoimmune diseases, such as RA. However, it is clear that TLRs are involved in the pathogenesis of certain inflammatory and autoimmune diseases, but it is not yet understood, if and how the TLRs participate in the initiation of these diseases.

As research in the field of signal transduction by the TLRs continues, the differences among all the pathways induced by TLRs and their association in the pathogenesis of inflammatory and/or autoimmune diseases will be elucidated. This knowledge will hopefully lead to the development of new and successful therapies for the regulation of inflammation and the treatment of devastating diseases such as RA, SLE, CD, UC, and atherosclerosis.

ACKNOWLEDGMENTS

We would like to thank Pearl Gray for her help in the preparation of the manuscript.

REFERENCES

1. Gay NJ, Keith FJ. Drosophila Toll and IL-1 receptor. Nature 1991; 351(6325): 355–6.
2. Hashimoto C, Hudson KL, Anderson KV. The Toll gene of Drosophila, required for dorsal-ventral embryonic polarity, appears to encode a transmembrane protein. Cell 1988; 52(2): 269–79.
3. Dower SK, Kronheim SR, March CJ et al. Detection and characterization of high affinity plasma membrane receptors for human interleukin 1. J Exp Med 1985; 162(2): 501–15.
4. Bird TA, Gearing AJ, Saklatvala J. Murine interleukin 1 receptor. Direct identification by ligand blotting and purification to homogeneity of an interleukin 1-binding glycoprotein. J Biol Chem 1988; 263(24): 12063–9.
5. Urdal DL, Call SM, Jackson JL, Dower SK. Affinity purification and chemical analysis of the interleukin-1 receptor. J Biol Chem 1988; 263(6): 2870–7.
6. Dinarello CA. The interleukin-1 family: 10 years of discovery. FASEB J 1994; 8(15): 1314–25.
7. Dinarello CA. Biologic basis for interleukin-1 in disease. Blood 1996; 87(6): 2095–147.
8. Lemaitre B, Nicolas E, Michaut L, Reichhart JM, Hoffmann JA. The dorsoventral regulatory gene cassette spatzle/Toll/cactus controls the potent antifungal response in Drosophila adults. Cell 1996; 86(6): 973–83.
9. Medzhitov R, Preston-Hurlburt P, Janeway CA Jr. A human homologue of the Drosophila Toll protein signals activation of adaptive immunity. Nature 1997; 388(6640): 394–7.
10. Rock FL, Hardiman G, Timans JC, Kastelein RA, Bazan JF. A family of human receptors structurally related to Drosophila Toll. Proc Natl Acad Sci U S A 1998; 95(2): 588–93.
11. Hoshino K, Takeuchi O, Kawai T et al. Cutting edge: Toll-like receptor 4 (TLR4)-deficient mice are hyporesponsive to lipopolysaccharide: evidence for TLR4 as the Lps gene product. J Immunol 1999; 162(7): 3749–52.

12. Qureshi ST, Lariviere L, Leveque G et al. Endotoxin-tolerant mice have mutations in Toll-like receptor 4 (Tlr4). J Exp Med 1999; 189(4): 615–25.

13. Poltorak A, He X, Smirnova I et al. Defective LPS signaling in C3H/HeJ and C57BL/10ScCr mice: mutations in Tlr4 gene. Science 1998; 282(5396): 2085–8.

14. Agnese DM, Calvano JE, Hahm SJ et al. Human toll-like receptor 4 mutations but not CD14 polymorphisms are associated with an increased risk of gram-negative infections. J Infect Dis 2002; 186(10): 1522–5.

15. Arbour NC, Lorenz E, Schutte BC et al. TLR4 mutations are associated with endotoxin hyporesponsiveness in humans. Nat Genet 2000; 25(2): 187–91.

16. Lorenz E, Mira JP, Frees KL, Schwartz DA. Relevance of mutations in the TLR4 receptor in patients with gram-negative septic shock. Arch Intern Med 2002; 162(9): 1028–32.

17. Kurt-Jones EA, Popova L, Kwinn L et al. Pattern recognition receptors TLR4 and CD14 mediate response to respiratory syncytial virus. Nat Immunol 2000; 1(5): 398–401.

18. Travassos LH, Girardin SE, Philpott DJ et al. Toll-like receptor 2-dependent bacterial sensing does not occur via peptidoglycan recognition. EMBO Rep 2004; 5(10): 1000–6.

19. Alexopoulou L, Holt AC, Medzhitov R, Flavell RA. Recognition of double-stranded RNA and activation of NF-kappaB by Toll-like receptor 3. Nature 2001; 413(6857): 732–8.

20. Hemmi H, Kaisho T, Takeuchi O et al. Small anti-viral compounds activate immune cells via the TLR7 MyD88-dependent signaling pathway. Nat Immunol 2002; 3(2): 196–200.

21. Heil F, Hemmi H, Hochrein H et al. Species-specific recognition of single-stranded RNA via toll-like receptor 7 and 8. Science 2004; 303(5663): 1526–9.

22. Lee J, Chuang TH, Redecke V et al. Molecular basis for the immunostimulatory activity of guanine nucleoside analogs: activation of Toll-like receptor 7. Proc Natl Acad Sci U S A 2003; 100(11): 6646–51.

23. Lund JM, Alexopoulou L, Sato A et al. Recognition of single-stranded RNA viruses by Toll-like receptor 7. Proc Natl Acad Sci U S A 2004; 101(15): 5598–603.

24. Hemmi H, Takeuchi O, Kawai T et al. A Toll-like receptor recognizes bacterial DNA. Nature 2000; 408(6813): 740–5.

25. Bauer S, Kirschning CJ, Hacker H et al. Human TLR9 confers responsiveness to bacterial DNA via species-specific CpG motif recognition. Proc Natl Acad Sci U S A 2001; 98(16): 9237–42.

26. Hayashi F, Smith KD, Ozinsky A et al. The innate immune response to bacterial flagellin is mediated by Toll-like receptor 5. Nature 2001; 410(6832): 1099–103.

27. Yarovinsky F, Zhang D, Andersen JF et al. TLR11 activation of dendritic cells by a protozoan profilin-like protein. Science 2005; 308(5728): 1626–9.

28. Ohashi K, Burkart V, Flohe S, Kolb H. Cutting edge: heat shock protein 60 is a putative endogenous ligand of the toll-like receptor-4 complex. J Immunol 2000; 164(2): 558–61.

29. Vabulas RM, Ahmad-Nejad P, da Costa C et al. Endocytosed HSP60s use toll-like receptor 2 (TLR2) and TLR4 to activate the toll/interleukin-1 receptor signaling pathway in innate immune cells. J Biol Chem 2001; 276(33): 31332–9.

30. Vabulas RM, Ahmad-Nejad P, Ghose S et al. HSP70 as endogenous stimulus of the Toll/interleukin-1 receptor signal pathway. J Biol Chem 2002; 277(17): 15107–12.

31. Vabulas RM, Braedel S, Hilf N et al. The endoplasmic reticulum-resident heat shock protein Gp96 activates dendritic cells via the Toll-like receptor 2/4 pathway. J Biol Chem 2002; 277(23): 20847–53.

32. Okamura Y, Watari M, Jerud ES et al. The extra domain A of fibronectin activates Toll-like receptor 4. J Biol Chem 2001; 276(13): 10229–33.

33. Biragyn A, Ruffini PA, Leifer CA et al. Toll-like receptor 4-dependent activation of dendritic cells by beta-defensin 2. Science 2002; 298(5595): 1025–9.

34. Smiley ST, King JA, Hancock WW. Fibrinogen stimulates macrophage chemokine secretion through toll-like receptor 4. J Immunol 2001; 167(5): 2887–94.

35. Johnson GB, Brunn GJ, Kodaira Y, Platt JL. Receptor-mediated monitoring of tissue well-being via detection of soluble heparan sulfate by Toll-like receptor 4. J Immunol 2002; 168(10): 5233–9.

36. Termeer C, Benedix F, Sleeman J et al. Oligosaccharides of hyaluronan activate dendritic cells via toll-like receptor 4. J Exp Med 2002; 195(1): 99–111.

37. Gao B, Tsan MF. Endotoxin contamination in recombinant human heat shock protein 70 (Hsp70) preparation is responsible for the induction of tumor necrosis factor alpha release by murine macrophages. J Biol Chem 2003; 278(1): 174–9.

38. Kariko K, Ni H, Capodici J, Lamphier M, Weissman D. mRNA is an endogenous ligand for Toll-like receptor 3. J Biol Chem 2004; 279(13): 12542–50.

39. Leadbetter EA, Rifkin IR, Hohlbaum AM et al. Chromatin-IgG complexes activate B cells by dual engagement of IgM and Toll-like receptors. Nature 2002; 416(6881): 603–7.

40. Jiang D, Liang J, Fan J et al. Regulation of lung injury and repair by Toll-like receptors and hyaluronan. Nat Med 2005; 11(11): 1173–9.

41. O'Neill LA. TLRs play good cop, bad cop in the lung. Nat Med 2005; 11(11): 1161–2.

42. Choe J, Kelker MS, Wilson IA. Crystal structure of human toll-like receptor 3 (TLR3) ectodomain. Science 2005; 309(5734): 581–5.

43. Bell JK, Botos I, Hall PR et al. The molecular structure of the Toll-like receptor 3 ligand-binding domain. Proc Natl Acad Sci U S A 2005; 102(31): 10976–80.

44. Weber AN, Tauszig-Delamasure S, Hoffmann JA et al. Binding of the Drosophila cytokine Spatzle to Toll is direct and establishes signaling. Nat Immunol 2003; 4(8): 794–800.

45. Weber AN, Moncrieffe MC, Gangloff M, Imler JL, Gay NJ. Ligand-receptor and receptor-receptor interactions act in concert to activate signaling in the Drosophila toll pathway. J Biol Chem 2005; 280(24): 22793–9.

46. Xu Y, Tao X, Shen B et al. Structural basis for signal transduction by the Toll/interleukin-1 receptor domains. Nature 2000; 408(6808): 111–15.

47. Bonnert TP, Garka KE, Parnet P et al. The cloning and characterization of human MyD88: a member of an IL-1 receptor related family. FEBS Lett 1997; 402(1): 81–4.

48. Li S, Strelow A, Fontana EJ, Wesche H. IRAK-4: a novel member of the IRAK family with the properties of an IRAK-kinase. Proc Natl Acad Sci U S A 2002; 99(8): 5567–72.

49. Kollewe C, Mackensen AC, Neumann D et al. Sequential autophosphorylation steps in the interleukin-1 receptor-associated kinase-1 regulate its availability as an adapter in interleukin-1 signaling. J Biol Chem 2004; 279(7): 5227–36.

50. Cao Z, Xiong J, Takeuchi M, Kurama T, Goeddel DV. TRAF6 is a signal transducer for interleukin-1. Nature 1996; 383(6599): 443–6.

51. Deng L, Wang C, Spencer E et al. Activation of the IkappaB kinase complex by TRAF6 requires a dimeric ubiquitin-conjugating enzyme complex and a unique polyubiquitin chain. Cell 2000; 103(2): 351–61.

52. Wang C, Deng L, Hong M et al. TAK1 is a ubiquitin-dependent kinase of MKK and IKK. Nature 2001; 412(6844): 346–51.

53. Kobayashi K, Hernandez LD, Galan JE et al. IRAK-M is a negative regulator of Toll-like receptor signaling. Cell 2002; 110(2): 191–202.

54. Wesche H, Gao X, Li X et al. IRAK-M is a novel member of the Pelle/interleukin-1 receptor-associated kinase (IRAK) family. J Biol Chem 1999; 274(27): 19403–10.

55. Hardy MP, O'Neill LA. The murine IRAK2 gene encodes four alternatively spliced isoforms, two of which are inhibitory. J Biol Chem 2004; 279(26): 27699–708.

56. Honda K, Yanai H, Negishi H et al. IRF-7 is the master regulator of type-I interferon-dependent immune responses. Nature 2005; 434(7034): 772–7.

57. Uematsu S, Sato S, Yamamoto M et al. Interleukin-1 receptor-associated kinase-1 plays an essential role for Toll-like receptor (TLR)7- and TLR9-mediated interferon-{alpha} induction. J Exp Med 2005; 201(6): 915–23.

58. Kawai T, Sato S, Ishii KJ et al. Interferon-alpha induction through Toll-like receptors involves a direct interaction of IRF7 with MyD88 and TRAF6. Nat Immunol 2004; 5(10): 1061–8.

59. Takaoka A, Yanai H, Kondo S et al. Integral role of IRF-5 in the gene induction programme activated by Toll-like receptors. Nature 2005; 434: 243–9.

60. Fitzgerald KA, Palsson-McDermott EM, Bowie AG et al. Mal (MyD88-adapter-like) is required for Toll-like receptor-4 signal transduction. Nature 2001; 413(6851): 78–83.

61. Horng T, Barton GM, Medzhitov R. TIRAP: an adapter molecule in the Toll signaling pathway. Nat Immunol 2001; 2(9): 835–41.

62. Yamamoto M, Sato S, Hemmi H et al. Role of adapter TRIF in the MyD88-independent Toll-like receptor signaling pathway. Science 2003; 301: 640–3.

63. Hoebe K, Du X, Georgel P et al. Identification of Lps2 as a key transducer of MyD88-independent TIR signalling. Nature 2003; 424: 743–8.

64. Yamamoto M, Sato S, Hemmi H et al. TRAM is specifically involved in the Toll-like receptor 4-mediated MyD88-independent signaling pathway. Nat Immunol 2003; 4(11): 1144–50.

65. O'Neill LA, Fitzgerald KA, Bowie AG. The Toll-IL-1 receptor adapter family grows to five members. Trends Immunol 2003; 24(6): 286–9.

66. Yamamoto M, Sato S, Hemmi H et al. Essential role for TIRAP in activation of the signalling cascade shared by TLR2 and TLR4. Nature 2002; 420(6913): 324–9.

67. Horng T, Barton GM, Flavell RA, Medzhitov R. The adapter molecule TIRAP provides signalling specificity for Toll-like receptors. Nature 2002; 420(6913): 329–33.

68. Kagan JC, Medzhitov R. Phosphoinositide-mediated adapter recruitment controls Toll-like receptor signaling. Cell 2006; 125(5): 943–55.

69. Fitzgerald KA, Chen ZJ. Sorting out Toll signals. Cell 2006; 125(5): 834–6.

70. Fitzgerald KA, McWhirter SM, Faia KL et al. IKKepsilon and TBK1 are essential components of the IRF3 signaling pathway. Nat Immunol 2003; 4(5): 491–6.

71. Fitzgerald KA, Rowe DC, Barnes BJ et al. LPS-TLR4 signaling to IRF-3/7 and NF-kappaB involves the toll adapters TRAM and TRIF. J Exp Med 2003; 198(7): 1043–55.

72. Yamamoto M, Sato S, Mori K et al. Cutting edge: a novel Toll/IL-1 receptor domain-containing adapter that preferentially activates the IFN-beta promoter in the Toll-like receptor signaling. J Immunol 2002; 169(12): 6668–72.

73. Oshiumi H, Matsumoto M, Funami K, Akazawa T, Seya T. TICAM-1, an adapter molecule that participates in Toll-like receptor 3-mediated interferon-beta induction. Nat Immunol 2003; 4(2): 161–7.

74. Sato S, Sugiyama M, Yamamoto M et al. Toll/IL-1 receptor domain-containing adapter inducing IFN-beta (TRIF) associates with TNF receptor-associated factor 6 and TANK-binding kinase 1, and activates two distinct

transcription factors, NF-kappa B and IFN-regulatory factor-3, in the Toll-like receptor signaling. J Immunol 2003; 171(8): 4304–10.

75. Jiang Z, Mak TW, Sen G, Li X. Toll-like receptor 3-mediated activation of NF-kappaB and IRF3 diverges at Toll-IL-1 receptor domain-containing adapter inducing IFN-beta. Proc Natl Acad Sci U S A 2004; 101(10): 3533–8.

76. Meylan E, Burns K, Hofmann K et al. RIP1 is an essential mediator of Toll-like receptor 3-induced NF-kappa B activation. Nat Immunol 2004; 5(5): 503–7.

77. Cusson-Hermance N, Khurana S, Lee TH, Fitzgerald KA, Kelliher MA. Rip1 mediates the Trif-dependent toll-like receptor 3- and 4-induced NF-{kappa}B activation but does not contribute to interferon regulatory factor 3 activation. J Biol Chem 2005; 280(44): 36560–6.

78. Covert MW, Leung TH, Gaston JE, Baltimore D. Achieving stability of lipopolysaccharide-induced NF-kappaB activation. Science 2005; 309(5742): 1854–7.

79. Oshiumi H, Sasai M, Shida K et al. TICAM-2: a bridging adapter recruiting to Toll-like receptor 4 TICAM-1 that induces interferon-beta. J Biol Chem 2003; 278: 49751–62.

80. McGettrick AF, Brint EK, Palsson-McDermott EM et al. Trif-related adapter molecule is phosphorylated by PKC{varepsilon} during Toll-like receptor 4 signaling. Proc Natl Acad Sci U S A 2006; 103(24): 9196–201.

81. Rowe DC, McGettrick AF, Latz E et al. The myristoylation of TRIF-related adapter molecule is essential for Toll-like receptor 4 signal transduction. Proc Natl Acad Sci U S A 2006; 103(16): 6299–304.

82. Wietek C, Miggin SM, Jefferies CA, O'Neill LA. Interferon regulatory factor-3-mediated activation of the interferon-sensitive response element by Toll-like receptor (TLR) 4 but not TLR3 requires the p65 subunit of NF-kappa. J Biol Chem 2003; 278(51): 50923–31.

83. Carly M, Goodbody R, Schröder M, et al. The human adaptor SARM negatively regulates adaptor protein TRIF-dependent Toll-like receptor signalling. Nat Immunol 2006; 7(10): 1074-81.

84. Edfeldt K, Swedenborg J, Hansson GK, Yan ZQ. Expression of toll-like receptors in human atherosclerotic lesions: a possible pathway for plaque activation. Circulation 2002; 105(10): 1158–61.

85. Bsibsi M, Ravid R, Gveric D, van Noort JM. Broad expression of Toll-like receptors in the human central nervous system. J Neuropathol Exp Neurol 2002; 61(11): 1013–21.

86. Cario E, Podolsky DK. Differential alteration in intestinal epithelial cell expression of toll-like receptor 3 (TLR3) and TLR4 in inflammatory bowel disease. Infect Immun 2000; 68(12): 7010–17.

87. Abreu MT, Thomas LS, Arnold ET et al. TLR signaling at the intestinal epithelial interface. J Endotoxin Res 2003; 9(5): 322–30.

88. Radstake TR, Roelofs MF, Jenniskens YM et al. Expression of toll-like receptors 2 and 4 in rheumatoid synovial tissue and regulation by proinflammatory cytokines interleukin-12 and interleukin-18 via interferon-gamma. Arthritis Rheum 2004; 50(12): 3856–65.

89. Roelofs MF, Joosten LA, Abdollahi-Roodsaz S et al. The expression of toll-like receptors 3 and 7 in rheumatoid arthritis synovium is increased and costimulation of toll-like receptors 3, 4, and 7/8 results in synergistic cytokine production by dendritic cells. Arthritis Rheum 2005; 52(8): 2313–22.

90. van der Heijden IM, Wilbrink B, Tchetverikov I et al. Presence of bacterial DNA and bacterial peptidoglycans in joints of patients with rheumatoid arthritis and other arthritides. Arthritis Rheum 2000; 43(3): 593–8.

91. Gaston JS. Heat shock proteins and arthritis – new readers start here. Autoimmunity 1997; 26(1): 33–42.

92. Poole AR, Dieppe P. Biological markers in rheumatoid arthritis. Semin Arthritis Rheum 1994; 23(6 Suppl 2): 17–31.

93. Noble PW, McKee CM, Cowman M, Shin HS. Hyaluronan fragments activate an NF-kappa B/I-kappa B alpha autoregulatory loop in murine macrophages. J Exp Med 1996; 183(5): 2373–8.

94. Li M, Carpio DF, Zheng Y et al. An essential role of the NF-kappa B/Toll-like receptor pathway in induction of inflammatory and tissue-repair gene expression by necrotic cells. J Immunol 2001; 166(12): 7128–35.

95. Brentano F, Schorr O, Gay RE, Gay S, Kyburz D. RNA released from necrotic synovial fluid cells activates rheumatoid arthritis synovial fibroblasts via Toll-like receptor 3. Arthritis Rheum 2005; 52(9): 2656–65.

96. Deng GM, Nilsson IM, Verdrengh M, Collins LV, Tarkowski A. Intra-articularly localized bacterial DNA containing CpG motifs induces arthritis. Nat Med 1999; 5(6): 702–5.

97. Liu ZQ, Deng GM, Foster S, Tarkowski A. Staphylococcal peptidoglycans induce arthritis. Arthritis Res 2001; 3(6): 375–80.

98. Zare F, Bokarewa M, Nenonen N et al. Arthritogenic properties of double-stranded (viral) RNA. J Immunol 2004; 172(9): 5656–63.

99. Joosten LA, Koenders MI, Smeets RL et al. Toll-like receptor 2 pathway drives streptococcal cell wall-induced joint inflammation: critical role of myeloid differentiation factor 88. J Immunol 2003; 171(11): 6145–53.

100. Choe JY, Crain B, Wu SR, Corr M. Interleukin 1 receptor dependence of serum transferred arthritis can be circumvented by toll-like receptor 4 signaling. J Exp Med 2003; 197(4): 537–42.

101. Lau CM, Broughton C, Tabor AS et al. RNA-associated autoantigens activate B cells by combined B cell antigen receptor/Toll-like receptor 7 engagement. J Exp Med 2005; 202(9): 1171–7.

102. Pisitkun P, Deane JA, Difilippantonio MJ et al. Autoreactive B cell responses to RNA-related antigens

due to TLR7 gene duplication. Science 2006; 312(5780): 1669–72.

103. Subramanian S, Tus K, Li QZ et al. A Tlr7 translocation accelerates systemic autoimmunity in murine lupus. Proc Natl Acad Sci U S A 2006; 103(26): 9970–5.

104. Radstake TR, Franke B, Hanssen S, et al. The Toll-like receptor-4 Asp299Gly functional variant is associated with decreased rheumatoid arthritis disease susceptibility but does not influence disease severity and/or outcome. Arthritis Rheum 2004; 50: 999–1001.

105. Kilding R, Akil M, Till S et al. A biologically important single nucleotide polymorphism within the toll-like receptor-4 gene is not associated with rheumatoid arthritis. Clin Exp Rheumatol 2003; 21(3): 340–2.

106. Sanchez E, Orozco G, Lopez-Nevot MA, Jimenez-Alonso J, Martin J. Polymorphisms of toll-like receptor 2 and 4 genes in rheumatoid arthritis and systemic lupus erythematosus. Tissue Antigens 2004; 63(1): 54–7.

107. Kiechl S, Lorenz E, Reindl M et al. Toll-like receptor 4 polymorphisms and atherogenesis. N Engl J Med 2002; 347(3): 185–92.

108. Ameziane N, Beillat T, Verpillat P et al. Association of the Toll-like receptor 4 gene Asp299Gly polymorphism with acute coronary events. Arterioscler Thromb Vasc Biol 2003; 23(12): e61–4.

109. Yang IA, Holloway JW, Ye S. TLR4 Asp299Gly polymorphism is not associated with coronary artery stenosis. Atherosclerosis 2003; 170(1): 187–90.

110. Netea MG, van Deuren M, Kullberg BJ, Cavaillon JM, Van der Meer JW. Does the shape of lipid A determine the interaction of LPS with Toll-like receptors? Trends Immunol 2002; 23(3): 135–9.

111. Franchimont D, Vermeire S, El Housni H et al. Deficient host-bacteria interactions in inflammatory bowel disease? The toll-like receptor (TLR)-4 Asp299gly polymorphism is associated with Crohn's disease and ulcerative colitis. Gut 2004; 53(7): 987–92.

112. Torok HP, Glas J, Tonenchi L, Mussack T, Folwaczny C. Polymorphisms of the lipopolysaccharide-signaling complex in inflammatory bowel disease: association of a mutation in the Toll-like receptor 4 gene with ulcerative colitis. Clin Immunol 2004; 112(1): 85–91.

113. Rudofsky G Jr, Reismann P, Witte S et al. Asp299Gly and Thr399Ile genotypes of the TLR4 gene are associated with a reduced prevalence of diabetic neuropathy in patients with type 2 diabetes. Diabetes Care 2004; 27(1): 179–83.

114. Yang IA, Barton SJ, Rorke S et al. Toll-like receptor 4 polymorphism and severity of atopy in asthmatics. Genes Immun 2004; 5(1): 41–5.

115. Kang TJ, Chae GT. Detection of Toll-like receptor 2 (TLR2) mutation in the lepromatous leprosy patients. FEMS Immunol Med Microbiol 2001; 31(1): 53–8.

116. Bochud PY, Hawn TR, Aderem A. Cutting edge: a Toll-like receptor 2 polymorphism that is associated with lepromatous leprosy is unable to mediate mycobacterial signaling. J Immunol 2003; 170(7): 3451–4.

117. Lorenz E, Mira JP, Cornish KL, Arbour NC, Schwartz DA. A novel polymorphism in the toll-like receptor 2 gene and its potential association with staphylococcal infection. Infect Immun 2000; 68(11): 6398–401.

118. Lee EY, Yim JJ, Lee HS et al. Dinucleotide repeat polymorphism in intron II of human Toll-like receptor 2 gene and susceptibility to rheumatoid arthritis. Int J Immunogenet 2006; 33(3): 211–15.

119. Hawn TR, Verbon A, Lettinga KD et al. A common dominant TLR5 stop codon polymorphism abolishes flagellin signaling and is associated with susceptibility to legionnaires' disease. J Exp Med 2003; 198(10): 1563–72.

120. Hawn TR, Wu H, Grossman JM et al. A stop codon polymorphism of Toll-like receptor 5 is associated with resistance to systemic lupus erythematosus. Proc Natl Acad Sci U S A 2005; 102(30): 10593–7.

121. Epinat JC, Gilmore TD. Diverse agents act at multiple levels to inhibit the Rel/NF-kappaB signal transduction pathway. Oncogene 1999; 18(49): 6896–909.

122. O'Neill LA. Therapeutic targeting of Toll-like receptors for inflammatory and infectious diseases. Curr Opin Pharmacol 2003; 3(4): 396–403.

123. Signal pharmaceuticals, Inc. Quinazoline analogs and related compounds and methods for treating inflammatory conditions. No 199901441 (1999).

124. Kopp E, Ghosh S. Inhibition of NF-kappa B by sodium salicylate and aspirin. Science 1994; 265(5174): 956–9.

125. Kwok BH, Koh B, Ndubuisi MI, Elofsson M, Crews CM. The anti-inflammatory natural product parthenolide from the medicinal herb Feverfew directly binds to and inhibits IkappaB kinase. Chem Biol 2001; 8(8): 759–66.

126. Wahl C, Liptay S, Adler G, Schmid RM. Sulfasalazine: a potent and specific inhibitor of nuclear factor kappa B. J Clin Invest 1998; 101(5): 1163–74.

127. Weber CK, Liptay S, Wirth T, Adler G, Schmid RM. Suppression of NF-kappaB activity by sulfasalazine is mediated by direct inhibition of IkappaB kinases alpha and beta. Gastroenterology 2000; 119(5): 1209–18.

128. Manna SK, Mukhopadhyay A, Aggarwal BB. Leflunomide suppresses TNF-induced cellular responses: effects on NF-kappa B, activator protein-1, c-Jun N-terminal protein kinase, and apoptosis. J Immunol 2000; 165(10): 5962–9.

129. O'Neill LA. Targeting signal transduction as a strategy to treat inflammatory diseases. Nat Rev Drug Discov 2006; 5(7): 549–63.

130. Spano JP, Bay JO, Blay JY, Rixe O. Proteasome inhibition: a new approach for the treatment of malignancies. Bull Cancer 2005; 92(11): E61–6, 945–52.

131. Dumas J, Hatoum-Mokdad H, Sibley R et al. 1-Phenyl-5-pyrazolyl ureas: potent and selective p38 kinase inhibitors. Bioorg Med Chem Lett 2000; 10(18): 2051–4.

132. Dumas J, Sibley R, Riedl B et al. Discovery of a new class of p38 kinase inhibitors. Bioorg Med Chem Lett 2000; 10(18): 2047–50.

133. English JM, Cobb MH. Pharmacological inhibitors of MAPK pathways. Trends Pharmacol Sci 2002; 23(1): 40–5.

134. Lasa M, Abraham SM, Boucheron C, Saklatvala J, Clark AR. Dexamethasone causes sustained expression of mitogen-activated protein kinase (MAPK) phosphatase 1 and phosphatase-mediated inhibition of MAPK p38. Mol Cell Biol 2002; 22(22): 7802–11.

135. Ogawa S, Lozach J, Benner C et al. Molecular determinants of crosstalk between nuclear receptors and toll-like receptors. Cell 2005; 122(5): 707–21.

136. Herlaar E, Brown Z. p38 MAPK signalling cascades in inflammatory disease. Mol Med Today 1999; 5(10): 439–47.

137. Liverton NJ, Butcher JW, Claiborne CF et al. Design and synthesis of potent, selective, and orally bioavailable tetrasubstituted imidazole inhibitors of p38 mitogen-activated protein kinase. J Med Chem 1999; 42(12): 2180–90.

138. McLay LM, Halley F, Souness JE et al. The discovery of RPR 200765A, a p38 MAP kinase inhibitor displaying a good oral anti-arthritic efficacy. Bioorg Med Chem 2001; 9(2): 537–54.

139. Badger AM, Griswold DE, Kapadia R et al. Disease-modifying activity of SB 242235, a selective inhibitor of p38 mitogen-activated protein kinase, in rat adjuvant-induced arthritis. Arthritis Rheum 2000; 43(1): 175–83.

140. Dominguez C, Powers DA, Tamayo N. p38 MAP kinase inhibitors: many are made, but few are chosen. Curr Opin Drug Discov Devel 2005; 8(4): 421–30.

141. Bowie A, O'Neill LA. The interleukin-1 receptor/Toll-like receptor superfamily: signal generators for pro-inflammatory interleukins and microbial products. J Leukoc Biol 2000; 67(4): 508–14.

142. Harte MT, Haga IR, Maloney G et al. The poxvirus protein A52R targets Toll-like receptor signaling complexes to suppress host defense. J Exp Med 2003; 197(3): 343–51.

143. McCoy SL, Kurtz SE, Macarthur CJ, Trune DR, Hefeneider SH. Identification of a peptide derived from vaccinia virus A52R protein that inhibits cytokine secretion in response to TLR-dependent signaling and reduces in vivo bacterial-induced inflammation. J Immunol 2005; 174(5): 3006–14.

10

Cadherin-11 mediates synovial lining organization: a new therapeutic target in inflammatory arthritis

Erika H Noss and Michael B Brenner

Introduction • Overview of cadherins • Cadherins in the synovium • Cadherins in cancer: implications for pannus behavior in inflammatory arthritis • Cadherins and inflammation • Cadherins as therapeutic targets in rheumatic diseases • Acknowledgments • References

INTRODUCTION

Cell-to-cell adhesion is vital for the formation and maintenance of all tissues. However, little is known about cell-to-cell interactions important in the synovial lining. Recently, expression of a cadherin superfamily member, cadherin-11, was identified on fibroblast-like synoviocytes (FLS). *In vitro* experiments demonstrated that the presence of cadherin-11 on FLS or a fibroblast cell line was sufficient to form a lining layer reminiscent of the synovium. The synovial lining in cadherin-11-deficient mice is hypoplastic, confirming the importance of this molecule in development of the synovium. Furthermore, cadherin-11 was necessary for the elaboration of both inflammation and cartilage erosions in a mouse model of inflammatory arthritis. As will be discussed in this chapter, these studies suggest that cadherin-11 on FLS plays a critical role in synovial inflammation and cartilage erosion, and may serve as a unique therapeutic target in the management of rheumatoid arthritis (RA). This review seeks to provide initial insights into how cadherin-11 modulates FLS behavior and emphasizes how cadherin function in development and cancer biology offers clues to its role in synovial pathology.

OVERVIEW OF CADHERINS

Several families of molecules are important for cell-to-cell or cell-to-matrix adhesion. Typically, β_1 integrins mediate cell-to-matrix adhesion while integrins, selectins, immunoglobulin superfamily molecules, nectins, and cadherins mediate cell-to-cell adhesion.[1–3] Early investigations divided cell adhesion systems into calcium-dependent and calcium-independent mechanisms.[4] Calcium-dependent cell-to-cell adhesion is mediated by cadherins, which are expressed in nearly all tissues. Cadherin binding is generally homophilic, meaning a cadherin of one type binds to a cadherin of the same type on a neighboring cell.[5] Although a given cell may express several different cadherins, patterns of cadherin expression are tissue-restricted.[6] Cadherin expression is particularly enriched in adherens junctions, specialized areas of cell-to-cell contact that connect to the internal actin cytoskeleton.[7]

Cadherin structure

Classic cadherins (the main focus of this review) belong to a family which includes the classic cadherins, desmogleins, desmocollins, protocadherins, and flamingo (or seven-pass) cadherins.[6,8] This superfamily is defined by the presence of extracellular cadherin repeats consisting of approximately 110 amino acids that fold into a 7-stranded β-sandwich structurally similar to the immunoglobulin domain.[6,9] Classic cadherins are glycosylated single-pass type I transmembrane proteins consisting of five extracellular cadherin repeats with a conserved cytoplasmic tail. The N-terminal extracellular cadherin repeats (or ectodomains) are separated from each other by conserved calcium binding sites. Calcium binding rigidifies the extended, chain-like cadherin structure and provides partial protection against protease digestion.[10,11] Cadherin binding specificity is determined largely by the N-terminal first ectodomain.[9,10,12] Multiple crystal structures have shown that binding occurs through formation of a strand dimer, where a conserved tryptophan from one cadherin inserts into a conserved hydrophobic pocket of an adjacent molecule.[11,13–15] This interaction occurs reciprocally between the two cadherins of adjacent cells in a two-fold symmetric, 'ball and socket' topology (*trans* binding). Other interactions between cadherins on the same cell can also occur (*cis* binding).[16,17] Clustering of cadherins by *cis* interactions with subsequent transition to *trans* binding is postulated to be important for regulation of cadherin adhesion.[10,12]

The C-terminal cytoplasmic tail contains two conserved binding sites for catenins, molecules that regulate cadherin turnover and attachment to the actin cytoskeleton (Figure 10.1).[12] More distally, β-catenin binds at the catenin binding sequence and interacts with α-catenin. Dissociation of α-catenin from the cadherin complex may act as a molecular switch, allowing α-catenin to bind to actin, inhibiting extension of actin fibers.[18,19] α-Catenin also binds to several other proteins important in regulation of actin cytoskeleton formation, including α-actinin, formin, and ZO-1.[7] More membrane proximal in the cadherin cytoplasmic tail is the p120 catenin binding region, also referred to as the conserved membrane proximal domain. Its binding is thought to be important for regulating cadherin transport, clustering, and interaction with various signaling cascades including src family kinases and small Rho GTPases.[20–23] Phosphorylation of cadherins and associated catenins regulates the stability of cadherin–catenin complexes, modulating the adhesive capacity of a cell.[24]

Classic cadherins are further divided into two subgroups: type I (including cadherins E, N, P, R, M) and type II (including cadherins

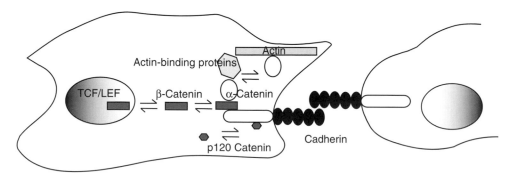

Figure 10.1 Interaction of cadherins with catenins is important for the formation of cell-to-cell contacts. Cadherin binding is classically homophillic, with cadherins of one type binding to a cadherin of the same type on an adjacent cell. Catenins bind to cadherins through conserved cytoplasmic tail binding motifs and are important for regulating cadherin complex turnover and linkage to the actin cytoskeleton. β-Catenin links α-catenin to the cadherin molecule, but cytosolic β-catenin can also translocate to the nucleus where it interacts with the TCF/LEF family of transcription factors. α-Catenin interacts with actin both directly and via binding to several proteins that regulate actin cytoskeleton turnover. P120 catenin binds more proximally to the cadherin tail and is thought to play a role in regulating complex stability and interactions with cell signaling pathways.

VE, 6, 7, 9, 10, 11, 12, 18, 19, 20).[6] Type I cadherins have only one conserved tryptophan located at the second amino acid position (Trp2) in the first ectodomain that participates in strand dimer formation. In contrast, type II cadherins have two tryptophans (Trp2 and Trp4). As a consequence, the hydrophobic pocket accommodating the tryptophans is larger in type II cadherins.[14] Type I cadherins also have a conserved histidine, alanine, valine (HAV) sequence in the first ectodomain that is not present in type II molecules. Interestingly, while type II cadherins have more homologous first ectodomain sequences compared with type I molecules, they also have greater variability in the intervening regions between the catenin binding motifs.[6,14] These structural distinctions between type I and type II cadherins suggest ways that cadherin structure may modify function, both in terms of binding specificity and cytoplasmic interactions.

Functional roles for cadherins

The importance of cadherins was first shown in morphogenetic studies. Initial observations correlated spatiotemporal expression of different cadherins with cellular migrations that lead to new tissue layer formation during embryonic development.[4] There are now many examples in which disruption of specific cadherin adhesions by various methods, including expression of dominant negative constructs and gene ablation, results in stage-specific failure of embryogenesis.[25-28] Observations from development studies indicate that cadherins are critical for cell sorting and subsequent tissue morphogenesis. *In vitro* experiments modeling this show that two cell lines expressing different cadherins or different levels of the same cadherin will separate into distinct, cell line-specific aggregates over time.[29,30] Simplistically, expression of like cadherins merges cell populations into a common structure, while loss or disconcordance of cadherin expression allows cells to migrate and form separate structures.[31]

Cadherins play a role in many critical processes that depend on cell-to-cell contacts.[5,12,32] Beyond their role in development, cadherins continue to be crucial in the controlled growth and turnover of adult tissues, including the maintenance of epithelial and endothelial junctions.[12,33] Cadherins are critically involved in cellular rearrangements necessary for the movement of cells over one another (intercellular motility). Such movements are important for separation of tissue layers, maintenance of tissue boundaries, intercalation of cells into tissue masses, formation of neuronal synapses, and regeneration of lining layers.

CADHERINS IN THE SYNOVIUM

Cadherins in normal synovium

The synovium is a delicate, lacy structure that lines the joint cavity, providing lubrication and nutrients to the articular cartilage.[34] It consists of a lining layer a few cells thick that rests on a looser connective tissue sublining. The synovial lining consists of two cell types, type A macrophage-like synoviocytes (MLS) and type B fibroblast-like synoviocytes (FLS).[35] Accordingly, the lining is neither an epithelial nor an endothelial structure and lacks a true basement membrane. However, FLS produce an organized extracellular matrix (ECM) that supports the lining layer, in which MLS and FLS make connections with each other and the underlying ECM. The nature of these connections has not been clearly defined.[1] Histological studies have shown that certain integrin/integrin-counter receptor subunits are expressed by synoviocytes.[36-39] It has been proposed that vascular cell adhesion molecule 1 (VCAM)-1 and intercellular cell adhesion molecule 1 (ICAM-1) on FLS may be important for mediating binding to MLS through their respective integrin ligands.[40-42]

Given the importance of cadherins in cell-to-cell interactions in other tissues, it was postulated that cadherins might play a role in the synovium. Using degenerative oligonucleotides corresponding to the highly conserved cadherin cytoplasmic tail, cadherin-11 was isolated from RA-FLS.[43] Cadherin-11 (initially named OB-cadherin) is a type II cadherin that was first cloned from both human and mouse osteoblast lines and was found to be highly homologous between these two species, differing in only 17 amino acids.[44,45] Cadherin-11 expression has been demonstrated in brain, lung, kidney, pericardium, testis, prostate, uterus, placenta, colon, and growth plate cartilage, but not in the liver, spleen, thymus, skeletal muscle, or normal skin.[43–52] Cadherin-11-deficient mice are known to have both reduced bone density in the calavaria and femoral metaphyses and enhanced long-term neuronal potentiation in the hippocampus, leading to reduced fear and anxiety responses.[53,54]

Using cell lines derived from synovial tissues, expression of cadherin-11 on human FLS was confirmed by northern, western, and flow cytometric analysis. No substantial expression of cadherin-11 was detected on CD45-positive bone marrow lineage cells (e.g. macrophages) in disaggregated synovial specimens, indicating cadherin-11 expression is principally on FLS.[43] Histological studies on normal, osteoarthritic, and RA synovium showed prominent cadherin-11 staining in the lining layer with rare cadherin-11-reactive cells noted in the sublining region.[43] Unlike prior reports,[55,56] no staining for epithelial (E)-cadherin was noted in the synovium, although more recently, neuronal (N)-cadherin FLS expression has also been demonstrated (unpublished observations).

The presence of cadherin-11 on FLS suggests that this molecule is important for mediating cell-to-cell contacts in the synovium. Confocal and immunoprecipitation studies established that FLS cadherin-11 is found predominantly at sites of cell-to-cell contacts and co-localizes with the molecules necessary for cadherin function: α-catenin, β-catenin, p120 catenin, and actin.[57] Moreover, cadherin-11 expression proved sufficient to organize a lining layer structure in three-dimensional culture systems. FLS dispersed in Matrigel™, a basement membrane-like ECM, formed a spontaneous lining at the media–matrix border over time in culture, similar to that of the synovial lining at the junction with the joint fluid space.[57] Formation of this lining *in vitro* was blocked by a cadherin-11-Fc fusion protein. Furthermore, cadherin-11 transfection into L cells, a fibroblast line that lacks its own cadherins but expresses catenins, confers upon these cells a similar ability to form a lining. The role of cadherin-11 in synovial lining formation, first suggested *in vitro*, has now been confirmed *in vivo*. Histologic examination of synovial joints from mice lacking functional cadherin-11 revealed the synovial lining to be hypoplastic.[58] By trichrome staining, the ECM underlying what cells were present was markedly reduced. Taken together, both *in vivo* mouse and *in vitro* mouse and human studies provide compelling evidence that cadherin-11 is a critical mediator of cell-to-cell interactions necessary for FLS-mediated synovial lining layer formation.

Cadherins in inflammatory arthritis

RA is a polyarticular inflammatory arthritis characterized by transformation of the synovial lining from a thin layer that respects other joint structures into a hyperplastic tissue mass, or pannus, capable of extending into the joint space and eroding cartilage and bone.[34] Inflammatory cells infiltrate the synovial sublining and produce proinflammatory cytokines, chemokines, and growth factors that stimulate synovial lining hyperplasia, resulting in a marked increase in both the numbers and activation of MLS and FLS.[59] In turn, synoviocytes release additional cytokines, chemokines, and growth factors that help sustain inflammation and produce enzymes that are capable of degrading ECM, destroying cartilage and bone.

Using the murine KxB/N serum transfer model of inflammatory arthritis,[60,61] the role of cadherin-11 was tested by inducing arthritis in both cadherin-11-deficient and wild-type mice Remarkably, compared with wild-type, cadherin-11-deficient mice developed substantially less arthritis by clinical measures and histologic examination.[58] Both a monoclonal antibody against cadherin-11 and a cadherin-11-Fc fusion protein inhibited the formation of arthritis, confirming that cadherin-11 modulates synovial inflammation.[58] Furthermore, cadherin-11-deficient mice were uniquely protected from direct cartilage erosion by the synovial pannus. The reduced hyperplastic synovial lining reaction that did occur in cadherin-11-deficient mice was disorganized and lacked the cellular compaction seen in the pannus of wild-type mice. In contrast to the lack of cartilage erosion in cadherin-11-deficient mice, the extent of bone erosion, mediated by osteoblast activation, was similar to wild-type arthritic mice. Therefore, cadherin-11 on FLS appears to have dual actions in inflammatory arthritis, contributing to both the underlying inflammatory response and FLS-mediated cartilage destruction.

CADHERINS IN CANCER: IMPLICATIONS FOR PANNUS BEHAVIOR IN INFLAMMATORY ARTHRITIS

The mechanisms by which cadherin-11 regulates synovial biology in health and inflammation are now under active investigation. Several lines of evidence indicate that cadherins may have a role in promoting cell motility and invasion. In particular, changes in cadherin expression in many tumors have been correlated with increased tumor invasiveness.[6] Examination of the role of cadherins in cancer may provide insights into how cadherin-11 functions in inflammatory arthritis.

The inflamed synovium becomes hyperplastic, forming a pannus that erodes into both articular cartilage and underlying bone in a manner somewhat analogous to a locally invasive tumor.[59] Cultured RA FLS, but not osteoarthritic or normal FLS, maintain the ability to invade cartilage implants in SCID mice, suggesting an underlying dysregulation of FLS in RA.[62] Although RA FLS are not tumor cells, they do display some characteristics of transformed cells.[34] These characteristics include anchorage-independent growth,[63] somatic mutations in the tumor suppression gene p53,[64] and possible origin from oligoclonal precursors.[65] As described earlier, the absence of cadherin-11 in mouse inflammatory arthritis results in a disorganized synovium that fails to crawl onto and degrade cartilage. How cadherin-11 modulates the ability of synovium to erode cartilage is not known. However, cadherins are known to impact the ability of cancer cells to invade and metastasize. Given that both cancer and inflamed synovium reflect cellular changes that permit aberrant tissue invasion, examination of the role of cadherins in cancer cell motility and invasion may provide insights into how cadherin-11 influences the invasive behavior of FLS.

Changes in cadherin expression and function are a hallmark of epithelial-to-mesenchymal transition (EMT), which is important both in embryonic development and in carcinoma formation. EMT is a process by which epithelial cells dissolve cell-to-cell contacts and lose apical-basal polarity, transforming into mesenchymal cells that are able to migrate. A hallmark of EMT is loss of E-cadherin function.[66] The first EMT in development occurs during gastrulation, where up-regulation of the Snail family of transcription factors represses E-cadherin expression and promotes migration of the developing mesoderm and endoderm from the epiblast. In tumor cells, EMT may be either partial or complete and requires a series of changes, including oncogenic transformation of ras, src, or receptor tyrosine kinases along with autocrine/paracrine signaling loops.[67,68] Several autocrine growth factors have been implicated, including transforming growth factor-β (TGF-β), platelet derived growth factor (PDGF), and fibroblast growth factors (FGF). In addition, multiple signaling loops are activated, including Wnt, Notch, Hedgehog, and nuclear factor kappa B (NF-κB), some of which lead to re-expression of development transcription factors such as Snail or its related family member, Slug.

Importantly, loss of E-cadherin expression or function is associated with several types of epithelial cell-derived tumors, including breast, skin, gastric, pancreatic, lung, and cervical cancers. Further, loss of E-cadherin also often correlates with increased invasiveness.[6,69–71] Expression of E-cadherin, by maintaining epithelial cell-to-cell contacts, is thought to act as a brake on invasion of cells into the underlying stroma. For example, in a mouse model of pancreatic β cell carcinogenesis, forced expression of E-cadherin resulted in arrest of tumor development while expression of a dominant negative form of E-cadherin induced early invasion and metastasis.[71]

Further investigations suggest that development of an invasive phenotype in epithelial carcinomas may not simply be due to loss of E-cadherin, but also to the inappropriate expression of mesenchymal cadherins such as N-cadherin and cadherin-11. In one histologic study of prostate cancer, increased tumor grade correlated with both decreased expression of E-cadherin and increased expression of both N-cadherin and cadherin-11.[52] Interestingly, certain tumor areas contained cells expressing both E-cadherin and N-cadherin, suggesting a transition state between the loss of an epithelial phenotype and acquisition of a mesenchymal phenotype. Correlation of N-cadherin expression with invasive phenotype has also been seen in breast cancer and melanoma.[72–74] Transfection of N-cadherin or cadherin-11 into breast cancer cell lines increased their motility and invasiveness *in vitro*, regardless of expression of E-cadherin.[75,76] In a mouse mammary tumor model, injection of one of these N-cadherin-expressing transfectants resulted in widespread metastasis not seen with the original cell line.[75] Similarly, transfection of cadherin-11 into the L-cell fibroblast cell line increased the motility.[21]

It is not fully clear how expression of N-cadherin or cadherin-11 may increase tumor invasiveness. It has been proposed that expression of these mesenchymal cadherins might promote increased interactions of tumor cells with the underlying stromal cells, helping overcome one barrier to invasion.[72] Alternatively, these cadherins might uniquely influence other pathways that promote invasion. One possibility is through direct interactions with growth factor receptors. For example, N-cadherin has been shown to associate with an FGF receptor, and breast cancer lines transfected with N-cadherin dramatically up-regulated matrix metalloproteinase (MMP)-9 expression when treated with FGF-2.[75] These results suggested that N-cadherin, by causing a sustained activation of an FGF receptor, promoted production of a protease capable of degrading ECM, leading to increased invasive capacity. In fibroblast cultures, increasing cadherin-11 contacts as cells became confluent resulted in dramatically increased expression of the angiogenic factor vascular endothelial growth factor (VEGF)-D,[77] providing another example where cadherins influenced that growth factor/growth factor receptor pathways.

Another possible way by which cadherins may influence invasion is through coordinated regulation of cadherin and integrin function to promote increased attachment to the ECM and its degradation by integrin-associated proteases.[78,79] Many examples of 'cross-talk' between cadherins and integrins have been described. For instance, integrin-mediated binding of fibronectin-coated beads to bovine aortic endothelial cell monolayers rapidly disassembled vascular endothelial (VE)–cadherin adherens junctions via increased catenin phosphorylation by activated src kinase.[80] It was postulated that integrin-mediated signals may be important in triggering disruption of cadherin contacts necessary to allow angiogenesis. In a skin cancer model, disruption of cadherin complexes with dominant negative E-cadherin construct in transformed human keratinocytes was shown to actually up-regulate α-2, α-3, and β-1 integrin expression, allowing tumor cells to be preferentially retained at the basement membrane when implanted onto the skin of nude mice.[81] Finally, siRNA knockdown of the integrin signaling molecules Fak and paxillin in HeLa cells resulted in both the impairment of robust collagen adhesions and formation of N-cadherin cell-to-cell contacts due to a failure to down-regulate activity of the small GTPase molecule, Rac1, at the cell periphery.[82]

The synovium is a mesenchymal tissue that expresses cadherin-11 and N-cadherin, and cadherin-11 appears necessary for FLS to invade into cartilage during inflammatory arthritis. Given the striking effects of mesenchymal cadherin-11 and N-cadherin in tumor cell behavior, it seems likely that cadherin-11 may similarly influence the invasive and destructive behavior of the synovial pannus in RA. Thus cadherins may influence cartilage invasion by FLS through modulation of their expression or adhesive activity, via changes in integrin function, by their association with growth factors, or through other undetermined mechanisms that remain to be characterized.

CADHERINS AND INFLAMMATION

Given that cadherin-11 plays a role in forming FLS-to-FLS contacts, it was unexpected that the inflammatory response in K/BxN serum transfer arthritis was strikingly impaired in cadherin-11-deficient mice. This observation suggests a role for cadherin-11 in the modulation of inflammation. One explanation for this finding may be that cadherin-11-deficient FLS are an ineffective scaffold, providing poor organization and support to infiltrating inflammatory cells. Impairment of the ability to remodel cell-to-cell contacts may prevent the ability of a tissue to recruit or sequester inflammatory cells. In a mouse sepsis model, disruption of VE–cadherin adherens junctions through expression of a dominant-negative cadherin construct prevented neutrophil accumulation in the lung, possibly through modulation of endothelial ICAM-1 function.[83] Furthermore, although cadherins classically bind to other cadherins, heterotypic interactions with non-cadherin ligands on subtypes of immune cells have been reported. One such interaction includes binding of intestinal T lymphocytes to E-cadherin via integrin αEβ7, which may have a role in localization of this T-cell subset to the gut mucosa.[84] More recently, binding of the NK cell receptor killer cell lectin-like receptor G1 (KLRG1) to E-, R-, and N-cadherin has been reported.[85,86] This interaction was shown to inhibit both NK cell killing as well as the acquisition of effector CD8+ memory T-cell function. It is possible that similar types of heterotypic interactions may be important in synovial inflammation.

In addition, there is a growing appreciation that FLS produce cytokines (e.g. interleukin (IL)-1, IL-6, IL-15), chemoattractants (e.g. IL-8, monocyte chemoattractant protein-1), and growth factors (e.g. PDGF, VEGF) that may contribute to synovial inflammation.[87] Impaired synovial hyperplasia in cadherin-11-deficient mice may decrease the amount of some mediators by impairing FLS recruitment, activation, or proliferation. In fact, in cancer cells lines, N-cadherin ligation has been shown to have an anti-apoptotic action by increasing Bcl-2 expression through activation of Akt/protein kinase B[88] or by sequestering procaspase-8, preventing its recruitment to death-inducing signaling complexes.[89]

Moreover, several major points of intersection exist between cadherins and gene transcription pathways. For example, when not bound to the cadherin cytoplasmic tail, β-catenin can translocate into the nucleus as a transcription factor in association with T-cell factor/lymphoid enhancer factor (TCF/LEF) family members (Figure 10.1).[90,91] TCF/LEF-induced transcription has been shown to up-regulate a diverse number of proteins, including c-myc, cyclin D1, and MMP-7.[90] β-Catenin is central to coordination of canonical Wnt signaling pathways. Wnts are important regulators of cellular proliferation and differentiation, and they have been implicated in increasing RANKL and fibronectin synthesis in RA FLS.[92] Binding of Wnts to their receptors, the Frizzled homologs, increases the cytosolic pool of free β-catenin available to translocate to the nucleus and bind to TCF/LEF. Thus, the amount of cytosolic β-catenin is tightly controlled, with free β-catenin being rapidly translocated into the nucleus or targeted for degradation. Regulated disassembly of cadherin complexes may potentially release a large pool of previously sequestered β-catenin into the cytosol, increasing TCF/LEF gene transcription.

Other points of intersection between cadherin complexes and both the NF-κB and mitogen-activated protein kinase (MAPK) signaling pathways have been described in mice with epidermal ablation of p120 catenin and α-catenin expression, respectively.[33,93] Both NF-κB and MAPK pathways are critical in the regulation of synovial inflammation, increasing expression of cytokines, proteases, and cell adhesion molecules.[59,94] Ablation of p120 catenin expression in mouse epidermis did not affect epidermal barrier function.[93] Instead, these mice developed progressive skin inflammation with hyperkeratosis and chronic wasting. Keratinocytes lacking p120 catenin had increased nuclear translocation of NF-κB with associated increased transcription of NF-κB-regulated genes such as TNF-α, IL-1β, and IL-6. Ablation of α-catenin, on the other hand, did result in dramatic defects in skin and limb formation.[33] α-Catenin–deficient epidermis displayed hyperproliferation with defects in epithelial polarity, and knockout keratinocytes displayed sustained activation of the Ras-MAPK cascade due to aberration in growth factor responses. Both examples highlight that cadherin–catenin complexes may interact with signaling pathways that control many cellular functions, including cellular proliferation and inflammatory responses. Whether the role of cadherin-11 in inflammatory arthritis is to maintain a scaffold that promotes inflammation or directly influences the production of inflammatory mediators will be an important goal of future work.

CADHERINS AS THERAPEUTIC TARGETS IN RHEUMATIC DISEASES

Cadherin-11 is expressed on FLS in the synovium and is important in the ability of these cells to form a lining layer structure. Compared with wild-type mice, cadherin-11-deficient mice challenged with K/BxN serum are resistant to the development of arthritis and protected against cartilage erosion. These observations suggest that the synovium is not just a bystander, but rather an active participant in the joint inflammatory response. Similar to the effect seen in cadherin-11-deficient mice, treatment of B6 mice with either an anti-cadherin-11 monoclonal antibody or a cadherin-11-Fc-fusion protein can block the initiation of arthritis, suggesting that molecules directed against cadherins may become a new class of therapeutics that can specifically target the behavior of FLS.

Treatment of RA over the last decade has been revolutionized by the development of biotherapeutic agents against different components of the immune system, including proinflammatory cytokines (e.g. the TNF inhibitors), B cells (rituximab), and T-cell costimulation (abatacept). Although RA is a disease caused by immune dysregulation, joint destruction is ultimately a result of bone and cartilage erosions, mediated by activation of osteoclasts and synovial pannus. Recently, it was shown that inhibition of the RANK-RANKL pathway can specifically inhibit bone erosions independent of inflammation by blocking osteoclast activity.[95] Furthermore, in mouse arthritis models, cotreatment with agents that block both inflammation and bone erosion had an additive effect in blocking joint destruction.[96] These results suggest that new classes of therapeutics independent from those that target the immune system may be valuable in targeting effector pathways that directly mediate joint destruction.

Currently, no therapies exist that that are designed primarily to protect cartilage. Cadherin-11 represents a new potential therapeutic target directed against FLS that may both reduce inflammation and uniquely protect against cartilage erosion. Ideally, agents will continue to be developed against all components of the synovial response: inflammatory cells, synovial pannus, and activated osteoclasts

---

Table 10.1 Targets for therapies in RA

Inflammation
Proinflammatory cytokines: anti-TNF-α, IL-1Ra, anti-IL6
B cells: anti-CD20
T-cell costimulation: CTLA-4-Ig

Bone erosions
Activated osteoclasts: anti-RANKL, osteoprotegrin

Cartilage erosions
FLS in the synovial pannus: anti-cadherin-11

(Table 10.1). Ultimately, combinations of agents that target these three classes of cells (inflammatory cells, FLS, and osteoclasts) may provide the safest and most effective treatment to prevent long-term joint destruction in RA.

ACKNOWLEDGMENTS

Many thanks to Dr Sandeep K. Agarwal for his critical reading of this manuscript.

REFERENCES

1. Agarwal SK, Brenner MB. Role of adhesion molecules in synovial inflammation. Curr Opin Rheumatol 2006; 18: 268–76.
2. Petruzzelli L, Takami M, Humes HD. Structure and function of cell adhesion molecules. Am J Med 1999; 106: 467–76.
3. Sakisaka T, Takai Y. Biology and pathology of nectins and nectin-like molecules. Curr Opin Cell Biol 2004; 16: 513–21.
4. Takeichi M. The cadherins: cell-cell adhesion molecules controlling animal morphogenesis. Development 1988; 102: 639–55.
5. Gumbiner BM. Cell adhesion: the molecular basis of tissue architecture and morphogenesis. Cell 1996; 84: 345–57.
6. Nollet F, Kools P, van Roy F. Phylogenetic analysis of the cadherin superfamily allows identification of six major subfamilies besides several solitary members. J Mol Biol 2000; 299: 551–72.
7. Kobielak A, Fuchs E. Alpha-catenin: at the junction of intercellular adhesion and actin dynamics. Nat Rev Mol Cell Biol 2004; 5: 614–25.
8. Yagi T, Takeichi M. Cadherin superfamily genes: functions, genomic organization, and neurologic diversity. Genes Dev 2000; 14: 1169–80.

9. Patel SD, Chen CP, Bahna F et al. Cadherin-mediated cell-cell adhesion: sticking together as a family. Curr Opin Struct Biol 2003; 13: 690–8.

10. Leckband D, Prakasam A. Mechanism and Dynamics of Cadherin Adhesion. Annu Rev Biomed Eng 2006 (Epub ahead of print).

11. Pertz O, Bozic D, Koch AW et al. A new crystal structure, Ca2+ dependence and mutational analysis reveal molecular details of E-cadherin homoassociation. Embo J 1999; 18: 1738–47.

12. Gumbiner BM. Regulation of cadherin-mediated adhesion in morphogenesis. Nat Rev Mol Cell Biol 2005; 6: 622–34.

13. Boggon TJ, Murray J, Chappuis-Flament S et al. C-cadherin ectodomain structure and implications for cell adhesion mechanisms. Science 2002; 296: 1308–13.

14. Patel SD, Ciatto C, Chen CP et al. Type II cadherin ectodomain structures: implications for classical cadherin specificity. Cell 2006; 124: 1255–68.

15. Shapiro L, Fannon AM, Kwong PD et al. Structural basis of cell-cell adhesion by cadherins. Nature 1995; 374: 327–37.

16. Brieher WM, Yap AS, Gumbiner BM. Lateral dimerization is required for the homophilic binding activity of C-cadherin. J Cell Biol 1996; 135: 487–96.

17. Chitaev NA, Troyanovsky SM. Adhesive but not lateral E-cadherin complexes require calcium and catenins for their formation. J Cell Biol 1998; 142: 837–46.

18. Drees F, Pokutta S, Yamada S et al. Alpha-catenin is a molecular switch that binds E-cadherin-beta-catenin and regulates actin-filament assembly. Cell 2005; 123: 903–15.

19. Yamada S, Pokutta S, Drees F et al. Deconstructing the cadherin-catenin-actin complex. Cell 2005; 123: 889–901.

20. Chen X, Kojima S, Borisy GG et al. p120 catenin associates with kinesin and facilitates the transport of cadherin-catenin complexes to intercellular junctions. J Cell Biol 2003; 163: 547–57.

21. Kiener HP, Stipp CS, Allen PG et al. The cadherin-11 cytoplasmic juxtamembrane domain promotes alpha-catenin turnover at adherens junctions and intercellular motility. Mol Biol Cell 2006; 17: 2366–76.

22. Reynolds AB, Roczniak-Ferguson A. Emerging roles for p120-catenin in cell adhesion and cancer. Oncogene 2004; 23: 7947–56.

23. Xiao K, Allison DF, Buckley KM et al. Cellular levels of p120 catenin function as a set point for cadherin expression levels in microvascular endothelial cells. J Cell Biol 2003; 163: 535–45.

24. Lilien J, Balsamo J. The regulation of cadherin-mediated adhesion by tyrosine phosphorylation/dephosphorylation of beta-catenin. Curr Opin Cell Biol 2005; 17: 459–65.

25. Larue L, Ohsugi M, Hirchenhain J et al. E-cadherin null mutant embryos fail to form a trophectoderm epithelium. Proc Natl Acad Sci U S A 1994; 91: 8263–7.

26. Luo Y, Radice GL. N-cadherin acts upstream of VE-cadherin in controlling vascular morphogenesis. J Cell Biol 2005; 169: 29–34.

27. Takeichi M. Morphogenetic roles of classic cadherins. Curr Opin Cell Biol 1995; 7: 619–27.

28. Radice GL, Rayburn H, Matsunami H et al. Developmental defects in mouse embryos lacking N-cadherin. Dev Biol 1997; 181: 64–78.

29. Duguay D, Foty RA, Steinberg MS. Cadherin-mediated cell adhesion and tissue segregation: qualitative and quantitative determinants. Dev Biol 2003; 253: 309–23.

30. Nose A, Nagafuchi A, Takeichi M. Expressed recombinant cadherins mediate cell sorting in model systems. Cell 1988; 54: 993–1001.

31. Takeichi M. Cadherins: a molecular family important in selective cell-cell adhesion. Annu Rev Biochem 1990; 59: 237–52.

32. Keller R. Shaping the vertebrate body plan by polarized embryonic cell movements. Science 2002; 298: 1950–4.

33. Vasioukhin V, Bauer C, Degenstein L et al. Hyperproliferation and defects in epithelial polarity upon conditional ablation of alpha-catenin in skin. Cell 2001; 104: 605–17.

34. Lee DM, Kiener HP, Brenner MB. Synoviocytes. In: Harris ED, Budd RC, Genovese MC et al. eds. Kelley's Textbook of Rheumatology, 7th edn. Philadelphia: Elsevier Saunders, 2005: 175-88.

35. Barland P, Novikoff AB, Hamerman D. Electron microscopy of the human synovial membrane. J Cell Biol 1962; 14: 207–20.

36. Nikkari L, Haapasalmi K, Aho H et al. Localization of the alpha v subfamily of integrins and their putative ligands in synovial lining cell layer. J Rheumatol 1995; 22: 16–23.

37. Pirila L, Aho H, Roivainen A et al. Identification of alpha6beta1 integrin positive cells in synovial lining layer as type B synoviocytes. J Rheumatol 2001; 28: 478–84.

38. Rinaldi N, Barth TF, Weis D et al. Loss of laminin and of the laminin receptor integrin subunit alpha 6 in situ correlates with cytokine induced down regulation of alpha 6 on fibroblast-like synoviocytes from rheumatoid arthritis. Ann Rheum Dis 1998; 57: 559–65.

39. Rinaldi N, Weis D, Brado B et al. Differential expression and functional behaviour of the alpha v and beta 3 integrin subunits in cytokine stimulated fibroblast-like cells derived from synovial tissue of rheumatoid arthritis and osteoarthritis in vitro. Ann Rheum Dis 1997; 56: 729–36.

40. Ishikawa H, Hirata S, Andoh Y et al. An immunohistochemical and immunoelectron microscopic study of adhesion molecules in synovial pannus formation in rheumatoid arthritis. Rheumatol Int 1996; 16: 53–60.

41. Shang XZ, Lang BJ, Issekutz AC. Adhesion molecule mechanisms mediating monocyte migration through synovial fibroblast and endothelium barriers: role for

CD11/CD18, very late antigen-4 (CD49d/CD29), very late antigen-5 (CD49e/CD29), and vascular cell adhesion molecule-1 (CD106). J Immunol 1998; 160: 467–74.

42. Wilkinson LS, Edwards JC, Poston RN et al. Expression of vascular cell adhesion molecule-1 in normal and inflamed synovium. Lab Invest 1993; 68: 82–8.

43. Valencia X, Higgins JM, Kiener HP et al. Cadherin-11 provides specific cellular adhesion between fibroblast-like synoviocytes. J Exp Med 2004; 200: 1673–9.

44. Hoffmann I, Balling R. Cloning and expression analysis of a novel mesodermally expressed cadherin. Dev Biol 1995; 169: 337–46.

45. Okazaki M, Takeshita S, Kawai S et al. Molecular cloning and characterization of OB-cadherin, a new member of cadherin family expressed in osteoblasts. J Biol Chem 1994; 269: 12092–8.

46. Hinz B, Pittet P, Smith-Clerc J et al. Myofibroblast development is characterized by specific cell-cell adherens junctions. Mol Biol Cell 2004; 15: 4310–20.

47. Kawaguchi J, Takeshita S, Kashima T et al. Expression and function of the splice variant of the human cadherin-11 gene in subordination to intact cadherin-11. J Bone Miner Res 1999; 14: 764–75.

48. MacCalman CD, Furth EE, Omigbodun A et al. Regulated expression of cadherin-11 in human epithelial cells: a role for cadherin-11 in trophoblast-endometrium interactions? Dev Dyn 1996; 206: 201–11.

49. Matsusaki T, Aoyama T, Nishijo K et al. Expression of the cadherin-11 gene is a discriminative factor between articular and growth plate chondrocytes. Osteoarthritis Cartilage 2006; 14: 353–66.

50. Munro SB, Turner IM, Farookhi R et al. E-cadherin and OB-cadherin mRNA levels in normal human colon and colon carcinoma. Exp Mol Pathol 1995; 62: 118–22.

51. Shibata T, Ochiai A, Gotoh M et al. Simultaneous expression of cadherin-11 in signet-ring cell carcinoma and stromal cells of diffuse-type gastric cancer. Cancer Lett 1996; 99: 147–53.

52. Tomita K, van Bokhoven A, van Leenders GJ et al. Cadherin switching in human prostate cancer progression. Cancer Res 2000; 60: 3650–4.

53. Kawaguchi J, Azuma Y, Hoshi K et al. Targeted disruption of cadherin-11 leads to a reduction in bone density in calvaria and long bone metaphyses. J Bone Miner Res 2001; 16: 1265–71.

54. Manabe T, Togashi H, Uchida N et al. Loss of cadherin-11 adhesion receptor enhances plastic changes in hippocampal synapses and modifies behavioral responses. Mol Cell Neurosci 2000; 15: 534–46.

55. Gibson KA, Kumar RK, Tedla N et al. Expression of the alphaEbeta7 integrin by mast cells in rheumatoid synovium. J Rheumatol 2000; 27: 2754–60.

56. Trollmo C, Nilsson IM, Sollerman C et al. Expression of the mucosal lymphocyte integrin alpha E beta 7 and its ligand E-cadherin in the synovium of patients with rheumatoid arthritis. Scand J Immunol 1996; 44: 293–8.

57. Kiener HP, Lee DM, Agarwal SK et al. Cadherin-11 induces rheumatoid arthritis fibroblast-like synoviocytes to form lining layers in vitro. Am J Pathol 2006; 168: 1486–99.

58. Lee DM, Kiener HP, Agarwal SK et al. Cadherin-11 in synovial lining formation and pathology in arthritis. Science 2007; 315: 1006–10.

59. Firestein GS. Evolving concepts of rheumatoid arthritis. Nature 2003; 423: 356–61.

60. Kouskoff V, Korganow AS, Duchatelle V et al. Organ-specific disease provoked by systemic autoimmunity. Cell 1996; 87: 811–22.

61. Matsumoto I, Staub A, Benoist C et al. Arthritis provoked by linked T and B cell recognition of a glycolytic enzyme. Science 1999; 286: 1732–5.

62. Muller-Ladner U, Kriegsmann J, Franklin BN et al. Synovial fibroblasts of patients with rheumatoid arthritis attach to and invade normal human cartilage when engrafted into SCID mice. Am J Pathol 1996; 149: 1607–15.

63. Lafyatis R, Remmers EF, Roberts AB et al. Anchorage-independent growth of synoviocytes from arthritic and normal joints. Stimulation by exogenous platelet-derived growth factor and inhibition by transforming growth factor-beta and retinoids. J Clin Invest 1989; 83: 1267–76.

64. Yamanishi Y, Boyle DL, Rosengren S et al. Regional analysis of p53 mutations in rheumatoid arthritis synovium. Proc Natl Acad Sci U S A. 2002; 99: 10025–30.

65. Imamura F, Aono H, Hasunuma T et al. Monoclonal expansion of synoviocytes in rheumatoid arthritis. Arthritis Rheum 1998; 41: 1979–86.

66. Thiery JP. Epithelial-mesenchymal transitions in tumour progression. Nat Rev Cancer 2002; 2: 442–54.

67. Avizienyte E, Frame MC. Src and FAK signalling controls adhesion fate and the epithelial-to-mesenchymal transition. Curr Opin Cell Biol 2005; 17: 542–7.

68. Huber MA, Kraut N, Beug H. Molecular requirements for epithelial-mesenchymal transition during tumor progression. Curr Opin Cell Biol 2005; 17: 548–58.

69. Cowin P, Rowlands TM, Hatsell SJ. Cadherins and catenins in breast cancer. Curr Opin Cell Biol 2005; 17: 499–508.

70. Foty RA, Steinberg MS. Cadherin-mediated cell-cell adhesion and tissue segregation in relation to malignancy. Int J Dev Biol 2004; 48: 397–409.

71. Perl AK, Wilgenbus P, Dahl U et al. A causal role for E-cadherin in the transition from adenoma to carcinoma. Nature 1998; 392: 190–3.

72. Hazan RB, Qiao R, Keren R et al. Cadherin switch in tumor progression. Ann NY Acad Sci 2004; 1014: 155–63.

73. Nagi C, Guttman M, Jaffer S et al. N-cadherin expression in breast cancer: correlation with an aggressive histologic variant—invasive micropapillary carcinoma. Breast Cancer Res Treat 2005; 94: 225–35.

74. Sanders DS, Blessing K, Hassan GA et al. Alterations in cadherin and catenin expression during the biological progression of melanocytic tumours. Mol Pathol 1999; 52: 151–7.

75. Hazan RB, Phillips GR, Qiao RF et al. Exogenous expression of N-cadherin in breast cancer cells induces cell migration, invasion, and metastasis. J Cell Biol 2000; 148: 779–90.

76. Nieman MT, Prudoff RS, Johnson KR et al. N-cadherin promotes motility in human breast cancer cells regardless of their E-cadherin expression. J Cell Biol 1999; 147: 631–44.

77. Orlandini M, Oliviero S. In fibroblasts Vegf-D expression is induced by cell-cell contact mediated by cadherin-11. J Biol Chem 2001; 276: 6576–81.

78. Brunton VG, MacPherson IR, Frame MC. Cell adhesion receptors, tyrosine kinases and actin modulators: a complex three-way circuitry. Biochim Biophys Acta 2004; 1692: 121–44.

79. Friedl P, Wolf K. Tumour-cell invasion and migration: diversity and escape mechanisms. Nat Rev Cancer 2003; 3: 362–74.

80. Wang Y, Jin G, Miao H et al. Integrins regulate VE-cadherin and catenins: dependence of this regulation on Src, but not on Ras. Proc Natl Acad Sci U S A 2006; 103: 1774–9.

81. Zhang W, Alt-Holland A, Margulis A et al. E-cadherin loss promotes the initiation of squamous cell carcinoma invasion through modulation of integrin-mediated adhesion. J Cell Sci 2006; 119: 283–91.

82. Yano H, Mazaki Y, Kurokawa K et al. Roles played by a subset of integrin signaling molecules in cadherin-based cell-cell adhesion. J Cell Biol 2004; 166: 283–95.

83. Orrington-Myers J, Gao XP, Kouklis P et al. Regulation of lung neutrophil recruitment by VE-cadherin. Am J Physiol Lung Cell Mol Physiol 2006; 291: L764–71.

84. Cepek KL, Shaw SK, Parker CM et al. Adhesion between epithelial cells and T lymphocytes mediated by E-cadherin and the alpha E beta 7 integrin. Nature 1994; 372: 190–3.

85. Grundemann C, Bauer M, Schweier O et al. Cutting edge: identification of E-cadherin as a ligand for the murine killer cell lectin-like receptor G1. J Immunol 2006; 176: 1311–15.

86. Ito M, Maruyama T, Saito N et al. Killer cell lectin-like receptor G1 binds three members of the classical cadherin family to inhibit NK cell cytotoxicity. J Exp Med 2006; 203: 289–95.

87. Ritchlin C. Fibroblast biology. Effector signals released by the synovial fibroblast in arthritis. Arthritis Res 2000; 2: 356–60.

88. Tran NL, Adams DG, Vaillancourt RR et al. Signal transduction from N-cadherin increases Bcl-2. Regulation of the phosphatidylinositol 3-kinase/Akt pathway by homophilic adhesion and actin cytoskeletal organization. J Biol Chem 2002; 277: 32905–14.

89. Gwak GY, Yoon JH, Yu SJ et al. Anti-apoptotic N-cadherin signaling and its prognostic implication in human hepatocellular carcinomas. Oncol Rep 2006; 15: 1117–23.

90. Huelsken J, Behrens J. The Wnt signalling pathway. J Cell Sci 2002; 115: 3977–8.

91. Nelson WJ, Nusse R. Convergence of Wnt, beta-catenin, and cadherin pathways. Science. 2004; 303: 1483–7.

92. Sen M. Wnt signalling in rheumatoid arthritis. Rheumatology (Oxford) 2005; 44: 708–13.

93. Perez-Moreno M, Davis MA, Wong E et al. p120-catenin mediates inflammatory responses in the skin. Cell 2006; 124: 631–44.

94. Sweeney SE, Firestein GS. Rheumatoid arthritis: regulation of synovial inflammation. Int J Biochem Cell Biol 2004; 36: 372–8.

95. Pettit AR, Ji H, von Stechow D, et al. TRANCE/RANKL knockout mice are protected from bone erosion in a serum transfer model of arthritis. Am J Pathol 2001; 159: 1689–99.

96. Zwerina J, Hayer S, Tohidast-Akrad M et al. Single and combined inhibition of tumor necrosis factor, interleukin-1, and RANKL pathways in tumor necrosis factor-induced arthritis: effects on synovial inflammation, bone erosion, and cartilage destruction. Arthritis Rheum 2004; 50: 277–90.

11

TNF-α

Marc Feldmann and Ravinder N Maini

Introduction • Cytokines and RA • Cytokine expression in rheumatoid synovium • Cytokine gene regulation in synovium • Studies in animal models confirm that TNF-α is a good therapeutic target in arthritis • What controls up-regulated TNF-α production in RA patients? • Biological role of TNF: lessons learned from TNF blockade in the clinic • References

INTRODUCTION

The mechanisms of autoimmune disease are quite diverse. In some diseases, antibodies are of major importance in driving the pathogenesis of the disease; these include myasthenia gravis disease, Graves' disease, Goodpasture's syndrome, and autoimmune hemolytic anemia.[1,2] In others T cells appear to be more important; these include multiple sclerosis and type I diabetes.[3,4] However, in human diseases the mechanisms are usually complex, and there are usually huge gaps in our knowledge. For diseases where antibodies are important, there is often clear-cut evidence; for example, improvement upon removing the antibody by plasmapheresis (e.g. in Goodpasture's syndrome), or mother-to-fetus transfer of disease due to transfer of pathogenic antibody. In other instances, if antibody-mediated pathology is not clearly defined, it is assumed that T cells are important. However, in human diseases, in contrast to animal models, the data needed to establish this point are usually circumstantial. In animal models transfer of T cells or antibody is possible to verify mechanisms. Collagen-induced arthritis, a model of rheumatoid arthritis (RA), is transferable by both T cells and antibodies.[5] However, other models differ. K/BxN arthritis is transferable by serum or purified antibodies to glucose-6-phosphate isomerase.[6]

Tumor necrosis factor (TNF)-α transgenic arthritis is transferable in the absence of T or B cells, as it can be back-crossed to T- and B-cell deficit RAG knockout mice.[7] Hence studies in animal models are inherently incapable of providing definitive answers as to the pathogenesis of complex heterogeneous multigenic diseases, such as RA.

For RA the mechanism of disease has been the subject of many different hypotheses with the role of T cells emphasized by some,[8–10] and that of antibody and B cells,[11] and of synovial fibroblast-like cells by others.[12,13] These conflicting hypotheses reflect the fact that there is much left to learn about pathogenic processes, let alone how these processes are engaged by the causative 'etiological' interactions of genes and environment.

The first attempts to evaluate directly the role of T cells in human autoimmune diseases such as RA by using therapeutic monoclonal antibodies to CD4 were not successful, and so failed to confirm their role.[14,15] However, CTLA-4-Ig (abatacept) has proved to be efficacious in RA[16] and more encouraging results appear to be forthcoming for non-lytic antibodies to CD4,[17] and possibly to CD3,[18] and concepts are emerging that might explain the failure of the early anti-CD4 experiments. These include the removal of CD4+ regulatory T cells, many of which

Cytokines
Short range protein mediators
Involved in: immunity,
inflammation, cell growth,
differentiation, repair, fibrosis
Produced in response to
'stress'
About 150 currently defined,
probably ~300 in total

**Proinflammatory cytokines
drive inflammation
(e.g. TNF, IL-1, IL-6, GM-CSF)**
Induce activation and
accumulation of leukocytes
These produce mediators
which cause pain, swelling,
stiffness and initiate tissue
damage

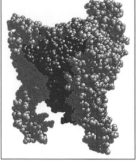

TNF-α bound to receptor

Figure 11.1 Cytokines as mediators of inflammation.

express CD25.[19] This may also explain the failure of interleukin (IL)-2 toxin to be beneficial.[20] Furthermore, while lytic antibodies to CD4 were very effective in reducing CD4+ counts in blood, this was not the case in terms of synovial T cells.[21,22]

CYTOKINES AND RA

Our work which led up to defining TNF-α as a useful therapeutic target is based on considering concepts of the pathogenesis of autoimmune disease. In 1983 we published a hypothesis based on immunohistological analysis of diseased tissue, overexpressing major histocompatibility complex (MHC) class II, suggesting that autoimmune disease involved up-regulation of antigen presentation.[23] The only molecules known at the time to up-regulate MHC class II expression were cytokines such as interferon (IFN)-γ, and thus we postulated that local cytokine production was a critical early step in the pathogenesis of autoimmunity (Figure 11.1). Our concept was based mostly on thyroid disease, but was also compatible with diabetes and RA,[24-26] in which up-regulation of MHC class I and II has also been noted. This hypothesis attracted a lot of attention and experimental support. Thus it was found that transgenic mice[27] expressing IFN-γ in the islets of Langerhans under the control of the insulin promoter developed an autoimmune diabetes. In contrast, transgenic mice expressing MHC class I antigen in the islets had islet damage,[28] but this was due to an autoimmune response. Subsequently transgenic mice overexpressing IFN-γ in many sites were found to develop local inflammatory autoimmune disease in the eye and CNS (Figure 11.2).[29,30]

To explore these hypothetical mechanisms of autoimmunity, and to investigate whether our concept was correct, we performed a number of studies in human systems. The first set of experiments was performed using thyroid tissue taken at operation from Graves' disease patients. With this tissue our colleague Marco Londei was able to clone autoreactive T cells from the thyroid tissue that recognized, and were restimulated, by thyroid epithelial cells from diseased

Up-regulation of HLA-DR in rheumatoid synovium

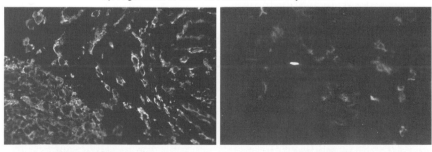

Rheumatoid arthritis   Osteoarthritis

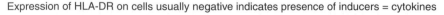

Expression of HLA-DR on cells usually negative indicates presence of inducers = cytokines

Figure 11.2 Sections of synovial tissue labeled with rabbit anti-HLA-DR antibody and using FITC-labeled anti-rabbit as second antibody. (Klareskog L et al. Proc Natl Acad Sci U S A 1982; 79: 3632–6.)

patients[31] or normal thyroid epithelial cells induced to express HLA class II. This result was interesting and controversial as it demonstrated that an epithelial cell, once it was induced by cytokines, was able to stimulate already activated T cells. Influenza-specific T-cell clones were also able to be stimulated by thyroid epithelial cells,[32] if these were appropriately HLA matched. Proinflammatory cytokine expression in Graves' disease tissue[33] was detectable and cytokine injection induced thyroiditis, and so the outline of this concept of autoimmune induction was established. However, attempts to use this information for patient benefit failed, as there is not much 'unmet medical need' in Graves' disease as judged by the pharmaceutical industry and hence no commercial interest. In RA there was also evidence of a local immune and inflammatory response as judged by the nature of the cell infiltrate, and up-regulated MHC expression. In contrast there was a significant unmet medical need, and also the opportunity to study the disease tissue at various stages, including at the height of the local disease process, which is not possible in most human diseases.

CYTOKINE EXPRESSION IN RHEUMATOID SYNOVIUM

Cytokines, short-range protein messenger molecules involved in immunity, inflammation, fibrosis, repair, etc., were first cloned in the early 1980s. With the cloning of cDNA for cytokines, assays specific for these molecules were developed; for example, detection of mRNA by northern blotting. Detection of the protein was made possible by the generation of specific monoclonal and polyclonal antibodies generated using the cytokine proteins obtained in pure form by expression from cDNA. Hence the function of cytokines could now be studied *in vivo* and *in vitro*, in the absence of contaminating signals. This led to a rapid expansion in cytokine research, which is still ongoing, and to the deeper understanding of multiple biological processes of high relevance to arthritis, including inflammation, immunity, and cell proliferation. Based on this understanding, the use of cytokines and anti-cytokines in medicine has been established. Initially this involved the use

of hemopoietic factors, such as erythropoietin (EPO)[34] and granulocyte colony-stimulating factor (G-CSF),[35] and the IFNs.[36,37]

Synovial joints, which are relatively acellular in health, with a lining layer of fibroblast-like cells and macrophages, are infiltrated by a massive accumulation of blood-borne cells in RA. These cells are chiefly T lymphocytes (20–30%) and macrophages (30–40%), with B lymphocytes, plasma cells, and dendritic cells.[38] To sustain this new tissue mass, angiogenesis is a prominent feature.[39–41] As multiple activated cell types are present in this tissue, it is not surprising that using appropriate technology it is found that there is abundant cytokine expression in the rheumatoid synovium (Table 11.1).

Cytokine analysis in RA engaged a number of research groups, assaying different aspects in various ways. The initial groups studied cytokines in synovial fluid. IL-1 was the first cytokine to be detected in RA, using a bioassay, by Fontana et al.[42] Other groups studied cytokine mRNA expression by *in situ* hybridization,[43] whereas the approach in our laboratory was to look for local mRNA expression by blotting.[44] The rationale for this was that locally produced cytokines were most likely to be important in the disease process. Having detected a plethora of cytokine mRNAs by *in situ* hybridization or blotting, it was important to establish that the relevant proteins were, indeed, synthesized in the synovium. Several approaches were useful. Immunostaining of biopsies was successful,[45] as were assays of cytokine protein in

---

Table 11.1 Many cytokines are produced in rheumatoid synovium

Proinflammatory
e.g. IL-1, IL-6, TNF-α, IL-12, IL-15, IL-17, IL-18,
  IFN-γ, IL-2, OncoM, GM-CSF
Anti-inflammatory
e.g. IL-10, IL-1Ra, TGF-β, IL-11, IL-13
Chemokines
e.g. IL-8, MIP-1α, MCP-1, RANTES, ENA-78, GROa
Growth factors
e.g. VEGF, PDGF, FGF

Almost all cytokines are present in RA synovium except IL-4

synovial fluids.[46–48] We also found that short-term unstimulated cultures of cells dissociated from the whole synovial membrane (a complex cell mixture) yielded cytokine-rich supernatants for assay.[38,44] These studies using multiple approaches verified that a great number of proinflammatory cytokines such as IL-1, TNF-α, IL-6, GM-CSF, and IL-8 were locally produced.[44,49–51] This was found in essentially all the rheumatoid synovial membrane samples assayed regardless of the duration of disease or its treatment.

In normal circumstances proinflammatory cytokines are expressed for a short period of time in response to extrinsic stimuli such as lipopolysaccharide (LPS). Thus their consistent presence in biopsies or operative samples suggested that, unlike normal stimulation, cytokine synthesis in rheumatoid synovial tissue may be 'constitutive'. This was also the first clue that cytokines may be important, as their production was dysregulated compared with normal cells in culture. However, analysis of the results also revealed that there were a number of proinflammatory cytokines such as TNF-α, IL-1, IL-6, and GM-CSF with closely related biological properties in active rheumatoid synovium. This raised the question as to which, if any, might be rate limiting, and hence might be a useful therapeutic target. If the concepts generated thus far *in vitro* were correct, then blocking a single cytokine might not be useful, as the proinflammatory activity would still be driven by the remaining proinflammatory cytokines.

We, and others, also studied the expression of anti-inflammatory cytokines such as IL-10, IL-1ra, and transforming growth factor(TGF)-β in rheumatoid synovium.[51–54] This was relevant, as it was possible that the chronic inflammation of RA was due to anti-inflammatory cytokines not being expressed there, and the proinflammatory mediators not being counterbalanced by anti-inflammatory mediators. The production of anti-inflammatory mediators such as IL-10, TGF-β1, soluble TNF receptor, IL-1 receptor antagonist, and IL-11 in rheumatoid synovium was found to be considerably up-regulated.[51–54] For example, levels of up to 1 ng/ml of IL-10 were found in rheumatoid synovial cultures. These quantities were found to be biologically significant from

neutralizing antibody studies, using anti-IL-10 in synovial cultures, in a mirror image of the anti-TNF-α work described below. It was found that anti-IL-10 antibody augmented the amounts of TNF-α and IL-1 produced by the synovial cultures 2–3-fold.[51] Thus the IL-10 endogenously produced was partially down-regulating the major proinflammatory cytokines. In a converse set of experiments it was shown that adding IL-10 to synovial cultures was anti-inflammatory, suggesting that IL-10 might be a useful therapeutic agent. This was indeed the case in animal models,[55] but in humans the therapeutic effect at tolerable doses was modest.[56]

The amounts of TGF-β1 are high in synovial culture, approximately 10 ng/ml.[57] It appears that this is a plateau level, as adding more has an insignificant effect on production. As the immunoregulatory effects of TGF-β are moderately long-lived *in vitro*, it is not possible to demonstrate any worsening of cytokine in synovial cultures on its neutralization, and so its role in the pathogenesis of RA is still not understood. In animal models there is convincing evidence that TGF-β has both proinflammatory and anti-inflammatory roles,[58] and regrettably the profibrotic effects of TGF-β1 have halted its use in clinical trials.[59]

The production of anti-inflammatory mediators in rheumatoid synovium appears to be partly under the regulation of the proinflammatory mediators, as blocking TNF-α partly inhibited production of IL-10, solTNF-R, and IL-1ra.[44,51] This appears to be also true *in vivo*, as judged by clinical trial data, most dramatically for IL-1ra,[60] somewhat less so for solTNF-R and IL-10. The implications of this are not fully understood, but it may explain why blocking TNF-α exerts only a temporary effect in patients due to the concomitant down-regulation of the IL-10, IL-1ra, and solTNF-R homeostatic mechanisms in the disequilibrium of cytokines, as shown in Figure 11.3.

Other anti-inflammatory cytokines appear to be poorly expressed. The presence of IL-4 in rheumatoid synovial tissue is occasional, and most studies do not report it.[61] This may be of relevance to the Th1 preponderance that is reported in rheumatoid patients, as IL-4 is the most potent cytokine skewing towards the

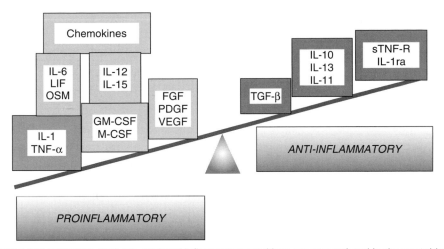

Figure 11.3 Cytokine disequilibrium. Both pro- and anti-inflammatory cytokines are up-regulated in rheumatoid synovium but the balance is in favor of proinflammatory cytokines promoting inflammation. (Reproduced with permission from Feldmann M, Brennan FM, Maini RN. Cell 1996; 85(3): 307–10.)

Th2 phenotype and inhibiting Th1 cells. IL-13 is reported to be present in some studies,[62] but not others.[63] The inconsistent results are not understood, but the heterogeneity of RA is well known.

CYTOKINE GENE REGULATION IN SYNOVIUM

To test if the pathology in RA is due to the dysregulated and prolonged production of cytokines, dissociated cell cultures of rheumatoid synovium were used to study cytokine regulation in the diseased tissue. The cells were found to reaggregate rapidly, and produced proinflammatory cytokines such as TNF-α, IL-1, and IL-6 continuously over the 6- or 7-day period that they were studied before the cell composition changed from its original mixture.[38,44] This culture system generated an *in vitro* model for studying the proinflammatory gene regulation in synovium and evaluating whether it was indeed abnormal or prolonged.

Faced with a plethora of candidate cytokines, the problem was which cytokine to study first. The properties of TNF-α and IL-1 are consistent with many features of RA. Because IL-1 (also described in the 1970s as 'catabolin') had been demonstrated to be involved in damage to the joints in a variety of experimental situations,[64–66] and hence presumably in RA, our colleague Fionula Brennan studied IL-1 regulation by

TNF-α in these dissociated rheumatoid synovium cell cultures. It was found that adding neutralizing anti-TNF-α antibodies (polyclonal at the time)[67] at the beginning of cultures abrogated their IL-1 production, assessed at protein or mRNA level (Figure 11.4). This was not the case for the IL-1 produced by osteoarthritic synovium. These data provided the first clue that TNF-α might be of particular importance in the mechanism of inflammation. Subsequent experiments revealed the widespread regulatory effects of anti-TNF-α antibody in synovial cultures, e.g. down-regulating other proinflammatory cytokines, such as IL-6, GM-CSF, and IL-8.[68–70]

The simplest interpretation for the widespread effects of anti-TNF on multiple cytokines is that TNF-α is at the apex of a proinflammatory 'cascade'. This concept is illustrated in Figure 11.5. The results raised the possibility that blocking TNF-α, just one of the multitude of proinflammatory cytokines, might, by its downstream effect on other cytokines, have a major influence on the complex disease process. Hence these results suggested that blocking TNF-α might be therapeutically useful, and this idea was subsequently tested.

It is important to stress that this work involved the use of mixed unpurified synovial cultures, and not cultured rheumatoid synovial

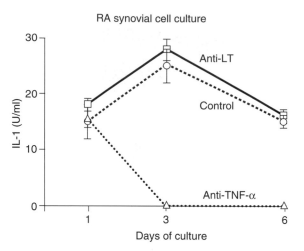

Approach
Operative sample synovium, active RA cells isolated, placed in 'tissue culture'

Observation
Spontaneous production of many mediators of disease – cytokines, enzymes, etc.

Experiment
Antibody to TNF inhibits production of other proinflammatory cytokines

Figure 11.4 IL-1 synthesis is down-regulated in cultures of synovial tissue from patients with RA but not osteoarthritis. (Reproduced with permission from Brennan FM et al. Lancet 1989; 2: 244–7.)

fibroblasts. Most studies prior to this time had focused on rheumatoid synovial fibroblasts, but we felt that these cells, undoubtedly important, were not representative of the complexity in the cell mixture synovium, and did not reflect the

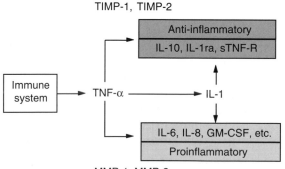

Figure 11.5 Cytokine cascade in RA. Pro- and anti-inflammatory cytokines interact in a 'network' or 'cascade'. (Adapted with permission from Feldmann M, Brennan FM, Maini RN. Cell 1996; 85(3): 307–10.)

important contribution of blood-borne cells capable of driving inflammation and immunity.

STUDIES IN ANIMAL MODELS CONFIRM THAT TNF-α IS A GOOD THERAPEUTIC TARGET IN ARTHRITIS

A number of studies in animal models have yielded consistent data indicating that TNF-α is intimately involved in the generation of arthritis. The properties of TNF-α are consistent with this concept.[71,72] One set of important studies has come from George Kollias' laboratory.[73] Beutler and Cerami[71] had reported that the 3' untranslated region of TNF-α was rich in A and U nucleotides. This AU-rich motif, AUUUA, was found in a great number of cytokines and proto-oncogenes. Shaw and Kamen[74] demonstrated that this motif reduced the half-life of mRNA, and it was shown that it was involved in macrophage expression. Kollias' group made transgenic mice that expressed a human TNF-α gene lacking the 3' untranslated region of TNF, replacing it with a β globin 3' untranslated region. This led to many lines of mice with dysregulated and up-regulated TNF-α production, and the transgenic mice were all found to develop an erosive arthritis, with some lines also having inflammatory bowel disease and skin inflammation.[75] This rather local inflammation was a different phenotype from the diffuse inflammation of the TGF-β1 knockouts.[76] It is still not clear why the joints in these mice are the major site of inflammation, despite many years of subsequent studies.

A different but complementary set of studies came from neutralizing TNF-α after disease onset in mice with a disease resembling RA. Injection of collagen type II into genetically susceptible mouse strains such as DBA/1 yielded an erosive arthritis with histological features resembling human RA.[77] Anti-TNF-α antibody injected at adequate doses (but not at low dose) after disease onset was found to ameliorate disease activity. The degree of footpad swelling, a measure of inflammation, the clinical score (production of degree of inflammation by number of affected paws), as well as the histology, all assessments of disease, were improved. Histologically there was less leukocyte infiltration

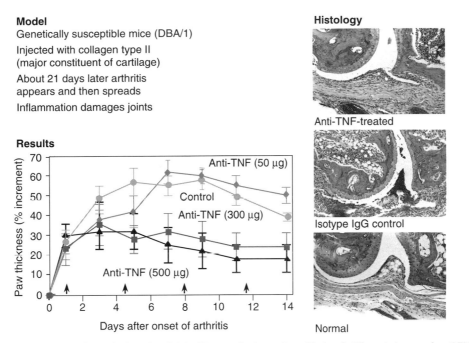

Figure 11.6 Animal model of collagen-induced arthritis. The graph shows the effects of different doses of anti-TNF on clinical progression of established arthritis. Arrows indicate time of injections of anti-TNF. Paw width was measured using callipers and increase in thickness expressed as a percentage compared with baseline. Histology: paraffin sections of paws were stained with hematoxylin. Bottom, normal joint; middle, severe arthritis; top, mouse treated with anti-TNF. (Reproduced with permission from Williams RO, Feldmann M, Maini RN. Proc Natl Acad Sci U S A 1992; 89: 9784–8.)

of the joints, less damage to cartilage, and less erosion of bone (Figure 11.6).

Similar studies in this model were reported within a few months of each other by the late Jeanette Thorbecke's group,[78] Richard Williams of our group,[79] and Pierre Piguet's group.[80] These animal studies were an important part of establishing the rationale for testing anti-TNF-α in human RA.

Proinflammatory cytokines, especially TNF-α, are very rapidly produced after stimulation, for example, by the ubiquitous LPS. Hence it was of importance to verify that the studies performed with human synovial tissue *in vitro* reflected the situation *in vivo*. A key experiment was to freeze biopsy tissue from joints within minutes of its extraction. In these few minutes TNF-α synthesis could not take place, and hence TNF-α expression *in vivo* could be inferred from these studies with fresh frozen tissue. A representative analysis is shown in Figure 11.7. These studies showed that TNF was expressed before removal

from the body,[45] as were TNF receptors.[81] These studies provided a rationale for anti-TNF-α therapy in RA (Table 11.2). With hindsight it is evident that the actions of TNF-α mimic many processes occurring in RA (Figure 11.8).

WHAT CONTROLS UP-REGULATED TNF-α PRODUCTION IN RA PATIENTS?

An understanding of the control of TNF-α production at sites of inflammation is a very interesting question, with considerable impact on therapeutic strategies for the future. This question can be studied at multiple levels. At the cellular level there is agreement that it is macrophages that make most of the TNF-α in rheumatoid synovium. But what drives them to do it? This has been studied in cellular terms and it has been reported that an atypical subset of T cells, which behave like T cells activated not by antigen but by cytokines, were important in inducing TNF-α in cell–cell contact mechanisms.[82]

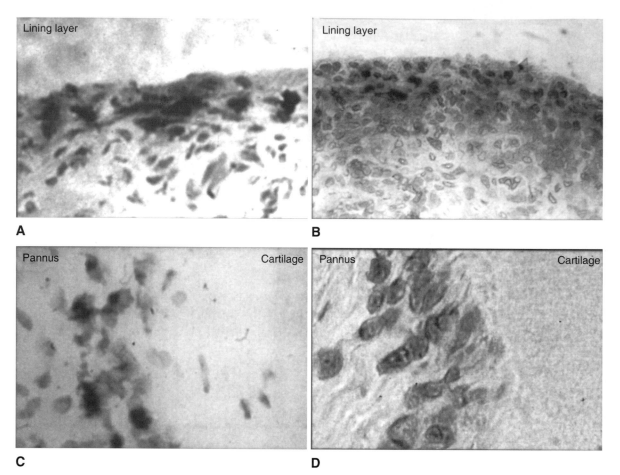

Figure 11.7 TNF-α (left panels) and p55 TNFR (right panels) colocalization was demonstrated by immunohistology in synovial lining layer (a, b) and at the cartilage–pannus junction (c, d). (Adapted with permission from Chu et al. Arthritis Rheum 1989; 34: 1125–32 and Delewan et al. Arthritis Rheum 1992; 35: 1170–8.)

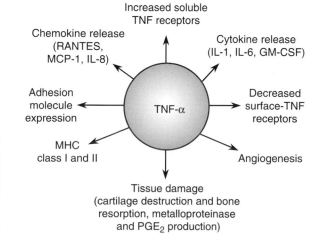

Figure 11.8 TNF-α actions relevant to the pathogenesis of rheumatoid arthritis.

Table 11.2 Rationale for anti-TNF-α therapy in rheumatoid arthritis

1. Dysregulated cytokine network in RA synovium is dependent on TNF-α
2. TNF-α/TNF receptor up-regulated in synovium
3. Animal model of RA responds very well to anti-TNF-α administered after disease onset

In molecular terms, a number of studies have suggested that IL-15[83] and IL-18[84] might be 'upstream' of TNF-α. It has also been proposed that IL-17 produced by T cells and expressed in RA joints may play an important role in the regulation of synthesis of TNF-α and IL-1, and in potentiating their activation on multiple pathways implicated in inflammation and bone destruction.[85–87] These studies are promising, but are by no means conclusive, as they are difficult to perform in synovial tissue. Nevertheless, these molecules might be therapeutic targets.

In terms of intracellular mechanisms, a number of pathways have been reported to regulate TNF-α production. The best studied is the p38 MAP kinase,[88] others include the other MAP kinases p42/44 ERK[89] and JNK[90] stress-activated kinase. Other interesting pathways include the NF-κB pathway[91,92] and the phosphotidyl inositol 3 kinase pathway.[92] However, in all these cases, these pathways control many biological processes, and so there may be costs in terms of safety in their excessive blockade.

BIOLOGICAL ROLE OF TNF: LESSONS LEARNED FROM TNF BLOCKADE IN THE CLINIC

Cytokine regulation

The rapid reduction in C-reactive protein and IL-6 concentrations in blood following TNF blockade in RA following infliximab was the first signal that gave plausibility to the key role that TNF played in the regulation of cytokines in RA.[93] Comparison of a high and low dose of TNF blocking agent and placebo injections[94] conclusively demonstrated that this biological effect was dose-related, superimposed on a diurnal variation of elevated IL-6 concentrations and associated with trapping of neutralized TNF by the monoclonal antibody in the circulation.[60] Serum levels of other cytokines which have been reported to decrease in serum include: IL-18, TNF,[95] IL-13,[96] possibly IL-7,[97] and a selective diminution of IL-15, but not of serum IL-16, IL-17, and GM-CSF measured at 14 and 30 weeks.[98] However, in arthroscopically obtained synovial biopsies the immunohistochemical measurement of IL-15 varied above or below baseline biopsy values without any correlation with clinical efficacy or simultaneous expression of TNF.[99]

The proposed role of TNF in regulating IL-1 predicted by preclinical experiments has been more difficult to substantiate because of low circulating levels,[67,60] but was shown by using a sensitive immunoassay on sequential blood samples on a subpopulation of patients in the same clinical trial.[100] IL-1ra and solTNF-R concentrations, the endogenously produced inhibitors of IL-1 and TNF, which are up-regulated in RA were shown to be also reduced following infliximab in this study.[60] As suggested earlier, this may partly explain why anti-TNF therapy rarely induces drug-free remission of established chronic disease.

Measurement of blood levels of cytokines and inhibitors is clearly subject to the availability of reagents and kits and the sensitivity, specificity, and accuracy of the assays are not always well established. In many instances blood levels are lower than that found in the joint and although more accessible for serial sampling than serial joint biopsies, the expression of cytokines in the diseased joints is arguably more important in evaluating their role in disease. These factors limit our current knowledge on the precise molecular relationships and interactions between pro- and anti-inflammatory pathways in the rheumatoid joint. However, the impact of TNF blockade on the cytokine network remains an important field of study in the quest for new cytokine therapeutic targets that will complement anti-TNF therapy in the future.

Inflammation, cell recruitment, and blood vessels

The reduction of joint swelling and tenderness that is a feature of TNF blockade is mirrored by a reduction in the cellularity of the synovial membrane.[101] The probability that this is a result of reduced angiogenesis, cell recruitment, and deactivation of an adhesive inflamed vasculature with active cell trafficking into the synovial tissue is supported by a number of observations. Whilst lymphocytes in the joints are depleted following infliximab therapy, circulating lymphocyte counts increase simultaneously with a decrease in blood levels of markers of turnover of adhesion molecules soluble E-selectin and soluble ICAM-1.[102] In addition there is a reduction in the blood levels of the major angiogenic factor VEGF.[41] Serial biopsies of synovial tissue before and after anti-TNF therapy show reduction of adhesion molecules E-selectin (specific for the endothelium), ICAM-1, and VCAM-1,[101] as well as a number of chemokines, notably IL-8 and MCP-1.[103] Gamma-camera imaging of [111]indium-labelled polymorphonuclear cells re-injected into RA patients with active disease and subsequently repeated at 2 weeks following a single infusion of infliximab clearly demonstrate ~50% reduction in the uptake of radioactivity in the knee and hand joints.[103] Other imaging techniques such as gadolinium-enhanced magnetic resonance imaging (MRI) and colour Doppler ultrasonic examination reveal diminished vascularity and inflammation.[104,105] These data strongly support the hypothesis that reduced cell recruitment and vascularity are major contributors to the anti-inflammatory action of TNF blockade.

The further possibility that cellularity may be reduced due to anti-TNF-induced apoptosis in RA has been proposed by Klareskog's group.[106] In their study, two markers of apoptosis, TUNEL and caspase-3 staining, in synovial macrophages was found to be induced after infliximab and etanercept treatment for 8 weeks. However, the proposed role of cell death induced by TNF blockade is debated and could not be documented by Tak and colleagues in synovial biopsies from RA patients repeatedly taken at baseline, 48 hours and 28 days after infliximab.[107]

Endothelial function has been investigated before and after anti-TNF therapy in RA. In the first of these from Steffan Gay's group, flow-mediated vasodilation was improved after 12 weeks as measured by high-resolution ultrasound examination of the brachial artery.[108] Using brachial ultrasonography another group reported vasodilatory responses improved for the first 4 weeks following every infusion every 8 weeks through a full year of observations.[109] Increased stiffness of the aorta attributed to chronic inflammation in RA patients compared with controls has been demonstrated; in a small subset of RA patients from this study, aortic stiffness measured by aortic pulse-wave velocity

was reduced significantly from baseline at 4 and 8 weeks after anti-TNF therapy.[110] These data suggest that anti-TNF therapy may prove to be of benefit in ameliorating inflammation-related atherosclerosis and endothelial dysfunction that contribute to an increase in cardiovascular risk in RA. This hypothesis is currently being examined in long-term follow-up of cohorts of treated patients.

Bone and cartilage protection

The protective effect of all three currently licensed anti-TNF biologics on progression of structural damage of joints has been documented in clinical trials, especially when used in combination with methotrexate.[111–113] The precise mechanisms that are responsible for the protective effect are not clearly defined, but it seems likely that several pathways and cellular effects are implicated.[114] These range from a reduction in the production of metalloproteinases by synoviocytes, reduction in recruitment of monocyte precursors, and a reduction in the production of key molecules such as M-CSF, IL-1, and RANK-ligand that are involved in the differentiation and destructive potential of osteoclasts. Reversal by anti-TNF therapy of suppression of the anabolic activity of osteoblasts and chondrocytes which compromises bone and cartilage matrix repair further contributes to restoring the imbalance between damage and repair. Observations supporting these concepts in studies in RA include demonstration of reduction by anti-TNF agents of matrix metalloproteinases,[115] increase in osteoprotegerin, the decoy receptor which binds to RANK-ligand and reduces osteoclastogenesis, and normalization of the stoichiometry of osteoprotegerin and RANK-ligand in favor of homeostasis following TNF blockade.[116, 117]

Improvement in radiographic progression of structural damage in a proportion of patients in anti-TNF therapy[111–113] raises the intriguing possibility of reversal of structural damage in a proportion of patients due to healing. Indeed repair of joints following TNF blockade has been demonstrated in the TNF transgenic mouse model of RA,[118] but as yet it has not been possible to document this conclusively by imaging of joints or pathological examination of tissues in anti-TNF-treated patients.

Anti-TNF therapy restores impaired T-cell function

Suppressed effector T-cell function reflected by impaired skin delayed hypersensitivity reaction and *in vitro* responses to recall antigens and mitogens has long been recognized as a feature of severe RA. The mechanisms that underlie the abnormality are currently being explored and there is evidence that TNF may, at least in part, explain these defects. Prolonged exposure to TNF of T-cell hybridoma clones leads to hyporesponsiveness to T-cell receptor signaling associated with down-regulation of TCR-ζ chain expression and impairment of distal signaling pathways.[119–121] Down-regulation of CD28 expression on exposure to TNF[122] is also described and will lead to impairment of the second signal required for T-cell activation. More recent work has focused on regulatory T cells that modulate effector T-cells function, induce tolerance, and prevent autoimmunity. The presence of regulatory CD4+ T cells (Tregs) with the characteristic phenotype (CD4+CD25hiFox P3+) has been demonstrated in peripheral blood and joints of RA patients.[123,124] However unlike normal Tregs the ability of RA Tregs to suppress proliferative response of and cytokine secretion by effector T cells (CD4+CD25−Fox P3−) has been found to be impaired.[125,126] Since exposure of human Tregs from healthy donors to TNF *in vitro* induces a similar impaired functional defect,[126] it has been hypothesized that the observed Treg abnormality in RA is dependent on a TNF-rich milieu.

It is therefore of great interest that the expected biological effects of TNF on T cells are reversed by TNF blockade. Thus anti-TNF therapy has been found to restore effector T-cell responses to antigens such as tuberculin PPD and collagen II[127, 128] restore expression of CD28,[129] and to reverse the impaired functional capacity of Tregs to suppress proliferation and cytokine secretion by CD4+CD25-effector T cells.[125,126]

These data overall suggest that aside from its direct proinflammatory action, TNF plays an important role in maintaining chronic autoimmune inflammatory disease. Although anti-TNF appears to restore Treg function, the relatively rare induction of long-lasting remission in established RA, in the absence of continuation of anti-TNF therapy, suggests that other homeostatic mechanisms remain resistant to the therapeutic intervention. The preliminary findings that anti-TNF-induced remission is more frequently observed in early RA and maintained without anti-TNF[130,131] points to a potentially reversible mechanism providing a biological explanation for the hypothetical therapeutic 'window of opportunity' in early disease.

REFERENCES

1. Weetman AP. Graves' disease. N Engl J Med 2000; 343: 1236–48

2. Salama AD, Levy JB, Lightstone L, Pusey CD. Goodpasture's disease. Lancet 2001; 385: 1374.

3. Steinman L. Multiple sclerosis: a co-ordinated immunological attack against myelin in the central nervous system. Cell 1996; 85: 299–302.

4. Tisch R, McDevitt H. Insulin dependent diabetes mellitus. Cell 1996; 85: 291–7.

5. Muller-Ladner U, Gay RE, Gay S. Activation of synoviocytes. Curr Opin Rheumatol 2000; 12: 186–94.

6. Kouskoff V, Korganow A-S, Duchatelle V et al. Organ-specific disease provoked by systemic autoimmunity. Cell 1996; 87: 811–22.

7. Plows D, Kontogeorgos G, Kollias G. Mice lacking mature T and B lymphocytes develop arthritis lesions after immunization with type II collagen. J Immunol 1999; 162: 1018–23.

8. Coakley G, Iqbal M, Brooks D et al. CD8+, CD57+ T cells from healthy elderly subjects suppress neutrophil development *in vitro*: implications for the neutropenia of Felty's and large granular lymphocyte syndromes. Arthritis Rheum 2000; 43: 834–43.

9. Seckinger P, Isaaz S, Dayer JM. A human inhibitor of tumor necrosis factor alpha. J Exp Med 1988; 167: 1511–16.

10. Cope AP. Exploring the pathogenesis of rheumatoid arthritis in transgenic and mutant mice. Curr Dir Autoimmun 2001; 3: 64–93.

11. Edwards JC, Cambridge G, Abrahams VM. Do self-perpetuating B lymphocytes drive human autoimmune disease? Immunology 1999; 97: 188–96.

12. Yamanishi Y, Firestein GS. Pathogenesis of rheumatoid arthritis: the role of synoviocytes. Rheum Dis Clin North Am 2001; 27: 355–71.

13. Pap T, Aupperle KR, Gay S et al. Invasiveness of synovial fibroblasts is regulated by p53 in the SCID mouse *in vivo* model of cartilage invasion. Arthritis Rheum 2001; 44: 676–81.

14. Moreland L, Pratt P, Mayes M. Minimal efficacy of a depleting chimaeric anti-CD4 (cM-T412) in treatment of

patients with refractory rheumatoid arthritis (RA) receiving concomitant methotrexate (MTX). Arthritis Rheum 1993; 36: 39.

15. Van de Lubbe PA, Dijkmans BAC, Markusse HM et al. A randomized double-blind, placebo-controlled study of CD4 monoclonal antibody therapy in early rheumatoid arthritis. Arthritis Rheum 1995; 38: 1097–106.

16. Kremer JM, Westhovens R, Leon M et al. Treatment of rheumatoid arthritis by selective inhibition of T-cell activation with fusion protein CTLA4Ig. N Engl J Med 2003; 13: 1907–15.

17. Schulze-Koops H, Davis LS, Haverty TP et al. Reduction of Th1 cell activity in the peripheral circulation of patients with rheumatoid arthritis after treatment with a non-depleting humanized monoclonal antibody to CD4. J Rheumatol 1998; 25: 2065–76.

18. Chatenoud L, Thervet E, Primo J, Bach JF. Anti CD3 antibody induces long-term remission of overt autoimmunity in nonobese diabetic mice. Proc Natl Acad Sci USA 1994; 91: 123–7.

19. Shevach EM, McHugh RS, Piccirillo CA, Thornton AM. Control of T cell activation by CD4+ CD25+ suppressor T cells. Immunol Rev 2001; 182: 58–67.

20. Strom TB, Kelley VR, Murphy JR et al. Interleukin-2 receptor-director therapies: antibody- or cytokine-based targeting molecules. Ann Rev Med 1993; 44: 343–53.

21. Moreland LW, Heck LWJ, Koopman WJ. Biologic agents for treating rheumatoid arthritis. Concepts and progress. Arthritis Rheum 1997; 40: 397–409.

22. Williams RO, Mason LJ, Feldmann M, Maini RN. Synergy between anti-CD4 and anti-tumor necrosis factor in the amelioration of established collagen-induced arthritis. Proc Natl Acad Sci USA 1994; 91: 2762–6.

23. Bottazzo GF, Pujol-Borrell R, Hanafusa T, Feldmann M. Role of aberrant HLA-DR expression and antigen presentation in induction of endocrine autoimmunity. Lancet 1983; 2: 1115–19.

24. Pujol-Borrell R, Todd I, Londei M et al. Inappropriate major histocompatibility complex class II expression by thyroid follicular cells in thyroid autoimmune disease and by pancreatic beta cells in type I diabetes. Mol Biol Med 1986; 3: 159–65.

25. Janossy G, Panayai G, Duke O et al. Rheumatoid arthritis: a disease of T-lymphocyte/macrophage immunoregulation. Lancet 1981; ii: 839–41.

26. Klareskog L, Forsum U, Scheynius A et al. Evidence in support of a self perpetuating HLA-DR dependent delayed type cell reaction in rheumatoid arthritis. Proc Natl Acad Sci U S A 1982; 72: 3632–6.

27. Sarvetnick N, Shizuru J, Liggitt D et al. Loss of pancreatic islet tolerance induced by beta-cell expression of interferon-gamma. Nature 1990; 346: 844–7.

28. Allison J, Campbell IL, Morahan G et al. Diabetes in transgenic mice resulting from over-expression of class I histocompatibility molecules in pancreatic beta cells. Nature 1988; 333: 529–33.

29. Geiger K, Howes E, Gallina M et al. Transgenic mice expressing IFN-gamma in the retina develop inflammation of the eye and photoreceptor loss. Invest Ophthalmol Vis Sci 1994; 35: 2667–81.

30. Antel JP, Owens T. Immune regulation and CNS autoimmune disease. J Neuroimmunol 1999; 100: 181–90.

31. Londei M, Bottazzo GF, Feldmann M. Human T-cell clones from autoimmune thyroid glands: specific recognition of autoiogous thyroid cells. Science 1985; 228: 85–89.

32. Londei M, Lamb JR, Bottazzo GF, Feldmann M. Epithelial cells expressing aberrant MHC class II determinants can present antigen to cloned human T cells. Nature 1984; 312: 639–41.

33. Grubeck-Loebenstein B, Buchan G, Chantry D et al. Analysis of intrathyroidal cytokine production in thyroid autoimmune disease: thyroid follicular cells produce IL-1 alpha and interleukin-6. Scand J Rheum 1989; 77: 324–30.

34. Cody J. Recombinant human erythropoietin for chronic renal failure anaemia in pre-dialysis patients. Cochrane Database Sys Rev 2001; 4: CD003266.

35. Morstyn G, Foote MA, Walker T, Molineux T. Filgrastim (r-metHuG-CSF) in the 21st century: SD/01. Acta Haematol 2001; 105: 151–5.

36. Herrine SK. Approach to the patient with chronic hepatitis C virus infection. Ann Intern Med 2002; 136: 747–57.

37. Bagnato F, Pozzilli C, Scagnolari C et al. A one year study on the pharmacodynamic profile of interferon-beta 1a in MS. Neurology 2002; 59: 1409–11.

38. Brennan FM, Chantry D, Jackson AM et al. Cytokine production in culture by cells isolated from the synovial membrane. J Autoimmun 1989; 2 (Suppl): 177–86.

39. Brenchley PEC. Antagonising angiogenesis in rheumatoid arthritis. Ann Rheum Dis 2001; 60 (Suppl 3): 71–4.

40. Koch AE. The role of angiogenesis in rheumatoid arthritis: recent developments. Ann Rheum Dis 2000; 59 (Suppl 1): 65–71.

41. Paleolog EM, Young S, Stark AC et al. Modulation of angiogenic vascular endothelial growth factor by tumor necrosis factor alpha and interleukin-1 in rheumatoid arthritis. Arthritis Rheum 1998; 41: 1258–65.

42. Fontana A, Hengartner H, Weber E et al. Interleukin 1 activity in the synovial fluid of patients with rheumatoid arthritis. Rheumatol Int 1982; 2: 49–53.

43. Wood NC, Symons JA, Dickens E, Duff GW. In situ hybridization of IL-6 in rheumatoid arthritis. Clin Exp Immunol 1992; 87: 183–9.

44. Feldmann M, Brennan FM, Maini RN. Role of cytokines in rheumatoid arthritis. Annu Rev Immunol 1996; 14: 397–440.

45. Chu CQ, Field M, Feldmann M, Maini RN. Localization of tumor necrosis factor a in synovial tissues and at the cartilage–pannus junction in patients with rheumatoid arthritis. Arthritis Rheum 1991; 34: 1125–32.

46. Hopkins SJ, Humphreys M, Jayson MI. Cytokines in synovial fluid. I. The presence of biologically active and immunoreactive IL-1. Clin Exp Immunol 1988; 72: 422–7.

47. Saxne T, Palladino MA Jr, Heinegard D et al. Detection of tumor necrosis factor α but not tumor necrosis factor β in rheumatoid arthritis synovial fluid and serum. Arthritis Rheum 1988; 31: 1041–5.

48. Arend WP, Dayer JM. Cytokines and cytokine inhibitors or antagonists in rheumatoid arthritis. Arthritis Rheum 1990; 33: 305–15.

49. Koch AE, Kunkel SL, Harlow LA et al. Enhanced production of monocyte chemoattractant protein-1 in rheumatoid arthritis. J Clin Invest 1992; 90: 772–9.

50. Brennan FM, Zachariae CO, Chantry D et al. Detection of interleukin 8 biological activity in synovial fluids from patients with rheumatoid arthritis and production of interleukin 8 mRNA by isolated synovial cells. Eur J Immunol 1990; 20: 2141–4.

51. Katsikis PD, Chu CQ, Brennan FM et al. Immunoregulatory role of interleukin 10 in rheumatoid arthritis. J Exp Med 1994; 179: 1517–27.

52. Wahl SM, Allen JB, Wong HL et al. Antagonistic and agonistic effects of transforming growth factor-β and IL-1 in rheumatoid synovium. J Immunol 1990; 145: 2514–19.

53. Fava R, Olsen N, Keski-Oja J et al. Active and latent forms of transforming growth factor b activity in synovial effusions. J Exp Med 1989; 169: 291–6.

54. Arend WP. Interleukin-1 receptor antagonist. Adv Immunol 1993; 54: 167–227.

55. Walmsley M, Katsikis PD, Abney E et al. Interleukin-10 inhibition of the progression of established collagen-induced arthritis. Arthritis Rheum 1996; 39: 495–503.

56. Maini RN, Paulus H, Breedveld FC et al. rHUIL-10 in subjects with active rheumatoid arthritis (RA): a phase I and cytokine response study. Arthritis Rheum 1997; 40 (Suppl): S224.

57. Brennan FM, Chantry D, Turner M et al. Transforming growth factor-β in rheumatoid arthritis synovial tissue: lack of effect on spontaneous cytokine production in joint cell cultures. Clin Exp Immunol 1990; 81: 278–85.

58. Allen JB, Manthey CL, Hand AR et al. Rapid onset synovial inflammation and hyperplasia induced by transforming growth factor b. J Exp Med 1990; 171: 231–47.

59. Gambaro G, Weigert C, Ceol M, Schleicher ED. Inhibition of transforming growth factor-beta 1 gene overexpression as a strategy to prevent fibrosis. Contrib Nephrol 2001; 131: 107–13.

60. Charles P, Elliott MJ, Davis D et al. Regulation of cytokines, cytokine inhibitors, and acute-phase proteins following anti-TNF-alpha therapy in rheumatoid arthritis. J Immunol 1999; 163: 1521–8.

61. Simon AK, Seipelt E, Sieper J. Divergent T-cell cytokine patterns in inflammatory arthritis. Proc Natl Acad Sci U S A 1994; 91: 8562–6.

62. Isomaki P, Luukkainen R, Toivanen P, Punnonen J. The presence of interleukin-13 in rheumatoid synovium and its antiinflammatory effects on synovial fluid macrophages from patients with rheumatoid arthritis. Arthritis Rheum 1996; 39: 1693–702.

63. Woods JM, Haines GK, Shah MR et al. Low level production of interleukin-13 in synovial fluid and tissue from patients with arthritis. Clin Immunol Immunopathol 1997; 85: 210–20.

64. Fell HB, Jubb RW. The effect of synovial tissue on the breakdown of articular cartilage in organ culture. Arthritis Rheum 1977; 20: 1359–71.

65. Dingle JT, Saklatvala J, Hembry R et al. A cartilage catabolic factor from synovium. Biochem J 1979; 184: 177–80.

66. Saklatvala J, Sarsfield SJ, Townsend Y. Purification of two immunologically different leucocyte proteins that cause cartilage resorption lymphocyte activation and fever. J Exp Med 1985; 162: 1208–15.

67. Brennan FM, Chantry D, Jackson A et al. Inhibitory effect of TNF alpha antibodies on synovial cell interleukin-1 production in rheumatoid arthritis. Lancet 1989; 2: 244–7.

68. Butler DM, Maini RN, Feldmann M, Brennan FM. Modulation of proinflammatory cytokine release in rheumatoid synovial membrane cell cultures. Comparison of monoclonal anti-TNFα antibody with the IL-1 receptor antagonist. Eur Cytokine Netw 1995; 6: 225–30.

69. Haworth C, Brennan FM, Chantry D et al. Expression of granulocyte-macrophage colony-stimulating factor in rheumatoid arthritis: regulation by tumor necrosis factor-alpha. Eur J Immunol 1991; 21: 2575–9.

70. Alvaro-Garcia JM, Zvaifler NJ, Brown CB et al. Cytokines in chronic inflammatory arthritis. VI. Analysis of the synovial cells involved in granulocyte-macrophage colony stimulating factor production and gene expression in rheumatoid arthritis and its regulation by IL-1 and TNFα. J Immunol 1991; 146: 3365–71.

71. Beutler B, Cerami A. Cachectin: more than a tumor necrosis factor. N Engl J Med 1987; 316: 379–85.

72. Vassalli P. The pathophysiology of tumor necrosis factors. Annu Rev Immunol 1992; 10: 411.

73. Keffer J, Probert L, Cazlaris H et al. Transgenic mice expressing human tumour necrosis factor: a predictive genetic model of arthritis. EMBO J 1991; 10: 4025–31.

74. Shaw G, Kamen R. A conserved AU sequence from the 3' untranslated region of GM-CSF mRNA mediates selective mRNA degradation. Cell 1986; 46: 659.

75. Douni E, Akassoglou K, Alexopoulou L et al. Transgenic and knockout analyses of the role of TNF in immune regulation and disease pathogenesis. J Inflamm 1995–96; 47: 27–38.

76. Christ M, McCartney-Francis NL, Kulkarni AB et al. Immune dysregulation in TGF-beta 1-deficient mice. J Immunol 1994; 153: 1936–46.

77. Holmdahl R, Andersson M, Goldschmidt TJ et al. Type II collagen autoimmunity in animals and provocations leading to arthritis. Immunol Rev 1990; 118: 193–232.

78. Thorbecke GJ, Shah R, Leu CH et al. Involvement of endogenous tumor necrosis factor alpha and transforming growth factor beta during induction of collagen type II arthritis in mice. Proc Natl Acad Sci USA 1992; 89: 7375–9.

79. Williams RO, Feldmann M, Maini RN. Anti-tumor necrosis factor ameliorates joint disease in murine collagen-induced arthritis. Proc Natl Acad Sci U S A 1992; 89: 9784–8.

80. Piguet PF, Grau GE, Vesin C et al. Evolution of collagen arthritis in mice is arrested by treatment with anti-tumour necrosis factor (TNF) antibody or a recombinant soluble TNF receptor. Immunology 1992; 77: 510–14.

81. Deleuran BW, Chu CQ, Field M et al. Localization of tumor necrosis factor receptors in the synovial tissue and cartilage–pannus junction in patients with rheumatoid arthritis. Implications for local actions of tumor necrosis factor alpha. Arthritis Rheum 1992; 35: 1170–8.

82. Brennan FM, Hayes AL, Ciesielski CJ et al. Evidence that rheumatoid arthritis synovial T cells are similar to cytokine-activated T cells. Arthritis Rheum 2002; 46: 31–41.

83. McInnes IB, Leung BP, Sturrock RD et al. Interleukin-15 mediates T cell-dependent regulation of tumor necrosis factor-alpha production in rheumatoid arthritis. Nat Med 1997; 3: 189–95.

84. Gracie JA, Forsey RJ, Chan WL et al. A proinflammatory role for IL-18 in rheumatoid arthritis. J Clin Invest 1999; 104: 1393–401.

85. Lubberts E, Koenders MI, van den Berg. The role of T cell interleukin-17 in conducting destructive arthritis: lessons from animal models. Arthritis Res Ther 2005; 7: 29–37.

86. Dong C. Diversification of T-helper-cell lineages: finding the family root of IL-17-producing cells. Nature Rev Immunol 2006; 6: 329–33.

87. McKenzie BS, Kastelein RA, Cua DJ. Understanding the IL-23-IL-17 immune pathway. Trends Immunol 2006; 27: 17–23.

88. Saklatvala J, Dean J, Finch A. Protein kinase cascades in intracellular signalling by interleukin-I and tumour necrosis factor. Biochem Soc Symp 1999; 64: 63–77.

89. Schett G, Tohidast-Akrad M, Smolen JS et al. Activation, differential localization and regulation of the stress-activated protein kinases, extracellular signal-regulated kinase, c-JUN N-terminal kinase, and p38 mitogen-activated protein kinase, in synovial tissue and cells in rheumatoid arthritis. Arthritis Rheum 2000; 43: 2501–12.

90. Derijard B, Hibi M, Wu IH et al. JNK1: a protein kinase stimulated by UV light and Ha-Ras that binds and phosphorylates the c-Jun activation domain. Cell 1994; 76: 1025–37.

91. Foxwell B, Browne K, Bondeson J et al. Efficient adenoviral infection with IkBa reveals that macrophage tumor necrosis factor a production in rheumatoid arthritis is NF-kB dependent. Proc Natl Acad Sci U S A 1998; 95: 8211–15.

92. Bondeson J, Foxwell B, Brennan F, Feldmann M. Defining therapeutic targets by using adenovirus: blocking NF-kB inhibits both inflammatory and destructive mechanisms in rheumatoid synovium but spares anti-inflammatory mediators. Proc Natl Acad Sci U S A 1999; 96: 5668–73.

93. Elliott MJ, Maini RN, Feldmann M et al. Treatment of rheumatoid arthritis with chimeric monoclonal antibodies to tumour necrosis factor α. Arthritis Rheum 1993; 36: 1681–90.

94. Elliott MJ, Maini RN, Feldmann M et al. Randomised double blind comparison of a chimaeric monoclonal antibody to tumour necrosis factor α (cA2) versus placebo in rheumatoid arthritis. Lancet 1994; 344: 1105–10.

95. van Oosterhout M, Levarht EW, Sont JK et al. Clinical efficacy of infliximab plus methotrexate in DMARD naive and DMARD refractory rheumatoid arthritis is associated with decreased synovial expression of TNF alpha and IL18 but not CXCL12. Ann Rheum Dis 2005; 64: 537–43.

96. Tokayer A, Carsons SE, Choksi B et al. High levels of interleukin 13 in rheumatoid arthritis sera are modulated by tumor necrosis factor antagonist therapy: association with dendritic cell growth activity. J Rheumatol 2002; 29: 454–61.

97. Van Roon JAG, Wenting-van Wijk M, Jahangier N et al. IL-7 stimulates T cell dependent TNF production by monocytes and persists upon anti-TNF therapy of RA patients. Arthritis Rheum 2005; 52: S274 (abstract).

98. Kageyama Y, Takahashi M, Torikai E et al. Treatment with anti-TNF-alpha antibody infliximab reduces serum IL-15 levels in patients with rheumatoid arthritis. Clin Rheumatol 2006; 26: 505–9.

99. Ernestam S, Af Klint E, Catrina AI et al. Synovial expression of IL-15 in rheumatoid arthritis is not influenced by blockade of tumour necrosis factor. Arthritis Res Ther 2005; 28: R18.

100. Lorenz HM, Grunke M, Hieronymus T. *In vivo* blockade of tumor necrosis factor-alpha in patient with rheumatoid arthritis: longterm effects after repeated infusion of chimeric monoclonal antibody cA2. J Rheumatol 2000; 27: 304–10.

101. Tak PP, Taylor PC, Breedveld FC et al. Decrease in cellularity and expression of adhesion molecules by anti-tumor necrosis factor α monoclonal antibody treatment in patients with rheumatoid arthritis. Arthritis Rheum, 1996; 39: 1077–81.

102. Paleolog EM, Hunt M, Elliott MJ et al. Deactivation of vascular endothelium by monoclonal anti-tumor necrosis factor α antibody in rheumatoid arthritis. Arthritis Rheum 1996; 39: 1082–91.

103. Taylor PC, Peters AM, Paleolog E et al. Reduction of chemokines levels and leukocytes traffic to joints by tumor necrosis factor α blockade in patients with rheumatoid arthritis. Arthritis Rheum 2000; 43: 38–47.

104. Kalden-Nemeth D, Grebmeier J, Antoni C et al. NMR monitoring of rheumatoid arthritis patients receiving anti-TNF-α monoclonal antibody therapy. Rheumatol Int 1997; 16: 249–55.

105. Taylor PC, Steuer A, Gruber J et al. Comparison of ultrasonographic assessment of synovitis and joint vascularity with radiological evaluation in a randomized, placebo-controlled study of infliximab therapy in early rheumatoid arthritis. Arthritis Rheum 2004; 50: 1107–16.

106. Catrina AI, Trollmo C, af Klint E et al. Evidence that anti-tumor necrosis factor therapy with both etanercept and infliximab induces apoptosis in macrophages, but not lymphocytes, in rheumatoid arthritis joints: extended report. Arthritis Rheum 2005, 52: 61–72.

107. Smeets TJ, Kraan MC, van Loon ME et al. Tumor necrosis factor alpha blockade reduces the synovial cell infiltrates early after initiation of treatment, but apparently not by induction of apoptosis in synovial tissue. Arthritis Rheum 2003; 48: 2155–62.

108. Hurimann D, Forster A, Noll G et al. Anti-tumor necrosis factor-alpha treatment improves endothelial function in patients with rheumatoid arthritis. Circulation 2002; 106: 2184–7.

109. Gonzales-Juanatey, C, Testa A, Garcia-Castelo A et al. Active but transient improvement of endothelial function in rheumatoid arthritis patients undergoing long-term treatment with anti-tumor necrosis factor alpha antibody. Arthritis Rheum 2004; 51: 447–50.

110. Maki-Petaja KM, Hall FC, Booth AD et al. Rheumatoid arthritis is associated with increased aortic pulse-wave velocity, which is reduced by anti-tumor necrosis factor-alpha therapy. Circulation 2006; 114: 1185–92.

111. Lipsky PE, van der Heijde D, St Clair EW et al. Infliximab and methotrexate in the treatment of rheumatoid arthritis. N Engl J Med 2000; 343: 1594–1602.

112. Klareskog L, van der Heijde D, de Jager P et al. Therapeutic effect of the combination of etanercept and methotrexate compared with each treatment alone in patients with rheumatoid arthritis: double-blind randomised controlled trial. Lancet 2004; 363: 675–81.

113. Breedveld FC, Weisman MH, Kavanaugh AF et al. The Premier Study a multicenter, randomized, double-blind clinical trial of combination therapy with adalimumab plus methotrexate versus methotrexate alone or adalimumab alone in patients with early, aggressive rheumatoid arthritis who had not had previous methotrexate treatment. Arthritis Rheum 2006; 54: 36–37.

114. Schett G, Hayer S, Zwerina J et al. Mechanisms of disease: the link between RANKL and arthritic bone disease. Nat Clin Pract Rheumatol 2005; 1: 47–54.

115. Brennan FM, Browne KA, Green PA et al. Reduction of serum matrix metalloproteinase 1 and matrix metalloproteinase 3 in RA patients following anti-TNFα cA2 therapy. Br J Rheumatol 1997; 36: 643–650.

116. Catrina AI, af Klint E, Ernestam S et al. Anti-tumor necrosis factor therapy increases synovial osteoprotegerin expression in rheumatoid arthritis. Arthritis Rheum 2006; 54: 76–81.

117. Ziolkowska M, Kurowska M, Radzikowska A et al. High levels of osteoprotegerin and soluble receptor activator of nuclear factor kappa B ligand in serum of rheumatoid arthritis patients and their normalization after anti-tumor necrosis factor alpha treatment. Arthritis Rheum 2002; 46: 1744–53.

118. Shealy DJ, Wooley PH, Emmell E et al. Anti-TNF α antibody allows healing of joint damage in polyarthritic transgenic mice. Arthritis Res 2002; 4: R7.

119. Isomaki P, Panesar M, Annenkov A et al. Prolonged exposure of T cells to TNF down-regulates TCR zeta and expression of the TCR/CD3 complex at the cell surface. J Immunol 2001; 166: 5497–507.

120. Clark JM, Annenkov AE, Panesar M et al. T cell receptor zeta reconstitution fails to restore response of T cells rendered hyporesponsive by tumor necrosis factor alpha. Proc Natl Acad Sci U S A 2004; 101: 1696–701.

121. Cope AP, Liblau RS, Yang XD et al. Chronic tumor necrosis factor alters T cell responses by attenuating T cell receptor signalling. J Exp Med 1997; 185: 1573–84.

122. Bryl E, Vallejo AN, Weyand C et al. Down-regulation of CD28 expression by TNF-α. J Immunol 2001; 167: 3231–8.

123. Cao D, van Vollenhoven R, Klareskog L et al. CD25brightCD4+ regulatory T cells are enriched in

inflamed joints of patients with chronic rheumatic disease. Arthritis Res Ther 2004; 6: R335–46.

124. Cao D, Borjesson O, Larsson P et al. FOXP3 identifies regulatory CD25bright CD4+ T cells in rheumatic joints. Scand J Immunol 2006; 63: 444–52.

125. Ehrenstein MR, Evans JG, Singh A et al. Compromised function of regulatory T cells in rheumatoid arthritis and reversal by anti-TNF α therapy. J Exp Med 2004; 200: 273–6.

126. Valencia X, Stephens G, Goldbach-Mansky R et al. TNF downmodulates the function of human CD4+CD25hi T-regulatory cells. Blood 2006; 108: 253–61.

127. Cope AP, Londei M, Chu NR et al. Chronic exposure to tumor necrosis factor (TNF) *in vitro* impairs the activation of T cells through the T cell receptor/CD3 complex; reversal *in vivo* by anti-TNF antibodies in patient with rheumatoid arthritis. J Clin Invest 1994; 94: 749–60.

128. Berg L, Lampa J, Rogberg S et al. Increased peripheral T cell reactivity to microbial antigens and collagen type II in rheumatoid arthritis after treatment with soluble TNFa receptors. Ann Rheum Dis 2001; 60: 133–9.

129. Bryl E, Vallejo AN, Matteson EL et al. Modulation of CD28 expression with anti-tumor necrosis factor a therapy in rheumatoid arthritis. Arthritis Rheum 2005; 52: 2996–3003.

130. Quinn MA, Conaghan PG, O'Connor PJ et al. Very early treatment with infliximab in addition to methotrexate in early, poor-prognosis rheumatoid arthritis reduces magnetic resonance imaging evidence of synovitis and damage, with sustained benefit after infliximab withdrawal: results from a twelve-month randomized, double-blind, placebo-controlled trial. Arthritis Rheum 2005; 52: 27–35.

131. Goekoop-Ruiteman YP, de Vries-Bouwstra JK, Allaart CF et al. Clinical and radiographic outcomes of four different treatment strategies in patients with early rheumatoid arthritis (the BeSt study): a randomized, controlled trial. Arthritis Rheum 2005; 11: 3381–90.

12

Update on interleukin-6

Norihiro Nishimoto and Tadamitsu Kishimoto

Introduction • Pathological significance of IL-6 in immunological disorders • Clinical studies of tocilizumab in RA • Clinical studies with tocilizumab in systemic-onset juvenile idiopathic arthritis (soJIA) • Clinical studies with tocilizumab in Castleman's disease • Conclusion • References

INTRODUCTION

Rheumatoid arthritis (RA) is a common autoimmune disease characterized by persistent synovitis with synovial cell proliferation and emergence of rheumatoid factors. The disease is often refractory to conventional therapy using various disease-modifying anti-rheumatic drugs (DMARDs) including methotrexate and low-dose corticosteroids. If the synovial inflammation continues, inflammatory cytokines are constitutively produced at the synovium that induce proliferation of vascular endothelial cells and synovial cells and activation of osteoclasts, as well as production of proteases. These processes result in destruction of cartilage and bone in the affected joints, leading to permanent disability.

Introduction of tumor necrosis factor (TNF) inhibitors into the clinic has revolutionized the treatment of RA not only by their much greater efficacy against the signs and symptoms of RA than conventional DMARDs but also by their capability to prevent joint destruction. The therapeutic goal for RA is now shifting from the control of symptoms to induction of remission. However, about 30–40 % of the patients with RA do not respond clinically to TNF inhibitors. Even among responders, the majority experience only partial improvement in disease activity.[1]

Furthermore, anti-TNF treatment often causes emergence of serious infections including tuberculosis.[2] Therefore, more effective and safe drugs are still urgently needed. Interleukin-6 (IL-6) is one of the target cytokines whose functions need to be blocked if such treatment is to succeed.

In the last edition we described the potential of anti-IL-6 therapy for immune inflammatory diseases including RA, utilizing a humanized anti-IL-6 receptor (IL-6R) antibody, tocilizumab (previously known as MRA or myeloma receptor antibody). In this chapter, we give an update on the development of anti-IL-6 therapy.

PATHOLOGICAL SIGNIFICANCE OF IL-6 IN IMMUNOLOGICAL DISORDERS

Multiple biological activities of IL-6 explain well the signs and symptoms of RA, and a series of experiments using animal models of arthritis have provided us with evidence that blocking IL-6 may be effective in the treatment of RA, as we previously described.[3] Briefly, IL-6 is involved in proliferation and differentiation of immunocompetent cells and osteoclast differentiation. IL-6 causes signs and symptoms of RA such as leukocytosis and fever, as well as abnormal laboratory findings such as hypergammaglobulinemia, increase in rheumatoid factors, thrombocytosis, increase in serum acute phase proteins such as C-reactive protein (CRP), fibrinogen, α1-antitrypsin, and serum amyloid A (SAA), as well as decrease in serum albumin. IL-6-deficient (IL-6[−/−]) mice are resistant to collagen-induced arthritis (CIA)[4,5] as well as antigen-induced arthritis (AIA).[6] IL-6 blockade with rat anti-mouse IL-6R monoclonal antibody inhibited the development of CIA in DBA/1J mice.[7] In addition, tocilizumab treatment decreased the incidence and the severity of CIA in cynomolgus monkeys,[8] whose IL-6R is recognized by tocilizumab.

The multiple biological actions of IL-6 are mediated by a unique receptor system which consists of two functional proteins: an 80 kDa ligand-binding chain (IL-6R, CD126) and a 130 kDa non-ligand-binding but signal-transducing chain (gp130, CD130) (Figure 12.1).[9] The soluble form of IL-6R (sIL-6R), lacking the intracytoplasmic portion of IL-6R, is found in serum and body fluids, including synovial fluid, and is also capable of signal transduction as a ligand-binding receptor. When IL-6 binds to the cell surface IL-6R

or the sIL-6R, the complex induces the homodimerization of gp130 and forms a high-affinity functional receptor complex of IL-6, IL-6R, and gp130. Note that the IL-6 signal can be transduced into cells as long as they express gp130. This process of signaling mediated by sIL-6R is called trans-signaling and plays a pathologically important role in RA and other rheumatic diseases because the target cells in the affected joints such as synovial fibroblasts, vascular endothelial cells, and osteoclasts express little IL-6R on their cell surface.[10] Tocilizumab recognizes both membrane-binding and soluble IL-6R and inhibits signal transduction of IL-6.

In the pathology of RA, there have been two important advances related to IL-6 biology since the last edition. One is on angiogenesis and the other is on iron metabolism.

IL-6 and vascular endothelial growth factor

Hyperplasia of synovial tissues in RA patients requires an increase in angiogenesis, which is necessary to oxygenate the growing tissue,

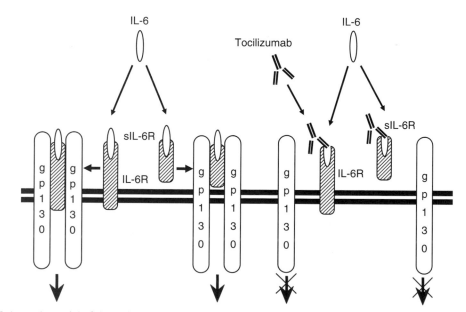

Figure 12.1 Schematic model of the IL-6 receptor system. The IL-6 receptor (IL-6R) system consists of two functional proteins: a ligand-binding IL-6R and a 130 kDa non-ligand-binding but signal-transducing gp130. The soluble form of IL-6R (sIL-6R) is found in serum and body fluids and is also capable of mediating signaling into cells. IL-6 binds to cell surface IL-6R or sIL-6R, the complex induces the homodimerization of gp130 and mediates signaling into cells (left side). Tocilizumab blocks the binding of IL-6 to both cell surface IL-6R and sIL-6R (right side).

as in a tumor. Vascular endothelial growth factor (VEGF), a potent angiogenic factor, is responsible not only for angiogenesis[11,12] but also for the induction of vascular permeability and inflammation.[11,13] Patients with RA show higher VEGF levels in serum and synovial fluids than those with osteoarthritis (OA) or other arthritides.[12] Serum VEGF levels correlate with disease activity and radiologic progression in patients with RA.[14] VEGF is mainly produced by the synovial cells in the affected joints but the regulation of VEGF production has not been fully understood.

When IL-6 and sIL-6R were added to cultured synovial cells, they increased VEGF production but the effect was not remarkable. However, IL-6, synergistically with IL-1β or TNF, augmented VEGF production from synovial cells, while there was no synergistic effect between IL-1β and TNF (Figure 12.2A).[15] Therefore, IL-6 is a pivotal cytokine that induces VEGF production synergistically with IL-1β or TNF, and blockade of IL-6 action inhibits VEGF production more effectively than inhibitors of IL-1 and TNF.[15] Indeed, serum VEGF levels were normalized by tocilizumab treatment (Figure 12.2B).

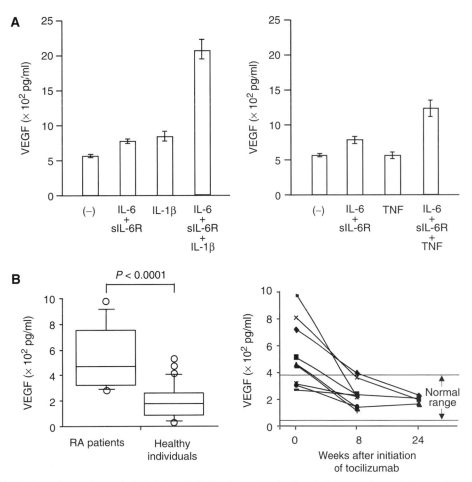

Figure 12.2 Regulation of vascular endothelial growth factor (VEGF) production by inflammatory cytokines. (A) IL-6, in the presence of sIL-6R, augmented the production of VEGF synergistically with IL-1 or TNF. RA synovial fibroblasts were cultured for 72 hours with IL-6/sIL-6R (100 ng/ml), IL-1β (5 ng/ml), and/or TNF (10 ng/ml). VEGF levels in the supernatants were determined by enzyme-linked immunosorbent assay (ELISA). Data from Nakahara et al.[15] (B) Tocilizumab therapy normalized serum VEGF levels in patients with rheumatoid arthritis (RA). VEGF levels were assayed by ELISA. Serum VEGF levels are significantly higher in RA patients than those of healthy controls. The serum VEGF levels were normalized with tocilizumab treatment. Data from Nakahara et al.[15]

IL-6 and hepcidin on anemia of chronic inflammation

The other advance is related to anemia of chronic inflammation, which considerably influences the quality of life of RA patients. Hepcidin is an iron regulatory peptide hormone which controls extracellular iron concentrations by binding to and inducing the degradation of the cellular iron exporter, ferroportin.[16] Hepcidin suppresses iron absorption from duodenal enterocytes and recycling of iron from senescent erythrocytes by macrophages while inducing iron storage in hepatocytes. Hepcidin is synthesized by hepatocytes under regulation by iron concentrations, hypoxia, anemia, and inflammatory cytokines. Among the cytokines, IL-6 is a potent inducer of hepcidin and excessive hepcidin production stimulated by IL-6 is responsible for anemia of chronic inflammation.[17,18] IL-1 is also capable of inducing hepcidin production[19] but TNF is not. Therefore, IL-6 blockade may provide a clinical benefit in the treatment of anemia of chronic inflammation when compared with TNF inhibitors.

IL-6 and anemia in collagen-induced arthritis

Involvement of IL-6 in the anemia of chronic inflammation has been investigated in the animal models in collaboration with Shin Nippon Biomedical Laboratories, Ltd. We have demonstrated a negative correlation between serum CRP levels and erythrocyte counts in cynomolgus monkeys with CIA (Figure 12.3A).

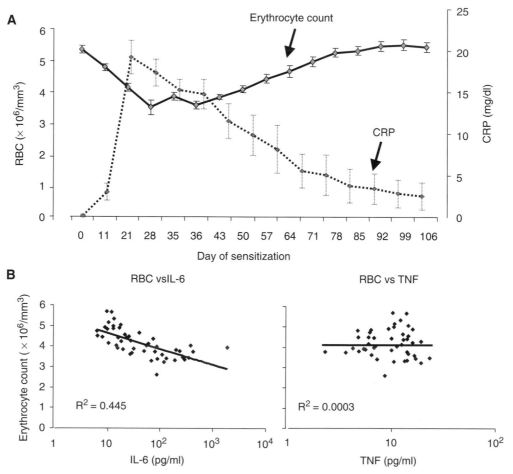

Figure 12.3 Anemia in cynomolgus monkeys with collagen-induced arthritis (CIA). (A) Negative correlation between CRP levels and erythrocyte counts in cynomolgus monkeys with CIA. (B) Erythrocyte counts correlate negatively with serum IL-6 levels but not with serum TNF levels. IL-6 vs erythrocyte counts (left side); TNF vs erythrocyte counts (right side).

Furthermore, serum IL-6 levels have been shown to correlate negatively with erythrocyte counts (Figure 12.3B), while there was no correlation between serum TNF levels and erythrocyte counts. This finding supports the previous report that IL-6 but not TNF induces hepcidin. IL-6 may be responsible for the anemia associated with CIA.

We need to know if serum hepcidin levels are decreased by IL-6 blockade in order to confirm that hepcidin is indeed responsible for the anemia of patients with immune inflammatory diseases including RA.

IL-6 and new animal models of arthritis

SKG mice spontaneously develop T-cell-mediated chronic autoimmune arthritis with a high rheumatoid factor titer. The joints affected in this mouse model are similar to those of human RA and the incidence is also higher in female than male mice. This evidence suggests that these mice may offer a new model of human RA.[20] Genetic introduction of IL-6 deficiency into SKG mice completely suppresses the development of arthritis, although either IL-1 or TNF deficiency only retards the onset of arthritis and partially reduces its incidence and severity.[21] Therefore, IL-6 is the most important factor in the arthritis of this model.

Mice with a point mutation of Tyr-759 in gp130 of IL-6R system subunit, a binding site of the src homology 2 domain-bearing protein tyrosine phosphatase (SHP)-2, have been shown to develop autoimmune arthritis through insufficient clonal selection of T cells in the thymus and increase in autoreactive antibodies.[22] The evidence shows that excess signaling through gp130 may result in the development of arthritis.

Both of these experiments again confirm the involvement of IL-6 in the development of arthritis.

CLINICAL STUDIES OF TOCILIZUMAB IN RA

Phase I/II trials with tocilizumab in patients with RA

Phase I/II trials of tocilizumab have been conducted both in the UK and in Japan. In the UK study, a single administration, randomized, double-blind, placebo-controlled, dose-escalation trial was conducted in 45 patients with active RA.[23] In the Japanese study, an open-label, multi-dose trial was conducted in 15 RA patients.[24]

Pharmacokinetics were investigated, especially in the Japanese phase I/II trial.[24] Tocilizumab 2, 4, or 8 mg/kg body weight was administered to patients with active RA every 2 weeks for 6 weeks. The serum tocilizumab concentration decreased in a non-linear manner over time within the dose range 2–8 mg/kg. The half-life ($t_{1/2}$) of tocilizumab in serum increased with repeated doses and as the dose level increased. The $t_{1/2}$ after the third dose of 8 mg/kg reached 241.8 ± 71.4 hours, which resembles the $t_{1/2}$ of human IgG. The mean area under the serum concentration/time curve (AUC) increased as the dose increased and the value (mean $\pm$ SD) was 10.66 ± 4.07 mg*hour/ml in the 8 mg/kg groups.

Serum CRP and SAA levels were completely normalized as long as tocilizumab was detectable in the serum, indicating that IL-6 is essential for the production of CRP and SAA *in vivo*. These acute phase protein levels could be used as surrogate markers to indicate that the tocilizumab concentration is adequate to block IL-6 activity.[24]

In the UK, 45 patients with active RA were sequentially allocated to receive a single intravenous dose of either 0.1, 1, 5 or 10 mg/kg of tocilizumab or placebo.[23] Two weeks after the treatment, a significant treatment difference was observed between 5 mg/kg tocilizumab and placebo, with five patients (55.6%) in the tocilizumab cohort and none in the placebo cohort achieving American College of Rheumatology (ACR) 20 response criteria (improvement of 20% or more in disease activity). In the Japanese study, repeated treatment with tocilizumab at intravenous doses up to 8 mg/kg biweekly administration was well tolerated and no serious adverse events were observed.[24] After 6 weeks of treatment, 60% of patients achieved ACR20 and after 24 weeks, 86%. These results encouraged us to move into phase II trials with tocilizumab in RA patients.

Phase II trials with tocilizumab in patients with RA

The safety and efficacy of tocilizumab treatment was evaluated in multi-center, double-blind, randomized, placebo-controlled phase II trials in RA patients both in Japan and Europe.[25,26]

In the Japanese study, 164 patients with refractory RA were randomized to receive either placebo, 4 or 8 mg/kg of tocilizumab intravenously every 4 weeks for a total of 3 months and clinical responses were evaluated using ACR criteria.[25] Tocilizumab treatment significantly improved all measures of disease activity in the ACR core set and a dose-response relationship was observed between the 4 and 8 mg/kg groups (Figure 12.4). The ACR50 and ACR70 responses in the 8 mg/kg group were also significantly higher than those in the placebo group. Efficacy was also evaluated using the Disease Activity Score 28 joint count (DAS28) categories and the incidence of 'good or moderate' response was 91% in the 8 mg/kg group, as compared with 72% ($p = 0.012$) in the 4 mg/kg group and 19% ($p < 0.001$) in the placebo group. Tocilizumab treatment also improved laboratory findings such as hemoglobin levels, platelet counts, serum levels of CRP, fibrinogen, SAA, albumin, and rheumatoid factors. Tocilizumab treatment significantly improved bone metabolism, suggesting that IL-6 blockade may prevent the osteoporosis of RA.

Concerning safety, the overall incidences of adverse events were 56, 59, and 51% in the placebo, 4, and 8 mg/kg groups, respectively, and there was no dose dependency. One patient died of reactivation of chronic active Epstein–Barr virus (EBV) infection and consequent hemophagocytosis syndrome after receiving a single dose of 8 mg/kg tocilizumab. Retrospectively, it was discovered that she had Hodgkin's disease with increased EBV DNA in plasma before enrollment to the study but was not excluded.[27]

Amongst laboratory findings, an increase in total cholesterol level was frequently reported (44%) in the tocilizumab groups. However, mean total cholesterol levels did not continue to increase with repeated dosing and became stable at about the upper limit of the normal range. High-density lipoprotein (HDL) cholesterol levels also increased and consequently the atherogenic index (total cholesterol – HDL cholesterol/HDL cholesterol) did not change throughout the study period. No cardiovascular complications were observed in association with the increase in the total cholesterol. Mild to moderate increases in liver function tests were also observed in 14 of 109 patients (12.8%) in the tocilizumab groups. There was no increase in antinuclear antibodies or anti-DNA antibodies. These data indicate that tocilizumab treatment is generally well tolerated and shows clinical benefit.[25]

A phase II study has also been conducted in Europe (CHARISMA study).[26] A total of 359 patients with active RA, with an incomplete

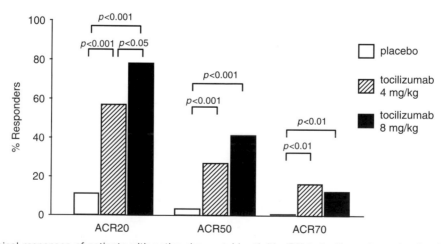

Figure 12.4 Clinical responses of patients with active rheumatoid arthritis (RA) to tocilizumab or placebo. RA patients were administered either placebo or 4 or 8 mg/kg tocilizumab every 4 weeks for a total of 3 months and the clinical responses were evaluated using ACR criteria. Data from Nishimoto et al.[25]

response to methotrexate at doses of 10 mg/week or above for at least 6 months, were randomized to receive tocilizumab or tocilizumab placebo every 4 weeks for a total of 12 weeks together with 10–25 mg/week of methotrexate or methotrexate placebo. Patients were randomized to receive 2, 4, or 8 mg/kg tocilizumab either as monotherapy, or in combination with methotrexate, or methotrexate monotherapy. Tocilizumab 8 mg/kg monotherapy and a combination of tocilizumab 8 mg/kg and methotrexate both yielded statistically significantly higher responses than methotrexate alone, as evaluated by DAS28 change from baseline. However, there was no statistically significant difference between tocilizumab 8 mg/kg monotherapy and 8 mg/kg plus methotrexate.

Phase III trials with tocilizumab in patients with RA

A phase III, randomized, controlled trial was performed in Japan to investigate the ability of tocilizumab to inhibit radiographic progression of joint damage in patients with active RA.[28] This trial demonstrated the superiority of tocilizumab monotherapy over conventional DMARDs in retarding radiographic progression as well as in reducing RA signs and symptoms.

This series of clinical studies clearly indicates the benefit of blocking IL-6 signaling using tocilizumab in the treatment of patients with RA.

CLINICAL STUDIES WITH TOCILIZUMAB IN SYSTEMIC-ONSET JUVENILE IDIOPATHIC ARTHRITIS (SOJIA)

soJIA is one of the most destructive and distressing diseases of childhood.[29] The clinical manifestations include quotidian fever, rheumatoid rash, arthritis, pericarditis, and hepatosplenomegaly, and the patients frequently progress to macrophage activation syndrome. Long-term administration of systemic corticosteroids is often mandatory and prolonged use of corticosteroids leads to multiple adverse effects such as growth suppression, spinal compression fractures, cataracts, etc. Although the etiology of the disease remains unknown, overproduction of IL-6 has been thought to be responsible for the

systemic manifestations and abnormal laboratory findings.[30,31] Increases in serum levels of IL-6 and sIL-6R have been reported to be closely related with disease activity in soJIA.[32,33]

The safety and efficacy of tocilizumab have been investigated in children with soJIA refractory to conventional therapy including methotrexate and corticosteroids.[34]

A phase II study involving intra-patient dose escalation was conducted in Japan in 11 children with active soJIA.[35] All patients received an initial dose of 2 mg/kg tocilizumab every 2 weeks. If the CRP value was more than 1.5 mg/dl at least 5 days after the first or second administration of tocilizumab, the dose was increased to 4 mg/kg for the next three doses. If 4 mg/kg failed to stabilize CRP levels, 8 mg/kg tocilizumab was administered every 2 weeks for a total of 3 doses. Patients included eight boys and three girls, mean age was 8.5 years and the mean disease duration was 4.2 years. At enrollment, patients were receiving corticosteroids at a mean dose of 13.7 mg. Tocilizumab was well tolerated in all patients and quickly ameliorated signs, symptoms, and laboratory abnormalities in all 11 patients. Three patients responded to treatment with 2 mg/kg tocilizumab, five patients to 4 mg/kg, and three patients to 8 mg/kg. Tocilizumab reduced both the frequency and severity of fever episodes and normalized CRP and ESR in all patients. Hemoglobin and albumin were also normalized.

The efficacy of tocilizumab was assessed using the JIA core set of six response variables including (1) global assessment of the severity of disease including febrile episodes and physical findings, (2) global assessment of overall well-being by the patient or parent, (3) functional ability (Childhood Health Assessment Questionnaire (C-HAQ) score), (4) number of joints with active arthritis, (5) number of joints with limited range of motion, and (6) ESR. Two weeks after the third stable dose of tocilizumab, 10 of 11 (91%) had a 50% improvement (JIA50 response), and 7 of 11 (64%) achieved a 70% improvement (JIA70 response) in core set criteria at the last observation. No patients withdrew during the study period and there were no serious adverse events.

The long-term safety and efficacy of tocilizumab were also assessed over 3 years in the same patients.[36] In this extension trial, 10 of 11 patients achieved a 70% improvement in JIA core set criteria. Moreover, doses of corticosteroids were successfully tapered without disease flares. Surprisingly, the most serious complication of soJIA, growth impairment, was improved during the course of the long-term study. Together with growth recovery, bone mineral density improved during treatment.

Woo et al. reported the results of an open-label trial with single infusions of tocilizumab at three dose levels (2, 4, 8 mg/kg) in Caucasian children with severe soJIA.[37] No dose-limiting toxicity was observed. Eleven of 18 patients achieved a 30% improvement and eight achieved a 50% improvement in JIA core set variables. Clinical improvement in these children was sustained for up to 8 weeks after the single dose of tocilizumab.

The results of both Japanese and European studies indicate that tocilizumab therapy is well tolerated and provides clinical benefit in patients with soJIA.

CLINICAL STUDIES WITH TOCILIZUMAB IN CASTLEMAN'S DISEASE

Castleman's disease is a benign lymphoproliferative disease characterized by chronic inflammatory manifestations and immunological disorders related to overproduction of IL-6.[38–41]

A multicenter prospective study was undertaken to evaluate the safety and efficacy of tocilizumab in patients with multicentric Castleman's disease in Japan.[42] In this study, 8 mg/kg of tocilizumab was administered biweekly for 16 weeks. Adjustments in dose and treatment interval were allowed for each patient in an extension phase after 16 weeks. Tocilizumab consistently improved lymphadenopathy and all the inflammatory parameters within 16 weeks. Hemoglobin, albumin, total cholesterol, HDL cholesterol and body mass index (BMI) all increased significantly and chronic inflammatory symptoms were successfully managed over 60 weeks.[42] Tocilizumab treatment was well tolerated and significantly improved chronic inflammatory symptoms and wasting in these patients. Tocilizumab was approved as an orphan drug for Castleman's disease in Japan in 2005.

CONCLUSION

There has been considerable progress in the clinical study of tocilizumab in immune inflammatory diseases. Clinical trials are now being conducted worldwide. However, the mechanism by which IL-6 blockade exerts its therapeutic effect is still not fully understood. In order fully to establish anti-IL-6 therapy, we need to elucidate the mechanism of action. The outcome of long-term treatment is also very important in assessing the therapeutic value of a new drug, especially in the case of a therapeutic agent for chronic inflammatory diseases such as RA.

The efficacy of tocilizumab has been demonstrated in the treatment of inflammatory diseases including soJIA and Castleman's disease, as well as RA. Further studies are required to fully establish the safest and most effective ways to use anti-IL-6 therapy in these refractory diseases.

REFERENCES

1. Olsen NJ, Stein CM. New drugs for rheumatoid arthritis. N Engl J Med 2004; 350: 2167–79.
2. Keane J, Gershon S, Wise RP et al. Tuberculosis associated with infliximab, a tumor necrosis factor alpha-neutralizing agent. N Engl J Med 2001; 345: 1098–104.
3. Nishimoto N, Yoshizaki K, Kishimoto T. Interleukin-6. In: Smolen J, Lipsky P, eds. Targeted Therapy in Rheumatology. London: Martin Dunitz, 2003: 231–41.
4. Alonzi T, Fattori E, Lazzaro D et al. Interleukin-6 is required for the development of collagen-induced arthritis. J Exp Med 1998; 187: 461–8.
5. Sasai M, Saeki Y, Ohshima S et al. Delayed onset and reduced severity of collagen-induced arthritis in interleukin-6-deficient mice. Arthritis Rheum 1999; 42: 1635–43.
6. Ohshima S, Saeki Y, Mima T et al. Interleukin 6 plays a key role in the development of antigen-induced arthritis. Proc Natl Acad Sci U S A 1998; 95: 8222–6.
7. Takagi N, Mihara M, Moriya Y et al. Blockage of interleukin-6 receptor ameliorates joint disease in murine collagen-induced arthritis. Arthritis Rheum 1998; 41: 2117–21.
8. Mihara M, Kotoh M, Nishimoto N et al. Humanized antibody to human interleukin-6 receptor inhibits the development of collagen arthritis in cynomolgus monkeys. Clin Immunol 2001; 98: 319–26.
9. Kishimoto T, Akira S, Taga T. Interleukin-6 and its receptor: a paradigm for cytokines. Science 1992; 258: 593–7.

10. Scheller J, Ohnesorge N, Rose-John S. Interleukin-6 trans-signalling in chronic inflammation and cancer. Scand J Immunol 2006; 63: 321–9.

11. Paleolog E M. Angiogenesis: a critical process in the pathogenesis of RA – a role for VEGF? Br J Rheumatol 1996; 35: 917–20.

12. Koch AE, Harlow LA, Haines GK et al. Vascular endothelial growth factor: a cytokine modulating endothelial function in rheumatoid arthritis. J Immunol 1994; 152: 4149–56.

13. Keck PJ, Hauser SD, Krivi G et al. Vascular permeability factor, an endothelial cell mitogen related to PDGF. Science 1989; 246: 1309–12.

14. Ballara S, Taylor PC, Reusch P et al. Raised serum vascular endothelial growth factor levels are associated with destructive change in inflammatory arthritis. Arthritis Rheum 2001; 44: 2055–64.

15. Nakahara H, Song J, Sugimoto M et al. Anti-interleukin-6 receptor antibody therapy reduces vascular endothelial growth factor production in rheumatoid arthritis. Arthritis Rheum 2003; 48: 1521–9.

16. Nemeth E, Ganz T. Regulation of iron metabolism by hepcidin. Annu Rev Nutr 2006; 26: 323–42.

17. Nemeth E, Valore EV, Territo M et al. Hepcidin, a putative mediator of anemia of inflammation, is a type II acute-phase protein. Blood 2003; 101: 2461–3.

18. Nemeth E, Rivera S, Gabayan V et al. IL-6 mediates hypoferremia of inflammation by inducing the synthesis of the iron regulatory hormone hepcidin. J Clin Invest 2004; 113: 1271–6.

19. Lee P, Peng H, Gelbart T et al. Regulation of hepcidin transcription by interleukin-1 and interleukin-6. Proc Natl Acad Sci U S A 2005; 102: 1906–10.

20. Sakaguchi N, Takahashi T, Hata H et al. Altered thymic T-cell selection due to a mutation of the ZAP-70 gene causes autoimmune arthritis in mice. Nature 2003; 426: 454–60.

21. Hata H, Sakaguchi N, Yoshitomi H et al. Distinct contribution of IL-6, TNF-alpha, IL-1, and IL-10 to T cell-mediated spontaneous autoimmune arthritis in mice. J Clin Invest 2004; 114: 582–8.

22. Atsumi T, Ishihara K, Kamimura D et al. A point mutation of Tyr-759 in interleukin 6 family cytokine receptor subunit gp130 causes autoimmune arthritis. J Exp Med 2002; 196: 979–90.

23. Choy EH, Isenberg DA, Garrood T et al. Therapeutic benefit after blocking interleukin-6 activity in rheumatoid arthritis with an anti-interleukin-6 receptor monoclonal antibody. Arthritis Rheum 2002; 46: 3143–50.

24. Nishimoto N, Yoshizaki K, Maeda K et al. Toxicity, pharmacokinetics, and dose finding study of repetitive treatment with humanized anti-interleukin 6 receptor antibody, MRA, in rheumatoid arthritis – Phase I/II clinical study. J Rheumatol 2003; 30: 1426–35.

25. Nishimoto N, Yoshizaki K, Miyasaka N et al. Treatment of rheumatoid arthritis with humanized anti-interleukin-6 receptor antibody: a multicenter, double-blind, placebo-controlled trial. Arthritis Rheum 2004; 50: 1761–9.

26. Maini RN, Taylor PC, Szechinski J et al. Double-blind randomized controlled clinical trial of the interleukin-6 receptor antagonist, tocilizumab, in European patients with rheumatoid arthritis who had an incomplete response to methotrexate. Arthritis Rheum 2006; 54: 2817–29.

27. Ogawa J, Harigai M, Akashi T et al. Exacerbation of chronic active Epstein–Barr virus infection in a patient with rheumatoid arthritis receiving humanized anti-interleukin-6 receptor antibody. Ann Rheum Dis 2006; 65: 1667–9.

28. Nishimoto N, Hashimoto J, Miyasaka N et al. Study of active controlled monotherapy used for rheumatoid arthritis, an IL-6 inhibitor (SAMSRI):-Evidence of clinical and radiographic benefit from an x-ray reader-blinded randomized controlled trial of tocilzumab. Ann Rheum Dis 2007 Jun 8[Epub ahead of print].

29. Petty RE, Cassidy JT. Chronic arthritis. In: Cassidy JT, Petty RE, eds. Textbook of Pediatric Rheumatology, 4th ed. Philadelphia: WB Sanders, 2001: 214–321.

30. de Benedetti F, Martini A. Is systemic juvenile rheumatoid arthritis an interleukin-6 mediated disease? J Rheumatol 1998; 25: 203–7.

31. Yokota S. Interleukin-6 as a therapeutic target in systemic-onset juvenile idiopathic arthritis. Curr Opin Rheumatol 2003; 15: 581–6.

32. Keul R, Heinrich PC, Muller-newen G et al. A possible role for soluble IL-6 receptor in the pathogenesis of systemic onset juvenile chronic arthritis. Cytokine 1998; 10: 729–34.

33. Fife MS, Ogilvie EM, Kelberman D et al. Novel IL-6 haplotypes and disease association. Genes Immun 2005; 6: 367–70.

34. Grom AA, Passo M. Macrophage activation syndrome in systemic juvenile rheumatoid arthritis. J Pediatr 1996; 129: 750–4.

35. Yokota S, Miyamae T, Imagawa T et al. Therapeutic efficacy of humanized recombinant anti-interleukin-6 receptor antibody in children with systemic-onset juvenile idiopathic arthritis. Arthritis Rheum 2005; 52: 818–25.

36. Yokota S, Miyamae T, Kurosawa R et al. Long-term treatment of systemic-onset juvenile idiopathic arthritis (soJIA) with humanized anti-IL-6 receptor monoclonal antibody, tocilizumab (Actemra). Arthritis Rheum 2005; 52 (Suppl): S725: 1956

37. Woo P, Wilkinson N, Prieur AM et al. Open label phase II trial of single, ascending doses of MRA in Caucasian children with severe systemic juvenile idiopathic arthritis: proof of principle of the efficacy of IL-6 receptor

blockade in this type of arthritis and demonstration of prolonged clinical improvement. Arthritis Res Ther 2005; 7: R1281–8.

38. Castleman B, Iverson L, Menendez VP. Localized mediastinal lymphnode hyperplasia resembling thymoma. Cancer 1956; 9: 822–30.

39. Keller AR, Hochholzer L, Castleman B. Hyalin-vascular and plasma-cell types of giant lymph node hyperplasia of the mediastinum and other locations. Cancer 1972; 29: 670–83.

40. Yoshizaki K, Matsuda T, Nishimoto N et al. Pathogenic significance of interleukin-6(IL-6/BSF-2) in Castleman's disease. Blood 1989; 74: 1360–7.

41. Nishimoto N, Sasai M, Shima Y et al. Improvement in Castleman's disease by humanized anti-IL-6 receptor antibody therapy. Blood 2000; 95: 56–61.

42. Nishimoto N, Kanakura Y, Aozasa K et al. Humanized anti-interleukin-6 receptor antibody treatment of multicentric Castleman's disease. Blood 2005; 106: 2627–32.

13

Interleukin-13

Marion Kasaian and Mary Collins

INTRODUCTION

Interleukin-13 (IL-13) is a type I cytokine that has emerged as a critical regulator of inflammatory immune responses.[1] It has been well characterized as a Th2 cytokine, and data from both human studies and animal models implicate IL-13 as a key mediator in the pathogenesis of asthma and in protective immune responses to parasite infection. Additional studies suggest that IL-13 may also have roles in other autoimmune and inflammatory conditions. In this chapter, we explore the biology of IL-13, and highlight data that suggest a role for IL-13 in rheumatic diseases and other autoimmune and chronic inflammatory diseases.

IL-13 AND IL-13 RECEPTORS

IL-13 was first identified in 1993 from a subtractive library screen of activated human T cells, in a search for new members of the cytokine family.[2] The gene for IL-13 is located within a 150 kb cytokine gene cluster on human chromosome 5q31. This region also contains the IL-5 gene, located 114 kb centromeric to the IL-13 gene, and the IL-4 gene located 12.6 kb telomeric to the IL-13 gene. Genes encoding granulocyte/ macrophage colony-stimulating factor (GM-CSF) and IL-3 are also located centromeric to IL-5 in the same region (Genbank NT_034772). The IL-4 and IL-13 genes are transcribed from the same strand on chromosome 5q31, and the genes encoding IL-5, IL-13, and IL-4 are transcribed in cells responding to shared stimuli.[3] IL-13 is preferentially expressed by activated Th2 cells, together with the Th2 cytokines IL-4 and IL-5.[4] In addition to T cells, IL-13 is produced by activated natural killer (NK) T cells, mast cells, and basophils,[5-7] cells which are also implicated in Th2-mediated immune responses.

IL-13 is a 15 kd monomeric four helix bundle cytokine that shares 30% amino acid identify with IL-4, its closest homolog.[2,8,9] Both IL-4 and IL-13 mediate their activity by binding to a shared receptor comprising the IL-4Rα chain and the IL-13Rα1 chain.[10] This receptor complex is expressed on B cells, monocytes, epithelial cells, endothelial cells, fibroblasts, and smooth muscle cells, which are direct cellular targets for IL-13.[1,11] IL-13 binds the IL-13Rα1 chain with a moderate affinity (Kd approx 40 nM),[12] but has no detectable affinity for the IL-4Rα chain. A higher affinity is detected for IL-13 binding to the IL-13Rα1/IL-4R complex, with a Kd of 500 pM.[12] The NMR structures indicate that IL-4 and

IL-13 share significant structural homology, and both cytokines interact with the shared IL-4R chain in a similar orientation.[13,14] A second IL-13 receptor, IL-13Rα2, has high affinity for IL-13, with a Kd of 2.5 nM, but as evidence of down-stream signaling has been lacking, it has been characterized as a 'decoy', binding to IL-13 and sequestering it from IL-13Rα1.[15–17] Recent evidence, however, suggests that IL-13Rα2 may be involved in mediating the profibrotic activity of IL-13.[18] A unique receptor complex exists for IL-4 and comprises the IL-4Rα chain and the gamma common cytokine receptor. This IL-4Rγc receptor complex binds only to IL-4, and cells bearing this receptor complex, such as T cells, do not respond to IL-13.

BIOLOGICAL ACTIVITY OF IL-13 ON CELL LINES *IN VITRO*

Heterodimerization of cell surface IL-13Rα1 and IL-4Rα receptor chains initiates IL-13 signaling via recruitment of Jak kinases, Jak1, Jak2, and Tyk2, resulting in the phosphorylation of the transcription factor, STAT6, a critical step in IL-13- and IL-4-dependent signaling.[19] Signaling pathways downstream of IL-13 receptor engagement are shown in Figure 13.1. In addition to STAT6, the IL-13Rα1/IL-4Rα complex can trigger phosphorylation of IRS1/2, recruitment of the adaptor protein Grb2, and activation of the PI3kinase pathway.[20,21] IL-13 also induces STAT1 and STAT3 phosphorylation and activation, which

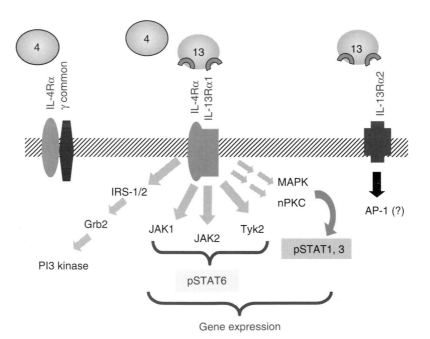

Figure 13.1 IL-13 receptors and signaling pathways. IL-13 and IL-4 can interact with a receptor form comprising the IL-13Rα1 and IL-4Rα subunits. Tyk2 is associated with IL-13Rα1. JAK1 and JAK2 are associated with IL-4Rα. Receptor engagement results in phosphorylation of Tyk2 or JAK1 and JAK2, which in turn phosphorylate STAT6. Phospho STAT6 migrates to the nucleus, where it induces transcription of IL-13-responsive genes. STAT1 and STAT3 may also be involved in IL-13 signaling pathways. Regulation of STAT3 by serine phosphorylation may be downstream of IL-13-induced MAPK activation, and involve a novel PKC isoform (nPKC). Receptor engagement also leads to phosphorylation of IRS1/2, recruitment of the adaptor protein Grb2, and activation of the PI3kinase pathway. IL-4, but not IL-13, can interact with cells through the IL-4Rα/γ common receptor complex. The IL-13Rα2 chain is thought to function primarily as a non-signaling decoy receptor, but recent evidence suggests potential activation of the AP-1 signaling pathway.[18]

have been implicated in responses of B cells, monocytes, and fibroblasts to IL-4 and IL-13 through the shared receptor.[22-24] Regulation of STAT3 by serine phosphorylation may be downstream of IL-13-induced mitogen-activated protein kinase (MAPK) activation, and involve a novel protein kinase C (PKC) isoform.[25] Roles for p38, JNK, and ERK have recently been implicated in IL-13-induced eotaxin production, independent of STAT6.[26-28] Finally, recent data suggest that IL-13Rα2 may trigger activator protein (AP)-1-mediated downstream events under appropriate conditions.[18]

EFFECTS OF IL-13 ON IMMUNE AND STRUCTURAL CELLS

The IL-13Rα1–IL-4Rα complex is expressed on B cells, where it drives immunoglobulin production, most notably IgE switch recombination, and can potentiate proliferative responses.[1,29] The receptor is also expressed on monocytes, where IL-13 induces expression of activation markers, including CD23 and major histocompatibility complex (MHC) class II.[8] IL-13 also stimulates arginase activity in monocytes,[30] resulting in depletion of arginine, down-regulation of inducible nitric oxide synthase (iNOS) expression, reduced NO production, and impaired macrophage cytotoxic function.[31,32] Furthermore, IL-13 is a major activator and inducer of transforming growth factor (TGF)-β production from monocytes.[33] Like IL-13, TGF-β induces collagen production and fibrosis, and debate exists over whether the profibrotic activity of these cytokines is independent,[34] or whether TGF-β mediates and amplifies the profibrotic activity of IL-13.[18,33] In conjunction with M-CSF or GM-CSF, IL-13 stimulates dendritic cell (DC) differentiation from monocytes,[35,36] resulting in loss of IL-13Rα1 expression upon monocyte maturation.[37]

Fibroblasts, epithelial cells, endothelial cells, and smooth muscle cells also express the IL-13 receptor. In response to IL-13, fibroblasts undergo increased adhesion marker expression,[38] chemokine production,[39] collagen synthesis,[40,41] differentiation to myofibroblasts,[42] expansion,[43,44] and contractile activity.[45] Epithelial cells respond to IL-13 by producing eotaxin,[46] and undergoing differentiation to mucus-secreting cells.[47] Endothelial cells up-regulate expression of vascular cell adhesion molecule (VCAM),[48] and IL-13 potentiates angiogenesis in response to soluble VCAM.[49] On smooth muscle cells, IL-13 induces vascular endothelial growth factor (VEGF) release,[50] arginase expression,[51] hypercontractility,[52] and generation of chemokines.[53-55]

IL-13 IN PARASITE IMMUNITY

IL-13 plays a critical role in defense against internal parasites. It is responsible for the STAT6-dependent expulsion of *Nippostrongylus brasiliensis* and other gastrointestinal nematodes in murine models, through induction of mucus secretion, intestinal muscle contractility, and other expulsion mechanisms.[1,56] Although IL-4 may play a similar role, IL-13 appears to be the critical cytokine *in vivo*, as mice lacking IL-13 are susceptible to severe infection.[57,58] With other parasites, however, a Th2 response can promote disease pathology. In appropriate mouse strains, IL-13 confers susceptibility to the extracellular parasite *Leishmania major*, or the helminth *Schistosoma mansoni*, by driving the hepatic fibrosis that ultimately leads to mortality.[59] The profibrotic effect of IL-13 is mediated through direct and indirect mechanisms. IL-13 can directly induce fibroblast differentiation[60] and the release of extracellular matrix glycoproteins,[40,41,61] but also acts indirectly by promoting the release and activation of additional profibrotic agents, including TGF-β.[33,62] IL-13 neutralization has therapeutic benefit in these models, associated with reduced hepatic fibrosis, whereas IL-13 overexpression accelerates pathology.[63-65] Similarly, in humans infected with *Schistosoma*, levels of fibrosis correlate strongly with the antigen-induced release of IL-13 from peripheral blood mononuclear cells (PBMCs).[66,67]

IL-13 IN ASTHMA

Extensive evidence supports a major role for IL-13 in driving asthma pathology. *In vitro*, IL-13 induces many cellular responses relevant to asthma, including B cell IgE production,[68] generation of eosinophil chemoattractants,[69] maturation of mucus-secreting goblet cells,[70] production of extracellular matrix proteins and myofibroblast differentiation reminiscent of remodeling,[42] and enhanced contractility of airway smooth muscle cells in response to cholinergic agonists.[71] In animal models, administration of exogenous IL-13,[72,73] or transgenic overexpression of IL-13[74,75] triggers asthmatic changes, including airway hyperresponsiveness, lung inflammation, and mucus secretion. Conversely, neutralization of IL-13 or IL-13 deficiency effectively reduces asthmatic changes in several animal models of respiratory disease.[73,76–78] IL-13 is a potent profibrotic cytokine.[79] IL-13 overexpression in the lung directly promotes lung fibrosis,[74,75] resulting in changes that are not easily reversible upon withdrawal of the cytokine.[80] Nevertheless, therapeutic dosing with IL-13 neutralizing antibody has been shown to halt further progression of fibrosis in OVA-sensitized mice following lung challenge,[81] and to partially reduce fibrosis in a chronic antigen challenge model of asthma,[82] and in a bleomycin-induced model of pulmonary fibrosis.[83] In humans, IL-13 can be found in bronchoalveolar lavage (BAL) fluid of asthmatics following lung allergen challenge,[84–86] and has been localized to mast cells infiltrating the airway smooth muscle layer in bronchial biopsies from asthmatics.[87] The association of IL-13 with asthma is confirmed and strengthened by observations that polymorphisms in genes encoding IL-13,[88] IL-13 receptor components,[89,90] or the IL-13R-associated signaling molecule STAT6,[91] are all associated with increased risk of atopic disease in human populations. In addition to asthma, a role for IL-13 has been implicated in chronic obstructive pulmonary disease (COPD), as mice with targeted overexpression of IL-13 in the lung are prone to development of emphysema, mucus, and inflammation reminiscent of this disease.[92]

IL-13 IN TUMOR IMMUNITY

In some mouse models, NK T cells producing IL-13 have been found to suppress tumor surveillance mechanisms mediated by cytotoxic T lymphocytes (CTL),[5,93] such that IL-13 neutralization reduces metastases and is associated with

therapeutic benefit.[94] In other models, however, IL-13 promotes immune surveillance against tumors, and is associated with reduced tumorigenicity.[95] A subset of human brain cancers and other solid tumors express high levels of IL-13Rα2, and it has been proposed that these tumors be targeted by IL-13 conjugated toxins.[96,97]

IL-13 is constitutively produced by Reed-Sternberg (RS) cells in Hodgkin's lymphoma.[98] Expression of IL-13Rα1 by these cells suggests that the cyokine may act as an autocrine growth factor,[99] and targeting IL-13 has proved to be an effective strategy for blocking growth of RS cells *in vitro* and *in vivo* following implantation into NOD/SCID mice.[100] Fibrosis is a common feature of Hodgkin's lymphoma lesions, and may be due in part to production of profibrotic agents such as IL-13 by the RS cells.[101] In support of this, IL-13 levels are higher in Hodgkin's disease lesions characterized by nodular sclerosis, as opposed to those of mixed cellularity.[98]

IL-13 IN RHEUMATIC DISEASE

Elevated serum levels of IL-13 have been reported in rheumatic diseases, including RA,[102–105] Sjögren's syndrome,[103] systemic lupus erythematosus (SLE),[103] systemic sclerosis,[103] scleroderma,[106] and psoriatic arthritis.[107] These data, together with our understanding of the biology of IL-13, suggest that IL-13 may either be contributing to the disease process or to repair mechanisms in a number of rheumatic diseases.

Several studies have reported the overexpression of IL-13 in rheumatoid synovial fluid.[104,105,108,109] A similar overexpression of IL-4 is not typically seen,[105] and elevated IL-13 levels are not seen in every study.[110,111] Interestingly, in a study examining synovial fluid aspirates taken from patients with a disease duration of less than 3 months, elevation of synovial IL-13 was the most robust predictor of which patients would go on to develop RA.[108] In contrast, synovial aspirates from patients with established RA did not exhibit elevated IL-13.[108] Synovial fluid from these early RA patients also had elevated levels of IL-2, IL-4, epidermal growth factor (EGF), fibroblast growth factor (βFGF) and IL-17, as compared with synovial fluid from patients that did not develop RA or from established RA patients.

Thus, IL-13 may contribute to early stage RA, but its role may change during the disease course.

Treatment of RA patients with the tumor necrosis factor (TNF)-α antagonist, etanercept (Enbrel®), has been shown to reduce levels of circulating IL-13 in a study measuring IL-13 in serum samples obtained from 20 patients 2–4 weeks after the initiation of treatment.[104] Treatment with the TNF-α-neutralizing antibody, infliximab, however, had no effect on serum IL-13 levels;[112] in a different study in which IL-13 levels were measured 4 weeks after two infusions of infliximab and in which five of eight patients had improved disease scores by ACR20 criteria.[112] Thus, the effect of TNF-α inhibition on serum IL-13 levels requires additional evaluation. It would be of particular interest to examine the impact of TNF-α blockade on IL-13 levels in very early RA patients.

Although elevated IL-13 levels are found in the rheumatoid synovium, Th2 cells, the prototypic producers of IL-13, are not present in large numbers.[113] Instead, synovial T cells appear to be committed to a Th1 phenotype,[114,115] raising the possibility that mast cells are the major IL-13-producing cell type at the site of tissue damage. Increased mast cell numbers and mast cell activation have long been described in synovial tissue, and at sites of involvement of other rheumatic diseases.[116–118] Mast cell-derived proinflammatory mediators, including TNF-α, IL-1β, and prostaglandin E_2 (PGE$_2$), have been implicated in exacerbation of tissue damage.[119,120] In animal models, RA can be induced by immune complexes, in a manner that may be dependent on mast cells,[121,122] and mast cell-deficient mice are protected from disease.[121,123] Mast cells are potent producers of IL-13 upon activation through cross-linking of cell surface FcεRI[124,125] or FcγRI.[126] The presence of activated mast cells in the rheumatoid synovium implicates them as likely contributors to IL-13 generation in RA.

ANTI-INFLAMMATORY EFFECTS OF IL-13 IN RHEUMATOID ARTHRITIS

In the proinflammatory, Th1-skewed environment of the rheumatoid lesion, the presence of IL-13 may represent an attempt by the immune system to limit damage caused by the disease. An anti-inflammatory effect of IL-13 in RA (summarized in Figure 13.2) is supported by *in vitro* observations that IL-13 abrogates expression of the proinflammatory cytokines, IL-1β,[105,127] IL-17,[128] IL-6,[129] and TNF-α[105] by rheumatoid synovial explants or synovial fluid macrophages. Overexpression of IL-13 in synovial tissue explants and synovial fibroblasts *in vitro* reduces spontaneous production of the proinflammatory

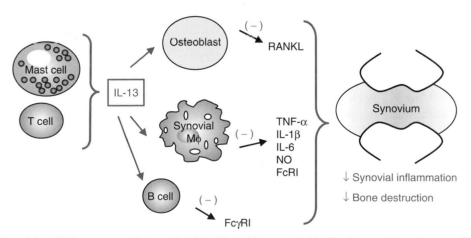

Figure 13.2 Potential anti-inflammatory effects of IL-13 in RA. IL-13, generated by T cells or activated mast cells, may reduce RANKL production by osteoblasts, thus ameliorating bone erosion. IL-13 also acts on synovial macrophages to down-regulate production of the proinflammatory mediators TNF-α, IL-1β, IL-6, and NO. IL-13 may also limit C′-mediated damage by down-regulating expression of FcγRI on synovial macrophages and B cells.

cytokines TNF-α and IL-1β, several chemokines, and PGE$_2$.[130] Furthermore, IL-13 down-regulates production of NO or hyaluronic acid (HA), indicators of oxidative stress, by RA synovial cells in response to the combination of TNF-α, IL-1β, and interferon-γ (IFN-γ).[131,132]

In addition to effects on inflammation, the presence of IL-13 in the rheumatoid synovium may protect against bone resorption. RANK and its ligand, RANKL, contribute to osteoclast differentiation and bone loss in RA, in balance with the protective decoy receptor, osteoprotegerin (OPG).[133,134] Antagonism of this system using antibody to RANKL,[135,136] or exogenously administered OPG,[137] has shown therapeutic benefit in treating human osteoporosis, and preserves bone in animal models of RA,[138,139] IL-13 has the capacity to inhibit bone resorption,[140–142] an effect which may be mediated by reduced expression of RANKL on osteoblasts,[143,144] or increased production of OPG.[143,144]

IL-4 may have a protective role against RANKL-mediated osteoclastogenesis in mice, through interaction with IL-4Rα, and downstream STAT6 activation.[145] In accordance with this, RANKL-induced osteoclast generation from macrophages of STAT6-deficient mice was not antagonized by IL-4,[145] whereas osteoclast generation from macrophages of mice with constitutively active STAT6 was impaired *in vitro* and *in vivo*.[146] In humans, a polymorphism in the IL-4Rα chain has been reported to be associated with enhanced susceptibility to the development of bone erosions in RA.[147] The I50V IL-4 Ralpha polymorphism results in reduced responses to IL-4 in human B cells, including STAT6 phosphorylation, CD23 up-regulation, and IgE production,[148] and in human T cells as evidenced by reduced STAT6 phosphorylation, GATA3 induction, and induction of IL-12Rβ2.[147] The effect of these polymorphisms on signaling by IL-13 in human B cells or macrophages has not been reported to date. As the IL-4Rα is required for IL-13 responses, however, this polymorphism could reduce STAT6 phosphorylation in response to IL-13 as well as IL-4, potentially leading to exaggerated osteoclast generation and bone resorption.

IL-13 may also limit pathogenic effects of complement activation. In the presence of TNF-α, IL-13 down-regulates expression and function of activating Fcγ receptors,[149] and synovial FcγRI expression was reduced in rats given intra-articular injections of adenovirus-expressing IL-13.[150] Rats administered IL-13 by intratracheal instillation are protected from immune complex-mediated lung injury[151] and *in vitro*, IL-13 protects porcine endothelial cells from complement-mediated damage.[152] Thus, IL-13 may exert anti-inflammatory effects through dampening of complement activation and complement-mediated injury.

ANIMAL MODELS OF ARTHRITIS SUPPORT A PROTECTIVE ROLE FOR IL-13

Overexpression of IL-13 in animal models of arthritis has been shown to ameliorate disease. This has been shown in both the DBA/I collagen-induced arthritis model,[153] and in mice expressing a human TNF-α-transgene.[154] Direct intra-articular administration of adenovirus expressing rat IL-13 ameliorated disease symptoms and pathology in a rat adjuvant-induced arthritis model (AIA).[155] In a mouse model of immune complex-mediated arthritis (ICA), inflammation in the joint was enhanced following intra-articular injection of an adenoviral vector encoding IL-13, but chondrocyte death, a correlate of cartilage destruction, was diminished.[150] The effects were thought to be secondary to IL-13-induced down-regulation of FcγRI expression in the synovium,[150] a mechanism which could limit tissue damage mediated by immune complexes.

PRO-INFLAMMATORY EFFECTS OF IL-13 IN RHEUMATOID ARTHRITIS

Although it has clear anti-inflammatory effects, there is also evidence for proinflammatory activities of IL-13 in the rheumatoid synovium, summarized in Figure 13.3. In the presence of IL-13 or IL-4, production of the proinflammatory cytokines IL-12[156] or TNF-α[157] by anti-CD40-stimulated synovial macrophages is enhanced, suggesting that under certain conditions of activation, IL-13 may exacerbate inflammatory responses. This is supported by evidence that IL-13 up-regulates VCAM-1 expression on rheumatoid fibroblast-like synoviocytes, in synergy with TNF-α.[158] Expression of VCAM-1 on synovial

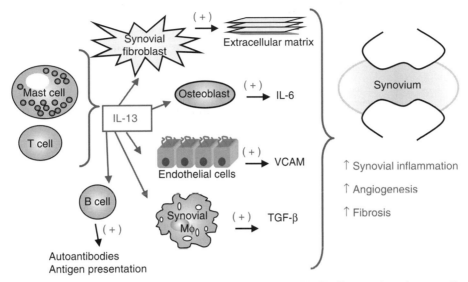

Figure 13.3 Potential proinflammatory effects of IL-13 in RA. IL-13, generated by T cells or activated mast cells, may stimulate production of collagen and other extracellular matrix proteins by synovial fibroblasts. IL-13 may induce production of the proinflammatory cytokine, IL-6, by osteoblasts. On endothelial cells, IL-13 up-regulates VCAM expression, promoting the influx of VLA4-expressing lymphocytes. IL-13 also triggers production of the profibrotic cytokine, TGF-β, by synovial macrophages, and stimulates B-cell antibody production and antigen presentation.

fibroblasts is a hallmark of RA, and is thought to be critical for the influx of VLA4-expressing inflammatory cells to the joint.[159] Furthermore, IL-13 and IL-4 appear to have anti-apoptotic effects on rheumatoid synoviocytes *in vitro*, suggesting that these cytokines may contribute to the synovial hyperplasia seen in RA.[160]

In RA, IL-6 is a key proinflammatory cytokine that contributes to osteoclast formation, inflammation, and autoantibody production.[161,162] Osteoblasts express IL-13 receptor and respond to IL-13 with increased production of IL-6.[163,164] IL-13 also induces IL-6 production from human lung fibroblasts,[38] keratinocytes,[165] and microglial cells,[166] but may reduce IL-6 generation from synovial macrophages[129] and other hematopoietic cell types.[167] By stimulating osteoblast production of IL-6, IL-13 may promote inflammation, osteoclast development, and bone erosion in RA.

Through its induction of antibody production, elevated IL-13 may be associated with high levels of rheumatoid factor or autoantibodies in RA and other rheumatic diseases.[103,106,168] Compounding this are potential effects of IL-13 on expression of Fc receptors or complement receptors. IL-13 induces expression of CR1 and CR3 on neutrophils, enhancing their production of the inflammatory mediator, PGE$_2$, following phagocytosis.[169] In contrast to those of healthy subjects, DCs derived from peripheral blood monocytes of RA patients failed to up-regulate expression of the inhibitory FcγRII in response to IL-13.[170] Thus, IL-13 may contribute to a chronic state of immune activation in the context of a complex autoimmune environment.

IL-13 AND SCLERODERMA

In patients with localized scleroderma or systemic sclerosis, IL-13 levels are elevated in serum.[103,106,171–173] In different studies, circulating IL-13 levels have been found to correlate with sedimentation rate,[172] levels of C-reactive protein (CRP),[172] titers of SSA/Ro antibody,[103] and the severity of SSc capillaroscopic features.[173] Although no difference in the number of IL-13-producing cells was found in peripheral blood,[174] alveolar macrophages from patients with systemic sclerosis secrete high levels of IL-13,[175] and the elevated serum IL-13 suggests a role for the cytokine in supporting the fibrosis and microvascular lesions that characterize this disease.[173]

In a mouse model of scleroderma induced by subcutaneous injections of bleomycin, IL-13-protein and IL-13-producing cells were found at the lesion site, along with increased expression of IL-13Rα1 and IL-13Rα2.[176] Similar findings were reported in a model of bleomycin-induced pulmonary fibrosis, in which IL-13 neutralization effectively blocked fibrotic changes.[83,177] In the tightskin mouse (TSK/+) model of scleroderma, IL-4Rα-deficient animals had reduced transcription of the profibrotic cytokine, TGF-β, and were protected from development of fibrosis,[178] implicating involvement of IL-4, IL-13, and/or STAT6. Thus, in scleroderma and systemic sclerosis, the profibrotic effects of IL-13 may prevail over its anti-inflammatory activities, leading to exacerbation of the disease.

IL-13 AND PSORIATIC ARTHRITIS

IL-13 levels were examined in the serum and synovial fluid of patients with psoriatic arthritis.[107] Although modest elevation was observed in the levels of IL-13 in synovial fluid of patients with psoriatic arthritis as compared with that of patients with osteoarthritis, this elevation was not as profound as that seen in RA patients. This suggests that IL-13 may be less important in psoriatic arthritis than in RA.

IL-13 AND SLE

IL-13 levels have been reported to be elevated in the serum of patients with SLE.[103,179] A comparison of IL-12 and IL-13 serum levels in SLE patients suggests that higher IL-13/IL-12 ratios may correlate with elevated IgM rheumatoid factor (RF) and IgM anti-cardiolipin serum autoantibodies.[180] The role of IL-13 in enhancing immunoglobulin production suggests that IL-13 could contribute to the elevated autoantibody levels that are characteristic of SLE patients. Additional studies are needed to clarify whether IL-13 contributes significantly to the pathology of SLE.

IL-13 AND INFLAMMATORY BOWEL DISEASE

The expression of IL-13 correlates with disease progression in animal models of ulcerative colitis (UC).

Mice deficient for the cytokine IL-10 develop spontaneous colitis, and expression of IL-13 and IL-4 by activated lamina propria cells from these mice increases with the progression of the spontaneous colitis observed in this model.[181] Experimental colitis can be induced by intrarectal administration of oxazalone to primed mice, with an ensuing colitis that is similar to human UC. Activated lamina propria mononuclear cells from mice in which colitis is induced express higher levels of Th2 cytokines, including IL-13.[182] The predominant source of IL-13 in this model was found to be NK T cells, and depletion of NK T cells resulted in prevention of disease. Neutralization of IL-13 using mouse IL-13Rα2-Fc prevented the development of colitis in this model, underscoring the pathogenic role of IL-13.[182] In human inflammatory bowel disease, lamina proprial cells from patients with UC produce more IL-13, whereas lamina proprial cells from Crohn's disease patients produce higher levels of IFN-γ. IL-13 is produced by NK T cells in UC patients, similar to the results found in the mouse model of UC.[183,184] Both IL-4Rα and IL-13Rα1 are expressed on colonic enterocytes in both UC and control intestinal samples, and these data support a role for IL-13 in driving the mucosal abnormalities associated with UC.[184]

CONCLUSIONS

IL-13 is made by T cells of the Th2 phenotype, as well as by NK T cells, mast cells, and basophils. IL-13 can have potent pro- and anti-inflammatory effects *in vitro* and *in vivo*. A growing body of evidence continues to implicate IL-13 in the pathology of human asthma. Whether IL-13 contributes in a major way to the pathology of rheumatic and inflammatory diseases beyond asthma is still being explored, although some data implicate IL-13 in other inflammatory diseases. Levels of serum IL-13 are elevated in multiple rheumatic diseases, including RA, SLE and systemic sclerosis. The precise contribution of IL-13 to the course of these diseases is unclear. Correlation of a polymorphism in the IL-4Rα chain with an increased susceptibility to erosive bone disease suggests that IL-13 may modulate the pathology in the joints of RA patients. Limited studies have been done to follow the levels of IL-13 in serum after treatment with disease-modifying anti-rheumatic drug (DMARD) therapies in RA. These studies will be of interest, as they could allow linkage of IL-13 levels with clinical outcome and therapeutic modalities. Further studies will also be of interest to confirm and explore the elevated IL-13 in the synovium of early-onset RA patients, and to determine if detection of IL-13 expression may be of diagnostic significance. IL-13 has also been shown to have a profibrotic role, which is thought to be important in the immune response against certain parasites. Additional data support a role for IL-13 in the fibrotic lung disease associated with chronic asthma. Very limited studies have been done to examine IL-13 in systemic sclerosis, in which fibrosis contributes significantly to disease pathology. IL-13 has been shown to contribute to disease pathology in animal models of UC, and evaluation of tissue samples from UC patients indicates that IL-13 is highly expressed in lamina proprial cells from these patients. Translation of these data into clinical studies may lead to the identification of new therapeutic modalities based upon modulation of IL-13 in inflammatory diseases.

ACKNOWLEDGMENT

The authors thank Dr Divya Chaudhary for helpful discussions.

REFERENCES

1. Wynn TA. IL-13 effector functions. Annu Rev Immunol 2003; 21: 425–56.
2. Minty A, Chalon P, Derocq JM et al. Interleukin-13 is a new human lymphokine regulating inflammatory and immune responses. Nature 1993; 362(6417): 248–50.
3. Ansel KM, Djuretic I, Tanasa B et al. Regulation of Th2 differentiation and Il4 locus accessibility. Annu Rev Immunol 2006; 24: 607–56.
4. Crane IJ, Forrester JV. Th1 and Th2 lymphocytes in autoimmune disease. Crit Rev Immunol 2005; 25(2): 75–102.
5. Terabe M, Matsui S, Noben-Trauth N et al. NKT cell-mediated repression of tumor immunosurveillance by IL-13 and the IL-4R-STAT6 pathway. Nat Immunol 2000; 1(6): 515–20.
6. Gibbs BF, Haas H, Falcone FH et al. Purified human peripheral blood basophils release interleukin-13 and preformed interleukin-4 following immunological activation. Eur J Immunol 1996; 26(10): 2493–8.
7. Burd PR, Thompson WC, Max EE et al. Activated mast cells produce interleukin 13. J Exp Med 1995; 181(4): 1373–80.
8. McKenzie AN, Culpepper JA, de Waal Malefyt R et al. Interleukin 13, a T-cell-derived cytokine that regulates human monocyte and B-cell function. Proc Natl Acad Sci U S A 1993; 90(8): 3735–9.
9. Zurawski SM, Vega F Jr., Huyghe B et al. Receptors for interleukin-13 and interleukin-4 are complex and share a novel component that functions in signal transduction. EMBO J 1993; 12(7): 2663–70.
10. Hershey GK, IL-13 receptors and signaling pathways: an evolving web. J Allergy Clin Immunol 2003; 111(4): 677–90;
11. Gauchat JF, Schlagenhauf E, Feng NP et al. A novel 4-kb interleukin-13 receptor alpha mRNA expressed in human B, T, and endothelial cells encoding an alternate type-II interleukin-4/interleukin-13 receptor. Eur J Immunol 1997; 27(4): 971–8.
12. Andrews AL, Holloway JW, Puddicombe SM et al. Kinetic analysis of the interleukin-13 receptor complex. J Biol Chem 2002; 277(48): 46073–8.
13. Eisenmesser EZ, Horita DA, Byrd RA. Secondary structure and backbone resonance assignments for human interleukin-13. J Biomol NMR 2001; 19(1): 93–4.
14. Moy FJ, Diblasio E, Wilhelm J et al. Solution structure of human IL-13 and implication for receptor binding. J Mol Biol 2001; 310(1): 219–30.
15. Bernard J, Treton D, Vermot-Desroches C et al. Expression of interleukin 13 receptor in glioma and renal cell carcinoma: IL13Ralpha2 as a decoy receptor for IL13. Lab Invest 2001; 81(9): 1223–31.
16. Feng N, Lugli SM, Schnyder B et al. The interleukin-4/interleukin-13 receptor of human synovial fibroblasts: overexpression of the nonsignaling interleukin-13 receptor alpha2. Lab Invest 1998; 78(5): 591–602.
17. Wood N, Whitters MJ, Jacobson BA et al. Enhanced interleukin (IL)-13 responses in mice lacking IL-13 receptor alpha 2. J Exp Med 2003; 197(6): 703–9.
18. Fichtner-Feigl S, Strober W, Kawakami K et al. IL-13 signaling through the IL-13alpha2 receptor is involved in induction of TGF-beta1 production and fibrosis. Nat Med 2006; 12(1): 99–106.
19. Murata T, Puri RK, Comparison of IL-13- and IL-4-induced signaling in EBV-immortalized human B cells. Cell Immunol 1997; 175(1): 33–40.
20. Kelly-Welch AE, Hanson EM, Boothby MR et al. Interleukin-4 and interleukin-13 signaling connections maps. Science 2003; 300(5625): 1527–8.
21. Jiang H, Harris MB, Rothman P. IL-4/IL-13 signaling beyond JAK/STAT. J Allergy Clin Immunol 2000; 105(6 Pt 1): 1063–70.

22. Umeshita-Suyama R, Sugimoto R, Akaiwa M et al. Characterization of IL-4 and IL-13 signals dependent on the human IL-13 receptor alpha chain 1: redundancy of requirement of tyrosine residue for STAT3 activation. Int Immunol 2000; 12(11): 1499–509.

23. Roy B, Bhattacharjee A, Xu B et al. IL-13 signal transduction in human monocytes: phosphorylation of receptor components, association with Jaks, and phosphorylation/activation of Stats. J Leukoc Biol 2002; 72(3): 580–9.

24. Doucet C, Jasmin C, Azzarone B. Unusual interleukin-4 and -13 signaling in human normal and tumor lung fibroblasts. Oncogene 2000; 19(51): 5898–905.

25. Xu B, Bhattacharjee A, Roy B et al. Interleukin-13 induction of 15-lipoxygenase gene expression requires p38 mitogen-activated protein kinase-mediated serine 727 phosphorylation of Stat1 and Stat3. Mol Cell Biol 2003; 23(11): 3918–28.

26. Peng Q, Matsuda T, Hirst SJ. Signaling pathways regulating interleukin-13-stimulated chemokine release from airway smooth muscle. Am J Respir Crit Care Med 2004; 169(5): 596–603.

27. Lee PJ, Zhang X, Shan P et al. ERK1/2 mitogen-activated protein kinase selectively mediates IL-13-induced lung inflammation and remodeling in vivo. J Clin Invest 2006; 116(1): 163–73.

28. Moore PE, Church TL, Chism DD et al. IL-13 and IL-4 cause eotaxin release in human airway smooth muscle cells: a role for ERK. Am J Physiol Lung Cell Mol Physiol 2002; 282(4): L847–53.

29. Defrance T, Carayon P, Billian G et al. Interleukin 13 is a B cell stimulating factor. J Exp Med, 1994; 179(1): 135–43.

30. Rodriguez PC, Zea AH, DeSalvo J et al. L-arginine consumption by macrophages modulates the expression of CD3 zeta chain in T lymphocytes. J Immunol 2003; 171(3): 1232–9.

31. Cosentino G, Soprana E, Thienes CP et al. IL-13 downregulates CD14 expression and TNF-alpha secretion in normal human monocytes. J Immunol 1995; 155(6): 3145–51.

32. El-Gayar S, Thuring-Nahler H, Pfeilschifter J et al. Translational control of inducible nitric oxide synthase by IL-13 and arginine availability in inflammatory macrophages. J Immunol 2003; 171(9): 4561–8.

33. Lee CG, Homer RJ, Zhu Z et al. Interleukin-13 induces tissue fibrosis by selectively stimulating and activating transforming growth factor beta(1). J Exp Med 2001; 194(6): 809–21.

34. Kaviratne M, Hesse M, Leusink M et al. IL-13 activates a mechanism of tissue fibrosis that is completely TGF-beta independent. J Immunol 2004; 173(6): 4020–9.

35. Hart PH, Bonder CS, Balogh J et al. Differential responses of human monocytes and macrophages to IL-4 and IL-13. J Leukoc Biol 1999; 66(4): 575–8.

36. Ahn JS, Agrawal B. IL-4 is more effective than IL-13 for in vitro differentiation of dendritic cells from peripheral blood mononuclear cells. Int Immunol 2005; 17(10): 1337–46.

37. Hart PH, Bonder CS, Balogh J et al. Diminished responses to IL-13 by human monocytes differentiated in vitro: role of the IL-13Ralpha1 chain and STAT6. Eur J Immunol 1999; 29(7): 2087–97.

38. Doucet C, Brouty-Boye D. Pottin-Clemenceau C et al., IL-4 and IL-13 specifically increase adhesion molecule and inflammatory cytokine expression in human lung fibroblasts. Int Immunol 1998; 10(10): 1421–33.

39. Terada N, Hamano N, Nomura T et al. Interleukin-13 and tumour necrosis factor-alpha synergistically induce eotaxin production in human nasal fibroblasts. Clin Exp Allergy 2000; 30(3): 348–55.

40. Oriente A, Fedarko NS, Pacocha SE et al. Interleukin-13 modulates collagen homeostasis in human skin and keloid fibroblasts. J Pharmacol Exp Ther 2000; 292(3): 988–94.

41. Jinnin M, Ihn H, Yamane K et al. Interleukin-13 stimulates the transcription of the human alpha2(I) collagen gene in human dermal fibroblasts. J Biol Chem 2004; 279(40): 41783–91.

42. Hashimoto S, Gon Y, Takeshita I et al. IL-4 and IL-13 induce myofibroblastic phenotype of human lung fibroblasts through c-Jun NH2-terminal kinase-dependent pathway. J Allergy Clin Immunol 2001; 107(6): 1001–8.

43. Jakubzick C, Choi ES, Kunkel SL et al. Impact of interleukin-13 responsiveness on the synthetic and proliferative properties of Th1- and Th2-type pulmonary granuloma fibroblasts. Am J Pathol 2003; 162(5): 1475–86.

44. Ingram JL, Rice AB, Geisenhoffer K et al. IL-13 and IL-1β promote lung fibroblast growth through coordinated up-regulation of PDGF-AA and PDGF-Ralpha. FASEB J, 2004; 18(10): 1132–4.

45. Liu X, Kohyama T, Wang H et al. Th2 cytokine regulation of type I collagen gel contraction mediated by human lung mesenchymal cells. Am J Physiol Lung Cell Mol Physiol 2002; 282(5): L1049–56.

46. Matsukura S, Stellato C, Georas SN et al. Interleukin-13 upregulates eotaxin expression in airway epithelial cells by a STAT6-dependent mechanism. Am J Respir Cell Mol Biol 2001; 24(6): 755–61.

47. Kuperman DA, Huang X, Koth LL et al. Direct effects of interleukin-13 on epithelial cells cause airway hyperreactivity and mucus overproduction in asthma. Nat Med 2002; 8(8): 885–9.

48. Schnyder B, Lugli S, Feng N, et al. Interleukin-4 (IL-4) and IL-13 bind to a shared heterodimeric complex on endothelial cells mediating vascular cell adhesion molecule-1 induction in the absence of the common gamma chain. Blood 1996; 87(10): 4286–95.

49. Fukushi J, Ono M, Morikawa W et al. The activity of soluble VCAM-1 in angiogenesis stimulated by IL-4 and IL-13. J Immunol 2000; 165(5): 2818–23.

50. Faffe DS, Flynt L, Bourgeois K et al. Interleukin-13 and interleukin-4 induce vascular endothelial growth factor release from airway smooth muscle cells: role of vascular endothelial growth factor genotype. Am J Respir Cell Mol Biol 2006; 34(2): 213–18.

51. Wei LH, Jacobs AT, Morris SM Jr et al. IL-4 and IL-13 upregulate arginase I expression by cAMP and JAK/STAT6 pathways in vascular smooth muscle cells. Am J Physiol Cell Physiol 2000; 279(1): C248–56.

52. Akiho H, Blennerhassett P, Deng Y et al. Role of IL-4, IL-13, and STAT6 in inflammation-induced hypercontractility of murine smooth muscle cells. Am J Physiol Gastrointest Liver Physiol 2002; 282(2): G226–32.

53. Hirst SJ, Hallsworth MP, Peng Q et al. Selective induction of eotaxin release by interleukin-13 or interleukin-4 in human airway smooth muscle cells is synergistic with interleukin-1beta and is mediated by the interleukin-4 receptor alpha-chain. Am J Respir Crit Care Med 2002; 165(8): 1161–71.

54. Faffe DS, Whitehead T, Moore PE et al. IL-13 and IL-4 promote TARC release in human airway smooth muscle cells: role of IL-4 receptor genotype. Am J Physiol Lung Cell Mol Physiol 2003; 285(4): L907–14.

55. Bouchelouche K, Andresen L, Alvarez S et al. Interleukin-4 and 13 induce the expression and release of monocyte chemoattractant protein 1, interleukin-6 and stem cell factor from human detrusor smooth muscle cells: synergy with interleukin-1beta and tumor necrosis factor-alpha. J Urol 2006; 175(2): 760–5.

56. Finkelman FD, Shea-Donohue T, Morris SC et al. Interleukin-4- and interleukin-13-mediated host protection against intestinal nematode parasites. Immunol Rev 2004; 201: 139–55.

57. Urban JF Jr, Noben-Trauth N, Donaldson DD, et al., IL-13, IL-4Ralpha, and Stat6 are required for the expulsion of the gastrointestinal nematode parasite Nippostrongylus brasiliensis. Immunity 1998; 8(2): 255–64.

58. Mohrs M, Ledermann B, Kohler G et al. Differences between IL-4- and IL-4 receptor alpha-deficient mice in chronic leishmaniasis reveal a protective role for IL-13 receptor signaling. J Immunol 1999; 162(12): 7302–8.

59. Noben-Trauth N, Paul WE, Sacks DL. IL-4- and IL-4 receptor-deficient BALB/c mice reveal differences in susceptibility to Leishmania major parasite substrains. J Immunol 1999; 162(10): 6132–40.

60. Doucet C, Brouty-Boye D, Pottin-Clemenceau C et al. Interleukin (IL) 4 and IL-13 act on human lung fibroblasts. Implication in asthma. J Clin Invest 1998; 101(10): 2129–39.

61. Jinnin M, Ihn H, Asano Y et al. Upregulation of tenascin-C expression by IL-13 in human dermal fibroblasts via the phosphoinositide 3-kinase/Akt and the protein kinase C signaling pathways. J Invest Dermatol 2006; 126(3): 551–60.

62. Wen FQ, Kohyama T, Liu X et al. Interleukin-4- and interleukin-13-enhanced transforming growth factor-beta2 production in cultured human bronchial epithelial cells is attenuated by interferon-gamma. Am J Respir Cell Mol Biol 2002; 26(4): 484–90.

63. Fallon PG, Richardson EJ, McKenzie GJ et al. Schistosome infection of transgenic mice defines distinct and contrasting pathogenic roles for IL-4 and IL-13: IL-13 is a profibrotic agent. J Immunol 2000; 164(5): 2585–91.

64. Mentink-Kane MM, Cheever AW, Thompson RW et al. IL-13 receptor alpha 2 down-modulates granulomatous inflammation and prolongs host survival in schistosomiasis. Proc Natl Acad Sci U S A 2004; 101(2): 586–90.

65. Chiaramonte MG, Cheever AW, Malley JD et al. Studies of murine schistosomiasis reveal interleukin-13 blockade as a treatment for established and progressive liver fibrosis. Hepatology 2001; 34(2): 273–82.

66. Alves Oliveira LF, Moreno EC, Gazzinelli G et al. Cytokine production associated with periportal fibrosis during chronic schistosomiasis mansoni in humans. Infect Immun 2006; 74(2): 1215–21.

67. de Jesus AR, Magalhaes A, Miranda DG, et al., Association of type 2 cytokines with hepatic fibrosis in human Schistosoma mansoni infection. Infect Immun 2004; 72(6): 3391–7.

68. de Vries JE, Punnonen J, Cocks BG et al. Regulation of the human IgE response by IL4 and IL13. Res Immunol 1993; 144(8): 597–601.

69. Chibana K, Ishii Y, Asakura T et al. Up-regulation of cysteinyl leukotriene 1 receptor by IL-13 enables human lung fibroblasts to respond to leukotriene C4 and produce eotaxin. J Immunol 2003; 170(8): 4290–5.

70. Laoukili J, Perret E, Willems T et al. IL-13 alters mucociliary differentiation and ciliary beating of human respiratory epithelial cells. J Clin Invest 2001; 108(12): 1817–24.

71. Grunstein MM, Hakonarson H, Leiter J et al. IL-13-dependent autocrine signaling mediates altered responsiveness of IgE-sensitized airway smooth muscle. Am J Physiol Lung Cell Mol Physiol 2002; 282(3): L520–8.

72. Wills-Karp M, Luyimbazi J, Xu X et al. Interleukin-13: central mediator of allergic asthma. Science 1998; 282(5397): 2258–61.

73. Grunig G, Warnock M, Wakil AE et al. Requirement for IL-13 independently of IL-4 in experimental asthma. Science 1998; 282(5397): 2261–3.

74. Zhu Z, Homer RJ, Wang Z et al. Pulmonary expression of interleukin-13 causes inflammation, mucus hypersecretion, subepithelial fibrosis, physiologic abnormalities, and eotaxin production. J Clin Invest 1999; 103(6): 779–88.

75. Fallon PG, Emson CL, Smith P et al. IL-13 overexpression predisposes to anaphylaxis following antigen sensitization. J Immunol 2001; 166(4): 2712–16.

76. Tekkanat KK, Maassab HF, Cho DS et al. IL-13-induced airway hyperreactivity during respiratory syncytial virus infection is STAT6 dependent. J Immunol 2001; 166(5): 3542–8.

77. Blease K, Jakubzick C, Westwick J et al. Therapeutic effect of IL-13 immunoneutralization during chronic experimental fungal asthma. J Immunol 2001; 166(8): 5219–24.

78. Walter DM, McIntire JJ, Berry G et al. Critical role for IL-13 in the development of allergen-induced airway hyperreactivity. J Immunol 2001; 167(8): 4668–75.

79. Wynn TA. Fibrotic disease and the T(H)1/T(H)2 paradigm. Nat Rev Immunol 2004; 4(8): 583–94.

80. Fulkerson PC, Fischetti CA, Hassman LM et al. Persistent effects induced by IL-13 in the lung. Am J Respir Cell Mol Biol 2006; 35: 337–46.

81. Yang G, Li L, Volk A et al. Therapeutic dosing with anti-interleukin-13 monoclonal antibody inhibits asthma progression in mice. J Pharmacol Exp Ther 2005; 313(1): 8–15.

82. Kumar RK, Herbert C, Webb DC et al. Effects of anticytokine therapy in a mouse model of chronic asthma. Am J Respir Crit Care Med 2004; 170(10): 1043–8.

83. Belperio JA, Dy M, Burdick MD et al. Interaction of IL-13 and C10 in the pathogenesis of bleomycin-induced pulmonary fibrosis. Am J Respir Cell Mol Biol 2002; 27(4): 419–27.

84. Huang SK, Xiao HQ, Kleine-Tebbe J et al. IL-13 expression at the sites of allergen challenge in patients with asthma. J Immunol 1995; 155(5): 2688–94.

85. Batra V, Musani AI, Hastie AT et al. Bronchoalveolar lavage fluid concentrations of transforming growth factor (TGF)-beta1, TGF-beta2, interleukin (IL)-4 and IL-13 after segmental allergen challenge and their effects on alpha-smooth muscle actin and collagen III synthesis by primary human lung fibroblasts. Clin Exp Allergy 2004; 34(3): 437–44.

86. Prieto J, Van Der Ploeg I, Roquet A et al. Cytokine mRNA expression in patients with mild allergic asthma following low dose or cumulative dose allergen provocation. Clin Exp Allergy 2001; 31(5): 791–800.

87. Brightling CE, Symon FA, Holgate ST et al. Interleukin-4 and -13 expression is co-localized to mast cells within the airway smooth muscle in asthma. Clin Exp Allergy 2003; 33(12): 1711–16.

88. Vercelli D. Genetics of IL-13 and functional relevance of IL-13 variants. Curr Opin Allergy Clin Immunol 2002; 2(5): 389–93.

89. Gao PS, Mao XQ, Hopkin JM et al. Functional significance of polymorphisms of the interleukin-4 and interleukin-13 receptors in allergic disease. Clin Exp Allergy 2000; 30(12): 1672–5.

90. Shirakawa I, Deichmann KA, Izuhara I et al. Atopy and asthma: genetic variants of IL-4 and IL-13 signalling. Immunol Today 2000; 21(2): 60–4.

91. Tamura K, Suzuki M, Arakawa H et al. Linkage and association studies of STAT6 gene polymorphisms and allergic diseases. Int Arch Allergy Immunol 2003; 131(1): 33–8.

92. Zheng T, Zhu Z, Wang Z et al. Inducible targeting of IL-13 to the adult lung causes matrix metalloproteinase- and cathepsin-dependent emphysema. J Clin Invest 2000; 106(9): 1081–93.

93. Ahlers JD, Belyakov IM, Terabe M et al. A push-pull approach to maximize vaccine efficacy: abrogating suppression with an IL-13 inhibitor while augmenting help with granulocyte/macrophage colony-stimulating factor and CD40L. Proc Natl Acad Sci U S A 2002; 99(20): 13020–5.

94. Park JM, Terabe M, van den Broeke LT et al. Unmasking immunosurveillance against a syngeneic colon cancer by elimination of CD4+ NKT regulatory cells and IL-13. Int J Cancer 2005; 114(1): 80–7.

95. Ma HL, Whitters MJ, Jacobson BA et al. Tumor cells secreting IL-13 but not IL-13Ralpha2 fusion protein have reduced tumorigenicity in vivo. Int Immunol 2004; 16(7): 1009–17.

96. Kioi M, Kawakami K, Puri RK, Analysis of antitumor activity of an interleukin-13 (IL-13) receptor-targeted cytotoxin composed of IL-13 antagonist and Pseudomonas exotoxin. Clin Cancer Res 2004; 10(18 Pt 1): 6231–8.

97. Husain SR, Puri RK. Interleukin-13 receptor-directed cytotoxin for malignant glioma therapy: from bench to bedside. J Neurooncol 2003; 65(1): 37–48.

98. Ohshima K, Akaiwa M, Umeshita R et al. Interleukin-13 and interleukin-13 receptor in Hodgkin's disease: possible autocrine mechanism and involvement in fibrosis. Histopathology 2001; 38(4): 368–75.

99. Skinnider BF, Kapp U, Mak TW. The role of interleukin 13 in classical Hodgkin lymphoma. Leuk Lymphoma 2002; 43(6): 1203–10.

100. Trieu Y, Wen XY, Skinnider BF et al. Soluble interleukin-13Ralpha2 decoy receptor inhibits Hodgkin's lymphoma growth in vitro and in vivo. Cancer Res 2004; 64(9): 3271–5.

101. Aldinucci D, Lorenzon D, Olivo K et al. Interactions between tissue fibroblasts in lymph nodes and Hodgkin/Reed-Sternberg cells. Leuk Lymphoma 2004; 45(9): 1731–9.

102. Stabler T, Piette JC, Chevalier X et al. Serum cytokine profiles in relapsing polychondritis suggest monocyte/macrophage activation. Arthritis Rheum 2004; 50(11): 3663–7.

103. Spadaro A, Rinaldi T, Riccieri V et al. Interleukin-13 in autoimmune rheumatic diseases: relationship with the autoantibody profile. Clin Exp Rheumatol 2002; 20(2): 213–16.

104. Tokayer A, Carsons SE, Chokshi B et al. High levels of interleukin 13 in rheumatoid arthritis sera are modulated by tumor necrosis factor antagonist therapy: association with dendritic cell growth activity. J Rheumatol 2002; 29(3): 454–61.

105. Isomaki P, Luukkainen R, Toivanen P et al. The presence of interleukin-13 in rheumatoid synovium and its antiinflammatory effects on synovial fluid macrophages from patients with rheumatoid arthritis. Arthritis Rheum 1996; 39(10): 1693–702.

106. Hasegawa M, Sato S, Nagaoka T et al. Serum levels of tumor necrosis factor and interleukin-13 are elevated in patients with localized scleroderma. Dermatology 2003; 207(2): 141–7.

107. Spadaro A, Rinaldi T, Riccieri V et al. Interleukin 13 in synovial fluid and serum of patients with psoriatic arthritis. Ann Rheum Dis 2002; 61(2):174-6.

108. Raza K, Falciani F, Curnow SJ et al. Early rheumatoid arthritis is characterized by a distinct and transient synovial fluid cytokine profile of T cell and stromal cell origin. Arthritis Res Ther 2005; 7(4): R784–95.

109. Hitchon CA, Alex P, Erdile LB et al. A distinct multicytokine profile is associated with anti-cyclical citrullinated peptide antibodies in patients with early untreated inflammatory arthritis. J Rheumatol 2004; 31(12): 2336–46.

110. Kotake S, Schumacher HR Jr, Yarboro CH et al. In vivo gene expression of type 1 and type 2 cytokines in synovial tissues from patients in early stages of rheumatoid, reactive, and undifferentiated arthritis. Proc Assoc Am Physicians 1997; 109(3): 286–301.

111. Furuzawa-Carballeda J, Alcocer-Varela J. Interleukin-8, interleukin-10, intercellular adhesion molecule-1 and vascular cell adhesion molecule-1 expression levels are higher in synovial tissue from patients with rheumatoid arthritis than in osteoarthritis. Scand J Immunol 1999; 50(2): 215–22.

112. Pittoni V, Bombardieri M, Spinelli FR et al. Anti-tumour necrosis factor (TNF) alpha treatment of rheumatoid arthritis (infliximab) selectively down regulates the production of interleukin (IL) 18 but not of IL12 and IL13. Ann Rheum Dis 2002; 61(8): 723–5.

113. Skapenko A, Leipe J, Lipsky PE et al. The role of the T cell in autoimmune inflammation. Arthritis Res Ther 2005; 7 (Suppl 2): S4–S14.

114. Isomaki P, Luukkainen R, Lassila O et al. Synovial fluid T cells from patients with rheumatoid arthritis are refractory to the T helper type 2 differentiation-inducing effects of interleukin-4. Immunology 1999; 96(3): 358–64.

115. Berner B, Akca D, Jung T et al. Analysis of Th1 and Th2 cytokines expressing CD4+ and CD8+ T cells in rheumatoid arthritis by flow cytometry. J Rheumatol 2000; 27(5): 1128–35.

116. Mican JM, Metcalfe DD. Arthritis and mast cell activation. J Allergy Clin Immunol 1990; 86 (4 Pt 2): 677–83.

117. Malone DG, Wilder RL, Saavedra-Delgado AM et al. Mast cell numbers in rheumatoid synovial tissues. Correlations with quantitative measures of lymphocytic infiltration and modulation by antiinflammatory therapy. Arthritis Rheum 1987; 30(2): 130–7.

118. Buckley MG, Walters C, Wong WM et al. Mast cell activation in arthritis: detection of alpha- and beta-tryptase, histamine and eosinophil cationic protein in synovial fluid. Clin Sci (Lond) 1997; 93(4): 363–70.

119. Woolley DE, Tetlow LC. Mast cell activation and its relation to proinflammatory cytokine production in the rheumatoid lesion. Arthritis Res 2000; 2(1): 65–74.

120. Woolley DE, The mast cell in inflammatory arthritis. N Engl J Med 2003; 348(17): 1709–11.

121. Lee DM, Friend DS, Gurish MF et al. Mast cells: a cellular link between autoantibodies and inflammatory arthritis. Science 2002; 297(5587): 1689–92.

122. Nigrovic PA, Lee DM. Mast cells in inflammatory arthritis. Arthritis Res Ther 2005; 7(1): 1–11.

123. Huang M, Berry J, Kandere K et al. Mast cell deficient W/W(v) mice lack stress-induced increase in serum IL-6 levels, as well as in peripheral CRH and vascular permeability, a model of rheumatoid arthritis. Int J Immunopathol Pharmacol 2002; 15(3): 249–254.

124. Toru H, Pawankar R, Ra C et al. Human mast cells produce IL-13 by high-affinity IgE receptor cross-linking: enhanced IL-13 production by IL-4-primed human mast cells. J Allergy Clin Immunol 1998; 102(3): 491–502.

125. Kobayashi H, Okayama Y, Ishizuka T et al. Production of IL-13 by human lung mast cells in response to Fcepsilon receptor cross-linkage. Clin Exp Allergy 1998; 28(10): 1219–27.

126. Okayama Y, Hagaman DD, Metcalfe DD. A comparison of mediators released or generated by IFN-gamma-treated human mast cells following aggregation of Fc gamma RI or Fc epsilon RI. J Immunol 2001; 166(7): 4705–12.

127. Hart PH, Ahern MJ, Smith MD et al. Regulatory effects of IL-13 on synovial fluid macrophages and blood monocytes from patients with inflammatory arthritis. Clin Exp Immunol 1995; 99(3): 331–7.

128. Chabaud M, Durand JM, Buchs N et al. Human interleukin-17: A T cell-derived proinflammatory cytokine produced by the rheumatoid synovium. Arthritis Rheum 1999; 42(5): 963–70.

129. Morita Y, Yamamura M, Kawashima M et al. Differential in vitro effects of IL-4, IL-10, and IL-13 on proinflammatory cytokine production and fibroblast proliferation in rheumatoid synovium. Rheumatol Int 2001; 20(2): 49–54.

130. Woods JM, Katschke KJ Jr, Tokuhira M et al. Reduction of inflammatory cytokines and prostaglandin E2 by

IL-13 gene therapy in rheumatoid arthritis synovium. J Immunol 2000; 165(5): 2755–63.

131. Borderie D, Hilliquin P, Hernvann A et al. Inhibition of inducible NO synthase by TH2 cytokines and TGF beta in rheumatoid arthritic synoviocytes: effects on nitrosothiol production. Nitric Oxide 2002; 6(3): 271–82.

132. Chenevier-Gobeaux C, Morin-Robinet S, Lemarechal H et al. Effects of pro- and anti-inflammatory cytokines and nitric oxide donors on hyaluronic acid synthesis by synovial cells from patients with rheumatoid arthritis. Clin Sci (Lond) 2004; 107(3): 291–6.

133. Wada T, Nakashima T, Hiroshi N et al. RANKL-RANK signaling in osteoclastogenesis and bone disease. Trends Mol Med 2006; 12(1): 17–25.

134. Kostenuik PJ. Osteoprotegerin and RANKL regulate bone resorption, density, geometry and strength. Curr Opin Pharmacol 2005; 5(6): 618–25.

135. McClung MR, Lewiecki EM, Cohen SB et al. Denosumab in postmenopausal women with low bone mineral density. N Engl J Med 2006; 354(8): 821–31.

136. Bekker PJ, Holloway DL, Rasmussen AS et al. A single-dose placebo-controlled study of AMG 162, a fully human monoclonal antibody to RANKL, in postmenopausal women. J Bone Miner Res 2004; 19(7): 1059–66.

137. Hamdy NA, Osteoprotegerin as a potential therapy for osteoporosis. Curr Rheumatol Rep, 2006; 8(1):50-4.

138. Saidenberg-Kermanac'h N, Corrado A, Lemeiter D et al. TNF-alpha antibodies and osteoprotegerin decrease systemic bone loss associated with inflammation through distinct mechanisms in collagen-induced arthritis. Bone 2004; 35(5): 1200–7.

139. Zwerina J, Hayer S, Tohidast-Akrad M et al. Single and combined inhibition of tumor necrosis factor, interleukin-1, and RANKL pathways in tumor necrosis factor-induced arthritis: effects on synovial inflammation, bone erosion, and cartilage destruction. Arthritis Rheum 2004; 50(1): 277–90.

140. Ahlen J, Andersson S, Mukohyama H et al. Characterization of the bone-resorptive effect of interleukin-11 in cultured mouse calvarial bones. Bone 2002; 31(1): 242–51.

141. Onoe Y, Miyaura C, Kaminakayashiki T et al. IL-13 and IL-4 inhibit bone resorption by suppressing cyclooxygenase-2-dependent prostaglandin synthesis in osteoblasts. J Immunol 1996; 156(2): 758–64.

142. Ura K, Morimoto I, Watanabe K et al. Interleukin (IL)-4 and IL-13 inhibit the differentiation of murine osteoblastic MC3T3-E1 cells. Endocr J 2000; 47(3): 293–302.

143. Palmqvist P, Lundberg P, Persson E et al. Inhibition of hormone and cytokine-stimulated osteoclastogenesis and bone resorption by interleukin-4 and interleukin-13 is associated with increased osteoprotegerin and decreased RANKL and RANK in a STAT6-dependent pathway. J Biol Chem 2006; 281(5): 2414–29.

144. Nakashima T, Kobayashi Y, Yamasaki S et al. Protein expression and functional difference of membrane-bound and soluble receptor activator of NF-kappaB ligand: modulation of the expression by osteotropic factors and cytokines. Biochem Biophys Res Commun 2000; 275(3): 768–75.

145. Abu-Amer Y. IL-4 abrogates osteoclastogenesis through STAT6-dependent inhibition of NF-kappaB. J Clin Invest 2001; 107(11): 1375–85.

146. Hirayama T, Dai S, Abbas S et al. Inhibition of inflammatory bone erosion by constitutively active STAT-6 through blockade of JNK and NF-kappaB activation. Arthritis Rheum 2005; 52(9): 2719–29.

147. Prots I, Skapenko A, Wendler J et al. Association of the IL4R single-nucleotide polymorphism I50V with rapidly erosive rheumatoid arthritis. Arthritis Rheum 2006; 54(5): 1491–500.

148. Mitsuyasu H, Yanagihara Y, Mao XQ et al. Cutting edge: dominant effect of Ile50Val variant of the human IL-4 receptor alpha-chain in IgE synthesis. J Immunol 1999; 162(3): 1227–31.

149. Liu Y, Masuda E, Blank MC et al. Cytokine-mediated regulation of activating and inhibitory Fc gamma receptors in human monocytes. J Leukoc Biol 2005; 77(5): 767–76.

150. Nabbe KC, van Lent PL, Holthuysen AE et al. Local IL-13 gene transfer prior to immune-complex arthritis inhibits chondrocyte death and matrix-metalloproteinase-mediated cartilage matrix degradation despite enhanced joint inflammation. Arthritis Res Ther 2005; 7(2): R392–401.

151. Mulligan MS, Warner RL, Foreback JL et al. Protective effects of IL-4, IL-10, IL-12, and IL-13 in IgG immune complex-induced lung injury: role of endogenous IL-12. J Immunol 1997; 159(7): 3483–9.

152. Grehan JF, Levay-Young BK, Fogelson JL et al. IL-4 and IL-13 induce protection of porcine endothelial cells from killing by human complement and from apoptosis through activation of a phosphatidylinositide 3-kinase/Akt pathway. J Immunol 2005; 175(3): 1903–10.

153. Bessis N, Boissier MC, Ferrara P et al. Attenuation of collagen-induced arthritis in mice by treatment with vector cells engineered to secrete interleukin-13. Eur J Immunol 1996; 26(10): 2399–403.

154. Bessis N, Chiocchia G, Kollias G et al. Modulation of proinflammatory cytokine production in tumour necrosis factor-alpha (TNF-alpha)-transgenic mice by treatment with cells engineered to secrete IL-4, IL-10 or IL-13. Clin Exp Immunol 1998; 111(2): 391–6.

155. Woods JM, Amin MA, Katschke KJ Jr et al. Interleukin-13 gene therapy reduces inflammation, vascularization, and bony destruction in rat adjuvant-induced arthritis. Hum Gene Ther 2002; 13(3): 381–93.

156. Mottonen M, Isomaki P, Luukkainen R et al. Regulation of CD154-induced interleukin-12 production in synovial fluid macrophages. Arthritis Res 2002; 4(5): R9.

157. Harigai M, Hara M, Nakazawa S et al. Ligation of CD40 induced tumor necrosis factor-alpha in rheumatoid arthritis: a novel mechanism of activation of synoviocytes. J Rheumatol 1999; 26(5): 1035–43.

158. Croft D, McIntyre P, Wibulswas A et al. Sustained elevated levels of VCAM-1 in cultured fibroblast-like synoviocytes can be achieved by TNF-alpha in combination with either IL-4 or IL-13 through increased mRNA stability. Am J Pathol 1999; 154(4): 1149–58.

159. Carter RA, Wicks IP. Vascular cell adhesion molecule 1 (CD106): a multifaceted regulator of joint inflammation. Arthritis Rheum 2001; 44(5): 985–94.

160. Relic B, Guicheux J, Mezin F et al. Il-4 and IL-13, but not IL-10, protect human synoviocytes from apoptosis. J Immunol 2001; 166(4): 2775–82.

161. Wong PK, Campbell IK, Egan PJ et al. The role of the interleukin-6 family of cytokines in inflammatory arthritis and bone turnover. Arthritis Rheum 2003; 48(5): 1177–89.

162. Nishimoto N, Kishimoto T. Inhibition of IL-6 for the treatment of inflammatory diseases. Curr Opin Pharmacol 2004; 4(4): 386–91.

163. Rifas L, Cheng SL. IL-13 regulates vascular cell adhesion molecule-1 expression in human osteoblasts. J Cell Biochem 2003; 89(2): 213–19.

164. Frost A, Jonsson KB, Brandstrom H et al. Interleukin (IL)-13 and IL-4 inhibit proliferation and stimulate IL-6 formation in human osteoblasts: evidence for involvement of receptor subunits IL-13R, IL-13Ralpha, and IL-4Ralpha. Bone 2001; 28(3): 268–74.

165. Derocq JM, Segui M, Poinot-Chazel C et al. Interleukin-13 stimulates interleukin-6 production by human keratinocytes. Similarity with interleukin-4. FEBS Lett 1994; 343(1): 32–6.

166. Sebire G, Delfraissy JF, Demotes-Mainard J et al. Interleukin-13 and interleukin-4 act as interleukin-6 inducers in human microglial cells. Cytokine 1996; 8(8): 636–41.

167. Guzdek A, Stalinska K, Guzik K et al. Differential responses of hematopoietic and non-hematopoietic cells to anti-inflammatory cytokines: IL-4, IL-13 and IL-10. J Physiol Pharmacol 2000; 51(3): 387–99.

168. Szodoray P, Alex P, Dandapani V et al. Apoptotic effect of rituximab on peripheral blood B cells in rheumatoid arthritis. Scand J Immunol 2004; 60(1-2): 209–18.

169. Yu CL, Huang MH, Kung YY et al. Interleukin-13 increases prostaglandin E2 (PGE2) production by normal human polymorphonuclear neutrophils by enhancing cyclooxygenase 2 (COX-2) gene expression. Inflamm Res 1998; 47(4): 167–73.

170. Radstake TR, Nabbe KC, Wenink MH et al. Dendritic cells from patients with rheumatoid arthritis lack the interleukin 13 mediated increase of Fc gamma RII expression, which has clear functional consequences. Ann Rheum Dis 2005; 64(12): 1737–43.

171. Sato S, Hasegawa M, Takehara K. Serum levels of interleukin-6 and interleukin-10 correlate with total skin thickness score in patients with systemic sclerosis. J Dermatol Sci 2001; 27(2): 140–6.

172. Hasegawa M, Fujimoto M, Kikuchi K et al. Elevated serum levels of interleukin 4 (IL-4), IL-10, and IL-13 in patients with systemic sclerosis. J Rheumatol 1997; 24(2): 328–32.

173. Riccieri V, Rinaldi T, Spadaro A et al. Interleukin-13 in systemic sclerosis: relationship to nailfold capillaroscopy abnormalities. Clin Rheumatol 2003; 22(2): 102–6.

174. Fujii H, Hasegawa M, Takehara K et al. Abnormal expression of intracellular cytokines and chemokine receptors in peripheral blood T lymphocytes from patients with systemic sclerosis. Clin Exp Immunol 2002; 130(3): 548–56.

175. Hancock A, Armstrong L, Gama R et al. Production of interleukin 13 by alveolar macrophages from normal and fibrotic lung. Am J Respir Cell Mol Biol 1998; 18(1): 60–5.

176. Matsushita M, Yamamoto T, Nishioka K. Upregulation of interleukin-13 and its receptor in a murine model of bleomycin-induced scleroderma. Int Arch Allergy Immunol 2004; 135(4): 348–56.

177. Jakubzick C, Choi ES, Joshi BH et al. Therapeutic attenuation of pulmonary fibrosis via targeting of IL-4- and IL-13-responsive cells. J Immunol 2003; 171(5): 2684–93.

178. Bhogal RK, Stoica CM, McGaha TL et al. Molecular aspects of regulation of collagen gene expression in fibrosis. J Clin Immunol 2005; 25(6): 592–603.

179. Morimoto S, Tokano Y, Kaneko H et al. The increased interleukin-13 in patients with systemic lupus erythematosus: relations to other Th1-, Th2-related cytokines and clinical findings. Autoimmunity 2001; 34(1): 19–25.

180. Spadaro A, Scrivo R, Bombardieri M et al. Relationship of interleukin-12 and interleukin-13 imbalance with class-specific rheumatoid factors and anticardiolipin antibodies in systemic lupus erythematosus. Clin Rheumatol 2003; 22(2): 107–11.

181. Spencer DM, Veldman GM, Banerjee S et al. Distinct inflammatory mechanisms mediate early versus late colitis in mice. Gastroenterology 2002; 122(1): 94–105.

182. Heller F, Fuss IJ, Nieuwenhuis EE et al. Oxazolone colitis, a Th2 colitis model resembling ulcerative colitis, is mediated by IL-13-producing NK-T cells. Immunity 2002; 17(5): 629–38.

183. Fuss IJ, Heller F, Boirivant M et al. Nonclassical CD1d-restricted NK T cells that produce IL-13 characterize an atypical Th2 response in ulcerative colitis. J Clin Invest 2004; 113(10): 1490–7.

184. Heller F, Florian P, Bojarski C et al. Interleukin-13 is the key effector Th2 cytokine in ulcerative colitis that affects epithelial tight junctions, apoptosis, and cell restitution. Gastroenterology 2005; 129(2): 550–64.

14

Biology of interleukin-15

Iain B McInnes, Foo Y Liew and J Alastair Gracie

Introduction • Structure of IL-15 • Biology of IL-15 and its receptor • Bioactivities of IL-15 • Conclusions
• Acknowledgments • References

INTRODUCTION

Interleukin-15 (IL-15) is a cytokine with quaternary structural similarities to IL-2.[1,2] IL-15 is widely expressed in the immune system, mediating regulatory and effector function in a variety of processes of relevance to both innate and adaptive arms of the immune response. The frequent description of IL-15 expression in inflammatory and autoimmune disorders has increased interest in elucidating its basic biology to properly facilitate targeting in the clinic. This chapter will review the basic biology of IL-15, highlighting particularly those properties and functions of relevance to human pathology.

STRUCTURE OF IL-15

IL-15 is a 4-alpha helix cytokine with structural similarity (but not primary sequence homology) with IL-2. Initial descriptions placed IL-15 close to IL-2 in terms of function but it is now recognized that IL-15 has wider distribution and functional effects. IL-15 gene is present on human chromosome 4q31 and mouse chromosome 8.[3] The human gene contains nine exons and eight introns that are variously utilized to generate distinct mRNA products that in turn account for altered intracellular trafficking of the mature protein and thereby effector function.

BIOLOGY OF IL-15 AND ITS RECEPTOR

IL-15 mRNA is broadly expressed throughout numerous normal human tissues and cell types, including activated monocytes, dendritic cells, and fibroblasts[4,5] (Table 14.1). However, IL-15 mRNA expression is not synonymous with protein detection in tissues, reflecting tight regulatory control of translation and secretion (Figure 14.1).[6] IL-15 is subject to significant post-transcriptional regulation. IL-15 mRNA 5'-untranslated region (UTR) contains 12 AUG triplets that significantly reduce the efficiency of translation. Deletion of this AUG-rich 5'UTR sequence in the HuT-102 cell line permits significant constitutive IL-15 secretion.[7] Similarly, replacement of the 48-amino acid signal peptide with that of IL-2 or CD33 induces significantly higher levels of IL-15 production in transfected cells.[8,9] A third regulatory element in the C-terminus region has also been proposed since FLAG fusion proteins exhibit higher levels of secretion than native construct.[8] Two isoforms of IL-15 are generated through this process. Secreted IL-15 is derived from a long signalling peptide (LSP) containing a 48-amino acid leader sequence, whereas a second isoform which contains a short signalling peptide (SSP) of 21-amino acids is retained within the cell and has been localized to non-endoplasmic regions in both cytoplasmic

Table 14.1 Expression of IL-15 in tissues

Cell types in which IL-15 has been identified

Macrophage/monocyte
Dendritic cells
T lymphocytes
Bone marrow stromal cells – primary culture/lines
Thymic epithelium
Epithelial tissues
    Fetal intestine
    Kidney
    Keratinocytes
    Fetal skin
    Retinal pigment
Renal proximal tubule cells
Fibroblasts
Chondrocytes
Astrocytes

and nuclear compartments.[10–14] Altered glycosylation of the IL-15 48-amino acid isoform may further regulate intracellular trafficking. Ultimately, cell membrane expression may be crucial in mediating extracellular function rather than secretion. The significance of nuclear expression is unclear but may constitute part of an endogenous regulatory feedback loop. The physiologic implications of this regulatory structure are also still unclear but clearly provide an intracellular pool of mRNA that can readily generate cytokine in the event of acute challenge without attendant delay in translational regulation.

Factors that drive endogenous IL-15 release are as yet poorly understood. The IL-15 promoter contains a variety of transcription sites in its 5′ regulatory region that are typica l of many proinflammatory cytokines, including NF-κB, NF-IL-6, myb, GCF, αIFN-2, IRF-E and γ-IRE.[4,5,15–17] However, it has proved difficult to establish consistent IL-15 secretion *in vitro* in most systems investigated to date. Factors demonstrated thus far to induce IL-15 secretion by human cells are diverse and include human herpesvirus 6 and 7, *Mycobacterium leprae, Mycobacterium tuberculosis, Staphylococcus aureus*, lipopolysaccharide (LPS), and ultraviolet irradiation.[18–23]

IL-15 binds a specific heterotrimeric receptor (IL-15R) that is widely distributed and which

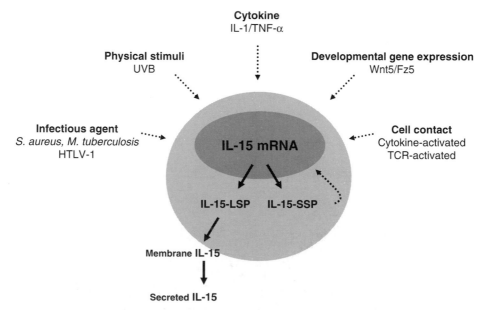

Figure 14.1 Various stimuli increase IL-15 mRNA expression, which is the dominant species since translation is tightly regulated (see text). Protein expression is in two forms – IL-15 long signaling peptide (IL-15-LSP) and IL-15 short signaling peptide (IL-15-SSP), which traffic in distinct pathways within the cell. Membrane IL-15 expression is reported primarily on macrophages where it likely has functional activity. Secreted IL-15 is found in only a limited set of culture conditions, usually in primary cultures from cells actvated *in vivo*, e.g. RA synovial tissues.

consists of a β chain (shared with IL-2) and the common γ chain, together with a unique α chain (IL-15α). IL-15Rα is a type I transmembrane receptor that is structurally related to the IL-2Rα chain. Its genomic location in humans is chromosome 10 and in mice, chromosome.[2] IL-15 binds IL-15Rα-chain with very high affinity – Ka greater than 10^{-11} M^{-1} in the absence of the β/γ chain complex.[24] This has functional implications for *in vivo* function and renders recombinant soluble receptor a useful probe for IL-15 expression and function in experimental systems. The domain structure is of interest in that it contains a sushi domain that is essential for cytokine binding and a long intracellular domain that suggests the potential for signaling capability independent of receptor complex formation. A further intriguing feature of IL-15–receptor interactions is their dependence upon ionic interactions rather than hydrophobic interactions that characterize most cytokine receptor binding.[25,26] The receptor is alternatively spliced to yield eight isoforms; those that lack exon 2 are unable to bind IL-15,[4,27–30] but may offer competitive inhibition of complex assembly with β/γ chains. Intriguingly, IL-15Rα (probably via an exon 2 coding region) and SSP-IL-15 localize to the nuclear membrane/nucleus, the functional implications of which are as yet unknown. It is possible that nuclear IL-15/IL-15Rα complexes act at the transcriptional level to limit IL-15 expression and thereby offer negative feedback within the cell.[31]

Recently a native soluble form of IL-15Rα chain has been detected that is shed from membrane molecule via a protease-dependent mechanism Thus far, only the tumor necrosis factor (TNF) converting enzyme (ADAM17) has been implicated in this process, although other protease interactions may also exist.[32] The function of such soluble receptor could reside in binding of free extracellular IL-15 and thereby act as a feedback inhibitor. However, one report documents enhanced activity of IL-15 in the presence of recombinant sushi domain of sIL-15Ra mediated via β/γ chain complexes, thereby suggesting agonist properties for the soluble receptor analogous to those reported for IL-6, sIL-6R, and gp130.[33] These observations place some doubt on the utility of soluble

receptor containing complexes as therapeutic agents at this time.

Understanding of the precise signaling pathways implicated in IL-15 effector function has been considerably expanded in recent years, in particular concerning their propensity to activate distinct cell types. In lymphocytes and probably other leukocytes except mast cells, the IL-15Rαβγ complex signals through JAK1/3 and STAT3/5.[4,5] Additional signaling through *src*-related tyrosine kinases and Ras/Raf/MAPK to fos/jun activation is also proposed. Further implicated pathways include those of the Bcl-related proteins, accounting for the regulation of apoptosis ascribed to IL-15 in a variety of cell types. IL-15Rα also appears to signal in the absence of βγ chain expression. The cytoplasmic tail of IL-15Rα contains regions homologous to TRAF2 binding domains, analogous to CD40, and may compete with TNFRI for TRAF2 binding.[5,34] Further studies have shown that IL-15Rα can associate with Syk kinase mediating regulatory function in human B-cell lines and in neutrophils.[35] Finally, IL-15Rα may exhibit some promiscuity in co-signaling with receptors from other receptor superfamilies, as has been described for a variety of receptors recently, e.g. epidermal growth factors. Thus in fibroblasts, the receptor tyrosine kinase, Axl, associates with IL-15Rα that in turn leads to activation of PI3K and Akt and thereby Bcl-2/Bcl-x_L.[36] By this means IL-15 may mediate rather diverse effects dependent upon the ambient receptor complement expressed on target cells and the relative expression of other cytokine and growth factor levels in an inflammatory milieu.

Further signaling potential exists whereby membrane IL-15 and IL-15Rα complexes may interact with β/γ chain on adjacent cells forming a *trans* signaling complex.[37] This pathway may be of particular importance in the expansion of CD8 T-cell subsets. It is also notable that IL-15 contains two sites at which IL-15Rα binding is possible, raising the possibility of one cytokine molecule binding two IL-15Rα chains allowing trans presentation of IL-15 to a hetrotrimeric IL-15 receptor complex on a recipient cell with the possibility of generating bi-directional signaling.[5]

An intriguing mechanism of immune regulation lies in direct signaling via the IL-15 molecule itself via reverse signaling. Thus, as described for members of the TNF superfamily, it is proposed that IL-15 is membrane expressed as an integral membrane protein, perhaps via its long signal peptide. Thereafter ligation of membrane IL-15 leads to serine phosphorylation of IL-15 itself and activation of mitogen-activated protein kinases (ERK1/2 and p38), and focal activated kinase. A further report has implicated a similar mechanism leading to activation of the small Rho-family GTPase Rac3. These pathways in turn are implicated in monocyte activation chemokine release and adhesion.[38,39]

BIOACTIVITIES OF IL-15

Commensurate with the broad expression of IL-15R, diverse proinflammatory activities have been attributed to IL-15 (Table 14.2). Key effects are discussed below.

T cells

T cells up-regulate IL-15Rα as an early feature of activation. IL-15 induces proliferation of mitogen-activated CD4+ and CD8+ T cells, T-cell clones, and γδT cells, with release of soluble IL-2Rα, and enhances cytotoxicity both in CD8+ T cells and lymphokine-activated killer cells.[4,40–42] Induction of numerous membrane activation markers has been observed including CD69, FasL, CD40L, TNFRII, and CD25,[43,44] primarily on CD45RO+ but not CD45RA+ T-cell subsets.[43] IL-15 exhibits T-cell chemokinetic activity [45,46] and induces adhesion molecule (e.g. intercellular adhesion molecule (ICAM)-3) redistribution.[47] It further induces chemokine (CC-, CXC-, and C-type) and chemokine receptor (CC but not CXC) expression on T cells.[48] Thus, IL-15 can recruit T cells and, thereafter, modify homo- or heterotypic cell–cell interactions within inflammatory sites.

IL-15 is generally considered to favor differentiation of type 1 responses. IL-15 primes naive CD4+ T cells from TCR transgenic mice for subsequent interferon (IFN)-γ expression, but not IL-4 production.[49] Antigen-specific responses in T cells from human immunodeficiency virus (HIV)-infected patients in the presence of high-dose IL-15 exhibit increased IFN-γ production.[50] Similarly IL-15 induces IFN-γ/IL-4 ratios which

Table 14.2 Biologic effects of IL-15	
Cell type	Key effects
T lymphocyte	• Activation/proliferation • Cytokine production Th/c1 and Th/c2 • Cytotoxicity • Chemokinesis • Cytoskeletal rearrangement • Adhesion molecule expression • Reduced apoptosis
B lymphocyte	• Ig production • Proliferation
NK cell	• Cytotoxicity • Cytokine production • Reduced apoptosis • Lineage development
Macrophage	• Dose-dependent effect on activation • Membrane expression – ?costimulation
Osteoclast	• Maturation • Calcitonin receptor
Dendritic cell	• Maturation • Activation
Neutrophil	• Activation • Cytoskeletal rearrangement • Cytokine release • Reduced apoptosis

favor Th1 dominance in mitogen-stimulated human T cells.[51] However, IL-15 induces IL-5 production from allergen-specific human T-cell clones, implying a positive role in Th2-mediated allergic responses.[52] Moreover, administration of soluble IL-15-IgG2b fusion protein in murine hypersensitivity models clearly implicates IL-15 in Th2 lesion development.[53] In contrast, IL-15 expression in type 2 associated atopic dermatitis patients was significantly lower than that in normal or psoriasis patients.[54] It is also now established that IL-15 has the capacity to expand IL-17-expressing T cells – in particular synovial T cells release large concentrations of IL-17 in response to IL-15 *in vitro*.[55] However, the relative role of IL-15 in comparison to IL-6, transforming growth factor (TGF)-β and IL-23p19 in expansion of Th17 cells in mice and particularly in humans is still unclear.[56]

A prominent role in T-cell memory is now established, especially for the CD8 compartment. IL-15 induces CD8[+] T-cell expansion *in vivo*.[57] IL-15Rα-deficient mice exhibit lymphopenia due to reduced proliferation and homing of mature lymphocytes, particularly of the CD8[+] subset. A key role in the development of several cell lineages of the innate immune response such as natural killer (NK) cells was also confirmed.[58] Similar abnormalities are observed in IL-15-deficient mice.[59] T-cell-independent hematopoietic IL-15Rα signals are vital for poly I:C induced bystander responses in CD8[+] T cells further suggest a vital role in maintaining memory responses.[60] Studies in IL-15 transgenic mice infected with *Listeria monocytogenes* further support a role for IL-15 in generating long-term antigen specific memory in the CD8[+] compartment.[61] Recent reports have extended these observations to include CD4[+] T cells,[62,63] suggesting that such effects may have broader consequence.

NK cells

IL-15 plays a fundamental role in thymic development of T-cell and, particularly, NK-cell lineages. Thus, IL-15, IL-15Rα, IL-15Rβ, IRF-1, and JAK3 gene targeted mouse strains all exhibit either deficiency or absence of NK-cell development and function. IL-15 induces NK-cell activation, measured either by direct cytotoxicity, antibody-dependent cellular cytotoxicity, or production of cytokines.[64–66] IL-15 acts as an NK-cell survival factor *in vivo* by maintaining Bcl-2 expression.[67–70] It has recently been directly implicated in promoting NK-cell-mediated shock in mice.[69] The effects of IL-15 in the NK-cell compartment have recently been comprehensively reviewed.[71]

Macrophages

Macrophages bind IL-15 with high affinity via expression of IL-15Rα/β/γ. IL-15 may function as an autocrine regulator of macrophage activation, such that low levels of IL-15 suppress whereas higher levels enhance proinflammatory monokine production.[72] The latter includes TNF-α, IL-1, and IL-6, together with the chemokines IL-8 and MCP-1.[72,73] Moreover, since human macrophages constitutively express bioactive membrane-bound IL-15, such autocrine effects are likely of early importance during macrophage activation. LPS or granulocyte/macrophase colony-stimulating factor (GM-CSF) rapidly induce translocation of preformed IL-15 stores to the plasma membrane of blood-derived CD14[+] macrophages where it is able to sustain T-cell proliferation.[74] This membrane expression may represent a major effector pathway for IL-15. Thus, IL-15-LSP that is secreted only at low levels is more efficient in viral host defence than is IL-15 engineered to be secreted at high levels.[75] IL-15 appears to directly enhanced macrophage effector function. IL-15 has been implicated in *M. leprae*-induced monocyte maturation.[76] IL-15 increases phorbol myristate acetate (PMA)-activated macrophage clearance of *Leishmania infantum* via an IL-12-dependent mechanism.[77] Similarly IL-15 is implicated in immune clearance of *M. tuberculosis* in a murine macrophage-dependent model.[78] In a variety of autoimmune models IL-15 expression has been closely linked to macrophage activation in part mediated via sustaining T cell–macrophage interactions.[79]

Dendritic cells

IL-15, together with GM-CSF, has recently been shown to support the maturation of monocytes into dendritic cells (CD1a[+], DR[+], CD14[-]) that could be further matured by LPS, TNF-α or CD-40L into CD83[+], DC-LAMP[+] cells.[80] A proportion of these cells expressed E-cadherin and CCR6, reminiscent of Langerhans cells. Moreover, DCs from common-γ chain-deficient mice exhibit reduced IL-12 and nitric oxide (NO) release that was shown in IL-15-deficient mice to be dependent primarily upon IL-15.[81] IL-15 is implicated in IL-2 release from mDCs,[82] and DC survival is regulated to some extent by an IL-15-dependent mechanism.[83] IL-15 has therefore been proposed as a critical component in the initiation of delayed-type hypersensitivity (DTH) immune responses *in vivo*. Together these data suggest that IL-15 may operate at an early stage to promote DC maturation and functional activation.

Neutrophils

Neutrophils express IL-15Rα and IL-15 can induce neutrophil activation and cytoskeletal rearrangement.[84,85] Thus IL-15 enhances neutrophil phagocytosis, increases *de novo* protein mRNA and protein synthesis (e.g. cytokines and chemokines), and resists progression of apoptosis. The latter appears to operate via a variety of mechanisms including induction of IL-1R synthesis and release, maintenance of myeloid differentiation factor-1 expression, and reduction of caspase 1 and caspase 3 activity, in turn modifying Bax expression.[5,86] Notably IL-15 mediates increased phagocytosis via a Syk-kinase-dependent mechanism (see above). The functional importance of these observations has been confirmed in particular using *in vitro* responses to *Candida albicans*. Their wider significance in autoimmune or inflammatory disease states is less clear at present.

Eosinophils and mast cells

IL-15 regulates survival of eosinophils. The precise mechanisms whereby this is mediated remain unclear but likely involve elaboration of GM-CSF production with consequent NF-κB nuclear translocation in an autocrine manner.[87] That mast cells have the potential to respond to IL-15 has long been recognized, not least in the original description of a novel IL-15R X on this lineage.[88] Whereas the identity of this receptor remains unclear, and subsequent studies have shown IL-15Rα on mast cells, there is now a significant literature to support a role for IL-15 in promoting effector function. Thus IL-15 enhances proliferation of bone marrow-derived mast cells, and as with other lineages delays apoptosis induced by coincident withdrawal of essential growth factors such as IL-3. This pathway appears to be mediated in part via Bcl-K$_L$ and local release of IL-4.[89] The concentrations required for these effects are high *in vitro* and their relevance *in vivo* remains unclear.

Osteoclasts

Addition of IL-15 to rat bone marrow cultures induces osteoclast development and up-regulates calcitonin receptor expression.[90]

Fibroblasts

Fibroblasts grown from a variety of tissues express IL-15, which may be of functional relevance to the capacity of host tissues to modulate evolving immune responses therein. IL-15 effector function in the context of immune-mediated pathology is considered in Chapter x. Membrane IL-15 is considered capable of promoting NK-cell and T-cell activation.[91,92] In potential autocrine regulatory loops IL-15 is also able to sustain fibroblast survival via modulation of Bcl-2 and Akt/PI3K-dependent pathways.[36]

CONCLUSIONS

IL-15 and its receptor are expressed on a wide range of hemopoietic and non-hemopoietic cell types. IL-15 thus provides a pathway whereby host tissues can contribute to the early phase of immune responses, providing enhancement of polymorphonuclear and NK-cell responses, and subsequently T-cell responses. Such activity may facilitate chronic rather than self-limiting inflammation should IL-15 synthesis be dysregulated. This subject will be addressed in Chapter x in this volume.

ACKNOWLEDGMENTS

The support of the Nuffield Foundation (Oliver Bird Fund), the Wellcome Trust, and the Arthritis Research Campaign (UK) is acknowledged.

REFERENCES

1. Grabstein KH, Eisenman J, Shanebeck K et al. Cloning of a T cell growth factor that interacts with the beta chain of the interleukin-2 receptor. Science 1994; 264: 965–8.
2. Bamford R, Grant A, Burton J et al. The interleukin (IL) 2 receptor {beta} chain is shared by IL-2 and a cytokine, provisionally designated IL-T, that stimulates T-cell proliferation and the induction of lymphokine-activated killer cells. Proc Natl Acad Sci USA 1994; 91: 4940–4.
3. Anderson DM, Johnson L, Glaccum MB et al. Chromosomal assignment and genomic structure of Il15. Genomics 1995; 25: 701–6.
4. Waldmann TA, Tagaya Y. The multifaceted regulation of Interleukin-15 expression and the role of this cytokine in NK cell differentiation and host response to intracellular pathogens. Annu Rev Immunol 1999; 17: 19–49.
5. Budagian V, Bulanova E, Paus R, Bulfone-Paus S. IL-15/IL-15 receptor biology: a guided tour through

an expanding universe. Cytokine Growth Factor Rev 2006; 17: 259–80.

6. Bamford RN, DeFilippis AP, Azimi N et al. The 5′ untranslated region, signal peptide, and the coding sequence of the carboxyl terminus of IL-15 participate in its multifaceted translational control. J Immunol 1998; 160: 4418–26.

7. Bamford RN, Battiata AP, Burton JD et al. Interleukin (IL) 15/IL-T production by the adult T-cell leukemia cell line HuT-102 is associated with a human T-cell lymphotrophic virus type I R region/IL-15 fusion message that lacks many upstream AUGs that normally attenuate IL-15 mRNA translation. Proc Natl Acad Sci USA 1996; 93: 2897–2902.

8. Onu A, Pohl T, Krause H, Bulfone-Paus S. Regulation of IL-15 secretion via the leader peptide of two IL-15 isoforms. J Immunol 1997; 158: 255–62.

9. Meazza R, Verdiani S, Biassoni R et al. Identification of a novel interleukin-15 (IL-15) transcript isoform generated by alternative splicing in human small cell lung cancer cell lines. Oncogene 1996; 12: 2187–92.

10. Tagaya Y, Kurys G, Thies TA et al. Generation of secretable and nonsecretable interleukin 15 isoforms through alternate usage of signal peptides. Proc Natl Acad Sci USA 1997; 94: 14444–9.

11. Nishimura H, Washizu J, Nakamura N et al. Translational efficiency is up-regulated by alternative exon in murine IL-15 mRNA. J Immunol 1998; 160: 936–42.

12. Gaggero A, Azzarone B, Andrei C et al. Differential intracellular trafficking, secretion and endosomal localization of two IL-15 isoforms. Eur J Immunol 1999; 29: 1265–74.

13. Nishimura H, Fujimoto A, Tamura N et al. A novel autoregulatory mechanism for transcriptional activation of the IL-15 gene by a nonsecretable isoform of IL-15 generated by alternative splicing, FASEB J 2005; 19, 19–28.

14. Dubois S, Magrangeas F, Lehours P et al. Natural splicing of exon 2 of human interleukin-15 receptor achain mRNA results in shortened form with a distinct pattern of expression. J Biol Chem 1999; 274: 26978–84.

15. Azimi N, Brown K, Bamford RN et al. Human T cell lymphotropic virus type I Tax protein trans-activates interleukin 15 gene transcription through an NF-kappa B site. Proc Natl Acad Sci USA 1998; 95: 2452–7.

16. Washizu J, Nishimura H, Nakamura N et al. The NF-kappaB binding site is essential for transcriptional activation of the IL-15 gene. Immunogenetics 1998; 48: 1–7.

17. Pereno R, Giron-Michel J, Gaggero A et al. IL-15/IL-15Rα intracellular trafficking in human melanoma cells and signal transduction through the IL-15Rα. Oncogene 2000; 19: 5153–62.

18. Flamand L, Stefanescu I, Menezes J. Human herpesvirus-6 enhances natural killer cell cytotoxicity via IL-15. J Clin Invest 1996; 97: 1373–81.

19. Atedzoe BN, Ahmad A, Menezes J. Enhancement of natural killer cell cytotoxicity by the human herpesvirus-7 via IL-15 induction. J Immunol 1997; 159: 4966–72.

20. Jullien D, Sieling PA, Uyemura K et al. IL-15, an immunomodulator of T cell responses in intracellular infection. J Immunol 1997; 158: 800–6.

21. Carson WE, Ross ME, Baiocchi RA et al. Endogenous production of interleukin 15 by activated human monocytes is critical for optimal production of interferon-gamma by natural killer cells in vitro. J Clin Invest 1995; 96: 2578–82.

22. Chehimi J, Marshall JD, Salvucci O et al. IL-15 enhances immune functions during HIV infection. J Immunol 1997; 158: 5978–87.

23. Mohamadzadeh M, Takashima A, Dougherty I et al. Ultraviolet B radiation up-regulates the expression of IL-15 in human skin. J Immunol 1995; 155: 4492–6.

24. Giri JG, Kumaki S, Ahdieh M et al. Identification and cloning of a novel IL-15 binding protein that is structurally related to the alpha chain of the IL-2 receptor. EMBO J 1995; 14: 3654–63.

25. Wang X, Rickert M, Garsia KC. Structure of the quaternary complex of interleukin-2 with its α, β and γχ receptors. Science 2005; 310: 1159–63.

26. Lorenzen I, Dingley AJ, Jacques Y, Grötzinger J. The structure of the IL-15α-receptor and its implication for ligand binding. J Biol Chem 2006; 281: 6642–7.

27. Waldmann T, Tagaya Y, Bamford R. Interleukin-2, interleukin-15, and their receptors. Int Rev Immunol 1998; 16: 205–26.

28. Tagaya Y, Bamford RN, DeFilippis AP, Waldmann TA. IL-15: a pleiotropic cytokine with diverse receptor/signaling pathways whose expression is controlled at multiple levels. Immunity 1996; 4: 329–36.

29. Anderson DM, Kumaki S, Ahdieh M et al. Functional characterization of the human interleukin-15 receptor alpha chain and close linkage of IL15RA and IL2RA genes. J Biol Chem 1995; 270: 29862–9.

30. Tagaya Y, Burton JD, Miyamoto Y, Waldmann TA. Identification of a novel receptor/signal transduction pathway for IL-15/T in mast cells. EMBO J 1996; 15: 4928–39.

31. Dubois S, Magrangeas F, Lehours P et al. Natural splicing of exon 2 of human interleukin-15 receptor α chain mRNA results in shortened form with a distinct pattern of expression. J Biol Chem 1999; 274: 26978–84.

32. Budagian V, Bulanova E, Orinska Z et al. Natural soluble interleukin-15Rα is generated by cleavage that involves the tumor necrosis factor-a-converting enzyme (TACE/ADAM17). J Biol Chem 2004; 279: 40368–75.

33. Mortier E, Quemener A, Vusio P et al. Soluble IL-15Rα sushi as a selective and potent agonist of IL-15 action through IL-15Rβ/γ: hyper-agonist IL-15-IL-15Rα fusion proteins. J Biol Chem 2005; 281: 1612–19.

34. Bulfone-Paus S, Bulanova E, Pohl T et al. Death deflected: IL-15 inhibits TNF-alpha-mediated apoptosis in fibroblasts by TRAF2 recruitment to the IL-15Ralpha chain. FASEB J 1999; 13: 1575–85.

35. Bulanova E, Budagian V, Pohl T et al. The IL-15Rα chain signals through association with Syk in human B cells. J Immunol 2001; 170: 5045–55.

36. Budagian V, Bulanova E, Orinska Z et al. A promiscuous liaison between IL-15 receptor and Axl receptor tyrosine kinase in cell death control. EMBO J 2005; 24: 4260–70.

37. Dubois S, Mariner J,Waldmann TA, Tagaya Y. IL-15Ra recycles and presents IL-15 in trans to neighboring cells. Immunity 2002; 17: 537– 47.

38. Budagian V, Bulanova E, Orinska Z et al. Reverse signaling through membrane-bound interleukin-15. J Biol Chem 2004; 279: 42192–201.

39. Neely GG, Epelman S, Ma LL et al. Monocytes surface-bound IL-15 can function as an activating receptor and participate in reverse signaling. J Immunol 2004; 172: 4225–34.

40. Nishimura H, Hiromatsu K, Kobayashi N et al. IL-15 is a novel growth factor for murine gamma delta T cells induced by Salmonella infection. J Immunol 1996; 156: 663–9.

41. Korholz D, Banning U, Bonig H et al. The role of interleukin-10 (IL-10) in IL-15-mediated T-cell responses. Blood 1997; 90: 4513–21.

42. Treiber-Held S, Stewart DM, Kurman CC, Nelson DL. IL-15 induces the release of soluble IL-2Ralpha from human peripheral blood mononuclear cells. Clin Immunol Immunopathol 1996; 79: 71–8.

43. Kanegane H, Tosato G. Activation of naive and memory T cells by interleukin-15. Blood 1996; 88: 230–5.

44. Mottonen M, Isomaki P, Luukkainen R et al. Interleukin-15 up-regulates the expression of CD154 on synovial fluid T cells. Immunology 2000; 100: 238–44.

45. Wilkinson PC, Liew FY. Chemoattraction of human blood T lymphocytes by interleukin-15. J Exp Med 1995; 181: 1255–9.

46. Al-Mughales J, Blyth TH, Hunter JA, and Wilkinson PC. The chemoattractant activity of rheumatoid synovial fluid for human lymphocytes is due to multiple cytokines. Clin Exp Immunol 1996; 106: 230–6.

47. Nieto M, del Pozo MA, Sanchez-Madrid F. Interleukin-15 induces adhesion receptor redistribution in T lymphocytes. Eur J Immunol 1996; 26: 1302–7.

48 Perera LP, Goldman CK, Waldmann TA. IL-15 induces the expression of chemokines and their receptors in T lymphocytes. J Immunol 1999; 162: 2606–12.

49. Seder RA. High-dose IL-2 and IL-15 enhance the in vitro priming of naive CD4 T cells for IFN-gamma but have differential effects on priming for IL-4. J Immunol 1996; 156: 2413–22.

50. Seder RA, Grabstein KH, Berzofsky JA, and McDyer JF. Cytokine interactions in human immunodeficiency virus-infected individuals: roles of interleukin (IL)-2, IL-12, and IL-15. J Exp Med 1995; 182: 1067–77.

51 Borger P, Kauffman HF, Postma DS et al. Interleukin-15 differentially enhances the expression of interferon-gamma and interleukin-4 in activated human (CD4) T lymphocytes. Immunology 1999; 96: 207–14.

52. Mori A, Suko M, Kaminuma O et al. IL-15 promotes cytokine production of human T helper cells. J Immunol 1996; 156: 2400–5.

53. Ruckert R, Herz U, Paus R et al. IL-15-IgG2b fusion protein accelerates and enhances a Th2 but not a Th1 immune response in vivo, while IL-2-IgG2b fusion protein inhibits both. Eur J Immunol 1998; 28: 3312–20.

54. Ong PY, Hamid QA, Travers JB et al. Decreased IL-15 may contribute to elevated IgE and acute inflammation in atopic dermatitis. J Immunol 2002; 168: 505–10.

55. Ziolkowska M, Koc A, Luszczykiewicz G et al. High levels of IL-17 in rheumatoid arthritis patients: IL-15 triggers in vitro IL-17 production via cyclosporin A-sensitive mechanism. J Immunol 2000; 164: 2832–8.

56. Weaver CT, Harrington LE, Mangan PR, Gavrieli M, Murphy KM. Th17: an effector CD4 T cell lineage with regulatory T cell ties. Immunity 2006; 24: 677–88.

57. Tough DF, Zhang X, Sprent J. An IFN-gamma-dependent pathway controls stimulation of memory phenotype CD8+ T cell turnover in vivo by IL-12, IL-18, and IFN-gamma. J Immunol 2001; 166: 6007–11.

58. Lodolce JP, Boone DL, Chai S, et al. IL-15 receptor maintains lymphoid homeostasis by supporting lymphocyte homing and proliferation. Immunity 1998; 9: 669–76.

59. Kennedy MK, Glaccum M, Brown SN et al. Reversible defects in natural killer and memory CD8 T cell lineages in interleukin 15-deficient mice. J Exp Med 2000; 191: 771–80.

60. Lodolce JP, Burkett PR, Boone DL et al. T cell-independent interleukin 15R{alpha} signals are required for bystander proliferation. J Exp Med 2001; 194: 1187–94.

61. Yajima T, Nishimura H, Ishimitsu R et al. Overexpression of IL-15 in vivo increases antigen-driven memory CD8+ T cells following a microbe exposure. J Immunol 2002; 168: 1198–203.

62. Geginat J, Sallusto F, Lanzavecchia A. Cytokine-driven proliferation and differentiation of human naive, central memory, and effector memory CD4+ T cells. J Exp Med 2001; 194: 1711–20.

63. Carson WE, Giri JG, Lindemann MJ et al. Interleukin (IL) 15 is a novel cytokine that activates human natural killer

cells via components of the IL-2 receptor. J Exp Med 1994; 180: 1395–403.

64. Warren HS, Kinnear BF, Kastelein RL, Lanier LL. Analysis of the costimulatory role of IL-2 and IL-15 in initiating proliferation of resting (CD56dim) human NK cells. J Immunol 1996; 156: 3254–9.

65. Cavazzana-Calvo M, Hacein-Bey S, de Saint Basile G et al. Role of interleukin-2 (IL-2), IL-7, and IL-15 in natural killer cell differentiation from cord blood hematopoietic progenitor cells and from gamma c transduced severe combined immunodeficiency X1 bone marrow cells. Blood 1996; 88: 3901–9.

66. Mrozek E, Anderson P, Caligiuri MA. Role of interleukin-15 in the development of human CD56 natural killer cells from CD34 hematopoietic progenitor cells. Blood 1996; 87: 2632–40.

67. Yu H, Fehniger TA, Fuchshuber P et al. Flt3 ligand promotes the generation of a distinct CD34+ human natural killer cell progenitor that responds to interleukin 15. Blood 1998; 92: 3647–57.

68. Carson WE, Fehniger TA, Haldar S et al. A potential role for interleukin-15 in the regulation of human natural killer cell survival. J Clin Invest 1997; 99: 937–43.

69. Carson WE, Yu H, Dierksheide J et al. A fatal cytokine-induced systemic inflammatory response reveals a critical role for NK cells. J Immunol 1999; 162: 4943–51.

70. Fehniger TA, Caligiuri MA. Interleukin 15: biology and relevance to human disease. Blood 2001; 97: 14–32.

71. Ma A, Koka R, Burkett P. Diverse functions of IL-2, IL-15, and IL-7 in lymphoid homeostasis. Annu Rev Immunol. 2006; 24: 657–79.

72. Alleva DG, Kaser SB, Monroy MA et al. IL-15 functions as a potent autocrine regulator of macrophage proinflammatory cytokine production: evidence for differential receptor subunit utilization associated with stimulation or inhibition. J Immunol 1997; 159: 2941–51.

73. Musso T, Calosso L, Zucca M et al. Human monocytes constitutively express membrane-bound, biologically active, and interferon-gamma-upregulated interleukin-15. Blood 1999; 93: 3531–9.

74. Neely GG, Robbins SM, Amankwah EK et al. Lipopolysaccharide-stimulated or granulocyte-macrophage colony-stimulating factor-stimulated monocytes rapidly express biologically active IL-15 on their cell surface independent of new protein synthesis. J Immunol 2001; 167: 5011–17.

75. Perera LP, Goldman CK, Waldmann TA. Comparative assessment of virulence of recombinant vaccinia viruses expressing IL-2 and IL-15 in immunodeficient mice. Proc Natl Acad Sci USA 2001; 98: 5146–51.

76. Krutzik SR, Tan B, Li H et al. TLR activation triggers the rapid differentiation of monocytes into macrophages and dendritic cells. Nat Med 2005; 11: 653–60.

77. D'Agostino P, Milano S, Arcoleo F et al. Interleukin-15, as interferon-gamma, induces the killing of *Leishmania infantum* in phorbol-myristate-acetate-activated macrophages increasing interleukin-12. Scand J Immunol 2004; 60: 609–14.

78. Maeurer MJ, Trinder P, Hommel G et al. Interleukin-7 or interleukin-15 enhances survival of *Mycobacterium tuberculosis*-infected mice. Infect Immun 2000; 68: 2962–70.

79. McInnes IB, Gracie JA. Interleukin-15: a new cytokine target for the treatment of inflammatory diseases. Curr Opin Pharmacol 2004; 4: 392–7.

80. Mohamadzadeh M, Berard F, Essert G et al. Interleukin 15 skews monocyte differentiation into dendritic cells with features of Langerhans cells. J Exp Med 2001; 194: 1013–20.

81. Ohtcki T, Suzue K, Maki C et al. Critical role of IL-15-IL-15R for antigen-presenting cell functions in the innate immune response. Nat Immunol 2001; 2: 1138–43.

82. Feau S, Facchinetti V, Granucci F et al. Dendritic cell-derived IL-2 production is regulated by IL-15 in humans and in mice. Blood 2005; 105: 697–702.

83. Dubois SP, Waldmann TA, Müller J. Survival adjustment of mature dendritic cells by IL-15. Proc Natl Acad Sci U S A 2005; 102: 8662–7.

84. Girard D, Paquet ME, Paquin R, Beaulieu AD. Differential effects of interleukin-15 (IL-15) and IL-2 on human neutrophils: modulation of phagocytosis, cytoskeleton rearrangement, gene expression, and apoptosis by IL-15. Blood 1996; 88: 3176–84.

85. Girard D, Boiani N, Beaulieu AD. Human neutrophils express the interleukin-15 receptor alpha chain (IL-15Ralpha) but not the IL-9Ralpha component. Clin Immunol Immunopathol 1998; 88: 232–40.

86. Bouchard A, Ratthe C, Girard D. Interleukin-15 delays human neutrophils apoptosis by intracellular events and not via extracellular factors: role of Mcl-1 and decreased activity of caspase-3 and caspase-8. J Leukoc Biol 2004; 75: 893–900.

87. Hoontrakoon R, Chu WH, Gardai SJ et al. Interleukin-15 inhibits spontaneous apoptosis in human eosinophils via autocrine production of granulocyte macrophage-colony stimulation factor and nuclear factor-κB activation. Am J Respir Cell Mol Biol 2002; 26: 404–12.

88. Tagaya Y, Bamford RN, DeFilippis AP, Waldmann TA. IL-15: a pleiotropic cytokine with diverse receptor/signaling pathways whose expression is controlled at multiple levels. Immunity 1996; 4: 329–36.

89. Masuda A, Matsuguchi T, Yamaki K, Hayakawa T, Yoshikai Y. Interleukin-15 prevents mouse mast cell apoptosis through STAT6-mediated Bcl-xL expression. J Biol Chem 2001; 276: 26107–13.

90. Ogata Y, Kukita A, Kukita T et al. A novel role of IL-15 in the development of osteoclasts: inability to replace its activity with IL-2. J Immunol 1999; 162: 2754–60.

91. Briard D, Brouty-Boye D, Azzarone B, Jasmin C. Fibroblasts from human spleen regulate NK cell differentiation from blood CD34+ progenitors via cell surface IL-15. J Immunol 2002; 168: 4326–32.

92. Rappl G, Kapsokefalou A, Heuser C et al. Dermal fibroblasts sustain proliferation of activated T cells via membrane-bound interleukin-15 upon long-term stimulation with tumor necrosis factor-α. J Invest Dermatol 2001; 116: 102–9.

15

Interleukin-17: a new target in arthritis

Pierre Miossec, Myew-Ling Toh and Saloua Zrioual

Introduction • Discovery and structure of IL-17 • IL-17 receptors and mode of action • Control of IL-17 with biotechnology tools • Waiting for a treatment • References

INTRODUCTION

The favorable clinical results obtained with tumor necrosis factor (TNF)-α inhibitors have clearly demonstrated the contribution of cytokines to inflammation and destruction in rheumatoid arthritis (RA). As some patients do not respond and the effect of TNF-α inhibition is suspensive, additional cytokines can be considered as new targets. Interleukin (IL)-17 is now considered because of its proinflammatory and joint destructive properties (Figure 15.1). In addition, its production by T cells would clarify the contribution of T-cell subsets to arthritis. At the same time, it remains to be clarified why it took 10 years to move from the identification of the role of IL-17 to planning clinical trials with the appropriate tools. After a summary of the classical knowledge on IL-17, we will focus on the new aspects regarding IL-17 obtained since our previous review on the subject in 2003.[1]

DISCOVERY AND STRUCTURE OF IL-17

In 1995/96, researchers at Immunex, Seattle[2] and at Schering-Plough, Lyon France[3] defined effects of the new cytokine IL-17, by demonstrating its effects on mesenchymal cells, including synoviocytes, such as the induction of various inflammatory cytokines. Later a systematic gene bank analysis found sequences with four cysteine residues, characteristic of IL-17, in other proteins subsequently classified as IL-17 family members.[4] They are now listed as IL-17A to F. IL-17E is IL-25, implicated in Th2 allergic reactions and has anti-inflammatory properties.[5,6] IL-17F is the closest to IL-17A, with a 50% sequence homology, and appears to share a number of properties with IL-17A, although its role in inflammation and related diseases remains to be investigated in more detail. Accordingly, we will focus on these two members, unless indicated.

IL-17 RECEPTORS AND MODE OF ACTION

As for other cytokines, IL-17 acts through cell membrane receptors. A mouse IL-17 receptor was isolated, first followed by the description of the human counterpart.[7,8] Comparison of known sequences and protein structures indicated that the IL-17 receptor is a member of a new family.[7] In contrast to the restricted production of IL-17 by T cells, its receptor is widely expressed on almost any cell type. However, receptor affinity assays demonstrated that the isolated IL-17 receptor interacts with IL-17 with low affinity. Such low affinity suggested that additional chains may be associated with the IL-17 receptor. However, the soluble form of this low affinity chain is a potent inhibitor of IL-17 function. Patent issues are probably the reason why additional research on IL-17 receptors took so long.

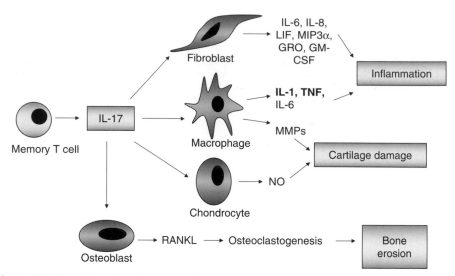

Figure 15.1 Effects of IL-17 on interactions between cells and cytokines associated with destruction in rheumatoid arthritis.

Recently, the IL-17 receptor complex has been clarified in the mouse. It is composed of the combination of two chains: IL-17RA and IL-17RC.[9] The two chains bind IL-17A and F with different affinities. It was suggested that IL-17RA is the receptor for IL-17A and IL-17RC for IL-17F, but this remains unclear.

Intracellular signaling molecules have been identified and their pharmacological control is the target of active research. IL-17 shares many signal transduction pathways with IL-1 and TNF-α. In particular, JNK, TRAF-6, p38, and NF-kB are key signaling molecules downstream of IL-17 receptor binding, implicated in the biological effects of IL-17.[10,11] These pathways have been identified in mesenchymal cells such as synoviocytes,[12] chondrocytes,[13] osteoblasts, and myoblasts. In the development of experimental autoimmune encephalomyelitis, results in IL-17-deficient mice suggest that protein kinase C (PKC) theta is implicated in the regulation of IL-17 in T-cell function.[14]

Source of IL-17

IL-17 was first described as a CD4+ T-cell product. Although eosinophils were shown to be the source of IL-17 in bronchial secretions in asthma,[15] the contribution of eosinophil-derived IL-17 over that from T cells is unknown.

Classification of IL-17 in the classical Th1/Th2 balance has advanced recently, at least in the mouse. The first step came from the isolation of IL-23 and the separation of its properties from those of IL-12. In experimental models ofencephalomyelitis, it was demonstrated that interferon (IFN)-γ was induced by IL-12 and not IL-23.[16] Conversely, IL-23 was found to be a key factor for induction of IL-17. Anti-IL-23 antibody treatment reduced systemic and local levels of IL-17 in the experimental encephalomyelitis.[17] Similar effects are observed in other experimental models of inflammatory and autoimmune diseases.[18,19] In contrast to the potent anti-inflammatory effects of IL-23 inhibition, *in vitro* murine studies demonstrate relatively weak stimulatory effects of IL-23 on IL-17 production. Recent papers indicate that transforming growth factor (TGF)-β and IL-6 have much more potent effects compared with IL-23.[20] In addition there is a regulatory balance between Th17 cells and regulatory T cells. IL-6 and TGF-β induce Th17 cells, whereas IL-6 inhibits the generation of Foxp3-positive regulatory T cells induced by TGF-β.[20]

New understanding of the Th1/Th2 balance came from the identification of a new lineage of murine CD4+ T cells characterized by IL-17 secretion and thus named Th IL-17 or Th17 (Figure 15.2). In addition, IL-17 production was shown to be inhibited by IFN-γ. The divergent

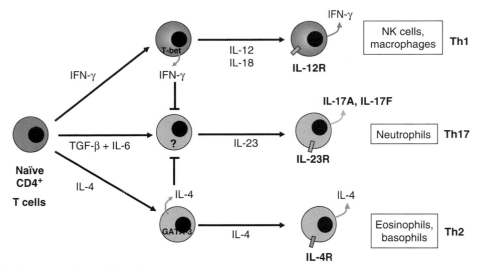

Figure 15.2 Th17: a new subset of Th cells.

effect of IL-12 in induction of IFN-γ versus IL-23 in induction of IL-17 was then extended to human *in vitro* studies.[21]

Transcription factors have been associated with the development of CD4+ T-cell subsets. T bet and STAT1 are required for Th1 cell development, whereas GATA-3 and STAT6 are required for the development of Th2 cells. The transcription factors required for the development of Th17 remain to be clarified. Although T bet and STAT1 are not required for the initial production of IL-17, T bet is needed for an optimal production of IL-17 in response to IL-23.[17] However, opposite results have been published showing a negative effect of T bet.[22]

The morphology of IL-17-producing T cells is of interest to understand its biology. This unusual aspect was first observed by staining IL-17-positive cells in the RA synovium.[23] The positive cells resembled plasma cells with a remote nucleus indicating potent secretory activity. Similar morphology was observed in activated T cells from peripheral blood and lymph nodes. Following polyclonal activation, IL-17-positive cells lose T-cell receptor and CD3 membrane markers but retain the CD4 membrane marker. A parallel can be drawn between B cells, which have lost their B-cell membrane receptor when they start producing soluble immunoglobulins as plasma cells. It is unclear whether these cells are terminally differentiated and will thus subsequently die, or whether they can revert to a more common T-cell phenotype with possibly different secretory functions.

Interactions between IL-17 and other proinflammatory cytokines

IL-17 was described by its ability to induce the production of IL-6 and IL-8 by fibroblasts.[3] When IL-1, IL-17, and TNF-α are compared for effects on IL-6 production, IL-1 is clearly the most potent followed by TNF-α, whereas IL-17 is poorly active. The most interesting aspect of these studies is the additive and often synergistic effects observed when combining IL-1 or TNF-α with IL-17.[24] These synergistic effects with TNF-α were observed in all mesenchymal cells tested, first with synoviocytes,[24] then with chondrocytes,[25,26] osteoblasts,[27,28] and myoblasts.[29] Similarly, it appears that IL-17F is poorly active alone and acts in synergy with TNF-α (unpublished observations).

The mechanisms responsible for such synergy are not fully understood. However, when low concentrations of cytokines, which reflect more directly the *in vivo* situation, are used in combination, a very potent effect on transcription factor activation is observed in mesenchymal cells such as synoviocytes, osteoblasts, or myoblasts.[29–31] In addition, cytokine combinations result in recruitment of additional transcription factors not activated when cytokines are used alone, even at optimal concentrations.

Furthermore, these cytokines interact with each other at the level of production. IL-17 increases the production of IL-1 and TNF-α by monocytes.[32] Thus low concentrations of IL-17 will increase the proinflammatory properties of these monocyte-derived cytokines. The widespread expression of IL-1 and TNF-α, in contrast to the restricted expression of IL-17 by T cells, would suggest that IL-17 has a regulatory role in fine tuning of the inflammatory response.[33]

IL-17 in arthritis

Demonstration of the presence of IL-17 in RA was carried out using a bioassay where synoviocytes were exposed to RA synovium supernatants in the presence of an anti-IL-17 blocking antibody.[34] This resulted in a 70% inhibition of the IL-6-inducing activity present in these supernatants. Thus in 1999 in RA, bioactive IL-17 had been identified, studies demonstrated that it interacted with other key proinflammatory cytokines, and finally its proinflammatory effects could be inhibited by a neutralizing antibody ready for drug development. Direct addition of exogenous IL-17 to RA synovium pieces increased IL-6 production, whereas that of a neutralizing anti-IL-17 antibody reduced it. The same results were observed with juxta-articular bone samples, indicating the local production of IL-17 inside bone, and its contribution to destruction. Furthermore, some of the IL-17-producing cells in synovium, and possibly in bone, express RANK ligand (RANKL) and contribute to destruction through RANK interactions on osteoclasts. In addition, IL-17 increases RANKL expression in mesenchymal cells including synoviocytes.[35] Recently, the presence of IL-17-positive cells in RA synovium was predictive of joint damage at 2 years.[36]

IL-17 has differential effects on the production of chemokines, which regulate cell migration to the RA synovium. Synergy is again observed between IL-1, TNF-α, and IL-17 in induction of synoviocyte MIP3α (now renamed CCL20), a chemokine involved in the migration of memory T cells and immature dendritic cells (DCs).[37] This can be inhibited by the anti-inflammatory cytokines IL-4 and IL-13. Similar results are observed for the production of CXC chemokines involved in the migration of neutrophils. In contrast, IL-17 inhibits TNF-α-induced production of CC chemokines such as RANTES involved in the migration of mononuclear cells.[38]

On DCs in RA synovium, there is a defect in DC maturation with a relative accumulation of immature DCs.[39] IL-17 interacts with IL-1 and TNF-α to favor DC migration, acting in synergy to induce the production of CCL20/MIP-3α.[37] CCL20-producing cells are located in the lining layer and perivascular infiltrates in close association with CD1a immature DCs. Addition of exogenous IL-17 to synovium explants increases CCL20 production. Conversely, specific soluble receptors for IL-1, IL-17, and TNF-α inhibit CCL20 production to various degrees but maximal inhibition is obtained only with combination of these inhibitors.

Proinflammatory cytokines produced by RA synovium have destructive patterns. As for IL-1 and TNF-α, IL-17 increases the spontaneous production of metalloproteases (MMPs) by synoviocytes, IL-1 again being more potent. Addition of IL-4, IL-13, and IL-10 to synoviocyte cultures reduces the spontaneous production of MMP-1 and induces TIMP-1 production by synoviocytes stimulated with IL-17 and/or IL-1β. In the presence of anti-IL-17 blocking antibody, MMP-1 production and collagenase activity by RA synovium is reduced with a decrease of type I collagen C-telopeptide fragments (CTX) released in the supernatants.[40] From these results, IL-17 appears to contribute to both the inflammatory and destructive aspects of RA.

In chondrocytes, IL-17 induces prostaglandin E_2 (PGE_2) and nitric oxide (NO) production by cartilage explants in an IL-1 independent but LIF-dependent fashion.[26,41,42] IL-17 increased collagenase-3 production as for IL-1, mainly through AP-1 activation.

In osteoblasts, IL-17 induces IL-6 production.[43] As in chondrocytes, but only in combination with TNF-α, IL-17 induces NO production in osteoblastic cells by an NF-κB-dependent mechanism.[44] During cell interactions between osteoblasts and osteoclast precursors, the presence of IL-17 induces osteoclastogenesis.[45] IL-17 and other cytokines stimulating osteoclastogenesis, such as IL-1β and TNF-α, increase the expression of RANKL with a concomitant decrease in osteoprotegerin (OPG) expression in osteoblasts/stromal cells.[46] IL-17-producing T cells express the membrane form and secrete the soluble form of RANKL.[47] These biological aspects identified IL-17 as a new key cytokine involved in bone resorption.[27] In the context of RA, T cells in juxta-articular bone are the source of IL-17, which then acts locally to destroy bone.[48]

The results observed with isolated cells were extended by using *ex vivo* models with synovial explants and *in vivo* animal models. In these human *ex vivo* models, addition of IL-17 enhances IL-6 production and collagen destruction and inhibits collagen synthesis by RA synovium explants.[49] In isolated mouse cartilage explants, IL-17 increases cartilage proteoglycan loss and inhibits its synthesis.[48,50] On human RA bone explants, IL-17 also increases bone resorption and decreases formation.[48] Suppression of bone-derived endogenous IL-17 with specific inhibitors results in a protective effect on bone destruction. Conversely, intra-articular administration of IL-17 into a normal mouse joint induces cartilage degradation. These effects are IL-1-independent, as the IL-17 effect is still observed in IL-1-deficient mice.[51] Furthermore, in line with RA chronicity, the continuous administration of IL-17 by gene therapy leads to massive inflammation with a mononuclear cell infiltrate and massive bone and cartilage destruction.[52] Such bone but not cartilage destruction can be prevented with OPG. In collagen-induced arthritis, it is important to oppose arthritis induction in naïve conditions where IL-17 contribution is TNF-dependent as opposed to the chronic phase where such dependency is lost.[53]

In conclusion, the contributions of IL-17 derived from synovium and bone marrow T cells to joint destruction are strong arguments for the control of IL-17 in the treatment of RA.

CONTROL OF IL-17 WITH BIOTECHNOLOGY TOOLS

At the time of its discovery, two specific IL-17 inhibitors, a human anti-IL-17A monoclonal antibody (MAb) and a soluble receptor (sR) for mouse IL-17A, were already available to be tested *in vitro* and in animal models. Later new MAbs against the protein and the receptor and a sR for human IL-17A were obtained.

The use of these tools in animal and in *ex vivo* human models has provided the rationale for IL-17 inhibition in RA or other inflammatory diseases (Figure 15.3). In animal models, soluble IL-17 receptor and anti-IL-17 antibody treatment reduces severity, and joint damage.[54–56] In RA synovium and bone *ex vivo* models, addition of IL-17 inhibition reduces inflammation and destruction. As IL-1, TNF-α and IL-17 have many additive and/or synergistic effects *in vitro*, it was of interest to test whether their combined inhibition with sR would lead to an enhanced effect on *ex vivo* models of synovium inflammation and bone destruction, where RA synovium and bone explants are cultured in the presence of etanercept, the TNF-α p75 sR alone, and in combination with type II IL-1 sR and IL-17 sR.[57] In synovium, all three sR used alone decrease IL-6 production by approximately one-third and that of CTX by one-half. Combinations are more effective, inhibiting IL-6 production and collagen degradation by up to 70%. Similar results are obtained with bone explants. These results support the concept of combination therapy in the clinic, which may increase the percentage of responding patients as well as the degree of individual patient response.

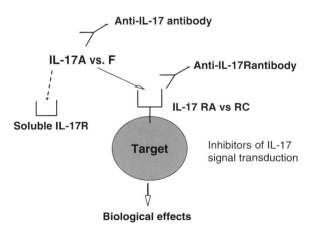

Figure 15.3 Specific inhibitors of IL-17 proteins and receptors.

IL-17 function is also inhibited by Th2 cytokines, which control IL-1 and TNF-α at the same time. Administration of IL-4 to mice with arthritis through gene therapy prevents bone erosion and diminishes the formation of osteoclast-like cells.[58] MRNA and protein levels of IL-17 and RANKL are markedly suppressed, leading to reduced osteoclast activation and finally bone destruction.

When selecting the available biotechnology products for trials, the respective contribution of IL-17F over IL-17A and that of IL-17RA over IL-17RC remain to be clarified.

Possible side effects

Inhibition of TNF has been associated with side effects. The most severe were infections, mostly with intracellular bacteria. Tuberculosis was the most common manifestation mostly, through reactivation.

The role of IL-17 in host defense appears to be different from that of TNF. IL-17 has a major effect on neutrophils. IL-17 induces the maturation of CD34 hematopoietic lymphoid and myeloid progenitors.[59] In the same way, IL-17 induces neutrophil accumulation in infected lungs. In addition, IL-17 activates neutrophils to produce chemokines and hematopoietic growth factors.[60] Mice deficient in the IL-17 receptor have an increased sensitivity and mortality to lung bacterial infection, suggesting a mechanism for CD4 T-cell defects associated with bacterial pneumonia.[61] In RA, the immune defect associated with TNF-α inhibition could be related to a role for IL-17 to control opportunistic infections such as tuberculosis. In this case, inhibition of TNF-α modifies the synergy of the cytokines acting on or produced by T cells.

These effects of IL-17 on host defense have to be considered carefully when inhibition of IL-17 is considered in patients where systemic immune defenses are already altered. Regarding potential side effects associated with IL-17 inhibition, blocking of IL-17 in humans may have limitations by reducing innate and T-cell-mediated immunity. This may affect the host defense, increasing the risk of neutrophils well as T-cell-mediated infections.[62] Results in models of tumor growth are too contradictory to evaluate

a possible risk in solid tumors and lymphomas when blocking IL-17.

WAITING FOR A TREATMENT

Regarding the contribution of T cells to RA, results with IL-17 have clarified this once highly discussed issue.[63] This proinflammatory cytokine is produced in the RA synovial membrane, by an infiltrating CD4+ T-cell subset. When in contact with synoviocytes, IL-17-producing T cells have an increased ability to favor destruction and to block repair activity. Furthermore, IL-17 produced by T lymphocytes from bone marrow contributes locally to juxta-articular bone destruction. Finally, IL-17 acts in synergy or additively with TNF-α and IL-1, increasing their production and action. Accordingly, inhibition of IL-17 could be beneficial in human RA, as has been demonstrated in many experimental models of RA. Tools for treatment are already available. A business strategic decision is needed to move forward. Combination therapy with the current cytokine inhibitors may be of interest to increase the rate and duration of response.

REFERENCES

1. Miossec P. Interleukin-17 in rheumatoid arthritis: if T cells were to contribute to inflammation and destruction through synergy. Arthritis Rheum 2003; 48: 594–601.
2. Yao Z, Painter SL, Fanslow Wc et al. Human IL-17: a novel cytokine derived from T cells. J Immunol 1995; 155: 5483–6.
3. Fossiez F, Djossou O, Chomarat P et al. T cell interleukin-17 induces stromal cells to produce proinflammatory and hematopoietic cytokines. J Exp Med 1996; 183: 2593–603.
4. Aggarwal S, Gurney AL. IL-17: prototype member of an emerging cytokine family. J Leukoc Biol 2002; 71: 1–8.
5. Starnes T, Broxmeyer HE, Robertson MJ, Hromas R. Cutting edge: IL-17D, a novel member of the IL-17 family, stimulates cytokine production and inhibits hemopoiesis. J Immunol 2002; 169: 642–6.
6. Owyang AM, Zaph C, Wilson EH et al. Interleukin 25 regulates type 2 cytokine-dependent immunity and limits chronic inflammation in the gastrointestinal tract. J Exp Med 2006; 203: 843–9.
7. Yao Z, Fanslow WC, Seldin MF et al. Herpesvirus Saimiri encodes a new cytokine, IL-17, which binds to a novel cytokine receptor. Immunity 1995; 3: 811–21.

8. Yao Z, Spriggs MK, Derry JM et al. Molecular characterization of the human interleukin (IL)-17 receptor. Cytokine 1997; 9: 794–800.

9. Toy D, Kugler D, Wolfson M et al. Cutting edge: interleukin 17 signals through a heteromeric receptor complex. J Immunol 2006; 177: 36–9.

10. Hwang SY, Kim JY, Kim KW et al. IL-17 induces production of IL-6 and IL-8 in rheumatoid arthritis synovial fibroblasts via NF-kappaB- and PI3-kinase/Akt-dependent pathways. Arthritis Res Ther 2004; 6: R120–8.

11. Schwandner R, Yamaguchi K, Cao Z. Requirement of tumor necrosis factor receptor-associated factor (TRAF)6 in interleukin 17 signal transduction. J Exp Med 2000; 191: 1233–40.

12. Kehlen A, Thiele K, Riemann D, Langner J. Expression, modulation and signalling of IL-17 receptor in fibroblast-like synoviocytes of patients with rheumatoid arthritis. Clin Exp Immunol 2002; 127: 539–46.

13. Shalom-Barak T, Quach J, Lotz M. Interleukin-17-induced gene expression in articular chondrocytes is associated with activation of mitogen-activated protein kinases and NF-kappaB. J Biol Chem 1998; 273: 27467–73.

14. Tan SL, Zhao J, Bi C et al. Resistance to experimental autoimmune encephalomyelitis and impaired IL-17 production in protein kinase C theta-deficient mice. J Immunol 2006; 176: 2872–9.

15. Molet S, Hamid Q, Davoine F et al. IL-17 is increased in asthmatic airways and induces human bronchial fibroblasts to produce cytokines. J Allergy Clin Immunol 2001; 108: 430–8.

16. Cua DJ, Sherlock J, Chen Y et al. Interleukin-23 rather than interleukin-12 is the critical cytokine for autoimmune inflammation of the brain. Nature 2003; 421: 744–8.

17. Chen Y, Langrish CL, McKenzie B et al. Anti-IL-23 therapy inhibits multiple inflammatory pathways and ameliorates autoimmune encephalomyelitis. J Clin Invest 2006; 116: 1317–26.

18. Langrish CL, Chen Y, Blumenschein WM et al. IL-23 drives a pathogenic T cell population that induces autoimmune inflammation. J Exp Med 2005; 201: 233–40.

19. Yen D, Cheung J, Scheerens H et al. IL-23 is essential for T cell-mediated colitis and promotes inflammation via IL-17 and IL-6. J Clin Invest 2006; 116: 1310–16.

20. Bettelli E, Carrier Y, Gao W et al. Reciprocal developmental pathways for the generation of pathogenic effector TH17 and regulatory T cells. Nature 2006; 441: 235–8.

21. Hoeve MA, Savage ND, de Boer T et al. Divergent effects of IL-12 and IL-23 on the production of IL-17 by human T cells. Eur J Immunol 2006; 36: 661–70.

22. Mathur AN, Chang HC, Zisoulis DG et al. T-bet is a critical determinant in the instability of the IL-17-secreting T-helper phenotype. Blood. 2006; 108: 1595–601.

23. Page G, Sattler A, Kersten S et al. Plasma cell-like morphology of Th1-cytokine-producing cells associated with the loss of CD3 expression. Am J Pathol 2004; 164: 409–17.

24. Chabaud M, Fossiez F, Taupin JL, Miossec P. Enhancing effect of IL-17 on IL-1-induced IL-6 and leukemia inhibitory factor production by rheumatoid arthritis synoviocytes and its regulation by Th2 cytokines. J Immunol 1998; 161: 409–14.

25. Martel-Pelletier J, Mineau F, Jovanovic D, Di Battista JA, Pelletier JP. Mitogen-activated protein kinase and nuclear factor kappaB together regulate interleukin-17-induced nitric oxide production in human osteoarthritic chondrocytes: possible role of transactivating factor mitogen-activated protein kinase-activated proten kinase (MAPKAPK). Arthritis Rheum 1999; 42: 2399–409.

26. LeGrand A, Fermor B, Fink C et al. Interleukin-1, tumor necrosis factor alpha, and interleukin-17 synergistically up-regulate nitric oxide and prostaglandin E2 production in explants of human osteoarthritic knee menisci. Arthritis Rheum 2001; 44: 2078–83.

27. Van bezooijen RL, Farih-Sips HC, Papapoulos SE, Lowik CW. Interleukin-17: a new bone acting cytokine in vitro. J Bone Miner Res 1999; 14: 1513–21.

28. Shen F, Hu Z, Goswami J, Gaffen SL. Identification of common transcriptional regulatory elements in interleukin-17 target genes. J Biol Chem. 2006; 281: 24138–48.

29. Chevrel G, Page G, Granet C et al. Interleukin-17 increases the effects of IL-1beta on muscle cells: arguments for the role of T cells in the pathogenesis of myositis. J Neuroimmunol 2003; 137: 125–33.

30. Granet C, Miossec P. Combination of the pro-inflammatory cytokines IL-1, TNF-alpha and IL-17 leads to enhanced expression and additional recruitment of AP-1 family members, Egr-1 and NF-kappaB in osteoblast-like cells. Cytokine 2004; 26: 169–77.

31. Granet C, Maslinski W, Miossec P. Increased AP-1 and NF-kappaB activation and recruitment with the combination of the proinflammatory cytokines IL-1beta, tumor necrosis factor alpha and IL-17 in rheumatoid synoviocytes. Arthritis Res Ther 2004; 6: R190–8.

32. Jovanovic DV, Di Battista JA, Martel-Pelletier J et al. IL-17 stimulates the production and expression of proinflammatory cytokines, IL-beta and TNF-alpha, by human macrophages. J Immunol 1998; 160: 3513–21.

33. Katz Y, Nadiv O, Beer Y. Interleukin-17 enhances tumor necrosis factor alpha-induced synthesis of interleukins 1,6, and 8 in skin and synovial fibroblasts: a possible role as a 'fine-tuning cytokine' in inflammation processes. Arthritis Rheum 2001; 44: 2176–84.

34. Chabaud M, Durand JM, Buchs N et al. Human interleukin-17: a T cell-derived proinflammatory cytokine produced by the rheumatoid synovium. Arthritis Rheum 1999; 42: 963–70.

35. Page G, Miossec P. RANK and RANKL expression as markers of dendritic cell-T cell interactions in paired samples of rheumatoid synovium and lymph nodes. Arthritis Rheum 2005; 52: 2307–12.

36. Kirkham BW, Lassere MN, Edmonds JP et al. Synovial membrane cytokine expression is predictive of joint damage progression in rheumatoid arthritis: a two-year prospective study (the DAMAGE study cohort). Arthritis Rheum 2006; 54: 1122–31.

37. Chabaud M, Page G, Miossec P. Enhancing effect of IL-1, IL-17, and TNF-alpha on macrophage inflammatory protein-3alpha production in rheumatoid arthritis: regulation by soluble receptors and Th2 cytokines. J Immunol 2001; 167: 6015–20.

38. Schnyder B, Schnyder-Candrian S, Pansky A et al. IL-17 reduces TNF-induced Rantes and VCAM-1 expression. Cytokine 2005; 31: 191–202.

39. Page G, Lebecque S, Miossec P. Anatomic localization of immature and mature dendritic cells in an ectopic lymphoid organ: correlation with selective chemokine expression in rheumatoid synovium. J Immunol 2002; 168: 5333–41.

40. Chabaud M, Garnero P, Dayer JM et al. Contribution of interleukin 17 to synovium matrix destruction in rheumatoid arthritis. Cytokine 2000; 12: 1092–9.

41. Attur MG, Patel RN, Abramson SB, Amin AR. Interleukin-17 up-regulation of nitric oxide production in human osteoarthritis cartilage. Arthritis Rheum 1997; 40: 1050–3.

42. Cai L, Yin JP, Starovasnik MA et al. Pathways by which interleukin 17 induces articular cartilage breakdown in vitro and in vivo. Cytokine 2001; 16: 10–21.

43. Rifas L, Avioli LV. A novel T cell cytokine stimulates interleukin-6 in human osteoblastic cells. J Bone Miner Res 1999; 14: 1096–103.

44. Van Bezooijen RL, Papapoulos SE, Lowik CW. Effect of interleukin-17 on nitric oxide production and osteoclastic bone resorption: is there dependency on nuclear factor-kappaB and receptor activator of nuclear factor kappaB (RANK)/RANK ligand signaling? Bone 2001; 28: 378–86.

45. Kotake S, Udagawa N, Takahashi N et al. IL-17 in synovial fluids from patients with rheumatoid arthritis is a potent stimulator of osteoclastogenesis. J Clin Invest 1999; 103: 1345–52.

46. Nakashima T, Kobayashi Y, Yamasaki S et al. Protein expression and functional difference of membrane-bound and soluble receptor activator of NF-kappaB ligand: modulation of the expression by osteotropic factors and cytokines. Biochem Biophys Res Commun 2000; 275: 768–75.

47. Romas E, Gillespie MT, Martin TJ. Involvement of receptor activator of NFkappaB ligand and tumor necrosis factor-alpha in bone destruction in rheumatoid arthritis. Bone 2002; 30: 340–6.

48. Chabaud M, Lubberts E, Joosten L, van Den Berg W, Miossec P. IL-17 derived from juxta-articular bone and synovium contributes to joint degradation in rheumatoid arthritis. Arthritis Res 2001; 3: 168–77.

49. Chabaud M, Aarvak T, Garnero P, Natvig JB, Miossec P. Potential contribution of IL-17-producing Th(1)cells to defective repair activity in joint inflammation: partial correction with Th(2)-promoting conditions. Cytokine 2001; 13: 113–18.

50. Lubberts E, Joosten LA, van de Loo FA, van den Gersselaar LA, van den Berg WB. Reduction of interleukin-17-induced inhibition of chondrocyte proteoglycan synthesis in intact murine articular cartilage by interleukin-4. Arthritis Rheum 2000; 43: 1300–6.

51. Lubberts E, Joosten LA, Oppers B et al. IL-1-independent role of IL-17 in synovial inflammation and joint destruction during collagen-induced arthritis. J Immunol 2001; 167: 1004–13.

52. Lubberts E, Joosten LA, van de Loo FA et al. Overexpression of IL-17 in the knee joint of collagen type II immunized mice promotes collagen arthritis and aggravates joint destruction. Inflamm Res 2002; 51: 102–4.

53. Koenders MI, Lubberts E, van de Loo FA et al. Interleukin-17 acts independently of TNF-alpha under arthritic conditions. J Immunol 2006; 176: 6262–9.

54. Bush KA, Farmer KM, Walker JS, Kirkham BW. Reduction of joint inflammation and bone erosion in rat adjuvant arthritis by treatment with interleukin-17 receptor IgG1 Fc fusion protein. Arthritis Rheum 2002; 46: 802–5.

55. Lubberts E, Koenders MI, Oppers-Walgreen B et al. Treatment with a neutralizing anti-murine interleukin-17 antibody after the onset of collagen-induced arthritis reduces joint inflammation, cartilage destruction, and bone erosion. Arthritis Rheum 2004; 50: 650–9.

56. Koenders MI, Lubberts E, Oppers-Walgreen B et al. Blocking of interleukin-17 during reactivation of experimental arthritis prevents joint inflammation and bone erosion by decreasing RANKL and interleukin-1. Am J Pathol 2005; 167: 141–9.

57. Chabaud M, Miossec P. The combination of tumor necrosis factor alpha blockade with interleukin-1 and interleukin-17 blockade is more effective for controlling synovial inflammation and bone resorption in an ex vivo model. Arthritis Rheum 2001; 44: 1293–303.

58. Lubberts E, Joosten LA, Chabaud M et al. IL-4 gene therapy for collagen arthritis suppresses synovial IL-17 and osteoprotegerin ligand and prevents bone erosion. J Clin Invest 2000; 105: 1697–710.

59. Schwarzenberger P, La Russa V, Miller A et al. IL-17 stimulates granulopoiesis in mice: use of an alternate,

novel gene therapy-derived method for in vivo evaluation of cytokines. J Immunol 1998; 161: 6383–9.

60. Jones CE, Chan K. Interleukin-17 stimulates the expression of interleukin-8, growth-related oncogene-alpha, and granulocyte-colony-stimulating factor by human airway epithelial cells. Am J Respir Cell Mol Biol 2002; 26: 748–53.

61. Ye P, Rodriguez FH, Kanaly S et al. Requirement of interleukin 17 receptor signaling for lung CXC chemokine and granulocyte colony-stimulating factor expression, neutrophil recruitment, and host defense. J Exp Med 2001; 194: 519–27.

62. Benchetrit F, Ciree A, Vives V et al. Interleukin-17 inhibits tumor cell growth by means of a T-cell-dependent mechanism. Blood 2002; 99: 2114–21.

63. Firestein GS, Zvaifler NJ. How important are T cells in chronic rheumatoid synovitis?: II. T cell-independent mechanisms from beginning to end. Arthritis Rheum 2002; 46: 298–308.

16

The role of interleukin-18 in inflammation

Charles A Dinarello

Summary • Introduction • IL-18 as an immunoregulatory cytokine • Acknowkedgments • References

SUMMARY

Several autoimmune diseases are thought to be mediated, in part, by interleukin (IL)-18. Many are those with associated elevated interferon-γ (IFN-γ) levels such as systemic lupus erythematosus (SLE), macrophage-activation syndrome, rheumatoid arthritis (RA), Crohn's disease, and psoriasis, as well as graft versus host disease (GVHD). In addition, ischemia, including acute renal failure in humans, appears to involve IL-18. Animal studies also support the concept that IL-18 is a key player in models of lupus erythematosus, atherosclerosis, GVHD, and hepatitis. Unexpectedly, IL-18 plays a role in appetite control and the development of obesity. IL-18 is a member of the IL-1 family; IL-1β and IL-18 are closely related, and both require the intracellular cysteine protease caspase-1 for biological activity. The IL-18 binding protein, a naturally occurring, specific inhibitor of IL-18, neutralizes IL-18 activities and has been shown to be safe in patients. Other options for reducing IL-18 activities are inhibitors of caspase-1, human monoclonal antibodies (mAbs) to IL-18, soluble IL-18 receptors, and anti-IL-18 receptor (mAbs).

INTRODUCTION

IL-18 is a member of the IL-1 family of cytokines and is structurally related to IL-1β.[1] Recently, a new member of the IL-1 family, IL-33, has been reported. Structurally IL-33 is closely related to IL-18,[2] but unlike IL-18, IL-33 binds to its own receptor, ST2, a long-time orphan receptor in the IL-1 family of cytokines.[2] The IL-1β and the IL-18 precursors require caspase-1 for cleavage, activity and release.[3–5] Therefore, anti-proteases that inhibit caspase-1 reduce the processing and release of IL-1β as well as IL-18. Now, IL-33 can be added to the list of members of the IL-1, which require caspase-1 for processing and release.[2] However, it is important to note that IL-18 is not a recapitulation of the biology or clinical significance of IL-1 or similar to the biological activity of IL-33; in fact, IL-18 is a unique cytokine exhibiting inflammatory as well as immunoregulatory processes distinct from IL-1β or IL-33. For example, IL-1β is not required for IFN-γ production, whereas IL-18 is required.[6] Initially considered primarily a Th1 polarizing cytokine, IL-18 is also relevant to Th2 diseases.[7] As discussed in this chapter, animal models reveal that targeting IL-18 holds promise for the treatment of autoimmune and inflammatory diseases.

IL-18 AS AN IMMUNOREGULATORY CYTOKINE

The importance of IL-18 as an immunoregulatory cytokine is derived from its prominent biological property of inducing IFN-γ. IL-18 was first described in 1989 in the serum following an injection of endotoxin into mice pretreated with *Proprionibacterium acnes* and shown to induce IFN-γ; however, at that time many investigators concluded that the serum factor was nothing but IL-12. With a great deal of diligence, the putative IFN-γ-inducing factor activity was purified from thousands of mouse livers and the N-terminal amino acid sequence revealed a unique cytokine, not IL-12. With molecular cloning of 'IFN-γ-inducing factor' in 1995,[1] the name was changed to IL-18. Surprisingly, the new cytokine was related to IL-1 and particularly to IL-1β. Both cytokines, lacking signal peptides, are first synthesized as inactive precursors, and neither is secreted via the Golgi. Following cleavage by caspase-1, the active 'mature' cytokines are released. Macrophages and dendritic cells (DCs) are the primary sources for active IL-18, but the IL-18 precursor is found constitutively expressed in epithelial cells throughout the body. Previously, it was thought that inhibition of caspase-1 as a therapeutic target was specific for reducing the activity of IL-1β but it became clear that IL-18 activity would also be affected. In fact, any phenotypic characteristic of caspase-1-deficient mice undergoing inflammatory challenges must be differentiated as due to reduced IL-1β or IL-18 activity. For example, the IL-1β-deficient mouse is susceptible to models of colitis, whereas the caspase-1-deficient mouse is resistant;[8] antibodies to IL-18 are protective, whereas the IL-1 receptor antagonist is not.[8,9]

Because of its role in the production of IFN-γ, T-cell polarization is a characteristic of IL-18, whereas IFN-γ induction is not a prominent characteristic of IL-1. IL-18 exhibits characteristics of other proinflammatory cytokines, such as increases in cell adhesion molecules, nitric oxide (NO) synthesis, and chemokine production. A unique property of IL-18 is the induction of Fas ligand (FasL). The induction of fever, an important clinical property of IL-1, tumor necros factor (TNF)-α, and IL-6, is not a property of IL-18. Injection of IL-18 into mice, rabbits, or humans does not produce fever.[10,11] Unlike IL-1 and TNF-α, IL-18 does not induce cyclooxygenase-2 and hence there is no production of prostaglandin E_2 (PGE_2).[12,13] IL-18 has been administered to humans for the treatment of cancer to increase the activity and expansion of cytotoxic T cells. Although the results of clinical trials are presently unknown, several preclinical studies reveal the benefit of IL-18 administration in certain models of rodent cancer. Not unexpectedly and similar to several cytokines, the therapeutic focus on IL-18 has shifted from its use as an immune stimulant to inhibition of its activity.

Because IL-18 can increase IFN-γ production, blocking IL-18 activity in autoimmune diseases is potentially an attractive therapeutic target. However, anti-IL-12 has been shown to reduce the severity of Crohn's disease as well as psoriasis. Therefore, IL-12 can induce IFN-γ in the absence of IL-18. However, there are many models of IL-18 activity independent of IFN-γ. For example, we have recently reported a new cytokine, IL-32, which was discovered in the total absence of IL-12 or IFN-γ.[14] Furthermore, a model of inhibition of proteoglycan synthesis is IL-18-dependent but IFN-γ-independent.[15] In addition, IL-18-dependent melanoma metastasis to the liver is IFN-γ-independent.[16] The results of preclinical studies and the targeting of IL-18 to treat autoimmune and inflammatory diseases will be discussed in this chapter.

Role of IL-18 in the loss of insulin-producing β cells

Several studies report that the levels of IL-18 in various transplant models, as well as in kidney transplant patients, correlate with graft failure. Using mice that overproduce IL-18BP as diabetic islet graft recipients, it was reported that IL-18 indeed plays a role in the damage inflicted upon transplanted islets. In view of the wide distribution of IL-18 producer cells, it was essential to identify the cellular sources of damaging IL-18. To address this issue directly, islets from IL-18-deficient mice were transplanted into wild-type recipient mice, resulting in a greater survival compared with wild-type islets transplanted into wild-type mice.[17] This finding supports the concept of local endogenous islet IL-18 being sufficient to promote β cell injury during islet transplantation. In fact, lack of islet-derived IL-18 from grafted islets resulted in a similar outcome to that obtained by reduced activity of IL-18 in mice transgenic for IL-18BP, suggesting that host-derived IL-18 plays a negligible role in islet graft failure.[17]

Therapeutic strategies for reducing IL-18 activities

The strategies for reducing IL-18 activity include neutralizing anti-IL-18 mAbs, caspase-1 inhibitors, and blocking antibodies to the IL-18 receptor chains. Caspase-1 inhibitors are oral agents and presently in clinical trials in RA a reduction in the signs and symptoms of the disease has been observed. Caspase-1 inhibitors prevent the release of active IL-1β and IL-18 and therefore may derive clinical benefit by reducing the activities of both cytokines.[3,4,18] A naturally occurring IL-18 binding protein (IL-18BP) was discovered in 1999; IL-18BP is effective in neutralizing IL-18 activity.[19] IL-18BP is not a soluble form of either chain of the IL-18 receptor but rather a constitutively secreted, high affinity, and specific inhibitor of IL-18.[20,21] IL-18BP is currently in clinical trials for the treatment of RA and severe psoriasis. Although the results of these trials have not been published, in phase I and phase II clinical trials IL-18BP was safe even at the highest doses in over 6 weeks of treatment.

Caspase-1 and non-caspase-1 processing of IL-18

The importance of caspase-1 in inflammation has been revealed in patients with mutations in the NALP3 gene locus, which participates in the conversion of procaspase-1 to active caspase-1. Single amino acid point mutations in the gene product result in increased processing and release of IL-1β.[22] Clinical manifestations include mental retardation, hearing loss, exquisite sensitivity to cold, and deforming arthritis.[23] Some patients have extremely high levels of serum amyloid A protein with renal deposits and terminal renal failure; within a few days of IL-1 blockade using the IL-1 receptor antagonist, these patients exhibit a near total reversal in both the symptoms and the biochemical abnormalities of the disease.[24] It remains likely that IL-18 also contributes to disease in these patients.

The non-caspase-1 enzyme associated with processing both the IL-1β and the IL-18 precursors is proteinase-3 (PR-3).[25] Agonistic autoantibodies to PR-3 are pathological in Wegener's granulomatosis and may contribute to the non-caspase-1 cleavage of the IL-18 precursor and IFN-γ production in this disease. Epithelial cells stimulated with PR-3 in the presence of endotoxin release active IL-18 into the supernatant.[26] Since lactate dehydrogenase activity is not released, the appearance of active IL-18 is not due to cell leakage or death. Injecting mice with recombinant FasL results in hepatic damage, which is IL-18-dependent.[27] However, FasL-mediated cell death is IL-18-dependent, caspase-1-independent,[27] but ischemia-reperfusion injury resulting in cell death is via an IL-18- and caspase-1-dependent pathway.[28,29]

P2X7 receptor targeting

The P2X7 receptor is involved in the secretion of IL-1β as well as IL-18.[30–32] Stimulation of this receptor by ATP is a well-described event in the release of IL-1β as well as IL-18. A tyrosine derivative named KN-62 exhibits selective P2X7 receptor-blocking properties.[33] In a study of small molecule inhibitors of this receptor, analogs of KN-62-related compounds were characterized for their ability to affect the human P2X7 receptor on monocyte-derived human macrophages.[33] Although several analogs inhibited the secretion of IL-1β, no data exist on the effect of these inhibitors on IL-18 secretion.[33] Unlike IL-1β, the secretion of IL-18 has mostly been studied *in vivo* in mice that have been treated with *Cryptosporidium parvum*,[4] rather than *in vitro*. *In vitro*, the release of IL-18 requires the presence of activated T cells.[34,35]

Targeting the IL-18 receptors

Antibodies to either chain of the IL-18 receptor complex are attractive options for treating IL-18-mediated diseases. The IL-18 receptor chains (IL-18Rα and IL-18Rβ) are members of the IL-1 receptor family. The binding sites for IL-18 to the IL-18 receptor α chain are similar to those for IL-1 binding to the IL-1 receptor type I.[36–38] Two sites bind to the ligand binding chain (IL-18Rα) and a third site binds to the IL-18Rβ chain, also called the signal transducing chain. The intracellular chains of the IL-18 receptors contain the Toll domains, which are essential for initiating signal transduction (see Figure 16.1).

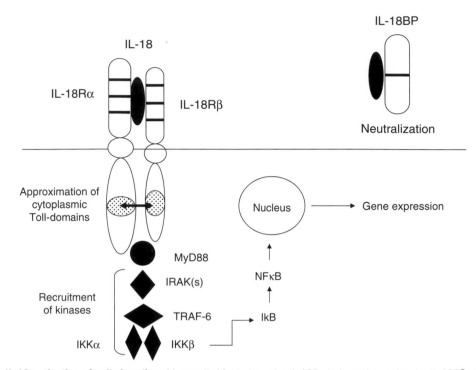

Figure 16.1 IL-18 activation of cell signaling. Mature IL-18 binds to the IL-18R chain and recruits the IL-18Rβ chain, resulting in the formation of a heterodimeric complex. As a result of the formation of the extracellular complex, the intracellular chains also form a complex which brings the Toll domains of each receptor chain into close proximity. Although poorly understood, the close proximity of the Toll domains recruits the intracellular protein MyD88 to the receptor chains. MyD88 is common to cells activated by IL-1, IL-18, and TLR-4 ligands (endotoxins). Following MyD88 recruitment, there is a rapid phosphorylation of the IL-1 receptor activating kinases (IRAKs). There are four IRAK proteins. Depending on the cell type, other kinases have been reported to undergo phosphorylation. These are the TNF receptor activating factor (TRAF)-6 and inhibitory kappa B kinases (IKK) α and β (not shown). Phosphorylation of IKK results in the phosphorylation of IkB and translocation of NF-κB to the nucleus. However, this is not observed uniformly in all cell types and there are distinct differences in NF-κB activation in different cells stimulated with IL-18.[13] In addition, IL-18-activated cells phosphorylate mitogen-activating protein kinase (MAPK) p38. In IL-18-activated cells, new genes are expressed and translated. Those shown in the figure represent the proinflammatory genes. Preventing IL-18-induced cellular activation is accomplished by the presence of IL-18BP. IL-18BP is present in the extracellular milieu as a constitutively expressed protein where it can bind and neutralize IL-18, thus preventing activation of the cell surface receptors. In addition, formation of inactive complexes of IL-18BP with IL-18 and the IL-18Rβ chain deprives the cell of the participation of IL-18Rβ chain in activating the cell.

The Toll domains of the IL-18 receptors are similar to the same domains of the Toll-like receptors, which recognize various microbial products, viruses, and nucleic acids. As a therapeutic option, however, commercial antibodies generated to the IL-18 receptor α and β chains are 100-fold less effective in neutralizing IL-18 activity compared with the IL-18BP.[39] Nevertheless, the development of blocking antibodies to IL-18 receptor chains remains a viable therapeutic option, since an antibody to the type I IL-1 receptor chain is in clinical trials in RA.

Unless converted into a fusion protein in somewhat the same manner as that of other soluble cytokine receptors, it is unlikely that the soluble form of the monomeric form of the IL-18Rα is a candidate therapeutic agent due to its low affinity. Another member of the IL-1 family (IL-1F), IL-1F7,[40] may be the naturally occurring receptor antagonist of IL-18. IL-1F7 binds to the IL-18Rα chain with a high affinity but this binding does not recruit the IL-18Rβ chain. The occupancy of the IL-18Rα without formation of the heterodimer with the IL-18Rβ is the same mechanism by which the IL-1 receptor antagonist prevents the activity of IL-1. But IL-1F7 does not affect the activity of IL-18[41,42] and the biological significance of IL-1F7 binding to the IL-18Rα remains unclear. However, in the presence of low concentrations of IL-18BP, IL-1F7 reduces the activity of IL-18.[43]

Deficiency in IL-18 and IL-18 receptor reveal distinctly opposing phenotypes

An unexpected finding surfaced upon transplantation of islets from IL-18R-deficient mice into wild-type recipient mice.[17] It was anticipated that implantation of islets that lack IL-18R would result in a similar protected phenotype to that of IL-18 deficient islets. However, graft failure in IL-18R-deficient islets was accelerated compared with islets from wild-type donors.[17] Remarkably, the median survival time of IL-18R-deficient islets grafted into a wild-type diabetic host was 9 days, whereas the median survival time of IL-18-deficient islets in a wild-type host was 14.5 days.[17] One explanation is that excess IL-18 from IL-18R-deficient islets exits into the surrounding host tissue where it triggers the production of IL-18-induced injurious mediators. In fact, IL-18R-deficient islets spontaneously produce twofold greater IL-18 levels. IL-18R-deficient splenocytes also produced more IL-18 than wild-type cells. However, isolated IL-18R-deficient macrophages, although unresponsive to IL-18, produced more TNF-α than wild-type macrophages *in vitro*. This finding challenges the underlying assumption that the IL-18R is specific to the IL-18 pathway, and prompted further dissection of the differences between IL-18- and IL-18R-deficient cells.

Alternate signaling of IL-18R

The unexpected increase in islet failure, observed in wild-type mice transplanted with islets from IL-18R-deficient mice, was associated with increased spontaneous production of IL-18 from IL-18R-deficient islets and splenocytes, and of TNF-α from macrophages. Splenocytes from 18R-deficient mice stimulated *in vitro* by concanavalin A (ConA), Toll-like receptor-2 engagement, or by anti-CD3 antibodies consistently produced more proinflammatory cytokines compared with wild-type, whereas IL-18-deficient cells produced less than wild-type.[17] For example, IL-18R-deficient splenocytes released nearly threefold greater TNF-α and MIP-1α than IL-18-deficient cells upon stimulation by *Staphylococcus epidermidis*.

The divergence of responses between IL-18R- and IL-18-deficient cells is unexplained. More likely, the data suggest the existence of an IL-18-independent inhibitory pathway that converges with the IL-18 pathway at the IL-18R. Accordingly, in cells deficient in the receptor, a putative inhibitory signal, along with the proinflammatory IL-18 signal pathway, is absent. Gutcher et al. also provided clear evidence that an IL-18-independent engagement of IL-18R exists.[44] In murine experimental autoimmune encephalomyelitis (EAE), IL-18-deficient mice are susceptible to disease progression whereas IL-18R-deficient mice are protected. As such, these investigators concluded that there are two distinct pathways converging on the IL-18R: one signal requires IL-18 and the other involves an unknown ligand.

The study comparing islet survival in IL-18- and 18R-deficient mice differs from the EAE model in several aspects. Islets from mice deficient in IL-18 or IL-18R implanted into a wild-type animal allows for responses of an intact immune system to the genetically altered cells. In the EAE, altered immune system responses are inherent to the knockout gene. Additionally, in the transplanted islet, early responding cells, such as macrophages, most probably mediate damage; the EAE model provides insights into mechanisms of cell-mediated, autoimmune processes. Nevertheless, with striking similarity to data presented here, deficiency in IL-18R chain confers an opposite phenotype to that observed in IL-18 deficiency.

Whether the convergence upon IL-18Rα chain involves a second ligand or a novel receptor accessory chain is presently unknown. IL-1F7, a member of IL-1 family with significant sequence homology with IL-18, binds to IL-18BP and IL-18Rα chain.[41,43] Upon binding to IL-18R, IL-1F7 does not induce IFN-γ production and exhibits no apparent competition with IL-18.[41] The combination of IL-18BP and IL-1F7 results in greater inhibition of IL-18 activity compared with IL-18BP alone, conferring on IL-1F7 the property of a naturally occurring modulator of IL-18 activity.[41] For any signal in the IL-1 family of receptors to occur, an accessory chain is recruited, the binding of which in this case would result in inhibition of IL-18 activity. Whether the accessory chain is the established IL-18Rβ chain or a novel receptor chain is yet undetermined. Indeed, it was reported that mixing IL-1F7 with soluble IL-18Rα and IL-18Rβ chains did not result in a ternary complex, as formed in the presence of IL-18 and the same receptor subunits. Therefore, we speculate that the accessory receptor chain recruited for IL-1F7 is novel. This model provides a mechanism by which lack of IL-18Rα chain results in the loss of a negative signal, accompanied by the appearance of a heightened inflammatory response.

IL-18 binding protein

The discovery of the IL-18BP took place during the search for the extracellular (soluble) receptors for IL-18 in human urine. Nearly all the soluble cytokine receptors are found in human urine.[45] For example, the TNF p75 soluble receptor, used widely for the treatment of RA, ankylosing spondylitis, and psoriasis, was initially purified and sequenced using ligand-specific affinity chromatography.[46] In searching for IL-18 soluble receptors, IL-18 was covalently bound to a matrix and highly concentrated human urine, donated by Italian nuns, was passed over the matrix and eluted with acid to disrupt the ligand (in this case IL-18) for its soluble receptors. Unexpectedly, instead of the elution of soluble forms of the cell surface IL-18 receptors, the IL-18BP

was discovered.[19] This was due to the higher affinity of the IL-18BP for the ligand compared with the soluble receptors.

The IL-18BP is a constitutively secreted protein, with a high affinity (400 pM) binding to IL-18. There is very limited amino acid sequence homology between IL-18BP and the cell surface IL-18 receptors; IL-18BP lacks a transmembrane domain and contains only one Ig-like domain.[21,47] IL-18BP shares many characteristics with the soluble form of the IL-1 type II receptor in that both function as decoys to prevent the binding of their respective ligands to the signaling receptor chains.[48] In fact, there is limited amino acid homology between IL-18BP and the IL-1 receptor type II, suggesting a common ancestor. In humans, IL-18BP is highly expressed in spleen and the intestinal tract, both immunologically active tissues.[19] Alternate mRNA splicing of IL-18BP results in four isoforms.[19,21] Of considerable importance is that the prominent 'a' isoform is present in the serum of healthy humans at a 20-fold molar excess compared with IL-18.[20] This level of IL-18BP may contribute to a default mechanism by which a Th1 response to foreign organisms is blunted to reduce triggering an autoimmune response to a routine infection. The promoter for IL-18BP contains two IFN-γ response elements [49] and constitutive gene expression for IL-18BP is IFN-γ-dependent,[50] suggesting a compensatory feedback mechanism. Thus elevated levels of IFN-γ stimulate more IL-18BP in an attempt to reduce IL-18-mediated IFN-γ production. For example, in mice deficient in IFN regulatory factor-1, a transcription factor for IFN-γ, low to absent tissue levels of IL-18BP are found compared with wild-type mice.[51] These IFN regulatory factor-1 deficient mice are exquisitely sensitive to colitis but when treated with exogenous IL-18BP, exhibit reduced disease.[52]

Viral IL-18BP

The most convincing evidence that IL-18 is a major player in inflammatory conditions and that IL-18BP is functional in combating inflammation comes from a natural experiment in humans. *Molluscum contagiosum* is a common viral infection of the skin often seen in children and in individuals with HIV-1 infection.

The infection is characterized by raised but bland eruptions; there are large numbers of viral particles in the epithelial cells of the skin but histologically there are few inflammatory or immunologically active cells in or near the lesions. Clearly, the virus fails to elicit an inflammatory or immunological response. A close amino acid similarity exists between human IL-18BP and a gene found in various members of the Poxviruses. The greatest homology is with *Molluscum contagiosum*.[19,53,54] The viral genes encoding for viral IL-18BP have been expressed and the recombinant proteins neutralize mammalian IL-18 activity.[53,.54] The ability of viral IL-18BP to reduce the activity of mammalian IL-18 likely explains the lack of inflammatory and immune cells in the infected skin and the blandness of the lesions. One may conclude from this natural experiment of *Molluscum contagiosum* infection that blocking IL-18 reduces immune and inflammatory processes such as the function of DCs and inflammatory cells.

IL-18:IL-18BP imbalance in macrophage-activating syndrome

Also known as hemophagocytic syndrome, macrophage-activating syndrome (MAS) is characterized by an uncontrolled and poorly understood activation of Th1 lymphocytes and macrophages. In a study of 20 patients with MAS secondary to infections, autoimmune disease, lymphoma, or cancer, the concentrations of circulating IL-18, IL-18BP, IFN-γ, and IL-12 were determined and matched with clinical parameters. Evidence of stimulation of macrophages and natural killer (NK) cells was highly increased in MAS but not in control patients. Most importantly, concentrations of IL-18BP were only moderately elevated, resulting in a high level of biologically active free IL-18[20] in MAS (4.6-fold increase compared with controls ($p < 0.001$). Others have reported marked expression of IL-18 in fatal MAS.[55] Free IL-18 but not IL-12 concentrations significantly correlated with clinical status and the biological markers of MAS such as anemia, hypertriglyceridemia, and hyperferritinemia, and also with markers of Th1 lymphocyte or macrophage activation such as elevated concentrations of IFN-γ, soluble IL-2,

and TNF receptor concentrations. Therefore, treatment of life-threatening MAS with IL-18BP is a logical therapeutic intervention to correct the severe IL-18:IL-18BP imbalance resulting in Th1 lymphocyte and macrophage activation.

Neutralizing antibodies to IL-18

Although there are no clinical trials of neutralizing antibodies to IL-18, preclinical studies have employed IL-18 antibodies to reduce IL-18 activity in animal models of disease. The results of these studies are shown in Table 16.1. Assuming that neutralizing antibodies to IL-18 are developed and tested in human diseases, what are the anticipated differences between a neutralizing antibody and a neutralizing soluble receptor or a binding protein such as IL-18BP? First, to evaluate such differences, the agent with the highest affinity is preferable. From a pharmacokinetic viewpoint, a long half-life is preferable. One can increase the binding affinity for a ligand by converting a soluble receptor or binding protein to a divalent fusion protein. However, the danger here is the increased risk of creating a novel epitope for antibody production. The advantage of mAbs is that they are human and the risk of developing antibodies to a human antibody is reduced significantly. At first glance, one would conclude that high affinity human antibodies to IL-18 are preferable to the IL-18BP. However, if a divalent fusion protein of IL-18BP has a high affinity and is not immunogenic, the next issue is a comparison of the half-life of a mAb to that of a fusion protein. Here the issue is one of safety. A short half-life is preferential for rapid cessation of therapy in the event of a life-threatening infection, whereas long half-life antibodies exert their effects of suppressing host defense for weeks. In fact, the large body of evidence for comparing infections associated with anti-TNF-α mAbs (infliximab or adalimumab) to the soluble TNF p75 receptor fusion protein (etanercept) may, in part, be due to differences in half-life as well as mechanism of action.[56] In the case of neutralizing IL-18, the suppression of IFN-γ is of concern for host defense against intracellular organisms such as *Mycobacterium tuberculosis*.[57]

Table 16.1 Reduction in disease severity with blocking of endogenous IL-18 activity

Disease model	Intervention	Outcome
Acute DSS-induced colitis	anti-IL-18 antibodies[9]; IL-18BP[84]	↓ clinical disease; ↓ TNFα, IFNγ, IL-1, MIP-1,2
Chronic DSS-induced colitis	casp-1 KO[8]	↓ IL-1β, IFNγ and CD3 cells
TNBS colitis colitis-induced colitis	IL-18BP[85]	↓ clinical disease; ↓ cytokines
CD62/CD4 T-cell-induced colitis	adenoviral antisense IL-18[86]	↓ clinical disease; ↓ mucosal IFNγ
Streptococcal wall-induced arthritis	IL-18 antibodies[15]	↑ cartilage proteoglycan synthesis ↓ inflammation;
Collagen-induced arthritis	IL-18BP; IL-18[59]; Ad-viral IL-18BP[87]	↓ clinical disease; ↓ cytokines
Collagen-induced arthritis	IL-18 deficient mice[58]	↓ clinical disease; ↓ cytokines
Graft versus host disease	anti-18[65]	↓ CD8+-mediated mortality
Lupus prone mice	IL-18 vaccination[60]	↓ mortality; ↓ nephritis
Allergic airway hyperresponsiveness	IL-18 vaccination [88]	↓ bronchocontriction
Experimental myasthenia gravis	anti- IL-18[89]	↓ clinical disease
Autoimmune encephalomyelitis	casp-1 KO[90]; casp-1 inhibition[90]	↓ clinical disease; ↓ IFNγ
Con-A-induced hepatitis	anti-18[91]; IL-18BP[27]; IL-18BP-Tg[92]	↓ liver enzymes
Fas-mediated hepatic failure	IL-18 deficient mice[93]; IL-18BP[27]	↓ liver necrosis
Pseudomonas exotoxin-A hepatitis	IL-18BP[27]	↓ liver enzymes; ↓ IFNγ
IL-12-induced IFNγ	anti-18[94]; casp-1 KO[94]	↓ IFNγ
Endotoxin-induced IFNγ	anti-18[1, 95]; IL-18BP[19, 27]; casp-1 KO	↓ IFNγ
LPS-induced hepatic necrosis	anti-IL-18 monoclonal [1, 95]; IL-18BP[27]	↓ necrosis; ↓ TNFα; ↓ FasL
LPS -induced lung neutrophils	IL-18[95]	↑ survival; ↓ myeloperoxidase
Melanoma hepatic metastasis	IL-18BP [16, 96]	↓ metastatic foci; ↓ VCAM-1
Ischemia-induced hepatic failure	anti-18[97]	↓ apoptosis; ↓ NFκB
Ischemia-induced acute renal failure	anti-IL-18 polyclonal [29]; casp-1 KO[29]	↓ creatinine; ↓ urea
Ischemic myocardial dysfunction	IL-18BP[28]; casp-1 inhibition[28]	↑ myocardial contractility
LPS-induced myocardial suppression	anti-IL-18 polyclonal [72]	↑ heart contractility; ↓ IL-1β
Atherosclerosis in ApoE KO mice	IL-18BP[77]	↓ plaques; ↓ infiltrates ↑ vessel collagen
Islet allograft rejection	IL-18 deficient [17]	↓ rejection

Blocking IL-18 in disease models

As with any cytokine, its role in a particular disease process is best assessed by employing specific neutralization of the cytokine in a complex disease model. Although mice deficient in IL-18 have been generated and tested for the development of autoimmune diseases,[58] any reduction in severity may be due to a reduction in the immune response such as antigens or the sensitization process itself and does not address the effect of IL-18 on established disease. IL-18 neutralization in wild-type mice is effective in reducing collagen-induced arthritis[59] as well as inflammatory arthritis.[15] Inflammatory arthritis is of particular relevance since this is a model of cartilage loss due to decreased proteoglycan

synthesis and is independent of IFN-γ. IL-18 contributes to the lupus-like disease in mice[60] via IFN-γ production. There are other models based on a reduction in IL-18 activity in wild-type mice. Caspase-1-deficient mice provide useful models for disease[6,29] but here the effect may be on IL-1β, IL-18, or both.

Most investigations initially focused on IL-18 in Th1-mediated diseases in which IFN-γ plays a prominent role. However, it soon became clear that blocking IL-18 resulted in reduction of disease severity in models where IFN-γ has no significant role or in mice deficient in IFN-γ. For example, IL-18-mediated loss of cartilage synthesis in arthritis models is IFN-γ-independent.[15] Prevention of melanoma metastases is IL-18-dependent but IFN-γ-independent,[16] and similar findings exist for ischemia-reperfusion injury in the heart, kidney, and liver. Table 16.1 lists various animal models of Th1-, Th2-, and non-immune-mediated disease where the effect of reducing endogenous IL-18 activities has been reported.

IL-18 in Th1-like diseases

In driving the Th1 response, IL-18 appears to act in association with IL-12 or IL-15, as IL-18 alone does not induce IFN-γ. The effect of IL-12 is, in part, to increase the expression of IL-18 receptors on T lymphocytes, thymocytes, and NK cells.[7,61,62] It appears that the role of IL-18 in the polarization of the Th1 response is dependent on IFN-γ and IL-12 receptor β2 chain expression. The production of IFN-γ by the combination of IL-18 plus IL-12 is an example of true synergism in cytokine biology, similar to the synergism of IL-1 and TNF-α in models of inflammation. Since IFN-γ is the 'signature' cytokine of CD4[+] and CD8[+] T cells as well as NK cells, a great deal of the biology of IL-18 is considered to be due to IFN-γ production. DCs deficient in the IFN-γ transcription factor T bet exhibit impaired IFN-γ production after stimulation with IL-18 plus IL-12.[63] IL-18 is constitutively present in monocytes and monocyte-derived type 1 DCs. Thus, IFN-γ induced by the combination of IL-12 plus IL-18 appears to be via the T bet transcription factor.

Graft versus host disease

IFN-γ plays a major pathological role in this disease due to its Th1-inducing properties and the generation of cytotoxic T cells. Using a cohort of 157 patients who received unrelated donor bone marrow transplantation and developed GVHD, a polymorphism in the IL-18 promoter (G137C, C607A, G656T) was identified and associated with statistically significantly decreased risk of death.[64] One hundred days after the transplant, the mortality in patients with this polymorphism was 23% compared with 48% in those patients without the polymorphism and after 1 year the mortality was 36% versus 65%, respectively. The probability of the survival was twofold in patients with this haplotype.[64] In the case of GVHD in mice, paradoxical effects of IL-18 have been reported depending on whether the disease is CD4[+] or CD8[+] T-cell-mediated. In humans, T cells are responsible for the disease following allogeneic bone marrow transplantation. Administration of IL-18 to recipient mice increased survival in CD4[+]-mediated disease but resulted in worsening in the CD8[+]-mediated disease.[65] Neutralizing anti-IL-18 mAbs significantly reduced CD8[+]-mediated mortality.[65] Administration of IL-18 reduces the severity of the disease by inducing the production of Th2 cytokines.[66] The importance of IL-18 in GVHD was also demonstrated in mice deficient in the IL-18 receptor α chain (Table 16.2). Other models of disease in mice deficient in this receptor chain are listed in Table 16.2.

Table 16.2 Studies on IL-18 receptor deficient mice[1]

Model	Observation	Reference
Th1 response	↓ IFNγ production; ↓ cytotoxicity	98
IL-18/IL-2-induced lung injury	↓ lethality	99
Graph vs. Host Disease	↓ disease severity	100
Lupus-prone mice	↓ disease lethality; ↓ nephritis	101
NK-mediated cytotoxicty in vivo[2]	↓ cytotoxicty	102
dextran sulphate sodium colitis	↑ disease and lethality	103
Islet allograft rejection	↑ rejection	17

[1] Unless stated otherwise, IL-18 receptor deficient mice lack the IL-18Rα chain.
[2] Mice are deficient in IL-18 receptor beta chain

IL-18 and Th2 diseases

The combination of IL-18 plus IL-12 suppresses IgE synthesis via IFN-γ production and suggests a role for IL-18 in Th2 polarization. For example, in models of allergic asthma, injecting IL-12 plus IL-18 suppresses IgE synthesis, eosinophilia, and airway hyperresponsiveness, as reviewed by Nakanishi et al.[7] In contrast, the administration of IL-18 *alone* enhanced basophil production of IL-4 and histamine and increased serum IgE levels in wild-type and IL-4-deficient mice.[67] Overexpression of mature IL-18 in the skin results in worsening of allergic and non-allergic cutaneous inflammation via Th2 cytokines.[68] Mice overexpressing IL-18 or overexpressing caspase-1 develop an atopic-like dermatitis with mastocytosis and the presence of Th2 cytokines. Elevated serum IgE was also present in these mice.[69] Although IL-18 remains a Th1 cytokine, there are increasing reports showing a role for IL-18 in promoting Th2-mediated diseases.[70] Upon neutralization of IL-18 in cocultures of type 1 DCs with allogeneic naive T lymphocytes the Th1/Th2 phenotype was not affected, whereas anti-IL-12 down-regulated the Th1 response.[71] In fact, IL-18 receptors were expressed on DCs of the type 2 lineage, suggesting a Th2 response.[71]

IL-18 and the heart

Unexpectedly, IL-18 is an important cytokine in myocardial ischemia reperfusion injury, a model of acute infarctions, where it functions to decrease the contractile force of the heart. It appears that the role of IL-18 in myocardial dysfunction is independent of IFN-γ but likely related to the induction of FasL. Human heart tissue contains preformed IL-18 in macrophages and endothelial cells.[28] Upon reducing IL-18 activity with either IL-18BP or a caspase-1 inhibitor, the functional impairment of the ischemia-reperfusion injury was reduced.[28] A neutralizing anti-IL-18 polyclonal antibody resulted in near prevention of endotoxin-induced myocardial suppression in mice and myocardial IL-1β levels were also reduced.[72] Using caspase-1-deficient mice subjected to ligation of the left anterior decending coronary artery as a model for myocardial infarction, significantly lower mortality was observed in the deficient mice compared with the wild-type mice.[73] Caspase-1-deficient mice also had lower levels of IL-18, metalloproteinase (MMP)-3 activity, and myocyte apoptosis following the injury. In humans, myocardial tissue steady-state levels of IL-18, IL-18Rα chain, and IL-18BP mRNA and their respective protein levels were measured in patients with end-stage heart failure. Circulating plasma and myocardial tissue levels of IL-18 were increased in the patients compared with age-matched healthy subjects.[74] However, mRNA levels of IL-18 BP were decreased in the failing myocardium. In fact, plasma IL-18 levels were significantly higher in patients who died compared with levels in survivors.[74]

There is increasing evidence that IL-18 contributes to atherosclerosis. Unlike the IFN-γ-independent role of IL-18 in ischemic heart disease, the atherosclerotic process involves infiltration of the arterial wall by macrophages and T cells and IFN-γ has been identified in the plaque and considered essential for the disease.[75] Human atherosclerotic plaques from the coronary arteries exhibit increased IL-18 and IL-18 receptors compared with non-diseased segments of the same artery.[76] The post-caspase-1 cleavage IL-18 was found to colocalize with macrophages, whereas IL-18 receptors were expressed on endothelial and smooth muscle cells. The localization of IL-18 and IL-18 receptors in smooth muscle cells is an unexpected but important finding for the pathogenesis of atherosclerosis.[75,76]

Atherosclerotic arterial lesions with infiltrating, lipid-laden macrophages as well as T cells develop spontaneously in male apolipoprotein E (apoE)-deficient mice fed a normal diet. When injected for 30 days with IL-18, these mice exhibited a doubling of the lesion size without a change in serum cholesterol.[75] There was also a fourfold increase in infiltrating T cells. However, when apoE-deficient mice were back-crossed into IFN-γ-deficient mice, the IL-18-induced increase in lesion size was not observed.[75] Although exogenous administration of IL-18 worsened the disease, such an experimental design can be related to the dose of IL-18. Therefore, reduction of natural levels of IL-18 in the apoE-deficient mice is a more rigorous assessment for a role of IL-18 in atherosclerosis. Using apoE-deficient mice and overexpression of IL-18BP by transfection with an IL-18BP-containing plasmid, reduced numbers of infiltrating macrophages and T cells as well as decreases in cell death and lipid content of the plaques were found.[77] In addition, increases in smooth muscle cells and collagen content suggested a stable plaque phenotype with prevention of progression in this well-established model of human coronary artery disease.

IL-18 and renal ischemia

Like myocardial ischemia-reoxygenation, there is an unexpected role in renal ischemia for IL-18, which is independent of T cells and IFN-γ. Clinically, loss of renal function in patients with septic shock contributes to mortality significantly. IL-18 was measured in patients with acute renal failure as well as patients with poor renal function. There was a remarkably high level of urinary IL-18 compared with other renal diseases ($p < 0.001$).[78] IL-18 was also elevated in the urine of patients with delayed function of cadaveric transplants.[78] The conclusion of the study was that urinary IL-18 is a marker for proximal tubular injury in acute renal failure.

In a large clinical study in intensive care units (ICUs), the level of IL-18 in the urine of patients correlated with the development of renal failure more than creatinine as a predictor of impending renal failure.[79] More impressively, based on IL-18 urine levels, it was possible to predict mortality in the ICU by 48 hours, a time period nearly 2 days before other indicators of impending death. These findings in humans are consistent with animal studies. Using a reversible model of acute renal failure, mice deficient in caspase-1 were protected[29] which was due to impaired processing of the IL-18 precursor by caspase-1. Furthermore, wild-type mice were also protected by a preinfusion of neutralizing anti-IL-18 polyclonal antibodies.[29] Protection was not afforded by administration of the IL-1 receptor antagonist and therefore the model reflects the role of IL-18 rather than IL-1β processing. Although the mechanism for the role of IL-18 in causing acute renal failure remains

unclear, it is not related to a decrease in neutrophilic infiltration.

Cardiopulmonary bypass often results in acute renal failure. In 20 patients who developed acute renal failure following bypass surgery, serial urine samples were evaluated for IL-18 levels and compared to 35 matched control patients also undergoing cardiopulmonary bypass but without acute renal injury. Acute renal injury was defined as an increase in serum creatinine of 50% or greater. The findings were remarkable in that elevated creatinine levels occurred 48–72 hours after bypass surgery whereas urine IL-18 was statistically significantly increased 4–6 hours after the end of surgery.[80] Peak levels of urinary IL-18 were 25-fold greater 12 hours after surgery and remained elevated for 48 hours. Multivariate analysis of elevated urinary IL-18 and urinary neutrophil gelatinase-associated lipocalin, also elevated 25-fold early in acute renal failure, revealed that these two markers were independently associated with number of days of acute renal injury. These studies suggest that that elevated urinary IL-18 levels predict acute renal injury after bypass surgery and may be used as a reliable biomarker rather than serum creatinine.[80]

IL-18 deficiency triggers overeating, obesity, and insulin resistance

Although mice deficient in IL-18 are resistant to various exogenous challenges, an unexpected observation was that as mice aged, they gained significantly more weight than wild-type control mice. By 6 months of age, IL-18-deficient mice were 18.5% heavier than age-and sex-matched wild-type mice, and by 12 months they were 38.1% heavier.[81] The difference in weight was due to more body fat. Basic metabolic rate and core temperature were not different between the two strains but increased food intake accounted for the weight gain. Not unexpectedly, leptin levels were higher in the IL-18-deficient mice and leptin levels correlated with body weight but there was no evidence that fat mice deficient in IL-18 were resistant to leptin.[81] IL-6 levels were similar in the two groups. The islets of the IL-18-deficient mice exhibited normal architecture but were larger than those of wild-type mice.

Histological examination of major organs did not reveal significant difference but the aorta of the IL-18-deficient mice contained lipid deposits characteristic of atherosclerosis.[81]

Mice deficient in IL-18 at 6 months of age exhibited elevated fasting glucose compared with wild-type controls, although at 3 months of age there were no differences between the two groups. Glucose tolerance testing was abnormal in the IL-18-deficient mice and consistent with insulin resistance. Mice deficient in the α chain of the IL-18 receptor also exhibited similar increases in weight at 6 months as well as elevated plasma fasting glucose and insulin resistance. In addition, mice overexpressing the natural inhibitor of IL-18, IL-18BP, over-ate, gained weight, and were hyperglycemic.[81] The administration of recombinant murine IL-18 to the IL-18-deficient mice reversed insulin resistance. The rise in glucose was prevented by the administration of recombinant IL-18 to either the wild-type or the IL-18-deficient mice but not the IL-18 receptor-deficient mice.

The mechanism for the increased eating in mice deficient in IL-18, deficient in the IL-18 receptor, or in transgenic mice overexpressing the IL-18BP, appears to be a defect in the control of food intake by the hypothalamic satiety center. Insulin resistance in the liver and muscle were due to the obese condition. Of importance is the observation that unlike IL-1β, IL-18 does not cause fever[10,82] and does not induce COX-2.[13] Phosphorylation of STAT3 was defective in mice deficient in IL-18. Nevertheless, recombinant IL-18 administered intracerebrally inhibited food intake and, in addition, recombinant IL-18 reversed hyperglycemia in mice deficient for IL-18, through activation of STAT3 phosphorylation.[81] Hepatic genes for glucose neogenesis were increased in mice deficient in IL-18, possibly due to the phosphorylation of STAT3. In mice deficient for IL-18, there was less constitutive phosphorylation of STAT3 in the liver. Since IL-18 is constitutively expressed in health in mice and humans,[83] the decrease in STAT3 phosphorylation may be due to the lack of IL-18 in these mice. These findings indicate a new role of IL-18 in the homeostasis of energy intake and insulin sensitivity.

ACKNOWLEDGMENTS

These studies are supported by NIH grants AI-15614 and HL-68743 and the Colorado Cancer Center.

REFERENCES

1. Okamura H, Tsutsui H, Komatsu T et al. Cloning of a new cytokine that induces interferon-γ. Nature 1995; 378: 88–91.
2. Schmitz J, Owyang A, Oldham E et al. IL-33, an interleukin-1-like cytokine that signals via the IL-1 receptor-related protein ST2 and induces T helper type 2-associated cytokines. Immunity 2005; 23(5): 479–90.
3. Ghayur T, Banerjee S, Hugunin M et al. Caspase-1 processes IFN-gamma-inducing factor and regulates LPS-induced *IFN*-gamma production. Nature 1997; 386(6625): 619–23.
4. Gu Y, Kuida K, Tsutsui H et al. Activation of interferon-γ inducing factor mediated by interleukin-1β converting enzyme. Science 1997; 275: 206–9.
5. Mariathasan S, Newton K, Monack DM et al. Differential activation of the inflammasome by caspase-1 adaptors ASC and Ipaf. Nature 2004; 430(6996): 213–18.
6. Fantuzzi G, Puren AJ, Harding MW, Livingston DJ, Dinarello CA. IL-18 regulation of IFN-γ production and cell proliferation as revealed in interleukin-1β converting enzyme-deficient mice. Blood 1998; 91: 2118–25.
7. Nakanishi K, Yoshimoto T, Tsutsui H, Okamura H. Interleukin-18 is a unique cytokine that stimulates both Th1 and Th2 responses depending on its cytokine milieu. Cytokine Growth Factor Rev 2001; 12(1): 53–72.
8. Siegmund B, Lehr HA, Fantuzzi G, Dinarello CA. IL-1beta -converting enzyme (caspase-1) in intestinal inflammation. Proc Natl Acad Sci U S A 2001; 98(23): 13249–54.
9. Siegmund B, Fantuzzi G, Rieder F et al. Neutralization of interleukin-18 reduces severity in murine colitis and intestinal IFN-γ and TNF-α production. Am J Physiol Regul Integr Comp Physiol 2001; 281(4): R1264–73.
10. Gatti S, Beck J, Fantuzzi G, Bartfai T, Dinarello CA. Effect of interleukin-18 on mouse core body temperature. Am J Physiol Regul Integr Comp Physiol 2002; 282(3): R702–9.
11. Li S, Goorha S, Ballou LR, Blatteis CM. Intracerebroventricular interleukin-6, macrophage inflammatory protein-1 beta and IL-18: pyrogenic and PGE(2)-mediated? Brain Res 2003; 992(1): 76–84.
12. Reznikov LL, Kim SH, Westcott JY et al. IL-18 binding protein increases spontaneous and IL-1-induced prostaglandin production via inhibition of IFN-gamma. Proc Natl Acad Sci U S A 2000; 97(5): 2174–9.

13. Lee JK, Kim SH, Lewis EC et al. Differences in signaling pathways by IL-1beta and IL-18. Proc Natl Acad Sci U S A 2004; 101(23): 8815–20.

14. Kim SH, Han SY, Azam T, Yoon DY, Dinarello CA. Interleukin-32: a cytokine and inducer of TNFalpha. Immunity 2005; 22(1): 131–42.

15. Joosten LA, van De Loo FA, Lubbers E et al. An IFN-gamma-independent proinflammatory role of IL-18 in murine streptococcal cell wall arthritis. J Immunol 2000; 165(11): 6553–8.

16. Carrascal MT, Mendoza L, Valcarcel M et al. Interleukin-18 binding protein reduces b16 melanoma hepatic metastasis by neutralizing adhesiveness and growth factors of sinusoidal endothelium. Cancer Res 2003; 63(2): 491–7.

17. Lewis EC, Dinarello CA. Responses of IL-18 and IL-18 receptor deficient pancreatic islets differ with convergence of positive and negative signals for the IL-18 receptor. Proc Natl Acad Sci U S A 2006; 103: 16852–7.

18. Randle JC, Harding MW, Ku G, Schonharting M, Kurrle R. ICE/Caspase-1 inhibitors as novel anti-inflammatory drugs. Expert Opin Investig Drugs 2001; 10(7): 1207–9.

19. Novick D, Kim S-H, Fantuzzi G et al. Interleukin-18 binding protein: a novel modulator of the Th1 cytokine response. Immunity 1999; 10: 127–36.

20. Novick D, Schwartsburd B, Pinkus R et al. A novel IL-18BP ELISA shows elevated serum IL-18BP in sepsis and extensive decrease of free IL-18. Cytokine 2001; 14(6): 334–42.

21. Kim S-H, Eisenstein M, Reznikov L et al. Structural requirements of six naturally occurring isoforms of the interleukin-18 binding protein to inhibit interleukin-18. Proc Natl Acad Sci U S A 2000; 97: 1190–5.

22. Agostini L, Martinon F, Burns K et al. NALP3 forms an IL-1β processing inflammasome with increased activity in Muckle-Wells auto-inflammatory disorder. Immunity 2004; 20: 319–25.

23. Aganna E, Martinon F, Hawkins PN et al. Association of mutations in the NALP3/CIAS1/PYPAF1 gene with a broad phenotype including recurrent fever, cold sensitivity, sensorineural deafness, and AA amyloidosis. Arthritis Rheum 2002; 46(9): 2445–52.

24. Hawkins PN, Lachmann HJ, Aganna E, McDermott MF. Spectrum of clinical features in Muckle-Wells syndrome and response to anakinra. Arthritis Rheum 2004; 50: 607–12.

25. Coeshott C, Ohnemus C, Pilyavskaya A et al. Converting enzyme-independent release of TNFα and IL-1β from a stimulated human monocytic cell line in the presence of activated neutrophils or purified proteinase-3. Proc Natl Acad Sci U S A 1999; 96: 6261–6.

26. Sugawara S, Uehara A, Nochi T et al. Neutrophil proteinase 3-mediated induction of bioactive IL-18 secretion by human oral epithelial cells. J Immunol 2001; 167(11): 6568–75.

27. Faggioni R, Cattley RC, Guo J et al. IL-18-binding protein protects against lipopolysaccharide-induced lethality and prevents the development of Fas/Fas ligand-mediated models of liver disease in mice. J Immunol 2001; 167(10): 5913–20.

28. Pomerantz BJ, Reznikov LL, Harken AH, Dinarello CA. Inhibition of caspase 1 reduces human myocardial ischemic dysfunction via inhibition of IL-18 and IL-1beta. Proc Natl Acad Sci U S A 2001; 98(5): 2871–6.

29. Melnikov VY, Ecder T, Fantuzzi G et al. Impaired IL-18 processing protects caspase-1-deficient mice from ischemic acute renal failure. J Clin Invest 2001; 107(9): 1145–52.

30. Perregaux DG, McNiff P, Laliberte R, Conklyn M, Gabel CA. ATP acts as an agonist to promote stimulus-induced secretion of IL-1 beta and IL-18 in human blood. J Immunol 2000; 165(8): 4615–23.

31. Solle M, Labasi J, Perregaux DG et al. Altered cytokine production in mice lacking P2X(7) receptors. J Biol Chem 2001; 276(1): 125–32.

32. Laliberte RE, Eggler J, Gabel CA. ATP treatment of human monocytes promotes caspase-1 maturation and externalization. J Biol Chem 1999; 274(52): 36944–51.

33. Baraldi PG, del Carmen Nunez M, Morelli A et al. Synthesis and biological activity of N-arylpiperazine-modified analogues of KN-62, a potent antagonist of the purinergic P2X7 receptor. J Med Chem 2003; 46(8): 1318–29.

34. Gardella S, Andrei C, Costigliolo S, et al. Interleukin-18 synthesis and secretion by dendritic cells are modulated by interaction with antigen-specific T cells. J Leukoc Biol 1999; 66(2): 237–41.

35. Gardella S, Andrei C, Poggi A, Zocchi MR, Rubartelli A. Control of interleukin-18 secretion by dendritic cells: role of calcium influxes. FEBS Lett 2000; 481(3): 245 8.

36. Kato Z, Jee J, Shikano H et al. The structure and binding mode of interleukin-18. Nat Struct Biol 2003; 10(11): 966–71.

37. Azam T, Novick D, Bufler P et al. Identification of a critical Ig-like domain in IL-18 receptor alpha and characterization of a functional IL-18 receptor complex. J Immunol 2003; 171(12): 6574–80.

38. Casadio R, Frigimelica E, Bossu P et al. Model of interaction of the IL-1 receptor accessory protein IL-1RAcP with the IL-1beta/IL-1R(I) complex. FEBS Lett 2001; 499(1–2): 65–8.

39. Reznikov LL, Kim SH, Zhou L et al. The combination of soluble IL-18Rα and IL-18Rβ chains inhibits IL-18-Induced IFN-γ. J Interferon Cytokine Res 2002; 22(5): 593–601.

40. Kumar S, McDonnell PC, Lehr R et al. Identification and initial characterization of four novel members of the interleukin-1 family. J Biol Chem 2000; 275(14): 10308–14.

41. Pan G, Risser P, Mao W et al. IL-1H, an interleukin 1-related protein that binds IL-18 receptor/IL- 1Rrp. Cytokine 2001; 13(1): 1–7.

42. Kumar S, Hanning CR, Brigham-Burke MR et al. Interleukin-1F7B (IL-1H4/IL-1F7) is processed by caspase-1 and mature IL-1F7B binds to the IL-18 receptor but does not induce IFN-gamma production. Cytokine 2002; 18(2): 61–71.

43. Bufler P, Azam T, Gamboni-Robertson F et al. A complex of the IL-1 homologue IL-1F7b and IL-18-binding protein reduces IL-18 activity. Proc Natl Acad Sci U S A 2002; 99(21): 13723–8.

44. Gutcher I, Urich E, Wolter K, Prinz M, Becher B. Interleukin 18-independent engagement of interleukin 18 receptor-alpha is required for autoimmune inflammation. Nat Immunol 2006; 7(9): 946–53.

45. Novick D, Engelmann H, Wallach D et al. Purification of soluble cytokine receptors from normal human urine by ligand-affinity and immunoaffinity chromatography. J Chromatogr 1990; 510: 331–7.

46. Engelmann H, Novick D, Wallach D. Two tumor necrosis factor-binding proteins purified from human urine. Evidence for immunological cross-reactivity with cell surface tumor necrosis factor receptors. J Biol Chem 1990; 265(3): 1531–6.

47. Kim SH, Azam T, Novick D et al. Identification of amino acid residues critical for biological activity in human interleukin-18. J Biol Chem 2002; 14: 14.

48. Dinarello CA. The many worlds of reducing interleukin-1. Arthritis Rheum 2005; 52(7): 1960–7.

49. Hurgin V, Novick D, Rubinstein M. The promoter of IL-18 binding protein: activation by an IFN-gamma-induced complex of IFN regulatory factor 1 and CCAAT/enhancer binding protein beta. Proc Natl Acad Sci U S A 2002; 99(26): 16957–62.

50. Paulukat J, Bosmann M, Nold M et al. Expression and release of IL-18 binding protein in response to IFN-γ. J Immunol 2001; 167(12): 7038–43.

51. Fantuzzi G, Reed D, Qi M et al. Role of interferon regulatory factor-1 in the regulation of IL-18 production and activity. Eur J Immunol 2001; 31(2): 369–75.

52. Siegmund B, Sennello JA, Lehr HA et al. Interferon regulatory factor-1 as a protective gene in intestinal inflammation: role of TCR gamma delta T cells and interleukin-18-binding protein. Eur J Immunol 2004; 34(9): 2356–64.

53. Xiang Y, Moss B. Correspondence of the functional epitopes of poxvirus and human interleukin-18-binding proteins. J Virol 2001; 75(20): 9947–54.

54. Xiang Y, Moss B. Determination of the functional epitopes of human interleukin-18- binding protein by site-directed mutagenesis. J Biol Chem 2001; 276(20): 17380–6.

55. Maeno N, Takei S, Imanaka H et al. Increased interleukin-18 expression in bone marrow of a patient with systemic juvenile idiopathic arthritis and unrecognized macrophage-activation syndrome. Arthritis Rheum 2004; 50(6): 1935–8.

56. Dinarello CA. Differences between anti-tumor necrosis factor-alpha monoclonal antibodies and soluble TNF receptors in host defense impairment. J Rheumatol Suppl 2005; 74: 40–7.

57. Ottenhoff TH, Verreck FA, Lichtenauer-Kaligis EG et al. Genetics, cytokines and human infectious disease: lessons from weakly pathogenic mycobacteria and salmonellae. Nat Genet 2002; 32(1): 97–105.

58. Wei XQ, Leung BP, Arthur HM, McInnes IB, Liew FY. Reduced incidence and severity of collagen-induced arthritis in mice lacking IL-18. J Immunol 2001; 166(1): 517–21.

59. Plater-Zyberk C, Joosten LA, Helsen MM et al. Therapeutic effect of neutralizing endogenous IL-18 activity in the collagen-induced model of arthritis. J Clin Invest 2001; 108(12): 1825–32.

60. Bossu P, Neumann D, Del Giudice E et al. IL-18 cDNA vaccination protects mice from spontaneous lupus-like autoimmune disease. Proc Natl Acad Sci U S A 2003; 100(24): 14181–6.

61. Kim SH, Reznikov LL, Stuyt RJ et al. Functional reconstitution and regulation of IL-18 activity by the IL- 18R beta chain. J Immunol 2001; 166(1): 148–54.

62. Neumann D, Martin MU. Interleukin-12 upregulates the IL-18Rβ chain in BALB/c thymocytes. J Interferon Cytokine Res 2001; 21(8): 635–42.

63. Lugo-Villarino G, Maldonado-Lopez R, Possemato R, Penaranda C, Glimcher LH. T-bet is required for optimal production of IFN-gamma and antigen-specific T cell activation by dendritic cells. Proc Natl Acad Sci U S A 2003; 100(13): 7749–54.

64. Cardoso SM, DeFor TE, Tilley LA et al. Patient interleukin-18 GCG haplotype associates with improved survival and decreased transplant-related mortality after unrelated-donor bone marrow transplantation. Br J Haematol 2004; 126(5): 704–10.

65. Min CK, Maeda Y, Lowler K et al. Paradoxical effects of interleukin-18 on the severity of acute graft-versus-host disease mediated by CD4+ and CD8+ T-cell subsets after experimental allogeneic bone marrow transplantation. Blood 2004; 104(10): 3393–9.

66. Reddy P, Ferrara JL. Role of interleukin-18 in acute graft-vs-host disease. J Lab Clin Med 2003; 141(6): 365–71.

67. Hoshino T, Yagita H, Ortaldo JR, Wiltrout RH, Young HA. In vivo administration of IL-18 can induce IgE production through Th2 cytokine induction and up-regulation of CD40 ligand (CD154) expression on CD4+ T cells. Eur J Immunol 2000; 30(7): 1998–2006.

68. Kawase Y, Hoshino T, Yokota K et al. Exacerbated and prolonged allergic and non-allergic inflammatory

cutaneous reaction in mice with targeted interleukin-18 expression in the skin. J Invest Dermatol 2003; 121(3): 502–9.

69. Konishi H, Tsutsui H, Murakami T et al. IL-18 contributes to the spontaneous development of atopic dermatitis-like inflammatory skin lesion independently of IgE/stat6 under specific pathogen-free conditions. Proc Natl Acad Sci U S A 2002; 99(17): 11340–5.

70. Nakanishi K, Yoshimoto T, Tsutsui H, Okamura H. Interleukin-18 regulates both Th1 and Th2 responses. Annu Rev Immunol 2001; 19: 423–74.

71. Kaser A, Kaser S, Kaneider NC et al. Interleukin-18 attracts plasmacytoid dendritic cells (DC2s) and promotes Th1 induction by DC2s through IL-18 receptor expression. Blood 2004; 103(2): 648–55.

72. Raeburn CD, Dinarello CA, Zimmerman MA et al. Neutralization of IL-18 attenuates lipopolysaccharide-induced myocardial dysfunction. Am J Physiol 2002; 283(2): H650–7.

73. Friteau L, Francesconi E, Lando D, Dugas B, Damais C. Opposite effect of interferon-γ on PGE2 release from interleukin-1-stimulated human monocytes or fibroblasts. Biochem Biophys Res Commun 1988; 157(3): 1197–204.

74. Mallat Z, Heymes C, Corbaz A et al. Evidence for altered interleukin 18 (IL)-18 pathway in human heart failure. FASEB J 2004; 18(14): 1752–4.

75. Whitman SC, Ravisankar P, Daugherty A. Interleukin-18 enhances atherosclerosis in apolipoprotein E(−/−) mice through release of interferon-gamma. Circ Res 2002; 90(2): E34–8.

76. Gerdes N, Sukhova GK, Libby P et al. Expression of interleukin (IL)-18 and functional IL-18 receptor on human vascular endothelial cells, smooth muscle cells, and macrophages: implications for atherogenesis. J Exp Med 2002; 195(2): 245–57.

77. Mallat Z, Corbaz A, Scoazec A et al. Interleukin-18/interleukin-18 binding protein signaling modulates atherosclerotic lesion development and stability. Circ Res 2001; 89(7): E41–5.

78. Parikh CR, Jani A, Melnikov VY, Faubel S, Edelstein CL. Urinary interleukin-18 is a marker of human acute tubular necrosis. Am J Kidney Dis 2004; 43(3): 405–14.

79. Parikh CR, Abraham E, Ancukiewicz M, Edelstein CL. Urine IL-18 is an early diagnostic marker for acute kidney injury and predicts mortality in the intensive care unit. J Am Soc Nephrol 2005; 16: 3046–52.

80. Parikh CR, Mishra J, Thiessen-Philbrook H et al. Urinary IL-18 is an early predictive biomarker of acute kidney injury after cardiac surgery. Kidney Int 2006; 70(1): 199–203.

81. Netea MG, Joosten LA, Lewis E et al. Deficiency of interleukin-18 in mice leads to hyperphagia, obesity and insulin resistance. Nat Med 2006; 12(6): 650–6.

82. Stuyt RJ, Netea MG, Verschueren I et al. Interleukin-18 does not modulate the acute-phase response. J Endotoxin Res 2005; 11(2): 85–8.

83. Puren AJ, Fantuzzi G, Dinarello CA. Gene expression, synthesis and secretion of IL-1β and IL-18 are differentially regulated in human blood mononuclear cells and mouse spleen cells. Proc Natl Acad Sci U S A 1999; 96: 2256–61.

17

Interleukin-21

Rosanne Spolski and Warren J Leonard

Overview • Structural features of the IL-21/IL-21R system • Regulation of expression of IL-21 and the IL-21R • IL-21 effects on CD4+ T cell differentiation • IL-21 controls CD8+ T cell homeostasis and function • Analysis of IL-21R KO mice: role of IL-21 in B-cell function • IL-4 and IL-21 together appear to explain the B-cell defect in human XSCID • IL-21 is a critical regulator of Ig production even though it is pro-apoptotic • IL-21 augments functional development of NK cells • IL-21 negatively controls immune responses through effects on dendritic cells • IL-21: clinical implications for autoimmunity, allergy, and cancer • Conclusion • Acknowledgment • References

OVERVIEW

Interleukin-21 (IL-21) is a four α-helical bundle type I cytokine that is produced by CD4+ T cells and has actions on T, B, natural killer (NK), and myeloid cells.[1,2] IL-21 binds to a receptor that comprises IL-21R and the common cytokine receptor γ chain, γ_c, the protein that is mutated in patients with X-linked severe combined immunodeficiency (XSCID).[1,3] In XSCID, T cells and NK cells are absent or profoundly decreased in number and B cells are present but not functional. γ_c is also a component of the receptors for IL-2, IL-4, IL-7, IL-9, and IL-15 (Figure 17.1). The actions of all six γ_c family cytokines are summarized in Table 17.1. The defective T-cell and NK-cell development are due substantially to defective signaling by IL-7 and IL-15, respectively. We discuss herein that IL-21 is important for T, B, NK, and myeloid cell biology. Interestingly, depending on the target cell and stimulation context, IL-21 can be pro-apoptotic or can promote the differentiation and/or proliferation of target cells. In particular, IL-21 can potently augment T-cell proliferation and the expansion of CD8+ T cells, can drive B-cell differentiation to memory cells and terminally differentiated plasma cells, has anti-tumor

actions, and is implicated as playing a role in the development of autoimmunity. As such, IL-21 is a pleiotropic cytokine with diverse immunomodulatory actions. Although more development is needed, based on animal studies, IL-21 has the potential to be of clinical importance, where either increasing or decreasing its activities may be therapeutically useful depending on the clinical setting.

STRUCTURAL FEATURES OF THE IL-21/IL-21R SYSTEM

The IL-21 binding protein was first identified as a novel type I cytokine receptor that was discovered based on either genomic[4] or EST-based sequencing efforts.[5] Originally, it was also denoted as 'NILR' for novel interleukin receptor.[4] Based on its sequence, the protein was predicted to be a typical type I cytokine receptor containing four conserved cysteine residues and a WSXWS motif with an amino acid sequence that was most similar to the IL-2 receptor β chain. The IL-21R gene is located on human chromosome 16 and mouse chromosome 7 immediately downstream of the IL-4R gene. The ligand for this novel receptor protein was identified based on expression cloning[5] and found to be most similar

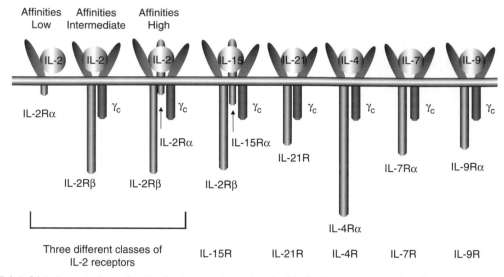

Figure 17.1 IL-21 belongs to the γ_c family of cytokines. Receptors in this family are composed of the common cytokine receptor γ chain as well as a receptor-specific chain. In the case of the IL-2 or IL-15 receptors, affinity is modulated by the presence or absence of a third chain, IL-2Rα or IL-15Rα.

Table 17.1 The actions of the six γ_c family cytokines

Cytokine	Receptor	CD4 T cell	CD8 T cell	B cell	NK cell	Myeloid cell
IL-2	γ_c, IL2Rβ, IL2Rα	Proliferation, Th2 differentiation, peripheral T reg survival	Proliferation	Proliferation, Ig production	Augments cytotoxic activity	Augments neutrophil activation
IL-4	γ_c, IL-4Rα or IL-13Rα and IL-4Rα	Th2 differentiation	Tc2 differentiation	Proliferation, isotype switch, plasma cell differentiation		Macrophage, basophil differentiation
IL-7	γ_c, IL-7Rα	Development, homeostasis	Development, homeostasis	Development (in the mouse)	Development or homeostasis	
IL-9	γ_c, IL-9Rα	Proliferation	Proliferation	Maturation		Mast cell development
IL-15	γ_c, IL-2Rβ, IL-15Rα	Proliferation	Homeostasis, memory, cytotoxic function		Proliferation, cytotoxic activity	Mast cell growth
IL-21	γ_c, IL-21R	Proliferation, cytokine induction	Proliferation, cytokine induction, cytotoxic function	Proliferation, isotype switch, plasma cell differentiation	Proliferation, cytotoxic activity	Suppresses antigen-presenting function of DCs

to IL-2, IL-4, and IL-15, which – along with IL-7 and IL-9 – share the common cytokine receptor γ chain, γ_c, as a critical receptor component.[6] Correspondingly, the IL-21 receptor contains IL-21R + γ_c.[7,8] As γ_c is encoded by the gene that is mutated in humans with XSCID,[9] it was predicted that defects in IL-21-mediated signaling might contribute to the defective lymphoid development and function in this disease.

Proximal signal transduction by IL-21 is similar to that for other γ_c family cytokines in that it activates the Janus family tyrosine kinases, Jak1 and Jak3 (Figure 17.2), with Jak1 binding to IL-21R[4] and Jak3 binding to γ_c.[1,10] These kinases in turn mediate IL-21-dependent activation primarily of STAT1 and STAT3 and to a lesser degree STAT5a and STAT5b.[4,5,11–13] This STAT protein activation profile distinguishes IL-21 from other γ_c-dependent cytokines that primarily activate

either STAT5a and STAT5b (IL-2, IL-7, IL-9, and IL-15)[1,14] or STAT6 (IL-4).[15,16]

REGULATION OF EXPRESSION OF IL-21 AND THE IL-21R

IL-21 is produced by CD4[+] T cells.[5] The IL-21R is known to be expressed on T, B, and NK cells, some myeloid cells, and on keratinocytes.[4,5,17–20] Within the lymphoid lineages, IL-21R expression is developmentally regulated. In the developing T-cell lineage, IL-21R appears as thymocytes transition from the immature CD4[−]CD8[−] double negative stage to the CD4[+]CD8[+] double positive stage and then increases in density on the most mature CD4[+] and CD8[+] single positive thymocytes.[17] A specific role for IL-21 in the process of thymic development remains to be determined, although the normal development

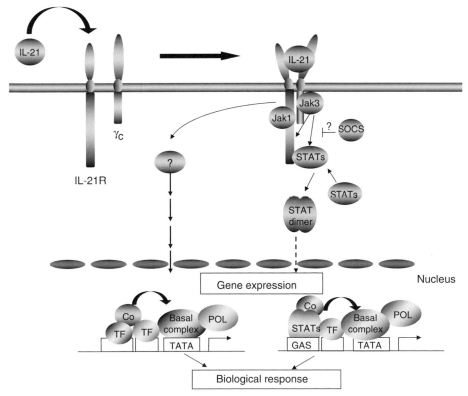

Figure 17.2 IL-21 signaling pathways. Upon IL-21 binding, IL-21R and γ_c interact with Jak1 and Jak3, respectively, which are activated and then phosphorylate STAT1, STAT3, and weakly STAT5, leading to STAT dimerization and translocation to the nucleus with subsequent binding to target gene regulatory elements. Further characterization of IL-21 signaling will lead to an understanding of potential targets for therapeutic inhibition of signaling.

of thymocytes in IL-21R knockout (KO) mice[21] suggests that this may be a redundant role. Within the B-cell lineage, IL-21R is also developmentally regulated, with receptor appearing as cells progress from the pro-B-cell stage to the immature B220[high]IgM[low] B-cell stage.[17] Although naïve peripheral T cells and B cells express detectable IL-21R, levels of expression are increased by signals through either the T-cell antigen receptor or the B-cell antigen receptor.[17,22] In the case of human T cells, induction of IL-21R mRNA levels is regulated in part by T-cell receptor (TCR) induced expression and dephosphorylation of the transcription factor Sp1.[22] IL-21R expression levels are also regulated by cytokine signals; interferon (IFN)-α reduces levels of IL-21R mRNA in both T cells and NK cells,[23] whereas IL-21 can increase IL-21R mRNA levels in T cells,[24] thus providing a mechanism for amplification of IL-21R signaling by IL-21 itself.

Although the genes encoding IL-21 and IL-2 are adjacent to each other, the regulation of IL-21 production in CD4[+] T cells differs from that of IL-2. Both cytokines are strongly induced by TCR signaling, but IL-21 can be induced by a calcium signal alone in human preactivated T cells, in contrast to IL-2 whose induction in these cells requires both a calcium signal and a signal through protein kinase C.[25] Nuclear factor of activated T cells (NFAT) binding sites have been identified as playing a role, in conjunction with other factors, in the transcriptional activation of the IL-21 gene.[25,26] The different mode of induction of IL-21 and IL-2 implies that they may play temporally distinct roles in the regulation of the immune response.

IL-21 EFFECTS ON CD4[+] T CELL DIFFERENTIATION

Although it is known that IL-21 is produced by CD4[+] T cells in response to specific antigen signals, the full range of its functional effects on naïve and activated CD4[+] T cells remain to be delineated. Evaluation of IL-21R KO mice revealed no abnormalities in either thymic or peripheral CD4[+] T-cell numbers or proliferative responses,[21] suggesting that any developmental or proliferative effects that IL-21 may have on the CD4[+] T-cell lineage are redundant with those of other cytokines. In addition to the absence of developmental effects for CD4[+] T cells in IL-21R KO mice, there were no differences in the levels of IFN-γ or IL-4 produced by either wild-type or IL-21R KO CD4[+] T cells in response to anti-CD3 stimulation.[21] Although in vitro experiments demonstrated that IL-21 could costimulate the proliferation of anti-CD3 activated peripheral T cells,[5] it is likely that these proliferative effects were primarily on the CD8[+] T cells, as naïve CD4[+] T cells exhibit very little proliferation in response to IL-21.[24] The presence of IL-21 in cultures of total splenocytes also had no effect on the production of Th1- or Th2-type cytokines.[27]

Several laboratories have examined the T-helper subset-specific expression of IL-21 and obtained distinct and ostensibly inconsistent results. For example, DNA array analysis of expression in Th1- and Th2-polarized CD4[+] T cells from human peripheral blood revealed IL-21 mRNA in Th1 but not in Th2 cells.[28] Nevertheless, IL-21 mRNA is expressed in a distinctive population of follicular CD4[+] T cells with a non-Th1/Th2 phenotype that function in B-cell help.[28] Although another study reported that IL-21 mRNA is produced by Th2- but not Th1-polarized murine CD4[+] T cells,[29] we reproducibly find IL-21 mRNA to be expressed by both Th1 and Th2 CD4[+] T cells polarized in vitro as well as in CD4[+] T cells that are strongly Th1-polarized in vivo (unpublished results). Although inclusion of IL-21 during the process of Th1 polarization was reported to reduce production of IFN-γ but not other Th1-type cytokines, IL-21 had no such inhibitory effect on fully polarized Th1 cells,[29] suggesting that it may play a role in precursor commitment. The delayed-type hypersensitivity (DTH) response is a classic Th1-mediated reaction: IL-21R KO mice exhibited stronger DTH responses and produced more IFN-γ than wild-type mice, implying a potential role for IL-21 in the down-regulation of these in vivo Th1 responses.[29] Nevertheless, another study showed that IL-21 could induce a number of genes involved in Th1 responses, including IFN-γ, IL-12Rβ2 and T bet.[12] Although more work is needed to clarify the lineage-specific expression and function of IL-21 for CD4[+] T cells, the overall data indicate that IL-21 can be

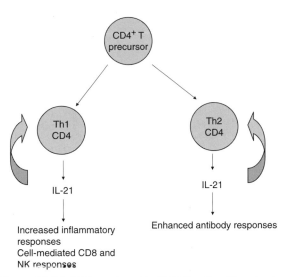

Figure 17.3 IL-21 is produced by CD4$^+$ T cells, with autocrine effects on CD4$^+$ T-cell function. T-cell receptor stimulation of the naïve CD4$^+$ T-cell precursor leads to the production of IL-21 along with other cytokines that induce differentiation into either Th1 cells, which function in the regulation of inflammation and cell-mediated responses, or Th2 cells, which regulate B-cell production of antibody. Both Th1 and Th2 subsets can produce IL-21, which mediates these diverse effects.

produced by both Th1 and Th2 cells (Figure 17.3), in part influenced by the specific experimental setting.

IL-21 CONTROLS CD8$^+$ T CELL HOMEOSTASIS AND FUNCTION

CD8$^+$ T-cell homeostatic proliferation is regulated *in vivo* by both IL-7 and IL-15.[30,31] It is now clear that IL-21 plays important roles in the regulation of both the proliferation and function of CD8$^+$ T cells. In the absence of a T-cell receptor signal, although IL-21 alone has no significant effect on *in vitro* CD8$^+$ T-cell proliferation, it has a strong synergistic effect on proliferation in combination with either IL-7 or IL-15 *in vitro*.[24] Significantly, both naïve and memory phenotype CD8$^+$ T cells can be expanded by the synergistic effect of IL-21 and IL-15, implying a potential role for IL-21 in both the induction phase and the memory phase of an immune response (Figure 17.4). Gene array analysis of CD8$^+$ T cells treated with either IL-21, IL-15, or the combination of these two cytokines revealed sets of genes that are either induced or repressed by the individual cytokines. Importantly, it also identified a set of genes that is induced or repressed only by the combination of IL-21 and

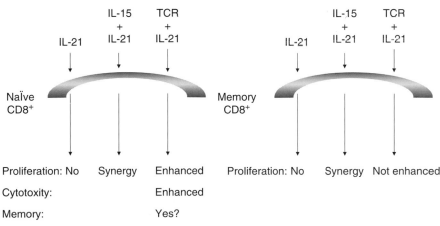

Figure 17.4 IL-21 effects on CD8$^+$ T cells depend on the developmental stage and on other cytokines. Although naïve CD8$^+$ T cells and CD8$^+$ memory T cells express the IL-21R, they do not proliferate in response to IL-21 alone. Both populations proliferate synergistically in response to the combination of IL-21 with IL-15. TCR signaling in the presence of IL-21 leads to enhanced proliferation as well as cytotoxic function in naïve CD8$^+$ T cells. Memory CD8$^+$ T-cell proliferation in response to TCR signals is not enhanced by IL-21. A role for IL-21 in memory cell formation has not been established.

IL-15, suggesting a possible molecular basis for the synergistic actions of these cytokines.[24] Additionally, IL-15 was found to up-regulate expression of the IL-21 receptor on CD8+ T cells,[32] thus enhancing the responses of naïve cells to IL-21 signals.

In contrast to the lack of proliferative responses of naïve CD8+ T cells to IL-21 alone, this cytokine has a significant effect on the *in vitro* expansion of antigen-primed CD8+ T cells. As compared with cells activated by peptide in the absence of IL-21, IL-21 led to a 20-fold expansion of human melanoma-specific T cells and also led to the generation of a population of high affinity antigen-specific CD8+ T cells that exhibit enhanced cytolytic activity.[33] Although IL-21 strongly enhances proliferative responses of antigen-primed naïve CD8+ T cells, it has no effect on the proliferation of antigen-primed memory phenotype CD8+ T cells,[33] suggesting a greater role for IL-21 in priming. Interestingly, among the γ_c-dependent cytokines, IL-21 uniquely can increase the expression of the CD28 costimulatory molecule on CD8 T cells.[32,33] Although IL-15-mediated proliferation leads to down-regulation of CD28, this down-regulation can be prevented by the inclusion of IL-21, suggesting a potential mechanism for the increased antigen responsiveness of IL-21-primed CD8+ T cells.

The specific role of IL-21 in the generation of a primary CD8+ T-cell immune response or in the maintenance of a CD8+ T-cell memory response remains to be fully delineated. Although IL-21R KO mice exhibit normal generation of both thymic and peripheral CD8+ T cells, these mice have significantly lower primary CD8+ T-cell responses to a vaccinia virus-encoded antigen,[24] suggesting a role for IL-21 either in the antigen-priming phase or in the expansion phase of this immune response.

In accord with these effects of IL-21 on the development of a functional CD8+ T-cell response, IL-21 plays a role in anti-tumor responses. A comparative study of the effects of IL-2, IL-15, and IL-21 on CD8+ T-cell-mediated anti-tumor responses demonstrated that IL-21 could lead to tumor rejection and long-term survival of the host, even when administered after full tumor development.[34] In these anti-tumor responses, IL-21 is most effective at inducing a persistent *in vivo* cytotoxic T-lymphocyte (CTL) population, in part due to reduced *in vivo* apoptosis of the CTL population. The molecular mechanism for this increased persistence of tumor antigen-specific CD8+ T cells remains to be determined. The synergistic effects of IL-15 and IL-21 on CD8+ T-cell proliferation and function also have been confirmed in an *in vivo* system in which mice with large established melanomas are treated with adoptively transferred tumor-specific CD8+ T cells, followed by treatment of the mice with cytokine.[24] The combination of IL-15 and IL-21 treatment results in the regression of a subset of these melanomas that is accompanied by the synergistic expansion of tumor-specific CD8+ T cells.

ANALYSIS OF IL-21R KO MICE: ROLE OF IL-21 IN B-CELL FUNCTION

IL-21R KO and wild-type mice have similar numbers of both immature and mature B cells, and mature B cells from both IL-21R KO and wild-type mice manifest equivalent proliferation in response to LPS or to treatment with anti-CD40 plus anti-IgM.[21] Thus, IL-21 signaling does not play an essential and non-redundant role for B-cell development or proliferation. However, IL-21 can influence B-cell function in a manner that depends on costimulatory signals. For example, IL-21 can promote the proliferation of B cells stimulated with anti-CD40, but it inhibits proliferation in B cells stimulated via the B-cell receptor plus IL-4.[5] The basis for these differential effects of IL-21 remains unknown.

Interestingly, an analysis of immunoglobulin levels revealed that naïve IL-21R KO mice exhibit lower levels of serum IgG1 but significantly higher levels of serum IgE than do wild-type mice, and immunization of these mice with T-cell-dependent antigens such as ovalbumin or keyhole limpet hemocyanin resulted in much lower levels of antigen-specific IgG1, IgG3, and IgG2b, as well as higher levels of IgE than are induced in wild-type mice.[21] The higher levels of IgE in the IL-21R KO mice were unexpected in light of the fact that the IL-21R KO mice do not show increased production of IL-4, which is known to be responsible for switching to the IgE isotype.[35] Moreover, it is unusual and perhaps unprecedented to find reduced IgG1 in a situation where IgE levels were increased, as these isotypes are usually regulated in parallel by IL-4.

Consistent with elevated IgE levels in IL-21R KO mice, IL-21 injection into mice during the course of antigen immunization diminishes antigen-specific IgE levels.[27] This is consistent with the observation that IL-21 inhibits the induction of germ-line Cε transcripts by LPS plus IL-4, suggesting a molecular mechanism by which IL-21 regulates IgE levels.[27] Interestingly, *in vitro* experiments with human peripheral blood B cells reveal that whereas IL-21 can inhibit the induction of IgE by mitogen- and IL-4-stimulated-cells, it increases IgE production in B cells stimulated with CD40 plus IL-4 signals.[36] Thus, the ability of IL-21 to influence IgE production also appears to be dependent on the specific costimulatory signals received by the B cell at the time of IL-21 exposure.

Although enhanced levels of IgE in the IL-21R KO mice suggest a negative regulatory role for IL-21 in IgE production, IL-4/IL-21R double KO (DKO) mice cannot produce antigen-specific IgE, indicating that the enhanced IgE levels in the IL-21R KO are indeed still dependent on IL-4.[21] Surprisingly, the levels of IgG1, IgG2a, IgG2b, and IgG3 are also essentially absent in the DKO mice as compared with either IL-4 or IL-21R KO mice, and IgM levels are also greatly reduced. Thus, the IL-4/IL-21R DKO mice exhibit a pan-hypogammaglobulinemia, suggesting that IL-21 and IL-4 have an important cooperative role in the regulation of immunoglobulin production.

IL-4 AND IL-21 TOGETHER APPEAR TO EXPLAIN THE B-CELL DEFECT IN HUMAN XSCID

The B-cell phenotype in these IL-4/IL-21R DKO mice is reminiscent of that observed in humans with XSCID. This suggests that the loss of signaling by IL-4 and IL-21 is responsible for the B-cell phenotype in humans with XSCID. XSCID patients lack T and NK cells but normal numbers of B cells develop. Mice lacking γc expression lack not only T and NK cells, but also B cells as a result of the critical role of IL-7 signaling for B-cell development in mice. In contrast, in humans, IL-7 is not essential for B-cell development. In the

IL-4/IL-21R DKO mice, because IL-7 signaling is intact, B cells could develop, allowing us to observe the effect of eliminating IL-4 and IL-21. Given the panhypogammaglobulinemia in the IL-4/IL-21R DKO mice, it appears that these are the dominant γc cytokines responsible for the B-cell defect in human XSCID.

IL-21 IS A CRITICAL REGULATOR OF IG PRODUCTION EVEN THOUGH IT IS PRO-APOPTOTIC

One of the most puzzling findings concerning IL-21 is its pro-apoptotic activity for B cells *in vitro*. This pro-apoptotic activity is modulated by the specific B-cell costimulatory signals, such that IL-21 induces a high level of apoptosis in B cells stimulated with either lipopolysaccharide (LPS) or anti-IgM, and significantly less apoptosis when stimulated with anti-CD40.[17,37,38] An increase in the pro-apoptotic factor, Bim, has been suggested to play a mechanistic role in the apoptotic activity of IL-21 on B cells.[17] The finding that IL-21 is pro-apoptotic is surprising in light of the anti-apoptotic activity of other γc-dependent cytokines such as IL-2 and IL-7.[39,40] Most importantly, the pro-apoptotic activity seems inconsistent with the results from the IL21R KO mice, indicating a crucial role for IL-21 in the generation of the immunoglobulin response.

To study IL-21 *in vivo*, we have used IL-21 transgenic mice and wild-type mice hydrodynamically transfected with IL-21 plasmid DNA.[38] In both cases, IL-21 can indeed induce apoptotic events in the naïve mature B-cell population, based on staining with annexin V, confirming the *in vitro* findings.[38] Surprisingly, in spite of the induction of apoptosis, in both the IL-21 transgenic and the IL-21 plasmid-injected mice, there is an increase in total B-cell numbers *in vivo*, rather than a decrease, with an increase in immature B cells, little if any change in mature B cells, and a marked increase in the generation of both post-switch B cells (B cells that no longer express IgD or IgM but instead express surface IgG) and plasma cells.[38]

The increase in plasma cells in IL-21 transgenic mice correlated with increased levels of serum IgM and IgG1, and correspondingly higher numbers of surface IgG1+ cells, demonstrating the functionality of these cells.[38] IL-21 has also been shown to induce plasma-cell differentiation in human B cells, including post-switch memory cells and naïve cord blood B cells, which typically are poorly responsive *in vitro*.[41] Isotype switching to IgG1 and IgG3 is also induced by IL-21 in human B cells.[42] Interestingly, although IL-21 and IL-4 cooperate in the generation of the antibody response based on studies with IL-4/IL-21R DKO mice, IL-4 and IL-21 can also exert reciprocal effects on the generation of post-switch cells *in vitro*, with IL-4 decreasing the numbers of IL-21-induced IgG1+ cells in the case of both murine and human B cells.[38,41] Moreover, whereas IL-4 is the classic inducer of CD23 (FcεRI) expression on B cells, IL-21 is a potent repressor of CD23 expression on mature B cells.[38] The positive effects of IL-21 on immunoglobulin production can be explained by the observation that IL-21 can induce expression of Blimp-1,[38] a transcription factor known to function as a master switch for the plasma cell program.[43] Surprisingly, IL-21 also induced

Bcl-6 mRNA and protein expression, in spite of the fact that Blimp-1 and Bcl-6 are each known to inhibit expression of the other protein and to lead to execution of either a plasma cell or a germinal center program in B cells.[43] It is possible that Blimp-1 and Bcl-6 are both induced by IL-21 but within different individual cells rather than being co-expressed.

A major goal is to understand the specific stage of the immune response at which IL-21 would preferentially promote apoptosis versus B-cell differentiation. The collective data suggest that in the absence of a T-cell signal, such as that provided by anti-CD40, IL-21 exerts a relatively weak signal for B cells stimulated through the B-cell receptor, with anti-IgM and in fact inhibits proliferation of cells stimulated with anti-IgM plus IL-4. However, when T-cell costimulation and B-cell receptor signals are combined, IL-21 has potent costimulatory effects on both B-cell proliferation and function (Figure 17.5). This suggests that the pro-apoptotic action of IL-21 may be a mechanism for eliminating incompletely activated autoreactive B cells.

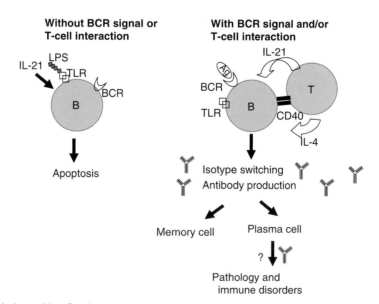

Figure 17.5 IL-21 can induce either B-cell apoptosis or plasma cell differentiation depending on costimulatory signals. In the absence of a B-cell receptor (BCR) signal or in the presence of a Toll-like receptor (TLR) signal such as LPS, IL-21 leads to B-cell apoptosis. In the presence of a BCR signal and additional T-cell derived signals or cytokines, IL-21 induces B-cell differentiation along the plasma cell or memory cell pathway, resulting in antibody production. Enhanced antibody production in response to IL-21 may lead to autoimmune disease.

IL-21 AUGMENTS FUNCTIONAL DEVELOPMENT OF NK CELLS

NK cell development, proliferation, and function are known to be dependent on γ_c-dependent cytokines, since γ_c KO mice lack mature NK cells.[44,45] IL-15 has been implicated in NK functional development, as mice deficient in IL-15 signaling have greatly reduced NK-cell numbers.[46,47] IL-21R KO mice have normal numbers of functional NK cells in peripheral lymphoid organs,[21,48] demonstrating that IL-21 does not play a non-redundant role in NK-cell development. However, early work indicated that IL-21 can accelerate the *in vitro* differentiation of bone marrow precursors to NK cells.[5] IL-21 alone is not sufficient to induce proliferation of immature NK cells but can act in concert with either IL-2 or IL-15.[49] Interestingly, increased proliferation is seen when low doses of IL-21 are added to IL-2 or IL-15, whereas higher doses of IL-21 inhibit proliferation.[49] This inhibitory effect on NK-cell proliferation was accompanied by phenotypic conversion to effector cytolytic cells, with higher levels of perforin and IFN-γ as well as enhanced cytolytic activity. The enhanced effector function is associated with increased apoptosis of NK cells[48,50] that can be blocked by the inclusion of other cytokines such as IL-15. The role of IL-21 in the NK-cell lineage thus involves effects on both proliferation and maturation, but the specific effect depends on the concentration of IL-21 as well as the presence of other cytokines (Figure 17.6).

The *in vivo* effects of IL-21 on NK-cell function have been confirmed in experiments wherein systemic expression of high levels of IL-21 was shown to inhibit the growth of pre-established melanomas.[51] NK activity against melanoma target cells was significantly increased after IL-21 delivery, and anti-tumor activity could be inhibited by the *in vivo* ablation of the NK-cell population.[51] Other studies have shown that NK cells activated through the NKG2D pathway are important in the IL-21 induced anti-tumor immunity and that this effect depends on perforin and is independent of the adaptive immune response.[52]

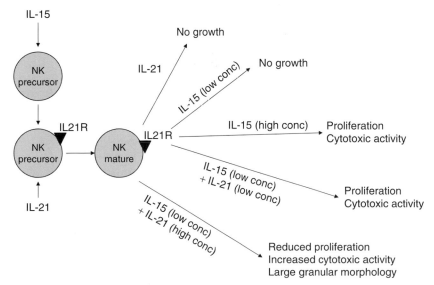

Figure 17.6 IL-21 plays a role in the proliferation and maturation of NK cells. IL-21R is present on NK precursors, and IL-21 in combination with other factors enhances the development of mature NK cells. Although IL-21 alone does not induce the proliferation of mature NK cells, in combination with IL-15 it can induce both proliferation and enhanced cytotoxic activity. However, higher concentrations of IL-21 in combination with IL-15, although leading to increased cytotoxic activity, also result in reduced proliferative responses.

IL-21 NEGATIVELY CONTROLS IMMUNE RESPONSES THROUGH EFFECTS ON DENDRITIC CELLS

Although most of the effects of IL-21 on immune responses are mediated by its actions on the lymphoid lineage, it is also clear that at least certain myeloid cells are targets for IL-21 and other γ_c-dependent cytokines. Although myeloid cell numbers in both γ_c KO and Jak3 KO mice are normal, dendritic cells (DCs) from these mice have increased survival in the absence of cytokines, suggesting that although signaling through γ_c-dependent cytokines is not required for development, these cytokines can negatively regulate DC survival and cytokine production.[53] This inhibitory effect is exemplified by the *in vitro* action of IL-21 on DC function. DCs can be expanded *in vitro* from bone marrow precursors in response to granulocyte/macrophage colony-stimulating factor (GM-CSF) and IL-4, and interestingly, the phenotypic and functional characteristics of DCs expanded in these cytokines in the additional presence of either IL-21 or IL-15 are markedly distinct.[18,19] Although IL-15-generated DCs express both IL-2Rβ and IL-2Rα, IL-21-generated DCs express neither of these receptor components. Moreover, unlike DCs expanded with IL-15, those expanded with IL-21 maintain an immature phenotype characterized by low levels of the chemokine receptor CCR7, low levels of major histocompatibility complex (MHC) class II, and increased antigen uptake. These DCs cannot be induced by lipopolysaccharide (LPS) stimulation to up-regulate surface antigens important for antigen presentation such as CD80, CD86, or MHC class II. Importantly, DCs expanded in the presence of IL-21 can inhibit antigen-specific T-cell proliferation, whereas those expanded with IL-15 preferentially stimulate T-cell responses.[18,19] These results suggest that the presence of IL-21 at the time of initiation of the immune response by antigen-presenting cells (APCs) may down-regulate T-cell responses. Interestingly, while IL-21 and IL-15 have distinct effects on DC function, these two cytokines have synergistic effects on both NK and CD8+ T cells. Therefore, the timing and the location of immune responses will likely be important with regard to whether IL-21 will have positive or negative regulatory effects.

IL-21: CLINICAL IMPLICATIONS FOR AUTOIMMUNITY, ALLERGY, AND CANCER

IL-21 controls immune processes through a complicated interaction of both positive and negative regulatory effects already known to occur within the lymphoid and myeloid lineage target cells. Consequently, there may be many scenarios in which either disruption or amplification of IL-21 signals will have clinical benefit. The ability of IL-21 to promote plasma cell differentiation suggests that aberrant IL-21/IL-21R signaling might contribute to the development of antibody-mediated autoimmune disorders. Overexpression of IL-21 has now been detected in three different autoimmune mouse models, the BXSB-*Yaa* mouse[38] which is a model for systemic lupus erythematosus (SLE), the *sanroque* mouse,[54] and the nonobese diabetic (NOD) mouse which is a model for autoimmune diabetes.[55] One of the genetic loci conferring the autoimmune phenotype in the NOD mouse is the *Idd3* locus, which contains both the IL-21 and the IL-2 genes,[56] and it is possible that mutations in this locus contribute directly to the higher level of IL-21 expression. It was suggested that high levels of IL-21 in the NOD mouse serve to amplify the homeostatic proliferation of an autoreactive CD8+ T-cell population.[55] However, IL-21 certainly might instead or additionally exert major actions on B cells in this setting. NOD mice also have markedly reduced B-cell numbers, which we speculate might result from the apoptotic effect of high IL-21 levels in the absence of costimulatory signals. BXSB-*Yaa* mice, which develop severe SLE, develop an age-dependent increase in the expression of IL-21 mRNA as well as serum IL-21 levels.[38] Of the other cytokines examined, only IL-10 mRNA was also increased. Corresponding to the increase in IL-21, these mice also had increased serum levels of IgG1, IgG2b, and IgG3. Higher levels of IL-21 in the disease state could be an initiating or amplifying signal for the accumulation of plasma cells and production of high levels of autoantibodies. Another mouse strain, the mutant *sanroque* mouse, has a defect in a

T-cell costimulatory pathway mediated by inducible costimulator (ICOS) which is accompanied by the overproduction of IL-21 and the development of a lupus-like pathology.[54] The functional link between overexpression of IL-21 and ICOS remains to be determined, although the co-expression of these two proteins in the follicular helper T subset that controls germinal center antibody responses[28] suggests that this may be the controlling cell subset. In each of these autoimmune models, it remains to be determined whether the disease phenotype can develop in the absence of IL-21. IL-21 might also play a role in the development or maintenance of the disease state in inflammatory bowel disease, given that elevated levels of IL-21 were detected at the site of inflammation in patients with Crohn's disease and IL-21 was responsible for enhanced Th1 cell function at these mucosal sites.[57]

Work in another autoimmune model system, experimental autoimmune encephalomyelitis (EAE), suggests a potential role for IL-21 in disease pathogenesis. When mice were treated with IL-21 before the induction of disease, they developed an exacerbated central nervous system inflammatory response and more severe disease symptoms which were the result of both B- and T-cell responses.[58] Circulating myelin-specific antibodies were significantly higher, and T cells from mice treated with IL-21 produced higher IFN-γ levels and could adoptively transfer the encephalitis to naïve mice. Interestingly, in this model system, the timing of IL-21 administration was critical, as IL-21 given after disease induction has no effect on the progress or severity of the disease.[58] The specific mechanism by which IL-21 exacerbates the disease remains to be determined, but an understanding of this mechanism will suggest potential targets for disruption of disease severity.

Although high levels of IL-21 appear to have the potential to either initiate or exacerbate various autoimmune diseases, the effects of IL-21 on B-cell differentiation and antibody production suggest scenarios in which elevation of IL-21 levels may be of use in the treatment of diseases such as allergy and asthma. The possibility that IL-21 can inhibit the production of IgE, overriding its usual control by Th2 cytokines, is suggested by experiments demonstrating that IL-21 treatment of antigen-primed mice decreased IgE production and reduced eosinophil migration into the airways.[27] The ability to modulate both antibody levels and cell migration suggests that IL-21 may play a role in the normal regulation of airway responses to antigen, and that modulating IL-21 levels might potentially control these cellular responses.

The potent anti-tumor effect of IL-21 in various mouse models hopefully can be translated to the clinical setting in a number of human cancers. Among the cytokines that have been used in tumor therapy, IL-21 has a unique effect on the persistence of tumor-specific CD8+ T cells, raising the possibility that it might be employed as a mechanism for inducing long-term tumor immunity.

CONCLUSION

Since the first reports of the discovery of IL-21 and IL-21R in 2000, this γ_c family cytokine system has been shown to be responsible for a remarkably broad range of actions on T, B, NK, and dendritic cells. It can induce proliferation and apoptosis, and has stimulatory and suppressive actions, depending on the target cell and its specific developmental or activation state. Although more work is needed, administering IL-21 or inactivating the action of IL-21 holds clinical promise in different settings. Inhibiting the action of IL-21 might prove useful for autoimmune disorders, whereas providing IL-21 may have anti-tumor effects; however, treatment for cancer would have to be undertaken with cognizance of the possibility of exacerbating autoimmune disorders. IL-21 is an exciting cytokine with pleiotropic actions on multiple lineages. Understanding how and when it exerts various effects *in vivo* are some of the major basic science challenges, with the goal that these can contribute to better moving IL-21 toward the clinical arena.

ACKNOWLEDGMENT

We thank Dr Jian-Xin Lin for critical comments and help in preparing figures.

REFERENCES

1. Leonard WJ. Cytokines and immunodeficiency diseases. Nat Rev Immunol 2001; 1: 200–8.

2. Leonard WJ, Spolski R. Interleukin-21: a modulator of lymphoid proliferation, apoptosis and differentiation. Nat Rev Immunol 2005; 5: 688–98.

3. Noguchi M, Nakamura Y, Russell SM et al. Interleukin-2 receptor gamma chain: a functional component of the interleukin-7 receptor. Science 1993; 262: 1877–80.

4. Ozaki K, Kikly K, Michalovich D, Young PR, Leonard WJ. Cloning of a type I cytokine receptor most related to the IL-2 receptor beta chain. Proc Natl Acad Sci U S A 2000; 97: 11439–44.

5. Parrish-Novak J, Dillon SR, Nelson A et al. Interleukin 21 and its receptor are involved in NK cell expansion and regulation of lymphocyte function. Nature 2000; 408: 57–63.

6. Leonard WJ, Lin JX. Cytokine receptor signaling pathways. J Allergy Clin Immunol 2000; 105: 877–88.

7. Asao H, Okuyama C, Kumaki S et al. Cutting edge: the common gamma-chain is an indispensable subunit of the IL-21 receptor complex. J Immunol 2001; 167: 1–5.

8. Habib T, Senadheera S, Weinberg K, Kaushansky K. The common gamma chain (gamma c) is a required signaling component of the IL-21 receptor and supports IL-21-induced cell proliferation via JAK3. Biochemistry 2002; 41: 8725–31.

9. Noguchi M, Yi H, Rosenblatt HM et al. Interleukin-2 receptor gamma chain mutation results in X-linked severe combined immunodeficiency in humans. Cell 1993; 73: 147–57.

10. Russell SM, Tayebi N, Nakajima H et al. Mutation of Jak3 in a patient with SCID: essential role of Jak3 in lymphoid development. Science 1995; 270: 797–800.

11. Bennett F, Luxenberg D, Ling V et al. Program death-1 engagement upon TCR activation has distinct effects on costimulation and cytokine-driven proliferation: attenuation of ICOS, IL-4, and IL-21, but not CD28, IL-7, and IL-15 responses. J Immunol 2003; 170: 711–18.

12. Strengell M, Sareneva T, Foster D, Julkunen I, Matikainen S. IL-21 up-regulates the expression of genes associated with innate immunity and Th1 response. J Immunol 2002; 169: 3600–5.

13. Strengell M, Matikainen S, Siren J et al. IL-21 in synergy with IL-15 or IL-18 enhances IFN-gamma production in human NK and T cells. J Immunol 2003; 170: 5464–9.

14. Lin JX, Mietz J, Modi WS, John S, Leonard WJ. Cloning of human Stat5B. Reconstitution of interleukin-2-induced Stat5A and Stat5B DNA binding activity in COS-7 cells. J Biol Chem 1996; 271: 10738–44.

15. Hou J, Schindler U, Henzel WJ et al. An interleukin-4-induced transcription factor: IL-4 Stat. Science 1994; 265: 1701–6.

16. Quelle FW, Shimoda K, Thierfelder W et al. Cloning of murine Stat6 and human Stat6, Stat proteins that are tyrosine phosphorylated in responses to IL-4 and IL-3 but are not required for mitogenesis. Mol Cell Biol 1995; 15: 3336–43.

17. Jin H, Carrio R, Yu A, Malek TR. Distinct activation signals determine whether IL-21 induces B cell costimulation, growth arrest, or Bim-dependent apoptosis. J Immunol 2004; 173: 657–65.

18. Brandt K, Bulfone-Paus S, Foster DC, Ruckert R. Interleukin-21 inhibits dendritic cell activation and maturation. Blood 2003; 102: 4090–8.

19. Brandt K, Bulfone-Paus S, Jenckel A et al. Interleukin-21 inhibits dendritic cell-mediated T cell activation and induction of contact hypersensitivity in vivo. J Invest Dermatol 2003; 121: 1379–82.

20. Distler JH, Jungel A, Kowal-Bielecka O et al. Expression of interleukin-21 receptor in epidermis from patients with systemic sclerosis. Arthritis Rheum 2005; 52: 856–64.

21. Ozaki K, Spolski R, Feng CG et al. A critical role for IL-21 in regulating immunoglobulin production. Science 2002; 298: 1630–4.

22. Wu Z, Kim HP, Xue HH et al. Interleukin-21 receptor gene induction in human T cells is mediated by T-cell receptor-induced Sp1 activity. Mol Cell Biol 2005; 25: 9741–52.

23. Strengell M, Julkunen I, Matikainen S. IFN-alpha regulates IL-21 and IL-21R expression in human NK and T cells. J Leukoc Biol 2004; 76: 416–22.

24. Zeng R, Spolski R, Finkelstein SE et al. Synergy of IL-21 and IL-15 in regulating CD8+ T cell expansion and function. J Exp Med 2005; 201: 139–48.

25. Kim HP, Korn LL, Gamero A M, Leonard WJ. Calcium-dependent activation of interleukin-21 gene expression in T cells. J Biol Chem 2005; 280: 25291–7.

26. Mehta DS, Wurster AL, Weinmann AS, Grusby MJ. NFATc2 and T-bet contribute to T-helper-cell-subset-specific regulation of IL-21 expression. Proc Natl Acad Sci U S A 2005; 102: 2016–21.

27. Suto A, Nakajima H, Hirose K et al. Interleukin 21 prevents antigen-induced IgE production by inhibiting germ line C(epsilon) transcription of IL-4-stimulated B cells. Blood 2002; 100: 4565–73.

28. Chtanova T, Tangye SG, Newton R et al. T follicular helper cells express a distinctive transcriptional profile, reflecting their role as non-Th1/Th2 effector cells that provide help for B cells. J Immunol 2004; 173: 68–78.

29. Wurster AL, Rodgers VL, Satoskar AR et al. Interleukin 21 is a T helper (Th) cell 2 cytokine that specifically inhibits the differentiation of naive Th cells into interferon gamma-producing Th1 cells. J Exp Med 2002; 196: 969–77.

30. Schluns KS, Kieper WC, Jameson SC, Lefrancois L. Interleukin-7 mediates the homeostasis of naive and memory CD8 T cells in vivo. Nat Immunol 2000; 1: 426–32.

31. Zhang X, Sun S, Hwang I. Tough DF, Sprent J. Potent and selective stimulation of memory-phenotype CD8+ T cells in vivo by IL-15. Immunity 1998; 8: 591–9.

32. Alves NL, Arosa FA, van Lier RA. IL-21 sustains CD28 expression on IL-15-activated human naive CD8+ T cells. J Immunol 2005; 175: 755–62.

33. Li Y, Bleakley M, Yee C. IL-21 influences the frequency, phenotype, and affinity of the antigen-specific CD8 T cell response. J Immunol 2005; 175: 2261–9.

34. Moroz A, Eppolito C, Li Q et al. IL-21 enhances and sustains CD8+ T cell responses to achieve durable tumor immunity: comparative evaluation of IL-2, IL-15, and IL-21. J Immunol 2004; 173: 900–9.

35. Kuhn R, Rajewsky K, Muller W. Generation and analysis of interleukin-4 deficient mice. Science 1991; 254: 707–10.

36. Wood N, Bourque K, Donaldson DD et al. IL-21 effects on human IgE production in response to IL-4 or IL-13. Cell Immunol 2004; 231: 133–45.

37. Mehta DS, Wurster AL, Whitters MJ et al. IL-21 induces the apoptosis of resting and activated primary B cells. J Immunol 2003; 170: 4111–18.

38. Ozaki K, Spolski R, Ettinger R et al. Regulation of B cell differentiation and plasma cell generation by IL-21, a novel inducer of Blimp-1 and Bcl-6. J Immunol 2004; 173: 5361–71.

39. Akashi K, Kondo M, von Freeden-Jeffry U, Murray R, Weissman IL. Bcl-2 rescues T lymphopoiesis in interleukin-7 receptor-deficient mice. Cell 1997; 89: 1033–41.

40. Otani H, Erdos M, Leonard WJ. Tyrosine kinase(s) regulate apoptosis and bcl-2 expression in a growth factor-dependent cell line. J Biol Chem 1993; 268: 22733–36.

41. Eltinger R, Sims GP, Failhurst AM et al. IL-21 induces differentiation of human naive and memory B cells into antibody-secreting plasma cells. J Immunol 2005; 175: 7867–79.

42. Pene J, Gauchat JF, Lecart S et al. Cutting edge: IL-21 is a switch factor for the production of IgG1 and IgG3 by human B cells. J Immunol 2004; 172: 5154–7.

43. Calame KL, Lin KI, Tunyaplin C. Regulatory mechanisms that determine the development and function of plasma cells. Annu Rev Immunol 2003; 21: 205–30.

44. DiSanto JP, Muller W, Guy-Grand D, Fischer A, Rajewsky K. Lymphoid development in mice with a targeted deletion of the interleukin 2 receptor gamma chain. Proc Natl Acad Sci U S A 1995; 92: 377–81.

45. Cao X, Shores EW, Hu-Li J et al. Defective lymphoid development in mice lacking expression of the common cytokine receptor gamma chain. Immunity 1995; 2: 223–38.

46. Lodolce JP, Boone DL, Chai S et al. IL-15 receptor maintains lymphoid homeostasis by supporting lymphocyte homing and proliferation. Immunity 1998; 9: 669–76.

47. Kennedy MK, Glaccum M, Brown SN et al. Reversible defects in natural killer and memory CD8 T cell lineages in interleukin 15-deficient mice. J Exp Med 2000; 191: 771–80.

48. Kasaian MT, Whitters MJ, Carter LL et al. IL-21 limits NK cell responses and promotes antigen-specific T cell activation: a mediator of the transition from innate to adaptive immunity. Immunity 2002; 16: 559–69.

49. Toomey JA, Gays F, Foster D, Brooks CG. Cytokine requirements for the growth and development of mouse NK cells in vitro. J Leukoc Biol 2003; 74: 233–42.

50. Brady J, Hayakawa Y, Smyth MJ, Nutt SL. IL-21 induces the functional maturation of murine NK cells. J Immunol 2004; 172: 2048–58.

51. Wang G, Tschoi M, Spolski R et al. In vivo antitumor activity of interleukin 21 mediated by natural killer cells. Cancer Res 2003; 63: 9016–22.

52. Takaki R, Hayakawa Y, Nelson A et al. IL-21 enhances tumor rejection through a NKG2D-dependent mechanism. J Immunol 2005; 175: 2167–73.

53. Yamaoka K, Min B, Zhou YJ, Paul WE, O'Shea JJ. Jak3 negatively regulates dendritic-cell cytokine production and survival. Blood 2005; 106: 3227–33.

54. Vinuesa CG, Cook MC, Angelucci C et al. A RING-type ubiquitin ligase family member required to repress follicular helper T cells and autoimmunity. Nature 2005; 435: 452–8.

55. King C, Ilic A, Koelsch K, Sarvetnick N. Homeostatic expansion of T cells during immune insufficiency generates autoimmunity. Cell 2004; 117: 265–77.

56. Denny P, Lord CJ, Hill NJ et al. Mapping of the IDDM locus Idd3 to a 0.35-cM interval containing the interleukin-2 gene. Diabetes 1997; 46: 695–700.

57. Monteleone G, Monteleone I, Fina D et al. Interleukin-21 enhances T-helper cell type I signaling and interferon-gamma production in Crohn's disease. Gastroenterology 2005; 128: 687–94.

58. Vollmer TL, Liu R, Price M et al. Differential effects of IL-21 during initiation and progression of autoimmunity against neuroantigen. J Immunol 2005; 174: 2696–701.

18

The biology of human interleukin-32

Charles A Dinarello and Soo-Hyun Kim

Introduction • Isoforms of IL-32 • Binding of human IL-32α to proteinase-3 • Production of IL-32 from human monocytes *in vitro* • Cooperation of monocytes with lymphocytes is necessary for full IL-32 production • IL-32 in arthritis • IL-32 in Crohn's disease • Acknowledgments • References

INTRODUCTION

Interleukin-32 (IL-32)[1] is a proinflammatory cytokine originally described as a transcript termed NK4 found in activated natural killer (NK) cells and T lymphocytes.[2] Although IL-32 is expressed at low levels in health, in disease conditions such as rheumatoid arthritis (RA), chronic obstructive pulmonary disease (COPD), Crohn's disease, and psoriasis, the expression increases markedly. IL-32 is a major transcript in gene array studies in epithelial cells stimulated with interferon (IFN)-γ *in vitro*. In mycobacterial infections, pulmonary macrophages contain IL-32 but macrophages from healthy lung tissue do not.

IL-32 was 're-discovered' during a search for IL-18-inducible genes independent of IL-12 or IL-15 costimulation. We generated a cell line that expressed both chains of the IL-18 receptor (IL-18 receptor α and β chains). In the absence of costimulants, IL-18 induced several expected proinflammatory genes in the human lung epithelial cell line A549. However, there was a high level of expression in transcript termed NK4. Upon expression of the recombinant form of the NK4 transcript, it became clear that NK4 encoded for a protein with many of the characteristics of proinflammatory cytokines.[1] For these reasons, the name was changed to IL-32. Although IL-32 was first reported as transcript in IL-2-activated NK and T cells, it appears that epithelial cells are a dominant and widespread source. In fact, the A549 cell line is a human lung carcinoma cell line. Others have reported the presence of mRNA for IL-32 in Epstein–Barr virus-infected lymphoma cells,[3] neuroblastoma cells,[4] and hematopoietic progenitor cells.[5] Primary human B cells, even when stimulated with IgM or anti-CD40, do not express significant levels of IL-32.[6] However, the cytokine is highly expressed in activated primary human T cells following stimulation with anti-CD3 or the combination of phorbol myristate acetate (PMA) and ionomycin.[6] Northern blot analysis of various human tissues from healthy subjects reveal low constitutive expression of steady-state levels of mRNA in the prostate, moderate in the thymus, small intestine, and colon, but high in the spleen and peripheral blood leukocytes.

ISOFORMS OF IL-32

In the case of human IL-32, six isoforms have been described. The original isoform of the NK4 transcript is presently termed IL-32γ. All isoforms have an intact first exon, which precedes the translational initiation site (ATG) found in the terminal end of the second isoform. Isoforms IL-32α, IL-32β, IL-32δ, and IL-32α each have a deletion in the carboxy end of the third exon. In contrast, IL-32γ has a complete exon 3 such that the third and fourth exons have no intronic sequences. IL-32ζ has no second or third exon; the ATG is part of the fourth exon. All isoforms have an intact fifth and sixth exon. With the exception of IL-32α, all isoforms have an intact seventh and eighth exon. In the case of IL-32α, there is a deletion in the seventh exon. The IL-32α isoform, although produced by most cell lines, has two large deletions, whereas IL-32γ has no deletions. Figure 18.1 illustrates the six isoforms of human IL-32 derived from alternate splicing.

BINDING OF HUMAN IL-32α TO PROTEINASE-3

In an attempt to isolate an IL-32α soluble receptor or binding protein, recombinant IL-32α was covalently immobilized on agarose and preparations of concentrated crude human urinary proteins were applied for chromatographic separation. A specific 30 kDa protein eluted from the column during acid washing and was identified by mass spectrometry as proteinase-3 (PR-3).[7] PR-3 is a neutrophil granule serine protease, exists as a soluble or membrane form, and is the major autoantigen for autoantibodies in the systemic vasculitic disease Wegener's granulomatosis. The affinity of IL-32α to PR-3 is 2.65 ± 0.4 nM. However, irreversible inactivation of PR-3 enzymatic activity did not significantly change binding to the cytokine. Nevertheless, limited cleavage of IL-32 yielded products consistent with PR-3 enzyme activity. Moreover, following limited cleavage by PR-3, IL-32α was more active than intact IL-32α in inducing macrophage inflammatory protein-2 in mouse macrophages and IL-8 in human peripheral blood mononuclear cells (PBMCs).[7] Therefore, PR-3 is a specific IL-32α binding protein, independent of its enzymatic activity, but limited cleavage of IL-32α by PR-3 enhances the activities of the cytokine. It is possible that specific inhibition of PR-3 activity to process IL-32 or neutralization of IL-32 by inactive PR-3 or its fragments may reduce the consequences of IL-32 in immune-regulated diseases.

PRODUCTION OF IL-32 FROM HUMAN MONOCYTES *IN VITRO*

Similar to other proinflammatory cytokines, the mechanisms for production *in vitro* from primary human cells provide important information for its production in disease. Whole human blood was stimulated with 1×10^7 microorganisms/ml of heat-killed *Mycobacterium tuberculosis*. IL-32 was primarily measured in the total cell lysate. Similar stimulation was observed when freshly isolated PBMCs were stimulated

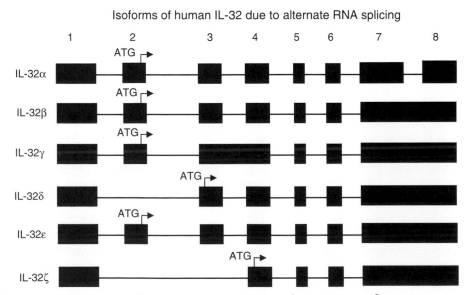

Figure 18.1 Six isoforms of human IL-32. Data are derived from Kim et al.[1] and Brown et al.[5]

with *M. tuberculosis*.[8] Interestingly, whereas endotoxin also moderately stimulated IL-32 production in PBMCs, stimulation with other Toll-like receptor (TLR) agonists such as Pam3Cys (TLR2), poly I:C (TLR3), flagellin (TLR5), or CpG (TLR9) did not induce IL-32 production. Similarly, stimulation of PBMCs with other heat-killed microorganisms such as *Staphylococcus aureus*, *Candida albicans* or *Aspergillus fumigatus* did not stimulate IL-32 production. No IL-32 was found in the adherent cells incubated with control medium. However, after 24 hours, IL-32 mRNA for the first four isoforms were present in the unstimulated PBMCs.

COOPERATION OF MONOCYTES WITH LYMPHOCYTES IS NECESSARY FOR FULL IL-32 PRODUCTION

When PBMCs isolated from healthy volunteers were stimulated with IFN-γ, IL-1β or tumor necrosis factor (TNF)-α, only IFN-γ induced IL-32. In the human epithelial cell line WISH, IFN-γ also stimulates IL-32.[1] Of all the cytokines, IFN-γ is essential for host defense against mycobacterial infection and therefore the ability of IFN-γ to induce IL-32 may be related to a role for IL-32 in anti-mycobacterial defense. One can conclude from large population studies that a well-contained granuloma containing live *M. tuberculosis* is not incompatible with long life as long as the patient's immune system is fully functional. A fully functional immune system includes cytokine production, particularly IFN-γ. Most notably, mutations in any of five genes that control IFN-γ production result in severe and life-threatening mycobacterial disease from birth.[9] These include the IFN-γ receptor type I and type II, the p40 chain of IL-12, the IL-12 receptor β1, and the intracellular transcription factor known as STAT1. These human studies are supported by a large body of animal studies showing failure to contain *M. tuberculosis* infection in mice treated with antibodies to or lacking production of IFN-γ.

When comparing total PBMCs, isolated adherent monocytes, or the non-adherent lymphocyte population following stimulation with *M. tuberculosis*, monocytes were the main source of IL-32.[8] However, the presence of lymphocytes was necessary for optimal release of IL-32, since there were significantly lower amounts of IL-32 from monocytes alone, compared with the mixed monocyte/lymphocyte population from PBMCs. In addition, monocyte-derived macrophages and dendritic cells (DCs) were also capable of producing moderate amounts of IL-32.

It was also reported that *M. tuberculosis* stimulates IL-32 through a caspase-1/IL-18/IFN-γ–dependent mechanism.[8] To investigate the pathway leading to the stimulation of IL-32 by *M. tuberculosis*, PBMCs were stimulated with the mycobacteria in the presence or absence of cytokine inhibitors. Inhibition of IL-18 and IL-1β processing by a caspase-1 inhibitor strongly decreased the production of IFN-γ and IL-32, but not that of TNF. To discern whether these effects were due to endogenous IL-18 or IL-1β, cells were stimulated with *M. tuberculosis* in the presence of the natural inhibitors of IL-18 and IL-1: IL-18 binding protein (IL-18BP) respectively. IL-18BP strongly decreased the production of IL-32 and IFN-γ stimulated by *M. tuberculosis*, whereas IL-1Ra had no effects.[8] To assess whether IL-32 production is mediated via intermediary IFN-γ release from lymphocytes, IFN-γ activity was blocked using anti-IFN-γ antibody.[8] Blockade of IFN-γ activity inhibited the production of IL-32, while also moderately affecting TNF synthesis. Thus *M. tuberculosis* stimulates the production of IL-32 through a caspase-1/IL-18/IFN-γ pathway.

IL-32 IN ARTHRITIS

In culture, synovial cells isolated from human biopsies take on a specialized stellate fibroblast-like form first reported by Krane and Dayer.[10] These fibroblast-like synoviocytes, termed synovial fibroblasts (SF), can be cultured from tissues of patients with RA as well as osteoarthritis. In general, steady-state mRNA in SF isolated from these two distinct arthritides express similar levels of cytokines, chemokines, and their respective receptors when cultured in the absence of exogenous stimulation.[11] However, constitutive expression is differentially observed between third passage SF from RA compared with FLS from biopsies of osteoarthritis.[11] In that study, synovial biopsies were obtained from eight patients with RA and nine patients with osteoarthritis. Gene array was performed with over 54 000 transcripts. The mean differential expression of IL-32 in RA compared with osteoarthritis was 3.85-fold greater ($p = 0.0073$).[11] Another differentially expressed gene was monocytes chemoattractant protein-1 (MCP-1, CCL2). MCP-1 expression was 2.5-fold greater in SF from RA compared with osteoarthritis ($p = 0.02$).[11] The authors argue that since the level of expression of inflammatory genes from SF are similar in RA and osteoarthritis, the differential increase in IL-32 may implicate a role for this cytokine in RA.[11] A similar argument was proposed for the high degree of expression of MCP-1. Since recombinant IL-32 stimulates chemokines from macrophagic cells *in vitro*,[1] the finding of both IL-32 and MCP-1 may be more than just coincidental.

Although the studies by Chiocchia and coworkers provide an important observation in differential gene expression of IL-32,[11] direct evidence for IL-32 in RA was reported by Joosten and colleagues.[12] IL-32 staining was observed in 25 of the 29 synovial biopsies; marked staining was predominantly found in the lining layer of the synovium.[12] The cells that were the most positive for IL-32 staining were macrophage-like cells. The percentage of RA patients with IL-32-positive biopsies was lower among the group showing little clinical arthritis compared with those with moderate or severe knee inflammation. Assessment scores for IL-32 in the lining were highly correlated with those for microscopic inflammation on routinely stained tissue sections ($r = 0.80$, $p < 0.0001$) and also with the acute phase reaction as measured by the erythrocyte sedimentation rate ($r = 0.71$, $p < 0.0001$). TNF-α was detectable in only 50% of the RA patients. In contrast IL-1β staining was observed in most synovial biopsies (90% of the RA patients), whereas IL-18 was detectable in 79% of the same synovial tissue samples. The levels of IL-32 and TNF-α expression in the same biopsies were strongly correlated ($r = 0.68$, $p < 0.004$ for lining). However, a greater association was found for IL-32 presence in the lining layers with the expression of IL-1β and IL-18 in the same biopsies ($r = 0.79$, $p < 0.0001$ for IL-1β and $r = 0.82$, $p < 0.0001$).

In a recent study, IL-32 steady-state gene expression was assessed in lymphoid tissues, as well as in stimulated peripheral T cells, monocytes, and B cells.[13] Similar to the studies of Netea et al.,[8] activated T cells were important for IL-32 mRNA expression in monocytes and B cells.[13] Not unexpectedly and similar to published observations,[1,12] TNF-α induced IL-32 mRNA expression in T cells, monocyte-derived DCs, and synovial fibroblasts. Also confirming previous studies,[11] steady-state IL-32 mRNA expression was high in the synovial tissues of RA patients,[13] as well as in synovial-infiltrated lymphocytes using *in situ* hybridization.[13]

Following administration of bone marrow cells overexpressing the human IL-32β isoform, splenocytes from the recipient mice exhibited increased TNF-α, IL-1β, and IL-6 production and secretion,[13] which was enhanced by the presence of endotoxin. In addition to increased production of TNF-α from splenocytes of IL-32β expressing mice, serum TNF-α levels were increased. TNF-α, IL-1β, and IL-6 expression were elevated as well as endotoxin-stimulated macrophages and DCs. In mice with bone marrow transplants of the human IL-32β isoform, there was worsening of the clinical score using collagen antibody-induced arthritis as well as in mice subjected to sulfonic acid-induced colitis.[13] Upon transfer of CD4+ T cells expressing IL-32β, there was a significant exacerbation of collagen-induced arthritis (CIA).[13] It was previously demonstrated that recombinant human IL-32 injected directly into the knee joints of wild-type mice resulted in a severe inflammatory infiltration but that the response to IL-32 was markedly reduced in mice deficient in TNF-α.[12] Using transfer of IL-32β-expressing cells with CIA, TNF-α blockade prevented the exacerbating effects of human IL-32β.[13] The authors concluded that IL-32 worsens the inflammatory responses of experimental arthritis and colitis and that the effects of IL-32 in these models of inflammation are due to TNF-α activity. However, blocking IL-1β or IL-6 in mice overexpressing IL-32 has yet to be determined.

IL-32 IN CROHN'S DISEASE

Activation of non-specific inflammatory responses (innate immunity) plays an essential role in host defense against invading organisms. In general, these responses include the induction of proinflammatory cytokines, which assist the host in eliminating the infection by non-immune mechanisms such as emigration of phagocytic cells and the production of toxic products to destroy the organisms. Indeed, bacterial products induce cytokines via pattern-recognition receptors for several bacterial products. The two most clinically relevant families of microbial receptors are the cell-surface TLRs and the intracellular nuclear oligomerization domain (NOD) receptor family. IL-32 acts in a synergistic manner with the NOD1- and NOD2-specific muropeptides of peptidoglycans for the release of IL-1β and IL-6 (3–10-fold increase).[14] In contrast, IL-32 did not influence the cytokine production induced via TLRs. The synergistic effect of IL-32 and the synthetic muramyl dipeptide (MDP) on cytokine production was absent in cells of patients with Crohn's disease bearing the NOD2 frame shift mutation,[14] demonstrating that the IL-32/MDP synergism depends on NOD2. This *in vitro* synergism between IL-32 and NOD2 ligands was consistent with a marked constitutive expression of IL-32 in human colon epithelial tissue. In addition, the potentiating effect of IL-32 on the cytokine production induced by the synthetic muropeptide FK-156 was absent in NOD1-deficient macrophages, supporting the interaction between IL-32 and NOD1 pathways.[14] Of importance, the synergism between IL-32 and MDP/NOD2 for the induction of IL-6 was dependent on the activation of caspase-1 and the secretion of IL-1β. Only additive effects of IL-32 and muropeptides were observed for TNF-α production. The modulation of intracellular NOD2 pathways by IL-32, but not the cell surface TLRs, as well as the marked expression of IL-32 in colon mucosa, suggest a role for IL-32 in the pathogenesis of Crohn's disease.

ACKNOWLEDGMENTS

The authors thank Drs Mihai G. Netea, Eli C. Lewis, Leo A. Joosten, Do-Young Yoon, Daniela Novick, Menchem Rubinstein, and Tania Azam for their contributions to the understanding of the biology of IL-IL-32. S-H.K was supported by NIH grants AI-15614, HL-68743 CA-04 6934, and a grant from Amgen, Inc.

REFERENCES

1. Kim SH, Han SY, Azam T, Yoon DY, Dinarello CA. Interleukin-32: a cytokine and inducer of TNFalpha. Immunity 2005; 22(1): 131–42.

2. Dahl CA, Schall RP, He HL, Cairns JS. Identification of a novel gene expressed in activated natural killer cells and T cells. J Immunol 1992; 148(2): 597–603.

3. Carter KL, Cahir-McFarland E, Kieff E. Epstein–Barr virus-induced changes in B-lymphocyte gene expression. J Virol 2002; 76(20): 10427–36.

4. Park GH, Choe J, Choo HJ et al. Genome-wide expression profiling of 8-chloroadenosine- and 8-chloro-cAMP-treated human neuroblastoma cells using radioactive human cDNA microarray. Exp Mol Med 2002; 34(3): 184–93.

5. Brown J, Matutes E, Singleton A et al. Lymphopain, a cytotoxic T and natural killer cell-associated cysteine proteinase. Leukemia 1998; 12(11): 1771–81.

6. Goda C, Kanaji T, Kanaji S et al. Involvement of IL-32 in activation-induced cell death in T cells. Int Immunol 2006; 18(2): 233–40.

7. Novick D, Rubinstein M, Azam T et al. Proteinase 3 is an interleukin-32 binding protein. Proc Natl Acad Sci U S A 2006; 103: 3316–21.

8. Netea MG, Azam T, Lewis EC et al. *Mycobacterium tuberculosis* induces interleukin-32 production through a caspase-1/IL-18/interferon-gamma-dependent mechanism. PLoS Med 2006; 3(8): e277.

9. Ottenhoff TH, Verreck FA, Lichtenauer-Kaligis EG et al. Genetics, cytokines and human infectious disease: lessons from weakly pathogenic mycobacteria and salmonellae. Nat Genet 2002; 32(1): 97–105.

10. Dayer JM, Graham R, Russell G, Krane SM. Collagenase production by rheumatoid synovial cells: stimulation by a human lymphocyte factor. Science 1977; 195(4274): 181–3.

11. Cagnard N, Letourneur F, Essabbani A et al. Interleukin-32, CCL2, PF4F1 and GFD10 are the only cytokine/chemokine genes differentially expressed by in vitro cultured rheumatoid and osteoarthritis fibroblast-like synoviocytes. Eur Cytokine Netw 2005; 16(4): 289–92.

12. Joosten LA, Netea MG, Kim SH et al. IL-32, a proinflammatory cytokine in rheumatoid arthritis. Proc Natl Acad Sci U S A 2006; 103(9): 3298–303.

13. Shoda H, Fujio K, Yamaguchi Y et al. Interactions between IL-32 and tumor necrosis factor alpha contribute to the exacerbation of immune-inflammatory diseases. Arthritis Res Ther 2006; 8(6): R166.

14. Netea MG, Azam T, Ferwerda G et al. IL-32 synergizes with nucleotide oligomerization domain (NOD) 1 and NOD2 ligands for IL-1β and IL-6 production through a caspase 1-dependent mechanism. Proc Natl Acad Sci U S A 2005; 102(45): 16309–14.

19

The interferons

Lars Rönnblom, Maija-Leena Eloranta and Gunnar Alm

Introduction • The IFN proteins and genes • Activation of type I IFN genes • Activation of the type II IFN (IFN-γ) gene • Activation of type III IFN genes • Cellular basis of type I and III IFN production • Mode of activation of type I IFN production in immature PDCs • The IFN receptors and their signaling pathways • Negative regulation of IFN signaling pathways • Genes, proteins, and cell functions regulated by IFNs • Activation of the type I IFN system in autoimmune diseases • A causative role for type I IFN in autoimmunity • Type II IFN (IFN-γ) in autoimmune diseases • An etiopathogenic mechanism for autoimmunity involving the type I IFN system • Therapeutic targets • Acknowledgments • References

INTRODUCTION

The interferons (IFNs) were the first cytokines to be discovered,[1] evaluated as therapeutic agents in viral infections and cancers, and produced on a large scale as recombinant proteins for clinical use.[2] The IFNs are defined by their ability to interfere with replication of viruses in cells via induction of new mRNA and protein synthesis. They are grouped into type I IFN, type II IFN, and type III IFN and are encoded by no less than 21 different genes in man. These three major classes of IFNs (I–III) act on separate receptors. The type I IFNs have been most extensively studied and constitute an important part of innate immunity against viral infections, but also act as a link to adaptive immunity via many effects on key immune cells, such as T cells, B cells, and dendritic cells (DCs). The inducers of type I IFN production (typically virus), the cells producing type I IFNs, the type I IFN genes and proteins, as well as the targets cells affected by the type I IFNs, can be defined as the type I IFN system. The type III IFNs may be included in this system, because of many similarities to type I IFN. Type II IFN (IFN-γ) on the other hand is more clearly separate, because it is typically produced by activated T and natural killer (NK) cells and differs in function compared with type I/III IFN (see below). Types I, II, and III IFNs have an extraordinarily wide range of effects on innate and adaptive immune responses and have attracted a great deal of interest because of their potentially pivotal role in development of autoimmune diseases, although type III IFNs have not been extensively studied in this respect. We here review the biology of the IFNs, with emphasis on their involvement in autoimmune diseases.

THE IFN PROTEINS AND GENES

The human IFN genes (including chromosomal location) and proteins (including their amino acid numbers and homologies) are listed in Table 19.1. The type I IFNs are encoded by a family of 17 genes, 13 genes for the different − IFN-α subtypes and single genes for IFN-β, -ω, -κ, and -ε.[3] The type I IFNs are all significantly homologous at the gene and protein sequence level. The type I IFN genes (designated as in Table 19.1) are located in the type I IFN locus on the short arm of chromosome 9 at 9p21.3, distributed over a 400 kb stretch. The gene for IFN-κ

Table 19.1 Human type I, II, and III interferon (IFN) genes and proteins

IFN type	Genes	Gene locus	Proteins[a]	Size (amino acids)	Sequence homologies
I	IFNA1, 2, 4, 5, 6, 7, 8, 10, 13, 14, 16, 17, 21	9p21.3	IFN-α1, 2, 4, 5, 6, 7, 8, 10, 13, 14, 16, 17, 21 (n = 13)	165–166	> 75%[b]
I	IFNB1	9p21.3	IFN-β	166	30%
I	IFNE1	9p21.3	IFN-ε	185	30%
I	IFNK	9p21.2	IFN-κ	180	30%
I	IFNW1	9p21.3	IFN-ω	172–174	75%
II	IFNG	12q15	IFN-γ	146	NS
III	IL29, IL28A, IL28B	19q13.2	IFN-λ1, 2, 3, (IL-29, IL-28A, IL-28B)	175–181	> 80%[b] (low to IFN-α)

NS, not significant.

[a]IFN-α1 and IFN-α13 have identical amino acid sequences.

[b]Homologies between IFN-α subtypes and between IFN-λ subtypes. Homologies to IFN-α.

(*IFNK*) is however located slightly outside the type I IFN locus, at 9p21.2. The type I IFN genes lack introns, except for *IFNK*, which has one intron. The type I IFN genes are mainly silent in cells, but their expression can be induced in cells, for example, by viral infection (see below). However, IFN-κ has been reported to be expressed in resting keratinocytes.[4]

Type II IFN, also termed IFN-γ, is encoded by the gene *IFNG* that contains three introns and is located on chromosome 12 (12q15). There is no significant homology with type I or III IFNs at DNA or protein levels (Table 19.1).

The type III IFNs consist of three genes (*IL29, IL28A, IL28B*) and corresponding proteins, which are highly homologous. The genes are located at chromosome 19 (19q13.2) and contain five exons. The type III IFNs were identified and described as IL-29, IL-28A, and IL-28B, or IFN-λ1, IFN-λ2, and IFN-λ3 in independent publications.[5,6] Their designation as type III IFNs[7] is appropriate since they display antiviral activity, are induced by viruses, display a weak homology with type I IFN, and act via a separate receptor.

ACTIVATION OF TYPE I IFN GENES

Expression of type I IFN genes is typically induced by viruses, but some bacteria and protozoa are also IFN-inducers. The critical first step is here the activation of Toll-like receptors (TLRs) or intracellular sensors by microbial DNA or RNA molecules, which leads to phosphorylation and activation of several transcription factors that bind to positive regulatory domains (PRDs), located 5′ of the transcription initiation sites in type I IFN genes (Figure 19.1).[8,9] These transcription factors include the IFN regulatory factors (IRFs) IRF-3, IRF-5, and IRF-7, which interact with virus-responsive elements (VREs) in PRDs. The VREs consist of repeats of GAAANN motifs and are essential for type I IFN gene expression. However, several other transcription factors are also involved and they include IRF-1 and IRF-2. In the IFN-β gene (*IFNB1*), which has been most extensively studied, the PRDI and PRDIII elements contain such VREs. However, a PRDII element also interacts with NF-κB. The NF-κB and IRF-3/IRF-7 interact with the transcription factors ATF-2/c-Jun and HMGI(Y) and form an enhanceosome that causes expression of the genes. IRF-3, IRF-7, and IRF-5 are also involved in induced expression of IFN-α genes via formation of enhanceosomes.

The mode of action of the TLRs in the activation of type I IFN (and other genes) is complicated, but has been significantly unraveled in recent years (see Chapter 9).[8,10–12] TLR3 is commonly viewed to have an endosomal localization in cells and mediates type I IFN production induced by double-stranded RNA (dsRNA).

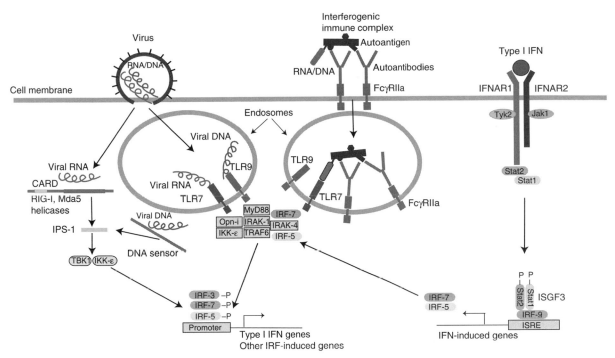

Figure 19.1 Activation of type I IFN genes in immature plasmacytoid dendritic cells (PDCs), also termed natural IFN-producing cells (NIPCs), by virus or immune complexes containing RNA or DNA molecules. Endosomal TLR7 (recognizing single-stranded RNA) and TLR9 (recognizing CpG-DNA) are activated by endocytosis of virus, or after FcγRIIa-mediated endocytosis of immune complexes. Via assembly of a MyD88-associated signaling complex with multiple adaptors and kinases, the IRFs (IRF-3, -5, -7) are activated by phosphorylation. Then, type I IFN genes, as well as (not shown; see text) genes for several proinflammatory cytokines ('IRF-induced genes') are expressed. Nucleic acids introduced into the cytoplasm, at least viral dsRNA or dsDNA, can be recognized, e.g. by RIG-I and Mda5 helicases (dsRNA), and as yet unidentified sensors (dsDNA). Such cytoplasmic RNA/DNA recognition pathways converge via a common adapter protein (IPS-1) that mediates activation of the kinases TBK1 and IKKε, resulting in activation of IRFs and type I IFN gene transcription. Genes involved in TLR-mediated activation are up-regulated by type I IFN, including IRF-5/7 and TLR7, forming the basis of an endogenous enhancing loop by which type I IFN increases its own production and that of several proinflammatory cytokines (the priming phenomenon). Not shown is the capacity of TLR3 to mediate induction of type I IFN expression by dsRNA and of TLR4 to activate IFN-β gene transcription.

TLR3 uses TRIF (and not MyD88, see below) as the adapter, and the further signaling pathways involve activation of IRF-3 (and perhaps IRF-7), NF-κB and ATF2/c-Jun transcription factors, and eventually expression of genes encoding both IFN-α and -β and proinflammatory cytokines (see Chapter 9). TLR4 is a receptor for bacterial lipopolysaccharide (LPS), but also certain viral proteins, and is present on the cell surface. Upon TLR4 ligation, the genes for IFN-β and several proinflammatory cytokines are induced via signaling pathways involving the final activation of especially transcription factors IRF-3 and NF-κB (see Chapter 9).

TLR7 and TLR8 bind and become activated by single-stranded RNA (ssRNA), while TLR9 in contrast is activated by unmethylated CpG-rich DNA (Figure 19.1). These TLRs then recruit the MyD88 adapter protein that subsequently interacts with a set of molecules that include TRAF6, IRAK1, IRAK4, osteopontin (Opn-i), and the IκB kinase-α (IKK-α).[8,11] This complex recruits and phosphorylates IRF-5 and IRF-7. In addition there are pathways that result in activation of NF-κB and ATF2/c-Jun, as described for TLR3 (see Chapter 9). This causes strong induction of IFN-α and proinflammatory cytokines.[8,11] In the mouse, data indicate that IRF-5 is responsible for

TLR-mediated expression of proinflammatory cytokines, while IRF-7 is required for induction of type I IFN.[8] The situation may differ in human cells, where IRF-5 has been shown to mediate type I IFN induction.[13] As further discussed below, the type I IFN production mediated by TLR7 and TLR9 occurs principally in immature plasmacytoid dendritic cells (PDCs), also termed natural type I IFN-producing cells (NIPC).

There are also TLR-independent intracellular pathways mediating type I IFN production induced by nucleic acids that enter the cytosol (Figure 19.1). One involves the protein kinase R (PKR) that is activated by dsRNA.[14] However, the two RNA helicases RIG-I and Mda5 appear more important in the intracellular recognition of dsRNA.[11] These CARD-containing helicases use the mitochondria-associated adapter MAVS (also termed IPS-1, VISA or Cardif) and possibly other adapters such as RIP1 and FADD to activate the kinases TBK1 and IKKε. This results in phosphorylation of IRF-3 and IRF-7 and thus type I IFN expression. Also, intracellular dsDNA can trigger activation of IRF-3 and NF-κB via TBK1 and IKKε, leading to production of type I IFN and proinflammatory cytokines,[15,16] but the actual sensors are not RIG-I or Mda5 and therefore remain to be defined.

Consequently, several endosomal TLR-dependent and intracellular TLR-independent mechanisms are involved in the triggering of production of type I IFN and proinflammatory cytokines by microbial DNA and RNA. Importantly, they also mediate responses to mammalian-derived DNA and RNA and are therefore of considerable interest in autoimmune diseases (see below).

ACTIVATION OF THE TYPE II IFN (IFN-γ) GENE

The production and action of IFN-γ has been extensively reviewed.[17] The main IFN-γ producers are cytotoxic and helper T cells, as well as NK cells (Figure 19.2). However, other cells such as DCs, mast cells, B cells, and macrophages can also produce IFN-γ. In fact, even the NIPCs/PDCs, the principal type I IFN producers, have been reported to produce IFN-γ.[18] The IFN-γ gene contains binding sites for several transcription factors in the regulatory region upstream of

the start of transcription. They include AP-1, CREB/ATF, NFAT, T bet, NF-κB, as well as the signal tranducers and activator of transcription (STAT) factors 1, 4, and 5, but not the IRFs that are involved in type I IFN gene expression (Figure 19.2). This spectrum partly explains why IFN-γ genes are induced by several cytokines, such as IL-2, IL-12, IL-15, IL-18, IL-21, IL-23, IL-27, and type I IFN, alone or in combinations.[9,17] IL-12 and IL-18 are active alone, but the IFN-γ-inducing capacity is markedly enhanced when they are combined. Furthermore, monocytes/macrophages/DCs can be activated via, for example, TLR7, to produce IL-12, which in turn acts on NK cells to induce IFN-γ production and cell proliferation, and this is enhanced by exposure of these cells to IL-2 or type I IFN.[19] However, both NK cells and memory T cells express TLR7, and at least the latter cells can also be activated by TLR7 agonists to produce IFN-γ.[20] Thus, production of type I IFN, IL-12, and several proinflammatory cytokines is coordinated with production of IFN-γ by NK cells. This may be an important event, because type I and II IFNs have synergistic actions in several systems (see below).

In the activation of the IFN-γ production by NK cells, the interaction of NK-cell receptors NKG2D with the ligands MICA/MICB and of TNFRSF18 with the ligand TNFSF18 (GITRL) are important (Figure 19.2). For T cells, interaction of their T-cell receptor (TCR) with ligand major histocompatibility complex (MHC)–peptide complexes, CD2 molecules with ligand CD58, or TNFRSF15 with ligand TNFSF15 contribute to the activation of IFN-γ production. The fact that all mentioned ligands can be expressed by myeloid or plasmacytoid DCs, which also produce IFN-γ-inducing cytokines, is the basis for important cross-talk whereby activated DCs promote IFN-γ production.[21,22] This has functional implications, in that type I–III IFNs are produced concomitantly.

ACTIVATION OF TYPE III IFN GENES

Type III IFN (IFN-λ1-3; IL-28A/28B/29) production is triggered by viruses, and the mechanisms of activation appear similar to those for type I IFN, involving TLRs and activation of

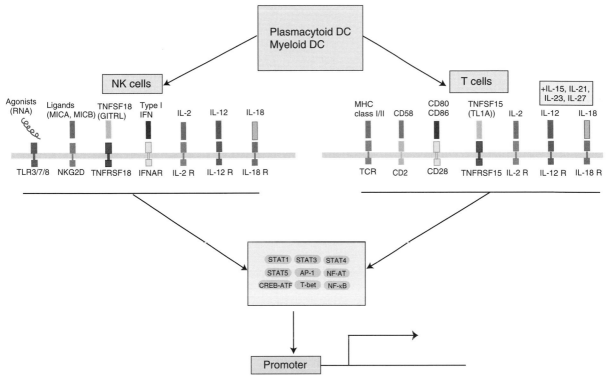

Figure 19.2 Activation of type II IFN (IFN-γ) genes in NK cells and T cells. The activation is dependent on interaction of these cells with, for example, activated plasmacytoid or myeloid DCs. Such DCs produce cytokines (e.g. IL-12, IL-15, IL-18, IL-21, IL-27, type I IFN) and also express cell membrane molecules that activate IFN-γ genes in T and NK cells. The membrane molecules include MHC class I/II interacting with TCR, CD58 with CD2, CD80/86 with CD28, and MICA/MICB with NKG2D, as well as TNF superfamily members TNFSF15 and TNFSF18 that interact with corresponding receptors. NK cells and T cells also express TLRs that contribute to their activation. The regulation of the IFN-γ gene is complex, involving many transcription factors (See in the box), that in separate ways can cause gene expression.

NF-κB, IRF-3, and IRF-7.[23] Also, priming of cells with type I IFN dramatically increased both type I and III IFN expression, at least in part due to increased expression of IRF-7 and TLRs.[24]

CELLULAR BASIS OF TYPE I AND III IFN PRODUCTION

Many different types of cells can produce type I IFN, but in small quantities and mainly in response to certain RNA viruses, such as influenza and Sendai virus. This restricted response is most likely due to lack of components essential for efficient type I IFN gene expression. For instance, the transcription factors IRF-5 and IRF-7 are preferentially expressed in human cells of lymphoid origin and TLR7 and TLR9 in the principal IPC, the immature PDC.[8,11]

In man, monocytes/macrophages and myeloid/monocyte-derived DCs produce type I IFN in response to the dsRNA poly-IC and to certain RNA viruses,[24,25] and here the intracellular sensors RIG-I and Mda5 are involved.[26] These cells do express TLR3, 4, 7, and 8, but produce IL-12 instead of type I IFN upon exposure to TLR7/8 agonists.[24,25]

In contrast, the immature PDCs, also termed NIPCs, produce extremely large amounts of IFN-α (about 1×10^9 molecules in 12 hours) in response to many different microorganisms.[27,28] The NIPCs/PDCs are infrequent in the circulation, less than 1% of peripheral blood mononuclear cells, and can be recruited to sites of inflammation. The cells express, for instance, MHC class II, CD4, CD40, CD83, high levels of the IL-3 receptor (CD123), pre-Tα, λ5, and two specific markers termed blood DC antigen 2 (BDCA-2) and BDCA-4, but lack the costimulatory molecules CD80 and CD86. The BDCA-2 molecule is an endocytic type II C-type lectin, which can function as an antigen-capturing molecule.[29] The NIPCs/PDCs express the Fcγ receptor IIa (FcγRIIa),[30] the TLRs 1, 6, 7, 9, and 10,[31] and have high endocytotic activity. They also express the transcription factors IRF-1, -3, -4, -5, -7, and -8.[27,32] This explains in part the capacity of NIPCs/PDCs to sense a wide variety of molecules in the environment, especially nucleic acids, and respond to such potential danger signals by an extraordinarily high production of type I IFN and type III IFN. However, these cells can also produce other cytokines, including TNF-α and IL-6, and several chemokines, such as CXCL1-3, CXCL9-11, and CCL3-5.[27] They also produce IL-12 when costimulated by CD40L,[33,34] although this was not confirmed in a recent study.[35] NIPCs/PDCs rapidly die *in vitro*, unless stimulated by IL-3 or granulocyte/macrophage colony-stimulating factor (GM-CSF).[28] In contrast, the cytokines IL-10 and TNF-α inhibit IFN-α production by NIPCs/PDCs.[36] Immature PDCs express the chemokine receptors CXCR3 and CXCR4, as well as more uniquely the receptor for chemerin,[37,38] i.e. ChemR23. These receptors are important for directing the migration of the cells from blood to peripheral tissues and lymph nodes, when exposed to the ligands CXCL9–11, CXCL12, and chemerin, respectively. Activated and mature PDCs on the other hand express CCR7, important in migration from inflamed tissues via lymph vessels to regional lymph nodes.

MODE OF ACTIVATION OF TYPE I IFN PRODUCTION IN IMMATURE PDCs

Activation of the NIPCs/PDCs can occur by engagement of TLR7 and TLR9 or by intracellular mechanisms, as outlined above. The TLRs are located in the endosomes and endocytosis of the IFN-inducers is therefore required. Certain small molecules can directly activate endosomal TLRs, such as imidazoquinolines (e.g. Resiquimod

and Imiquimod), guanine nucleoside analogs (e.g. 7-allyl-8-oxoguanosine, i.e. Loxoribine), or short oligodeoxyribonucleotides (ODN) containing unmethylated CpG-dinucleotides.[11] Some viruses can also reach this endosomal compartment and trigger type I IFN production by exposing the TLR9 to DNA (e.g. herpes simplex virus) or TLR7 to RNA (e.g. influenza virus).[11] Single-stranded (ss) RNA with guanosine- and uridine-rich sequences, carried by liposomes, can also activate IFN-α production via interaction with TLR7.[39,40] Interestingly, both RNA- and DNA-containing immune complexes (ICs) induce IFN-α production by NIPCs/PDCs. Such interferogenic ICs are internalized by NIPCs/PDCs via FcγRIIa, reach the endosomes and activate the TLR7 and TLR9.[30,41,42] Importantly, apoptotic cells release material containing DNA and RNA that can trigger type I IFN production in NIPCs/PDCs, when combined with autoantibodies from patients with systemic lupus erythematosus (SLE) and Sjögren's syndrome (SpS).[43–45] Cells dying by necrosis release only RNA-containing material with interferogenic properties.[44] Both U1 snRNA and hY1RNA can induce type I IFN production and ICs consisting of autoantibodies and U1snRNP particles are able to induce type I IFN production specifically in NIPCs/PDCs via TLR7.[46–48] However, several other RNA species that associate with protein autoantigens are potential IFN-inducers when present in ICs. Accordingly, the same molecules that are released at cell death and constitute major autoantigens in SLE and several other systemic autoimmune diseases are also potent IFN-α-inducers and can act as endogenous adjuvants in the autoimmune process (see below).

THE IFN RECEPTORS AND THEIR SIGNALING PATHWAYS

The effects of the IFNs are mediated by three different receptors, type I IFN acting on the IFNAR, type II IFN (IFN-γ) on the IFNGR, and type III IFN on the IL28R.[49] The properties of the receptors and their signaling pathways are summarized in Table 19.2 and Figure 19.3. The IFNAR and IFNGR are displayed on most cell types, while IL28R have a more limited expression. They all consist of two chains that lack intrinsic

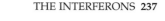

Table 19.2 The interferon (IFN) receptors

Receptor	Chains	Human gene locus	Janus kinases
Type I IFN	IFNAR1	21q22.11	Jak1, Tyk2
(IFNAR)	IFNAR2	21q22.11	
Type II IFN	IFNGR1	6q23-q24	Jak1, Jak2
(IFNGR)	IFNGR2	21q22.11	
Type III IFN	IL28RA	1p36.11	Jak1, Tyk2
(IL28R)	IL10RB	21q22.11	

kinase activity, are associated with Janus kinases (Jak), and use members of the STAT family as main regulators of gene expression.

The interaction of type I IFN with the IFNAR results in activation of the two receptor-associated tyrosine kinase 2 (Tyk2) and Jak1, phosphorylation of STAT1 and STAT2, and formation of a tri-molecular complex with IRF9. Such complexes, designated IFN-stimulated gene factor 3 (ISGF3), bind to IFN-stimulated response elements (ISREs) that are present in the promoters of a large number of genes. Phosphorylated STAT1 can also form homodimers that interact with the IFN-γ-activated sites (GAS), also present in the promoters of many genes. Several genes have both ISRE and GAS elements. However, at least in lymphoid cells, the IFNAR can also activate STAT3–6, which can form functionally relevant homodimers and heterodimers. The activated STAT proteins can interact with several other proteins, including p300 and CBP (CREB-binding-protein) that are important in regulating gene transcription. Besides the already complex Jak-STAT pathway, the IFNAR also can use the

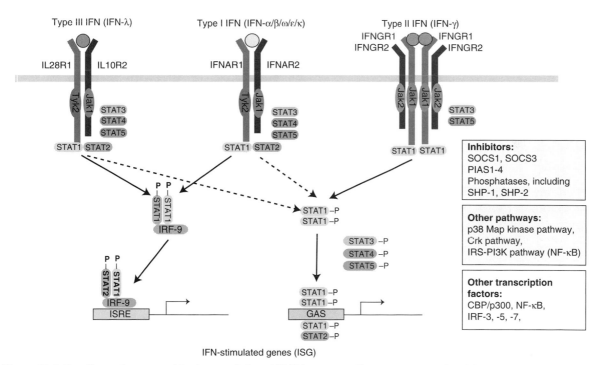

Figure 19.3 Signaling pathways used by the type I, II, and III IFN receptors. The receptor-associated Janus kinases, Jak1, Jak2, and Tyk2, are indicated as well as the involved signal transducers and activators of transcription (STAT) factors. STAT1 and STAT2 are typically activated by phosphorylation, STAT1 and STAT2 forming a tri-molecular complex with IRF-9 (ISGF3) that interacts with IFN-stimulated response element (ISRE) in promoters of IFN-stimulated genes. STAT1 dimers can interact with IFN-γ-activated sites (GAS). The signaling pathways and target genes of type I and III IFN are similar, partially overlapping those of the type II IFN (IFN-γ), e.g. via STAT1 dimer formations. The latter is less pronounced for type I and III IFN (broken lines) than for IFN-γ. In the STAT pathway, STAT3–5 are also activated as indicated. As indicated in boxes, several other pathways and transcription factors are described to be activated by IFNs, and receptor signals are modulated by members of the SOCS and PIAS families, as well as by phosphatases. For further details, see the text.

Crk- and the p38-MAPK pathways for some of the antiproliferative and antiviral effects of type I IFN. Furthermore, the insulin receptor substrate 1 (IRS1)/phosphatidyl-inositol 3-kinase (PI3K) signaling pathway is involved in, for example, IFN-α/β-mediated regulation of apoptosis and induced production of anti-inflammatory IL-1Ra and IL-10. IL28R, used by the three type III IFNs, has many similarities to IFNAR with respect to the Jak-STAT pathway, but many of its functions still remain to be clarified.[7] They may in fact differ from type I IFN in some respects.[50]

IFNGR, via Jak1 and Jak2, typically activates only STAT1, with the formation of STAT1 homodimers.[17] A less pronounced activation of STAT2 and formation of ISGF3 complexes has also been reported. Thus type I and II IFN functionally overlap, partly explaining the reported cross-talk between IFNAR and IFNGR.[49] Type II IFN can also activate other pathways, including the Crk and PI3K pathways.

NEGATIVE REGULATION OF IFN SIGNALING PATHWAYS

Cytokine signaling is controlled by several inhibitors (Figure 19.3), including constitutively expressed Src homology 2 (SH2) domain containing phosphatases (SHP), protein inhibitors of activated STAT (PIAS), and inducible suppressors of cytokine signalling (SOCS).[51,52] The mammalian SHPs act mainly by dephosphorylating signaling components in the pathways. The PIAS consist of four members, PIAS1, PIAS3, PIASx, and PIASy, that bind to STAT1, STAT3, STAT1 and STAT4, respectively. At least PIAS1 and PIAS3 act by preventing binding of STAT to DNA. Inhibition of STAT function by sumoylation is another recently demonstrated mechanism of action.

The SOCS family has seven members, which have SH2-domains, and can therefore bind to phosphotyrosine residues in receptors or Janus kinases. The expression of SOCS1 and SOCS3 is induced by type I and II IFN. Interestingly SOCS1 interacts with the IFNAR1 chain selectively, and inhibits the function of the IFNAR, probably by preventing binding and activation of Tyk2. Also SOCS3 can inhibit type I IFN signaling.[53]

GENES, PROTEINS, AND CELL FUNCTIONS REGULATED BY IFNs

The IFNs have several important functions in innate immunity, especially in the defense against viral infections. However, they also have prominent effects in adaptive immunity. The multitude of actions of the IFNs are due to their ability to increase the expression of hundreds of genes and down-regulate others.[54,55] Owing to the overlapping signaling pathways of type I-III IFN, their spectra of IFN-stimulated genes (ISGs) also partially overlap. The proteins corresponding to these ISGs have many effects on many different cell types (examples are provided in Table 19.3).

The ISGs include genes that encode proteins such as RIG-I and IRF-5/7, which are involved in expression of type I IFN genes. Other proteins are involved in inhibition of viral replication, e.g. 2,5-oligoadenylate synthetase (OAS), dsRNA-dependent protein kinase (PKR), RNase L and Mx protein. Type I IFNs also have antiproliferative effects mediated by, for example, up-regulation of p21 and p27, inhibitors of cyclin-dependent kinases. Type I IFN can promote apoptosis in several ways, e.g. by up-regulation of death receptors/ligands TRAIL/Apo2L and Fas/FasL, as well as by PI3K/mammalian target of rapamycin signaling pathways.[56] Type I IFNs precipitate apoptosis in virus-infected cells by up-regulation of dsRNA-activated protein kinase (PKR). A remarkable finding is that the IFN-inducible gene 15 (ISG15) protein conjugates to many cell proteins (including prominent ISGs, Jak, and STAT) and enhances the effects of type I IFN, although its mode of action is not clear.[57] Type I IFNs can also increase the CD69 expression and cytotoxic activity of NK cells.[58] Especially type II IFN can also induce expression of genes in, for example, monocytes/macrophages, such as inducible nitric oxide synthase (iNOS), resulting in generation of NO that is important in destruction of bacteria and viruses. Type I IFNs also increase expression of TLR3, TLR4, and TLR7.[23]

With regard to adaptive immunity, type I IFNs cause DC maturation and activation, with increased expression of MHC class I and II molecules, chemokines, and chemokine receptors, as

Table 19.3 Immunomodulatory effects of type I and type II IFN

Target cell	Effect
Many cells	Antiviral effects via induction of antiviral proteins. Directing cell migrations via induction of cell adhesion molecules (e.g. ICAM-1) and chemokines. Induction of apoptosis and inhibition of cell proliferation
DC	Survival, maturation, and activation. Enhanced antigen presentation, cross-presentation to Tc cells, and stimulation of Th1 and B cells via, e.g. increased expression of costimulatory molecules and MHC class I/II
PDC/NIPC	Prolonged survival, increased type I IFN production (type I IFN)
Monocyte/macrophage	Up-regulation of TLR2/3/4/7/8. Enhanced antimicrobial activity via increased NADPH oxidase and iNOS (mainly type II IFN). Differentiation to myeloid DC and inhibition of IL-12 production (mainly type I IFN)
Th cell	Enhanced Th1 differentiation via, e.g. increased expression of IL-12 receptor, IFN-γ, and T bet. Activation and survival of naive and memory T cells
Tc cell	Increased cytotoxic activity, prolonged survival
B cell	Enhanced activation and differentiation of plasmablasts to plasma cells, Ig class switch, and antibody production
NK cell	Enhanced cytotoxicity and IFN-γ production (mainly type I IFN)

ICAM-1, intracellular adhesion molecule-1; DC, dendritic cell; PDC, plasmacytoid dendritic cells; NIPCs; natural IFN-producing cells; MHC, major histocompatibility complex; TLR, Toll-like receptor; iNOS, inducible nitric oxide synthase; NK, natural killer.

well as costimulatory molecules such as CD80, CD86, the B lymphocyte stimulator (BLyS), and a proliferation-inducing ligand (APRIL).[59] This promotes development of helper T cells, which develop along the Th1 pathway, in part because of IFN-induced expression of IL-12 receptors and T bet.[60,61] Development of cytotoxic T cells is also stimulated by type I IFNs, due to an increase in DC cross-presentation[62] and inhibition of T cell apoptosis.[63,64] Type I IFNs also enhance B-cell activation, differentiation, antibody production, and Ig isotype class switching.[65–67] Furthermore, type I IFNs promote the production of several cytokines by NK cells and monocytes/macrophages/DCs, such as IFN-γ, IL-6, IL-10, and IL-15.[59] Interestingly, type I IFN also potentiates the effects of IFN-γ and IL-6[68,69] and shifts the actions of IL-10 from an anti-inflammatory to a more proinflammatory profile.[70]

Type II IFNs, that is IFN-γ, have many effects in common with type I IFNs, as extensively reviewed.[17] The type I and type II IFNs are, however, produced by different stimuli and by different cells in innate immunity, and may therefore be viewed as complementary IFNs with important functions in innate immunity.

In addition, they serve as a bridge between innate and adaptive immunity. They can be viewed as 'stress hormones' in the immune system, signaling danger and contributing to its activation during infections. However, as discussed below, this also entails an increased risk of immunization by autoantigens.

ACTIVATION OF THE TYPE I IFN SYSTEM IN AUTOIMMUNE DISEASES

The type I IFN system has especially in recent years been implicated in the pathogenesis of several autoimmune diseases (Table 19.4). Patients with SLE frequently display serum levels of IFN-α, which correlate to activity and severity of the disease, as well as to markers of immune activation that are considered important in the disease process.[36,59] The latter include serum levels of IL-10, complement activation, and titers of antibodies to dsDNA. High serum IFN-α levels also associate with fever and skin rashes in SLE. Blood leukocytes of SLE patients also have increased levels of the type I IFN-inducible protein MxA, indicating ongoing production of biologically active IFN, probably mostly IFN-α.

Table 19.4 Autoimmune diseases with evidence of activation of type I IFN system[a]

Disease
Systemic lupus erythematosus
Sjögren's syndrome
Dermatomyositis/polymyositis
Psoriasis
Systemic sclerosis
Insulin-dependent diabetes mellitus (type 1 diabetes)
Rheumatoid arthritis
Autoimmune hepatitis

[a]Expression of IFN-stimulated genes (the IFN signature) or other evidence of ongoing type I IFN production.

This is verified by gene array expression profiles in blood leukocytes and tissues from SLE patients, which demonstrate activation of many type I IFN-stimulated genes.[71–73] Type I IFN, and not IFN-γ, is responsible for this IFN signature,[74] but it cannot be excluded that type III IFN also contributes. The IFN signature appears to be associated with more active disease, recent onset, and severe disease manifestations. However, further longitudinal studies of the IFN signature in SLE patients are required to determine its value in predicting and monitoring disease flares and organ manifestations, as well as treatment response and outcome. The NIPCs/PDCs appear to be relevant type I IFN producers *in vivo* and can in fact be demonstrated in both the skin and lymph nodes from SLE patients.[75–78] They are probably recruited from blood, which shows a more than 70-fold reduction of the number of NIPCs/PDCs.[79] Here, the chemokine receptors CXCR3/CXCR4 on NIPCs/PDCs and the chemokines CXCL10/CXCL12 may be involved,[28] as well as the chemotactic agent chemerin that interacts with the ChemR23 receptor on NIPCs/PDCs.[37,38]

Increased serum levels of IFN-α and expression of IFN-α in pancreatic islets have been described in insulin-dependent diabetes mellitus.[80] Furthermore, expression of IFN-α genes in islets precedes the lymphocyte infiltration and islet cell destruction in experimental diabetes, which can be prevented by neutralizing anti-IFN-α antibodies. Also, increased IFN-α mRNA expression was found in liver biopsies from

patients with primary biliary cirrhosis.[81] In rheumatoid arthritis (RA), an infiltration of NIPCs/PDCs and expression of IFN-β and the type I IFN-inducible protein MxA can be detected in the synovium.[82,83] Patients with dermatomyositis have a typical IFN gene signature and IFN-α-producing NIPCs/PDCs in muscle tissue.[84,85]

In Sjögren's syndrome (pSS), IFN-α-producing cells[45] and PDCs[86] are present in minor salivary glands, which also have gene expression profiles with prominent up-regulation of type I IFN-stimulated genes.[86,87] Furthermore, the ability of pSS sera to form IFN-α-inducing ICs with apoptotic cell material was associated with both positive labial salivary gland score and, for example, dermatological, hematological, and pulmonary extraglandular disease manifestations. Patients with systemic sclerosis also have an IFN signature at the blood leukocyte level.[88] In psoriasis, patients show increased expression of IFN-α mRNA and IFN-induced proteins, as well as an infiltration of IFN-α-producing NIPCs/PDCs.[77,89,90] These NIPCs/PDCs and IFN-α were furthermore demonstrated to play an essential role in the development of psoriatic lesions in human skin in a xenograft model.[90] This landmark finding directly implicates type I IFN and NIPCs/PDCs in the pathogenesis of a human autoimmune disease.

A CAUSATIVE ROLE FOR TYPE I IFN IN AUTOIMMUNITY

Type I IFN, especially IFN-α and IFN-β, have been used for more than 25 years for therapy of several viral and malignant diseases in man.[2] Prominent side effects during IFN-α treatment are occurrence of autoantibodies and autoimmune disease.[91] For instance, as many as 19% of patients with malignant carcinoid tumors treated with IFN-α eventually developed autoimmune disease and even more often autoantibodies, including antinuclear and anti-dsDNA antibodies.[92] The types of autoimmunity include pernicious anemia, autoimmune thyroiditis and Grave's disease, autoimmune hepatitis, insulin-dependent diabetes mellitus, RA, polymyositis, vasculitis, and SLE.[93,94] This broad spectrum of autoimmune diseases may be explained by a genetic predisposition of individuals to develop a certain autoimmune disease, and that type I IFN acts as a trigger of a largely genetically determined autoimmune program. For instance, as many as 68% of patients with pre-existing anti-thyroid autoantibodies developed autoimmune thyroid disease during IFN-α treatment.[92] Several of the side effects seen during IFN-α therapy, such as fever, fatigue, myalgia, arthralgia, and leukopenia, are not autoimmune in nature. Such IFN-α-mediated effects may, however, also be relevant in certain autoimmune diseases. The existing data therefore indicate that type I IFN can initiate autoimmune reactions in man, and maybe even more efficiently enhance ongoing autoimmune processes and thereby precipitate clinically overt systemic and organ-specific autoimmune diseases.

It is well established that the genetic background is important in autoimmune diseases, and several genes are associated with increased susceptibility to develop SLE.[95] Genes related to type I IFN could be important, and recent studies in fact revealed single-nucleotide polymorphisms (SNPs) in the genes for tyrosine kinase 2 (Tyk2) and IFN regulatory factor 5 (IRF-5) that were associated with human SLE.[96,97] These two genes have important functions in the type I IFN system as described above. However, Tyk2 is also involved in the function of the receptors for several other cytokines that are thought to be important in SLE, such as IL-6 and IL-10.[98] As a TLR7/8/9-activated transcription factor, IRF-5 increases the expression of several other genes involved in cell signaling, apoptosis, cell cycle regulation, and immune activation.[99] Polymorphisms altering the function of Tyk2 and IRF-5 may therefore in many ways facilitate the development of an autoimmune disease such as SLE. Still, the association of Tyk2 and IRF-5 genes with SLE supports the contention that the type I IFN system has an important role in the etiopathogenesis of this disease. Several genes already reported to be associated with SLE may act via the type I IFN system, for instance, the gene encoding FcγRIIa, which is important in the activation of NIPCs/PDCs by interferogenic ICs, as well as genes for complement factors C1q and C-reactive protein, which contribute to clearance of apoptotic cells.[95]

A role for type I IFN in SLE is also supported by findings in murine SLE models.[59] Thus, administration of IFN-inducers or exogenous IFN-α/β to NZB and NZB/W mice worsens the disease. Furthermore, IFNAR knockout mice have a dramatically reduced SLE disease.[100,101] On the other hand, the absence of a functional IFNAR in MRL/lpr lupus mice results in aggravated lupus disease,[102] indicating important differences between experimental murine lupus models.

TYPE II IFN (IFN-γ) IN AUTOIMMUNE DISEASES

IFN-γ has well-established functions in immune responses, and has for many years been implicated in the etiology and pathogenesis of autoimmune diseases.[103] A few case reports have described a possible development of SLE during IFN-γ therapy in man. However, there is no clear evidence of increased levels of IFN-γ in tissues and serum in SLE patients, early reports of increased levels most likely being due to IFN-α.[104,105] Furthermore, the IFN signatures in SLE patients are due to type I IFN and not IFN-γ.[74] This is in contrast to the observations in MLR/lpr lupus mice, where a clear IFN-γ gene signature has been described.[106]

Lupus-prone mice with increased IFN-γ production have more severe lupus-like disease and deficiencies in either IFN-γ or IFNGR ameliorate the disease.[103] Also, neutralization of IFN-γ by anti-IFN-γ antibodies or soluble IFNGR inhibited lupus in (NZBxNZW)F1 mice.[107,108] Finally, the IFN-γ-inducing cytokines IL-12 and IL-18 accelerate murine lupus and neutralization of them inhibits disease.[109,110] Also in experimental diabetes, islet destruction can be associated with IFN-γ. Thus, expression of IFN-γ in β cells resulted in diabetes in normal mice,[111] while development of the disease in NOD mice was inhibited in IFNGR[-/-] mice, but accelerated by IFN-γ administration.[80] Several studies in murine RA models have demonstrated increased production of IFN-γ in inflamed joints, that administration of IFN-γ aggravates the arthritis, and that inhibition of IFN-γ action ameliorates the arthritis.[103] However, the opposite results have been found in other studies, possibly due to stimulatory effects of IFN-γ on the immunizing stage in the autoimmune process, but inhibitory effects on the inflammatory process.[103] Another example of IFN-γ-associated autoimmune disease is multiple sclerosis, where impaired IFN-γ function results in more severe disease in murine experimental allergic encephalomyelitis, while opposite results were seen in experimental autoimmune thyroiditis.[103] Most of these effects of IFN-γ are compatible with its fundamental role in the immune response, promoting, for example, development of Th1 and Tc cells, as well as B-cell production

of complement-fixing IgG antibodies with high affinity for Fcγ receptors.

AN ETIOPATHOGENIC MECHANISM FOR AUTOIMMUNITY INVOLVING THE TYPE I IFN SYSTEM

The type I IFN system may trigger and then maintain autoimmune processes by a vicious circle-like mechanism (Figure 19.4).[36,112,113] Infections by viruses or bacteria can start the first autoimmune reactions and production and

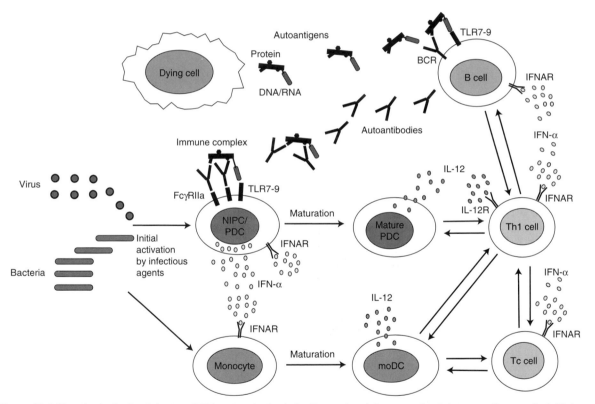

Figure 19.4 Hypothetical role of the type I IFN system in the induction and maintenance of autoimmune disease. An initial production of autoantibodies can occur during viral or bacterial infections, in part due to induced production of immunostimulatory type I IFN and other cytokines induced by microbial components (e.g. nucleic acids). Such autoantibodies can form immune complexes (ICs) with autologous DNA or RNA and associated proteins, released by apoptotic or necrotic cells. These ICs act as endogenous inducers of production of type I IFN and other cytokines (e.g. IL-12 and chemokines) in NIPCs/PDCs via interaction of RNA/DNA with Toll-like receptors 7–9 (TLR7–9) and autoantibodies with Fcγ receptor IIa (FcγRIIa) (see Figure 19.1). The ICs can also also stimulate autoantibody-producing B cells via combined interaction with TLR7–9 and with B-cell receptors (BCRs) specific for IC components. Type I IFN, especially IFN-α, has many immunostimulatory actions that include promotion of maturation of monocyte-derived DCs (moDC), development of T-helper type 1 (Th1) cells and cytotoxic T (Tc) cells, as well as activation of B cells (double arrows indicate cell interactions). More autoantibodies and interferogenic ICs consequently form, resulting in continued IFN-α production and IFN-mediated immunostimulation. The autoimmune process is thus maintained by a mechanism with the features of a vicious circle.

action of type I IFN by NIPCs/PDCs is important here, as outlined above, but obviously other costimulatory cytokines such as IL-12 and IFN-γ are important. In fact, autoantibodies against, for example, RNA- and DNA-binding proteins, often appear during viral infections,[114] indicating loss of self-tolerance to ubiquitous cellular autoantigens. Possible mechanisms include functional maturation of DCs, molecular mimicry, T-cell epitope spreading, and bystander activation of T cells, facilitated by type I IFN and other inflammatory stimuli as described in the fertile field hypothesis.[115] Mechanisms involving molecular mimicry can explain the linkage of Epstein–Barr virus (EBV) to SLE, because the EBNA-1 viral protein cross-reacts with the major autoantigens Sm B', Sm D1, and Ro60.[116] Autoantibodies directed to nucleic acid-associated proteins or nucleic acids have also been detected in individuals long before development of SLE.[117] When such autoantibodies are available, they can form ICs by combining with apoptotic or necrotic cell material that contains interferogenic DNA or RNA. Such ICs are continuously formed and can activate the TLR7/9 of NIPCs/PDCs and could thus cause a prolonged production of type I IFN in the absence of exogenous inducers, such as virus or bacteria. Obviously, other cytokines produced besides type I IFN are also relevant, including type III IFN, chemokines, IL-6, and IL-12 (see above). The activated NIPCs/PDCs can in this way promote autoimmunity by enhancing DC maturation, T-cell activation, and stimulation of B cells (see above). Autoreactive B cells can also be more directly activated by DNA- or RNA-associated autoantigens via combined interaction with BCR and either TLR9 (DNA) or TLR7 (RNA), a process markedly enhanced by IFN-α.[118,119] This will selectively enhance production of autoantibodies that can form interferogenic ICs. More immunogenic and IFN-inducing material can be generated by increased apoptosis or necrosis (e.g. due to infections and ultraviolet light), and both increased apoptosis and decreased clearance of apoptotic cell material are seen in SLE.[120] Furthermore, type I IFN can increase both apoptosis[56,121] and the expression of autoantigens.[122] It has also been proposed that MHC class I up-regulation caused by type I IFN in tissues makes them a target for autoimmune attack by cytotoxic T cells.[123]

A process with features of a vicious circle is therefore established, which maintains the autoimmune process by continuously exposing the immune system to endogenous type I IFN-inducers and to the type I IFN (and other cytokines) produced by the NIPCs/PDCs. This causes activation of more autoimmune T and B cells, and further production of autoantibodies that form interferogenic ICs. The activity of the vicious circle is also increased by recruitment of new NIPCs/PDCs to tissues by chemokines and priming of these cells by, e.g. type I IFN. The priming by type I IFN is essential for activation of NIPCs/PDCs and B cells, and the activity of the vicious circle may decrease if type I IFN production subsides. Activation of the latter (e.g. during viral infections) may then reactivate the vicious circle, explaining disease flares observed in SLE patients during infections. On the other hand cytokines that limit the activity of NIPCs/PDCs, especially IL-10 and TNF-α, may serve as a beneficial negative feedback mechanism in SLE.[124] The activities in the vicious circle described above most likely occur in the lymphoid organs.

While our hypothesis was originally proposed to explain part of the etiology and pathogenesis of SLE, a similar model has also been suggested to operate in pSS.[45,125] Here, it is envisioned that the vicious circle also operates in the major target organs, i.e. the salivary and lacrimal glands, especially in connection with lymphocytic foci.

A major feature of this vicious circle hypothesis is the formation of ICs with autologous RNA or DNA that act as TLR7/8/9-dependent activators of NIPCs/PDCs. Whether interferogenic IC is always the cause of the type I IFN production remains to be determined. However, the fact that NIPCs/PDCs are activated in psoriasis patients that lack detectable antibodies to RNA or DNA and associated protein autoantigens indicates that other endogenous type I IFN-inducers exist.

THERAPEUTIC TARGETS

The connection between the type I IFN system and autoimmune disease suggests that down-regulation of this system could be a therapeutic approach and many potential therapeutic targets exist (Table 19.5). In fact, two effective therapeutic agents in SLE, chloroquine and glucocorticoids, inhibit IFN-α production by NIPCs/PDCs[126,127] and down-regulate the IFN signature,[128] but have many other effects. The foremost therapeutic target in SLE may be IFN-α, and a humanized monoclonal anti-IFN-α antibody that neutralizes all IFN-α subtypes has been developed.[129] Another therapeutic option is soluble IFNAR that binds to and neutralizes type I IFN.[130] The NIPCs/PDCs could also be directly targeted by human monoclonal antibodies (mAbs) to their specific marker BDCA-2, and ligation of this molecule inhibits their IFN-α production.[29,131] The NIPCs/PDCs must also enter lymphoid organs through the high endothelial venulae or inflamed peripheral tissues such as skin and intestinal mucosa via vascular endothelial cells. Here, blockade of the action of relevant chemotactic agents are potential therapeutic targets, including the interaction of chemerin, and the chemokines CXCL10 (IP-10) and CXCL12 (SDF-1) with their receptors. Other possible therapeutic approaches include elimination of the DNA or RNA in endogenous IFN-α-inducers, and DNase treatment has already been tried in SLE patients, but without clear therapeutic effect.[132] Perhaps RNase should be added to destroy RNA-containing inducers as well. The tolerogen LPJ 394 that reduces the level of anti-dsDNA antibodies in SLE has only a moderate effect on disease activity,[133] not surprisingly considering that other autoantibody specificities are important in interferogenic ICs. There are several ways to prevent the action of interferogenic ICs on NIPCs/PDCs, including blockade of FcγRIIa by specific antibodies[30] and inhibition of TLRs by oligodeoxyribonucleotide (ODN) or oligoribonucleotide (ORN) TLR antagonists.[134] Signaling molecules downstream of the TLRs, such as MyD88, IRAK-1, IRAK-4, IRF-5, and IRF-7, are also potential therapeutic targets, especially those with kinase activity. The IFNAR may also be targeted by antagonists, for instance antibodies blocking receptor interaction with type I IFN.[135] Signaling molecules used by the IFNAR are also possible targets, inhibitors of Tyk2 being one example. Finally, the induced expression of type I IFN-stimulated genes (ISGs) could be blocked by, for example, histone deacetylase inhibitors.[136,137]

Consequently, there are many therapeutic target molecules in the type I IFN system.

Table 19.5 Therapeutic targets within the type I IFN system

Target	Type of drug	Effect
Interferogenic RNA or DNA	Nucleases	Eliminate IFN-inducing nucleic acids
Autoantibodies	Tolerogen/B-cell depletion	Inhibit formation of interferogenic immune complexes
Fcγ receptor IIa	Antagonist	Inhibit uptake of interferogenic immune complexes
Type I IFN	Soluble IFN receptors or neutralizing antibodies	Eliminate biologically active IFN
Type I IFN receptor	Antagonist	Prevent interaction of IFN with receptors
Type I IFN receptor associated kinases	Tyrosine kinase (Tyk2, Jak1) inhibitors	Inhibit signaling from type I IFN (and other) receptors
Toll-like receptors (TLR) 7–9	Inhibitory ORN or ODN	Inhibit binding of stimulatory nucleic acids
TLR7–9 associated kinases (e.g. IRAK-1, -4)	Serine/threonine kinase inhibitors	Inhibit activation of transcription factors IRF-5 and IRF-7
IFN-inducible genes	Histone deacetylase inhibitors	Inhibit IFN-stimulated gene transcription
Plasmacytoid dendritic cells (PDCs)	Anti-BDCA-2 antibodies	Inhibit production of IFN by PDCs
Plasmacytoid dendritic cells (PDCs)	Chemokine and chemerin antagonists	Prevent PDCs homing to tissues

ORN, oligoribonucleotide; ODN, oligodeoxyribonucleotide.

Several of these molecules have many other functions in the immune system and inhibition of their action can have additional beneficial effects, besides those on the type I IFN system. The results of the clinical trials aiming at down-regulating the activity of the type I IFN system will therefore be of great interest, because they will provide the crucial proof that this system indeed has a pivotal role in human autoimmune disease. Therapeutic agents that are developed to inhibit the activity of the type I IFN system may in fact be of value in many autoimmune diseases (cf. Table 19.5). However, given the important role of the IFN system in the normal immune response, such treatment may increase the susceptibility to infectious agents. For the future, the roles of type II IFN (IFN-γ) and type III IFN also remain to be considered in the etiopathogenesis of autoimmunity and explored as therapeutic targets.

ACKNOWLEDGMENTS

This work was supported in part by grants from the Swedish Research Council, the Swedish Rheumatism Foundation, the King Gustaf V 80-year Foundation, and the Uppsala University Hospital Research and Development Fund.

REFERENCES

1. Isaacs A, Lindenmann J. Virus interference. I. The interferon. Proc R Soc B 1957; 147: 258–67.
2. Brassard DL, Grace MJ, Bordens RW. Interferon-α as an immunotherapeutic protein. J Leukoc Biol 2002; 71: 565–81.
3. Hardy MP, Owczarek CM, Jermiin LS et al. Characterization of the type I interferon locus and identification of novel genes. Genomics 2004; 84: 331–45.
4. LaFleur DW, Nardelli B, Tsareva T et al. Interferon-κ, a novel type I interferon expressed in human keratinocytes. J Biol Chem 2001; 276: 39765–71.
5. Kotenko SV, Gallagher G, Baurin VV et al. IFN-λs mediate antiviral protection through a distinct class II cytokine receptor complex. Nat Immunol 2003; 4: 69–77.
6. Sheppard P, Kindsvogel W, Xu W et al. IL-28, IL-29 and their class II cytokine receptor IL-28R. Nat Immunol 2003; 4: 63–8.
7. Dumoutier L, Tounsi A, Michiels T et al. Role of the interleukin (IL)-28 receptor tyrosine residues for antiviral and antiproliferative activity of IL-29/interferon-λ 1: similarities with type I interferon signaling. J Biol Chem 2004; 279: 32269–74.
8. Honda K, Yanai H, Takaoka A et al. Regulation of the type I IFN induction: a current view. Int Immunol 2005; 17: 1367–78.
9. Malmgaard L. Induction and regulation of IFNs during viral infections. J Interferon Cytokine Res 2004; 24: 439–54.
10. Kawai T, Akira S. TLR signaling. Cell Death Differ 2006; 13: 816–25.
11. Kawai T, Akira S. Innate immune recognition of viral infection. Nat Immunol 2006; 7: 131–7.
12. Mogensen TH, Paludan SR. Reading the viral signature by Toll-like receptors and other pattern recognition receptors. J Mol Med 2005; 83: 180–92.
13. Schoenemeyer A, Barnes BJ, Mancl ME et al. The interferon regulatory factor, IRF5, is a central mediator of Toll-like receptor 7 signaling. J Biol Chem 2005; 280: 17005–12.
14. Sledz CA, Holko M, de Veer MJ et al. Activation of the interferon system by short-interfering RNAs. Nat Cell Biol 2003; 5: 834–9.
15. Ishii KJ, Coban C, Kato H et al. A Toll-like receptor-independent antiviral response induced by double-stranded B-form DNA. Nat Immunol 2006; 7: 40–8.
16. Stetson DB, Medzhitov R. Recognition of cytosolic DNA activates an IRF3-dependent innate immune response. Immunity 2006; 24: 93–103.
17. Schroder K, Hertzog PJ, Ravasi T et al. Interferon-γ: an overview of signals, mechanisms and functions. J Leukoc Biol 2004; 75: 163–89.
18. Bendriss-Vermare N, Burg S, Kanzler H et al. Virus overrides the propensity of human CD40L-activated plasmacytoid dendritic cells to produce Th2 mediators through synergistic induction of IFN-γ and Th1 chemokine production. J Leukoc Biol 2005; 78: 954–66.
19. Hart OM, Athie-Morales V, O'Connor GM et al. TLR7/8-mediated activation of human NK cells results in accessory cell-dependent IFN-γ production. J Immunol 2005; 175: 1636–42.
20. Caron G, Duluc D, Fremaux I et al. Direct stimulation of human T cells via TLR5 and TLR7/8: flagellin and R-848 up-regulate proliferation and IFN-γ production by memory CD4+ T cells. J Immunol 2005; 175: 1551–7.
21. Gerosa F, Gobbi A, Zorzi P et al. The reciprocal interaction of NK cells with plasmacytoid or myeloid dendritic cells profoundly affects innate resistance functions. J Immunol 2005; 174: 727–34.
22. Hanabuchi S, Watanabe N, Wang YH et al. Human plasmacytoid predendritic cells activate NK cells through glucocorticoid-induced tumor necrosis factor receptor-ligand (GITRL). Blood 2006; 107: 3617–23.
23. Österlund P, Veckman V, Siren J et al. Gene expression and antiviral activity of alpha/beta interferons and interleukin-29 in virus-infected human myeloid dendritic cells. J Virol 2005; 79: 9608–17.

24. Siren J, Pirhonen J, Julkunen I et al. IFN-α regulates TLR-dependent gene expression of IFN-α, IFN-β, IL-28, and IL-29. J Immunol 2005; 174: 1932–7.

25. Ito T, Amakawa R, Kaisho T et al. Interferon-α and interleukin-12 are induced differentially by Toll-like receptor 7 ligands in human blood dendritic cell subsets. J Exp Med 2002; 195: 1507–12.

26. Kato H, Takeuchi O, Sato S et al. Differential roles of MDA5 and RIG-I helicases in the recognition of RNA viruses. Nature 2006; 441: 101–5.

27. Fitzgerald-Bocarsly P. Natural interferon-α producing cells: the plasmacytoid dendritic cells. Biotechniques 2002; 33: S16–S29.

28. Colonna M, Trinchieri G, Liu YJ. Plasmacytoid dendritic cells in immunity. Nat Immunol 2004; 5: 1219–26.

29. Dzionek A, Sohma Y, Nagafune J et al. BDCA-2, a novel plasmacytoid dendritic cell-specific type II C-type lectin, mediates antigen capture and is a potent inhibitor of interferon α/β induction. J Exp Med 2001; 194: 1823–34.

30. Båve U, Magnusson M, Eloranta ML et al. FcγRIIa is expressed on natural IFN-α-producing cells (plasmacytoid dendritic cells) and is required for the IFN-α production induced by apoptotic cells combined with lupus IgG. J Immunol 2003; 171: 3296–302.

31. Hornung V, Rothenfusser S, Britsch S et al. Quantitative expression of Toll-like receptor 1-10 mRNA in cellular subsets of human peripheral blood mononuclear cells and sensitivity to CpG oligodeoxynucleotides. J Immunol 2002; 168: 4531–7.

32. Takauji R, Iho S, Takatsuka H et al. CpG-DNA-induced IFN-α production involves p38 MAPK-dependent STAT1 phosphorylation in human plasmacytoid dendritic cell precursors. J Leukoc Biol 2002; 72: 1011–19.

33. Cella M, Facchetti F, Lanzavecchia A et al. Plasmacytoid dendritic cells activated by influenza virus and CD40L drive a potent Th1 polarization. Nat Immunol 2000; 1: 305–10.

34. Krug A, Rothenfusser S, Hornung V et al. Identification of CpG oligonucleotide sequences with high induction of IFN-α/β in plasmacytoid dendritic cells. Eur J Immunol 2001; 31: 2154–63.

35. Ito T, Kanzler H, Duramad O et al. Specialization, kinetics, and repertoire of type 1 interferon responses by human plasmacytoid predendritic cells. Blood 2006; 107: 2423–31.

36. Rönnblom L, Eloranta ML, Alm GV. The type I interferon system in systemic lupus erythematosus. Arthritis Rheum 2006; 54: 408–20.

37. Vermi W, Riboldi E, Wittamer V et al. Role of ChemR23 in directing the migration of myeloid and plasmacytoid dendritic cells to lymphoid organs and inflamed skin. J Exp Med 2005; 201: 509–15.

38. Zabel BA, Silverio AM, Butcher EC. Chemokine-like receptor 1 expression and chemerin-directed chemotaxis distinguish plasmacytoid from myeloid dendritic cells in human blood. J Immunol 2005; 174: 244–51.

39. Heil F, Hemmi H, Hochrein H et al. Species-specific recognition of single-stranded RNA via Toll-like receptor 7 and 8. Science 2004; 303: 1526–9.

40. Diebold SS, Kaisho T, Hemmi H et al. Innate antiviral responses by means of TLR7-mediated recognition of single-stranded RNA. Science 2004; 303: 1529–31.

41. Means TK, Latz E, Hayashi F et al. Human lupus autoantibody-DNA complexes activate DCs through cooperation of CD32 and TLR9. J Clin Invest 2005; 115: 407–17.

42. Barrat FJ, Meeker T, Gregorio J et al. Nucleic acids of mammalian origin can act as endogenous ligands for Toll-like receptors and may promote systemic lupus erythematosus. J Exp Med 2005; 202: 1131–9.

43. Båve U, Alm GV, Rönnblom L. The combination of apoptotic U937 cells and lupus IgG is a potent IFN-α inducer. J Immunol 2000; 165: 3519–26.

44. Lövgren T, Eloranta ML, Båve U et al. Induction of interferon-α production in plasmacytoid dendritic cells by immune complexes containing nucleic acid released by necrotic or late apoptotic cells and lupus IgG. Arthritis Rheum 2004; 50: 1861–72.

45. Båve U, Nordmark G, Lövgren T et al. Activation of the type I interferon system in primary Sjögren's syndrome: a possible etiopathogenic mechanism. Arthritis Rheum 2005; 52: 1185–95.

46. Savarese E, Chae OW, Trowitzsch S et al. U1 small nuclear ribonucleoprotein immune complexes induce type I interferon in plasmacytoid dendritic cells through TLR7. Blood 2006; 107: 3229–34.

47. Vollmer J, Tluk S, Schmitz C et al. Immune stimulation mediated by autoantigen binding sites within small nuclear RNAs involves Toll-like receptors 7 and 8. J Exp Med 2005; 202: 1575–85.

48. Lövgren T, Eloranta ML, Kastner B et al. Induction of interferon-α by immune complexes or liposomes containing systemic lupus erythematosus and Sjögren's syndrome autoantigen-associated RNA. Arthritis Rheum 2006; 54: 1917–27.

49. Platanias LC. Mechanisms of type-I- and type-II-interferon-mediated signalling. Nat Rev Immunol 2005; 5: 375–86.

50. Ank N, West H, Bartholdy C et al. Lambda interferon (IFN-λ), a type III IFN, is induced by viruses and IFNs and displays potent antiviral activity against select virus infections in vivo. J Virol 2006; 80: 4501–9.

51. Wormald S, Hilton DJ. Inhibitors of cytokine signal transduction. J Biol Chem 2004; 279: 821–4.

52. Naka T, Fujimoto M, Tsutsui H et al. Negative regulation of cytokine and TLR signalings by SOCS and others. Adv Immunol 2005; 87: 61–122.

53. Vlotides G, Sorensen AS, Kopp F et al. SOCS-1 and SOCS-3 inhibit IFN-α-induced expression of the antiviral

proteins 2,5-OAS and MxA. Biochem Biophys Res Commun 2004; 320: 1007–14.

54. Kunzi MS, Pitha PM. Interferon targeted genes in host defense. Autoimmunity 2003; 36: 457–61.

55. Sarkar SN, Sen GC. Novel functions of proteins encoded by viral stress-inducible genes. Pharmacol Ther 2004; 103: 245–59.

56. Pokrovskaja K, Panaretakis T, Grander D. Alternative signaling pathways regulating type I interferon-induced apoptosis. J Interferon Cytokine Res 2005; 25: 799–810.

57. Liu YC, Penninger J, Karin M. Immunity by ubiquityla-tion: a reversible process of modification. Nat Rev Immunol 2005; 5: 941–52.

58. Romagnani C, Della Chiesa M, Kohler S et al. Activation of human NK cells by plasmacytoid den-dritic cells and its modulation by CD4+ T helper cells and CD4+ CD25hi T regulatory cells. Eur J Immunol 2005; 35: 2452–8.

59. Theofilopoulos AN, Baccala R, Beutler B et al. Type I interferons (α/β) in immunity and autoimmunity. Annu Rev Immunol 2005; 23: 307–35.

60. Hibbert L, Pflanz S, De Waal Malefyt R et al. IL-27 and IFN-α signal via Stat1 and Stat3 and induce T-Bet and IL-12Rβ2 in naive T cells. J Interferon Cytokine Res 2003; 23: 513–22.

61. Siren J, Sareneva T, Pirhonen J et al. Cytokine and con-tact-dependent activation of natural killer cells by influenza A or Sendai virus-infected macrophages. J Gen Virol 2004; 85: 2357–64.

62. Le Bon A, Etchart N, Rossmann C et al. Cross-priming of CD8+ T cells stimulated by virus-induced type I interferon. Nat Immunol 2003; 4: 1009–15.

63. Marrack P, Kappler J, Mitchell T. Type I interferons keep activated T cells alive. J Exp Med 1999; 189: 521–30.

64. Zhang X, Sun S, Hwang I et al. Potent and selective stimulation of memory-phenotype CD8+ T cells in vivo by IL-15. Immunity 1998; 8: 591–9.

65. Jego G, Palucka AK, Blanck JP et al. Plasmacytoid den-dritic cells induce plasma cell differentiation through type I interferon and interleukin 6. Immunity 2003; 19: 225–34.

66. Braun D, Caramalho I, Demengeot J. IFN-α/β enhances BCR-dependent B cell responses. Int Immunol 2002; 14: 411–19.

67. Le Bon A, Schiavoni G, D'Agostino G et al. Type I inter-ferons potently enhance humoral immunity and can promote isotype switching by stimulating dendritic cells in vivo. Immunity 2001; 14: 461–70.

68. Mitani Y, Takaoka A, Kim SH et al. Cross talk of the interferon-α/β signalling complex with gp130 for effec-tive interleukin-6 signalling. Genes Cells 2001; 6: 631–40.

69. Takaoka A, Mitani Y, Suemori H et al. Cross talk between interferon-γ and -α/β signaling components in

caveolar membrane domains. Science 2000; 288: 2357–60.

70. Sharif MN, Tassiulas I, Hu Y et al. IFN-α priming results in a gain of proinflammatory function by IL-10: implications for systemic lupus erythematosus patho-genesis. J Immunol 2004; 172: 6476–81.

71. Baechler EC, Gregersen PK, Behrens TW. The emerging role of interferon in human systemic lupus erythematosus. Curr Opin Immunol 2004; 16: 801–7.

72. Peterson KS, Huang JF, Zhu J et al. Characterization of heterogeneity in the molecular pathogenesis of lupus nephritis from transcriptional profiles of laser-captured glomeruli. J Clin Invest 2004; 113: 1722–33.

73. Kirou KA, Lee C, George S et al. Activation of the interferon-α pathway identifies a subgroup of systemic lupus erythematosus patients with distinct serologic features and active disease. Arthritis Rheum 2005; 52: 1491–503.

74. Kirou KA, Lee C, George S et al. Coordinate overex-pression of interferon-α-induced genes in systemic lupus erythematosus. Arthritis Rheum 2004; 50: 3958–67.

75. Blomberg S, Eloranta ML, Cederblad B et al. Presence of cutaneous interferon-α producing cells in patients with systemic lupus erythematosus. Lupus 2001; 10: 484–90.

76. Farkas L, Beiske K, Lund-Johansen F et al. Plasmacytoid dendritic cells (natural interferon- α/β-producing cells) accumulate in cutaneous lupus erythematosus lesions. Am J Pathol 2001; 159: 237–43.

77. Wollenberg A, Wagner M, Gunther S et al. Plasmacytoid dendritic cells: a new cutaneous dendritic cell subset with distinct role in inflammatory skin dis-eases. J Invest Dermatol 2002; 119: 1096–102.

78. Rönnblom L, Alm GV. The natural interferon-α produc-ing cells in systemic lupus erythematosus. Hum Immunol 2002; 63: 1181–93.

79. Cederblad B, Blomberg S, Vallin H et al. Patients with systemic lupus erythematosus have reduced numbers of circulating natural interferon-α-producing cells. J Autoimmun 1998; 11: 465–70.

80. Stewart TA. Neutralizing interferon alpha as a thera-peutic approach to autoimmune diseases. Cytokine Growth Factor Rev 2003; 14: 139–54.

81. Takii Y, Nakamura M, Ito M et al. Enhanced expression of type I interferon and Toll-like receptor-3 in primary biliary cirrhosis. Lab Invest 2005; 85: 908–20.

82. Lande R, Giacomini E, Serafini B et al. Characterization and recruitment of plasmacytoid dendritic cells in syn-ovial fluid and tissue of patients with chronic inflam-matory arthritis. J Immunol 2004; 173: 2815–24.

83. van Holten J, Smeets TJ, Blankert P, Tak PP. Expression of interferon β in synovial tissue from patients wih rheumatoid arthritis: comparison with patients with osteoarthritis and reactive arthritis. Ann Rheum Dis 2006; 64: 1780–82.

84. Tezak Z, Hoffman EP, Lutz JL et al. Gene expression profiling in DQA1*0501+ children with untreated dermatomyositis: a novel model of pathogenesis. J Immunol 2002; 168: 4154–63.

85. Greenberg SA, Pinkus JL, Pinkus GS et al. Interferon-α/β-mediated innate immune mechanisms in dermatomyositis. Ann Neurol 2005; 57: 664–78.

86. Gottenberg JE, Cagnard N, Lucchesi C et al. Activation of IFN pathways and plasmacytoid dendritic cell recruitment in target organs of primary Sjögren's syndrome. Proc Natl Acad Sci U S A 2006; 103: 2770–5.

87. Hjelmervik TO, Petersen K, Jonassen I et al. Gene expression profiling of minor salivary glands clearly distinguishes primary Sjögren's syndrome patients from healthy control subjects. Arthritis Rheum 2005; 52: 1534–44.

88. Tan FK, Zhou X, Mayes MD et al. Signatures of differentially regulated interferon gene expression and vasculotrophism in the peripheral blood cells of systemic sclerosis patients. Rheumatology (Oxford) 2006; 45: 694–702.

89. van der Fits L, van der Wel LI, Laman JD et al. In psoriasis lesional skin the type I interferon signaling pathway is activated, whereas interferon-α sensitivity is unaltered. J Invest Dermatol 2004; 122: 51–60.

90. Nestle FO, Conrad C, Tun-Kyi A et al. Plasmacytoid predendritic cells initiate psoriasis through interferon-α production. J Exp Med 2005; 202: 135–43.

91. Gota C, Calabrese L. Induction of clinical autoimmune disease by therapeutic interferon-α. Autoimmunity 2003; 36: 511–18.

92. Rönnblom LE, Alm GV, Öberg KE. Autoimmunity after alpha-interferon therapy for malignant carcinoid tumors. Ann Intern Med 1991; 115: 178–83.

93. Ioannou Y, Isenberg DA. Current evidence for the induction of autoimmune rheumatic manifestations by cytokine therapy. Arthritis Rheum 2000; 43: 1431–42.

94. Raanani P, Ben-Bassat I. Immune-mediated complications during interferon therapy in hematological patients. Acta Haematol 2002; 107: 133–44.

95. Tsao BP. Update on human systemic lupus erythematosus genetics. Curr Opin Rheumatol 2004; 16: 513–21.

96. Sigurdsson S, Nordmark G, Goring HH et al. Polymorphisms in the tyrosine kinase 2 and interferon regulatory factor 5 genes are associated with systemic lupus erythematosus. Am J Hum Genet 2005; 76: 528–37.

97. Graham RR, Kozyrev SV, Baechler EC et al. A common haplotype of interferon regulatory factor 5 (IRF5) regulates splicing and expression and is associated with increased risk of systemic lupus erythematosus. Nat Genet 2006; 38: 550–5.

98. Dean GS, Tyrrell-Price J, Crawley E et al. Cytokines and systemic lupus erythematosus. Ann Rheum Dis 2000; 59: 243–51.

99. Barnes BJ, Richards J, Mancl M et al. Global and distinct targets of IRF-5 and IRF-7 during innate response to viral infection. J Biol Chem 2004; 279: 45194–207.

100. Santiago-Raber ML, Baccala R, Haraldsson KM et al. Type-I interferon receptor deficiency reduces lupus-like disease in NZB mice. J Exp Med 2003; 197: 777–88.

101. Braun D, Geraldes P, Demengeot J. Type I interferon controls the onset and severity of autoimmune manifestations in lpr mice. J Autoimmun 2003; 20: 15–25.

102. Hron JD, Peng SL. Type I IFN protects against murine lupus. J Immunol 2004; 173: 2134–42.

103. Baccala R, Kono DH, Theofilopoulos AN. Interferons as pathogenic effectors in autoimmunity. Immunol Rev 2005; 204: 9–26.

104. Preble OT, Black RJ, Friedman RM et al. Systemic lupus erythematosus: presence in human serum of an unusual acid-labile leukocyte interferon. Science 1982; 216: 429–31.

105. Hooks JJ, Jordan GW, Cupps T et al. Multiple interferons in the circulation of patients with systemic lupus erythematosus and vasculitis. Arthritis Rheum 1982; 25: 396–400.

106. Liu J, Karypis G, Hippen KL et al. Genomic view of systemic autoimmunity in MRLlpr mice. Genes Immun 2006; 7: 156–68.

107. Jacob CO, van der Meide PH, McDevitt HO. In vivo treatment of (NZB X NZW)F1 lupus-like nephritis with monoclonal antibody to γ interferon. J Exp Med 1987; 166: 798–803.

108. Ozmen L, Roman D, Fountoulakis M et al. Experimental therapy of systemic lupus erythematosus: the treatment of NZB/W mice with mouse soluble interferon-gamma receptor inhibits the onset of glomerulonephritis. Eur J Immunol 1995; 25: 6–12.

109. Xu H, Kurihara H, Ito T et al. IL-12 enhances lymphoaccumulation by suppressing cell death of T cells in MRL-lpr/lpr mice. J Autoimmun 2001; 16: 87–95.

110. Bossu P, Neumann D, Del Giudice E et al. IL-18 cDNA vaccination protects mice from spontaneous lupus-like autoimmune disease. Proc Natl Acad Sci U S A 2003; 100: 14181–6.

111. Sarvetnick N, Shizuru J, Liggitt D et al. Loss of pancreatic islet tolerance induced by β-cell expression of interferon-γ. Nature 1990; 346: 844–7.

112. Rönnblom L, Alm GV. An etiopathogenic role for the type I IFN system in SLE. Trends Immunol 2001; 22: 427–31.

113. Rönnblom L, Eloranta ML, Alm GV. Role of natural interferon-α producing cells (plasmacytoid dendritic cells) in autoimmunity. Autoimmunity 2003; 36: 463–72.

114. Hunziker L, Recher M, Macpherson AJ et al. Hypergammaglobulinemia and autoantibody induction mechanisms in viral infections. Nat Immunol 2003; 4: 343–9.

115. Fujinami RS, von Herrath MG, Christen U et al. Molecular mimicry, bystander activation, or viral persistence: infections and autoimmune disease. Clin Microbiol Rev 2006; 19: 80–94.

116. McClain MT, Heinlen LD, Dennis GJ et al. Early events in lupus humoral autoimmunity suggest initiation through molecular mimicry. Nat Med 2005; 11: 85–9.

117. Arbuckle MR, McClain MT, Rubertone MV et al. Development of autoantibodies before the clinical onset of systemic lupus erythematosus. N Engl J Med 2003; 349: 1526–33.

118. Lau CM, Broughton C, Tabor AS et al. RNA-associated autoantigens activate B cells by combined B cell antigen receptor/Toll-like receptor 7 engagement. J Exp Med 2005; 202: 1171–7.

119. Rifkin IR, Leadbetter EA, Busconi L et al. Toll-like receptors, endogenous ligands, and systemic autoimmune disease. Immunol Rev 2005; 204: 27–42.

120. Gaipl US, Voll RE, Sheriff A et al. Impaired clearance of dying cells in systemic lupus erythematosus. Autoimmun Rev 2005; 4: 189–94.

121. Kirou KA, Vakkalanka RK, Butler MJ et al. Induction of Fas ligand-mediated apoptosis by interferon-α. Clin Immunol 2000; 95: 218–26.

122. Hueber W, Zeng D, Strober S et al. Interferon-α-inducible proteins are novel autoantigens in murine lupus. Arthritis Rheum 2004; 50: 3239–49.

123. Lang KS, Recher M, Junt T et al. Toll-like receptor engagement converts T-cell autoreactivity into overt autoimmune disease. Nat Med 2005; 11: 138–45.

124. Båve U, Vallin H, Alm GV et al. Activation of natural interferon-α producing cells by apoptotic U937 cells combined with lupus IgG and its regulation by cytokines. J Autoimmun 2001; 17: 71–80.

125. Nordmark G, Alm GV, Rönnblom L. Mechanism of disease: primary Sjögren's syndrome and the type I interferon system. Nat Clin Pract Rheum 2006; 2: 262–9.

126. Lebon P. Inhibition of herpes simplex virus type 1-induced interferon synthesis by monoclonal antibodies against viral glycoprotein D and by lysosomotropic drugs. J Gen Virol 1985; 66: 2781–6.

127. Shodell M, Shah K, Siegal FP. Circulating human plasmacytoid dendritic cells are highly sensitive to corticosteroid administration. Lupus 2003; 12: 222–30.

128. Bennett L, Palucka AK, Arce E et al. Interferon and granulopoiesis signatures in systemic lupus erythematosus blood. J Exp Med 2003; 197: 711–23.

129. Chuntharapai A, Lai J, Huang X et al. Characterization and humanization of a monoclonal antibody that neutralizes human leukocyte interferon: a candidate therapeutic for IDDM and SLE. Cytokine 2001; 15: 250–60.

130. McKenna SD, Vergilis K, Arulanandam AR et al. Formation of human IFN-β complex with the soluble type I interferon receptor IFNAR-2 leads to enhanced IFN stability, pharmacokinetics, and antitumor activity in xenografted SCID mice. J Interferon Cytokine Res 2004; 24: 119–29.

131. Blomberg S, Eloranta ML, Magnusson M et al. Expression of the markers BDCA-2 and BDCA-4 and production of interferon-α by plasmacytoid dendritic cells in systemic lupus erythematosus. Arthritis Rheum 2003; 48: 2524–32.

132. Davis JC Jr, Manzi S, Yarboro C et al. Recombinant human DNase I (rhDNase) in patients with lupus nephritis. Lupus 1999; 8: 68–76.

133. Alarcon-Segovia D, Tumlin JA, Furie RA et al. LJP 394 for the prevention of renal flare in patients with systemic lupus erythematosus: results from a randomized, double-blind, placebo-controlled study. Arthritis Rheum 2003; 48: 442–54.

134. Lenert PS. Targeting Toll-like receptor signaling in plasmacytoid dendritic cells and autoreactive B cells as a therapy for lupus. Arthritis Res Ther 2006; 8: 203.

135. Benizri E, Gugenheim J, Lasfar A et al. Prolonged allograft survival in cynomolgus monkeys treated with a monoclonal antibody to the human type I interferon receptor and low doses of cyclosporine. J Interferon Cytokine Res 1998; 18: 273–84.

136. Genin P, Morin P, Civas A. Impairment of interferon-induced IRF-7 gene expression due to inhibition of ISGF3 formation by trichostatin A. J Virol 2003; 77: 7113–19.

137. Chang HM, Paulson M, Holko M et al. Induction of interferon-stimulated gene expression and antiviral responses require protein deacetylase activity. Proc Natl Acad Sci U S A 2004; 101: 9578–83.

20

Osteoprotegerin

Allison R Pettit and Ellen M Gravallese

Introduction • RANKL and OPG: opposing actions in bone remodelling • RANKL-induced osteoclastogenesis in RA focal bone erosion • OPG treatment in animal models of arthritis • Comparison of OPG to other anti-resorptive therapies in arthritis models • OPG Therapy may also prevent systemic osteopenia/osteoporosis and juxta-articular osteopenia in RA • Will OPG be useful for preventing bone erosion in other forms of arthritis? • The utility of serum RANKL and OPG levels in predicting bone resorption • Targeting the RANKL/OPG cytokine system • Additional considerations • Conclusions • References

INTRODUCTION

Bone loss is associated with several diseases, most notably rheumatoid arthritis (RA). Focal bone erosions appear to be a very early feature of RA and are associated with disease severity and long-term functional impairment, making targeted therapy for focal bone erosion an important goal of treatment. Bone erosion occurs in other rheumatic diseases, including psoriatic arthritis (PsA). Therefore, clear delineation of the mechanisms of bone destruction in rheumatologic diseases is necessary for the development of effective therapies to prevent and control this disease process. The characterization of the central roles of receptor activator of NF-κB ligand (RANKL) and osteoprotegerin (OPG) in physiologic bone remodeling has facilitated many of the recent advances in our understanding of pathologic bone loss. OPG, initially described as a negative regulator of bone mass, was subsequently shown to effectively inhibit the formation and function of bone resorbing osteoclasts by functioning as a decoy receptor for RANKL. Therefore, pharmacologic blockade of RANKL by OPG, or agents mimicking the actions of OPG, is a logical strategy for regulating pathologic bone loss. Importantly, however, an optimal therapy for preventing pathologic bone destruction would block bone erosion in a targeted fashion without compromising general skeletal integrity.

We have previously provided an overview of the literature demonstrating the critical opposing roles of OPG and RANKL in regulating bone mass, as well as the evidence implicating RANKL as a key cytokine in the pathogenesis of focal bone erosion in RA.[1] Additionally, we discussed preliminary data examining the utility of OPG as a therapeutic agent in animal models of inflammatory arthritis and the potential contribution of other cytokines, particularly tumor necrosis factor (TNF) and interleukin (IL)-1, to osteoclastogenesis in inflammatory arthritis. Finally, we raised several caveats in the use of OPG as a targeted therapy for bone destruction, including the potential interaction with TNF-related apoptosis-inducing ligand (TRAIL). This chapter will provide an update of recent developments in our understanding of the regulation of bone resorption in RA and PsA, with a particular focus on blockade of RANKL as a targeted therapy for focal bone erosion and systemic osteoporosis in these diseases.

RANKL AND OPG: OPPOSING ACTIONS IN BONE REMODELLING

Physiologic bone remodelling is primarily achieved through the coordinated and balanced activity of osteoblasts, cells that form bone, and osteoclasts that resorb bone. In physiologic bone remodeling, 'coupling' between bone resorption and bone formation is achieved in part through the expression of RANKL and OPG by bone lining cells of the osteoblast lineage.[2] RANKL is an essential factor for osteoclastogenesis *in vivo*.[3–5] RANKL signals its biologic effects through receptor activator of NF-κB (RANK), a receptor expressed on the surface of myeloid lineage osteoclast precursor cells and mature osteoclasts, resulting in the activation of specific intracellular signaling pathways. Signaling downstream of RANK is mediated in part through the adaptor proteins TNF receptor-associate factor (TRAF)-2, TRAF-5, and TRAF-6, leading to activation of NF-κB, as well as the Akt and mitogen-activated protein kinase (MAPK) pathways.[6–9] Activator protein (AP)-1 is a transcription factor complex essential in the process of osteoclastogenesis that is activated downstream of RANK signaling by both TRAF-6-dependent and -independent pathways.[9–13] More recently, signaling through RANK has been demonstrated to activate nuclear factor of activated T cells c1 (NFATc1), which is a key transcriptional regulator of osteoclastogenesis.[13–15] The role of many of these signaling molecules and transcription factors in osteoclastogenesis has been confirmed by animal models in which these pathways have been genetically modified.[10,13,16–19] The evidence suggests that it is the combination of simultaneous activation of NFATc1, AP-1, and NF-κB by RANK that induces osteoclast differentiation and function (reviewed by Takayanagi).[20]

The RANKL–RANK interaction provides a very powerful signal for osteoclastogenesis, as it stimulates multiple stages of osteoclast differentiation and activity including maturation, migration, fusion, activity, and survival.[3,21–26] OPG, a soluble decoy receptor for RANKL, blocks all of the biologic effects of RANKL.[27–30] Thus, it is the balance between RANKL and OPG expression that determines the degree of osteoclast differentiation and function and ultimately the degree of bone resorption in a given setting.[31]

RANKL-INDUCED OSTEOCLASTOGENESIS IN RA FOCAL BONE EROSION

There is compelling evidence provided by animal studies implicating osteoclasts as the primary cell type responsible for focal bone erosion in inflammatory arthritis, and RANKL as a critical cytokine in osteoclast generation and activity at the erosion site.[32–36] This paradigm is also supported by evidence from studies in RA. Both RANKL and OPG are expressed in cells derived from RA synovial tissues[32,37–44] and osteoclasts have been demonstrated at sites of focal bone erosion in RA tissues.[37,45,46] An increase in the RANKL/OPG mRNA expression ratio has been demonstrated in RA synovial tissues, correlating with the degree of *in vitro* osteoclastogenesis and bone resorption.[42] The RANKL/OPG ratio is significantly higher in RA synovium compared with other inflammatory joint diseases and with osteoarthritis.[40,47] Additionally, this ratio correlates with disease activity.[40] We recently demonstrated expression of RANKL protein at sites of RA focal bone erosion, adjacent to RANK+ osteoclasts and their precursor cells,[44] as had been previously shown in the CIA (collagen-induced arthritis) model of inflammatory arthritis.[48] Additionally, OPG protein expression at these sites was limited, suggesting that in RA the RANKL/OPG balance contributes to the generation of a pro-osteoclastogenic microenvironment at the pannus–bone interface, resulting in focal bone erosion.[44] The exact cellular sources of RANKL and OPG at sites of focal bone erosion in RA have yet to be definitively identified. Osteoblast lineage cells,[46,49] T cells,[37,39,41] and synovial fibroblasts[37,38,41] are all possible cellular sources of RANKL at sites of RA focal bone erosion. Elucidation of the identity of the RANKL-expressing cells, as well as detailed characterization of the cellular composition in and adjacent to sites of focal bone erosion, are important to the further characterization of the pathogenic events involved in this process.

OPG TREATMENT IN ANIMAL MODELS OF ARTHRITIS

Studies investigating the pathogenesis of focal bone erosion in animal models of arthritis with differing induction and effector mechanisms have provided convincing evidence for the critical role of RANKL, and of osteoclasts, in focal bone erosion in inflammatory arthritis. OPG treatment in the rat adjuvant-induced arthritis model (AIA)[32] demonstrated only minimal loss of cortical and trabecular bone in OPG-treated animals compared with severe bone loss in untreated control animals. Accordingly, osteoclast numbers were also dramatically reduced in the joints of treated animals.[32] These observations were extended in a study from our own laboratory investigating the K/BxN serum transfer arthritis model in RANKL-deficient mice.[33] This study demonstrated that in the absence of RANKL there was a complete lack of osteoclasts and dramatic protection from bone erosion. As the serum transfer arthritis model bypasses direct T-cell involvement in inflammation, this experimental strategy avoided blocking the potential contributions of RANKL to arthritic inflammation. We accordingly observed equivalent levels of inflammation in both arthritic RANKL-deficient and arthritic control mice.[33] These findings were confirmed by the absence of osteoclast formation and focal bone erosion in arthritic c-fos-deficient mice. c-fos-deficient mice are osteopetrotic, as this transcription factor is required for the differentiation of osteoclast precursor cells to osteoclasts. When crossed with the human TNF transgenic (hTNFtg) mice that develop spontaneous inflammatory arthritis, arthritic c-fos$^{-/-}$hTNFtg mice were fully protected against bone destruction even though inflammation was demonstrated to be equivalent in arthritic c-fos$^{-/-}$hTNFtg and c-fos$^{+/+}$hTNFtg mice.[34] There was no difference in the composition of the cellular infiltrate or matrix metalloproteinase (MMP) production among these groups.[34] Similarly, arthritic RANK$^{-/-}$hTNFtg mice, also osteopetrotic due to a defect in osteoclastogenesis, demonstrated an absence of focal articular bone erosion in joints. However, the degree of bone erosion and inflammation in this study was not assessed in detail.[50]

Several additional studies have examined the use of OPG-Fc (referred to as OPG for the remainder of this chapter) as a treatment strategy for the prevention of focal bone erosion in various animal models of inflammatory arthritis. We previously reviewed several of these studies,

which demonstrated protection from bone erosion in hTNFtg arthritis[51] and CIA.[36] OPG-mediated protection from focal bone erosion has subsequently been confirmed in both AIA and CIA by more recent studies.[52,53] Additionally, RANKL protein expression was increased both in inflamed joints and systemically in both the CIA and AIA models in the early stages of arthritis. This increase in RANKL protein was associated with periarticular and systemic osteopenia in both of these inflammatory arthritis models.[52] A detailed kinetic and dose-ranging study of OPG therapy in the rat AIA model demonstrated that OPG protects from bone erosion in a dose- and schedule-dependent manner. Although most effective when given early in disease, OPG therapy was demonstrated to arrest bone erosion when given at any time during the evolution of arthritis.[54] OPG treatment had prolonged efficacy with regard to bone preservation and osteoclasts were eradicated even when OPG was given at peak of disease.[54,55] However, there was limited effect on bone integrity when OPG treatment was administered at disease peak due to the presence of pre-existing destruction.[55] These observations highlight the potential advantage of aggressive, early use of anti-resorptive therapies for preserving joint integrity in inflammatory arthritis.[56]

OPG therapy had no effect on the severity of inflammation in any of the animal models previously discussed.[32,36,51,54,55] This lack of effect of OPG treatment on the inflammatory process is somewhat surprising in view of the potential role that RANKL plays in adaptive immunity.[4,21,57,58] OPG treatment may cooperate with other disease-modifying agents to decrease inflammation, as was indicated by additive suppressive effects of OPG in combination with anti-TNF therapy in the hTNFtg arthritis model.[59] However, this observation was not corroborated by a study in the CIA animal model that also examined combination therapy with OPG plus anti-TNF and observed no additional decrease in inflammation with combination therapy compared to anti-TNF therapy alone.[60] The minimal effect of OPG treatment on inflammation is supported by a study that investigated the outcome of OPG therapy on cellular and humoral immune responses.[61] *In vivo* immune regulatory effects of OPG were shown to be mild and were predominantly limited to improved humoral responses in T-cell-dependent and -independent models of antibody-mediated immunity.[61] Although the evidence suggests that OPG treatment does not have a major effect on the immune response, this potential complication of long-term OPG treatment should continue to be monitored.

COMPARISON OF OPG TO OTHER ANTI-RESORPTIVE THERAPIES IN ARTHRITIS MODELS

Bisphosphonates, which inhibit osteoclast activity and survival, are the current standard therapy for systemic bone resorption. Several studies have examined the use of bisphosphonates in RA but with varying success.[62–65] Studies in animal models of arthritis have compared the efficacy of OPG and bisphosphonate treatment for the prevention of focal and systemic bone loss. One such study using the hTNFtg model demonstrated similar efficacy of OPG and pamidronate in reducing the size and number of bone erosions, with the combination of these therapies demonstrating additive effects on these disease outcomes.[51] Two studies, one in the rat CIA model[66] and one in the hTNFtg arthritis model,[67] demonstrated that the potent bisphosphonate zoledronic acid significantly prevented focal joint destruction when administered at disease onset. In the CIA study, zoledronic acid treatment reduced histologic and radiographic measures of focal bone erosion and juxta-articular bone loss, including decreased osteoclast surface and osteoclast number in inflamed joints.[66] In the hTNFtg study, focal bone erosions were reduced by 95% in animals treated with repeated doses of zoledronic acid and synovial osteoclast numbers were also significantly reduced.[67] Similarly, incadronate was demonstrated to suppress radiologic and histologic measures of joint destruction in established rat AIA in a dose-dependent manner.[68]

These studies support the hypothesis that bisphosphonate therapy is a viable treatment strategy for protection against joint damage in RA and that this protection is achieved through the reduction of osteoclast numbers at sites of arthritic inflammation.[66,67] A recent study in a small cohort of early RA patients demonstrated that hand and wrist erosions (measured by magnetic resonance imaging) were decreased by 61% in zoledronic acid-treated patients compared with the placebo group, supporting the proposition that bisphosphonate therapy can prevent focal bone erosion in RA.[69] However, a study investigating two models of hypercalcemia of malignancy demonstrated that OPG treatment was a more effective therapy than pamidronate or zoledronic acid with regard to preventing bone destruction, suggesting that OPG treatment, or other methods of directly targeting RANKL function, may be a superior therapeutic strategy.[70]

TNF and IL-1 are key regulators of inflammation in RA and have also been demonstrated to have both direct and indirect positive effects on osteoclast generation, function, and/or survival.[71–76] Induction of experimental arthritis in either RANKL-deficient[33] or RANK-deficient[50] mice suggests that the contribution of TNF and IL-1 to osteoclast generation or function in inflammatory arthritis cannot occur *in vivo* in the absence of RANKL induction of RANK-specific signaling pathways. Additionally, in collaboration with Dr Benoist and colleagues, we demonstrated that TNF is not required for bone erosion in the K/BxN serum transfer model of arthritis. In arthritic TNF-deficient or arthritic TNF receptor I/II-deficient mice, osteoclast-mediated bone erosion was present, and the degree of bone erosion was proportionate to the severity of inflammation.[77] These observations are supported by a more recent study, also using the K/BxN serum transfer model in TNF receptor I/II-deficient chimeric mice.[78] Taken together, these studies support the hypothesis that RANKL is required for the generation of osteoclasts and subsequent bone erosion in inflammatory arthritis.

Interestingly, recent evidence suggests that TNF mediates its pro-osteoclastogenic activity through IL-1-mediated up-regulation of RANKL expression.[79] Clinical trials using recombinant human IL-1 receptor antagonist demonstrated bone-sparing effects in RA patients and the ability to prevent the development of new bone erosions.[80] However, IL-1 blockade in the hTNFtg model is not as effective as TNF blockade at reducing osteoclast numbers or bone erosion.[59] This may reflect the nature of the animal model, which is TNF-driven, or the mechanism of action of the drug used, which requires greater than 95% IL-1 receptor occupancy to achieve effective blockade. Of note, therapy with both TNF- and IL-1-blocking agents in this model resulted in dramatic attenuation of all disease measures, including bone erosion.[59] Therefore, the anti-resorptive effects of these treatments may be a consequence of indirect mechanisms including reduced inflammation and subsequently reduced production of pro-osteoclastogenic factors or may be a combination of both direct and indirect actions. It is of major clinical interest to delineate the mechanism of the bone-sparing effects of anti-TNF and anti-IL-1 therapies in RA and compare and contrast these to the potential utility of OPG.

Recent studies in animal models of arthritis have undertaken detailed comparisons of monotherapy and combination therapy using OPG and/or anti-TNF and/or anti-IL-1 agents. In the hTNFtg arthritis model, Zwerina et al. initiated therapy at the onset of disease using either anti-TNF alone (infliximab), anti-IL-1 alone (anakinra), OPG alone (OPG-Fc), the three possible dual combinations of these agents, and triple therapy.[59] In this TNF-driven animal model, anti-TNF was the only monotherapy that inhibited inflammation (51% decrease), while anti-TNF in combination with either anti-IL-1 (91% decrease) or OPG (81% decrease) demonstrated additive effects resulting in dramatic reduction of inflammation.[59] Bone erosion and osteoclast numbers in inflamed joints were also assessed after mono-, dual or triple therapy. Anti-TNF showed greater reduction in bone erosion and osteoclast number than either OPG or anti-IL-1 mono-therapies. Additionally, OPG in combination with either anti-TNF or anti-IL-1 was equal to or less potent than anti-TNF alone. Dual therapy of anti-TNF plus anti-IL-1 and triple therapy completely blocked bone erosion and greatly reduced osteoclast formation.[59] The greater efficacy of anti-TNF therapy in this study may be a direct reflection of the pathogenic mechanism of the arthritis model being driven by overexpression of TNF. Additional studies in other arthritis models with varying disease

induction and effector mechanisms are needed to further elucidate the hierarchy of signals ultimately leading to focal bone erosion.

Two recent studies have addressed the question of whether combining either anti-TNF or OPG therapy with the bone anabolic action of parathyroid hormone (PTH) can improve bone structural outcomes in inflammatory arthritis. Strikingly, both studies showed that the combination of either anti-TNF or OPG with PTH in AIA, CIA, and hTNFtg arthritis models effectively ablated bone erosion and also resulted in bone repair.[53,81] This line of investigation is of obvious interest to the field of rheumatology and further investigation of the ability to prevent bone erosion while simultaneously inducing targeted bone repair is warranted.

OPG THERAPY MAY ALSO PREVENT SYSTEMIC OSTEOPENIA/OSTEOPOROSIS AND JUXTA-ARTICULAR OSTEOPENIA IN RA

Fewer studies have focused on the mechanisms and prevention of juxta-articular and systemic bone loss in animal models of arthritis. Evidence from investigation of systemic bone loss suggests that OPG therapy inhibits arthritis-associated systemic bone loss.[82–84] In the CIA and AIA models, OPG treatment initiated 4 days after disease onset prevented systemic osteopenia.[52] When given at disease onset, OPG completely prevented systemic bone loss in the hTNFtg arthritis model, an outcome that was not achieved by treatment with pamidronate or anti-TNF.[35] Additionally, OPG treatment initiated 5 weeks after disease onset was also effective in preventing further systemic bone loss in this arthritis model.[81] Similarly, treatment of the hTNFtg model with the potent bisphosphonate zoledronic acid demonstrated a significant protection against systemic bone loss.[67] This evidence supports the hypothesis that systemic bone loss in inflammatory arthritis models is also mediated by osteoclasts, and that targeting RANKL to prevent or arrest this disease process is a logical approach.

Notably, combination therapy with OPG plus PTH initiated 5 weeks after disease onset in the hTNFtg arthritis model demonstrated not only prevention of new bone erosion but complete reversal of systemic bone loss to normal levels of bone density. This effect was attributed to both a reduction of osteoclast numbers and stimulation of osteoblasts in treated animals, as demonstrated by histomorphometric measures of osteoclast and osteoblast number and function.[81] In contrast, this study demonstrated that OPG therapy alone had negative effects on the number of osteoblasts on the surface of bone within affected joints,[81] indicating a potential adverse skeletal outcome of OPG treatment.[85] These observations raise the concern that long-term inhibition of osteoclastogenesis may result in reduced skeletal integrity through decreased bone turnover, a possibility that will need to be closely monitored in future clinical trials using this therapeutic strategy.

Peri- or juxta-articular bone loss is an early feature of RA that occurs in trabecular bone adjacent to inflamed joints and often precedes focal bone erosion.[86] Five studies in animal models of arthritis have provided preliminary evidence to support the hypothesis that osteoclasts are also important cellular mediators of juxta-articular bone loss. Three separate studies in mouse or rat CIA demonstrated preservation of juxta-articular bone after treatment with either OPG[36,60] or zoledronic acid,[66] providing preliminary evidence that osteoclasts are mediating this process. Similarly, treatment of the rat AIA model from disease induction with either clodronate[87] or incadronate,[88] led to prevention of juxta-articular bone destruction. More detailed studies addressing whether this disease process is a result of RANKL-stimulated, osteoclast-mediated bone loss are needed. Specifically, detailed investigation (including bone mineral density (BMD) and histomorphometic assessment) of juxta-articular bone protection should be performed in several animal models of arthritis in the setting of RANKL signaling blockade.

WILL OPG BE USEFUL FOR PREVENTING BONE EROSION IN OTHER FORMS OF ARTHRITIS?

PsA also has associated arthritic focal bone destruction and, as in RA, bone erosion in PsA involves the aberrant generation and activation of osteoclasts. Osteoclasts have been demonstrated

in resorption pits at the pannus–bone interface in PsA tissues.[89] Additionally, robust RANKL protein expression was demonstrated in synovial lining cells, contrasting with OPG expression, which was reported to be minimal. Intriguingly, elevated numbers of RANK+ potential osteoclast precursor cells have been observed in both the peripheral blood and joint tissue samples containing synovium and bone from PsA patients.[89] The ability of TNF to increase the number of available osteoclast precursors is supported by studies in the hTNFtg animal model, which demonstrated that TNF signaling, but not signaling through RANK, is associated with a robust increase in splenic and circulating osteoclast precursors.[50,90] Of note, the number of peripheral potential osteoclast precursor cells was significantly reduced in PsA patients after anti-TNF therapy.[89] These results suggest that TNF may be contributing to bone erosion, at least in part, through increasing the number and availability of osteoclast precursor cells. It would also be of interest to determine if TNF-mediated mobilization of osteoclast precursor cells also occurs in other inflammatory arthritides, particularly RA. Few studies have directly investigated the mechanisms of bone destruction in other autoimmune diseases that have local and/or systemic bone destruction.[46,91–95] Delineation of these mechanisms will help determine whether osteoclast-targeted therapies will have 'universal' or disease-specific bone protective effects.

THE UTILITY OF SERUM RANKL AND OPG LEVELS IN PREDICTING BONE RESORPTION

The question has been raised as to whether serum RANKL and/or OPG levels can be used as markers of bone resorption activity in disease. In healthy subjects, OPG levels in serum are positively correlated with age, suggesting that there is a compensatory increase in OPG to protect against increased bone resorption in later life.[96–101] However, a study in a large healthy twin cohort indicated that serum RANKL and OPG levels have only a weak association with BMD.[102] In the setting of disease, the current data are conflicting. In postmenopausal osteoporosis, serum OPG levels have been found to be higher in osteoporotic women compared with controls,[98,103] negatively related to BMD,[104] unrelated to BMD,[96,105] positively associated with BMD,[106] and associated with vertebral fracture.[100,106] In contrast, serum RANKL levels are commonly undetectable in healthy and postmenopausal women,[106,107] and data suggest that RANKL serum levels are not correlated with age in either sex.[101,108]

In RA patients the positive association of OPG with age is lost, supporting the hypothesis that bone metabolism is altered in this disease.[93,108] Serum OPG and RANKL levels in RA have been shown to be elevated compared with healthy controls; however, the ratio of this receptor–ligand pair was similar in the two groups. Additionally, anti-TNF therapy normalized serum RANKL and OPG levels without altering the RANKL/OPG ratio.[108] Another study in long-standing RA and osteoarthritis (OA) observed no difference in RANKL or OPG serum levels between these disease groups.[109] In another study, serum OPG levels in OA were similar to healthy controls, while somewhat surprisingly, serum RANKL was higher in OA than in healthy controls.[110] Finally, elevated serum RANKL levels have been reported in and associated with severity in osteolytic diseases (including prosthesis aseptic loosening, giant cell tumors, osteitis, primary benign bone tumors, tumors of soft tissues, hematologic malignancies, primary malignant bone tumors, and bone metastases from other primary origins),[111,112] but no change in OPG was observed compared to healthy controls.[111] Overall, the data with regard to the prognostic value of either RANKL or OPG serum level as resorption indicators are contradictory. Further investigation is needed before the utility of serum OPG or RANKL levels as prognostic tests for bone resorption in rheumatologic and osteolytic diseases can be determined.

TARGETING THE RANKL/OPG CYTOKINE SYSTEM

RANKL is predicted to be an important therapeutic target in many diseases in which bone loss is a cardinal feature. As a 'proof of principle', an initial human trial in 2003 using OPG therapy to block RANKL in a cohort of postmenopausal women demonstrated that a single dose of OPG resulted in a sustained reduction in systemic markers of bone resorption.[113]

Additional strategies targeting RANKL that mimic that action of OPG have subsequently been investigated. Cheng et al. designed exocyclic peptidomimetics based on their ability to mimic OPG in computer modeling of the OPG–RANKL interaction. These small molecule OPG simulators inhibited in vitro osteoclastogenesis (although not as efficiently as OPG), in vitro bone resorption, and in vivo bone loss in the mouse ovariectomy model.[114] Onyia et al. used an alternative approach and successfully performed high through-put screening for small molecule stimulators of OPG expression. The most potent of these was able to stimulate OPG mRNA and protein expression in osteoblasts, prevent anabolic bone responses in vivo, decrease cancer metastases to bone in an animal model and, of particular relevance to this chapter, prevent bone destruction in the rat AIA model.[115] These studies support the hypothesis that small molecule regulators of RANKL and OPG will likely be a fruitful approach to drug design for prevention of bone destruction.

Denosumab (AMG 162), a human monoclonal antibody to RANKL, is currently under investigation as a therapeutic strategy for preventing bone loss. The anti-resorptive activity and safety of denosumab was recently evaluated in a cohort of postmenopausal women in a randomized, double-blind, placebo-controlled, single subcutaneous dose, dose escalation trial.[113] This study showed that denosumab was well tolerated, and resulted in a dose-dependent rapid and sustained decrease in systemic markers of bone resorption with a more delayed decrease in bone formation markers.[113] One advantage of denosumab is that it appears to have a significantly longer half-life than OPG in cynomolgus monkeys, suggesting that this therapy will require less frequent administration.[116] Further development and testing of this and other therapeutic strategies targeting osteoclasts are highly anticipated.

ADDITIONAL CONSIDERATIONS

The critical role of the RANKL/RANK/OPG cytokine-receptor system in physiologic bone remodelling raises the question of whether effective long-term inhibition of this pathway will have detrimental effects on the skeleton. Studies have yielded mixed results with regard to the possible detrimental outcome of targeting this pathway on fracture healing.[117–123] However, evidence does indicate that bone formation rates may be inhibited by OPG therapy,[113,124,125] likely as a result of loss of osteoclast–osteoblast coupling.[85] In particular, assessments of the accumulation of bone micro-damage and fracture healing need to be closely monitored in the setting of RANKL blockade.

The ability of OPG and other anti-RANKL therapies to protect against cartilage destruction in arthritis is still unclear. Evidence from studies in animal models of arthritis has provided conflicting observations. Protection from cartilage destruction after OPG treatment was observed in the rat AIA model.[32] We demonstrated partial protection from cartilage destruction in the serum transfer model in the absence of RANKL. However, detailed histologic analysis suggested that this was an indirect effect due to protection of underlying subchondral bone.[33] In the arthritic c-fos[−/−]hTNFtg model, detailed analysis (including quantitation of proteoglycan loss, cartilage destruction, and MMP expression) demonstrated no protection from cartilage destruction despite dramatic protection from focal bone erosion.[34] The expression of RANKL, RANK, and OPG mRNA and protein has been demonstrated in chondrocytes *in vivo* in some studies[126–128] but not confirmed in others.[129,130] However, stimulation of primary human chondrocytes with RANKL did not result in any changes in chondrocyte gene expression, NF-κB activity, or production of collagenase or nitric oxide,[127] indicating that RANKL does not directly activate chondrocytes *in vitro*. In the growth plate of OPG knockout (KO) mice, cartilage was demonstrated to be abnormal, an observation that was associated with the accumulation of TRAP-expressing osteoclast-like cells at the chondro-osseous junction. Electron microscopy demonstrated that these osteoclast-like cells formed resorption lacunae with clear zones, but not ruffled borders, on the cartilage matrix.[131] Theses cells are likely to be what has been referred to in the literature as 'chondroclasts'.[132] Interestingly, treatment of OPG KO with OPG partially rescued the growth plate defect in these

mice, suggesting that the RANKL/OPG system may control chondroclast generation and/or function.[131] Therefore, given the demonstration that chondrocytes may express RANKL and OPG *in vivo* and that OPG may inhibit chondroclast activity, OPG and/or anti-RANKL therapy may have a direct protective effect on cartilage by preventing chondroclast-mediated resorption. The exact functional role of RANKL and OPG in chondrocytes, if any, and the effects of RANKL blockade on cartilage require additional research.

Considerable evidence now suggests that OPG and RANKL may contribute to normal physiologic processes and disease in the vasculature. Although it is beyond the scope of this chapter to review this literature (for review see Collin-Osdoby),[133] it is important to point out that therapeutic agents targeting either OPG or RANKL activity may have direct effects on the vasculature. Further investigations of the biological role of the RANKL/RANK/OPG receptor–ligand system in vascular biology and disease are needed.

The ability of OPG to function as a decoy receptor for TRAIL[134] is a developing area of research and implicates OPG as a survival factor for tumors.[135,136] Of particular relevance, a recent study suggested that expression of OPG protects RA synovial fibroblasts from TRAIL-induced apoptosis *in vitro*.[137] The effect of OPG treatment on synovial hyperplasia in animal models of arthritis has not been specifically investigated and the potential for this therapy to have detrimental effects on synovial fibroblasts, particularly after long-term therapy, needs to be evaluated. Finally, continued monitoring of the immunologic consequence of altering RANKL signaling through RANK is required, although, at the current time the immune regulatory consequences of OPG therapy appear to be minimal.

CONCLUSIONS

The accumulated evidence strongly supports the hypothesis that the RANKL/RANK/OPG system is a dominant pathway in the generation and function of osteoclasts and in the process of bone erosion in RA. A similar mechanism is implicated in other diseases that have associated bone loss, but more definitive studies are required to substantiate this paradigm. Control of osteoclast differentiation and function in normal physiology and in disease is a highly complex interplay of positive and negative regulators. Blockade of upstream factors, as has been shown for TNF, could also regulate the process of focal bone erosion. While we have made many advances in our understanding of the mechanisms of bone destruction in rheumatologic disease, a more complete understanding of additional regulatory factors will be important in the prevention of this disease outcome. A future goal in this area of research is not only to halt bone destruction, but also to stimulate targeted bone repair and improve the joint structure and subsequent function in patients with inflammatory arthritis.

REFERENCES

1. Pettit AR, Gravellese EM. Osteoprotegerin. In: Lipsky PE, Smolen JS, eds. Targeted Therapies in Rheumatology. London: Martin Dunitz, 2003: 359–77.
2. Hofbauer LC, Khosla S, Dunstan CR et al. The roles of osteoprotegerin and osteoprotegerin ligand in the paracrine regulation of bone resorption. J Bone Miner Res 2000; 15(1): 2–12.
3. Lacey DL, Timms E, Tan HL et al. Osteoprotegerin ligand is a cytokine that regulates osteoclast differentiation and activation. Cell 1998; 93(2): 165–76.
4. Kong YY, Yoshida H, Sarosi I et al. OPGL is a key regulator of osteoclastogenesis, lymphocyte development and lymph-node organogenesis. Nature 1999; 397(6717): 315–23.
5. Yasuda H, Shima N, Nakagawa N et al. Osteoclast differentiation factor is a ligand for osteoprotegerin/osteoclastogenesis-inhibitory factor and is identical to TRANCE/RANKL. Proc Natl Acad Sci U S A 1998; 95(7): 3597–602.
6. Wong BR, Josien R, Lee SY et al. The TRAF family of signal transducers mediates NF-kappaB activation by the TRANCE receptor. J Biol Chem 1998; 273(43): 28355–9.
7. Darnay BG, Haridas V, Ni J, Moore PA, Aggarwal BB. Characterization of the intracellular domain of receptor activator of NF-kappaB (RANK). Interaction with tumor necrosis factor receptor-associated factors and activation of NF-kappab and c-Jun N-terminal kinase. J Biol Chem 1998; 273(32): 20551–5.
8. Kobayashi T, Walsh MC, Choi Y. The role of TRAF6 in signal transduction and the immune response. Microbes Infect 2004; 6(14): 1333–8.
9. David JP, Sabapathy K, Hoffmann O, Idarraga MH, Wagner EF. JNK1 modulates osteoclastogenesis through both c-Jun phosphorylation-dependent and -independent mechanisms. J Cell Sci 2002; 115(Pt 22): 4317–25.
10. Grigoriadis AE, Wang ZQ, Cecchini MG et al. c-Fos: a key regulator of osteoclast-macrophage lineage determination and bone remodeling. Science 1994; 266(5184): 443–8.
11. Fleischmann A, Hafezi F, Elliott C et al. Fra-1 replaces c-Fos-dependent functions in mice. Genes Dev 2000; 14(21): 2695–700.
12. Kenner L, Hoebertz A, Beil T et al. Mice lacking JunB are osteopenic due to cell-autonomous osteoblast and osteoclast defects. J Cell Biol 2004; 164(4): 613–23.
13. Ikeda F, Nishimura R, Matsubara T et al. Critical roles of c-Jun signaling in regulation of NFAT family and RANKL-regulated osteoclast differentiation. J Clin Invest 2004; 114(4): 475–84.
14. Takayanagi H, Kim S, Koga T et al. Induction and activation of the transcription factor NFATc1 (NFAT2) integrate RANKL signaling in terminal differentiation of osteoclasts. Dev Cell 2002; 3(6): 889–901.
15. Gohda J, Akiyama T, Koga T et al. RANK-mediated amplification of TRAF6 signaling leads to NFATc1 induction during osteoclastogenesis. EMBO J 2005; 24(4): 790–9.
16. Lomaga MA, Yeh WC, Sarosi I et al. TRAF6 deficiency results in osteopetrosis and defective interleukin-1, CD40, and LPS signaling. Genes Dev 1999; 13(8): 1015–24.
17. Naito A, Azuma S, Tanaka S et al. Severe osteopetrosis, defective interleukin-1 signalling and lymph node organogenesis in TRAF6-deficient mice. Genes Cells 1999; 4(6): 353–62.
18. Franzoso G, Carlson L, Xing L et al. Requirement for NF-kappaB in osteoclast and B-cell development. Genes Dev 1997; 11(24): 3482–96.
19. Steingrimsson E, Moore KJ, Lamoreux ML et al. Molecular basis of mouse microphthalmia (mi) mutations helps explain their developmental and phenotypic consequences. Nat Genet 1994; 8(3): 256–63.
20. Takayanagi H. Mechanistic insight into osteoclast differentiation in osteoimmunology. J Mol Med 2005; 83(3): 170–9.
21. Dougall WC, Glaccum M, Charrier K et al. RANK is essential for osteoclast and lymph node development. Genes Dev 1999; 13: 2412–24.
22. Li J, Sarosi I, Yan XQ et al. RANK is the intrinsic hematopoietic cell surface receptor that controls osteoclastogenesis and regulation of bone mass and calcium metabolism. Proc Natl Acad Sci U S A 2000; 97(4): 1566–71.
23. Jimi E, Akiyama S, Tsurukai T et al. Osteoclast differentiation factor acts as a multifunctional regulator in

murine osteoclast differentiation and function. J Immunol 1999; 163(1): 434–42.

24. Burgess TL, Qian Y, Kaufman S et al. The ligand for osteoprotegerin (OPGL) directly activates mature osteoclasts. J Cell Biol 1999; 145(3): 527–38.

25. Lacey DL, Tan HL, Lu J et al. Osteoprotegerin ligand modulates murine osteoclast survival in vitro and in vivo. Am J Pathol 2000; 157(2): 435–48.

26. Henriksen K, Karsdal M, Delaisse JM, Engsig MT. RANKL and vascular endothelial growth factor (VEGF) induce osteoclast chemotaxis through an ERK1/2-dependent mechanism. J Biol Chem 2003; 278(49): 48745–53.

27. Simonet WS, Lacey DL, Dunstan CR et al. Osteoprotegerin: a novel secreted protein involved in the regulation of bone density. Cell 1997; 89(2): 309–19.

28. Yasuda H, Shima N, Nakagawa N et al. Identity of osteoclastogenesis inhibitory factor (OCIF) and osteoprotegerin (OPG): a mechanism by which OPG/OCIF inhibits osteoclastogenesis in vitro. Endocrinology 1998; 139(3): 1329–37.

29. Shalhoub V, Faust J, Boyle WJ et al. Osteoprotegerin and osteoprotegerin ligand effects on osteoclast formation from human peripheral blood mononuclear cell precursors. J Cell Biochem 1999; 72(2): 251–61.

30. Hakeda Y, Kobayashi Y, Yamaguchi K et al. Osteoclastogenesis inhibitory factor (OCIF) directly inhibits bone-resorbing activity of isolated mature osteoclasts. Biochem Biophys Res Commun 1998; 251(3): 796–801.

31. Fazzalari NL, Kuliwaba JS, Atkins GJ, Forwood MR, Findlay DM. The ratio of messenger RNA levels of receptor activator of nuclear factor kappaB ligand to osteoprotegerin correlates with bone remodeling indices in normal human cancellous bone but not in osteoarthritis. J Bone Miner Res 2001; 16(6): 1015–27.

32. Kong YY, Feige U, Sarosi I et al. Activated T cells regulate bone loss and joint destruction in adjuvant arthritis through osteoprotegerin ligand. Nature 1999; 402(6759): 304–9.

33. Pettit AR, Ji H, von Stechow D et al. TRANCE/RANKL knockout mice are protected from bone erosion in a serum transfer model of arthritis. Am J Pathol 2001; 159(5): 1689–99.

34. Redlich K, Hayer S, Ricci R et al. Osteoclasts are essential for TNF-alpha-mediated joint destruction. J Clin Invest 2002; 110(10): 1419–27.

35. Schett G, Redlich K, Hayer S et al. Osteoprotegerin protects against generalized bone loss in tumor necrosis factor-transgenic mice. Arthritis Rheum. 2003; 48(7): 2042–51.

36. Romas E, Sims NA, Hards DK et al. Osteoprotegerin reduces osteoclast numbers and prevents bone erosion

in collagen-induced arthritis. Am J Pathol 2002; 161(4): 1419–27.

37. Gravallese EM, Manning C, Tsay A et al. Synovial tissue in rheumatoid arthritis is a source of osteoclast differentiation factor. Arthritis Rheum 2000; 43: 250–8.

38. Takayanagi H, Iizuka H, Juji T et al. Involvement of receptor activator of nuclear factor kappa-B ligand/osteoclast differentiation factor in osteoclastogenesis from synoviocytes in rheumatoid arthritis. Arthritis Rheum 2000; 43: 259–69.

39. Horwood NJ, Kartsogiannis V, Quinn JMW et al. Activated T lymphocytes support osteoclast formation in vitro. Biochem Biophys Res Commun 1999; 265(1): 144–50.

40. Crotti TN, Smith MD, Weedon H et al. Receptor activator NF-kappaB ligand (RANKL) expression in synovial tissue from patients with rheumatoid arthritis, spondyloarthropathy, osteoarthritis, and from normal patients: semiquantitative and quantitative analysis. Ann Rheum Dis 2002; 61(12): 1047–54.

41. Kotake S, Udagawa N, Hakoda M et al. Activated human T cells directly induce osteoclastogenesis from human monocytes: possible role of T cells in bone destruction in rheumatoid arthritis patients. Arthritis Rheum 2001; 44(5): 1003–12.

42. Haynes DR, Crotti TN, Loric M et al. Osteoprotegerin and receptor activator of nuclear factor kappaB ligand (RANKL) regulate osteoclast formation by cells in the human rheumatoid arthritic joint. Rheumatology (Oxford) 2001; 40(6): 623–30.

43. Vanderborght A, Linsen L, Thewissen M et al. Osteoprotegerin and receptor activator of nuclear factor-kappaB ligand mRNA expression in patients with rheumatoid arthritis and healthy controls. J Rheumatol 2004; 31(8): 1483–90.

44. Pettit AR, Walsh NC, Manning C, Goldring SR, Gravallese EM. RANKL protein is expressed at the pannus-bone interface at sites of articular bone erosion in rheumatoid arthritis. Rheumatology (Oxford) 2006; 45: 1068–76.

45. Bromley M, Woolley DE. Chondroclasts and osteoclasts at subchondral sites of erosion in the rheumatoid joint. Arthritis Rheum 1984; 27(9): 968–75.

46. Gravallese EM, Harada Y, Wang JT et al. Identification of cell types responsible for bone resorption in rheumatoid arthritis and juvenile rheumatoid arthritis. Am J Pathol 1998; 152(4): 943–51.

47. Fonseca JE, Cortez-Dias N, Francisco A et al. Inflammatory cell infiltrate and RANKL/OPG expression in rheumatoid synovium: comparison with other inflammatory arthropathies and correlation with outcome. Clin Exp Rheumatol 2005; 23(2): 185–92.

48. Lubberts E, Oppers-Walgreen B, Pettit AR et al. Increase in expression of receptor activator of nuclear

factor kappaB at sites of bone erosion correlates with progression of inflammation in evolving collagen-induced arthritis. Arthritis Rheum 2002; 46(11): 3055–64.

49. Kwan Tat S, Padrines M, Theoleyre S, Heymann D, Fortun Y. IL-6, RANKL, TNF-alpha/IL-1: interrelations in bone resorption pathophysiology. Cytokine Growth Factor Rev 2004; 15(1): 49–60.

50. Li P, Schwarz EM, O'Keefe RJ et al. RANK signaling is not required for TNFalpha-mediated increase in CD11(hi) osteoclast precursors but is essential for mature osteoclast formation in TNFalpha-mediated inflammatory arthritis. J Bone Miner Res 2004; 19(2): 207–13.

51. Redlich K, Hayer S, Maier A et al. Tumor necrosis factor alpha-mediated joint destruction is inhibited by targeting osteoclasts with osteoprotegerin. Arthritis Rheum 2002; 46(3): 785–92.

52. Stolina M, Adamu S, Ominsky M et al. RANKL is a marker and mediator of local and systemic bone loss in two rat models of inflammatory arthritis. J Bone Miner Res 2005; 20(10): 1756–65.

53. Schett G, Middleton S, Bolon B et al. Additive bone-protective effects of anabolic treatment when used in conjunction with RANKL and tumor necrosis factor inhibition in two rat arthritis models. Arthritis Rheum 2005; 52(5): 1604–11.

54. Campagnuolo G, Bolon B, Feige U. Kinetics of bone protection by recombinant osteoprotegerin therapy in Lewis rats with adjuvant arthritis. Arthritis Rheum 2002; 46(7): 1926–36.

55. Bolon B, Campagnuolo G, Feige U. Duration of bone protection by a single osteoprotegerin injection in rats with adjuvant-induced arthritis. Cell Mol Life Sci 2002; 59(9): 1569–76.

56. Breedveld FC, Han C, Bala M et al. Association between baseline radiographic damage and improvement in physical function after treatment of patients with rheumatoid arthritis. Ann Rheum Dis 2005; 64(1): 52–5.

57. Josien R, Li HL, Ingulli E et al. TRANCE, a tumor necrosis factor family member, enhances the longevity and adjuvant properties of dendritic cells in vivo. J Exp Med 2000; 191(3): 495–502.

58. Josien R, Wong BR, Li HL, Steinman RM, Choi Y. TRANCE, a TNF family member, is differentially expressed on T cell subsets and induces cytokine production in dendritic cells. J Immunol 1999; 162(5): 2562–8.

59. Zwerina J, Hayer S, Tohidast-Akrad M et al. Single and combined inhibition of tumor necrosis factor, interleukin-1, and RANKL pathways in tumor necrosis factor-induced arthritis: effects on synovial inflammation, bone erosion, and cartilage destruction. Arthritis Rheum 2004; 50(1): 277–90.

60. Saidenberg-Kermanac'h N, Corrado A, Lemeiter D et al. TNF-alpha antibodies and osteoprotegerin decrease systemic bone loss associated with inflammation through distinct mechanisms in collagen-induced arthritis. Bone 2004; 35(5): 1200–7.

61. Stolina M, Guo J, Faggioni R, Brown H, Senaldi G. Regulatory effects of osteoprotegerin on cellular and humoral immune responses. Clin Immunol 2003; 109(3): 347–54.

62. Valleala H, Laasonen L, Koivula MK et al. Two year randomized controlled trial of etidronate in rheumatoid arthritis: changes in serum aminoterminal telopeptides correlate with radiographic progression of disease. J Rheumatol 2003; 30(3): 468–73.

63. Hasegawa J, Nagashima M, Yamamoto M et al. Bone resorption and inflammatory inhibition efficacy of intermittent cyclical etidronate therapy in rheumatoid arthritis. J Rheumatol 2003; 30(3): 474–9.

64. Eggelmeijer F, Papapoulos SE, van Paassen HC et al. Increased bone mass with pamidronate treatment in rheumatoid arthritis. Results of a three-year randomized, double-blind trial. Arthritis Rheum 1996; 39(3): 396–402.

65. Maccagno A, Di Giorgio E, Roldan EJ, Caballero LE, Perez Lloret A. Double blind radiological assessment of continuous oral pamidronic acid in patients with rheumatoid arthritis. Scand J Rheumatol 1994; 23(4): 211–14.

66. Sims NA, Green JR, Glatt M et al. Targeting osteoclasts with zoledronic acid prevents bone destruction in collagen-induced arthritis. Arthritis Rheum 2004; 50(7): 2338–46.

67. Herrak P, Gortz B, Hayer S et al. Zoledronic acid protects against local and systemic bone loss in tumor necrosis factor-mediated arthritis. Arthritis Rheum 2004; 50(7): 2327–37.

68. Zhao H, Liu S, Huang D et al. The protective effects of incadronate on inflammation and joint destruction in established rat adjuvant arthritis. Rheumatol Int 2006; 26: 732–40.

69. Jarrett SJ, Conaghan PG, Sloan VS et al. Preliminary evidence for a structural benefit of the new bisphosphonate zoledronic acid in early rheumatoid arthritis. Arthritis Rheum 2006; 54(5): 1410–14.

70. Morony S, Warmington K, Adamu S et al. The inhibition of RANKL causes greater suppression of bone resorption and hypercalcemia compared with bisphosphonates in two models of humoral hypercalcemia of malignancy. Endocrinology 2005; 146(8): 3235–43.

71. Arend WP, Dayer J-M. Inhibition of the production and effects of interleukin-1 and tumor necrosis factor α in rheumatoid arthritis. Arthritis Rheum 1995; 38: 151–60.

72. Fuller K, Murphy C, Kirstein B, Fox SW, Chambers TJ. TNFalpha potently activates osteoclasts, through a

direct action independent of and strongly synergistic with RANKL. Endocrinology 2002; 143(3): 1108–18.

73. Lam J, Takeshita S, Barker JE et al. TNF-alpha induces osteoclastogenesis by direct stimulation of macrophages exposed to permissive levels of RANK ligand. J Clin Invest 2000; 106(12): 1481–8.

74. Jimi E, Nakamura I, Ikebe T et al. Activation of NF-kappaB is involved in the survival of osteoclasts promoted by interleukin-1. J Biol Chem 1998; 273(15): 8799–805.

75. Jimi E, Nakamura I, Duong LT et al. Interleukin 1 induces multinucleation and bone-resorbing activity of osteoclasts in the absence of osteoblasts/stromal cells. Exp Cell Res 1999; 247(1): 84–93.

76. Azuma Y, Kaji K, Katogi R, Takeshita S, Kudo A. Tumor necrosis factor-alpha induces differentiation of and bone resorption by osteoclasts. J Biol Chem 2000; 275(7): 4858–64.

77. Ji H, Pettit A, Ohmura K et al. Critical roles for interleukin 1 and tumor necrosis factor alpha in antibody-induced arthritis. J Exp Med 2002; 196(1): 77–85.

78. Kitaura H, Zhou P, Kim HJ et al. M-CSF mediates TNF-induced inflammatory osteolysis. J Clin Invest 2005; 115(12): 3418–27.

79. Wei S, Kitaura H, Zhou P, Ross FP, Teitelbaum SL. IL-1 mediates TNF-induced osteoclastogenesis. J Clin Invest 2005; 115(2): 282–90.

80. Watt I, Cobby M. Treatment of rheumatoid arthritis patients with interleukin-1 receptor antagonist: radiologic assessment. Semin Arthritis Rheum 2001; 30 (5 Suppl 2): 21–5.

81. Redlich K, Gortz B, Hayer S et al. Repair of local bone erosions and reversal of systemic bone loss upon therapy with anti-tumor necrosis factor in combination with osteoprotegerin or parathyroid hormone in tumor necrosis factor-mediated arthritis. Am J Pathol 2004; 164(2): 543–55.

82. Capparelli C, Morony S, Warmington K et al. Sustained antiresorptive effects after a single treatment with human recombinant osteoprotegerin (OPG): a pharmacodynamic and pharmacokinetic analysis in rats. J Bone Miner Res 2003; 18(5): 852–8.

83. Kostenuik PJ, Bolon B, Morony S et al. Gene therapy with human recombinant osteoprotegerin reverses established osteopenia in ovariectomized mice. Bone 2004; 34(4): 656–64.

84. Min H, Morony S, Sarosi I et al. Osteoprotegerin reverses osteoporosis by inhibiting endosteal osteoclasts and prevents vascular calcification by blocking a process resembling osteoclastogenesis. J Exp Med 2000; 192(4): 463–74.

85. Martin TJ, Sims NA. Osteoclast-derived activity in the coupling of bone formation to resorption. Trends Mol Med 2005; 11(2): 76–81.

86. Scott DL. Prognostic factors in early rheumatoid arthritis. Rheumatology (Oxford) 2000; 39 (Suppl 1): 24–9.

87. Oelzner P, Brauer R, Henzgen S et al. Periarticular bone alterations in chronic antigen-induced arthritis: free and liposome-encapsulated clodronate prevent loss of bone mass in the secondary spongiosa. Clin Immunol 1999; 90(1): 79–88.

88. Akiyama T, Mori S, Mashiba T et al. Incadronate disodium inhibits joint destruction and periarticular bone loss only in the early phase of rat adjuvant-induced arthritis. J Bone Miner Metab 2005; 23(4): 295–301.

89. Ritchlin CT, Haas-Smith SA, Li P, Hicks DG, Schwarz EM. Mechanisms of TNF-alpha- and RANKL-mediated osteoclastogenesis and bone resorption in psoriatic arthritis. J Clin Invest 2003; 111(6): 821–31.

90. Li P, Schwarz EM, O'Keefe RJ et al. Systemic tumor necrosis factor alpha mediates an increase in peripheral CD11bhigh osteoclast precursors in tumor necrosis factor alpha-transgenic mice. Arthritis Rheum 2004; 50(1): 265–76.

91. Mason T, Reed AM, Nelson AM et al. Frequency of abnormal hand and wrist radiographs at time of diagnosis of polyarticular juvenile rheumatoid arthritis. J Rheumatol 2002; 29(10): 2214–18.

92. Varsani H, Patel A, van Kooyk Y, Woo P, Wedderburn LR. Synovial dendritic cells in juvenile idiopathic arthritis (JIA) express receptor activator of NF-kappaB (RANK). Rheumatology (Oxford) 2003; 42(4): 583–90.

93. Franck H, Meurer T, Hofbauer LC. Evaluation of bone mineral density, hormones, biochemical markers of bone metabolism, and osteoprotegerin serum levels in patients with ankylosing spondylitis. J Rheumatol 2004; 31(11): 2236–41.

94. Petri M. Musculoskeletal complications of systemic lupus erythematosus in the Hopkins Lupus Cohort: an update. Arthritis Care Res 1995; 8(3): 137–45.

95. Grisar J, Bernecker PM, Aringer M et al. Ankylosing spondylitis, psoriatic arthritis, and reactive arthritis show increased bone resorption, but differ with regard to bone formation. J Rheumatol 2002; 29(7): 1430–6.

96. Khosla S, Arrighi HM, Melton LJ 3rd et al. Correlates of osteoprotegerin levels in women and men. Osteoporos Int 2002; 13(5): 394–9.

97. Oh KW, Rhee EJ, Lee WY et al. Circulating osteoprotegerin and receptor activator of NF-kappaB ligand system are associated with bone metabolism in middle-aged males. Clin Endocrinol (Oxf) 2005; 62(1): 92–8.

98. Oh KW, Rhee EJ, Lee WY et al. The relationship between circulating osteoprotegerin levels and bone mineral metabolism in healthy women. Clin Endocrinol (Oxf) 2004; 61(2): 244–9.

99. Szulc P, Hofbauer LC, Heufelder AE, Roth S, Delmas PD. Osteoprotegerin serum levels in men: correlation with age, estrogen, and testosterone status. J Clin Endocrinol Metab 2001; 86(7): 3162–5.

100. Fahrleitner-Pammer A, Dobnig H, Piswanger-Soelkner C et al. Osteoprotegerin serum levels in women: correlation with age, bone mass, bone turnover and fracture status. Wien Klin Wochenschr 2003; 115(9): 291–7.

101. Trofimov S, Pantsulaia I, Kobyliansky E, Livshits G. Circulating levels of receptor activator of nuclear factor-kappaB ligand/osteoprotegerin/macrophage-colony stimulating factor in a presumably healthy human population. Eur J Endocrinol 2004; 150(3): 305–11.

102. Abrahamsen B, Hjelmborg JV, Kostenuik P et al. Circulating amounts of osteoprotegerin and RANK ligand: genetic influence and relationship with BMD assessed in female twins. Bone 2005; 36(4): 727–35.

103. Yano K, Tsuda E, Washida N et al. Immunological characterization of circulating osteoprotegerin/osteoclastogenesis inhibitory factor: increased serum concentrations in postmenopausal women with osteoporosis. J Bone Miner Res 1999; 14(4): 518–27.

104. Rogers A, Saleh G, Hannon RA, Greenfield D, Eastell R. Circulating estradiol and osteoprotegerin as determinants of bone turnover and bone density in postmenopausal women. J Clin Endocrinol Metab 2002; 87(10): 4470–5.

105. Browner WS, Lui LY, Cummings SR. Associations of serum osteoprotegerin levels with diabetes, stroke, bone density, fractures, and mortality in elderly women. J Clin Endocrinol Metab 2001; 86(2): 631–7.

106. Mezquita-Raya P, de la Higuera M, Garcia DF et al. The contribution of serum osteoprotegerin to bone mass and vertebral fractures in postmenopausal women. Osteoporos Int 2005; 16(11): 1368–74.

107. Hawa G, Brinskelle-Schmal N, Glatz K, Maitzen S, Woloszczuk W. Immunoassay for soluble RANKL (receptor activator of NF-kappaB ligand) in serum. Clin Lab 2003; 49(9-10): 461–3.

108. Ziolkowska M, Kurowska M, Radzikowska A et al. High levels of osteoprotegerin and soluble receptor activator of nuclear factor kappa B ligand in serum of rheumatoid arthritis patients and their normalization after anti-tumor necrosis factor alpha treatment. Arthritis Rheum 2002; 46(7): 1744–53.

109. Skoumal M, Kolarz G, Haberhauer G et al. Osteoprotegerin and the receptor activator of NF-kappa B ligand in the serum and synovial fluid. A comparison of patients with longstanding rheumatoid arthritis and osteoarthritis. Rheumatol Int 2005; 26(1): 63–9.

110. Pulsatelli L, Dolzani P, Silvestri T et al. Soluble receptor activator of nuclear factor-kappaB Ligand (sRANKL)/ osteoprotegerin balance in ageing and age-associated diseases. Biogerontology 2004; 5(2): 119–27.

111. Grimaud E, Soubigou L, Couillaud S et al. Receptor activator of nuclear factor kappaB ligand (RANKL)/ osteoprotegerin (OPG) ratio is increased in severe osteolysis. Am J Pathol 2003; 163(5): 2021–31.

112. Terpos E, Szydlo R, Apperley JF et al. Soluble receptor activator of nuclear factor kappaB ligand-osteoprotegerin ratio predicts survival in multiple myeloma: proposal for a novel prognostic index. Blood 2003; 102(3): 1064–9.

113. Bekker PJ, Holloway DL, Rasmussen AS et al. A single-dose placebo-controlled study of AMG 162, a fully human monoclonal antibody to RANKL, in postmenopausal women. J Bone Miner Res 2004; 19(7): 1059–66.

114. Cheng X, Kinosaki M, Takami M et al. Disabling of receptor activator of nuclear factor-kappaB (RANK) receptor complex by novel osteoprotegerin-like peptidomimetics restores bone loss in vivo. J Biol Chem 2004; 279(9): 8269–77.

115. Onyia JE, Galvin RJ, Ma YL et al. Novel and selective small molecule stimulators of osteoprotegerin expression inhibit bone resorption. J Pharmacol Exp Ther 2004; 309(1): 369–79.

116. Kostenuik PJ. Osteoprotegerin and RANKL regulate bone resorption, density, geometry and strength. Curr Opin Pharmacol 2005; 5: 618–25.

117. Kon T, Cho TJ, Aizawa T et al. Expression of osteoprotegerin, receptor activator of NF-kappaB ligand (osteoprotegerin ligand) and related proinflammatory cytokines during fracture healing. J Bone Miner Res 2001; 16(6): 1004–14.

118. Yoshida H, Hayashi S, Kunisada T et al. The murine mutation osteopetrosis is in the coding region of the macrophage colony stimulating factor gene. Nature 1990; 345(6274): 442–4.

119. Flick LM, Weaver JM, Ulrich-Vinther M et al. Effects of receptor activator of NFkappaB (RANK) signaling blockade on fracture healing. J Orthop Res 2003; 21(4): 676–84.

120. Ulrich-Vinther M, Schwarz EM, Pedersen FS, Soballe K, Andreassen TT. Gene therapy with human osteoprotegerin decreases callus remodeling with limited effects on biomechanical properties. Bone 2005; 37: 751–8.

121. Ulrich-Vinther M, Andreassen TT. Osteoprotegerin treatment impairs remodeling and apparent material properties of callus tissue without influencing structural fracture strength. Calcif Tissue Int 2005; 76(4): 280–6.

122. Li C, Mori S, Li J et al. Long-term effect of incadronate disodium (YM-175) on fracture healing of femoral shaft in growing rats. J Bone Miner Res 2001; 16(3): 429–36.

123. Komatsubara S, Mori S, Mashiba T et al. Long-term treatment of incadronate disodium accumulates

microdamage but improves the trabecular bone microarchitecture in dog vertebra. J Bone Miner Res 2003; 18(3): 512–20.

124. Ross AB, Bateman TA, Kostenuik PJ et al. The effects of osteoprotegerin on the mechanical properties of rat bone. J Mater Sci Mater Med 2001; 12(7): 583–8.

125. Bekker PJ, Holloway D, Nakanishi A et al. The effect of a single dose of osteoprotegerin in postmenopausal women. J Bone Miner Res 2001; 16(2): 348–60.

126. Carda C, Silvestrini G, Gomez de Ferraris ME, Peydro A, Bonucci E. Osteoprotegerin (OPG) and RANKL expression and distribution in developing human craniomandibular joint. Tissue Cell 2005; 37(3): 247–55.

127. Komuro H, Olee T, Kuhn K et al. The osteoprotegerin/receptor activator of nuclear factor kappaB/receptor activator of nuclear factor kappaB ligand system in cartilage. Arthritis Rheum 2001; 44(12): 2768–76.

128. Silvestrini G, Ballanti P, Patacchioli F et al. Detection of osteoprotegerin (OPG) and its ligand (RANKL) mRNA and protein in femur and tibia of the rat. J Mol Histol 2005; 36(1-2): 59–67.

129. Mueller RJ, Richards RG. Immunohistological identification of receptor activator of NF-kappaB ligand (RANKL) in human, ovine and bovine bone tissues. J Mater Sci Mater Med 2004; 15(4): 367–72.

130. Nakamura H, Tsuji T, Hirata A, Yamamoto T. Localization of osteoprotegerin (OPG) on bone surfaces and cement lines in rat tibia. J Histochem Cytochem 2002; 50(7): 945–53.

131. Yamazaki H, Sasaki T. Effects of osteoprotegerin administration on osteoclast differentiation and trabecular bone structure in osteoprotegerin-deficient mice. J Electron Microsc (Tokyo) 2005; 54(5): 467–77.

132. Nordahl J, Andersson G, Reinholt FP. Chondroclasts and osteoclasts in bones of young rats: comparison of ultrastructural and functional features. Calcif Tissue Int 1998; 63(5): 401–8.

133. Collin-Osdoby P. Regulation of vascular calcification by osteoclast regulatory factors RANKL and osteoprotegerin. Circ Res 2004; 95(11): 1046–57.

134. Emery JG, McDonnell P, Burke MB et al. Osteoprotegerin is a receptor for the cytotoxic ligand TRAIL. J Biol Chem 1998; 273(23): 14363–7.

135. Nyambo R, Cross N, Lippitt J et al. Human bone marrow stromal cells protect prostate cancer cells from TRAIL-induced apoptosis. J Bone Miner Res 2004; 19(10): 1712–21.

136. Holen I, Cross SS, Neville-Webbe HL et al. Osteoprotegerin (OPG) expression by breast cancer cells in vitro and breast tumours in vivo – a role in tumour cell survival? Breast Cancer Res Treat 2005; 92(3): 207–15.

137. Miyashita T, Kawakami A, Nakashima T et al. Osteoprotegerin (OPG) acts as an endogenous decoy receptor in tumour necrosis factor-related apoptosis-inducing ligand (TRAIL)-mediated apoptosis of fibroblast- like synovial cells. Clin Exp Immunol 2004; 137(2): 430–6.

21

Update: inflammatory, angiogenic, and homeostatic chemokines and their receptors

Zoltán Szekanecz and Alisa E Koch

Introduction • Chemokines • Chemokine receptors • Chemokines and chemokine receptors in synovial inflammation and angiogenesis • Inflammatory, angiogenic and homeostatic chemokines: a well-justified classification? • Regulation of chemokine production during leukocyte recruitment • Chemokine targeting strategies • Conclusions • Acknowledgments • References

INTRODUCTION

Chemokines are small proteins exerting chemotactic activity towards cells, especially immune cells. Target cells express matching receptors for these mediators. Chemokines have been classified into supergene families with respect to their structure (see below).[1–14] Recently, chemokine/chemokine receptor pairs have also been functionally categorized as being 'homeostatic' (alternatively: constitutive, housekeeping or lymphoid), 'angiogenic/angiostatic', or 'inflammatory' (alternatively: inducible), although these functions often overlap.[7,12–14] Generally, all chemokines described in this chapter in context with arthritis may be considered to be 'inflammatory'. Many of these chemokines also promote or suppress angiogenesis. 'Homeostatic' chemokines usually play a role in B-cell recruitment, germinal center formation, and the development of lymphoid tissues under physiological conditions. However, the latter mediators have also been implicated in lymphoma- or inflammation-associated B-cell migration.[7,12–16]

Numerous aspects of chemokines and chemokine receptors in rheumatic diseases have been discussed recently.[2] Here, we will give an update on recent developments in chemokine research. Regarding the recent functional classification described above, we will primarily focus on inflammatory and angiogenic/angiostatic chemokines and their receptors, as these molecules are involved in the pathogenesis of arthritis. Among inflammatory rheumatic diseases, we picked rheumatoid arthritis (RA), a chronic inflammatory and destructive articular disease as a prototype, as the majority of chemokine studies have been performed in this disease and its animal models.[1–6]

First, we will give a brief overview of the chemokine and chemokine receptor subsets. Those inflammatory, angiogenic/angiostatic, and homeostatic chemokines and chemokine receptors will be discussed in more detail, which may be important in the pathogenesis of RA and thus may become targets for anti-chemokine therapy. As the last few years have seen a rapid development of studies on chemokine and chemokine receptor targeting, we will summarize data obtained in RA and in animal models of arthritis. Based on the great number of recent studies, it is very likely that the next few years will bring several new preclinical and clinical trials in this field.

CHEMOKINES

Chemokines are chemotactic cytokines involved in the migration of various cells into tissues. In RA, these mediators chemoattract inflammatory leukocytes, which cross the endothelial barrier and migrate into the synovial tissue (ST).[1–11,17,18] Chemokines have been classified into four distinct supergene families with respect to their structural similarities and differences. According to the location of cysteine (C) residues, these families are designated as CXC, CC, C, and CX_3C chemokines (Table 21.1).

Accordingly, the four chemokine receptor groups are CXCR, CCR, CR, and CX_3CR, respectively[1,3,4,9–11,19] (Table 21.2). Currently, there are more than 50 known chemokines and 19 chemokine receptors[1–12] (Tables 21.1 and Table 21.2). In 2000, a new classification system was introduced. Now chemokines are considered as chemokine ligands and, apart from their classical name (see later), each chemokine has been assigned a designation of CXCL, CCL, XCL, or CX_3CL1[1,5,11,19] (Tables 21.1 and Table 21.2). In this review, both the classical and the new designations will be used.

Table 21.1 The structural and functional classification of chemokines[a]

Family	Classical nomenclature	New nomenclature	Inflammatory	Angiogenic (+)/ angiostatic (−)	Homeostatic
CXC	Groα	CXCL1	+	+	
	Groβ	CXCL2			
	Groγ	CXCL3			
	PF4	CXCL4	+	−	
	ENA-78	CXCL5	+	+	
	GCP-2	CXCL6	+		
	CTAP-III	CXCL7	+	+	
	IL-8	CXCL8	+	+	
	Mig	CXCL9	+	−	
	IP-10	CXCL10	+	−	
	ITAC	CXCL11			+
	SDF-1α,β	CXCL12	+	+	+
	BCA-1	CXCL13	+		+
	—	CXCL16	+		+
CC	I-309	CCL1			+
	MCP-1	CCL2	+		
	MIP-1α	CCL3	+		
	MIP-1β	CCL4			
	RANTES	CCL5	+		
	MCP-3	CCL7	?[b]		
	MCP-2	CCL8	?[b]		
	Eotaxin	CCL11			+
	MCP-5	CCL12			
	MCP-4	CCL13			
	HCC-1	CCL14	?[b]		+
	HCC-2	CCL15	?[b]		+
	HCC-4	CCL16	?[b]		+
	TARC	CCL17			+
	PARC	CCL18			+
	ELC	CCL19	+		+
	MIP-3α	CCL20	+		+
	SLC (6Ckine)	CCL21	+		+

[a]See text for abbreviations.

[b]Only one study available supporting this.

Table 21.1 The structural and functional classification of chemokines—cont'd

Family	Classical nomenclature	New nomenclature	Inflammatory	Angiogenic (+)/ angiostatic (−)	Homeostatic
	MDC	CCL22			+
	MPIF-1	CCL23			+
	Eotaxin-2	CCL24			+
	Eotaxin-3	CCL26			+
	CTACK	CCL27			+
	MEC	CCL28			+
	LD78β	CCL3L1			
C	Lymphotactin	XCL1	+		
	SCM-1β	XCL2			
CX$_3$C	Fractalkine	CX$_3$CL1	+	+	

Table 21.2 Chemokine receptor–ligand pairs

Chemokine receptor	Chemokine ligand
CXC chemokine receptors	
CXCR1	IL-8/CXCL8, GCP-2/CXCL6
CXCR2	IL-8/CXCL8, ENA-78/CXCL5, Groα/CXCL1, Groβ/CXCL2, Groγ/CXCL3, CTAP-III/CXCL7, GCP-2/CXCL6
CXCR3	IP-10/CXCL10, PF4/CXCL4, Mig/CXCL9, ITAC/CXCL11
CXCR4 (fusin)	SDF-1/CXCL12
CXCR5	BCA-1/CXCL13
CXCR6	CXCL16
CC chemokine receptors	
CCR1	MIP-1α/CCL3, RANTES/CCL5, MCP-3/CCL7, HCC-1/CCL14, HCC-2/CCL15, HCC-4/CCL16, LD78β/CCL3L1, MPIF-1/CCL23
CCR2	MCP-1/CCL2, MCP-3/CCL7, MCP-4/CCL13, HCC-4/CCL16
CCR3	Eotaxin/CCL11, eotaxin-2/CCL24, eotaxin-3/CCL26, RANTES/CCL5, MCP-2/CCL8, MCP-3/CCL7, MCP-4/CCL13, HCC-2/CCL15, MEC/CCL28
CCR4	TARC/CCL17, MDC/CCL22, CKLF1
CCR5	MIP-1α/CCL3, MIP-1β/CCL4, RANTES/CCL5, LD78β/CCL3L1, MCP-2/CCL8, HCC-1/CCL14
CCR6	MIP-3α/CCL20
CCR7	MIP-3β/CCL19, SLC/6Ckine/CCL21
CCR8	I-309/CCL1
CCR9	TECK/CCL25
CCR10	CTACK/CCL27, MEC/CCL28
C chemokine receptors	
XCR1	Lymphotactin/XCL1, SCM-1β/XCL2
CX$_3$C chemokine receptors	
CX$_3$CR1	Fractalkine/CX$_3$CL1
Other	
DARC	Duffy antigen, some CC and CXC chemokines

See text for abbreviations.

CXC chemokines

In CXC chemokines, there are two conserved C residues separated by one unconserved amino acid.[1,10,11] There may be close relationship between the genetic or protein structure of these mediators and their function. For example, most CXC chemokines chemoattract neutrophils. Many genes coding these chemokines are clustered on chromosome 4q12-13.[11] However, the genes of some CXC chemokines, such as platelet factor 4 (PF4)/CXCL4 and interferon (IFN)-γ-inducible 10 kDa protein (IP-10)/ CXCL10, are located on different chromosomes, and these novel chemokines recruit lymphocytes and monocytes.[10,11] In addition, some CXC chemokines promote, while others inhibit angiogenesis.[4,20,21] In general, the angiogenic or angiostatic action of these mediators greatly depends on the ELR amino acid sequence. ELR-containing chemokines, such as interleukin-8 (IL-8)/CXCL8, epithelial-neutrophil activating protein-78 (ENA-78)/CXCL5, growth-regulated oncogene α (Groα)/CXCL1, and connective tissue-activating peptide-III (CTAP-III)/CXCL7 stimulate neovascularization. In contrast, CXC chemokines lacking the ELR sequence, such as PF4/CXCL4, IP-10/CXCL10, and monokine induced by IFN-γ (Mig)/CXCL9 are angiostatic.[4,20,21] However, there may be exceptions to the rule, as the ELR-lacking stromal cell-derived factor 1 (SDF-1)/ CXCL12 is angiogenic.[4,21]

Apart from being chemotactic for leukocytes, CXC chemokines are involved in a number of mechanisms underlying inflammation. These chemoattractants may also stimulate leukocyte integrin expression, L-selectin shedding, inflammatory cell adhesion, cytoskeleton reorganization, neutrophil degranulation, respiratory burst, and phagocytosis, as well as the production of matrix metalloproteinases (MMPs), leukotrienes, and platelet-activating factor.[10]

CC chemokines

These chemoattractants have adjacent conserved C residues.[9,11] CC chemokines stimulate monocyte chemotaxis, but some members of this subclass may also recruit lymphocytes. The genes of monocyte-chemoattracting CC chemokines have been clustered to chromosome 17q11.2. In contrast, genes of CC chemokines recruiting lymphocytes are generally located elsewhere.[1,3,9,11]

C and CX₃C chemokines

These two chemokine subsets have been described based on the special position of C residues.[3,4,22] The C family contains two members: lymphotactin/XCL1 and single C motif 1β (SCM-1β)/XCL2. The CX₃C subset contains a single member: fractalkine/CX₃CL1.[3,4,22–24] Lymphotactin is primarily involved in the migration of T lymphocyte subsets to inflammatory sites.[24] Fractalkine is chemotactic for mononuclear cells, but also serves as an adhesion molecule.[22,23]

CHEMOKINE RECEPTORS

Chemokines described above mediate their effects via 7-transmembrane domain receptors expressed on the target cells.[11] There is a redundancy between CXC and CC chemokine receptors and their ligands (Table 21.2). For example, CXCR2, CCR1, or CCR3 have numerous chemokine ligands. In contrast, CXCR6, CCR8, or CCR9 are specific receptors for one single ligand[1,3,11] (Table 21.2). There is only one C and CX₃C chemokine receptor for their respective chemokine ligands[22,23] (Table 21.2).

Again, there may be relationship between a certain chemokine receptor and the function of its ligand(s). Single-ligand receptors, such as CCR8 or CCR9, bind to chemokine ligands mostly exerting homeostatic functions (see later). In contrast, CXCR2, a receptor recognizing most ELR motif-containing CXC chemokines, plays a crucial role in inflammation and angiogenesis. Furthermore, CXCR3 is a receptor for most ELR-lacking, angiostatic CXC chemokines[1,3,11,20,21] (Table 21.2). Chemokine receptors have also been associated with various subtypes and histological variants of autoimmune inflammation. For example, RA, which is considered a Th1-type disease, is associated with CXCR3 and CCR5, while asthma, a known Th2-type disease, is rather associated with CCR3, CCR4, and CCR8.[11,25,26]

CHEMOKINES AND CHEMOKINE RECEPTORS IN SYNOVIAL INFLAMMATION AND ANGIOGENESIS

CXC chemokines

Among CXC chemokines, IL-8/CXCL8, ENA-78/CXCL5, Groα/CXCL1, CTAP-III/CXCL7, granulocyte chemotactic protein 2 (GCP-2)/CXCL6, IP-10/CXCL10, Mig/CXCL9, PF4/CXCL4, SDF-1/CXCL12, and B-cell activating chemokine 1 (BCA-1)/CXCL13 and, recently CXCL16, have been implicated in RA. Thus, these chemokines may be considered 'inflammatory'.[1–6,27–37]

We and others detected abundant IL-8/CXCL8 in the sera, synovial fluids (SF), and ST of RA patients.[27,32,38] ST macrophages, synovial lining cells, fibroblasts, and endothelial cells produce IL-8/CXCL8.[32,39,40] While macrophages constitutively express this chemokine, ST fibroblasts produce IL-8/CXCL8 upon stimulation with proinflammatory cytokines including tumor necrosis factor-α (TNF-α) or IL-1β.[32,41] Other chemokines, such as RANTES/CCL5, monocyte chemoattractant protein-1 (MCP-1)/CCL2, and SDF-1/CXCL12 also up-regulate IL-8/CXCL8 expression on RA ST fibroblasts.[42] The regulation of IL-8/CXCL8 production by ST fibroblasts is controlled by NF-κB.[43] In a recent study, an IL-8/CXCL8 binding site was discovered on EC syndecan-3. This site is selectively induced in RA, suggesting the role of chemokine–syndecan interactions during leukocyte trafficking into RA ST.[44] IL-8/CXCL8 exerts proinflammatory and angiogenic effects. When clinically involved and uninvolved joints of RA patients were compared using arthroscopy, IL-8/CXCL8 protein and gene expression were increased in the ST of the involved joints compared with the uninvolved joints of patients.[45] This chemokine induced synovial inflammation after an intra-articular injection of recombinant IL-8/CXCL8 into the rabbit knee joint. Synovial histology highly resembled human RA.[46] TNF-α blockade resulted in decreased neutrophil migration into the joints of RA patients, which was associated with diminished IL-8/CXCL8 in the ST.[47] IL-8/CXCL8 also regulates leukocyte adhesion and angiogenesis in RA. SF IL-8/CXCL8 levels were correlated with β_2 integrin expression on neutrophils.[48] Furthermore, the ELR-containing

IL-8/CXCL8 is chemotactic and mitogenic for vascular endothelial cells (ECs) *in vitro*.[20,21,49] ECs express CXCR2, a receptor for IL-8/CXCL8.[50,51]

ENA-78/CXCL5, similarly to IL-8/CXCL8, exerts chemotactic activity for neutrophils and promotes neovascularization.[10,21,40] Large amounts of ENA-78/CXCL5 have been detected in RA SF and ST.[31] RA ST fibroblasts constitutively secrete ENA-78/CXCL5. The basal production of this chemokine is further stimulated by TNF-α, IL-1, and IL-18.[31,52] In addition to fibroblasts, ST lining cells, interstitial macrophages, and ECs express ENA-78/CXCL5.[31] In rat adjuvant-induced arthritis (AIA), a rodent model for RA, the development of arthritis was associated with abundant ENA-78/CXCL5 production in the sera and later in the joints of rats.[53] ENA-78/CXCL5 exerts angiogenic activity in RA.[40]

Groα/CXCL1, a potent chemoattractant for neutrophils, has been detected in the SF and ST of RA patients.[28,41] The production of this chemokine by ST fibroblasts may be augmented by TNF-α or IL-1.[28,41] Groα/CXCL1 also enhances collagen deposition by RA fibroblasts and thus synovial fibrosis.[54] Not only fibroblasts, but also lining cells and macrophages express high amounts of Groα/CXCL1 in the ST.[28,55]

CTAP-III/CXCL7 is derived from human platelets.[56] This chemokine has been detected in the sera and ST of RA patients.[56,57] CTAP-III/CXCL7 stimulates the proliferation of ST fibroblasts and matrix synthesis.[56,57] Cytokines and growth factors including IL-1, basic fibroblast growth factor (bFGF), and epidermal growth factor (EGF) act in concert with CTAP-III/CXCL7 during proteoglycan synthesis.[56,57] CTAP-III/CXCL7 also induces angiogenesis.[1,56,57]

GCP-2/CXCL6 expression is up-regulated on RA ST fibroblasts via Toll-like receptor 2 (TLR2) signaling pathways.[58] There is abundant production of this chemokine in the RA SF.[58]

IP-10/CXCL10 may exert proinflammatory, but anti-angiogenic effects in RA.[1,20,59] IP-10/CXCL10 has been detected in the sera, SF, and ST of RA patients;[59,60] however, results regarding serum chemokine levels are rather controversial. One study showed the production of IP-10/CXCL10 to be similar to normal,[29] while another study found increased serum levels of this chemokine.[60] RA ST fibroblasts and macrophages express IP-10/CXCL10.[59] The induction of this chemokine on ST fibroblasts requires intercellular adhesion molecule 1 (ICAM-1) and β_2 integrins.[59] Thus, IP-10/CXCL10 may stimulate the ingress of Th1-type cells into the RA ST.[59] The ELR-lacking IP-10/CXCL10 suppresses neovascularization.[20,21]

Like IP-10/CXCL10, Mig/CXCL9 also mediates synovial inflammation, but inhibits angiogenesis.[20,21,55,60] This chemokine is present in RA SF and ST.[55,60,61] In the ST, primarily macrophages and synovial lining cells produce Mig/CXCL9.[55,60] Cultured ST fibroblasts produce Mig/CXCL9 upon stimulation with IFN-γ.[61] Mig/CXCL9 also lacks the ELR motif and thus it is angiostatic.[20,21]

There are elevated serum PF4/CXCL4 levels in RA patients.[62] Little is known about the role of this chemokine in inflammatory synovitis. PF4/CXCL4, similarly to IP-10/CXCL10 and Mig/CXCL9, lacks the ELR sequence and inhibits angiogenesis.[20,21]

SDF-1/CXCL12 is a specific ligand for CXCR4. This otherwise homeostatic chemokine has been implicated in T-cell, B-cell, and monocyte recruitment into the synovium.[33,34,63,64] SDF-1/CXCL12 is expressed by synovial ECs and this chemokine induces strong integrin-mediated adhesion of T cells to ICAM-1.[33] Direct cellular contact of cytokine-stimulated T cells with ST fibroblasts resulted in increased production of SDF-1/CXCL12 by the fibroblasts.[65] T cells are also able to migrate beneath RA ST fibroblasts. This process is termed pseudoemperipolesis. SDF-1/CXCL12 has been implicated in this process as well.[64] In a SCID mouse model, SDF-1/CXCL12 stimulated monocyte recruitment into human ST engrafted onto the mice.[63] A gene variant of SDF/CXCL12 has been associated with radiographic progression in RA.[66] SDF-1/CXCL12, despite lacking the ELR motif, promotes neovascularization.[67,68] RA ST fibroblasts abundantly produce SDF-1/CXCL12 under hypoxic conditions. In this situation, SDF-1/CXCL12 becomes immobilized on endothelial heparan sulfate, where this chemokine is able to promote angiogenesis and inflammation.[67,69]

The crucial role of B cells in the pathogenesis of RA has been acknowledged and B-cell targeting became a major issue in biological therapy of RA.[15,16,70] BCA-1/CXCL13 is the specific ligand for CXCR5, which is expressed on most mature B cells and a subset of T cells.[12] BCA-1/CXCL13 is a homeostatic chemokine involved in B-cell migration and the formation of germinal centers.[1,12,13] However, it is also expressed on follicular dendritic cells (DCs) in the RA ST.[71] In the ST, ECs and fibroblasts also produce BCA-1/CXCL13.[71] BCA-1/CXCL13 has recently been implicated in inflammatory lymphoid tissue organization and aggregate formation in the RA ST.[72]

Recently, we and others studied the possible role of CXCL16 in RA. CXCL16 may be considered a homeostatic chemokine as it mediates lymphocyte recruitment to lymph nodes. This chemokine is the single specific ligand for CXCR6. Markedly elevated CXCL16 levels were found in RA SF.[35] In the RA ST, lining cells and macrophages showed intense expression of this chemokine.[35,36] Monocytes begin to express CXCL16 upon differentiation into macrophages.[37] In the SCID mouse chimera model, CXCL16 recruited human mononuclear cells to the engrafted human RA ST.[35] CXCL16 recruits CXCR6-expressing RA SF T cells.[37]

Among CXC chemokines, SDF-1/CXCL12, BCA-1/CXCL13, and CXCL16 may be involved in lymphocyte recruitment under homeostatic or inflammatory conditions.[35–37,63–65,72]

CC chemokines

Among CC chemokines, MCP-1/CCL2, macrophage inflammatory protein 1α (MIP-1α)/CCL3, MIP-3α/CCL20, RANTES/CCL5, Epstein–Barr virus-induced gene 1 ligand chemokine (ELC)/CCL19, SLC/CCL21 and, recently, chemokine-like factor 1 (CKLF1) have been implicated in inflammatory mechanisms underlying RA.[1–6,72,73] According to one recent study, MCP-2/CCL8, MCP-3/CCL7, HCC-1/CCL14, HCC-2/CCL15, and HCC-4/CCL16 may also be involved in RA.[74]

MCP-1/CCL2 chemoattracts monocytes, T cells, natural killer (NK) cells, and basophils.[9,75,76] We and others have detected high amounts of this chemokine in RA sera and SF.[75,76] RA ST macrophages and fibroblasts produce MCP-1/CCL2.[41,75,76] TNF-α and IL-1 enhance the release of MCP-1/CCL2 by ST fibroblasts.[41,76]

IL-18 also induces MCP-1/CCL2 production by macrophages.[77] Among other triggering factors, hypoxia decreases,[78] while TLR2 ligands stimulate MCP-1/CCL2 expression by ST fibroblasts.[58] The injection of MCP-1/CCL2 into rabbit knees induced arthritis.[79]

MIP-1α/CCL3 chemoattracts various cell types including monocytes, T cells, B cells and NK cells, basophils, and eosinophils.[3,9] This chemokine has been detected in SF and ST of RA patients.[41,80] SF mononuclear cells, as well as ST fibroblasts and macrophages are main producers of MIP-1α/CCL3.[41,80] MIP-1α/CCL3 production is augmented by TNF-α, IL-1, and IL-15.[80,81]

MIP-3α/CCL20 is chemotactic for monocytes, T cells, B cells, and immature DCs.[1] This chemokine binds to its specific receptor, CCR6.[82] Abundant MIP-3α/CCL20 has been detected in RA SF and ST.[82–84] In the ST, mostly synovial lining cells and infiltrating mononuclear cells express this chemokine.[82] RA ST fibroblasts also produce this chemokine in response to TNF-α, IL-1, IL-17, and IL-18.[82–85]

RANTES/CCL5 exerts chemotactic activity towards monocytes, T cells, and NK cells, eosinophils, and basophils.[9,86] RANTES/CCL5 has been detected in RA peripheral blood and SF T cells, as well as in RA ST lining cells and macrophages.[55,87,88] TNF-α, IL-1, and IFN-γ augment RANTES/CCL5 production by ST fibroblasts.[41,89] Articular chondrocytes also express this chemokine.[90] RANTES/CCL5 is one of the mediators of RA SF-induced chemotactic activity for leukocytes.[91] RANTES/CCL5 is also involved in cytokine networks present in the RA ST, as it induces ST fibroblasts to produce IL-8/CXCL8 and IL-6.[42] A distinct polymorphism in the RANTES promoter gene has been associated with susceptibility to RA in the Chinese population.[92]

ELC/CCL19 is homeostatic; however, it acts similarly to SDF-1/CXCL12 and BCA-1/CXCL13 in RA. ELC/CCL19 is also a B-cell chemoattracting mediator, detected in RA ST.[93] These three chemokines may be involved in both homeostatic and inflammation-associated B-cell recruitment and in germinal center formation.[1,12,93]

SLC/CCL21 is another homeostatic chemokine involved in lymphoid tissue organization. Recently, the production of this chemokine has been associated with lymphoneogenesis and germinal center formation in RA.[72]

In a recent study, MCP-2/CCL8, MCP-3/CCL7, HCC-1/CCL14, HCC-2/CCL15, and HCC-4/CCL16 were detected in the RA ST, as well as in other types of arthritis for the first time. Among these chemokine ligands, HCC-2/CCL15 showed an increased expression in RA compared with osteoarthritis or reactive arthritis.[74]

CKLF1 is a cytokine chemotactic for various leukocytes and a functional ligand of CCR4. Its expression is up-regulated on activated CD4+ and CD8+ T cells, but not on CD19+ B cells in RA.[73]

C and CX₃C chemokines

Lymphotactin/XCL1 has been detected on CD8+, as well as CD4+/CD28− T cells in RA.[94] This chemokine stimulates T-cell accumulation into the RA joint and down-regulates MMP-2 production by RA ST fibroblasts.[24]

Fractalkine/CX₃CL1 plays a dual role, being chemotactic for monocytes and lymphocytes and also mediating cell adhesion.[22,25] High levels of this chemokine have been detected in RA SF.[25] SF monocytes, as well as ST macrophages, fibroblasts, ECs and DCs produce fractalkine/CX₃CL1 in RA.[25,95] Fractalkine/CX₃CL1 also recruits T cells into the RA joint.[42,95] Senescent CD4+ T cells accumulate in the RA joint. Fractalkine/CX₃CL1 enhances the adhesion of these T cells to synovial fibroblasts. In addition, this chemokine provides survival signals for and costimulates the production of proinflammatory cytokines by these T cells.[95] Recently, fractalkine/CX₃CL1 has been implicated in neovascularization and atherosclerosis. CX₃CR1-deficient mice showed attenuated development of atherosclerosis.[96] In humans, an M280/I249 polymorphism in the CX₃CR1 gene was associated with reduced cardiovascular risk.[97] Fractalkine/CX₃CL1 is also angiogenic.[98] As accelerated atherosclerosis and increased cardiovascular risk is the primary cause of death in RA patients, these results may have important clinical relevance.

Chemokine receptors

Among CXC chemokine receptors, CXCR1 and CXCR2 recognize the most important proinflammatory and pro-angiogenic CXC chemokines described above[1,3] (Table 21.2). Both CXCR1 and

CXCR2 are expressed on RA macrophages and neutrophils, as well as articular chondrocytes.[1,3,99] CXCR2, a receptor for most ELR-containing angiogenic chemokines, is expressed by ECs and thus plays a role in chemokine-induced angiogenesis.[50,51] CXCR3 may be the most important receptor in leukocyte homing into the RA ST. It is expressed in T-cell-rich areas of the inflamed ST.[25,26,100] CXCR3 marks a subset of T cells. Most T cells in the RA SF express this chemokine receptor.[101] The high expression of CXCR3 on SF T cells has been associated with a high IFN-γ/IL-4 ratio, suggesting a preferential Th1 over Th2 phenotype of these T cells.[102] Furthermore, high expression of CXCR3 in early RA ST has been associated with increased production of its ligand, Mig/CXCL9.[61] CXCR3 is also expressed on RA ST ECs and DCs.[100,103] As discussed above, CXCR4, the specific receptor for SDF-1/CXCL12, may play a role in the SDF-1/CXCL12-derived retention of lymphocytes within the RA ST.[33,34,74] CXCR5 expression is up-regulated in RA compared with non-RA ST. In RA, CXCR5 is expressed by T cells, B cells, macrophages, and ECs.[102] CXCR6, the specific receptor for CXCL16, is expressed by one-half of RA SF lymphocytes.[35] IL-15 stimulation up-regulates CXCR6 expression on T cells.[36] As described above, CXCR4, CXCR5, and CXCR6 bind their respective ligands, SDF-1/CXCL12, BCA-1/CXCL13, and CXCL16. Thus, these CXC chemokine receptors may play an important role in lymphocyte recruitment under both homeostatic and inflammatory conditions.[1,7,12,33-37]

Among CC chemokine receptors, CCR1 is abundantly expressed in the RA ST.[74,104] CCR5 shows strong expression on RA SF mononuclear cells, as well as RA ST T cells and fibroblasts.[25,26,74,105,106] CCR5 expression on ST T cells has been associated with a Th1-type cytokine profile.[101] CCR5, as well as CCR1, CCR2, and CCR3 is also expressed by articular chondrocytes.[99] CCR4 and CCR5 on lymphocytes are crucial for leukocyte recruitment into the RA joint.[103] There is an increasing body of evidence for the role of the truncated Δ32-CCR5 non-functional receptor allele in RA. There was no difference between the frequency of wild-type CCR5 genotype in RA and controls. However, while none of the RA patients had the homozygous Δ32-CCR5 genotype,

some control subjects expressed this genotype.[107,108] A recent meta-analysis confirmed that this polymorphism of CCR5 is protective against the development of RA.[108] In a comparative study on CC chemokine receptors, CCR expression was assessed on RA peripheral blood, SF, and ST monocyte/macrophages. Peripheral blood monocytes mainly express CCR1 and CCR2, suggesting that these receptors are involved in monocyte recruitment from the circulation. In contrast, CCR3 and CCR5 expression are up-regulated in RA SF, indicating that these CCRs may be important in monocyte retention in the joint.[104] The expression and signaling pathways of CCR1, CCR2, and CCR5 have been studied using the rat AIA model. Increases in tyrosine phosphorylation of these chemokine receptors were observed in the arthritic rats after day 14. CCR1 signaling was associated with Janus kinase 1 (JAK-1), signal transducer and activator of transcription 1 (STAT1) and STAT3; CCR2 was associated with JAK-2, STAT1 and STAT3; while CCR5 was associated with JAK-1, STAT1, and STAT3. Phosphorylated STAT1 and STAT3 were detected in ST lining cells, macrophages, and ECs in the arthritic joint.[109] Regarding other CCRs, RA articular chondrocytes express CCR3 and produce its ligand, RANTES/CCL5.[90,99] CCR6, the single receptor for MIP-3α/CCL20, has been detected on RA ST leukocytes.[82] Recently, a putative chemokine receptor, CCR-like receptor 2 (CCRL2) has been identified on RA SF neutrophils and macrophages.[110]

Regarding the C and CX$_3$C chemokine receptors, XCR1, the lymphotactin/XCL1 receptor, is expressed on ST lymphocytes, macrophages, and fibroblasts.[1,3] CX$_3$CR1, the fractalkine/CX$_3$CL1 receptor, has been detected on RA SF T cells and macrophages, as well as on RA ST macrophages and DCs.[23] Thus, CX$_3$CR1, as well as fractalkine/CX$_3$CL1, have been implicated in monocyte and lymphocyte ingress into the RA joint.[23]

As shown in Table 21.2, DARC cannot be classified into the four classical chemokine receptor subclasses. DARC, originally described on erythrocytes, binds the Duffy antigen, as well as some CXC and CC chemokines. Recently, DARC expression has been detected on RA ST ECs.[111]

INFLAMMATORY, ANGIOGENIC AND HOMEOSTATIC CHEMOKINES: A WELL-JUSTIFIED CLASSIFICATION?

As described above, chemokines have recently been functionally classified into these three subgroups.[7,12–14] As many functions of these chemokines overlap, it is debatable whether such classification is really justified. Several aspects of these chemokines are discussed above.

Numerous CXC and CC chemokines, as well as the C and CX₃C chemokines implicated in the pathogenesis of arthritis, are termed 'inflammatory chemokines'. These chemokines are expressed in inflamed tissues on stimulation by proinflammatory cytokines or during contact with pathogenic agents. Inflammatory chemokines, as described above, recruit mostly effector cells including monocytes, neutrophils, and effector T cells into tissues.[12] As described above and listed in Table 21.1, there is a great body of evidence suggesting the role of the CXC chemokines IL-8/CXCL8, ENA-78/CXCL5, Groα/CXCL1, CTAP-III/CXCL7, IP-10/CXCL10, Mig/CXCL9, PF4/CXCL4, GCP-2/CXCL6, SDF-1/CXCL12, BCA-1/CXCL13, and CXCL16 in RA. Among CC chemokines, MCP-1/CCL2, MIP-1α/CCL3, MIP-3α/CCL20, RANTES/CCL5, ELC/CCL19, and SLC/CCL21 have been implicated in leukocyte recruitment underlying inflammatory synovitis. Finally, the C chemokine lymphotactin/XCL1 and the CX₃C chemokine fractalkine/CX₃CL1 are also considered as arthritis-associated inflammatory chemokines[1–6,72,73] (Table 21.1). Accordingly, CXCR1 and CXCR2 binding most ELR-containing, CXCR3 recognizing ELR-lacking CXC chemokines, as well as CXCR4, CXCR5, and CXCR6, specific receptors for SDF-1/CXCL12, BCA-1/CXCL13, and CXCL16, respectively, are involved in the pathogenesis of RA[1–6,35–37] (Table 21.2). CCR1, CCR2, CCR3, CCR4, CCR5, and CCR6, as well as XCR1 and CX₃CR1, receptors mostly recognizing inflammatory chemokine ligands, have also been implicated in inflammatory synovitis[1–6] (Table 21.2).

All ELR-containing CXC chemokines described above, as well as the ELR-lacking SDF-1/CXCL12 promote angiogenesis in RA, thus, these mediators can be termed 'angiogenic chemokines'. In accordance, CXCR2 is the major chemokine receptor on ECs that mediates neovascularization. In contrast, the ELR-lacking IP-10/CXCL10, PF4/CXCL4, and Mig/CXCL9, as well as their receptor, CXCR3, suppress capillary formation, and thus these are 'angiostatic chemokines'. In addition, all these chemokines are also termed inflammatory[1–5,21] (Table 21.2).

'Homeostatic chemokines' are constitutively produced in discrete microenvironments of lymphoid or non-lymphoid tissues, such as in the skin or mucosa. These chemokines promote lymphocyte migration and recruitment into these tissues. Homeostatic chemokines mediate physiologic traffic of cells that belong to the adaptive immune system and are involved in antigen sampling and immune surveillance.[12,13] Among CXC chemokines, SDF-1/CXCL12, BCA-1/CXCL13, and CXCL16, as well as their respective receptors, CXCR4, CXCR5, and CXCR6, exert such effects.[1,12,13,35–37] Numerous CC chemokines including MDC/CCL22 and TARC/CCL17 binding to CCR4, ELC/CCL19 and SLC/CCL21 binding to CCR7, TECK/CCL25 binding to CCR9, CTACK/CCL27 and MEC/CCL28 binding to CCR10 have been implicated in the homeostasis of primary, secondary, and peripheral lymphoid tissues.[12,13] As discussed above, some data suggest that among these homeostatic chemokines SDF-1/CXCL12, BCA-1/CXCL13, CXCL16, ELC/CCL19, SLC/CCL21, and maybe others, are also involved in arthritis-associated inflammatory cell recruitment.[1,12,34–37,65,71,72,93] In many ways the synovium is similar to the skin- and mucosa-associated lymphoid tissues, which explains the involvement of otherwise homeostatic chemokines in synovial inflammation.[12,13,71]

REGULATION OF CHEMOKINE PRODUCTION DURING LEUKOCYTE RECRUITMENT

There is a temporal regulation of chemokine and chemokine receptor production in the inflamed synovium. We have assessed the temporal expression of CXC and CC chemokines relevant for the pathogenesis of arthritis in sera and joint homogenates of rats with AIA. The production of ENA-78/CXCL5 and MIP-1α/CCL3 showed a very early increase, preceding clinical symptoms. The abundant production of these chemokines occurred parallel with early inflammatory events, such as neutrophil recruitment and the production of acute phase reactants. In contrast, MCP-1/CCL2 was rather involved in the later phase of AIA.[112] When AIA rats were treated with a polyclonal antibody to ENA-78/CXCL5, antagonism of this chemokine also supported that ENA-78/CXCL5 is involved in the very early inflammatory events underlying AIA.[53] When we assessed the temporal regulation of chemokine receptors in rat AIA, CCR1 exhibited high constitutive expression on macrophages throughout the disease course. CCR5 expression was up-regulated on ST macrophages, correlating with macrophage CCR2 expression. In contrast, CCR2 on ECs was down-regulated during the progression of the disease. CCR3 expression on macrophages decreased during the course of AIA. CXCR4 expression was up-regulated on ECs, preceding the peak of inflammation. Thus, CCR2 and CCR5 may sustain inflammatory changes, while CCR2 and CCR3 may play a role in initial recruitment of leukocytes into the ST.[113]

A two-way regulatory network of proinflammatory cytokines and chemokines exists in the arthritic synovium.[3,4,114,115] As discussed above, some cytokines including TNF-α, IL-1, IL-6, IL-15, IL-18, and others may enhance, while others may suppress chemokine production.[3,4,31,41,76,115] For example, IL-8/CXCL8 secretion by RA ST fibroblasts is stimulated by the Th2-type IL-4 but inhibited by the Th1-type IFN-γ. In contrast, RANTES/CCL5 production is suppressed by IL-4 but augmented by IFN-γ.[89] These data suggest that the Th1/Th2 balance or imbalance may influence the local chemokine pattern in the ST. On the other hand, some chemokines may influence the release of other mediators.[3,53,116] For example, MIP-1α/CCL3 stimulates the synthesis of TNF-α, IL-1, and IL-6 by synovial macrophages.[3,116] Treatment of rat AIA with a polyclonal antibody to ENA-78/CXCL5 resulted in the inhibition of IL-1 expression in the ST.[53]

CD4+/CD28− T cells accumulating in RA resemble a functionally end-differentiated, non-dividing, short-lived effector memory T-cell subpopulation. These cells, when adoptively transferred into human RA synovium–SCID mouse chimeras, homed to both lymph nodes and the RA ST. Infiltrating T cells coexpressed the CCR5, CCR7, and CXCR4 chemokine receptors, and migrated in response to both the inflammatory chemokine RANTES/CCL5 and the homeostatic chemokine SDF-1/CXCL12. Thus, both inflammatory and homeostatic chemokines and their receptors are involved in the recruitment of this effector memory T-cell subset into the RA ST.[117]

TLRs may also be involved in the regulation of chemokine function. TLR2 ligands activate synovial fibroblasts. Peptidoglycan, a TLR2 ligand, stimulated, among others, IL-8/CXCL8, Groα/CXCL1, MCP-1/CCL2, MIP-1α/CCL3, and RANTES/CCL5 mRNA expression by these fibroblasts using an RT-PCR assay.[58]

The regulation of inflammatory cell recruitment into the ST also involves chemokine–adhesion molecule interactions. Leukocyte adhesion to synovial ECs occurs in several steps. An early, weaker adhesion termed 'rolling', occurring within the first hours, is mediated mostly by selectin adhesion receptors and their ligands. Rolling on ECs triggers leukocyte activation due to the interactions between chemokine receptors on leukocytes and proteoglycans on ECs. Activation-dependent, firm adhesion involves mostly integrins and their ligands, as well as junctional adhesion molecules (JAMs). These events involve the secretion of various chemokines. Transendothelial migration of leukocytes involving integrins occurs when secreted chemokines bind to EC heparan sulfate. Chemokines preferentially attract EC-bound leukocytes.[13,118,119] ECs themselves also produce a number of inflammatory mediators including chemokines, such as MCP-1/CCL2 and Groα/CXCL1.[2,4,119] Chemokine–adhesion molecule cross-talk described here may synchronize the sequence of events during leukocyte extravasation into the inflamed ST.

There may be distinct histological patterns of synovitis in RA, which may be associated with different chemokine profiles. There are at least two distinguishable histological types: some specimens show diffuse mononuclear cell infiltrates, while others are classified as 'follicular synovitis' showing the formation of germinal center-like structures. In a recent study, the serum levels of IL-8/CXCL8, MCP-1/CCL2, and RANTES/CCL5 were significantly higher in the follicular type in comparison with the diffuse histological variant.[120]

CHEMOKINE TARGETING STRATEGIES

Chemokines and chemokine receptors can be targeted in a number of ways. However, there is a limitation of human RA trials, therefore most available data were obtained in various experimental animal models of arthritis. In humans, disease-modifying anti-rheumatic drugs (DMARDs), currently used in the treatment of RA, may themselves influence chemokine production. Also, as there are interactions between proinflammatory cytokines and chemokines in the ST, anti-TNF-α therapy may also suppress inflammatory chemokine production. Apart from these indirect actions, direct chemokine and chemokine receptor targeting using antibodies to chemokines or synthetic chemokine inhibitors carried out mostly in experimental arthritis may be a feasible strategy and may become a part of biological therapy in the near future.[1–6]

Experimental arthritis

CXC chemokines and chemokine receptors

Numerous inflammatory chemokines and their receptors have been targeted in the last few years. Among CXC chemokines, neutralizing antibodies to IL-8/CXCL8 prevented leukocyte infiltration and arthritis in rabbits.[121] A neutralizing polyclonal anti-ENA-78/CXCL5 antibody was administered intravenously to rats using the AIA model. The antibody injected before the onset of arthritis attenuated the severity of the disease. Anti-ENA-78/CXCL5 also reduced the number of IL-1-immunoreactive cells in the ST lining layer. However, this antibody was unable to influence the disease course when injected during the later stages of arthritis.[53] The preventative administration of an anti-Groα/CXCL1 antibody delayed the onset and severity of murine collagen-induced arthritis (CIA).[122] IP-10/CXCL10 naked DNA vaccine induced the development of AIA in rats. These rats developed

protective immunity against arthritis. Adoptive transfer of self-specific anti-IP-10/CXCL10 or rabbit anti-rat IP-10/CXCL10 antibodies resulted in disease suppression.[123] A bioactive synthetic peptide derived from the angiogenesis inhibitor chemokine PF4/CXCL4 suppressed murine CIA, as well as arthritis-associated angiogenesis. Although the mechanism of action of this peptide remains unclear, treatment suppressed serum IL-1 levels in these animals.[30] Recently, an anti-CXCL16 monoclonal antibody (mAb) reduced the clinical arthritis score and suppressed leukocyte infiltration and bone destruction in murine CIA.[36]

A nonpeptide oral antagonist of the CXCR2 receptor inhibited IL-8/CXCL- or LPS-induced arthritis in rabbits.[124] CXCR2 gene-deficient mice exhibited leukocyte-deficient inflammatory responses in a murine model of inflammation.[125] In another study, the same mice showed less severe Lyme arthritis in comparison with wild-type animals.[126] TAK-779, an inhibitor of CXCR3 and CCR5, has been developed. As described above, both CXCR3 and CCR5 are involved in Th1-type cell recruitment to sites of inflammation. A synthetic antagonist inhibited the binding of CXCR3 and CCR5 to their respective ligands and suppressed chemokine-induced integrin activation.[127] AMD3100, a CXCR4 antagonist, inhibited CIA in IFN-γ-deficient mice.[128] Analogs of the 14-mer peptide T140 also act as CXCR4 antagonists. These compounds ameliorated the clinical severity of murine CIA.[129]

CC chemokines and their receptors

Passive immunization of mice with anti-MIP-1α/CCL3 postponed the onset and decreased the severity of CIA.[122] MIP-1α/CCL3 gene-deficient mice exhibit milder clinical and histology scores following the induction of CIA.[130] A neutralizing mAb to MCP-1/CCL2 reduced ankle swelling by 30% and significantly decreased the number of synovial ST macrophages in rat CIA.[131] An anti-MCP-1/CCL2 antibody also prevented the recruitment of ^{111}In-labeled T cells into the synovium in the rat model of streptococcal cell wall antigen (SCW)-induced arthritis.[132] A peptide inhibitor containing a 67 amino acid sequence of

MCP-1/CCL2 inhibited the development of arthritis in MRL-lpr mice.[133] An anti RANTES/ CCL5 antibody reduced mouse CIA.[134] KE-298, an experimental anti-rheumatic agent, inhibited both MCP-1/CCL2 and RANTES/CCL5 production, as well as the severity of rat AIA.[135]

Several CCR1 and CCR2 antagonists have been developed during the last few years, and some of them have been introduced to human trials as well.[136–140] Preclinical studies with CCR1-deficient mice have also been initiated.[137] Met-RANTES, a CCR1/CCR5 antagonist, suppressed the development of CIA in mice.[141] Preventatively administered Met-RANTES also reduced the severity of joint inflammation in rat AIA. In addition, Met-RANTES injected locally into the ankles of AIA rats reduced leukocyte infiltration of the joint. Met-RANTES also down-regulated CCR1 and CCR5 expression in the joint.[142] A nonpeptide CCR5 antagonist preventatively inhibited mouse CIA.[143] Rather surprisingly, in one study, CCR5 gene-deficient mice developed CIA to the same extent as wild-type animals.[144] However, in another study, CCR5 gene-deficient mice showed a significant reduction in the incidence of CIA, which was associated with significantly lower serum IgG levels and augmented IL-10 production by spleen cells.[145] Similar controversy was observed when using anti-CCR2 antibodies or CCR2 gene-deficient animals. Anti-CCR2 antibody administered during the initiation of murine CIA markedly improved the clinical symptoms, while blockade during the later stages of the disease rather aggravated both clinical and histologic signs of arthritis.[140] In addition, CCR2 gene-deficient mice developed more severe CIA than did wild-type controls.[140,144] These data suggest that suppressing the action of chemokine receptors using antibodies may give different results to chemokine receptor gene-deficient animal studies. Hence, CCR blockade using antibodies or other inhibitors may be promising for future therapies.

Adenoviral gene transfer may also be a useful method in chemokine targeting. The vaccinia virus expresses a 35 kDa soluble protein (35k), which inactivates a number of CC chemokines. A recombinant adenovirus containing 35k reduced migration of CCR5-transfected cells in response to RANTES/CCL5. This vector also suppressed chemotaxis of both CCR5-transfected cells and primary macrophages in mice.[146]

Other chemokines

An antibody to fractalkine/CX$_3$CL1 decreased clinical arthritis scores and reduced ST leukocyte infiltration and bone erosion in murine CIA.[147]

Combined chemokine blockade

Several recent studies have addressed the use of multiple chemokine blocking strategies. For example, a combination of MCP-1/CCL2 and Groα/CXCL1 inhibition with chemokine antagonists resulted in a greater extent of arthritis suppression than MCP-1/CCL2 blockade alone in a murine AIA model.[148] Rat AIA was diminished by DNA vaccination using chemokine DNA vaccines to MCP-1/CCL2, MIP-1α/CCL3, and RANTES/ CCL5.[149] In the rabbit LPS-induced arthritis model, the combination of anti-IL-8/CXCL8 and anti-Groα/CXCL1 antibodies resulted in a more pronounced inhibition of knee joint leukocyte infiltration than did either of the two antibodies alone.[150] Certainly, there may be increased toxicity using combined strategies, which may be an issue during future human trials.[1]

Human rheumatoid arthritis

Effects of anti-rheumatic agents on chemokines

Corticosteroids, such as dexamethasone, effectively suppressed IL-8/CXCL8 and MCP-1/ CCL2 production in RA.[151] Among non-steroidal anti-inflammatory drugs (NSAIDs), diclofenac and meloxicam reduced IL-8/CXCL8 production in rat antigen-induced arthritis.[152]

Regarding DMARDs, sulfasalazine inhibited IL-8/CXCL8, Groα/CXCL1, and MCP-1/CCL2 production by cultured RA ST explants.[153] Sulfapyridine inhibited the expression of IL-8/ CXCL8 and MCP-1/CCL2 on cytokine-treated EC.[154] In contrast, gold salts hardly had any effects on IL-8/CXCL8 or MCP-1/CCL2 synthesis.[151] A combination treatment of RA patients with methotrexate and leflunomide decreased MCP-1/ CCL2 expression in the ST. The reduction of plasma chemokine levels was associated with improvement in some clinical outcome measures.[155] Antioxidants, such as N-acetyl-L-cysteine and 2-oxothiazolidine-4-carboxylate, suppressed the synthesis of IL-8/CXCL8 and MCP-1/CCL2 mRNA by cytokine-treated isolated human synovial cells.[156]

Effects of anti-TNF-α biologicals on chemokine production

Infliximab, an anti-TNF-α mAb, reduced synovial expression of IL-8/CXCL8 and MCP-1/CCL2 in RA patients. Decreased chemokine release was associated with diminished inflammatory cell ingress into the RA ST.[47] In addition, infliximab decreased the expression of CCR3 and CCR5 on T cells. The expression of these chemokine receptors was higher on non-responders than on responders.[157] Treatment of RA patients with infliximab, as well as etanercept, a recombinant TNF-α receptor-immunoglobulin fusion protein, resulted in the sustained retention of CXCR3+ T cells in the circulation, which reflects a clearance of these cells from the ST.[158] Anti-TNF therapy also down-regulates CXCL16 expression on synovial macrophages.[37]

Direct chemokine and chemokine receptor targeting in humans

Antibodies to IL-8/CXCL8, ENA-78/CXCL5, and Groα/CXCL1, at least partially, neutralized RA SF-induced neutrophil chemotactic activity.[28] These *in vitro* studies suggest that these CXC chemokines could be therapeutically targeted in RA. Nevertheless, there has been one trial using an anti-IL-8/CXCL8 antibody in RA, but results of this trial were not published and the further development of this compound was terminated.[1]

Numerous small molecule CCR1 antagonists have recently been developed.[136–139] In a 2-week phase Ib study, one of these inhibitors decreased the number of ST macrophages.[139] One-third of the patients also fulfilled the ACR (American College of Rheumatology) 20% criteria for improvement.[139] CP-481,715, a selective CCR1 antagonist, inhibited monocyte chemotactic activity present in RA SF samples.[138] Some CCR2 inhibitors have also entered clinical trials.[140]

CONCLUSIONS

In this chapter, we have discussed the putative role of chemokines and their receptors in RA. There is a structural and a functional classification of chemokines. The former includes four groups: CXC, CC, C, and CX₃C chemokines. There is a redundancy and binding promiscuity between chemokine receptors and their ligands. Recently, a functional classification distinguishing between inflammatory, angiogenic/angiostatic, and homeostatic chemokines has been introduced. However, numerous effects of these chemokines overlap. For example, most inflammatory CXC chemokines containing the ELR motif also promote angiogenesis, while ELR-lacking, otherwise inflammatory chemokines suppress neovascularization. Numerous homeostatic chemokines, which are involved in lymphocyte recruitment and lymphoid tissue organization, may also play a role in B-cell migration underlying germinal center formation within the inflamed synovium. Anti-chemokine and anti-chemokine receptor targeting may be used therapeutically in the future biological therapy of arthritis. In addition to the clear clinical benefit, we can learn a lot from these trials about the actions of the targeted chemokines and their receptors. Today, most data in this field are obtained from experimental models of arthritis; however, results of some human trials have also become available. Thus, it is possible that a number of specific chemokine and chemokine receptor antagonists will be developed and administered to patients in the near future. Yet, some caveats must be considered based on experimental results. First, in many animal studies, anti-chemokine targeting was successful in a preventative manner, before the development of arthritis, rather than during the later course of the disease. Such 'preclinical prevention' would hardly be feasible in humans. In addition, many chemokine receptor antagonists are species-specific, therefore data obtained from animal models are difficult to translate to human use. Finally, cleavage of some chemokines by proteases may result in antagonistic, rather than agonistic effects on their receptors. Hopefully, these caveats will be clarified in the near future and at least some of the potential treatment modalities will be used to control inflammation and prevent joint destruction, and thus will benefit our patients.

ACKNOWLEDGMENTS

This work was supported by NIH grants AR-048267 and AI-40987 (A.E.K.), the William D. Robinson and Frederick Huetwell Endowed Professorship (A.E.K.), Funds from the Veterans' Administration (A.E.K.), and grant no. T048541 from the National Scientific Research Fund (OTKA) (Z.S.).

REFERENCES

1. Koch AE. Chemokines and their receptors in rheumatoid arthritis. Arthritis Rheum 2005; 52: 710–21.
2. Szekanecz Z, Kim J, Koch AE. Chemokines. In: Smolen JS, Lipsky PE, eds. Targeted Therapies in Rheumatology. London: Martin Dunitz, 2003: 345–58.
3. Szekanecz Z, Kim J, Koch AE. Chemokines and chemokine receptors in rheumatoid arthritis. Semin Immunol 2002; 399: 1–7.
4. Szekanecz Z, Koch AE. Chemokines and angiogenesis. Curr Opin Rheumatol 2001; 13: 202–8.
5. Szekanecz Z, Szucs G, Szanto S, Koch AE. Chemokines in rheumatic diseases. Curr Drug Targ 2006; 7: 91–102.
6. Kunkel SL, Lukacs N, Kasama T, Strieter RM. The role of chemokines in inflammatory joint disease. J Leukoc Biol 1996; 58: 6–12.
7. Vergunst CE, Tak PP. Chemokines: their role in rheumatoid arthritis. Curr Rheumatol Rep 2005; 7: 382–8.
8. Tarrant TK, Patel DD. Chemokines and leukocyte trafficking in rheumatoid arthritis. Pathophysiology 2006; 13: 1–14.
9. Taub DD. C-C chemokines – an overview. In: Koch AE, Strieter RM, eds. Chemokines in Disease. Austin: RG Landes Company, 1996: 27–54.
10. Walz A, Kunkel SL, Strieter RM. C-X-C chemokines – an overview. In: Koch AE, Strieter RM, eds. Chemokines in Disease. Austin: RG Landes Company, 1996: 1–25.
11. Zlotnik A, Yoshie O. Chemokines: a new classification system and their role in immunity. Immunity 2000; 12: 121–7.
12. Moser B, Loetscher P. Lymphocyte traffic control by chemokines. Nat Immunol 2001; 2: 123–8.
13. Kunkel EJ, Butcher EC. Chemokines and the tissue-specific migration of lymphocytes. Immunity 2002; 16: 1–4.
14. Trentin L, Cabrelle A, Facco, M et al. Homeostatic chemokines drive migration of malignant B cells in patients with non-Hodgkin lymphomas. Blood 2004; 104: 502–8.
15. Silverman GJ, Carson DA. Roles of B cells in rheumatoid arthritis. Arthritis Res Ther 2003; 5 (Suppl 4): 1–6.
16. De Vita S, Zaja F, Sacco S et al. Efficacy of selective B cell blockade in the treatment of rheumatoid arthritis. Arthritis Rheum 2002; 46: 2029–33.
17. Harris ED. Rheumatoid arthritis: pathophysiology and implications for therapy. N Engl J Med 1990; 332: 1277–87.
18. Oppenheim JJ, Zachariae COC, Mukaida N, Matsushima K. Properties of the novel proinflammatory supergene "intercrine" cytokine family. Annu Rev Immunol 1991; 9: 617–48.
19. Bacon K, Baggiolini M, Broxmeyer H et al. Chemokine/chemokine receptor nomenclature. J Interferon Cytokine Res 2002; 22: 1067–8.
20. Strieter RM, Polverini PJ, Kunkel SL et al. The functional role of the ELR motif in CXC chemokine-mediated angiogenesis. J Biol Chem 1995; 270: 27348–57.
21. Strieter RM, Kunkel SL, Shanafelt AB et al. The role of C-X-C chemokines in the regulation of angiogenesis. In: Koch AE, Strieter RM, eds. Chemokines in Disease. Austin: RG Landes Company, 1996: 195–209.
22. Bazan JF, Bacon KB, Hardiman G et al. A new class of membrane bound chemokine with a X3C motif. Nature 1997; 385: 640–4.
23. Ruth JH, Volin MV, Haines III GK et al. Fractalkine, a novel chemokine in rheumatoid arthritis and rat adjuvant-induced arthritis. Arthritis Rheum 2001; 44: 1568–81.
24. Borthwick NJ, Akbar AN, MacCormac LP et al. Selective migration of highly differentiated primed T cells, defined by low expression of CD45RB, across human umbilical vein endothelial cells: effects of viral infection on transmigration. Immunology 1997; 90: 272–80.
25. Loetscher P, Uguccioni M, Bordoli L et al. CCR5 is characteristic of Th1 lymphocytes. Nature 1998; 391: 344–5.
26. Qin S, Rottman JB, Myers P et al. The chemokine receptors CXCR3 and CCR5 mark subsets of T cells with a homing predilection for certain inflammatory sites. J Clin Invest 1998; 101: 746–50.
27. Hogan M, Sherry B, Ritchlin C et al. Differential expression of the small inducible cytokines groα and groβ by synovial fibroblasts in chronic arthritis: possible role in growth regulation. Cytokine 1994; 6: 61–9.
28. Koch AE, Kunkel SL, Shah MR et al. Growth related gene product alpha: a chemotactic cytokine for neutrophils in rheumatoid arthritis. J Immunol 1995; 155: 3660–6.
29. Narumi S, Tominaga Y, Tamaru M et al. Expression of IFN-inducible protein-10 in chronic hepatitis. J Immunol 1997; 158: 5536–44.
30. Wooley PH, Schaefer C, Whalen JD et al. A peptide sequence from platelet factor 4 (CT-112) is effective in

the treatment of type II collagen induced arthritis in mice. J Rheumatol 1997; 24: 890–8.

31. Koch AE, Kunkel SL, Harlow LA et al. Epithelial neutrophil activating peptide-78: a novel chemotactic cytokine for neutrophils in arthritis. J Clin Invest 1994; 94: 1012–18.

32. Koch AE, Kunkel SL, Burrows JC et al. Synovial tissue macrophage as a source of the chemotactic cytokine IL-8. J Immunol 1991; 147: 2187–95.

33. Buckley CD, Amft N, Bradfield PF et al. Persistent induction of the chemokine receptor CXCR4 by TGF-β 1 on synovial T cells contributes to their accumulation within the rheumatoid synovium. J Immunol 2000; 165: 3423–9.

34. Nanki T, Hayashida K, El-Gabalawy HS et al. Stromal cell-derived factor-1-CXC chemokine receptor 4 interactions play a central role in CD4+ T-cell accumulation in rheumatoid arthritis synovium. J Immunol 2000; 165: 6590–8.

35. Ruth JH, Haas CS, Park CC et al. CXCL16-mediated cell recruitment to rheumatoid arthritis synovial tissue and murine lymph nodes is dependent upon the MAPK pathway. Arthritis Rheum 2006; 54: 765–78.

36. Nanki T, Shimaoka T, Hayashida K et al. Pathogenic role of CXCL16-CXCR6 pathway in rheumatoid arthritis. Arthritis Rheum 2005; 52: 3004–14.

37. van der Voort R, van Lieshout AW, Toonen LW et al. Elevated CXCL16 expression by synovial macrophages recruits memory T cells into rheumatoid joints. Arthritis Rheum 2005; 52: 1381–91.

38. Endo H, Akahoshi T, Takagishi K et al. Elevation of interleukin-8 (IL-8) levels in joint fluids of patients with rheumatoid arthritis and the induction by IL-8 of leukocyte infiltration and synovitis in rabbit joints. Lymphokine Cytokine Res 1991; 10: 245–52.

39. Deleuran B, Lemche P, Kristensen M et al. Localisation of interleukin 8 in the synovial membrane, cartilage–pannus junction and chondrocytes in rheumatoid arthritis. Scand J Rheumatol 1994; 23: 2–7.

40. Koch AE, Volin MV, Woods JM et al. Regulation of angiogenesis by the C-X-C chemokines interleukin-8 and epithelial neutrophil activating peptide-78 in the rheumatoid joint. Arthritis Rheum 2001; 44: 31–40.

41. Hosaka S, Akahoshi T, Wada C, Kondo H. Expression of the chemokine superfamily in rheumatoid arthritis. Clin Exp Immunol 1994; 97: 451–7.

42. Nanki T, Nagasaka K, Hayashida K et al. Chemokines regulate IL-6 and IL-8 production by fibroblast-like synoviocytes from patients with rheumatoid arthritis. J Immunol 2001; 167: 5381–5.

43. Georganas C, Liu H, Perlman H et al. Regulation of IL-6 and IL-8 expression in rheumatoid arthritis synovial fibroblasts: the dominant role for NF-κB but not C/EBP β or c-jun. J Immunol 2000; 165: 7199–206.

44. Patterson AM, Gardner L, Shaw J et al. Induction of a CXCL8 binding site on endothelial syndecan-3 in rheumatoid synovium. Arthritis Rheum 2005; 52: 2331–42.

45. Kraan MC, Patel DD, Haringman JJ et al. The development of clinical signs of rheumatoid synovial inflammation is associated with increased synthesis of the chemokine CXCL8 (interleukin-8). Arthritis Res 2001; 3: 65–71.

46. Chen Y, Davidson BL, Marks RM. Adenovirus-mediated transduction of the interleukin 8 gene into synoviocytes. Arthritis Rheum 1994; 37: S304.

47. Taylor PC, Peters AM, Paleolog E et al. Reduction of chemokine levels and leukocyte traffic to joints by tumor necrosis factor alpha blockade in patients with rheumatoid arthritis. Arthritis Rheum 2000; 43: 38–47.

48. De Gendt CM, De Clerck LS, Bridts CH et al. Relationship between interleukin-8 and neutrophil adhesion molecules in rheumatoid arthritis. Rheumatol Int 1996; 16: 169–73.

49. Koch AE, Polverini PJ, Kunkel SL et al. Interleukin-8 as a macrophage-derived mediator of angiogenesis. Science 1992; 258: 1798–801.

50. Rot A, Hub E, Middleton J et al. Some aspects of IL-8 pathophysiology. III. Chemokine interaction with endothelial cells. J Leukoc Biol 1996; 59: 39–44.

51. Salcedo R, Ponce ML, Young HA et al. Human endothelial cells express CCR2 and respond to MCP-1: direct role of MCP-1 in angiogenesis and tumor progression. Blood 2000; 96: 34–40.

52. Morel JC, Park CC, Kumar P, Koch AE. Interleukin-18 induces rheumatoid arthritis synovial fibroblast CXC chemokine production through NFκB activation. Lab Invest 2001; 81: 1371–83.

53. Halloran MM, Woods JM, Strieter RM et al. The role of an epithelial neutrophil-activating peptide-78-like protein in rat adjuvant-induced arthritis. J Immunol 1999; 162: 7492–500.

54. Unemori EN, Amento EP, Bauer EA, Horuk R. Melanoma growth-stimulatory activity/GRO decreases collagen expression by human fibroblasts. J Biol Chem 1993; 268: 1338–42.

55. Konig A, Krenn V, Toksoy A et al. Mig, GRO alpha and RANTES messenger RNA expression in lining layer, infiltrates and different leucocyte populations of synovial tissue from patients with rheumatoid arthritis, psoriatic arthritis and osteoarthritis. Virchows Arch 2000; 436: 449–58.

56. Castor CW, Andrews PC, Swartz RD et al. The origin, variety, distribution, and biologic fate of connective tissue activating peptide-III isoforms: characteristics in patients with rheumatic, renal, and arterial disease. Arthritis Rheum 1993; 36: 1142–53.

57. Castor CW, Smith EM, Hossler PA et al. Detection of connective tissue activating peptide-III isoforms in

synovium from osteoarthritis and rheumatoid arthritis patients: patterns of interaction with other synovial cytokines in cell culture. Arthritis Rheum 1992; 35: 783–93.

58. Pierer M, Rethage J, Seibl R et al. Chemokine secretion of rheumatoid arthritis synovial fibroblasts stimulated by Toll-like receptor 2 ligands. J Immunol 2004; 172: 1256–65.

59. Hanaoka R, Kasama T, Muramatsu M et al. A novel mechanism for the regulation of IFN-γ inducible protein-10 expression in rheumatoid arthritis. Arthritis Res Ther 2003; 5: R74–81.

60. Patel DD, Zachariah JP, Whichard LP. CXCR3 and CCR5 ligands in the rheumatoid arthritis synovium. Clin Immunol 2001; 98: 39–45.

61. Tsubaki T, Takegawa S, Hanamoto H et al. Accumulation of plasma cells expressing CXCR3 in the synovial sublining regions of early rheumatoid arthritis in association with production of Mig/CXCL9 by synovial fibroblasts. Clin Exp Immunol 2005; 141: 363–71.

62. Yamamoto T, Chikugo T, Tanaka Y. Elevated plasma levels of β-thromboglobulin and platelet factor 4 in patients with rheumatic disorders and cutaneous vasculitis. Clin Rheumatol 2002; 21: 501–4.

63. Blades MC, Ingegnoli F, Wheller SK et al. Stromal cell-derived factor 1 (CXCL12) induces monocyte migration into human synovium transplanted onto SCID mice. Arthritis Rheum 2002; 46: 824–36.

64. Bradfield PF, Amft N, Vernon-Wilson E et al. Rheumatoid fibroblast-like synoviocytes overexpress the chemokine stromal cell-derived factor 1 (CXCL12) which supports distinct patterns and rates of CD4+ and CD8+ T cell migration within synovial tissue. Arthritis Rheum 2003; 48: 2472–82.

65. Burger D. Cell contact interactions in rheumatology. The Kennedy Institute for Rheumatology, London, UK, 1–2 June 2000. Arthritis Res 2000; 2: 472–6.

66. Joven B, Gonzalez N, Aguilar F et al. Association between stromal cell derived factor 1 chemokine gene variant and radiographic progression of rheumatoid arthritis. Arthritis Rheum 2005; 52: 354–6.

67. Pablos JL, Santiago B, Galindo M et al. Synoviocyte-derived CXCL12 is displayed on endothelium and induces angiogenesis in rheumatoid arthritis. J Immunol 2003; 170: 2147–52.

68. Salcedo R, Wasserman K, Young HA et al. Vascular endothelial growth factor and basic fibroblast growth factor induce expression of CXCR4 on human endothelial cells: in vivo neovascularization induced by stromal-derived factor-1alpha. Am J Pathol 1999; 154: 1125–35.

69. Santiago B, Baleux F, Palao G et al. CXCL12 is displayed by rheumatoid endothelial cells through its basic amino-terminal motif on heparan sulfate proteoglycans. Arthritis Res Ther 2006; 8: R43.

70. Edwards JCW, Cambridge G, Abrahams VM. Do self-perpetuating B lymphocytes drive human autoimmune disease? Immunology 1999; 97: 188–96.

71. Takemura S, Braun A, Crowson C et al. Lymphoid neogenesis in rheumatoid synovitis. J Immunol 2001; 167: 1072–80.

72. Manzo A, Paoletti S, Carulli M et al. Systematic microanatomical analysis of CXCL13 and CCL21 in situ production and progressive lymphoid organization in rheumatoid synovitis. Eur J Immunol 2005; 35: 1347–59.

73. Li T, Zhong J, Chen Y et al. Expression of chemokine-like factor 1 is upregulated during T lymphocyte activation. Life Sci 2006; 79: 519–24.

74. Haringman JJ, Smeets TJ, Reinders-Blankert P, Tak PP. Chemokine and chemokine receptor expression in paired peripheral blood mononuclear cells and synovial tissue of patients with rheumatoid arthritis, osteoarthritis and reactive arthritis. Ann Rheum Dis 2006; 65: 294–300.

75. Koch AE, Kunkel SL, Harlow LA et al. Enhanced production of monocyte chemoattractant protein-1 in rheumatoid arthritis. J Clin Invest 1992; 90: 772–9.

76. Villiger PM, Terkeltaub R, Lotz M. Production of monocyte chemoattractant protein-1 by inflamed synovial tissue and cultured synoviocytes. J Immunol 1992; 149: 722–7.

77. Yoo JK, Kwon H, Khil LY et al. IL-18 induces monocyte chemotactin protein-1 production in macrophages through the phosphatidylinositol 3-kinase/Akt and MEK/ERK1/2 pathways. J Immunol 2005; 175: 8280–6.

78. Safronova O, Nakahama K, Onodera M et al. Effect of hypoxia on MCP-1 gene expression induced by interleukin-1 in human synovial fibroblasts. Inflamm Res 2003; 52: 480–6.

79. Akahoshi T, Wada C, Endo H et al. Expression of monocyte chemotactic and activating factor in rheumatoid arthritis. Arthritis Rheum 1993; 36: 762–71.

80. Koch AE, Kunkel SL, Harlow LA et al. Macrophage inflammatory protein-1 alpha. A novel chemotactic cytokine for macrophages in rheumatoid arthritis. J Clin Invest 1994; 93: 921–8.

81. Wang CR, Liu MF. Regulation of CCR5 expression and MIP-1α production in CD4+ T cells from patients with rheumatoid arthritis. Clin Exp Immunol 2003; 132: 371–8.

82. Matsui T, Akahoshi T, Namai R et al. Selective recruitment of CCR6-expressing cells by increased production of MIP-3 alpha in rheumatoid arthritis. Clin Exp Immunol 2001; 125: 155–61.

83. Ruth JH, Morel JCM, Park, CC et al. MIP-3a expression in the rheumatoid joint. Arthritis Rheum 2000; 43 (Suppl 9): S78.

84. Schlenk J, Lorenz HM, Haas JP et al. Extravasation into synovial tissue induces CCL20 mRNA expression in

polymorphonuclear neutrophils in patients with rheumatoid arthritis. J Rheumatol 2005; 32: 2291–8.

85. Chabaud M, Page G, Miossec P. Enhancing effect of Il-1, IL-17 and TNF-α on macrophage inflammatory protein-3α production in rheumatoid arthritis. J Immunol 2001; 167: 6015–20.

86. Schall TJ, Bacon K, Toy KJ, Goeddel DV. Selective attraction of monocytes and T lymphocytes of the memory phenotype by cytokine RANTES. Nature 1990; 347: 669–71.

87. Robinson E, Keystone EC, Schall TJ et al. Chemokine expression in rheumatoid arthritis (RA): evidence of RANTES and macrophage inflammatory protein (MIP)-1 beta production by synovial T cells. Clin Exp Immunol 1995; 101: 398–407.

88. Volin MV, Shah MR, Tokuhira M et al. RANTES expression and contribution to monocyte chemotaxis in arthritis. Clin Immunol Immunopathol 1998; 89: 44–53.

89. Rathanaswami P, Hachicha M, Sadick M et al. Expression of the cytokine RANTES in human rheumatoid synovial fibroblasts. Differential regulation of RANTES and interleukin-8 genes by inflammatory cytokines. J Biol Chem 1993; 268: 5834–9.

90. Alaaeddine N, Olee T, Hashimoto S et al. Production of the chemokine RANTES by articular chondrocytes and role in cartilage degradation. Arthritis Rheum 2001; 44: 1633–43.

91. Stanczyk J, Kowalski ML, Grzegorczyk J et al. RANTES and chemotactic activity in synovial fluids from patients with rheumatoid arthritis and osteoarthritis. Mediators Inflamm 2005; 2005(6): 343–8.

92. Wang CR, Guo HR, Liu MF. RANTES promoter polymorphism as a genetic risk factor for rheumatoid arthritis in the Chinese. Clin Exp Rheumatol 2005; 23: 379–84.

93. Buckley CD. Why do leucocytes accumulate within chronically inflamed joints? Rheumatology (Oxford) 2003; 42: 1433–44.

94. Blaschke S, Middel P, Dorner BG et al. Expression of activation-induced, T cell-derived, and chemokine related cytokine/lymphotactin and its functional role in rheumatoid arthritis. Arthritis Rheum 2003; 48: 1858–72.

95. Sawai H, Park YW, Robertson J et al. T cell costimulation by fractalkine-expressing synoviocytes in rheumatoid arthritis. Arthritis Rheum 2005; 52: 1392–401.

96. Lesnik P, Haskell CA, Charo IF. Decreased atherosclerosis in CX3CR1 -/- mice reveals a role for fractalkine in atherogenesis. J Clin Invest 2003; 111: 333–40.

97. McDermott DH, Fong AM, Yang Q et al. Chemokine receptor mutant CX3CR1-M280 has impaired adhesive function and correlates with protection from cardiovascular disease in humans. J Clin Invest 2003; 111: 1241–50.

98. Volin MV, Woods JM, Amin MA et al. Fractalkine: a novel angiogenic chemokine in rheumatoid arthritis. Am J Pathol 2001; 159: 1521–30.

99. Borzi RM, Mazzetti I, Cattini L et al. Human chondrocytes express functional chemokine receptors and release matrix-degrading enzymes in response to C-X-C and C-C chemokines. Arthritis Rheum 2000; 43: 1734–41.

100. Garcia-Lopez MA, Sanchez-Madrid F, Rodriguez-Frade JM et al. CXCR3 chemokine receptor distribution in normal and inflamed tissues. Lab Invest 2001; 81: 409–18.

101. Wedderburn LR, Robinson N, Patel A et al. Selective recruitment of polarized T cells expressing CCR5 and CXCR3 to the inflamed joints of children with juvenile idiopathic arthritis. Arthritis Rheum 2000; 43: 765–74.

102. Schmutz C, Hulme A, Burman A et al. Chemokine receptors in the rheumatoid synovium: upregulation of CXCR5. Arthritis Res Ther 2005; 7: R217–29.

103. Ruth JH, Rottman JB, Katschke KJ Jr et al. Selective lymphocyte chemokine receptor expression in the rheumatoid joint. Arthritis Rheum 2001; 44: 2750–60.

104. Katschke KJ Jr, Rottman JB, Ruth JH et al. Differential expression of chemokine receptors on peripheral blood, synovial fluid and synovial tissue monocytes/macrophages in rheumatoid arthritis. Arthritis Rheum 2001; 44: 1022–32.

105. Mack M, Bruhl H, Gruber R et al. Predominance of mononuclear cells expressing the chemokine receptor CCR5 in synovial effusions of patients with different forms of arthritis. Arthritis Rheum 1999; 42: 981–8.

106. Suzuki N, Nakajima A, Yoshino S et al. Selective accumulation of CCR5+ T lymphocytes into inflamed joints in rheumatoid arthritis. Int Immunol 1999; 11: 553–9.

107. Gomez-Reino JJ, Pablos JL, Carreira PE et al. Association of rheumatoid arthritis with a functional chemokine receptor, CCR5. Arthritis Rheum 1999; 42: 989–92.

108. Prahalad S. Negative association between the chemokine receptor CCR5-Δ32 polymorphism and rheumatoid arthritis: a metaanalysis. Genes Immun 2006; 7: 264–8.

109. Shahrara S, Amin MA, Woods JM et al. Chemokine receptor expression and in vivo signaling pathways in the joints of rats with adjuvant-induced arthritis. Arthritis Rheum 2003; 48: 3568–83.

110. Galligan CL, Matsuyama W, Matsukawa A et al. Up-regulated expression and activation of the orphan chemokine receptor, CCRL2, in rheumatoid arthritis. Arthritis Rheum 2004; 50: 1806–14.

111. Patterson AM, Siddall H, Chamberlain G et al. Expression of the Duffy antigen/receptor for chemokines (DARC) by the inflamed synovial endothelium. J Pathol 2002; 197: 108–16.

112. Szekanecz Z, Halloran MM, Volin MV et al. Temporal expression of inflammatory cytokines and chemokines in rat adjuvant-induced arthritis. Arthritis Rheum 2000; 43: 1266–77.

113. Haas CS, Martinez RJ, Attia N et al. Chemokine receptor expression in rat adjuvant-induced arthritis. Arthritis Rheum 2005; 52: 3718–30.

114. Feldmann M, Brennan FM, Maini RN. Role of cytokines in rheumatoid arthritis. Annu Rev Immunol 1996; 14: 397–440.

115. Szekanecz Z, Strieter RM, Koch AE. Cytokines in rheumatoid arthritis: potential targets for pharmacological intervention. Drugs Aging 1998; 12: 377–390.

116. Fahey TJ, Tracey KJ, Tekamp-Olson P et al. Macrophage inflammatory protein 1 modulates macrophage function. J Immunol 1991; 148: 2764–9.

117. Zhang X, Nakajima T, Goronzy JJ, Weyand CM. Tissue trafficking patterns of effector memory CD4+ T cells in rheumatoid arthritis. Arthritis Rheum 2005; 52: 3839–49.

118. Butcher EC. Leukocyte-endothelial cell recognition: three (or more) steps to specificity and diversity. Cell 1991; 67: 1033–6.

119. Imhof BA, Aurrand-Lions M. Adhesion mechanisms regulating the migration of monocytes. Nat Rev Immunol 2004; 4: 432–44.

120. Klimiuk PA, Sierakowski S, Latosiewicz R et al. Histological patterns of synovitis and serum chemokines in patients with rheumatoid arthritis. J Rheumatol 2005; 32: 1666–72.

121. Akahoshi T, Endo H, Kondo H et al. Essential involvement of interleukin-8 in neutrophil recruitment in rabbits with acute experimental arthritis induced by lipopolysaccharide and interleukin-1. Lymphokine Cytokine Res 1994; 13: 113–16.

122. Kasama T, Strieter RM, Lukacs NW et al. Interleukin-10 expression and chemokine regulation during the evolution of murine type II collagen-induced arthritis. J Clin Invest 1995; 95: 2868–76.

123. Salomon I, Netzer N, Wildbaum G et al. Targeting the function of IFNγ-inducible protein 10 suppresses ongoing adjuvant arthritis. J Immunol 2002; 169: 2865–73.

124. Podolin PL, Bolognese BJ, Foley JJ et al. A potent and selective nonpeptide antagonist of CXCR2 inhibits acute and chronic models of arthritis in the rabbit. J Immunol 2002; 169: 6435–44.

125. Terkeltaub R, Baird S, Sears P et al. The murine homolog of the interleukin-8 receptor CXCR2 is essential for the occurrence of neutrophilic inflammation in the air pouch model of acute urate crystal-induced gouty synovitis. Arthritis Rheum 1998; 41: 900–9.

126. Brown CR, Blaho VA, Loiacono CM. Susceptibility to experimental Lyme arthritis correlates with KC and monocyte chemoattractant protein-1 production in joints and requires neutrophil recruitment via CXCR2. J Immunol 2003; 171: 893–901.

127. Gao P, Zhou XY, Yashiro-Ohtani Y et al. The unique target specificity of a nonpeptide chemokine receptor antagonist: selective blockade of two Th1 chemokine receptors CCR5 and CXCR3. J Leukoc Biol 2003; 73: 273–80.

128. Hatse S, Princen K, Bridger G et al. Chemokine receptor inhibition by AMD3100 is strictly confined to CXCR4. FEBS Lett 2002; 527: 255–62.

129. Tamamura H, Fujii N. The therapeutic potential of CXCR4 antagonists in the treatment of HIV infection, cancer metastasis and rheumatoid arthritis. Expert Opin Ther Targets 2005; 9: 1267–82.

130. Chintalacharuvu SR, Wang JX, Giaconia JM, Venkataraman C. An essential role for CCL3 in the development of collagen-induced arthritis. Immunol Lett 2005; 100: 202–4.

131. Ogata H, Takeya M, Yoshimura T et al. The role of monocyte chemoattractant protein-1 (MCP-1) in the pathogenesis of collagen-induced arthritis in rats. J Pathol 1997; 182: 106–14.

132. Schrier DJ, Schimmer RC, Flory CM et al. Role of chemokines and cytokines in a reactivation model of arthritis in rats induced by injection with streptococcal cell walls. Leukoc Biol 1998; 63: 359–63.

133. Gong JH, Ratkay LG, Waterfield JD, Clark-Lewis I. An antagonist of monocyte chemoattractant protein 1 (MCP-1) inhibits arthritis in the MRL-lpr mouse model. J Exp Med 1997; 186: 131–7.

134. Barnes DA, Tse J, Kaufhold M et al. Polyclonal antibody directed against human RANTES ameliorates disease in the Lewis rat adjuvant-induced arthritis model. J Clin Invest 1998; 101: 2910–19.

135. Inoue T, Yamashita M, Higaki M. The new antirheumatic drug KE-298 suppresses MCP-1 and RANTES production in rats with adjuvant-induced arthritis and in IL-1-stimulated synoviocytes of patients with rheumatoid arthritis. Rheumatol Int 2001; 20: 149–53.

136. Pease JR, Horuk R. CCR1 antagonists in clinical development. Expert Opin Investig Drugs 2005; 14: 785–96.

137. Saeki T, Naya A. CCR1 chemokine receptor antagonists. Curr Pharm Des 2003; 9: 1201–8.

138. Gladue RP, Tylaska LA, Brissette WH et al. CP-481,715, a potent and selective CCR1 antagonist with potential therapeutic implications for inflammatory diseases. J Biol Chem 2003; 278: 40473–80.

139. Haringman JJ, Kraan MC, Smeets TJM et al. Chemokine blockade and chronic inflammatory disease: proof of concept in patients with rheumatoid arthritis. Ann Rheum Dis 2003; 62: 715–21.

140. Quinones MP, Estrada CA, Kalkonde Y et al. The complex role of the chemokine receptor CCR2 in collagen-induced arthritis: implications for therapeutic targeting of CCR2 in rheumatoid arthritis. J Mol Med 2005; 83: 672–81.

141. Plater-Zyberk C, Hoogewerf AJ, Proudfoot AE et al. Effect of a CC chemokine receptor antagonist on collagen

induced arthritis in DBA/1 mice. Immunol Lett 1997; 57: 117–20.

142. Shahrara S, Proudfoot AE, Woods JM et al. Amelioration of rat adjuvant-induced arthritis by Met-RANTES. Arthritis Rheum 2005; 52: 1907–19.

143. Yang YF, Mukai T, Gao P et al. A non-peptide CCR5 antagonist inhibits collagen-induced arthritis by modulating T cell migration without affecting any collagen T cell responses. Eur J Immunol 2002; 32: 2124–32.

144. Quinones MP, Ahuja SK, Jimenez F et al. Experimental arthritis in CC chemokine receptor 2-null mice closely mimics severe human rheumatoid arthritis. J Clin Invest 2004; 113: 856–66.

145. Bao L, Zhu Y, Zhu J, Lindgren JU. Decreased IgG production but increased MIP-1β expression in collagen-induced arthritis in C-C chemokine receptor 5-deficient mice. Cytokine 2005; 31: 64–71.

146. Bursill CA, Cai S, Channon KM, Greaves DR. Adenoviral-mediated delivery of a viral chemokine binding protein blocks CC-chemokine activity in vitro and in vivo. Immunobiology 2003; 207: 187–96.

147. Nanki T, Urasaki Y, Imai T et al. Inhibition of fractalkine ameliorates murine collagen-induced arthritis. J Immunol 2004; 173: 7010–16.

148. Gong JH, Yan R, Waterfield JD, Clark-Lewis I. Post-onset inhibition of murine arthritis using combined chemokine antagonist therapy. Rheumatology (Oxford) 2004; 43: 39–42.

149. Youssef S, Maor G, Wildbaum G et al. C-C chemokine-encoding DNA vaccines enhance breakdown of tolerance to their gene products and treat ongoing adjuvant arthritis. J Clin Invest 2000; 106: 361–71.

150. Matsukawa A, Yoshimura T, Fujiwara K et al. Involvement of growth-related protein in LPS-induced rabbit arthritis. Lab Invest 1999; 79: 591–600.

151. Loetscher P, Dewald B, Baggiolini M, Seitz M. Monocyte chemoattractant protein 1 and interleukin 8 production by rheumatoid synoviocytes: effects of anti-rheumatic drugs. Cytokine 1994; 6: 162–70.

152. Lopez-Armada MJ, Sanchez-Pernaute O, Largo R et al. Modulation of cell recruitment by anti-inflammatory agents in antigen-induced arthritis. Ann Rheum Dis 2002; 61: 1027–30.

153. Volin MV, Campbell PL, Connors MA et al. The effect of sulfasalazine on rheumatoid arthritis synovial tissue chemokine production. Exp Mol Pathol 2002; 73: 84–92.

154. Volin MV, Harlow LA, Woods JM et al. Treatment with sulfasalazine or sulfapyridine, but not 5-aminosalicyclic acid, inhibits basic fibroblast growth factor-induced endothelial cell chemotaxis. Arthritis Rheum 1999; 42: 1927–35.

155. Ho CY, Wong CK, Li EK et al. Suppressive effect of combination treatment of leflunomide and methotrexate on chemokine expression in patients with rheumatoid arthritis. Clin Exp Immunol 2003; 133: 132–8.

156. Sato M, Miyazaki T, Nagaya T et al. Antioxidants inhibit tumor necrosis factor-alpha mediated stimulation of interleukin-8, monocyte chemoattractant protein-1, and collagenase expression in cultured human synovial cells. J Rheumatol 1996; 23: 432–8.

157. Nissinen R, Leirisalo-Repo M, Peltomaa R et al. Cytokine and chemokine receptor profile of peripheral blood mononuclear cells during treatment with infliximab in patients with active rheumatoid arthritis. Ann Rheum Dis 2004; 63: 681–7.

158. Aeberli D, Seitz M, Juni P, Villiger PM. Increase of peripheral CXCR3 positive T lymphocytes upon treatment of RA patients with TNF-alpha inhibitors. Rheumatology (Oxford) 2005; 44: 172–5.

22

New developments in NF-κB

Keith Brown, Estefania Claudio and Ulrich Siebenlist

INTRODUCTION

NF-κB is a ubiquitously expressed family of inducible dimeric transcription factors with five members: Rel (c-Rel), RelA (p65), RelB, NF-κB1 (p50/p105), and NF-κB2 (p52/p100). It recognizes a common consensus DNA sequence motif and regulates a large number of target genes, particularly those involved in the immune system and defence against pathogens, also those concerned with inflammation, injury, stress and the acute phase response. In unstimulated cells, homo- or heterodimers of family members bind IκB inhibitory proteins (the closely related IκBα, IκBβ and IκBε) and these retain the NF-κB dimers in the cytoplasm. p105 and p100 precursor proteins, which encode p50 and p52 in their N-terminal halves, behave as IκBs, containing ankyrin repeats in their C-terminal halves, similar to those of the smaller IκBs[1,2] (Figure 22.1). The activation of NF-κB through a variety of cell membrane receptors including TNFR, IL-1R, Toll, TCR, and BCR proceeds via phosphorylation, ubiquitination, and proteasomal degradation of IκBs. The phosphorylation occurs at dual serine residues in the N-terminus of IκBs and is catalyzed by a complex of IκB kinases (IKKs) α and β combined with the regulatory subunit NEMO (IKKγ). Phosphorylation by the activated IKK complex is predominantly by IKKβ. This triggers lysine 48 (K48)-linked polyubiquitination at adjacent lysine residues initiated by a specific ubiquitin E3 ligase complex Skp1/Cul1/F-box protein-β-TrCp. This is followed by proteolysis at the 26S proteasome. The free NF-κB dimers (most commonly the p50/p65 heterodimer) translocate to the nucleus, bind κB DNA sites and activate gene transcription. This pathway is termed the 'classical' pathway of NF-κB activation[1,2] (Figure 22.2).

Recently a new pathway for NF-κB activation that is dependent on IKKα was described[3] (Figure 22.3). The pathway is termed the 'alternative' pathway and is independent of IKKβ and NEMO.[4–6] The target for IKKα is NF-κB2/p100, which is phosphorylated at its C-terminus then K48-polyubiquitinated. Proteolysis of the C-terminal half of p100 follows and free p52 containing the Rel homology domain is released. p52 most commonly associates with RelB and activation of the alternative pathway results in nuclear translocation of this heterodimer and transcriptional activation of distinct target genes.[7] Stimuli which activate the alternative pathway include, Lymphotoxin β R (LTβR), BAFFR, RANK, and CD40[2,8,9] (Figure 22.3).

Such advances have been made in the last few years across a wide area of the NF-κB field that a selective approach to reviewing the field must be taken. This review therefore focuses on three burgeoning fields of research: the extensive involvement of ubiquitination in the regulation of the classical pathway of NF-κB activation; pioneering efforts to unravel early steps in the

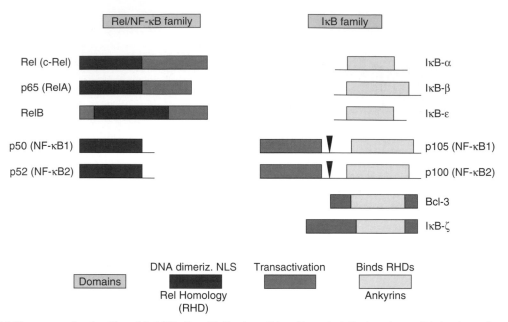

Figure 22.1 The mammalian families of Rel/NF-κB and IκB polypeptides. Characteristic domains and their primary functions are indicated. DNA, DNA binding; dimeriz., dimerization domain; RHD, Rel homology domain; NLS, nuclear localization sequence; Transactivation, transactivating domain, functions at nuclear target sites; Ankyrins, ankyrin repeat domain, functions by binding and inhibiting RHDs (Bcl-3 and IκBζ are exceptions since they do not function as classical inhibitors of NF-κB activity).

activation of the alternative pathway of NF-κB activation; and the striking advances made in translational research to dissect NF-κB's roles in inflammatory diseases, in particular, cancer and diabetes.

ADVANCES IN NF-κB REGULATION

The classical pathway

Ubiquitination and deubiquitination

While it has been known for several years that upon stimulation the classical pathway of NF-kB activation leads to IκB phosphorylation by the IKK complex followed by K48-linked polyubiquitination and proteolysis, recent studies have revealed a greater involvement of ubiquitination in the control of NF-κB. Ubiquitin ligases are activated by different upstream signaling pathways and act as regulators of IKK activation. The assembly of lysine 63 (K63) polyubiquitin chains provides platforms for the recruitment of IKK-activating complexes, a reaction that is counteracted by deubiquitinating enzymes. Furthermore, K48-ubiquitin conjugation targets upstream signaling mediators as well as nuclear NF-κB for post-inductive degradation to limit signaling.[10] Ea et al.[11] showed that polyubiquitination of RIP1 and polyubiquitin binding by NEMO are essential for the activation of IKK by tumor necrosis factor (TNF)-α. Based on their work and that of others they propose a model for IKK activation by TNF-α in which stimulation causes trimerization of TNF receptor 1 in the cell membrane and subsequent recruitment of signaling proteins, TRADD, TRAF2, TRAF5, and RIP1. The TRAF proteins recruit the Ubc13/ Uev1A E2 ubiquitin-conjugating enzyme to K63-polyubiquitinate RIP1. The polyubiquitin chains on RIP1 then interact with TAB2, a component of the TAK1 kinase complex, and with NEMO, thus resulting in recruitment of the IKK complex. TAK1 then phosphorylates and activates IKKβ. IκB is then phosphorylated, ubiquitinated, and degraded, allowing NF-κB to translocate to the nucleus to activate gene expression (Figure 22.2). TRAF2, TRAF5, and TRAF6 have been identified

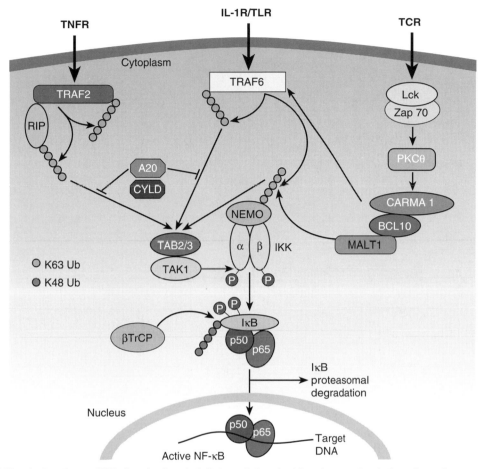

Figure 22.2 Classical pathway of NF-κB activation via IκB degradation. In this scheme, stimulation of membrane receptors with specific ligands leads to K63 polyubiquitination on TRAF2, TRAF6, RIP, and NEMO. The TAK kinase complex is recruited through association of the polyubiquitin chains with TAB2 and TAB3. Activated TAK1 may phosphorylate and activate IKKβ, which then phosphorylates IκB bound to cytosolic NF-κB, triggering its βTrCP-mediated K48 polyubiquitination and proteasome-mediated degradation. Liberated NF-κB then translocates to the nucleus (where further subunit modification and activation may occur) and transactivates target genes. CYLD and A20 are deubiquitinating enzymes that may block NF-κB activation by removal of K63 ubiquitinated chains from activated TRAFs, RIP, and NEMO. A20 may also terminate TNF-α-induced NF-κB activation by catalyzing the K48 ubiquitination of RIP, leading to its proteasomal degradation. See text for further details.

as possible candidates for upstream signaling by K63 ubiquitination.[10] All contain a RING domain that acts as an E3 ubiquitin ligase and K63 ubiquitin modifications of TRAF2 have been reported on TNF-α stimulation.[12]

Also, TRAF2 catalyses K63 polyubiquitination of RIP1.[13] Conclusive evidence of the physiologic significance of ubiquitination by TRAF2 in upstream signaling to NF-κB, however, remains elusive.[10,11,14] TRAF6 also acts as an E3 ubiquitin ligase and catalyzes the *in vitro* assembly of K63

polyubiquitin chains. It is autoubiquitinated and polyubiquitinates NEMO. TRAF6 is essential for IKK activation induced through the interleukin (IL)-1 receptor. If its ubiquitination function is blocked TRAF6 cannot mediate IKK activation.[10] In the T-cell receptor (TCR) signaling pathway to IKK and NF-κB, MALT1 has been suggested as a candidate ubiqitin E3 ligase. It carries out K63 ubiquitination of a carboxy-terminal lysine residue (lys 399) of NEMO. Mutation of this residue blocks IKK/NF-κB activation by BCL10.

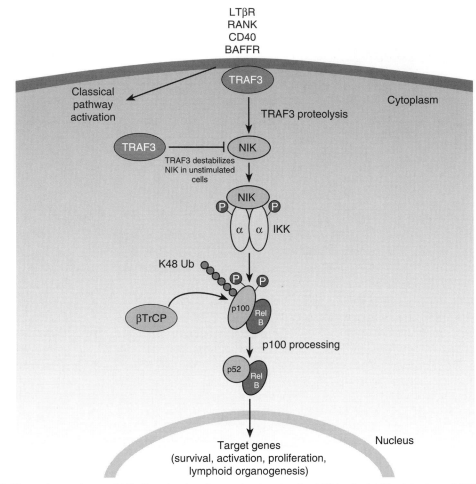

Figure 22.3 Alternative pathway of NF-κB activation. In unstimulated cells, NIK is destabilized by bound TRAF3. Activation through a subset of receptors of the TNFR superfamily including the B-cell activating factor receptor (BAFFR), CD40, RANK, and lymphotoxin β R (LTβR) leads to the recruitment of TRAF proteins (including TRAF3) to the receptor. TRAF3 (at least in some cell types) is degraded and active NIK is thus released. NIK then phosphorylates and activates IKK; it also recruits NF-κB2/p100 which is phosphorylated by IKKα. This triggers K48 polyubiquitination of p100 mediated by βTrCP E3 ubiquitin ligase and subsequent processing by the 26S proteasome to yield the mature subunit p52. Predominantly p52/RelB heterodimers are generated which migrate to the nucleus. The classical pathway of NF-κB activation is also activated through these receptors with some receptors (BAFFR) activating less strongly than others.

BCL10 is known to induce oligomerization of MALT1 which may enhance its E3 ligase activity.[10,15] BCL10 and MALT1 also induce E3 activity of TRAF6 and RNA interference studies suggest that TRAF2 and TRAF6 are necessary for IKK activation in Jurkat T cells following T-cell receptor (TCR) ligation[10] (Figure 22.2). Other lysine residues on NEMO are modified upon signaling by other stimuli. It has been suggested that different K63 ubiquitination sites on NEMO,

ubiquitinated in response to different signals, may integrate the various upstream signaling pathways by activating IKK, possibly via the TAK1/TAB complexes which are able to bind to K63-linked polyubiquitinated chains via the TAB proteins and activate IKK by the TAK1 IKK kinase[10] (Figure 22.2).

Several deubiquitinating enzymes (DUBs) have been identified which preferentially disassemble K63 poylubiquitin chains. One, CYLD, a ubiquitin-specific cysteine protease, is a tumor suppressor that is mutated in patients with familial cylindromatosis,[16] a condition that predisposes them to the development of benign tumors of the skin appendages. When overexpressed in transfected cells, CYLD physically interacts with NEMO and TRAF2 and inhibits the ubiquitination of TRAF2 and TRAF6, blocking the activation of NF-κB by Toll-like receptors (TLRs), IL1R and TNFR. Down-modulation of CYLD by RNAi or by mutation in the ubiquitin hydrolase domain resulted in constitutive ubiquitination of TRAF2 and increased inducible NF-κB activity, suggesting that CYLD functions as a negative regulator of NF-κB, perhaps by limiting the duration of IKK activity.[10,17–19] Reiley et al.[20] found that TNF-α induced rapid and transient NEMO-dependent phosphorylation of CYLD which is needed for TRAF2 ubiquitination and downstream activation. This suggests that phosphorylation of CYLD inactivates its deubiquitination activity and that site-specific phosphorylation of CYLD by IKK regulates its signaling function. However, the physical interactions reported above were observed with ectopic CYLD, NEMO, and TRAF2 and have not been seen with endogenous proteins. Also, a recent report suggested that in TNF-α-stimulated cells, CYLD down-modulation enhanced JNK but not IKK activation whereas it enhanced both upon CD40 stimulation.[21] Thus, at this time, the physiological role of CYLD in TNF-α-induced NF-κB regulation remains uncertain. It is possible that TNF-α/TRAF2-mediated polyubiquitination may preferentially activate JNK signaling, as suggested by Habelhah et al.[14]

Other DUB enzymes which regulate IKK have recently been reviewed.[10] The best studied, A20, inhibits IKK activity in two ways. Its N terminal domain contains a DUB function that removes K63 polyubiquitin chains from RIP and TRAF6, interfering with TNFR and TLR signaling to IKK and NF-κB and its C-terminal domain contains an E3 ubiquitin ligase function which mediates K48 polyubiquitination of RIP, triggering its proteasomal degradation.[13] A20 knockout results in termination of TNF-α-induced NF-κB activation, providing *in vivo* evidence for the role of this protein in negative regulation of NF-κB.[10,22]

The termination of NF-κB activation requires the resynthesis of IκBs degraded initially in response to signal. The IκB genes themselves are transcriptional targets of NF-κB. The IκBs, therefore, act in an autoregulatory feedback loop to limit the duration of NF-κB signaling.[2] Krappmann and Scheidereit[10] argue that additional feedback circuits must operate when upstream signaling is continuous, to augment the inhibition of NF-κB activation by resynthesized IκBs. They propose that selective ubiquitination provides multiple sites for feedback inhibition of NF-κB activation to operate. For example, RIP K48 ubiquitination and degradation is induced upon TNFR1 ligation[23] with A20 providing the ubiquitin ligase activity.[13] TRAF2 is also ubiquitinated and degraded with c-IAP1 acting as a ubiqitin ligase.[24] Both A20 and c-IAP1 are NF-κB targets thus activating an autoregulatory circuit able to shut down TNF signaling following its induction. Other examples of potential autoregulatory circuits involving ubiquitination have been reviewed by Krappmann and Scheidereit.[10]

SUMO modification

Protein modification by SUMO (small ubiquitin-like modifier) is an important regulatory mechanism for many cellular processes.[25,26] SUMO may regulate the NF-κB classical pathway in two ways.[26] Firstly, in response to activation signals, cytoplasmic IκBα undergoes polyubiquitination on lysines 21 and 22, targeting the protein for proteasomal degradation, releasing active NF-κB for translocation to the nucleus. IκBα can be modified by SUMO-1 on lysine 21, thus blocking ubiquitination and stabilizing the protein.[27] SUMO modification therefore leads to repression of NF-κB by formation of a fraction of IκBα that is unresponsive to signal. Secondly, in contrast to this negative regulation, it has recently been reported that SUMO modification is essential for activation of NF-κB by DNA damage signals.[26,28] SUMO conjugation to NEMO in response to genotoxic signals occurs only on IKK-free NEMO and is mediated in the nucleus by the SUMO E3-ligase, PIASy.[29] SUMO-modified NEMO accumulates in the nucleus.[28,29] Upon SUMO removal, NEMO is mono-ubiquitinated and shuttled back to the cytoplasm where it activates IKK and induces NF-κB. The mono-ubiquitination of NEMO is essential for its nuclear export and proceeds in the nucleus only after the phosphorylation on serine 85 of NEMO by the kinase, ATM (ataxia telangiectasia mutated).[30] In a model proposed by Wu et al.,[30] NEMO and ATM exit the nucleus together and, with the protein ELKS, form a cytosolic signaling complex with IKK to mediate NF-κB activation in response to genotoxic stimuli.

The alternative pathway

In the alternative pathway the upstream mechanism of IKKα activation is not well characterized. In response to signal, NF-κB-inducing kinase (NIK) is activated and phosphorylates and activates IKKα, which then phosphorylates p100, triggering its processing to p52[2,3,31–33] (Figure 22.3). How NIK is activated is uncertain. Only a very low level of NIK can be detected in unstimulated cells and it turns over rapidly. The mechanism responsible for rapid NIK turnover may involve TRAF3, as TRAF3 is known to negatively regulate BAFFR signaling to NF-κB in B lymphocytes.[34] TRAF3 is associated with BAFFR (a receptor which signals preferentially to the alternative pathway of NF-κB activation) and is bound to NIK in unstimulated cells where it induces NIK ubiquitination and proteolysis. Upon stimulation, through BAFFR or CD40, TRAF3 is degraded (how is not known) and NIK is stabilized and accumulates as a result of new synthesis.[33,35,36] It is possible that stimulation induces TRAF3 degradation only in some cell lines and it is unclear what other processes may play a role in NIK stabilization and activation.[33] Besides activating IKKα, NIK plays an additional role in p100 processing. It recruits IKKα to p100 in a kinase-independent manner and may phosphorylate p100 at C-terminal serine residues or recruit or modify other essential proteins for p100 processing.[32,33,37] The known receptors which activate the alternative pathway are members of a subgroup of the TNFR family: LTβR, BAFFR, RANK, and CD40. How they transduce their signals to NIK and IKKα is unclear as their receptor signaling domains resemble those of other TNFR family members.

Since they also activate the classical pathway, their intracellular signaling domains presumably possess sequence motifs which link them to the alternative pathway via NIK as well as to the classical pathway. Some light was shed on this question in the case of the BAFF receptor by the finding that mutation of a putative TRAF3-binding sequence motif of BAFFR (which preferentially induces the alternative pathway) PVPAT, abolished its interaction with TRAF3 and its ability to induce the alternative pathway. In contrast, its mutation to PVQET, a more typical TRAF-binding motif, rendered BAFFR able to induce strong classical NF-κB signaling. Also, the modified BAFFR associated more strongly and more rapidly with TRAF3. This suggests that the PVPAT motif is not only essential for BAFF signaling to TRAF but also determines its signaling specificity in induction of the alternative pathway.[38]

NF-κB IN INFLAMMATION AND DISEASE

Inflammation and NF-κB are closely connected. Inflammatory signals such as TNF-α activate NF-κB and NF-κB activates transcription of a number of proinflammatory genes, including IL-6 and TNF-α. Much progress has been made by several groups in characterizing NF-κB's involvement in inflammatory disease and in the contribution of chronic inflammation to the development of a variety of diseases including cancer, arthritis, atherosclerosis, and diabetes.[39] We review below the progress made in understanding the role of NF-κB and inflammation in two diseases: cancer and diabetes.

NF-κB in cancer

Certain chronic inflammatory diseases are associated with increased rates of cancer.[40,41] Examples of inflammation-driven cancers that have been studied in mouse models at the genetic and biochemical levels include colitis-associated cancer,[42] and genetically induced hepatic cancer (Mdr2 knockout mice).[43] Based on these studies it is proposed that activation of NF-κB by the classical pathway promotes inflammation-induced carcinogenesis. In other cancer models, including chemically induced skin and hepatic cancers, NF-κB had the opposite effect, inhibiting carcinogenesis.[44–47] Thus, depending on the cell type, NF-κB can either promote or inhibit carcinogenesis.

Colitis-associated cancer was induced in mice by injection of the procarcinogen, azoxymethane, and treatment with a gut inflammatory agent, dextran sulfate sodium salt (DSS).[42] Inhibition of NF-κB activation by inactivation of IKKβ in intestinal epithelial cells (enterocytes) resulted in fewer tumors in the treated mice but no change in tumor size. This suggested that IKKβ-dependent NF-κB in enterocytes contributes to tumor initiation or early promotion (rather than tumor growth and progression). Increased apoptosis of the IKKβ-deficient enterocytes including preneoplastic cells was noted following carcinogen/DSS treatment (probably due to defective induction of the anti-apoptotic NF-κB target, Bcl-XL). Thus, the tumor-promoting function of NF-κB in enterocytes depends on its anti-apoptotic effects on preneoplastic progenitors rather than on its activation of proinflammatory genes.[42] However, a second mechanism whereby NF-κB can affect tumor promotion depends on its induction of proinflammatory cytokines in myeloid cells. When IKKβ was deleted in myeloid cells which are not themselves transformed by carcinogen/DSS treatment but which are important for development of colitis-associated cancer, tumor size was decreased with some reduction also in tumor number.[42] The decrease in size was due to reduced proliferation of transformed epithelial cells. This proliferation depends on growth factors produced by myeloid cells. One of these is IL-6, encoded by an NF-κB target gene. Neutralizing antibodies to the IL-6 receptor inhibited tumor growth without affecting tumor number,[48] resembling somewhat the effect of myeloid-specific ablation of IKKβ. IKKβ-activated NF-κB therefore contributes to colitis-associated cancer in two ways: in enterocytes it activates anti-apoptotic genes and thereby suppresses the apoptotic elimination of preneoplastic cells and in myeloid cells it promotes the production of cytokines that act as growth factors for premalignant enterocytes.[41]

In inflammation-driven cholestatic cancer, caused by inactivation of the Mdr2 P-glycoprotein transporter,[49] chronic low grade liver inflammation

eventually leads to hepatocellular cancer at about 8 months of age. The initiating event in causation of the cancer is unknown, although the tumor stroma – like that in colitis-associated cancer – is an important source of tumor-promoting cytokines, here, TNF-α. As in the colitis model, inhibition of NF-κB (in this case, through expression of a non-degradable IκB 'super-repressor' active in hepatocytes) markedly reduced tumorigenesis.[43] How NF-κB is activated in this model is unknown but it appears to depend on production of TNF-α by non-parenchymal cells, i.e. Kupffer cells and endothelial cells. Inhibition of TNF-α signaling blocked activation of NF-κB in hepatocytes and early tumors and, like inhibition of NF-κB itself, increased hepatocyte apoptosis and reduced tumor number. Thus, in this model too, an important protumorigenic function of NF-κB is its anti-apoptotic role in promoting survival of premalignant or early neoplastic cells.[41] The role of NF-κB in inflammatory cells has not been fully investigated in this model but presumably is important for production of TNF-α and other cytokines. It should be noted that unlike the Mdr2 knockout model in which inhibition of NF-κB for the first 7 months of life did not reduce tumorigenesis, in the colitis-associated cancer model, most of the apoptotic death of IKKβ-deficient enterocytes occurred within a few days of exposure to carcinogen plus inflammatory agent, most likely due to inability to induce the anti-apoptotic factor Bcl-XL and higher expression of pro-apoptotic proteins.[40]

According to the models cited above NF-κB is a critical promoter of inflammation-linked cancers. However, strong evidence has recently emerged that it has the opposite effect in models of chemically induced skin and liver cancers. Maeda et al.[46] have described a tumor-suppressive role of IKKβ-dependent NF-κB activation in chemically induced hepatocarcinogenesis. They showed that while loss of NF-κB increased apoptosis (as was the case in the previously discussed models), in this case, compensatory proliferation of hepatocytes (including preneoplastic cells) stimulated by proinflammatory cytokines was instrumental in carcinogenesis. These authors used a mouse model with a hepatocyte-specific knockout of IKKβ, the predominant catalytic

certain cancers, diabetes, atherosclerosis, and autoimmune diseases. Considerable effort is presently being expended in the search for effective NF-κB inhibitors with tolerable toxicity for therapeutic use as anti-inflammatory and anti-cancer drugs. This is impeded by the difficulty of targeting NF-κB in pathological states because of the key importance of NF-κB in the physiology of healthy cells. Also, whether inhibition of NF-κB alone will suffice in treatment of these diseases or whether it can augment the efficacy of other treatments in combined therapy remains an open question. Further research to elucidate the molecular differences between the signaling of NF-κB to different target genes may assist us to answer this important question.

ACKNOWLEDGMENTS

The authors thank members of the Siebenlist laboratory for helpful discussions. Mary Rust is thanked for expert editorial assistance and Dr Anthony Fauci for his continued support.

REFERENCES

1. Brown K, Claudio E, Siebenlist U. NF-kappaB. In: Smolen JS, Lipsky PE, eds. Targeted Therapies in Rheumatology. London: Martin Dunitz, 2002: 381–401.

2. Hayden MS, Ghosh S. Signaling to NF-kappaB. Genes Dev 2004; 18: 2195–224.

3. Senftleben U, Cao Y, Xiao G et al. Activation by IKKalpha of a second, evolutionary conserved, NF-kappa B signaling pathway. Science 2001; 293: 1495–9.

4. Dejardin E, Droin NM, Delhase M et al. The lymphotoxin-beta receptor induces different patterns of gene expression via two NF-kappaB pathways. Immunity 2002; 17: 525–35.

5. Claudio E, Brown K, Park S, Wang H, Siebenlist U. BAFF-induced NEMO-independent processing of NF-kappa B2 in maturing B cells. Nat Immunol 2002; 3: 958–65.

6. Bonizzi G, Karin M. The two NF-kappaB activation pathways and their role in innate and adaptive immunity. Trends Immunol 2004; 25: 280–8.

7. Bonizzi G, Bebien M, Otero DC et al. Activation of IKKalpha target genes depends on recognition of specific kappaB binding sites by RelB:p52 dimers. EMBO J 2004; 23: 4202–10.

8. Cao Y, Bonizzi G, Seagroves TN et al. IKKalpha provides an essential link between RANK signaling and cyclin D1 expression during mammary gland development. Cell 2001; 107: 763–75.

9. Novack DV, Yin L, Hagen-Stapleton A et al. The IkappaB function of NF-kappaB2 p100 controls stimulated osteoclastogenesis. J Exp Med 2003; 198: 771–81.

10. Krappmann D, Scheidereit C. A pervasive role of ubiquitin conjugation in activation and termination of IkappaB kinase pathways. EMBO Rep 2005; 6: 321–6.

11. Ea CK, Deng L, Xia ZP, Pineda G, Chen ZJ. Activation of IKK by TNFalpha requires site-specific ubiquitination of RIP1 and polyubiquitin binding by NEMO. Mol Cell 2006; 22: 245–57.

12. Shi CS, Kehrl JH. Tumor necrosis factor (TNF)-induced germinal center kinase-related (GCKR) and stress-activated protein kinase (SAPK) activation depends upon the E2/E3 complex Ubc13-Uev1A/TNF receptor-associated factor 2 (TRAF2). J Biol Chem 2003; 278: 15429–34.

13. Wertz IE, O'Rourke KM, Zhou H et al. De-ubiquitination and ubiquitin ligase domains of A20 downregulate NF-kappaB signalling. Nature 2004; 430: 694–9.

14. Habelhah H, Takahashi S, Cho SG, Kadoya T, Watanabe T, Ronai Z. Ubiquitination and translocation of TRAF2 is required for activation of JNK but not of p38 or NF-kappaB. EMBO J 2004; 23: 322–32.

15. Lucas PC, Yonezumi M, Inohara N et al. Bcl10 and MALT1, independent targets of chromosomal translocation in malt lymphoma, cooperate in a novel NF-kappaB signaling pathway. J Biol Chem 2001; 276: 19012–19.

16. Bignell GR, Warren W, Seal S et al. Identification of the familial cylindromatosis tumour-suppressor gene. Nat Genet 2000; 25: 160–5.

17. Brummelkamp TR, Nijman SM, Dirac AM, Bernards R. Loss of the cylindromatosis tumour suppressor inhibits apoptosis by activating NF-kappaB. Nature 2003; 424: 797–801.

18. Kovalenko A, Chable-Bessia C, Cantarella G et al. The tumour suppressor CYLD negatively regulates NF-kappaB signalling by deubiquitination. Nature 2003; 424: 801–5.

19. Trompouki E, Hatzivassiliou E, Tsichritzis T et al. CYLD is a deubiquitinating enzyme that negatively regulates NF-kappaB activation by TNFR family members. Nature 2003; 424: 793–6.

20. Reiley W, Zhang M, Wu X, Granger E, Sun SC. Regulation of the deubiquitinating enzyme CYLD by IkappaB kinase gamma-dependent phosphorylation. Mol Cell Biol 2005; 25: 3886–95.

21. Reiley W, Zhang M, Sun SC. Negative regulation of JNK signaling by the tumor suppressor CYLD. J Biol Chem 2004; 279: 55161–7.

22. Lee EG, Boone DL, Chai S et al. Failure to regulate TNF-induced NF-kappaB and cell death responses in A20-deficient mice. Science 2000; 289: 2350–4.

23. Legler DF, Micheau O, Doucey MA, Tschopp J, Bron C. Recruitment of TNF receptor 1 to lipid rafts is essential for TNFα-mediated NF-kappaB activation. Immunity 2003; 18: 655–64.

24. Li X, Yang Y, Ashwell JD. TNF-RII and c-IAP1 mediate ubiquitination and degradation of TRAF2. Nature 2002; 416: 345–7.

25. Gill G. SUMO and ubiquitin in the nucleus: different functions, similar mechanisms? Genes Dev 2004; 18: 2046–59.

26. Hay RT. SUMO: a history of modification. Mol Cell 2005; 18: 1–12.

27. Desterro JM, Rodriguez MS, Hay RT. SUMO-1 modification of IkappaBalpha inhibits NF-kappaB activation. Mol Cell 1998; 2: 233–9.

28. Huang TT, Wuerzberger-Davis SM, Wu ZH, Miyamoto S. Sequential modification of NEMO/IKKgamma by SUMO-1 and ubiquitin mediates NF-kappaB activation by genotoxic stress. Cell 2003; 115: 565–76.

29. Mabb AM, Wuerzberger-Davis SM, Miyamoto S. PIASy mediates NEMO sumoylation and NF-kappaB activation in response to genotoxic stress. Nat Cell Biol 2006; 8: 986–93.

30. Wu ZH, Shi Y, Tibbetts RS, Miyamoto S. Molecular linkage between the kinase ATM and NF-kappaB signaling in response to genotoxic stimuli. Science 2006; 311: 1141–6.

31. Xiao G, Harhaj EW, Sun SC. NF-kappaB-inducing kinase regulates the processing of NF-kappaB2 p100. Mol Cell 2001; 7: 401–9.

32. Xiao G, Fong A, Sun SC. Induction of p100 processing by NF-kappaB-inducing kinase involves docking IκB kinase alpha (IKKα) to p100 and IKKα-mediated phosphorylation. J Biol Chem 2004; 279: 30099–105.

33. Xiao G, Rabson AB, Young W, Qing G, Qu Z. Alternative pathways of NF-kappaB activation: a double-edged sword in health and disease. Cytokine Growth Factor Rev 2006; 17: 281–93.

34. Xu LG, Shu HB. TNFR-associated factor-3 is associated with BAFF-R and negatively regulates BAFF-R-mediated NF-kappa B activation and IL-10 production. J Immunol 2002; 169: 6883–9.

35. Liao G, Zhang M, Harhaj EW, Sun SC. Regulation of the NF-kappaB-inducing kinase by tumor necrosis factor receptor-associated factor 3-induced degradation. J Biol Chem 2004; 279: 26243–50.

36. Qing G, Qu Z, Xiao G. Stabilization of basally translated NF-kappaB-inducing kinase (NIK) protein functions as a molecular switch of processing of NF-kappaB2 p100. J Biol Chem 2005; 280: 40578–82.

37. Liang C, Zhang M, Sun SC. beta-TrCP binding and processing of NF-kappaB2/p100 involve its phosphorylation at serines 866 and 870. Cell Signal 2006; 18: 1309–17.

38. Morrison MD, Reiley W, Zhang M, Sun SC. An atypical tumor necrosis factor (TNF) receptor-associated factor-binding motif of B cell-activating factor belonging to the TNF family (BAFF) receptor mediates induction of the noncanonical NF-kappaB signaling pathway. J Biol Chem 2005; 280: 10018–24.

39. Bottero V, Withoff S, Verma IM. NF-kappaB and the regulation of hematopoiesis. Cell Death Differ 2006; 13: 785–97.

40. Karin M, Greten FR. NF-kappaB: linking inflammation and immunity to cancer development and progression. Nat Rev Immunol 2005; 5: 749–59.

41. Karin M. Nuclear factor-kappaB in cancer development and progression. Nature 2006; 441: 431–6.

42. Greten FR, Eckmann L, Greten TF et al. IKKbeta links inflammation and tumorigenesis in a mouse model of colitis-associated cancer. Cell 2004; 118: 285–96.

43. Pikarsky E, Porat RM, Stein I et al. NF-kappaB functions as a tumour promoter in inflammation-associated cancer. Nature 2004; 431: 461–6.

44. van Hogerlinden M, Rozell BL, Ahrlund-Richter L, Toftgard R. Squamous cell carcinomas and increased apoptosis in skin with inhibited Rel/nuclear factor-κB signaling. Cancer Res 1999; 59: 3299–303.

45. van Hogerlinden M, Auer G, Toftgard R. Inhibition of Rel/Nuclear Factor-kappaB signaling in skin results in defective DNA damage-induced cell cycle arrest and Ha-ras- and p53-independent tumor development. Oncogene 2002; 21: 4969–77.

46. Maeda S, Kamata H, Luo JL, Leffert H, Karin M. IKKβ couples hepatocyte death to cytokine-driven compensatory proliferation that promotes chemical hepatocarcinogenesis. Cell 2005; 121: 977–90.

47. Sakurai T, Maeda S, Chang L, Karin M. Loss of hepatic NF-κ B activity enhances chemical hepatocarcinogenesis through sustained c-Jun N-terminal kinase 1 activation. Proc Natl Acad Sci U S A 2006; 103: 10544–51.

48. Becker C, Fantini MC, Schramm C et al. TGF-beta suppresses tumor progression in colon cancer by inhibition of IL-6 trans-signaling. Immunity 2004; 21: 491–501.

49. Mauad TH, van Nieuwkerk CM, Dingemans KP et al. Mice with homozygous disruption of the mdr2 P glycoprotein gene. A novel animal model for studies of nonsuppurative inflammatory cholangitis and hepatocarcinogenesis. Am J Pathol 1994; 145: 1237–45.

50. Maeda S, Chang L, Li ZW et al. IKKbeta is required for prevention of apoptosis mediated by cell-bound but not by circulating TNFalpha. Immunity 2003; 19: 725–37.

51. Deng Y, Ren X, Yang L, Lin Y, Wu X. A JNK-dependent pathway is required for TNFalpha-induced apoptosis. Cell 2003; 115: 61–70.

52. Kamata H, Honda S, Maeda S et al. Reactive oxygen species promote TNFalpha-induced death and sustained JNK activation by inhibiting MAP kinase phosphatases. Cell 2005; 120: 649–61.

53. Karin M. The regulation of AP-1 activity by mitogen-activated protein kinases. J Biol Chem 1995; 270: 16483–6.

54. Pham CG, Bubici C, Zazzeroni F et al. Ferritin heavy chain upregulation by NF-kappaB inhibits

TNFalpha-induced apoptosis by suppressing reactive oxygen species. Cell 2004; 119: 529–42.

55. Chang L, Kamata H, Solinas G et al. The E3 ubiquitin ligase itch couples JNK activation to TNFalpha-induced cell death by inducing c-FLIP(L) turnover. Cell 2006; 124: 601–13.

56. Dajee M, Lazarov M, Zhang JY et al. NF-kappaB blockade and oncogenic Ras trigger invasive human epidermal neoplasia. Nature 2003; 421: 639–43.

57. Zhang JY, Green CL, Tao S, Khavari PA. NF-kappaB RelA opposes epidermal proliferation driven by TNFR1 and JNK. Genes Dev 2004; 18: 17–22.

58. Wright G, Tan B, Rosenwald A et al. A gene expression-based method to diagnose clinically distinct subgroups of diffuse large B cell lymphoma. Proc Natl Acad Sci U S A 2003; 100: 9991–6.

59. Rosenwald A, Wright G, Leroy K et al. Molecular diagnosis of primary mediastinal B cell lymphoma identifies a clinically favorable subgroup of diffuse large B cell lymphoma related to Hodgkin lymphoma. J Exp Med 2003; 198: 851–62.

60. Rosenwald A, Wright G, Chan WC et al. The use of molecular profiling to predict survival after chemotherapy for diffuse large-B-cell lymphoma. N Engl J Med 2002; 346: 1937–47.

61. Alizadeh AA, Eisen MB, Davis RE et al. Distinct types of diffuse large-B-cell lymphoma identified by gene expression profiling. Nature 2000; 403: 503–11.

62. Staudt LM. Molecular diagnosis of the hematologic cancers. N Engl J Med 2003; 348: 1777–85.

63. Staudt LM, Dave S. The biology of human lymphoid malignancies revealed by gene expression profiling. Adv Immunol 2005; 87: 163–208.

64. Davis RE, Brown KD, Siebenlist U, Staudt LM. Constitutive nuclear factor kappaB activity is required for survival of activated B cell-like diffuse large B cell lymphoma cells. J Exp Med 2001; 194: 1861–74.

65. Lam LT, Davis RE, Pierce J et al. Small molecule inhibitors of IkappaB kinase are selectively toxic for subgroups of diffuse large-B-cell lymphoma defined by gene expression profiling. Clin Cancer Res 2005; 11: 28–40.

66. Savage KJ, Monti S, Kutok JL et al. The molecular signature of mediastinal large-B-cell lymphoma differs from that of other diffuse large-B-cell lymphomas and shares features with classical Hodgkin lymphoma. Blood 2003; 102: 3871–9.

67. Bargou RC, Leng C, Krappmann D et al. High-level nuclear NF-kappa B and Oct-2 is a common feature of cultured Hodgkin/Reed-Sternberg cells. Blood 1996; 87: 4340–7.

68. Bargou RC, Emmerich F, Krappmann D et al. Constitutive nuclear factor-kappaB-RelA activation is required for proliferation and survival of Hodgkin's disease tumor cells. J Clin Invest 1997; 100: 2961–9.

69. Cabannes E, Khan G, Aillet F, Jarrett RF, Hay RT. Mutations in the IkBa gene in Hodgkin's disease suggest a tumour suppressor role for IkappaBalpha. Oncogene 1999; 18: 3063–70.

70. Emmerich F, Meiser M, Hummel M et al. Overexpression of I kappa B alpha without inhibition of NF-kappaB activity and mutations in the I kappa B alpha gene in Reed-Sternberg cells. Blood 1999; 94: 3129–34.

71. Wood KM, Roff M, Hay RT. Defective IkappaBalpha in Hodgkin cell lines with constitutively active NF-kappaB. Oncogene 1998; 16: 2131–9.

72. Mathas S, Hinz M, Anagnostopoulos I et al. Aberrantly expressed c-Jun and JunB are a hallmark of Hodgkin lymphoma cells, stimulate proliferation and synergize with NF-kappa B. EMBO J 2002; 21: 4104–13.

73. Feuerhake F, Kutok JL, Monti S et al. NFkappaB activity, function, and target-gene signatures in primary mediastinal large B-cell lymphoma and diffuse large B-cell lymphoma subtypes. Blood 2005; 106: 1392–9.

74. Ngo VN, Davis RE, Lamy L et al. A loss-of-function RNA interference screen for molecular targets in cancer. Nature 2006; 441: 106–10.

75. Klover PJ, Zimmers TA, Koniaris LG, Mooney RA. Chronic exposure to interleukin-6 causes hepatic insulin resistance in mice. Diabetes 2003; 52: 2784–9.

76. Yuan M, Konstantopoulos N, Lee J et al. Reversal of obesity- and diet-induced insulin resistance with salicylates or targeted disruption of Ikkbeta. Science 2001; 293: 1673–7.

77. Cai D, Yuan M, Frantz DF et al. Local and systemic insulin resistance resulting from hepatic activation of IKK-beta and NF-kappaB. Nat Med 2005; 11: 183–90.

78. Arkan MC, Hevener AL, Greten FR et al. IKK-beta links inflammation to obesity-induced insulin resistance. Nat Med 2005; 11: 191–8.

79. Weil R, Israel A. Deciphering the pathway from the TCR to NF-kappaB. Cell Death Differ 2006; 13: 826–33.

80. Iwasaki A, Medzhitov R. Toll-like receptor control of the adaptive immune responses. Nat Immunol 2004; 5: 987–95.

81. Akira S, Takeda K. Toll-like receptor signalling. Nat Rev Immunol 2004; 4: 499–511.

23

Roles of the JAK-STAT signaling pathways in rheumatoid arthritis

Bradley J Bloom, Sam Zwillich, Anthony Milici and Paul Changelian

Introduction • Cytokines in RA • The JAK-STAT pathway • JAK-STAT inhibition in RA • Summary and conclusions • References

INTRODUCTION

Cytokine networks are an essential component of the pathophysiology of rheumatoid arthritis (RA). They involve an extremely complex series of interactions between cytokines and their respective receptors. The receptors then signal the affected cell to produce a variety of downstream substances that cause or regulate the inflammatory response, and related processes such as cartilage degradation and bone loss or deposition. Direct inhibition of individual cytokines such as tumor necrosis factor (TNF)-α and interleukin (IL)-1 have proven to be effective strategies in the treatment of RA, and in the case of TNF, have surpassed the efficacy of all previously known therapies. However, it is possible that the simultaneous inhibition of the effects of several cytokines would create an even more effective therapeutic strategy. Of course, this would need to be done in such a way as to not produce such broad immune suppression or other effects as to significantly increase the rate or types of adverse events when compared with currently accepted therapies.

One such strategy could be to inhibit the effectors of signal transduction that several cytokines have in common. A well-known pathway whose mechanism may be amenable to this multi-cytokine blocking approach is the Janus kinase system, which includes JAK-1, JAK-2, JAK-3, and Tyk-2. In particular, the heterodimeric/trimeric receptors for the cytokines IL-2, -4, -7, -9, -15, and -21 all share a common γ chain in their structure, and signal through the JAK-1 and -3/STAT (signal transducer and activator of transcription) pathways (Figures 23.1 and 23.2). JAK-3 is uniquely associated with downstream signaling of the common γ chain, and thus, inhibition of any step in this pathway could potentially lead to blockade of the effects of these important cytokines.[1] Further, inhibition of JAK-1 would also inhibit signaling by interferon (IFN)-γ, while inhibition of JAK-2 (through reduction of IL-6 signaling) could be useful in the treatment of RA, as IL-6 is a crucial mediator of inflammatory arthritis. Tyk-2 could also be an effective target for arthritis treatment. Tyk-2 is important to the signaling of interferons and IL-s 12 and -23. Furthermore, Tyk-2 knockout (KO) mice are resistant to the development of collagen-induced arthritis (CIA).[2] However, this pathway is relatively less elucidated than the other JAKs and therapies related to Tyk-2 are just now being developed.

On the other hand, important cytokines and growth factors, such as granulocyte/macrophage colony-stimulating factor (GM-CSF), erythropoietin, and thrombopoietin, also signal through JAK-2. Thus, a broad inhibition of this kinase

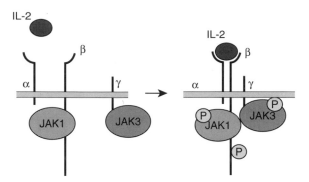

Figure 23.1 Cytokine/receptor interactions and the Janus kinases. When the JAK-related cytokines bind their respective receptors, this induces a conformational change in the receptor, leading to close association of JAKs 1 and 3, which are associated with the α and γ chains of the receptor, respectively. The JAKs then phospohorylate the receptor, enabling STAT recruitment.

could lead to significant problems with blunting of hematopoeisis.

This chapter will focus on: 1) the roles of the aforementioned cytokines in the immune response in general and RA specifically, 2) further definition of the JAK-STAT pathway and its role in cytokine signal transduction, and 3) potential strategies for blocking the effects of this pathway and its potential effects on RA disease activity.

CYTOKINES IN RA

The cytokines that effect their actions through their respective common γ chain-containing receptors, with the exception of IL-9, have been implicated to varying degrees in the pathogenesis of RA (Figure 23.2).

IL-2

IL-2 has been the subject of extensive research related to RA. IL-2 is primarily a proinflammatory cytokine which promotes the differentiation of T cells into so-called Th1 helper cells, which then also secrete IL-2. This amplified IL-2 response is among the key cytokines that activate macrophages, which in turn lead affected

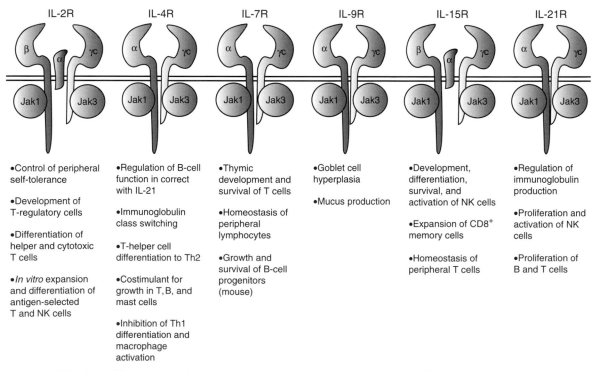

Figure 23.2 The six cytokine receptors that share a common γ chain and the downstream effects of their signaling. Reproduced with permission from Ivashkiv LB, Hu X. The JAK/STAT pathway in rheumatoid arthritis: pathogenic or protective? Arthritis Rheum 2003; 48: 2092–6.

cells such as fibroblasts and osteoclasts to cause the joint damage inherent in RA.

Indeed, strategies to inhibit the effects of IL-2 have been found to be effective in an experimental animal model, CIA, in rhesus monkeys. When daclizumab (anti-CD-25 mAb), a monoclonal antibody to the α subunit of the IL-2 receptor, was administered either prophylactically or therapeutically to these monkeys, it caused a significant decrease in clinical disease activity and markers of cartilage breakdown.[3]

In human RA, attempts have been made to correlate markers of the IL-2 pathway with disease activity. One study showed some weak correlations of serum levels of the soluble IL-2 receptor (IL-2R) with measures of disease activity, but they did not correlate with radiographic measures of joint damage.[4] A histopathologic study of rheumatoid synovium demonstrated that staining for significant amounts of IL-2R was a marker for a particular histologic finding, the presence of lymphocytic follicles, including germinal center-like structures.[5] This finding is estimated to occur in about one-third of patients with RA, and has been correlated with severe disease.

IL-15

IL-15 is presented next, as it bears great similarities in its effects to IL-2, and has homology of its β-receptor subunit in addition to the common γ chain. However, IL-15 does have some important distinctive features. First, some of its important functions may be executed by its membrane-bound form. Also, IL-15 appears to be particularly important in the maintenance of memory T cells. This observation implies that IL-15 may be key to maintenance of an immune response to recurrent and/or persistent exposure to antigen. While this is desirable in the case of microbial antigens, it is not desirable in the case of self-antigen (autoimmunity). Thus, it is possible that inhibition of IL-15 could increase the chance of deletion of memory T cells that are reactive to a putative causal self-antigen in RA. Combined with inhibiting its pleotropic IL-2-like effects on the proliferation and activation of lymphocytes, macrophages, and other cells in the joint (e.g. fibroblasts), this could provide a compelling rationale for IL-15 inhibition as a therapeutic strategy in RA.[6,7]

In fact, an initial, small open-label study of a mAb to IL-15 has been conducted. In this 12-week study, 63% of subjects achieved an ACR 20 response, 38% an ACR 50, and 20% an ACR 70. However, results must be interpreted with great caution as this study was only designed to observe safety and tolerability, and there was no placebo group for comparison.[6,8] A follow-up randomized, double-blind, placebo-controlled trial has also now been presented in abstract form. It appears to confirm the earlier response rates, although the proportion of ACR 20 responders was somewhat lower at the 14-week primary endpoint, leading to a failure to statistically separate from placebo at that time.[9] Nonetheless, the response rates seen in both studies are comparable to those seen with marketed biologic therapies for RA.

IL-4

IL-4 is classically thought of as an anti-inflammatory cytokine. It up-regulates the production of IL-1R antagonist, thus decreasing the deleterious effects of IL-1, and inhibits cartilage destruction by inhibiting TNF-induced release of metalloproteinases. Thus, it has always been theorized that IL-4 is beneficial to the treatment of RA. This, in fact, seemed to be confirmed by a study that introduced IL-4 into the joints of rats in the adjuvant-induced arthritis (AIA) model with an adenoviral vector. Whether introduced prophylactically or therapeutically, IL-4 significantly reduced joint inflammation and destruction in this model.[10]

However, there is also emerging evidence that in some ways IL-4 might promote arthritis. In one study, IL-4 was demonstrated to reduce apoptosis in synoviocytes, and thus promote synovial hyperplasia.[11] Furthermore, in another intriguing study, IL-4 KO mice did not develop the typical acute arthritis in a CIA model, but rather a chronic relapsing-remitting form of arthritis weeks later.[12]

IL-7

IL-7's primary role is to promote intra-thymic differentiation of lymphocytes and maintain the survival of peripheral naïve lymphocytes.[7] Circulating levels of IL-7 have been found to be relatively deficient in patients with active RA, and thus its role in RA has been questioned. Nonetheless, it does play potentially key roles in bone and joint physiology which implicate it in the pathogenesis of RA. For example, IL-7 also appears to play an important role in osteoclast differentiation, and thus may promote bone loss. Also, it increases activation of CD4+ T cells and monocytes/macrophages in RA synovium.[13–17]

IL-21

IL-21 is similar structurally to IL-2, -4, and -15, and is expressed by activated CD4+ T cells. It also is involved in the activation and expansion of natural killer (NK) cells and the costimulation and proliferation of B and T cells. Recently, the importance of this cytokine to promoting B-cell apoptosis has also been delineated.[18,19] Its expression is thought to be primarily limited to the immune system. The limited published studies of IL-21's role in RA to date in fact have confirmed through several independent methodologies that IL-21 is not expressed in RA synovium. However, its receptor (IL-21R) is highly expressed in the synovial lining layer. The significance of this is unclear. The authors of the aforementioned article theorize that it may play a role in excessive connective tissue deposition, as they have noted the same finding in the lungs of patients with pulmonary fibrosis and the skin of patients with systemic sclerosis. It is also unclear why IL-21 appears to be absent in the joint despite up-regulation of its receptor. It is theorized that perhaps this receptor has another ligand other than IL-21 that could be important to the development or perpetuation of RA.[20]

In short, the cytokines that signal through receptors with a common γ chain largely have effects that are already known to be essential in RA, or have begun to be implicated in RA through emerging data.

THE JAK-STAT PATHWAY

How then do these RA-related cytokines lead to the expression of other molecules key to the pathogenesis of this disease? This is through the JAK/STAT (signal transducers and activators of transcription) pathway.

In short, when the JAK-related cytokines bind their respective receptors, this induces a conformational change in the receptor, leading to close association of JAK-1 and JAK-3, which are associated with the α and γ chains of the receptor, respectively. The JAKs then phosphorylate the receptor, enabling STAT recruitment. The STATs in turn are phosphorylated, dimerize, and translocate to the nucleus, where they bind DNA and thereby regulate gene expression (Figure 23.3).

Seven distinct STAT molecules have been described. IL-4 signals primarily through STAT6, while the other common γ chain-associated cytokines signal primarily through STATs 3, 5a, and 5b. All of the other common γ chain-associated cytokines appear to regulate the expression of a similar profile of genes, although the overlap is less complete with IL-4, possibly due to its signaling through STAT6.[21]

JAK-STAT INHIBITION IN RA

We have reviewed the evidence implicating five important RA-related cytokines that act through the JAK/STAT pathway. It is thus logical that inhibition of this pathway could lead to a reduction in RA disease activity and associated joint destruction. Below we review the current direct evidence that JAK-3 and STATs are expressed in RA and that inhibition of these molecules could ameliorate this condition.

Walker et al. have recently demonstrated that in RA synovia (in this case exclusively from seropositive patients) there is a population of dendritic cells that intensely stains for JAK-3 and STATs 4 and 6. As dendritic cells are the primary antigen-presenting cells in RA and are key to perpetuation of inflammation, this further substantiates the role of JAK-3 and its signaling through STATs.[22]

It is thus reasonable to assume that inhibition of this pathway could lead to improvement of RA. It is possible that inhibition of selected STATs could be an attractive target for RA therapy. However, since the roles of the individual STATs have not been fully elucidated, and there seems to be some redundancy in signaling of proinflammatory cytokines through multiple STATs and other pathways, this may not be practical.

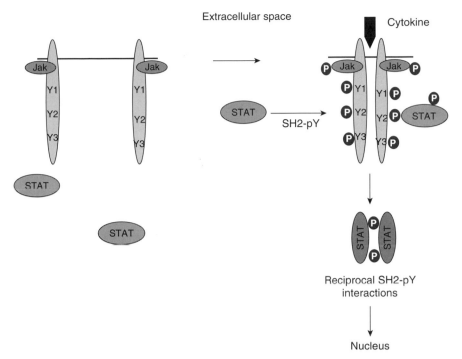

Figure 23.3 Cytokine activation of Janus-activated kinase/signal transducer and activator of transcription (JAK/STAT) pathway. Cytokine ligation and dimerization of plasma membrane receptors (shown in gray) result in activation of receptor-associated JAK kinase and phosphorylation (P) of receptor cytoplasmic domain tyrosine residues (Y1, Y2, Y3). Latent cytoplasmic STAT proteins are recruited to phosphorylated tyrosine residues via an SH2 domain-phosphotyrosine (SH2-pY) interaction. STATs are then phosphorylated on a conserved carboxy-terminus tyrosine, dimerize, and translocate to the nucleus to activate gene transcription. Reproduced with permission from Pesu M, Candotti F, Husa M et al. JaK-3 severe combined immunodeficiency, and a new class of immunosuppressive drugs. Immunol Rev, 2005; 203: 127–42.

Furthermore, some of the STATS that have been clearly implicated in RA inflammation (such as STAT3), also can be anti-inflammatory at times and it has been extremely difficult to synthesize molecules that inhibit protein–DNA interactions, the principal actions of STATs.

Agonists of proteins such as SOCS (suppressor of cytokine signaling) are also a promising strategy, as this protein is required in the activation of multiple STATs. SOCS agonists could block the proinflammatory effects of JAK-2-related cytokines such as IL-6 without having the potentially deleterious effects of direct inhibition of JAK-2 on hematopoiesis. Inhibition of JAK-3 itself could likely take care of many of the redundancies in the STAT pathway and produce a significant anti-inflammatory effect with minimal inhibition of anti-inflammatory cytokine effects.

An orally bioavailable inhibitor of JAK-3, CP-690,550 is now in clinical development. This inhibitor is effective in reducing allograft rejection in animal models of organ transplantation[23] and has been tested in two standard rodent models of RA, murine CIA and rat AIA.[24] In these latter experiments, CIA and AIA were induced in mice and rats using standard protocols and animals were dosed therapeutically with CP-690,550, up to 15 mg/kg/day, or vehicle control. Arthritis was scored clinically up to study end (28 days in mice and 14 days in rats) then animals were sacrificed and hind limbs were evaluated histologically. Serum CP-690,550 levels were determined at the time of sacrifice. CP-690,550 produced dose-dependent decreases in clinical scores in both models of RA, with ED50s of approximately 1.5 mg/kg/day. This corresponded to CP-690,550 serum levels of 5.8 ng/ml in mice (day 28) and 24 ng/ml in rats (day 14). In both RA models, all tested doses of CP-690,550 treatment resulted in a significant improvement in clinical scores, with >90% disease reduction observed at the 15 mg/kg/day dose. Histologic evidence of inflammation and joint damage was reduced by CP-690,550 in both RA models. In the CIA model, the histologically determined ED50 was approximately 6.5 mg/kg/day and in mice dosed at 15 mg/kg/day, all histologic parameters were equivalent to naïve mice.

The immunosuppressive activity of CP-690,550 was also assessed in a phase I study in 59 psoriasis patients given twice-daily doses of 5, 10, 20, 30 mg, 50 or 60 mg once daily, or placebo for 14 days.[25] All but the lowest CP-690,550 dose were associated with a significant percent reduction in modified Psoriasis Area and Severity Index on day 14. Reductions appeared to be correlated with drug exposure. CP-690,550 also improved Physician Global Assessments by 40–64% on day 14, in subject groups treated with the 20, 30, and 50 mg twice-daily doses. The medication was well tolerated. The combination of dramatic effects on an animal model of RA and a human immune-mediated disease are very preliminary, yet encouraging with regard to providing evidence for the potential promise of JAK-3 inhibition in RA. Thus, a phase 2A proof-of-concept study of CP-690,550 in patients with RA has recently been completed, with encouraging results [ref. Pending ACR abstract].

SUMMARY AND CONCLUSIONS

Available literature substantiates that an essential role for cytokine signaling is essential in the development and perpetuation of RA. Direct inhibition of single cytokines has already led to definitive improvements in the treatment of RA. It is theorized that interfering with common signaling pathways of multiple cytokines could produce at least an equally exuberant therapeutic effect. The JAK-STAT pathway is a prime example of that which could be amenable to producing such an effect. Of course, consideration must be given to the likelihood that deleterious effects could also ensue. Selective inhibition of JAK-3 in theory inhibits six cytokines important to immune regulation, five of which are felt to be implicated in the pathophysiology of RA. Use of the selective JAK-3 inhibitor, CP-690,550 has proven effective in animal models of transplantation and RA and now, preliminarily, in human psoriasis. Human arthritis studies are under way. Future study of the JAK-STAT pathway likely will provide further strategies for modulation of other steps in this pathway that may be beneficial in the treatment of rheumatoid arthritis.

REFERENCES

1. O'Shea JJ, Visconti R, Cheng TP, Gadina M. JAKs and STATs as therapeutic targets. Ann Rheum Dis 2000; 59 (Suppl 1): 115–18.
2. O'Shea JJ Targeting the Jak/STAT pathway for immunosuppression. Ann Rheum Dis 2004; 63 (Suppl 2): ii67–ii71.
3. Brok HP, Tekoppele JM, Hakimi J et al. Prophylactic and therapeutic effects of a humanized monoclonal antibody against the IL-2 receptor (daclizumab) on collagen induced arthritis (CIA) in rhesus monkeys. Clin Exp Immunol 2001; 124: 34–41.
4. Camilleri JP, Amos N, Williams BD et al. Serum soluble interleukin 2 receptor levels and radiological progression in early rheumatoid arthritis. J Rheumatol 2001; 28: 2576–8.
5. Klimiuk PA, Sierakowski S, Latosiewicz R et al. Interleukin 6, soluble interleukin-2 receptor, and soluble interleukin-6 receptor in the sera of patients with different histological patterns of rheumatoid synovitis. Clin Exp Rheumatol 2003; 21: 63–9.
6. Waldmann TA. Targeting the interleukin-15 system in rheumatoid arthritis. Arthritis Rheum 2005; 52: 2585–8.
7. Ma A, Koka R, Burkett P. Diverse functions of IL-2, IL-15, and IL-7 in lymphoid homeostasis. Annu Rev Immunol 2006; 24: 657–79.
8. Baslund B, Tvede N, Danneskiold-Samsoe B et al. Targeting interleukin-15 in patients with rheumatoid arthritis. Arthritis Rheum 2005; 52: 2686–92.
9. McInnes IMR, Zimmerman-Gorska I, Nayiager S, Baslund B, Baker N, Holloway D, Appleton B, Tsuji W. Safety and efficacy of a human monoclonal antibody to IL-15 (AMG 714) in patients with rheumatoid arthritis: results of a multi-center, randomized, double-blind, placebo-controlled trial. Ann Rheum Dis, 2006.
10. Woods JM, Katschke KJ, Volin MV et al. IL-4 adenoviral gene therapy reduces inflammation, proinflammatory cytokines, vascularization, and bony destruction in rat adjuvant-induced arthritis. J Immunol 2001; 166: 1214–22.
11. Relic B, Guicheux J, Mezin F et al. IL-4 and IL-13, but not IL-10, protect human synoviocytes from apoptosis. J Immunol 2001; 166: 2775–82.

12. Svennson L, Nandakumar KS, Johansson A, Jansson L, Holmdahl R. IL-4 deficient mice develop less acute but more chronic relapsing collagen-induced arthritis. Eur J Immunol 2002; 32: 2944–53.

13. Harada S, Yamamura M, Okamoto H et al. Production of interleukin-7 and interleukin-15 by fibroblast-like synoviocytes from patients with rheumatoid arthritis. Arthritis Rheum 1999; 42: 1508–16.

14. Ponchel F, Verburg RJ, Bingham SJ et al. Interleukin-7 deficiency in rheumatoid arthritis: consequences for therapy induced lymphopenia. Arthritis Res Ther 2005; 7: R80–92.

15. Toraldo G, Roggia C, Qian WP, Pacifici R, Weitzmann MN. IL-7 induces bone loss in vivo by induction of receptor activator of nuclear factor kappa-B ligand and tumor necrosis factor alpha from T cells. Proc Natl Acad Sci U S A 2003; 100: 125–30.

16. van Roon JAG, Glaudemans KA, Bijlsma JWJ, Lafeber FPJG. Interleukin 7 stimulates tumour necrosis factor alpha and Th1 cytokine production in joints of patients with rheumatoid arthritis. Ann Rheum Dis 2003; 62: 113–19.

17. van Roon JAG, Verweij MC, Wenting-van Wijk M et al. Increased intraarticular IL-7 in rheumatoid arthritis patients stimulates cell contact-dependent activation of CD4+ T cells and macrophages. Arthritis Rheum 2005; 52: 1700–10.

18. Mehta DS, Wurster AL, Whitters MJ et al. IL-21 induces the apoptosis of resting and activated primary B cells. J Immunol 2003; 170: 4111–18.

19. de Totero D, Meazza R, Zupo S et al. Interleukin-21 receptor (IL-21R) is up-regulated by CD40 triggering and mediates proapoptotic signals in chronic lymphocytic leukemia B cells. Blood 2006; 107: 3708–15.

20. Jungel A, Distler JH, Kurowska-Stolarska M et al. Expression of interleukin-21 receptor, but not interleukin-21, in synovial fibroblasts and synovial macrophages of patients with rheumatoid arthritis. Arthritis Rheum 2004; 50: 1468–76.

21. Kovanen PE, Rosenwald A, Fu J et al. Analysis of gamma-c family cytokine target genes. J Biol Chem 2003; 278: 5205–13.

22. Walker JG, Ahern MJ, Coleman M et al. Expression of JAK 3, STAT 1, STAT 4, and STAT 6 in inflammatory arthritis: unique JAK 3 and STAT 4 expression in dendritic cells in seropositive rheumatoid arthritis. Ann Rheum Dis 2006; 65: 149–56.

23. Changelian PS, Flanagan ME, Ball DJ et al. Prevention of organ allograft rejection by a specific janus kinase 3 inhibitor. Science 2003; 302: 875–8.

24. Milici AJ, A.L., Beckius GE, Gibbons CP, Perry BD, Fisher M, Kwansik Y, Zwillich SH, Changelian PS. Cartilage preservation by inhibition of Janus kinase 3 (JAK 3) in a murine collagen-induced arthritis (CIA) model and rat adjuvant arthritis (AA) model. Arthritis Rheum 2006. suppl.

25. Dose-dependent reduction in psoriasis severity as evidence of immunosuppressive activity of an oral JAK3 inhibitor in humans. Transplantation 2006; 82 (Suppl 2): 87.

24

Suppressor of cytokine signaling (SOCS) proteins as therapeutic targets in rheumatoid arthritis

Paul J Egan, Peter K Wong and Ian P Wicks

Introduction • SOCS proteins • SOCS-1 • SOCS-3 • Therapeutic potential of SOCS proteins for the treatment of RA • Acknowledgments • References

INTRODUCTION

Local synovial overproduction of proinflammatory cytokines appears to be a key pathogenic feature in the development of rheumatoid arthritis (RA). Cytokines such as tumor necrosis factor (TNF) and interleukin-1 (IL-1) have been shown to be important in disease progression, both in RA and in animal models of inflammatory arthritis. The central role of inflammatory cytokines in human RA has been exploited in the development of specific inhibitors which block the activity of proinflammatory cytokines by preventing binding to cognate receptors. Such agents are now widely used in the treatment of RA. However, approximately 40% of patients with RA fail to respond to treatment with TNF inhibitors, highlighting a large clinical need for new drugs. Another strategy for the development of novel therapeutics for the treatment of RA would be to target signal transduction pathways that are shared between a number of different cytokines. This approach would have the advantage of inhibiting multiple proinflammatory cytokines, potentially helping a larger proportion of patients. One family of proteins which may be useful therapeutic targets for the treatment of RA is the suppressor of cytokine signaling (SOCS) proteins.

SOCS PROTEINS

Although acute inflammatory responses induced by cytokine stimulation of cells are crucial for host defense against infection, uncontrolled inflammation can be deleterious for the host by causing tissue damage. For this reason, negative regulatory mechanisms exist to limit the extent of cytokine responses and tissue damage associated with host defense, and to return the body to normal homeostasis. One family of proteins that are involved in the negative regulation of inflammatory responses are the SOCS molecules.[1] These intracellular proteins are induced following cytokine stimulation and act in via classical negative feedbacks loop to inhibit signal transduction and control cytokine signaling. There are eight known SOCS proteins, SOCS1–7 and cytokine-inducible SH2-containing protein (CIS). SOCS proteins are characterized by a central SH2 domain and a C-terminal motif known as the SOCS box. SOCS-1 was originally identified independently by three groups through the ability to inhibit IL-6 signaling, using a screen for proteins able to bind the kinase region of Janus activated kinase (JAK)-2 and via homology of the SH2 domain to signal transducer and activator of transcription (STAT)-3.[2-4] SOCS-1 was identified as a protein that acted to negatively regulate the JAK-STAT pathway used by a number of cytokines for signal transduction. Subsequent database searches for homologous proteins identified other members of the SOCS family, as well as a range of proteins containing the SOCS box, clustered into additional protein families, including WSB proteins, which contain WD-40 repeats, SSB proteins, which contain SPRY domains, and ASB proteins, which contain ankyrin repeats.[5] However, to date these proteins, have not been shown to play a role in regulating cytokine signaling.

Initial studies on the ability of SOCS proteins to inhibit cytokine signaling reported that SOCS-1 was induced following stimulation with a wide variety of cytokines. These included cytokines that signal through the JAK-STAT pathway, including IL-2, IL-6, and interferon (IFN)-γ, as well as cytokines that utilize other signal transduction pathways, such as TNF.[2,6-8] In addition, SOCS-1 could be induced by other molecules, such as lipopolysaccharide (LPS).[9] Identification of cytokines inhibited by SOCS-1 was initially performed using *in vitro* overexpression systems. Collectively, these studies indicated that a wide variety of cytokines could be inhibited by SOCS-1, suggesting that SOCS proteins that SOCS proteins act more specifically to inhibit the activity. Subsequent experiments using SOCS-deficient mice have shown that SOCS proteins act more specifically but do inhibit the activity of a number of different cytokines.

SOCS proteins inhibit cytokine signaling in two ways (Figure 24.1). SOCS-1 and SOCS-3 inhibit the phosphorylation of STAT molecules

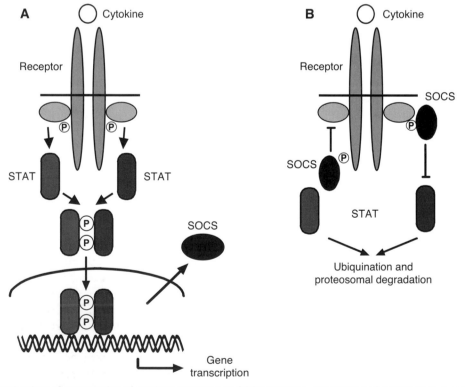

Figure 24.1 Mechanism of suppression of cytokine signaling by SOCS proteins. **(A)** Binding of cytokines to a cognate receptor initiates an intracellular signaling cascade, such as activation of the JAK-STAT signal transduction pathway. This results in transcription of target genes to bring about a biological response. Among the genes activated following cytokine signaling are *Socs1* and *Socs3*. **(B)** SOCS proteins bind to the receptor complex and inhibit STAT phosphorylation, either by binding to JAKs and inhibiting kinase activity, or by binding to the cytokine receptor itself, preventing recruitment of STATs to the receptor complex. SOCS proteins also target bound proteins for ubiquitination and proteosomal degradation via the SOCS box motif.

by activated JAKs. This can occur either through direct binding of SOCS-1 to JAKs, thereby inhibiting the catalytic domain, or by binding phosphorylated tyrosine residues on cytokine receptors, such as gp130, blocking recruitment of STAT molecules to the receptor complex. In both cases, phosphorylation of STATs is prevented, blocking translocation of activated STAT dimers to the nucleus. In addition, SOCS proteins are able to promote the degradation of bound proteins by ubiquination and proteosomal degradation.[10] This occurs through the binding of the SOCS box to elongins B and C, which are part of the E3 ubiquitin ligase complex. The SOCS box is essential for SOCS protein activity since deletion of the SOCS box from the protein results in marked loss of activity.[11]

The physiologic role of SOCS proteins has been determined by generating mice lacking individual SOCS proteins (Table 24.1). This approach has revealed strikingly different phenotypes, demonstrating that the SOCS proteins have specific and non-redundant functions *in vivo*. SOCS-1$^{-/-}$ mice are runted and die at around 2–3 weeks of age from an inflammatory syndrome in multiple organs and necrosis of the liver.[12,13] SOCS-2$^{-/-}$ mice are approximately 20% larger than their wild-type littermates due to

dysregulated growth hormone and insulin-like growth factor (IGF)-1 signaling.[14,15] Deletion of SOCS-3 results in embryonic lethality due to defects in placental development that arise as a result of defective leukemia inhibitory factor (LIF) signaling.[16,17] SOCS-4 and SOCS-5 have been implicated in the regulation of epidermal growth factor receptor signaling,[18,19] although SOCS-5$^{-/-}$ mice are phenotypically normal.[20] SOCS-6 binds to proteins associated with the insulin receptor signal transduction pathway and SOCS-6$^{-/-}$ mice were approximately 10% smaller than wild-type littermates. However, no defect in glucose homeostasis was observed in SOCS-6-deficient mice.[21] SOCS-7$^{-/-}$ mice developed mild growth retardation and approximately 50% of mice died within 15 weeks of age due to hydrocephalus. The biochemical basis for the development of hydrocephalus in the absence of SOCS-7 is not known.[22] CIS-deficient mice have been reported to have no phenotype,[16] although transgenic mice exhibit growth retardation, impairment of mammary gland development, and defects in IL-2 signaling, suggesting that CIS is involved in the regulation of STAT5 *in vivo*.[23]

Although much remains to be discovered about the physiologic roles of SOCS proteins, it is apparent that SOCS-1 and SOCS-3 are particularly active in the regulation of inflammatory responses. Mice deficient in either SOCS-1 or SOCS-3 spontaneously develop inflammation in multiple organs and eventually succumb to inflammatory syndromes. The biological functions of SOCS-1 and SOCS-3, however, are non-redundant, since the type of inflammatory responses these mice develop are different, due to regulation of a different panel of cytokines by SOCS-1 and SOCS-3, as discussed below.

SOCS-1

SOCS-1 was originally identified as an inhibitor of STAT1 phosphorylation. It is induced in response to a wide variety of stimuli, including cytokines such as IL-2, IL-4, IL-6, IL-10, granulocyte colony-stimulating factor (G-CSF), growth hormone, IFN-γ, TNF, and insulin, as well as other immunostimulatory molecules such as LPS[1]. SOCS-1 functions by binding to the catalytic

---

Table 24.1 Phenotypes of SOCS-deficient mice

Knockout	Phenotype	References
SOCS-1	Neonatal lethality due to monocytic infiltration into multiple organs, hepatocyte necrosis, and lymphopenia	12, 13
SOCS-2	Gigantism due to excessive response to growth hormone and IGF-1 signaling	14
SOCS-3	Mid-gestational lethality due to defective placental development	16, 17
SOCS-4	No knockout reported	
SOCS-5	No abnormality reported	20
SOCS-6	Mild growth retardation	21
SOCS-7	Mild growth retardation and development of hydrocephalus	22
CIS	No abnormality reported	16

domains of JAK molecules with high affinity, thereby inhibiting phosphorylation of STATs in a classical negative feedback loop.[3,4] Initial experiments designed to identify the cytokines inhibited by SOCS-1 focused on *in vitro* over-expression of SOCS-1 and as a result many cytokines were reported to be regulated by SOCS-1, including IL-2, IL-3, IL-4, IL-6, M-CSF, growth hormone, IGF-1, insulin, LIF, and ery-thropoietin.[1] Subsequent experiments, however, have established that the range of cytokines reg-ulated by SOCS-1 *in vivo* is more restricted. Data from experiments using cell lines transfected with SOCS-1 may therefore need to be re-interpreted due to possible artefacts from overexpression.

Mice deficient in SOCS-1 die within the first 2–3 weeks of age from a complex inflammatory phenotype. Lethality is associated with liver fail-ure due to leukocyte infiltration, fatty degenera-tion, and necrosis of hepatocytes. Mice also are runted, have a marked reduction in lymphoid cell development and develop inflammatory infiltrates in a variety of organs, including the lungs, skeletal muscle, pancreas, and spleen.[12,24] This syndrome was found to be dependent on dysregulated responsiveness to IFN-γ signaling, since SOCS-1$^{-/-}$ mice crossed onto an IFN-γ$^{-/-}$ background survived into adulthood without these features.[25] T cells and natural killer (NK) T cells were required as sources of IFN-γ for the development of the lethal inflammatory syndrome, since SOCS-1$^{-/-}$ RAG-2$^{-/-}$ double knockout mice remained healthy.[13] However, deficiency of SOCS-1 in T cells alone was not sufficient to induce spontaneous inflammation, since mice with a deletion of SOCS-1 specifically in T cells remained healthy.[26] In contrast, mice with deletions of SOCS-1 in both macrophages and T cells died between 7 and 30 weeks of age from splenomegaly and inflammatory infiltrates in multiple organs.[27] Liver necrosis, however, did not develop in these mice, as SOCS-1 was expressed normally in hepatocytes, resulting in normal responsiveness to IFN-γ signaling in these cells. Spontaneous inflammation in the absence of SOCS-1 is therefore dependent on both the production of IFN-γ by T cells and enhanced responsiveness to IFN-γ signaling by non-lymphoid cells.

Although SOCS-1$^{-/-}$ IFN-γ$^{-/-}$ mice survive until adulthood, long-term survival of these mice is impaired. Ageing SOCS-1$^{-/-}$ IFN-γ$^{-/-}$ mice develop inflammatory lesions in multiple organs, including the skin, gut, and lungs, and polycystic kidneys.[28] This indicates that SOCS-1 is also required for regulating signaling of other cytokines besides IFN-γ, including the cytokines that signal through the γc receptor, such as IL-2, IL-4, IL-7, IL-13, and IL-15. SOCS-1$^{-/-}$ IFN-γ$^{-/-}$ T cells showed enhanced proliferation when stimulated with IL-2 or IL-4 and prolonged STAT5 phosphorylation following stimulation with IL-2.[7,29] Since these cytokines are important in regulating T-cell development and homeosta-sis, disruption of SOCS-1-mediated cytokine signaling results in defective regulation of these processes.[26,30,31] SOCS-1 has also been shown to regulate IL-12 signaling, since SOCS-1$^{-/-}$ T cells were hyper-responsive following IL-12 stimula-tion.[32] SOCS-1 has also been shown to regulate cytokine responses mediated through other signal transduction pathways besides the JAK/ STAT pathway. These include the p38 mitogen-activated protein kinase (MAPK) pathway in response to TNF[8] and signal transduction initi-ated by binding of LPS to Toll-like receptor-4 (TLR4).[33,34] The latter occurs via the ability of SOCS-1 to induce the degradation of the TLR adaptor protein, Mal.[35]

SOCS-1 in arthritis

Development of inflammatory arthritis in either humans or animal models of the disease is a result of both local synovial inflammation in the affected joint and T-cell activation in the drain-ing lymph nodes. These processes require the involvement of multiple cell types, including macrophages, T cells, and dendritic cells and potentially require contributions from numer-ous cytokines known to be regulated by SOCS-1. We have used SOCS-1-deficient mice in a model of acute inflammatory arthritis to investigate the functions of SOCS-1 in regulating joint inflam-mation and T-cell activation *in vivo*.[36] This model is induced by intra-articular injection of methy-lated bovine serum albumin (mBSA) into the knee joints of mice, followed by daily subcutaneous injections of IL-1 over the next 3 days.[37,38] Arthritis develops in the injected knee joint and joint inflammation peaks on day 7 following the mBSA injection. This model replicates many features of human RA, including a requirement for joint macrophages, CD4[+] T-cell activation, and the production of inflammatory cytokines including TNF, GM-CSF, G-CSF, and IL-4. The model, however, is independent of B cells, CD8 T cells, and IFN-γ.[39,40] Since IFN-γ was not required for the development of disease, we were able to investigate the role of SOCS-1 in regulating inflammatory arthritis, by comparing the development of disease in SOCS-1[+/+] IFN-γ[−/−] and SOCS-1[−/−] IFN-γ[−/−] mice.

Induction of acute inflammatory arthritis in SOCS-1[−/−] IFN-γ[−/−] mice resulted in exacerbated synovial inflammation and increased joint destruction. This was characterized by an accumulation of activated macrophages and the formation of granulomas in the synovium. Activated macrophages and fibroblasts isolated from the inflamed synovium expressed a reporter gene under the control of the SOCS-1 promoter, indicating that SOCS-1 was being expressed in these cells. Significantly, synovial neutrophils and monocytes isolated following the development of arthritis had no reporter gene expression. This finding demonstrates that expression of SOCS-1 following induction of arthritis is not ubiquitous, but occurs in defined cell populations at distinct stages of activation and that SOCS-1 regulates differential responses to individual cytokines by each cell population. In wild-type mice, SOCS-1 was also localized by immunostaining to synovial granulomas and to pannus adjacent to the underlying bone, where activated macrophages accumulate. Collectively, these results show that SOCS-1 is a critical mediator of macrophage activation and that prolonged cytokine signaling in macrophages in the absence of SOCS-1 results in enhanced joint inflammation.

In addition to regulating the extent of synovial inflammation, SOCS-1 is also required to regulate T-cell activation in the draining lymph node. Following induction of acute inflammatory arthritis, SOCS-1[−/−] IFN-γ[−/−] mice developed lymphadenopathy in draining lymph nodes.

SOCS-1 reporter gene expression was also detected in activated, but not naive CD4[+] T cells. SOCS-1-deficient T cells were hyperproliferative to the immunizing antigen, mBSA, as well as to the T-cell mitogen, anti-CD3. Increased T-cell proliferation was seen in spite of the reported increase in apoptosis in SOCS-1-deficient T cells.[24]

SOCS-3

SOCS-3 is 35% homologous to SOCS-1 at the amino acid level. Like SOCS-1, SOCS-3 is induced by a wide range of cytokines, including IL-1, IL-2, IL-6, LIF, and TLR ligands. Although SOCS-3 also inhibits the JAK-STAT signaling pathway, it does this through a different mechanism to SOCS-1. Instead of binding directly to JAK molecules, SOCS-3 binds to phosphorylated tyrosine residues on activated cytokine receptors, such as gp130.[41] This prevents recruitment of STATs to the receptor complex, inhibiting the signal transduction cascade. Although SOCS-3 is homologous to SOCS-1 and also acts as a negative regulator of cytokine signaling, generation of mice lacking SOCS-3 has revealed distinct activities for SOCS-3, compared with SOCS-1, and has shown that these two molecules have non-redundant functions in vivo.

Nonspecific deletion of SOCS-3 results in mid-gestational embryonic lethality due to defective placental development.[16,17] Embryonic lethality has been shown to be due to prolonged LIF signaling, since placental development in SOCS-3[−/−] LIF[+/−] or SOCS-3[−/−] LIF[−/−] mice was normal, with mice born at expected Mendelian frequencies. Most neonatal mice, however, died shortly after birth.[42] Embryonic lethality has been overcome by using a conditional gene targeting strategy using cre recombinase and the loxP system to generate mice lacking SOCS-3 in defined tissue compartments. This has allowed the identification of the cytokines which are negatively regulated by SOCS-3 under physiological conditions in vivo. Mice lacking SOCS-3 in the liver showed prolonged STAT3 phosphorylation in hepatocytes following injection of IL-6, demonstrating that SOCS-3 negatively regulates IL-6 signaling in vivo.[43,44] IL-6 signaling occurs through the gp130 receptor, which is also shared by other cytokines, such as LIF, IL-11, IL-27, oncostatin M (OSM), ciliary neurotrophic factor (CNTF), and cardiotrophin (CT)-1, and SOCS-3 is able to regulate the signaling of these cytokines. Surprisingly, in addition to inducing IL-6-responsive genes following stimulation with IL-6, deletion of SOCS-3 also resulted in the induction of IFN-γ-responsive genes, through prolonged phosphorylation of STAT1.[43] The absence of SOCS-3 therefore results in qualitative as well as quantitative change to the response to IL-6 signaling, and results in the induction of anti-inflammatory effects that are not usually seen following IL-6 stimulation.[45] Generation of mice lacking SOCS-3 in hematopoietic and endothelial cells resulted in mice spontaneously developing neutrophilia, splenomegaly, and infiltration of neutrophils into multiple tissues. This defect was shown to be due to enhanced signaling to G-CSF, demonstrating that SOCS-3 is also required for the negative regulation of G-CSF signaling *in vivo*.[46]

SOCS-3 and arthritis

SOCS3 mRNA expression has been detected in synovial tissue taken from RA, but not osteoarthritis patients and this corresponds with increased expression of phosphorylated STAT3.[47] To evaluate the role of SOCS-3 in regulating the extent of synovial inflammation and joint destruction in animal models of inflammatory arthritis, we have used mice expressing conditional deletions of SOCS-3 in defined tissue compartments. Mice deficient in SOCS-3 in the hematopoietic and endothelial cell compartments (SOCS-3$^{-/\Delta vav}$) developed severe joint inflammation and tissue destruction following the induction of acute inflammatory arthritis.[48] Synovial inflammation was characterized by marked infiltration of neutrophils, accompanied by increased numbers of neutrophils in the bone marrow, peripheral blood, and spleen, and elevated levels of G-CSF in the serum. Since the absence of SOCS-3 results in hyper-responsiveness to G-CSF signaling, neutrophilia in mice lacking SOCS-3 was a result of both elevated levels of G-CSF produced as a result of exacerbated inflammatory arthritis and a heightened

sensitivity to G-CSF signaling. The neutrophilia seen in SOCS-3$^{-/\Delta vav}$ mice following induction of acute inflammatory arthritis did not develop in arthritic SOCS-1$^{-/-}$ IFN-γ$^{-/-}$ mice and neutrophils isolated from the synovium did not express a SOCS-1 reporter gene. In contrast, synovial granulomas, which were a prominent feature of inflammatory arthritis in SOCS-1$^{-/-}$ IFN-γ$^{-/-}$ mice, were absent in SOCS-3$^{-/\Delta vav}$ mice. This demonstrates that, although SOCS-1 and SOCS-3 are both necessary for the regulation of inflammatory arthritis, these molecules have non-redundant functions, due to regulation of different cytokines. This finding has implications for the use of SOCS proteins as therapeutic agents, since the effectiveness of SOCS proteins may depend on targeting expression to the particular cell populations that will provide the most clinical benefit.

In addition to severe synovitis, inflammatory arthritis in SOCS-3$^{-/\Delta vav}$ mice was characterized by the generation of increased numbers of osteoclasts and enhanced bone destruction. This was not seen in arthritic SOCS-1$^{-/-}$IFN-γ$^{-/-}$ mice, suggesting a specific role for endogenous SOCS-3 in the regulation of osteoclastogenesis. A potential mechanism for the enhanced osteoclastogenesis observed during joint inflammation was increased T-lymphocyte production of IL-17. IL-17 is important in the pathogenesis of bone destruction during RA by up-regulating osteoblast expression of receptor activator of NF-κB ligand (RANKL) relative to levels of the soluble decoy receptor osteoprotegerin (OPG). IL-17 also up-regulates G-CSF production by fibroblasts and endothelial cells, and elevated levels of G-CSF may promote osteoclast-mediated bone resorption. SOCS-3 has also recently been shown to regulate IL-23-mediated STAT3 phosphorylation and generation of Th cells that selectively produce IL-17 (Th17 cells).[49] Non-arthritic SOCS-3$^{-/\Delta vav}$ mice also had increased numbers of osteoclasts, with a corresponding 50% reduction in trabecular bone volume compared with wild-type littermate controls, suggesting that endogenous SOCS-3 normally inhibits osteoclastogenesis both basally and during inflammation. In contrast to our *in vivo* findings, however, overexpression of SOCS-3 in osteoclasts *in vitro* was reported to promote osteoclastogenesis, possibly via suppression of the inhibitory effects of IFN-β.[50] These findings suggest that the exact role of SOCS proteins in osteoclastogenesis remains to be determined.

There was comparatively more bone than cartilage destruction during mBSA/IL-1-induced arthritis in SOCS-3$^{-/\Delta vav}$ mice. This was not unexpected, as chondrocytes in SOCS-3$^{-/\Delta vav}$ mice expressed SOCS-3 normally, whereas osteoclasts, which are of hematopoietic lineage origin, lacked SOCS-3 following *Cre*-mediated deletion. Recent work has suggested that articular chondrocytes express SOCS-3 during inflammatory arthritis and that IL-1-induced expression of SOCS-3 may regulate IGF-1 – the major anabolic factor for cartilage homeostasis.[51] However, a more direct approach to examine the role of endogenous SOCS-3 in regulating cartilage differentiation and homeostasis will be to examine mice which have undergone chondrocyte-specific deletion of SOCS-3.

In addition to increased joint inflammation, the absence of SOCS-3 in T cells also contributed to exacerbated disease in SOCS-3$^{-/\Delta vav}$ mice. Draining lymph node T cells from arthritic SOCS-3$^{-/\Delta vav}$ mice had a marked increase in proliferation and IL-17 production following antigen-specific stimulation, and purified CD4$^+$ T cells from naive mice were hyperproliferative to anti-CD3 stimulation *in vitro*.[48] SOCS-3 has been implicated in the regulation of T-cell activation by binding to calcineurin and inhibiting activation of the transcription factor NF-AT.[52] SOCS-3 has also been reported to bind CD28 and inhibit the phosphorylation of PI3-K.[53] While SOCS-3 was expressed in naive T cells, expression was down-regulated after T-cell activation, allowing cell cycle progression.[54] In contrast, SOCS-1 was not expressed in naive T cells, but was up-regulated following activation.

THERAPEUTIC POTENTIAL OF SOCS PROTEINS FOR THE TREATMENT OF RA

Although SOCS-1 and SOCS-3 were originally thought to inhibit a wide variety of inflammatory cytokines, based on *in vitro* experiments, subsequent work using SOCS-deficient mice has shown more specific effects. Nevertheless, SOCS-1 and SOCS-3 are attractive candidates for

the development of novel therapeutic agents for the treatment of RA and other inflammatory conditions, since the cytokines regulated *in vivo* are important mediators of disease (Figure 24.2). The absence of SOCS-1 or SOCS-3 also results in marked exacerbation of joint inflammation in mouse models of RA, making a strong argument for the manipulation of SOCS proteins as a therapeutic strategy. Some issues, however, remain to be resolved. While mice lacking SOCS-1 or SOCS-3 develop exacerbated arthritis, would elevated levels of SOCS-1 or SOCS-3 in cells already expressing these proteins reduce disease? Second, since SOCS molecules are intracellular proteins, how might delivery into relevant cells within the joint be achieved?

Local delivery of SOCS-3 has been reported to be therapeutic in mouse models of inflammatory arthritis. Peri-articular injection of recombinant adenovirus expressing SOCS-3 was found to inhibit collagen-induced arthritis (CIA) in mice,[47] providing proof-of-principle evidence for locally elevated levels of SOCS proteins to treat inflammatory disease. Development and progression of CIA was inhibited for up to 50 days after injection of adenoviruses expressing SOCS-3. Of even greater clinical relevance, SOCS-3-expressing adenovirus was able to inhibit progression of established joint inflammation. *In vitro*, SOCS-3-expressing adenovirus inhibited proliferation and IL-6 production by synovial fibroblasts, providing a potential mechanism of action for the recombinant adenoviruses. Interestingly, SOCS-3-expressing adenovirus was more effective at preventing disease progression than viruses expressing a dominant negative STAT3. This suggests that SOCS-3 was not only suppressing gp130 and G-CSFR signaling (which both utilize STAT3), but was inhibiting additional signaling pathways. Furthermore, since adenoviruses are not able to efficiently infect myeloid cells, the therapeutic effect of SOCS-3-expressing adenoviruses would not have occurred via inhibition of neutrophil activity. The beneficial effects of SOCS-3 in this system were therefore most likely due to overexpression of SOCS-3 in synovial fibroblasts.

Although recombinant viruses are effective vectors for the delivery of SOCS proteins in animal models, there are numerous problems that would

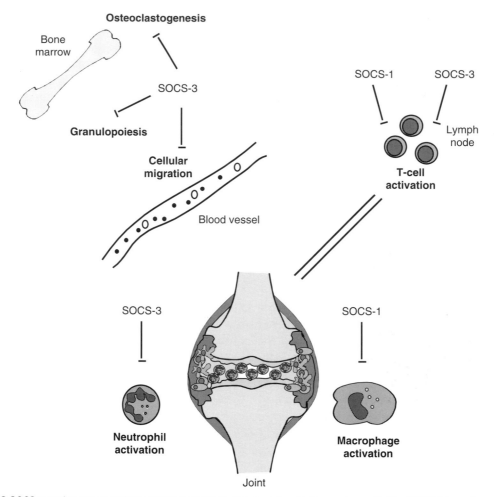

Figure 24.2 SOCS proteins act at multiple levels to regulate the severity of inflammatory arthritis. SOCS-1 is an important negative regulator of macrophage activation in the synovium. SOCS-3 regulates neutrophil production in the bone marrow, migration, and activation in the synovium. SOCS-3 also regulates the generation of osteoclasts and subsequent bone degradation following initiation of arthritis. Both SOCS-1 and SOCS-3 regulate the extent of T-cell activation in the draining lymph nodes.

need to be overcome before these agents could be used in clinical practice. These include potential issues with biosafety, stability of the vectors, and the generation of immune responses against the vectors. For this reason, alternative delivery strategies are needed. One promising approach is the generation of SOCS molecules that penetrate the cell membrane to access the intracellular compartment.[55] SOCS-3 was engineered to express a membrane-translocating motif, derived from the hydrophobic signal sequence of fibroblast growth factor 4. This resulted in a form of SOCS-3 that could be delivered into cells, while still retaining bioactivity. Remarkably, injection of cell-permeable SOCS3 could protect mice against the lethal effects of systemic inflammation induced by LPS or staphylococcal enterotoxin B, by reducing the production of inflammatory cytokines. Cell-permeable forms of SOCS proteins injected directly into arthritic joints could attenuate joint inflammation and represent a more effective delivery strategy than recombinant viruses. Another therapeutic approach that has been successfully used in a model of experimental allergic encephalomyelitis (EAE) was to use mimetic SOCS-1 peptides that could inhibit the kinase activity of JAK-2.[56] Administration of a lipopeptide based on the

SOCS-1 sequence was able to inhibit the development of EAE in mice and induce remission in mice with established disease. In addition to targeting cells at the site of inflammation, these strategies would also have the advantage of uptake by cells within the draining lymph nodes, which could inhibit the ongoing T-cell response to joint antigens, thereby further improving the efficacy of treatment.

Another possible therapeutic strategy is the use of drugs that up-regulate *in vivo* production of endogenous SOCS proteins. While there are currently few data on manipulation of SOCS expression, agonists of peroxisomal proliferator activated gamma nuclear receptor (PPAR-γ) have been shown to induce the expression of SOCS-1 and SOCS-3 mRNA *in vitro*.[57] Treatment of astrocytes and glial cells with a combination of rosiglitazone, an anti-diabetic agent, and 15-deoxy-Δ-12,14-prostaglandin J$_2$, which together are potent agonists of PPAR-γ, resulted in the induction of SOCS-1 and SOCS-3 mRNA and reduced phosphorylation of STAT1 and STAT3.[57] While the effect of drugs routinely used in the treatment of RA such as corticosteroids, methotrexate, or salazopyrine on SOCS expression is unclear, it is intriguing to speculate whether at least some of their therapeutic effect may be due to up-regulation of endogenous SOCS protein expression.

However, while manipulation of SOCS proteins may be a viable therapeutic goal for the treatment of a range of inflammatory conditions, a cautionary note is required. SOCS proteins regulate multiple signaling pathways and increased expression of SOCS proteins could result in significant side effects. While temporary overexpression of SOCS-3 had a beneficial effect on inflammatory arthritis,[47] prolonged overexpression of SOCS-3 in transgenic mice increased Th2 responses, including features of asthma in an airway hypersensitivity model.[58] These findings suggest that *in vivo* manipulation of SOCS proteins needs to be undertaken with great care and a firm understanding of SOCS biology. However, based on their ability to inhibit responses to numerous cytokines, SOCS-1 and SOCS-3 are attractive candidates for therapeutic intervention in RA and other chronic inflammatory diseases.

ACKNOWLEDGMENTS

This work was supported by the Reid Charitable Trusts, the National Health and Medical Research Council of Australia (project grant 305523), and Zenyth Therapeutics.

REFERENCES

1. Alexander WS. Suppressors of cytokine signalling (SOCS) in the immune system. Nat Rev Immunol 2002; 2: 410–16.
2. Starr R, Willson TA, Viney EM et al. A family of cytokine-inducible inhibitors of signalling. Nature 1997; 387: 917–21.
3. Endo TA, Masuhara M, Yokouchi M et al. A new protein containing an SH2 domain that inhibits JAK kinases. Nature 1997; 387: 921–4.
4. Naka T, Narazaki M, Hirata M et al. Structure and function of a new STAT-induced STAT inhibitor. Nature 1997; 387: 924–9.
5. Hilton DJ, Richardson RT, Alexander WS et al. Twenty proteins containing a C-terminal SOCS box form five structural classes. Proc Natl Acad Sci U S A 1998; 95: 114–19.
6. Sakamoto H, Yasukawa H, Masuhara M et al. A Janus kinase inhibitor, JAB, is an interferon-gamma-inducible gene and confers resistance to interferons. Blood 1998; 92: 1668–76.
7. Sporri B, Kovanen PE, Sasaki A et al. JAB/SOCS1/SSI-1 is an interleukin-2-induced inhibitor of IL-2 signalling. Blood 2001; 97: 221–6.
8. Morita Y, Naka T, Kawazoe Y et al. Signals transducers and activators of transcription (STAT)-induced STAT inhibitor-1 (SS-1)/suppressor of cytokine signalling-1 (SOCS-1) suppresses tumor necrosis factor α-induced cell death in fibroblasts. Proc Natl Acad Sci U S A 2000; 97: 5405–10.
9. Baetz A, Frey M, Heeg K et al. Suppressor of Cytokine Signalling (SOCS) proteins indirectly regulate Toll-like receptor signalling in innate immune cells. J Biol Chem 2004; 279: 54708–15.
10. Zhang JG, Farley A, Nicholson SE et al. The conserved SOCS box motif in suppressors of cytokine signaling binds to elongins B and C and may couple bound proteins to proteosomal degradation. Proc Natl Acad Sci U S A 1999; 96: 2071–6.
11. Zhang, JG, Metcalf D, Rakar S et al. The SOCS box of supressor of cytokine signaling-1 is important for inhibition of cytokine action in vivo. Proc Natl Acad Sci U S A 2001; 98: 13261–5.
12. Starr R, Metcalf D, Elefanty AG et al. Liver degeneration and lymphoid deficiencies in mice lacking suppressor of cytokine signaling-1. Proc Natl Acad Sci U S A 1998; 95: 14395–9.

13. Marine JC, Topham DJ, McKay C et al. SOCS1 deficiency causes a lymphocyte-dependent perinatal lethality. Cell 1999; 98: 609–16.

14. Metcalf D, Greenhalgh CJ, Viney EM et al. Gigantism in mice lacking suppressor of cytokine signalling-2. Nature 2000; 405: 1069–73.

15. Greenhalgh CJ, Rico-Bautista E, Lorentzon M et al. SOCS2 negatively regulates gowth hormone action in vitro and in vivo. J Clin Invest. 2005; 115: 397–406.

16. Marine JC, McKay C, Wang D et al. SOCS3 is essential in the regulation of fetal liver erythropoiesis. Cell 1999; 98: 617–27.

17. Roberts AW, Robb L, Raker S et al. Placental defects and embryonic lethality in mice lacking suppressor of cytokine signaling 3. Proc Natl Acad Sci U S A 2001; 98: 9324–9.

18. Nicholson SE, Metcalf D, Sprigg NS et al. Suppressor of cytokine signalling (SOCS)-5 is a potential negative regulator of epidermal growth factor signalling. Proc Natl Acad Sci U S A 2005; 102: 2328–33.

19. Kario E, Marmor MD, Adamsky K et al. Suppressors of cytokine signaling 4 and 5 regulate epidermal growth factor receptor signaling. J Biol Chem 2005; 280: 7038–48.

20. Brender C, Columbus R, Metcalf D et al. SOCS5 is expressed in primary B and T lymphoid cells but is dispensable for lymphocyte production and function. Mol Cell Biol 2004; 24: 6094–103.

21. Krebs DL, Uren RT, Metcalf D et al. SOCS-6 binds to insulin receptor substrate 4, and mice lacking the SOCS-6 gene exhibit mild growth retardation. Mol Cell Biol 2002; 22: 4567–78.

22. Krebs DL, Metcalf D, Merson TD et al. Development of hydrocephalus in mice lacking SOCS7. Proc Natl Acad Sci U S A 2004; 101: 15446–51.

23. Matsumoto A, Seki Y, Kubo M et al. Suppression of STAT5 functions in liver, mammary glands and T cells in cytokine-inducible SH2-containing protein 1 transgenic mice. Mol. Cell. Biol 1999; 19: 6396–407.

24. Naka T, Matsumoto T, Narazaki M et al. Accelerated apoptosis by augmented induction of Bax in SSI-1 (STAT-induced STAT inhibitor-1) deficient mice. Proc Natl Acad Sci U S A 1998; 95: 15577–82.

25. Alexander WS, Starr R, Fenner JE et al. SOCS1 is a critical inhibitor of interferon γ signalling and prevents the potentially fatal neonatal actions of this cytokine. Cell 1999; 98: 597–608.

26. Chong, MMW, Cornish AL, Darwiche R et al. Suppressor of Cytokine Signalling-1 is a critical regulator of interleukin-7-dependent CD8+ T cell differentiation. Immunity 2003; 18: 475–87.

27. Chong, MMW, Metcalf D, Jamieson E et al. Suppressor of cytokine signalling-1 in T cells and macrophages is critical for preventing lethal inflammation. Blood 2005; 2005: 1668–75.

28. Metcalf D, Mifsud S, Di Rago L et al. Polycystic kidneys and chronic inflammatory lesions are the delayed consequences of loss of the suppressor of cytokine signaling-1 (SOCS-1). Proc Natl Acad Sci U S A 2002; 99: 943–8.

29. Cornish AL, Chong MM, Davey GM et al. Suppressor of cytokine signaling-1 regulates signaling in response to interleukin-2 and γc-dependent cytokines in peripheral T cells. J Biol Chem 2003; 278: 22755–61.

30. Catlett IM, Hedrick SM. Suppressor of cytokine signaling 1 is required for the differentiation of CD4+ T cells. Nat. Immunol., 2005; 6: 715–21.

31. Davey GM, Starr R, Cornish AL et al. SOCS-1 regulates IL-15-driven homeostatic proliferation of antigen-naive CD8 T cells, limiting their autoimmune potential. J Exp Med 2005; 202: 1099–108.

32. Eyles JL, Metcalf D, Grusby MJ et al. Negative regulation of interleukin-12 signalling by suppressor of cytokine signalling-1. J Biol Chem 2002; 277: 43735–40.

33. Kinjyo I, Hanada T, Inagaki-Ohara K et al. SOCS1/JAB is a negative regulator of LPS- induced macrophage activation. Immunity 2002; 17: 583–91.

34. Nakagawa R, Naka T, Tsutsui H et al. SOCS-1 participates in negative regulation of LPS responses. Immunity 2002; 17: 677–87.

35. Mansell A, Smith R, Doyle SL et al. Suppressor of cytokine signalling 1 negatively regulates Toll-like receptor signaling by mediating Mal degradation. Nat Immunol 2006; 7: 148–55.

36. Egan PJ, Lawlor KE, Alexander WS et al. SOCS-1 regulates acute inflammatory arthritis and T cell activation. J Clin Invest 2003; 111: 915–24.

37. Staite ND, Richard KA, Aspar DG et al. Induction of an acute erosive monoarticular arthritis in mice by interleukin-1 and methylated bovine serum albumin. Arthritis Rheum 1990; 33: 253–60.

38. Lawlor KE, Campbell IK, O'Donnell K et al. Molecular and cellular mediators of interleukin-1-dependent acute inflammatory arthritis. Arthritis Rheum 2001; 44: 442–50.

39. Lawlor KE, Wong PK, Campbell IK et al. Acute CD4+ T lymphocyte-dependent interleukin-1-driven arthritis selectively requires interleukin-2 and interleukin-4, joint macrophages, granulocyte-macrophage colony stimulating factor, interleukin-6 and leukemia inhibitory factor. Arthritis Rheum 2005; 52: 3749–54.

40. Lawlor KE, Campbell IK, Metcalf D et al. Critical role for granulocyte colony-stimulating factor in inflammatory arthritis. Proc Natl Acad Sci U S A 2004; 101: 11398–403.

41. Nicholson SE, De Souza D, Fabri LJ et al. Suppressor of cytokine signalling-3 preferentially binds to the SHP-2-binding site on the shared cytokine receptor subunit gp130. Proc Natl Acad Sci U S A 2000; 97: 6493–8.

42. Robb L, Boyle K, Rakar S et al. Genetic reduction of embryonic leukemia-inhibitory factor production rescues placentation in SOCS3-null embryos but does not prevent inflammatory disease. Proc Natl Acad Sci U S A 2005; 102: 16333–8.

43. Croker BA, Krebs DL, Zhang JG et al. SOCS3 negatively regulates IL-6 signaling in vivo. Nat Immunol 2003; 4: 540–5.

44. Lang R, Pauleau A L, Parganas E et al. SOCS3 regulates the plasticity of gp130 signaling. Nat Immunol 2003; 4: 546–50.

45. Yasukawa H, Ohishi M, Mori H et al. IL-6 induces an anti-inflammatory response in the absence of SOCS3 in macrophages. Nat Immunol 2003; 4: 551–6.

46. Croker BA, Metcalf D, Robb L et al. SOCS3 is a critical physiological negative regulator of G-CSF signaling and emergency granulopoiesis. Immunity 2004; 20: 153–65.

47. Shouda T, Yoshida T, Hanada T et al. Induction of the cytokine signal regulator SOCS3/CIS3 as a therapeutic strategy for treating inflammatory arthritis. J Clin Invest 2001; 108: 1781–8.

48. Wong PKK, Egan PJ, Croker BA et al. SOCS-3 negatively regulates innate and adaptive immune mechanisms in acute IL-1-dependent inflammatory arthritis. J Clin Invest 2006; 116: 1571–81.

49. Chen Z, Laurence A, Kanno Y, et al. Selective regulatory function of SOCS3 in the formation of IL-17-secreting T cells. Proc Natl Acad Sci U S A 2006; 103: 8137–42.

50. Fox SW, Jaharul-Haque S, Lovibond AC et al. The possible role of TGF-β-induced Suppressors of Cytokine Signalling expression in osteoclast/macrophage lineage commitment in vitro. J Immunol 2003; 170: 3679–87.

51. Smeets RL, Veenbergen S, Arntz OJ et al. A novel role for suppressor of cytokine signalling 3 in cartilage destruction via induction of chondrocyte desensitization toward insulin-like growth factor. Arthritis Rheum 2006; 54: 1518–28.

52. Banerjee A, Banks AS, Nawijn MC et al. Suppressor of cytokine signaling 3 inhibits activation of NFATp. J Immunol 2002; 168: 4277–81.

53. Matsumoto A, Seki Y, Watanabe R et al. A role of suppressor of cytokine signaling 3 (SOCS3/CIS3/SSI3) in CD28-mediated interleukin 2 production. J Exp Med 2003; 197: 425–36.

54. Yu CR, Mahdi RM, Ebong S et al. Suppressor of cytokine signalling 3 regulates proliferation and activation of T-helper cells. J Biol Chem 2003; 278: 29752–9.

55. Jo D, Liu D, Yao S et al. Intracellular protein therapy with SOCS3 inhibits inflammation and apoptosis. Nat Med 2005; 8: 892–8.

56. Mujtaba MG, Flowers LO, Patel CB et al. Treatment of mice with the Suppressor of Cytokine Signaling-1 mimetic peptide, Tyrosine Kinase Inhibitor Peptide, prevents development of the acute form of experimental allergic encephalomyelitis and induces stable remission in the chronic relapsing/remitting form. J Immunol 2005; 175: 5077–86.

57. Park EJ, Park SY, Joe EH et al. 15d-PGJ2 and rosiglitazone suppress janus kinase-STAT inflammatory signalling through induction of suppressor of cytokine signalling 1 (SOCS1) and SOCS3 in glia. J Biol Chem 2003; 278: 14747–52.

58. Seki Y, Inoue H, Nagata N et al. SOCS-3 regulates onset and maintenance of TH2-mediated allergic responses. Nat Med 2003; 9: 1047–54.

25

Wnt signaling for targeted therapies in rheumatology

Kathleen T Rousche, Dolores Baksh and Rocky S Tuan

Wnt signaling pathways • Degenerative joint diseases • Wnt signaling in RA and OA • Current treatments for RA and OA • Conclusions • Acknowledgments • References

WNT SIGNALING PATHWAYS

Canonical Wnt signaling

The Wnt and Frizzled (Fz) gene families of signaling molecules were first discovered and characterized in *Drosophila*. Studies in the past several years have revealed the involvement of Wnt signaling in a number of different mammalian systems, influencing the developmental potential of a diverse pool of cells in these organisms.[1,2] Specifically, Wnt signaling has been shown to be a key regulator in stem cell renewal and differentiation.[3,4] For example, targeted disruption of Wnt signaling by loss of function mutation(s) or overexpression of components of the pathway are linked to dramatic phenotypes, as we have recently shown in mesenchymal stem cells (MSCs).[5,6]

Over 19 members of the Wnt family have been identified in mammals and, depending on the specific Wnt, signaling may proceed via canonical and/or non-canonical Wnt pathways[7,8] (Figure 25.1). Canonical Wnt signaling involves the binding of a Wnt ligand to a Fz receptor, and to the Wnt co-receptor, low-density lipoprotein-related protein 5 (LRP5) (Figure 25.1A). The binding of these components activates the cytoplasmic protein Disheveled (Dvl), leading to an inhibition of phosphorylation of β-catenin by glycogen synthase kinase-3β (GSK-β). β-Catenin is stabilized and subsequently translocates to the nucleus, where it binds with members of the T-cell factor (TCF) and lymphoid enhancer factor (LEF) transcription factor families, resulting in the enhanced expression of target genes, such as c-myc and cyclin D1.[9] In the absence of a Wnt ligand, β-catenin is phosphorylated by GSK-3β, in association with axin and adenomatous polyposis coli (APC), thus targeting β-catenin for ubiquitinylation and subsequent degradation by proteasomes.[1]

Non-canonical Wnt signaling

Early studies focusing on non-canonical Wnt signaling in *Drosophila* showed that Wnts, acting independently of β-catenin, were necessary to establish planar cell polarity (PCP), which is critical to embryonic axis development and convergent extension.[10–12] Vertebrates utilize a parallel pathway to that found in *Drosophila*, known as the Wnt/JNK (c-Jun N-terminal kinase) pathway that also regulates proper cell orientation and movements during gastrulation. In the PCP or Wnt/JNK pathway, signaling occurs via Dvl and progresses through activation of small GTPases, such as rac and rho, to JNK (Figure 25.1B). An additional non-canonical Wnt pathway is the Wnt/Ca^{2+} (calcium) pathway, in which intracellular Ca^{2+} is released, likely in a G protein-dependent manner, leading to the activation of

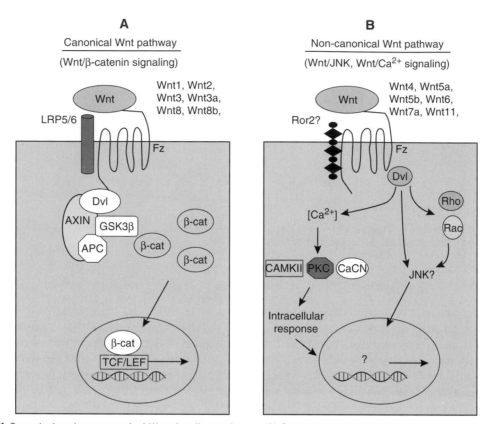

Figure 25.1 Canonical and non-canonical Wnt signaling pathways. (A) Canonical Wnt signaling is initiated following binding of Wnt to a specific Fz receptor and the Wnt co-receptor, LRP5/6. Receptor binding activates Dvl, leading to stabilization and subsequent translocation to the nucleus, and signaling proceeds following binding to TCF/LEF families of transcription factor members. (B) In vertebrates, non-canonical Wnt signaling occurs through the Wnt/Ca^{2+} or the Wnt/JNK pathway. In the Wnt/Ca^{2+} pathways, receptor binding is followed by an increase in intracellular Ca^{2+}, which leads to the activation of Ca^{2+}-sensitive enzymes and subsequent cellular response. In the Wnt/JNK pathway, signaling occurs via Dvl, and progresses through activation of small GTPases to JNK.

the Ca^{2+}-sensitive enzymes protein kinase C (PKC), Ca^{2+}-calmodulin-dependent kinase II (CAMKII), and calcineurin (CaCN).[13,14] The non-canonical Wnts, Wnt-4, -5A, and -11 activate the Wnt/Ca^{2+} pathway.[12] Non-canonical Wnt signaling also is initiated following the binding of a Wnt ligand to a Fz receptor, and recent evidence implicates the receptor orphan tyrosine kinase receptor (R or Z) as a potential co-receptor in this pathway.[15]

Activation of either the canonical or non-canonical Wnt pathway is dependent on the specific Wnt/Fz receptor combination, as well as the involvement of soluble Wnt mediators. Wnt inhibitory factor, secreted Fz-related proteins

(sFRPs), and dickkopfs (DKKs) are among the proteins that modulate Wnt signaling.[16] sFRPs share the CRD, or Wnt binding site of the Fzs, but lack the membrane-spanning segment, and thus have the capacity to act as potent Wnt inhibitors by blocking Wnt/Fz interaction. It is speculated that sFRPs may also serve a protective role by binding to Wnts and preventing their degradation. DKKs inhibit canonical Wnt signaling by binding to the LRP co-receptor.[17]

There is considerable interest in investigating the cross-talk between the canonical and non-canonical Wnt signaling pathways. In general, the pathways appear to antagonize one another, although certain Wnts are involved in both canonical and non-canonical signaling. A delicate balance of Wnts, and their receptors and mediators, is most likely responsible for controlling various cellular events, such as proliferation, cell fate decision, and differentiation, in which Wnts have been implicated in healthy and diseased states.

DEGENERATIVE JOINT DISEASES

Two of the most prevalent degenerative joint diseases in humans are rheumatoid arthritis (RA) and osteoarthritis (OA); affecting approximately 30 million people who are over 35 years of age.[18] Both diseases affect primarily the diarthrodial joints, and although the etiologies are significantly different, the end result consists of loss of joint mobility due to articular cartilage damage and pathogenic changes in the underlying bone.[17,18] RA and OA both affect the entire joint, including the cartilage, synovium, and bone. Although the two diseases progress differently with regard to the primary cell type involved, there is shared release of mediators implicated in joint destruction. Proinflammatory cytokines, including tumor necrosis factor (TNF)-α and interleukin (IL)-1β, along with matrix metalloproteinases (MMPs), are up-regulated in both RA and OA, and play major roles in tissue damage. Recent studies have implicated the Wnt proteins in the etiology of RA and OA. This is not surprising, as Wnts are critical to formation of the skeleton during embryonic development and are implicated in the regulation of adult bone homeostasis. It is interesting to speculate that aberrant Wnt and cytokine signaling may act synergistically in the compromised joint to potentiate disease progression. To date, the treatments for RA and OA are limited, and the development of suitable targeted therapies is greatly needed.

Rheumatoid arthritis

RA is considered to be a systemic inflammatory disease that affects 0.5–1% of the US population.[19] The disease is characterized by pathological changes in the synovium, which include inflammation of blood vessels in the joint cavity, followed by edema, and infiltration of inflammatory cells (e.g. macrophages, dendritic cells) into the synovium, where they coordinate antigen presentation and the induction of immune responses, leading to hyperplasia of the synovial lining and development of the pannus. In this cascade of disease onset, RA synovial cells, otherwise called fibroblast-like synoviocytes (FLSs), have been shown to play a central role in the progression of the disease through their uncontrolled proliferation, promotion of angiogenesis, and degradation of the cartilage extracellular matrix (ECM) macromolecules (e.g. collagen type II). The definitive cause of RA is not known, but it is likely that the anatomical and physiological features of diarthrodial joints render them targets of RA.

Role of fibroblast-like synoviocytes in RA

A great deal of knowledge has been gained with respect to the mediators of RA pathogenesis; however, the molecular mechanisms regulating and promoting sustained synovial hyperplasia and inflammation in RA have not been clearly elucidated. Much attention has been placed on FLSs in this regard, as these cells have been shown to be prevalent in the diseased area.[20] During disease onset and progression, the FLS population undergoes a proliferative phase and produces abnormal amounts of cytokines and chemokines such as IL-1β, IL-8, IL-15, and stromal-derived factor-1 (SDF-1), which can promote infiltration and activation of lymphocytes in the synovium, causing undesirable immune responses. Additionally, RA FLSs synthesize ECM proteins, including fibronectin and vascular endothelial molecules, such as VCAM-1, which can also facilitate lymphocyte recruitment and retention. RA FLSs also produce MMP enzyme precursors, such as pro-MMP3, that when activated may contribute to cartilage destruction by degrading ECM components, including collagens, gelatins, fibronectin, laminin, and proteoglycans.[21]

Osteoarthritis

OA, the most common form of arthritis, annually affects millions of people worldwide,[22] and is the leading cause of loss of mobility in the elderly.[23] OA is characterized by articular cartilage damage, loss of joint space, joint pain and stiffness, bony remodeling, and episodic local synovial inflammation.[18,23] One distinguishing feature that separates OA from other arthropathies is the presence of osteophytes in the joint. Osteophytes are indicative of new cartilage and bone development, and arise from either perichondrial progenitor cells or cells at the interface between the cartilage and the synovium.[24] This is of interest from a therapeutic perspective, as it supports the potential use of progenitor cells as a means to repair the damaged cartilage in OA. The risk factors for OA include age, obesity, and previous joint injury or surgery. In those affected, mechanical factors that may contribute to disease progression include misalignment, muscle weakness, or altered structural integrity of the joint.[23,25] There is no cure for OA and, in the latter stages, total joint replacement remains the treatment of choice for this widespread degenerative joint disease.

Role of chondrocytes in OA

Articular cartilage is the load-bearing tissue of the diarthrodial joints. It is composed of chondrocytes, which are responsible for the production of the ECM components essential for tissue integrity. While aberrant biochemical forces acting on the joint are the most common initiating factor in OA, the subsequent cellular response is what leads to the cartilage degradation that ensues. During OA, there is an imbalance between synthesis and degradation of matrix components by the chondrocytes. Cartilage degradation in OA is characterized by a two-phase response of the chondrocytes: a biosynthetic phase in which the chondrocytes secrete macromolecules in an effort to repair the tissue, and a degradative phase, where repair attempts fail and catabolic cytokines contribute to further matrix degradation and cartilage damage.[24] In OA, IL-1, TNF-α, IL-17, and IL-18 are produced by the chondrocytes and the synovium, resulting in increased MMP production and decreased synthesis of ECM components and MMP inhibitors. This in turn leads to the expression of other catabolic mediators such as proteases, chemokines, nitric oxide (NO), and prostaglandins that may contribute to further matrix degradation and apoptosis.[24,26]

WNT SIGNALING IN RA AND OA

Since Wnt proteins play a critical role in regulating chondrogenesis and limb development,[27,28] it is speculated that they may be involved in the pathogenesis of RA and OA. During tissue remodeling in the compromised joint, certain aspects of cartilage development are recapitulated, such as cell proliferation and synthesis of ECM components.[29] While the exact role(s) of Wnt signaling in the maintenance and destruction of cartilage observed in RA and OA remains largely unknown, recent studies have focused on mapping the expression pattern for the assignment of involvement of Wnts and their signaling components in pathogenesis.

In a study by Sen et al.,[30] Wnt1, Wnt5a, Wnt10b, Wnt11, Wnt13, and Fz2, Fz5, and Fz7 were found to be expressed in the synovial tissue harvested from OA patients. Similar expression levels were found in the synovium from RA patients, with the exception that Wnt5a and Fz5 were expressed in much higher levels in the RA synovium.[30] Another comprehensive analysis of Wnts in RA and OA tissues was also recently conducted by Nakamura et al.[18] Among the Wnts detected, Wnt7b mRNA and protein levels were up-regulated in the articular cartilage, bone, and synovium of RA and OA samples, and in the osteophytes of the OA tissue, compared with normal tissues. Wnt10b mRNA levels were also increased in RA and OA tissues.[18] Imai et al.[31] made a similar observation, noting that Wnt10b was most frequently expressed in RA synovium. Activation of the canonical pathway was suspected, as β-catenin levels were increased in Wnt10b-positive synovial fibroblasts. Furthermore, membrane-type MMP-1 (MT-MMP1), a cartilage degradation enzyme, was also expressed in these cells, as well as the pannus, and shown to be up-regulated in response to exogenous expression of Wnt10b.[31] In hMSCs, Wnt3a was shown to act through β-catenin to induce increases in MT-MMP1 expression.[32] Wnt 10b levels in synovial fibroblasts directly correlated with inflammatory cell infiltration, suggesting a possible role in the inflammatory events of RA.[31]

Recent studies have focused on the genetic basis of susceptibility to OA, and an association to the Fz-related protein gene, FRZB, has been identified.[33–35] The FRZB gene encodes for sFRP3, a known Wnt signaling antagonist, and functional FRZB variants have been identified that result from single nucleotide polymorphisms at highly conserved arginine residues and exhibit diminished capacity to effectively antagonize Wnt signaling.[34] sFRP3 is expressed in adult articular chondrocytes and appears to be involved in chondrocyte maturation,[36] and reduced sFRP3 activity may contribute to cartilage degradation in OA. sFRP1, sFRP3, and sFRP4 were shown to be expressed in both RA and OA tissues by Ijiri et al.,[37] but their expression levels were not significantly different from one another. In contrast, Imai et al.[31] reported elevated expression of sFRP1, sFRP3, and sFRP4 in OA versus RA synovium. Nakamura et al.[18] also reported a down-regulation of sFRP3 in OA synovium and cartilage, and in RA cartilage. sFRP-4 has been shown by James et al.[38] to be expressed at higher levels in OA cartilage compared with normal cartilage, and positive TUNEL staining in the same tissue sections suggested a potential role in apoptosis.

Although the results concerning expression of Wnts and their mediators in arthritic tissues in the studies described above are not in full agreement, a role for Wnt signaling components in disease progression is clearly indicated. The heterogeneity of the diseases and tissue types analyzed may explain the conflicting results, and it is likely that Wnt pathway activation is dependent on the stage of tissue degradation and disease progression.

Wnt pathway cross-talk in RA and OA

Given the central role that the inflammatory cytokines and growth factors play in joint development and the progression of RA and OA, many studies have focused on identifying how Wnt signaling may intersect with other signaling pathways implicated in joint destruction.

Wnts and cytokines, growth factors, and chemokines

Under normal conditions, chondrocytes express low levels of β-catenin.[39] However, β-catenin levels have been shown to be increased in OA and RA cartilage, and to contribute to the IL-1β-induced increase in cyclooxygenase-2 expression in chondrocytes.[40] Hwang et al.[41] showed that IL-1β induces the expression of Wnt5a and Wnt7a in cultured articular chondrocytes, concomitant with an increase in Wnt/β-catenin signaling. In particular, these studies showed that Wnt7a induced the dedifferentiation of chondrocytes by stimulation of β-catenin transcriptional activity, as observed by the inhibition of collagen type II expression. Transcriptional activity suppression using dominant-negative (dn) TCF-4 abolished this Wnt7a-induced dedifferentiation effect.[42] These results corroborate with those of Tufan et al.,[43,44] who showed that Wnt7a inhibits chondrogenesis both *in vivo* and *in vitro* via the sustained expression of N-cadherin and β-catenin induced by Wnt7a. Recent findings also suggest that the stimulation of β-catenin signaling accelerates the expression of collagen type X in chondrocytes, a marker of chondrocyte hypertrophy that is often associated with a related decrease in collagen type II expression.[42,45]

In RA tissues with increased levels of Wnt7b or in normal synovial cells transfected with Wnt7b, levels of TNF-α, IL-1β, and IL-6 were significantly increased, suggesting that Wnt7b may be involved in the pathogenesis of RA.[18] TNF-α has been shown to be up-regulated by Wnt10b in gastric carcinoma cells, and Wnts have been shown to stimulate IL-8 expression in human hepatocytes.[46] Results from a recent study provide evidence for the activation of the non-canonical Wnt signaling pathway by IL-1β. IL-1β treatment of articular chondrocytes resulted in the up-regulation of Wnt5a and down-regulation of Wnt11 expression. Chondrocytes treated with Wnt5a- and Wnt11-conditioned medium were also shown to have decreased and increased collagen type II expression, respectively. This observation of opposing Wnts effects is of interest, given the fact that both Wnt5a and Wnt11 are classified as non-canonical Wnts.

Interactions of transforming growth factor (TGF)-β, bone morphogenetic protein (BMP), fibroblast growth factor (FGF), and Wnt signaling pathways have been shown to be crucial in vertebrate limb development. The induction of DKK-1, a known Wnt antagonist, by BMP and FGF during limb development has been reported and may be mediated by Wnt ligands.[47]

TGF-β and Wnts share similar patterns of expression during various developmental events, and Wnt5a has been shown to mediate the chondro-stimulatory effects of TGF-β3.[48] In limb-bud mesenchyme and a chondrogenic cell line, canonical Wnt signaling was shown to inhibit chondrogenesis by interfering with BMP-2-induced expression of collagen type II and aggrecan through Twist1, a canonical transcription repressor.[49] In contrast, the overexpression of Wnt3a, a canonical Wnt, in C3H10T1/2 cells enhanced BMP-2-regulated chondrogenesis.[50] BMPs and TGF-β activation of canonical Wnt signaling also has been reported, with BMP-2 inducing Wnt1 and Wnt3a expression in C3H10T1/2 cells[51] and increasing Lef1 mRNA expression in C2C12 cells.[52] Smad 4 has been shown to interact indirectly with β-catenin,[50] and Smad 3 and Smad 4 directly with LEF1/TCF proteins in the nucleus to regulate gene expression.[53,54] TGF-β and Wnts can act together to enhance LEF1 transcriptional activity,[55] and have also been shown to have a synergistic effect on hMSC chondrogenic differentiation.[50,56,57]

During OA, significant levels of IGF-1, TGF-β, and BMPs are expressed in the joint, and likely act simultaneously with cytokines during attempts at cartilage remodeling and degradation. In articular chondrocytes, IL-1β and IL-6 have been shown to differentially regulate TGF-β synthesis.[58] TGF-β1 has been shown to inhibit IL-1β-induced cartilage degradation,[59] and both IGF-1 and osteogenic protein-1, a BMP family member, suppress IL-1β-induced MMP expression.[60] The present knowledge of the intimate relationship between Wnts and cytokines coupled with cytokine/growth factor interactions supports evidence for cross-talk among the Wnt, cytokine, and growth factor families of signaling proteins.

Wnts have been shown to stimulate the release of chemokines through β-catenin.[46] Chemokines closely resemble cytokines, and their role in the pathogenesis of RA and OA is under active investigation. Chemokines are highly expressed in RA, are produced by chondrocytes, and can stimulate the release of MMPs, leading to matrix degradation.[26,61] A recent study comparing FLSs derived from patients with OA and RA showed that the cells had nearly the same expression pattern for cytokines/chemokines and their receptors.[62] In RA, chemokines are associated with infiltration of immune cells into the joint, whereas in OA, chemokines may alter chondrocyte metabolism.[61] RA patients treated with a chemokine blocker have shown improvement over a 2-week period. The potential therapeutic application of blocking chemokine interaction with their receptors is currently under investigation. Chemokine machinery is present in normal and OA chondrocytes, but its involvement in OA is not well understood. Given that chemokines stimulate the release of MMPs, consistent with a role in joint tissue degradation under pathological conditions, the potential application of chemokine blockade is intriguing.[26,61]

These studies provide further evidence that the nature and regulation of cellular responses in joint tissues are dependent on the repertoire and levels of growth factors, Wnts, cyto/chemokines, and receptors expressed at a given time in the tissue. These findings support the notion that in the diseased joint, active tissue remodeling results from cellular responses mediated via several signaling pathways. Specifically, aberrant Wnt signaling may act to alter chondrocyte differentiation status, leading to matrix degradation and the onset of arthritis. Thus, modulation of Wnt signaling in response to cytokines, chemokines, and growth factors may lead to pathological changes in cartilage, representing potential cross-talk between the classical mediators of RA and OA and Wnt signaling (Figure 25.2).

Wnts and activation of downstream signaling pathways

Mitogen-activated protein kinase (MAPK), nuclear factor kappa B (NF-κB), and activating protein 1 (AP-1) are key intracellular signaling pathways that have been shown to be involved in cellular responses during development, normal tissue homeostasis, or tissue remodeling in the diseased state. Understanding which downstream targets are activated by Wnts and other signaling molecules is crucial to identifying points of pathway cross-talk. In human articular chondrocytes, JNK and p38 kinase pathways are activated in response to IL-1β and TNF-α.[63]

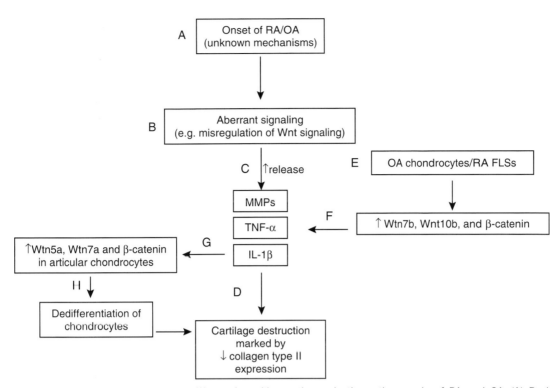

Figure 25.2 Potential interactions between Wnt and cytokine pathways in the pathogenesis of RA and OA. (A) During the progression of RA and OA, there is an up-regulation of inflammatory cytokines and select Wnt signaling molecules that leads to activation of downstream signaling pathways. (B) Aberrant signaling in either case may lead to cartilage destruction, resulting in loss of joint mobility and pathogenic changes to the bone. (C) In both RA and OA, there is shared release of IL-1β and TNF-α and MMPs, which may ultimately (D) lead to ECM degradation and cartilage damage. (E) OA chondrocytes and RA FLSs exhibit (F) increased levels of Wnt7b, Wnt10b, and β-catenin, which may lead to proinflammatory cytokine and MMP release. (G) IL-1β has been shown to induce Wnt5a and Wnt7a expression in articular chondrocytes, concomitant with an increase in β-catenin signaling which may (H) lead to chondrocyte dedifferentiation.

IL-1β- and TNF-α-induced MMP expression is regulated by JNK[64–66] and p38 kinase activity,[66,67] and regulation of MMP gene expression through PKC has also been reported.[68]

TGF-β activation of the MAPK signaling cascade promotes cartilage-specific gene expression. TGF-β-mediated MAPK signaling was shown to control Wnt7a gene expression and canonical Wnt signaling that is thought to regulate N-cadherin expression and cell adhesion during chondrogenesis of adult MSCs.[57] Wnt5a was found to mediate, through PKC-α and p38 MAPK activation, the chondrogenic effects of TGF-β3 on embryonic chick limb mesenchymal cells.[48] Hwang et al.[69] reported that Wnt3a induces chondrocyte dedifferentiation of MSCs through the β-catenin pathway and activation of

the AP-1 pathway. The dedifferentiation effect was a result of suppression of Sox-9, a major transcriptional regulator of collagen type II expression. In articular chondrocytes, IL-1β induced up- and down-regulation of Wnt 5a and Wnt11, respectively, and decreased and increased synthesis of ECM molecules. Furthermore, different signaling pathways were activated – Wnt5a activated JNK and Wnt 11 activated PKC – suggesting cartilage degradative and protective roles, respectively, for these non-canonical Wnts.[70]

NF-kB signaling has been shown to regulate chondrocyte apoptosis, a key event in cartilage degradation.[71] The activation of the NF-κB pathway is one of the key signaling pathways implicated in rheumatic diseases. Several reports have indicated that the activation of the transcriptional activator NF-κB in FLSs is a major inducer of proinflammatory cytokines, such as IL-1β and TNF-α[24,72] (Figure 25.2). However, the precise molecular mechanisms involving NF-κB activation leading to the activated phenotype of FLS in the rheumatoid joint has not been defined clearly. It has been reported recently that elevated signaling mediated by Wnt-Fz homologs in adult tissues is associated with various forms of proliferative disorders.[2] It is therefore plausible that activation of kinases, transcription factors, and cell growth/differentiation factors via the Wnt signaling pathway may direct changes in cell behavior in RA and OA pathogenesis. The concept is supported in part by the observations that several Wnt proteins and Fz receptors are highly expressed in synovial tissue of arthritic cartilage,[30] and the fact that Wnt inducible secreted protein 2 (WISP2) mRNA is detected at higher levels in RA synovium than in normal tissue.[73] It has been shown that Wnt5a signals through the PKC signaling pathway, and that the activation of PKC leads to NF-kB activation, resulting in the up-regulation of IL-6, IL-8, and IL-15.[30] In RA FLSs, overexpression of Wnt5a results in elevated IL-6, IL-8, and IL-15 secretion, suggesting that Wnt5a cross-talks with the NF-κB pathway via PKC, leading to secretion of proinflammatory cytokines.

Other mediators may also contribute to this cross-talk. That Wnt5a and Fz5 likely function as a ligand–receptor pair[74] and the fact that RA FLSs expressed high levels of Fz5 suggest that Wnt5a–Fz5 coupling activates RA FLSs, resulting in the secretion of proinflammatory cytokines.[75] In support, inhibition of the Wnt5a and Fz5 significantly decreased IL-6 and IL-15 expression in RA FLSs.[75] Sen et al.[76] showed that transfection of normal FLSs with Wnt1, a canonical Wnt, significantly up-regulated β-catenin-TCF/LEF activity, which led to the expression of pro-MMP-3. MMPs in their mature form enhance cartilage degradation by promoting the invasion of FLSs into cartilage.[77] Interestingly, transfection of RA FLSs with dnTCF-4 and sFRP-1 to antagonize canonical Wnt signaling down-regulated proMMP3. Therefore, constitutive Wnt signaling in FLSs may play a central role in the pathogenesis of RA.

CURRENT TREATMENTS FOR RA AND OA

Classically, RA and OA have been defined as inflammatory and degenerative joint diseases, respectively, and due to the nature of the differences in disease progression, treatment modalities for each have not significantly overlapped. Elucidation of the inflammatory events involved in RA has led to the development of several therapeutic treatments for RA – most of which target a single proinflammatory cytokine to slow disease progression, such as TNF-α or IL1-β – in particular anti-TNF-α agents and IL1-β receptor antagonists.[78,79] In addition, chemokine/chemokine receptor blocking agents are under clinical investigation for the treatment of RA.

For OA patients, non-pharmacological and pharmacological treatments are available for disease management, and focus primarily on treating the symptoms of OA. Current surgical procedures are aimed at lessening pain and restoring joint function, and total joint replacement remains the final treatment choice. There are no approved disease-modifying OA drugs that would concentrate on reversing cartilage destruction and promoting tissue regrowth. Although the initiating step in OA is often a biochemical agent or physical impact on the joint, the progression of the disease is regulated by the response of the chondrocyte – an up-regulation of proinflammatory cytokines that ultimately leads to cartilage destruction. Thus, even though RA progression is primarily through the FLSs, since RA and OA share common inflammatory mediators that lead to joint destruction, the use of therapies that share overlapping characteristics is feasible. Studies are underway to identify potential therapeutic targets for biological therapy for OA[79] that are similar to treatment strategies used for RA. Although cytokines and chemokines have been targeted, no specific therapy for the management of OA is accepted to date. Unfortunately, even with the treatments available for RA today, only 40% of patients respond to current therapies,[31] with the majority still exhibiting symptoms of RA. Thus, it appears that targeting a single cytokine may not be sufficient to effectively treat RA or OA, and that the development of new therapies is critical to the restoration of joint function and quality of life for those afflicted.

Wnt signaling pathway as a target for the development of therapeutic agents for RA and OA

Even with the therapeutic options targeting cytokines that have become available for the treatment of RA and are in the early trial stages for OA, there are currently no approved drugs that specifically target the cell types involved, i.e. chondrocytes and FLSs. From the evidence presented herein, showing enhanced Wnt activity in FLSs and chondrocytes during disease progression, strategic therapies targeting the Wnt signaling pathway may be an attractive alternative or adjunct to cytokine therapy.

Wnt binding to its cell surface receptor activates intracellular signaling cascades that may directly or indirectly result in one of a number of cellular responses, including cytokine/chemokine secretion, expression of MMPs, synthesis of matrix molecules, and regulation of growth factor responses. Thus, therapeutic intervention of joint destruction during RA and OA may be introduced at one or multiple steps in the Wnt signaling cascade.

Extracellular therapeutics may involve the systemic or intra-articular administration of soluble small molecules, including Wnt signaling antagonists such as sFRPs, receptor antagonists, or neutralizing antibodies may be used to inhibit Wnt binding to its Fz receptor. This would thereby prevent initiation of the Wnt signaling cascade and activation of the downstream signaling cascades that result in the expression of mediators of inflammation and cartilage degradation. Intracellular therapeutics may target the inhibition of Wnts and their receptors directly through the use of antisense oligonucleotides or siRNAs, or indirectly by interference of specific intermediates of Wnt signaling, such as β-catenin, and TCF/LEF transcription factors. Gene therapy using dominant-negative constructs, such as dnTCF, dnLEF, and dnβ-catenin, would block/suppress canonical signaling, and may also be employed to control disease progression (Figure 25.3).

Experimental results reported by Sen et al.[75,76] support the potential of these approaches. Overexpression of sFRP-1 or dnTCF-4 was shown to down-regulate proMMP expression in RA FLSs,[77] and blocking Wnt5a/Fz5 signaling using

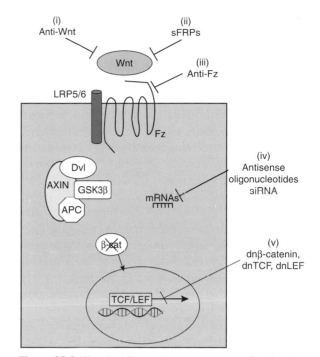

Figure 25.3 Wnt signaling pathway as a target for development of therapeutic agents for RA and OA. Extracellular and intracellular therapeutics targeting inhibition of the Wnt signaling cascade (primarily β-catenin), and subsequent activation of the downstream signaling that ultimately leads to cartilage degradation. Candidate therapeutics include antagonists for (i) Wnt and (ii) Wnt receptors, (iii) neutralizing antibodies, (iv) antisense oligonucleotides and siRNAs, and (v) gene therapy constructs.

neutralizing antibodies, antisense oligonucleotides, or dn expression vectors inhibited activation of FLSs, preventing proinflammatory cytokine secretion. In addition, inhibition of signaling through Fz5 decreased expression of the receptor activator of NF-κB ligand (RANKL).[75]

Blockade of canonical Wnt signaling to decrease cytokine and chemokine production may lead to decreased NO production and MMP expression, and ultimately a suppression of cartilage damage and disease progression. In addition to arresting joint destruction, effective therapeutic treatments should also promote the repair of the injured tissue. Given that the non-canonical and canonical Wnts have been shown to elicit opposing cellular responses, it is interesting to speculate that simultaneous stimulation and inhibition of the non-canonical and canonical Wnt pathways, respectively, may result in regeneration of the damaged tissue. Further development of Wnt-based therapies depends on understanding the complex sequence of molecular events in the Wnt cascades in the compromised joint, as well as in the affected joint the general efficacy of delivery methodologies, such as gene therapy, siRNA/RNAi, and neutralizing antibodies.

CONCLUSIONS

Great strides have been made toward gaining a better understanding of the molecular events involved in the progression of cartilage destruction in the joint. The evidence of the involvement of Wnts in the pathology of many diseases, including RA and OA, is the impetus for the development of therapies that target the components of the Wnt signaling pathway. A better understanding of the cross-talk between cytokine, growth factor, and Wnt signaling pathways is crucial to the development of novel therapeutics for rheumatic joint diseases.

ACKNOWLEDGMENTS

This work is supported by the Intramural Research Program of the National Institute of Arthritis, and Musculoskeletal and Skin Diseases, NIH (Z01 AR41131).

REFERENCES

1. Cadigan KM, Nusse R. Wnt signaling: a common theme in animal development. Genes Dev 1997; 11: 3286–305.
2. Logan CY, Nusse R. The Wnt signaling pathway in development and disease. Annu Rev Cell Dev Biol 2004; 20: 781–810.
3. Willert K, Brown JD, Danenberg E et al. Wnt proteins are lipid-modified and can act as stem cell growth factors. Nature 2003; 423: 448–52.
4. Moore KA. Recent advances in defining the hematopoietic stem cell niche. Curr Opin Hematol 2004; 11: 107–11.
5. Boland GM, Perkins G, Hall DJ et al. Wnt 3a promotes proliferation and suppresses osteogenic differentiation of adult human mesenchymal stem cells. J Cell Biochem 2004; 93: 1210–30.
6. Baksh D, G Boland, RS Tuan. Cross-talk between Wnt signaling pathways in human mesenchymal stem cells leads to functional antagonism during osteogenic differentiation. J Cell Biochem 2007 (in press).
7. Kuhl M, Sheldahl LC, Park M et al. The Wnt/Ca2+ pathway: a new vertebrate Wnt signaling pathway takes shape. Trends Genet 2000; 16: 279–83.
8. Du SJ, Purcell SM, Christian JL et al. Identification of distinct classes and functional domains of Wnts through expression of wild-type and chimeric proteins in Xenopus embryos. Mol Cell Biol 1995; 15: 2625–34.
9. He X, Semenov M, Tamai K et al. LDL receptor-related proteins 5 and 6 in Wnt/beta-catenin signaling: arrows point the way. Development 2004; 131: 1663–77.
10. McEwen DG, Peifer M. Wnt signaling: moving in a new direction. Curr Biol 2000; 10: R562–4.
11. Church VL, Francis-West P. Wnt signalling during limb development. Int J Dev Biol 2002; 46: 927–36.
12. Widelitz R. Wnt signaling through canonical and non-canonical pathways: recent progress. Growth Factors 2005; 23: 111–16.
13. Quaiser T, Anton R, Kuhl M. Kinases and G proteins join the Wnt receptor complex. Bioessays 2006; 28: 339–43.
14. Kuhl M. The WNT/calcium pathway: biochemical mediators, tools and future requirements. Front Biosci 2004; 9: 967–74.
15. Oishi I, Suzuki H, Onishi N et al. The receptor tyrosine kinase Ror2 is involved in non-canonical Wnt5a/JNK signalling pathway. Genes Cells 2003; 8: 645–54.
16. Bodine PV, Zhao W, Kharode YP et al. The Wnt antagonist secreted frizzled-related protein-1 is a negative regulator of trabecular bone formation in adult mice. Mol Endocrinol 2004; 18: 1222–37.
17. Sen M. Wnt signalling in rheumatoid arthritis. Rheumatology (Oxford) 2005; 44: 708–13.
18. Nakamura Y, Nawata M, Wakitani S. Expression profiles and functional analyses of Wnt-related genes in human joint disorders. Am J Pathol 2005; 167: 97–105.
19. Feldmann M, Maini RN. Anti-TNF alpha therapy of rheumatoid arthritis: what have we learned? Annu Rev Immunol 2001; 19: 163–96.
20. Takayanagi H, Oda H, Yamamoto S et al. A new mechanism of bone destruction in rheumatoid arthritis: synovial fibroblasts induce osteoclastogenesis. Biochem Biophys Res Commun 1997; 240: 279–86.
21. Zeisel MB, Druet VA, Wachsmann D et al. MMP-3 expression and release by rheumatoid arthritis fibroblast-like synoviocytes induced with a bacterial ligand of integrin alpha5beta1. Arthritis Res Ther 2005; 7: R118–26.
22. CDC. http://www.cdc.gov/arthritis/data_statistics/arthritis_related_statistics.htm.
23. Felson DT. Clinical practice. Osteoarthritis of the knee. N Engl J Med 2006; 354: 841–8.

24. Sandell LJ, Aigner T. Articular cartilage and changes in arthritis. An introduction: cell biology of osteoarthritis. Arthritis Res 2001; 3: 107–13.

25. Hunter DJ, Felson DT. Osteoarthritis. BMJ 2006; 332: 639–42.

26. Borzi RM, Mazzetti I, Marcu KB et al. Chemokines in cartilage degradation. Clin Orthop Relat Res 2004; (427 Suppl) S53–61.

27. Hartmann C, Tabin CJ. Wnt-14 plays a pivotal role in inducing synovial joint formation in the developing appendicular skeleton. Cell 2001; 104: 341–51.

28. DeLise AM, Fischer L, Tuan RS. Cellular interactions and signaling in cartilage development. Osteoarthritis Cartilage 2000; 8: 309–34.

29. Sandell LJ, Adler P. Developmental patterns of cartilage. Front Biosci 1999; 4: D731–42.

30. Sen M, Lauterbach K, El-Gabalawy H et al. Expression and function of wingless and frizzled homologs in rheumatoid arthritis. Proc Natl Acad Sci U S A 2000; 97: 2791–6.

31. Imai K, Morikawa M, D'Armiento J et al. Differential expression of WNTs and FRPs in the synovium of rheumatoid arthritis and osteoarthritis. Biochem Biophys Res Commun 2006; 345: 1615–20.

32. Neth P, Ciccarella M, Egea V et al. Wnt signaling regulates the invasion capacity of human mesenchymal stem cells. Stem Cells 2006; 24: 1892–903.

33. Loughlin J. Polymorphism in signal transduction is a major route through which osteoarthritis susceptibility is acting. Curr Opin Rheumatol 2005; 17: 629–33.

34. Loughlin J, Dowling B, Chapman K et al. Functional variants within the secreted frizzled-related protein 3 gene are associated with hip osteoarthritis in females. Proc Natl Acad Sci U S A 2004; 101: 9757–62.

35. Min JL, Meulenbelt I, Riyazi N et al. Association of the Frizzled-related protein gene with symptomatic osteoarthritis at multiple sites. Arthritis Rheum 2005; 52: 1077–80.

36. Enomoto-Iwamoto M, Kitagaki J, Koyama E et al. The Wnt antagonist Frzb-1 regulates chondrocyte maturation and long bone development during limb skeletogenesis. Dev Biol 2002; 251: 142–56.

37. Ijiri K, Nagayoshi R, Matsushita N et al. Differential expression patterns of secreted frizzled related protein genes in synovial cells from patients with arthritis. J Rheumatol 2002; 29: 2266–70.

38. James IE, Kumar S, Barnes MR et al. FrzB-2: a human secreted frizzled-related protein with a potential role in chondrocyte apoptosis. Osteoarthritis Cartilage 2000; 8: 452–63.

39. Ryu JH, Kim SJ, Kim SH et al. Regulation of the chondrocyte phenotype by beta-catenin. Development 2002; 129: 5541–50.

40. Kim SJ, Im DS, Kim SH et al. Beta-catenin regulates expression of cyclooxygenase-2 in articular chondrocytes. Biochem Biophys Res Commun 2002; 296: 221–6.

41. Hwang SG, Ryu JH, Kim IC et al. Wnt-7a causes loss of differentiated phenotype and inhibits apoptosis of articular chondrocytes via different mechanisms. J Biol Chem 2004; 279: 26597–604.

42. Akiyama H, Lyons JP, Mori-Akiyama Y et al. Interactions between Sox9 and beta-catenin control chondrocyte differentiation. Genes Dev 2004; 18: 1072–87.

43. Tufan AC, Daumer KM,Tuan RS. Frizzled-7 and limb mesenchymal chondrogenesis: effect of misexpression and involvement of N-cadherin. Dev Dyn 2002; 223: 241–53.

44. Tufan AC, Tuan RS. Wnt regulation of limb mesenchymal chondrogenesis is accompanied by altered N-cadherin-related functions. FASEB J 2001; 15: 1436–8.

45. Stanton LA, Sabari S, Sampaio AV et al. p38 MAP kinase signalling is required for hypertrophic chondrocyte differentiation. Biochem J 2004; 378: 53–62.

46. Levy L, Neuveut C, Renard CA et al. Transcriptional activation of interleukin-8 by beta-catenin-Tcf4. J Biol Chem 2002; 277: 42386–93.

47. Grotewold L, Ruther U. Bmp, Fgf and Wnt signalling in programmed cell death and chondrogenesis during vertebrate limb development: the role of Dickkopf-1. Int J Dev Biol 2002; 46: 943–7.

48. Jin EJ, Park JH, Lee SY et al. Wnt-5a is involved in TGF-beta3-stimulated chondrogenic differentiation of chick wing bud mesenchymal cells. Int J Biochem Cell Biol 2006; 38: 183–95.

49. Reinhold MI, Kapadia RM, Liao Z et al. The Wnt-inducible transcription factor Twist1 inhibits chondrogenesis. J Biol Chem 2006; 281: 1381–8.

50. Fischer L, Boland G, Tuan RS. Wnt-3A enhances bone morphogenetic protein-2-mediated chondrogenesis of murine C3H10T1/2 mesenchymal cells. J Biol Chem 2002; 277: 30870–8.

51. Rawadi G, Vayssiere B, Dunn F et al. BMP-2 controls alkaline phosphatase expression and osteoblast mineralization by a Wnt autocrine loop. J Bone Miner Res 2003; 18: 1842–53.

52. Vaes BL, Dechering KJ, Feijen A et al. Comprehensive microarray analysis of bone morphogenetic protein 2-induced osteoblast differentiation resulting in the identification of novel markers for bone development. J Bone Miner Res 2002; 17: 2106–18.

53. Nishita M, Hashimoto MK, Ogata S et al. Interaction between Wnt and TGF-beta signalling pathways during formation of Spemann's organizer. Nature 2000; 403: 781–5.

54. Westendorf JJ, Kahler RA, Schroeder TM. Wnt signaling in osteoblasts and bone diseases. Gene 2004; 341: 19–39.

55. Letamendia A, Labbe E, Attisano L. Transcriptional regulation by Smads: crosstalk between the TGF-beta and Wnt pathways. J Bone Joint Surg Am 2001; 83-A (Suppl 1): S31–S39.

56. Zhou S, Eid K, Glowacki J. Cooperation between TGF-beta and Wnt pathways during chondrocyte and adipocyte differentiation of human marrow stromal cells. J Bone Miner Res 2004; 19: 463–70.

57. Tuli R, Tuli S, Nandi S et al. Transforming growth factor-beta-mediated chondrogenesis of human mesenchymal progenitor cells involves N-cadherin and mitogen-activated protein kinase and Wnt signaling cross-talk. J Biol Chem 2003; 278: 41227–36.

58. Villiger PM, Kusari AB, ten Dijke P et al. IL-1 beta and IL-6 selectively induce transforming growth factor-beta isoforms in human articular chondrocytes. J Immunol 1993; 151: 3337–44.

59. Chandrasekhar S, Harvey AK. Transforming growth factor-beta is a potent inhibitor of IL-1 induced protease activity and cartilage proteoglycan degradation. Biochem Biophys Res Commun 1988; 157: 1352–9.

60. Im HJ, Pacione C, Chubinskaya S et al. Inhibitory effects of insulin-like growth factor-1 and osteogenic protein-1 on fibronectin fragment- and interleukin-1beta-stimulated matrix metalloproteinase-13 expression in human chondrocytes. J Biol Chem 2003; 278: 25386–94.

61. Vergunst CE, Tak PP. Chemokines: their role in rheumatoid arthritis. Curr Rheumatol Rep 2005; 7: 382–8.

62. Cagnard N, Letourneur F, Essabbani A et al. Interleukin-32, CCL2, PF4F1 and GFD10 are the only cytokine/chemokine genes differentially expressed by in vitro cultured rheumatoid and osteoarthritis fibroblast-like synoviocytes. Eur Cytokine Netw 2005; 16: 289–92.

63. Geng Y, Valbracht J, Lotz M. Selective activation of the mitogen-activated protein kinase subgroups c-Jun NH2 terminal kinase and p38 by IL-1 and TNF in human articular chondrocytes. J Clin Invest 1996; 98: 2425–30.

64. Han Z, Boyle DL, Chang L et al. c-Jun N-terminal kinase is required for metalloproteinase expression and joint destruction in inflammatory arthritis. J Clin Invest 2001; 108: 73–81.

65. Vincenti MP, Brinckerhoff CE. The potential of signal transduction inhibitors for the treatment of arthritis: is it all just JNK? J Clin Invest 2001; 108: 181–3.

66. Liacini A, Sylvester J, Li WQ et al. Inhibition of interleukin-1-stimulated MAP kinases, activating protein-1 (AP-1) and nuclear factor kappa B (NF-kappa B) transcription factors down-regulates matrix metalloproteinase gene expression in articular chondrocytes. Matrix Biol 2002; 21: 251–62.

67. Mengshol JA, Vincenti MP, Brinckerhoff CE. IL-1 induces collagenase-3 (MMP-13) promoter activity in stably transfected chondrocytic cells: requirement for Runx-2 and activation by p38 MAPK and JNK pathways. Nucleic Acids Res 2001; 29: 4361–72.

68. Reuben PM, Cheung HS. Regulation of matrix metalloproteinase (MMP) gene expression by protein kinases. Front Biosci 2006; 11: 1199–215.

69. Hwang SG, Yu SS, Lee SW et al. Wnt-3a regulates chondrocyte differentiation via c-Jun/AP-1 pathway. FEBS Lett 2005; 579: 4837–42.

70. Ryu JH, Chun JS. Opposing roles of WNT-5A and WNT-11 in interleukin-1beta regulation of type II collagen expression in articular chondrocytes. J Biol Chem 2006; 281: 22039–47.

71. Malemud CJ. Cytokines as therapeutic targets for osteoarthritis. BioDrugs 2004; 18: 23–35.

72. Ghosh P, Smith M. Osteoarthritis, genetic and molecular mechanisms. Biogerontology 2002; 3: 85–8.

73. Tanaka I, Morikawa M, Okuse T et al. Expression and regulation of WISP2 in rheumatoid arthritic synovium. Biochem Biophys Res Commun 2005; 334: 973–8.

74. He X, Saint-Jeannet JP, Wang Y et al. A member of the Frizzled protein family mediating axis induction by Wnt-5A. Science 1997; 275: 1652–4.

75. Sen M, Chamorro M, Reifert J et al. Blockade of Wnt-5A/frizzled 5 signaling inhibits rheumatoid synoviocyte activation. Arthritis Rheum 2001; 44: 772–81.

76. Sen M, Reifert J, Lauterbach K et al. Regulation of fibronectin and metalloproteinase expression by Wnt signaling in rheumatoid arthritis synoviocytes. Arthritis Rheum 2002; 46: 2867–77.

77. Pap T, Muller-Ladner U, Gay RE et al. Fibroblast biology. Role of synovial fibroblasts in the pathogenesis of rheumatoid arthritis. Arthritis Res 2000; 2: 361–7.

78. Goldblatt F, Isenberg DA. New therapies for rheumatoid arthritis. Clin Exp Immunol 2005; 140: 195–204.

79. Abramson SB, Yazici Y. Biologics in development for rheumatoid arthritis: relevance to osteoarthritis. Adv Drug Deliv Rev 2006; 58: 212–25.

26

Inflammatory mediators: update on cyclooxygenases and prostaglandin synthases

Leslie Crofford, Mohit Kapoor and Fumiaki Kojima

Introduction • Arachidonic acid metabolism • Cyclooxygenases • Prostaglandins • Terminal PG synthases • Lipoxygenases and leukotrienes • Non-steroidal anti-inflammatory drugs in RA • Future therapeutic targets • Summary • References

INTRODUCTION

Rheumatoid arthritis (RA) is a chronic autoimmune inflammatory disease of the synovial joints. It is characterized clinically by pain, swelling, stiffness, and deformity of affected joints due to infiltration and proliferation of synovial tissues and progressive joint destruction. This process can result in physical disability and premature death. Infiltrating cell types including macrophages, neutrophils, T and B cells release a plethora of proinflammatory mediators that change the phenotype of resident endothelial cells, synovial fibroblasts, chondrocytes, osteoblasts, and osteoclasts. Lipid mediators generated from metabolism of cell membrane arachidonic acid (AA), the eicosanoids, are stimulated by cytokines such as interleukin (IL)-1 and tumor necrosis factor (TNF)-α. Eicosanoid biosynthetic enzymes have been a central target for basic research and drug interventions in RA and other inflammatory conditions. Although drugs such as non-steroidal anti-inflammatory drugs (NSAIDs) that inhibit production of these lipid mediators have not been shown to alter progression of joint destruction in RA, they reduce pain, stiffness, and swelling associated with disease. Even in this era of potent biologic therapies, most patients continue to use NSAIDs. This chapter discusses the current understanding of the role and contribution of key mediators and enzymes from the AA metabolic pathway towards RA pathophysiology. In addition, the authors discuss the current and future therapeutic targets within the AA metabolic pathway to counteract the symptoms related to inflammation.

ARACHIDONIC ACID METABOLISM

The first step of AA metabolism is the release of free AA from cell membrane phospholipids by phospholipase (PL) A_2. AA is further metabolized by metabolic enzymes including cyclooxygenases (COXs), lipoxygenases (LOXs), and further sequential terminal synthase enzymes to generate a diverse range of metabolites including prostaglandins (PGs), thromboxanes (TXs), leukotrienes (LTs), hydroxyeicosatetraenoic acids (HETEs) and lipoxins (LXs) (Figure 26.1). These eicosanoids act via specific cell surface receptors on peripheral nociceptors, endothelial cells, and resident structural cells of the joint in an

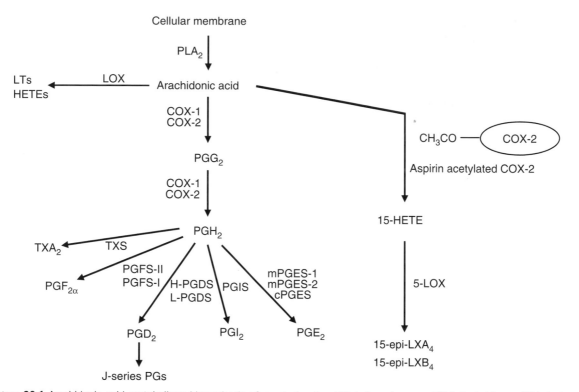

Figure 26.1 Arachidonic acid metabolism: biosynthesis of prostaglandins (PGs), thromboxanes (TXs), leukotrienes (LTs), hydroxy-eicosatetraenoic acids (HETEs), and lipoxins (LXs).

autocrine/paracrine fashion. Furthermore, these eicosanoids modulate leukocyte functions in complex ways.[1] Production of the different eicosanoids is cell type-dependent and changes over time, providing for their pleiotropic effects. For example, while some PGs clearly have pro-inflammatory properties, recent studies suggest that some AA-derived mediators including LXs and cyclopentenone PGs may contribute to resolution of inflammation by endogenous anti-inflammatory mechanisms.[2] Even proinflammatory PGs, such as PGE_2, inhibit some leukocyte functions.

CYCLOOXYGENASES

COX is the vital enzyme for the biosynthesis of PGH_2, the common substrate for bioactive PGs and TXs including PGE_2, PGD_2, $PGF_{2\alpha}$, PGI_2 (prostacyclin), and TXA_2. AA generated from

cell membrane phospholipids by PLA_2 in the initial step is converted to PGG_2, and then sequentially catalyzed to the unstable intermediate, PGH_2, by the peroxidase activity of COX.[3] To date, at least two major isozymes, COX-1 and COX-2, have been cloned and investigated.[4,5] COX-1 is expressed in most cell types and tissues constitutively and functions to maintain homeostasis.[6] Recently, a splice variant of COX-1 mRNA, retaining intron 1, and referred to by several names including COX-3, COX-1b or COX-1v, has been described.[7,8] However, this splice variant is described as occurring at relatively high levels in central nervous system tissues in mice, but the role of this splice variant in humans remains unclear.

COX-2 is induced in inflammatory cells and tissues in response to various proinflammatory cytokines, growth factors, and other mediators associated with inflammation,[9] suggesting a key role of COX-2 in the process of inflammation. High levels of COX-2 are observed in synovial tissues from patients with RA.[10–13] In cultured synovial fibroblasts from RA patients, COX-2 is up-regulated by inflammatory cytokines and other stimuli including IL-1, TNF-α, and phorbol myristate acetate and it is inhibited by glucocorticoids.[14–16] These observations regarding COX-2 expression in articular tissues are concordant with the clinical efficacy of COX-2 selective inhibitors in the treatment of RA.

The importance of COX-2 in various animal experimental models of arthritis has also been demonstrated. COX-2 inhibitors selective inhibitor, but not a COX-1 selective inhibitor, significantly reduced the severity of symptoms in rat adjuvant-induced arthritis (AIA) and mouse collagen-induced arthritis (CIA) models.[17–19] Furthermore, COX-2-deficient mice, but not COX-1-deficient mice, display a significant reduction in both clinical and histological signs of CIA.[20]

Apart from the PG biosynthetic pathway, recent studies have also shown that acetylation of COX-2 by aspirin triggers the generation of novel endogenous lipid mediators termed aspirin-triggered LXs (ATLs).[21] ATLs mediate endogenous stop signals which help in the resolution of inflammation. ATLs have been shown to limit neutrophil chemotaxis, adherence, and transmigration; inhibit superoxide anion generation; inhibit eosinophil migration; and decrease the production of proinflammatory mediators, including TNF-α and LTD_4, in various animal models of inflammation.[22–26] Apart from ATLs, aspirin treatment of human tissues *in vitro* and murine tissues *in vivo* has been shown to generate novel 17R-hydroxy series docosanoids which are also involved in limiting inflammation and promoting resolution.[27] These mediators are the oxygenated products derived from omega-3 polyunsaturated fatty acids. Since these novel mediators are generated during the resolution phase of inflammation, they have been termed as resolvins. The role of ATLs and resolvins in RA pathophysiology remains poorly understood; however, the anti-inflammatory mechanisms triggered by these endogenous mediators may prove to be fruitful in devising novel

therapeutic strategies for counteracting inflammation during RA.

PROSTAGLANDINS

PGE_2 is one of the major proinflammatory PGs in RA. High concentrations of PGE_2 are detectable in the synovial fluid of patients with RA.[28] PGE_2 production at sites of inflammation is correlated with the induction of COX-2. PGE_2 exerts its effects via four EP receptor subtypes, EP1, EP2, EP3, and EP4, which have a different intracellular signaling. Animal models of arthritis have given useful information on the role of EP receptor subtypes in PGE_2 signaling. EP4 receptor-deficient mice display reduction of incidence and severity of arthritis in the collagen antibody-induced arthritis (CAIA) model.[29] In CIA, combination of EP2 genetic deletion and EP4 pharmacological antagonism shows attenuation of arthritis in mice.[30] In addition, administration of neutralizing antibodies against PGE_2 results in reduction of carageenan-induced paw edema and AIA in the rat.[31] The efficacy of the specific neutralization of PGE_2 was indistinguishable from that of the NSAIDs, which block the production of all PGs. These data suggest that PGE_2 is a critical PG in the pathophysiology of inflammatory arthritis.

PGI_2 and its receptor (IP receptor) signaling also contribute towards the acute inflammatory responses including pain, vasodilation, and enhanced vascular permeability.[32] A recent study demonstrated that PGI_2 receptor (IP receptor)-deficient mice show the reduction of chronic inflammatory symptoms in CIA and CAIA models, suggesting the role of PGI_2 in addition to PGE_2 in chronic inflammation in the arthritic joint.[30]

In contrast to proinflammatory PGs, 15-deoxy-$\Delta^{12,14}$-PJG$_2$ (15d-PGJ$_2$), a metabolite of PGD$_2$, exerts anti-inflammatory effect, at least in part, through the activation of peroxisome proliferator-activated receptor gamma (PPAR-γ) in peripheral inflammation.[33] 15d-PGJ$_2$ inhibits expression of proinflammatory cytokines such as IL-1β and TNF-α in cultured synovial fibroblasts.[34] In addition, 15d-PGJ$_2$ inhibits the growth of synovial fibroblasts by facilitating apoptosis and reduces the inflammatory features such as pannus formation and mononuclear cell infiltration in a model of AIA.[35]

TERMINAL PG SYNTHASES

Various terminal enzymes that specifically catalyze the conversion of PGH_2 to each bioactive prostanoid downstream of COX have been cloned and characterized in recent years. These enzymes are termed PGE synthase (PGES) for PGE_2, PGDS for PGD_2, PGFS for $PGF_{2\alpha}$, PGIS for PGI_2, and TXS for TXA_2, respectively.[3,36] Isozymes of PLA_2, COX, and various terminal synthases appear to be functionally coupled by virtue of their co-regulated expression and subcellular localization that is based on the specific cell type and the presence or absence of pro- or anti-inflammatory stimuli.[37,38] Specific changes in PG production are therefore dependent on the extracellular milieu and in turn participate in the initiation or resolution of inflammation. Over time during an acute inflammatory process, PGE_2 biosynthesis gives way to PGD_2 and its anti-inflammatory metabolite, 15d-PGJ_2, that participate in resolution of inflammation as expression of PGES wanes.[2,39,40]

At least three forms of PGES – cytosolic PGES (cPGES), microsomal PGES (mPGES)-1, and mPGES-2 – have been cloned and characterized. These enzymes specifically catalyze the conversion of PGH_2 to PGE_2 in the final step of PGE_2 biosynthesis; however, their catalytic activity differs, with mPGES-1 being the most efficient.[41,42] cPGES and mPGES-2 are constitutively expressed in a wide variety of cells and tissues.[43,44] On the other hand, mPGES-1 is an inducible enzyme that shows coordinated induction with COX-2 under inflammatory conditions.[45,46] mPGES-1 is dramatically induced in parallel with COX-2 in cultured synovial fibroblasts from RA patients in response to stimulation by proinflammatory cytokines, IL-1β and TNF-α.[47,48] It has also been confirmed that mPGES-1 expression is inhibited by glucocorticoids. In addition, mPGES-1 is positively autoregulated by its product PGE_2 in synovial fibroblasts and chondrocytes though the activation of EP2 and EP4 receptors under IL-1β-stimulated condition.[41,49] mPGES-1 is expressed in synovial tissues of RA patients and the induction seems to be correlated

with the extent of disease activity of RA.[44,50] Induction of mPGES-1 is also observed in joint tissues of rat AIA.[51] In addition, mPGES-1-deficient mice exhibit reduction of inflammatory changes and histopathologic changes such as pannus formation and joint erosion in the CIA and CAIA models.[52,53] These data suggest that mPGES-1 may be a valid pharmacological target for the treatment of RA.

PGDS exists in two known isoforms, namely, lipocalin PGDS (L-PGDS) and hematopoietic PGDS (H-PGDS). H-PGDS is responsible for the production of PGD_2 and its metabolite 15d-PGJ_2 in peripheral inflammation.[39,54] It has been reported that retrovirally transfected PGDS cDNA can suppress inflammatory responses *in vivo*.[55-57] In conversion of PGH_2 to TXA_2 or PGI_2, TXS and PGIS act as specific terminal enzymes, respectively.[58,59]

LIPOXYGENASES AND LEUKOTRIENES

Apart from cyclooxygenases, AA can also be metabolized via LOX enzyme, which results in the production of HETEs and LTs. LOX enzymes including 15-LOX and 12-LOX generate 15-HETE and 12-HETE, respectively, by metabolizing AA, whereas 5-LOX metabolizes AA to yield LTs.[60] 5-LOX metabolism of AA produces an unstable metabolite, LTA_4, which is subsequently hydrolyzed by LTA_4 hydrolase (LTA_4H) to LTB_4, or LTC_4 by LTC_4 synthase in combination with reduced glutathione. LTC_4 is further converted to LTD_4 by γ-glutamyl leukotrienase (γ-GL) and γ-glutamyl transpeptidase (γ-GT), and subsequently converted to LTE_4 by dipeptidase.[61,62] The ability of 5-LOX to utilize endogenous arachidonate for the production of LTs is dependent on a helper protein termed 5-LOX activating protein (FLAP).

5-LOX and FLAP have been shown to be expressed in RA synovial fibroblasts.[63] Animal studies using mice deficient in FLAP have been shown to have reduced severity of CIA,[64] suggesting a role of 5-LOX and FLAP in the pathophysiology of arthritis. Among all LTs, LTB_4 is most likely to be involved in the pathophysiology of RA. LTB_4 mediates its effects via two known G protein-coupled receptors, namely BLT_1 and BLT_2. Elevated levels of LTB_4 have been reported in the serum of patients with RA.[65] It has been reported that neutrophils in the inflamed joints of RA patients are the major source of LTB_4 production.[66] Animal studies using a murine model of CIA have shown that inhibition of LTB_4 by MK886 (an inhibitor of LTB_4 synthesis) reduces proinflammatory cytokine production, disease severity, articular inflammation, and joint destruction.[67]

NON-STEROIDAL ANTI-INFLAMMATORY DRUGS IN RA

In 1971, Sir John Vane first demonstrated that the mechanism of action of aspirin and other NSAIDs is due to inhibition of COX and subsequent inhibition of PG production. Since then, NSAIDs have been extensively used for the management of pain, swelling, and stiffness in RA.[68] Non-selective or traditional NSAIDs are effective in the management of pain associated with RA but are associated with a number of gastrointestinal (GI) and renal side effects due to their inhibitory effects on both COX-1 and COX-2 activities, along with inhibition of PG and TX production.[69] Selective inhibitors of COX-2 (COXIBs) were therefore developed to overcome the GI side effects of non-selective NSAIDs. Although COXIBs are associated with reduced incidence of serious GI side effects, recent reports have demonstrated an increased risk for cardiovascular events associated with the inhibition of COX-2.[70 72] In the history of NSAIDs and COXIBs, more drugs have failed than succeeded. For example, of the three COXIBs indicated for the treatment of RA released since 1999, only one remains on the market. The current issues for COX inhibitors include ongoing GI risk that while reduced by strategies, including co-administration of proton pump inhibitors or misoprostol and use of COXIBs, have not eliminated serious GI events associated with these medications. Co-administration of low-dose aspirin, whose use is quite frequent in patients with RA, especially in light of the increased cardiovascular risk in this disease, increases GI toxicity. All of these drugs have renal effects including increased blood pressure, which may contribute to long-term issues with cardiovascular adverse events in RA. The cardiovascular issues continue to be troublesome

and it cannot be concluded from current data that any drug that inhibits COX-2, non-specific or specific, is free of cardiovascular adverse effects.

All these issues raise important questions regarding the balance of safety and efficacy of non-specific and COX-2-specific NSAIDs in the treatment of RA, and have led to a resurgence in efforts to discover alternate targets within the eicosanoid biosynthetic pathway. The fact that the COX isozymes sit relatively high up in the biosynthetic pathway and lead to inhibition of all PGs, makes inhibition of these enzymes rather crude tools if indeed the desire is to inhibit the production or action of only one PG or to block its actions. The current task at hand is to devise new therapeutic tools to control chronic inflammation associated with RA. More specific targeting of the eicosanoid pathway may allow for benefit, while minimizing risks.

FUTURE THERAPEUTIC TARGETS

Since the discovery of mPGES-1 as an inducible enzyme that results in marked increases in PGE_2 biosynthesis, the possibility of mPGES-1 as a therapeutic target in counteracting inflammation in diseases such as RA has been raised. Animal studies using mPGES-1-deficient mice reveal resistance to pain, arthritis, and fever, which are the important therapeutic properties of COX inhibitors.[52,53,73] No specific inhibitor of mPGES-1 enzyme is available at this time, but research is ongoing.

In evaluating the potential for mPGES-1 as a target, issues of safety advantages and efficacy disadvantages compared with currently available drugs must be considered. Recently reported cardiovascular side effects associated with the use of COXIBs emphasize the need to understand the potential consequences of mPGES-1 inhibition in this organ system. One of the hypotheses put forward to explain the cardiovascular effects of COX-2 inhibition is the loss of anti-thrombotic PGI_2 derived from endothelial COX-2, which plays a key role in the regulation of thrombogenesis.[74] Studies by our group and others suggest that inhibition of mPGES-1 may escape the cardiovascular side effects seen with inhibition of COX-2. Our recent study using mouse embryonic fibroblasts isolated from mice with genetically deleted mPGES-1 enzyme demonstrated that genetic deletion of mPGES-1 results in diversion in the production pattern from predominant PGE_2 to PGI_2, suggesting a shunting phenomenon within the AA metabolic pathway upon mPGES-1 genetic deletion, whereas pharmacological inhibition and genetic deletion of COX-2 resulted in dramatic decrease in the levels of not only PGE_2 but also PGI_2.[75] In addition, our results showed that mPGES-1 gene deletion causes elevation of nitrite levels, a stable metabolic product of nitric oxide (NO). PGI_2 and NO are potent vasodilators and are involved in the maintenance of vascular homeostasis, and clinical studies support their beneficial effects for the management of circulatory disorders.[76–79] To further support this, another recent study showed that genetic deletion of mPGES-1 depressed PGE_2 production, increased PGI_2 production, and had no effect on thromboxane biosynthesis in vivo. In addition, mPGES-1 deletion did not have any effect on thrombogenesis and blood pressure.[80] In view of the above results, mPGES-1 pharmacological inhibition may not be associated with the cardiovascular side effects seen with inhibition of COX-2 and continues to be an attractive target for counteracting inflammation during inflammatory diseases including RA. However, mPGES-1 is expressed in the kidney and may be important in renal homeostasis.[45,81] Furthermore, PGI_2 has its own proinflammatory properties, and increased prostacyclin production may counteract efficacy of mPGES-1 inhibition in patients with RA and other inflammatory disorders.

Other strategies would include inhibition of EP receptors; however, it is likely that both EP2 and EP4 would require inhibition and the effect of this strategy on the homeostatic properties of PGE_2 has not become clear as yet. Increasing production of anti-inflammatory lipid mediators or using these agents therapeutically may also provide benefits.

SUMMARY

As research progresses to provide evidence and better understanding of the specific eicosanoids involved in inflammation and anti-inflammation, targeted therapies specifically aimed at altering this balance will be possible. At present, inhibition of PGE_2 production seems most likely to come to fruition for the treatment of the pain and inflammation of RA. Promoting increased levels of anti-inflammatory eicosanoids may also prove to be a feasible strategy in the treatment of RA. At present, the potential adverse consequences and overall efficacy of alternate treatment strategies to COX inhibition remain unclear.

REFERENCES

1. Rocca B, Spain LM, Pure E et al. Distinct roles of prostaglandin H synthases 1 and 2 in T-cell development. J Clin Invest 1999; 103: 1469–77.
2. Hortelano S, Castrillo A, Alvarez AM, Bosca L. Contribution of cyclopentenone prostaglandins to the resolution of inflammation through the potentiation of apoptosis in activated macrophages. J Immunol 2000; 165: 6525–31.
3. Crofford LJ, Prostaglandin biology. Gastroenterol Clin North Am 2001;30: 863–76.
4. Xie WL, Chipman JG, Robertson DL, Erikson RL, Simmons DL. Expression of a mitogen-responsive gene encoding prostaglandin synthase is regulated by mRNA splicing. Proc Natl Acad Sci U S A 1991; 88: 2692–6.
5. Kujubu DA, Fletcher BS, Varnum BC, Lim RW, Herschman HR. TIS10, a phorbol ester tumor promoter-inducible mRNA from Swiss 3T3 cells, encodes a novel prostaglandin synthase/cyclooxygenase homologue. J Biol Chem 1991; 266: 12866–72.
6. Vane JR, Botting RM. Mechanism of action of anti-inflammatory drugs. Scand J Rheumatol Suppl 1996; 102: 9–21.
7. Chandrasekharan NV, Dai H, Roos KL et al. COX-3, a cyclooxygenase-1 variant inhibited by acetaminophen and other analgesic/antipyretic drugs: cloning, structure, and expression. Proc Natl Acad Sci U S A 2002; 99: 13926–31.
8. Qin N, Zhang SP, Reitz TL, Mei JM, Flores CM. Cloning, expression, and functional characterization of human cyclooxygenase-1 splicing variants: evidence for intron 1 retention. J Pharmacol Exp Ther 2005; 315: 1298–305.
9. Jones DA, Carlton DP, McIntyre TM, Zimmerman GA, Prescott SM. Molecular cloning of human prostaglandin endoperoxide synthase type II and demonstration of expression in response to cytokines. J Biol Chem 1993; 268: 9049–54.

10. Crofford LJ, COX-1 and COX-2, tissue expression: implications and predictions. J Rheumatol Suppl 1997; 49: 15–19.

11. Crofford LJ. COX-2 in synovial tissues. Osteoarthritis Cartilage 1999; 7: 406–8.

12. Siegle I, Ktein T, Backman JT et al. Expression of cyclooxygenase 1 and cyclooxygenase 2 in human synovial tissue: differential elevation of cyclooxygenase 2 in inflammatory joint diseases. Arthritis Rheum 1998; 41: 122–9.

13. Kang RY, Freire-Moar J, Sigal E, Chu CQ. Expression of cyclooxygenase-2 in human and an animal model of rheumatoid arthritis. Br J Rheumatol 1996; 35: 711–18.

14. Crofford LJ, Wilder RL, Ristimaki AP et al. Cyclooxygenase-1 and -2 expression in rheumatoid synovial tissues. Effects of interleukin-1 beta, phorbol ester, and corticosteroids. J Clin Invest 1994; 93: 1095–101.

15. Angel J, Berenbaum F, Le Denmat C et al. Interleukin-1-induced prostaglandin E2 biosynthesis in human synovial cells involves the activation of cytosolic phospholipase A2 and cyclooxygenase-2. Eur J Biochem 1994; 226: 125–31.

16. Sano, H, Hla T, Maier JA et al. In vivo cyclooxygenase expression in synovial tissues of patients with rheumatoid arthritis and osteoarthritis and rats with adjuvant and streptococcal cell wall arthritis. J Clin Invest 1992; 89: 97–108.

17. Chan CC, Boyes S, Brideau C et al. Rofecoxib [Vioxx, MK-0966; 4-(4′-methylsulfonylphenyl)-3-phenyl-2-(5H)-furanone]: a potent and orally active cyclooxygenase-2 inhibitor. Pharmacological and biochemical profiles. J Pharmacol Exp Ther 1999; 290: 551–60.

18. Ochi T, Goto T. Differential effect of FR122047, a selective cyclo-oxygenase-1 inhibitor, in rat chronic models of arthritis. Br J Pharmacol 2002; 135: 782–8.

19. Ochi T, Ohkubo Y, Mutoh S. Role of cyclooxygenase-2, but not cyclooxygenase-1, on type II collagen-induced arthritis in DBA/1J mice. Biochem Pharmacol 2003; 66: 1055–60.

20. Myers LK, Kang AH, Postlethwaite AE et al. The genetic ablation of cyclooxygenase 2 prevents the development of autoimmune arthritis. Arthritis Rheum 2000; 43: 2687–93.

21. Claria J, Serhan CN. Aspirin triggers previously undescribed bioactive eicosanoids by human endothelial cell-leukocyte interactions. Proc Natl Acad Sci U S A 1995; 92: 9475–9.

22. Devchand PR, Arita M, Hong S et al. Human ALX receptor regulates neutrophil recruitment in transgenic mice: roles in inflammation and host defense. FASEB J 2003; 17: 652–9.

23. Bandeira-Melo C, Bozza PT, Diaz BL et al. Cutting edge: lipoxin (LX) A4 and aspirin-triggered 15-epi-LXA4 block allergen-induced eosinophil trafficking. J Immunol 2000; 164: 2267–71.

24. Levy BD, Fokin VV, Clark JM et al. Polyisoprenyl phosphate (PIPP) signaling regulates phospholipase D activity: a 'stop' signaling switch for aspirin-triggered lipoxin A4. Faseb J 1999; 13: 903–11.

25. Wu SH, Lu C, Dong L et al. Lipoxin A4 inhibits TNF-alpha-induced production of interleukins and proliferation of rat mesangial cells. Kidney Int 2005; 68: 35–46.

26. McMahon B, Stenson C, McPhillips F et al. Lipoxin A4 antagonizes the mitogenic effects of leukotriene D4 in human renal mesangial cells. Differential activation of MAP kinases through distinct receptors. J Biol Chem 2000; 275: 27566–75.

27. Serhan CN, Hong S, Gronert K et al. Resolvins: a family of bioactive products of omega-3 fatty acid transformation circuits initiated by aspirin treatment that counter proinflammation signals. J Exp Med 2002; 196: 1025–37.

28. Egg D, Gunther R, Herold M, Kerschbaumer F. [Prostaglandins E2 and F2 alpha concentrations in the synovial fluid in rheumatoid and traumatic knee joint diseases]. Z Rheumatol 1980; 39: 170–5.

29. McCoy JM, Wicks JR, Audoly LP. The role of prostaglandin E2 receptors in the pathogenesis of rheumatoid arthritis. J Clin Invest 2002; 110: 651–8.

30. Honda T, Segi-Nishida E, Miyachi Y, Narumiya S, Prostacyclin-IP signaling and prostaglandin E2-EP2/EP4 signaling both mediate joint inflammation in mouse collagen-induced arthritis. J Exp Med 2006; 203: 325–35.

31. Portanova JP, Zhang Y, Anderson GD et al. Selective neutralization of prostaglandin E2 blocks inflammation, hyperalgesia, and interleukin 6 production in vivo. J Exp Med 1996; 184: 883–91.

32. Murata T, Ushikubi F, Matsuoka T et al. Altered pain perception and inflammatory response in mice lacking prostacyclin receptor. Nature 1997; 388: 678–82.

33. Marcus SL, Miyata KS, Zhang B et al. Diverse peroxisome proliferator-activated receptors bind to the peroxisome proliferator-responsive elements of the rat hydratase/dehydrogenase and fatty acyl-CoA oxidase genes but differentially induce expression. Proc Natl Acad Sci U S A 1993; 90: 5723–7.

34. Ji JD, Cheon H, Jun JB et al. Effects of peroxisome proliferator-activated receptor-gamma (PPAR-gamma) on the expression of inflammatory cytokines and apoptosis induction in rheumatoid synovial fibroblasts and monocytes. J Autoimmun 2001; 17: 215–21.

35. Kawahito Y, Kondo M, Tsubouchi Y et al. 15-Deoxy-delta (12,14)-PGJ(2) induces synoviocyte apoptosis and suppresses adjuvant-induced arthritis in rats. J Clin Invest 2000; 106: 189–97.

36. Urade Y, Watanabe K, Hayaishi O, Prostaglandin D, E, and F synthases. J Lipid Mediat Cell Signal 1995; 12: 257–73.

37. Ueno N, Murakami M, Tanioka T et al. Coupling between cyclooxygenase, terminal prostanoid synthase, and phospholipase A2. J Biol Chem 2001; 276: 34918–27.

38. Ueno N, Takegoshi Y, Kamei D, Kudo I, Murakami M. Coupling between cyclooxygenases and terminal prostanoid synthases. Biochem Biophys Res Commun 2005; 338: 70–6.

39. Gilroy DW, Colville-Nash PR, Willis D et al. Inducible cyclooxygenase may have anti-inflammatory properties. Nat Med 1999; 5: 698–701.

40. Ricote M, Li AC, Willson TM, Kelly CJ, Glass CK. The peroxisome proliferator-activated receptor-gamma is a negative regulator of macrophage activation. Nature 1998; 391: 79–82.

41. Kojima F, Kato S, Kawai S, Prostaglandin E synthase in the pathophysiology of arthritis. Fundam Clin Pharmacol 2005; 19: 255–61.

42. Sampey AV, Monrad S, Crofford LJ. Microsomal prostaglandin E synthase-1: the inducible synthase for prostaglandin E2. Arthritis Res Ther 2205; 7: 114–17.

43. Tanioka T, Nakatani Y, Semmyo N, Murakami M, Kudo I, Molecular identification of cytosolic prostaglandin E2 synthase that is functionally coupled with cyclooxygenase-1 in immediate prostaglandin E2 biosynthesis. J Biol Chem 2000; 275: 32775–82.

44. Murakami M, Nakashima K, Kamei D et al. Cellular prostaglandin E2 production by membrane-bound prostaglandin E synthase-2 via both cyclooxygenases-1 and -2. J Biol Chem 2003; 278: 37937–47.

45. Jakobsson PJ, Thoren S, Morgenstern R, Samuelsson B. Identification of human prostaglandin E synthase: a microsomal, glutathione-dependent, inducible enzyme, constituting a potential novel drug target. Proc Natl Acad Sci U S A 1999; 96: 7220–5.

46. Murakami M, Naraba H, Tanioka T et al. Regulation of prostaglandin E2 biosynthesis by inducible membrane-associated prostaglandin E2 synthase that acts in concert with cyclooxygenase-2. J Biol Chem 2000; 275: 32783–92.

47. Stichtenoth DO, Thoren S, Bian H et al. Microsomal prostaglandin E synthase is regulated by proinflammatory cytokines and glucocorticoids in primary rheumatoid synovial cells. J Immunol 2001; 167: 469–74.

48. Kojima F, Naraba H, Sasaki Y et al. Coexpression of microsomal prostaglandin E synthase with cyclooxygenase-2 in human rheumatoid synovial cells. J Rheumatol 2002; 29: 1836–42.

49. Kojima F, Naraba H, Sasaki Y et al. Prostaglandin E2 is an enhancer of interleukin-1beta-induced expression of membrane-associated prostaglandin E synthase in rheumatoid synovial fibroblasts. Arthritis Rheum 2003; 48: 2819–28.

50. Westman M, Korotkova M, Klint E et al. Expression of microsomal prostaglandin E synthase 1 in rheumatoid arthritis synovium. Arthritis Rheum 2004; 50: 1774–80.

51. Claveau D, Sirinyen M, Guay J et al. Microsomal prostaglandin E synthase-1 is a major terminal synthase that is selectively up-regulated during cyclooxygenase-2-dependent prostaglandin E2 production in the rat adjuvant-induced arthritis model. J Immunol 2003; 170: 4738–44.

52. Trebino CE, Stock JL, Gibbons CP et al. Impaired inflammatory and pain responses in mice lacking an inducible prostaglandin E synthase. Proc Natl Acad Sci U S A 2003; 100: 9044–9.

53. Kamei D, Yamakawa K, Takegoshi Y et al. Reduced pain hypersensitivity and inflammation in mice lacking microsomal prostaglandin e synthase-1. J Biol Chem 2004; 279: 33684–95.

54. Kanaoka Y, Ago H, Inagaki E et al. Cloning and crystal structure of hematopoietic prostaglandin D synthase. Cell 1997; 90: 1085–95.

55. Ando M, Murakami Y, Kojima F et al. Retrovirally introduced prostaglandin D2 synthase suppresses lung injury induced by bleomycin. Am J Respir Cell Mol Biol 2003; 28: 582–91.

56. Murakami Y, Akahoshi T, Aayoshi I et al. Inhibition of monosodium urate monohydrate crystal-induced acute inflammation by retrovirally transfected prostaglandin D synthase. Arthritis Rheum 2003; 48: 2931–41.

57. Kohno S, Endo H, Hashimoto A et al. Inhibition of skin sclerosis by 15deoxy Delta12,14-prostaglandin J2 and retrovirally transfected prostaglandin D synthase in a mouse model of bleomycin-induced scleroderma. Biomed Pharmacother 2006; 60: 18–25.

58. Zhang L, Chase MB, Shen RF. Molecular cloning and expression of murine thromboxane synthase. Biochem Biophys Res Commun 1993; 194: 741–8.

59. Miyata A, Hara S, Yokoyama C et al. Molecular cloning and expression of human prostacyclin synthase. Biochem Biophys Res Commun 1994; 200: 1728–34.

60. Williams KI, Higgs GA. Eicosanoids and inflammation. J Pathol 1998; 156: 101–10.

61. Peters-Golden M, Brock, T.G. 5-Lipoxygenase and FLAP. Prostaglandins Leukot Essent Fatty Acids 2003; 69: 99–109.

62. Samuelsson, B. The discovery of the leukotrienes. Am J Respir Crit Care Med 2000; 161: S2–6.

63. Bonnet C, Bertin P, Cook-Moreau J et al. Lipoxygenase products and expression of 5-lipoxygenase and 5-lipoxygenase-activating protein in human cultured synovial cells. Prostaglandins 1995; 50: 127–35.

64. Griffiths RJ, Smith MA, Roach ML et al. Collagen-induced arthritis is reduced in 5-lipoxygenase-activating protein-deficient mice. J Exp Med 1997; 185: 1123–9.

65. Sawazaki Y, [Leukotriene B4, leukotriene C4 and prostaglandin E2 in the serum, synovial fluid and synovium in patients with rheumatoid arthritis]. Nippon Ika Daigaku Zasshi 1989; 56: 559–64.

66. Moilanen E, Alanko J, Nissila M et al. Eicosanoid production in rheumatoid synovitis. Agents Actions 1989; 28: 290–7.

67. Canetti CA, Leung BP, Culshaws S et al. IL-18 enhances collagen-induced arthritis by recruiting neutrophils via TNF-alpha and leukotriene B4. J Immunol 2003; 171: 1009–15.

68. Crofford LJ, COX-2: where are we in 2003? – Specific cyclooxygenase-2 inhibitors and aspirin-exacerbated respiratory disease. Arthritis Res Ther 2003; 5: 25–7.

69. Meade EA, Smith WL, DeWitt DL. Differential inhibition of prostaglandin endoperoxide synthase (cyclooxygenase) isozymes by aspirin and other non-steroidal anti-inflammatory drugs. J Biol Chem 1993; 268: 6610–14.

70. Bresalier RS, Sandler RS, Quan H et al. Cardiovascular events associated with rofecoxib in a colorectal adenoma chemoprevention trial. N Engl J Med 2005; 352: 1092–102.

71. Solomon SD, McMurray JJ, Pfeffer MA et al. Cardiovascular risk associated with celecoxib in a clinical trial for colorectal adenoma prevention. N Engl J Med 2005; 352: 1071–80.

72. White WB, Faich G, Borer JS, Makuch RW. Cardiovascular thrombotic events in arthritis trials of the cyclooxygenase-2 inhibitor celecoxib. Am J Cardiol 2003; 92: 411–18.

73. Saha S, Engstrom L, Mackerlova L, Jakobsson PJ, Blomqvist A. Impaired febrile responses to immune challenge in mice deficient in microsomal prostaglandin E synthase-1. Am J Physiol Regul Integr Comp Physiol 2005; 288: R1100–7.

74. McAdam BF, Catella-Lawson F, Mardini IA et al. Systemic biosynthesis of prostacyclin by cyclooxygenase (COX)-2: the human pharmacology of a selective inhibitor of COX-2. Proc Natl Acad Sci U S A 1999; 96: 272–7.

75. Kapoor M, Kojima F, Qian M, Yang L, Crofford LJ. Shunting of prostanoid biosynthesis in microsomal prostaglandin E synthase-1 null embryo fibroblasts: regulatory effects on inducible nitric oxide synthase expression and nitrite synthesis. FASEB J 2006; 20: 2387–9.

76. Moncada S, Vane JR. Arachidonic acid metabolites and the interactions between platelets and blood-vessel walls. N Engl J Med 1979; 300: 1142–7.

77. Bunting S, Moncada S, Vane JR. The prostacyclin–thromboxane A2 balance: pathophysiological and therapeutic implications. Br Med Bull 1983; 39: 271–6.

78. Gibbons GH. Endothelial function as a determinant of vascular function and structure: a new therapeutic target. Am J Cardiol 1997; 79: 3–8.

79. Olschewski H, Walmrath D, Schermuly R et al. Aerosolized prostacyclin and iloprost in severe pulmonary hypertension. Ann Intern Med 1996; 124: 820–4.

80. Cheng Y, Wang M, Yu Y et al. Cyclooxygenases, microsomal prostaglandin E synthase-1, and cardiovascular function. J Clin Invest 2006; 116: 1391–9.

81. Schneider A, Zhang Y, Zhang M et al. Membrane-associated PGE synthase-1 (mPGES-1) is coexpressed with both COX-1 and COX-2 in the kidney. Kidney Int 2004; 65: 1205–13.

27

Complement and pregnancy loss

Jane E Salmon and V Michael Holers

Introduction • Complement cascade and tissue injury • Complement and fetal tolerance • Complement in mouse models of pregnancy loss • The alternative pathway as a target for anti-inflammatory therapies: pregnancy failure and beyond • References

INTRODUCTION

The journey from conception to birth is fraught with danger. It has been estimated that 50–70% of all conceptions fail. Complications that occur during pregnancy remain a serious clinical problem and the triggers and mediators of placental and fetal damage are poorly understood. Recurrent pregnancy loss affects 1–3% of couples.[1,2] Despite aggressive efforts to understand the basic biology underlying neonatal death and morbidity, their incidence has remained unchanged over the past 20–30 years. Furthermore, the well-established genetic, anatomic, endocrine, and infectious causes of fetal damage are not demonstrable in 50–60% of pregnancy complications, and more work is necessary to elucidate their pathogenesis.[2] In addition, preterm birth occurs in up to 10% of pregnancies, accounting for 70% of neonatal deaths and related neonatal morbidity, including neurological, respiratory, and metabolic complications in the newborn.[3,4] Intrauterine growth restriction (IUGR) occurs in up to 10% of infants born in the United States[5] and growth-restricted fetuses have higher mortality and morbidity rates than fetuses with weights > 10th percentile. While the insult to the fetus occurs *in utero*, the deleterious influence of IUGR contributes to long-term developmental delay, and a suboptimal intrauterine environment has been linked to metabolic disorders during adult life, including coronary artery disease, hypertension, hyperlipidemia, and insulin resistance.[6]

Although the causes of recurrent miscarriages and IUGR are poorly understood, an immune mechanism involving inappropriate and subsequently injurious recognition of the conceptus by the mother's immune system has been proposed. This misdirected immune response to fetus, placenta, or both, could yield a wide range of phenotypes including miscarriages early in pregnancy and IUGR later in pregnancy. Pregnancy constitutes a major challenge to the maternal immune system because it requires tolerance of fetal alloantigens encoded by paternal genes. Local factors at the maternal–fetal interface are required to maintain such tolerance and assure normal development of semiallogenic concepti.[7] The fetus is protected from maternal immune responses through mechanisms such as expression of HLA-G,[8] inhibitory T-cell costimulatory molecules,[9] and complement regulatory proteins by trophoblasts,[10] and by local maternal regulatory T cells[11] and production of the immunosuppressive enzyme indoleamine 2,3 dioxygenase.[12]

Murine models have recently been developed that have elucidated these protective mechanisms and excessive complement activation at the maternal–fetal interface has been observed when these mechanisms fail. We and others have identified a novel role for complement as an early effector in the pathway leading to pregnancy loss associated with placental inflammation.[13–15] Indeed, it appears that inhibition of complement activation is an absolute requirement for normal pregnancy,[10,16] and that in the antiphosphopholid syndrome overwhelming activation of complement triggered by antibodies deposited in placenta leads to fetal injury.[13,14] In addition to blocking effector molecules in the complement cascade, the alternative pathway of complement activation is emerging as a potential new target in the treatment of recurrent pregnancy loss.

COMPLEMENT CASCADE AND TISSUE INJURY

Activation of the complement cascade

The complement system, comprising over 30 proteins that act in concert to protect the host against invading organisms, initiates inflammation and tissue injury (Figure 27.1).[17,18] Activation of complement promotes chemotaxis of inflammatory cells, generates intracellular signaling events in local non-immune cells, and produces proteolytic fragments that enhance phagocytosis by polymorphonuclear leukocytes (PMNs) and monocytes. Lysis of cells and organisms identified as foreign is mediated by the formation of the membrane attack complex.

The classical pathway is activated when natural or elicited antibodies bind to antigen and unleash potent effectors associated with humoral responses in immune-mediated tissue damage. Activation of the classical pathway by natural antibodies plays a major role in the response to neoepitopes unmasked on ischemic endothelium, and thus may be involved in reperfusion injury.[19] In addition, the classical pathway is activated through the action of C-reactive protein

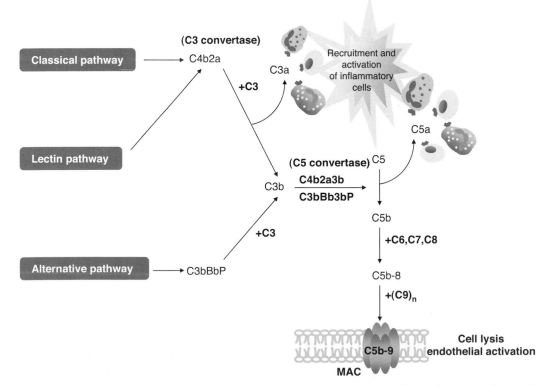

Figure 27.1 Complement cascade. Schematic diagram of the three complement activation pathways and the products they generate. From Hughes Syndrome, 2nd edn, Khamashta MA, Ed, 2006, page 396, chapter 31, by Girardi G and Salmon J, Figure 31.1. With kind permission of Springer Science and Business Media.

and serum amyloid P as they bind nuclear constituents released from necrotic or dying cells, or directly when apoptotic bodies derived from cells bind C1q.[20,21] The mannose-binding lectin (MBL) pathway is activated by MBL recognition of carbohydrates (often on infectious agents or as a specific form of carbohydrate designated G0 on the Fc domain of antibodies) or by the interaction with cytokeratin released from injured cells.[22] Following MBL binding, MBL-associated serine protease-2 (MASP-2) autoactivates and cleaves complement component 2 (C2) and C4 of the classical pathway, leading to the cleavage and activation of C3. Another associated protease, MASP-1, can directly cleave C3 and bypass the necessity for the classical pathway.[22]

Alternative pathway activation mechanisms differ in that they are initiated by the binding of spontaneously activated complement components to the surface of pathogens or self. The alternative pathway is activated through two processes. The first is an intrinsic mechanism called 'tickover' that involves the slow but continuous low grade hydrolysis of C3 and generates a conformationally altered form of C3 (designated C3(H$_2$O)) that is capable of binding factor B. Once factor B binding occurs, factor D can cleave factor B into Ba, which diffuses away, and Bb, which associates with C3(H$_2$O), and together they act as a protease to cleave and activate additional C3 molecules, generating C3a and C3b. C3b becomes fixed to targets through its thioester bond, factor B binds to this newly formed C3b and it is cleaved by factor D to Bb and Ba. C3bBb is stabilized by properdin, and acts as another C3 convertase, and the subsequently generated C3bBbC3b can then act as a C5 convertase. This pathway is antibody-independent and is triggered by the activity of factor B and properdin. Properdin promotes optimal rates of complement activation by virtue of its ability to bind and stabilize C3 and C5 convertases. Properdin, the only regulator of complement that amplifies its activation, is produced by T cells, monocytes/macrophages, and PMNs.

The second mechanism of alternative pathway activation is the 'amplification loop' (Figure 27.2). In this process, C3b that is formed by the action of the classical or lectin pathway-derived C3 convertases can bind factor B and lead to the formation

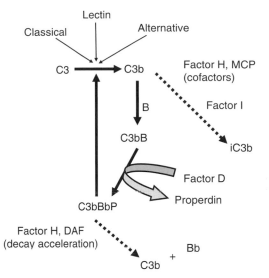

Figure 27.2 Details of alternative pathway amplification loop: components, activation, and regulatory steps. Independent of which pathway initiates C3 activation and C3b fixation to the target, factor B is able to bind C3b. This step is followed by cleavage of factor B by factor D into Bb and Ba, further C3 activation by proteolytic activity of C3b-associated Bb, and a continuous loop of activity that is stabilized by properdin. Serum factor H (a serum protein) and MCP/CD46 and DAF/ CD55 (membrane-bound proteins) provide a means to dampen and thus regulate activation of this amplification loop. Amount of complement activation is a sum of pro-activation (solid lines) and anti-activation (broken lines) effects.

of an alternative pathway C3 convertase, as described above. The alternative pathway is amplified at sites of tissue injury when inflammatory cells are recruited by effectors that may be generated by initial classical pathway activation. Necrotic cells fix complement, but more likely, a proinflammatory amplification loop results from alternative pathway activation by anaphylatoxin-responsive, infiltrating cells that secrete C3 and properdin to increase generation of complement cleavage products.

By means of these recognition and activation mechanisms, as well as the MBL pathway, the complement system identifies and responds to 'dangerous' situations presented by foreign antigens, pathogens, tissue injury, ischemia, apoptosis, and necrosis.[23] This capacity places the complement system at the center of many clinically important responses to foreign pathogens and, relevant to this chapter, to fetal injury mediated by cellular or humoral immune mechanisms.

Complement activities

The convergence of three complement activation pathways on the C3 protein results in a common pathway of effector functions (Figure 27.1). The initial step is generation of the fragments C3a and C3b. C3a, an anaphylatoxin that binds to receptors on leukocytes and other cells, causes activation and release of inflammatory mediators.[23] C3b and its further sequential cleavage fragments, iC3b and C3d, are ligands for complement receptors 1 and 2 (CR1 and CR2) and the β2 integrins, CD11b/CD18 and CD11c/CD18, present on a variety of inflammatory and immune accessory cells.[24,25] C3b attaches covalently to targets, followed by the assembly of C5 convertase with subsequent cleavage of C5 to C5a and C5b. C5a is a potent soluble inflammatory anaphylatoxic and chemotactic molecule that promotes recruitment and activation of neutrophils and monocytes and mediates endothelial cell activation through its receptor, C5aR (CD88), a member of the heptahelical seven transmembrane spanning protein family.[26,27] Binding of C5b to the target initiates the nonenzymatic assembly of the C5b-9 membrane attack complex (MAC). Insertion of C5b-9 MAC causes erythrocyte lysis through changes in intracellular osmolarity, while C5b-9 MAC damages nucleated cells primarily by activating specific signaling pathways through the interaction of the membrane-associated MAC proteins with heterotrimeric G proteins.[28,29]

In contrast to the somewhat uncertain role of C3 and the more proximal complement components, such as C1q, SAP, or C4, in promoting or protecting from autoimmune diseases like systemic lupus erythematosus (SLE), it is well accepted that activation of C5 and the insertion of MAC in the cell membrane results in a profound proinflammatory state affecting self-tolerance.[30] Thus, therapeutic strategies that target C5 and the more distal complement components, but leave C3 and the more proximal components unaffected, are an especially promising approach to complement inhibition.

The generation of C5a from C5 by C5 convertases is a major trigger of inflammation. Expression of C5aR, initially thought to be limited to neutrophils, monocytes, and eosinophils, has recently been shown to be more widespread and to include endothelial cells, liver parenchymal cells, vascular smooth muscle cells, bronchial epithelium, alveolar cells, mast cells, astrocytes, and human mesangial cells.[27] C5a binding on endothelial cells results in increased expression of P-selectin,[31] production of MIP-2, a potent neutrophil chemotactic factor, and MCP-1, involved in recruitment of monocytes and lymphocytes.[32] The release of chemokines in the presence of C5a leads to increased transmigration of neutrophils and amplification of inflammatory-mediated tissue damage.

Incorporation of C5b-9 MAC into cell membranes, a step absolutely dependent on C5 activation, also has pronounced effects on cell function. MAC binding activates several signal transduction pathways, resulting in increased arachidonic acid mobilization, generation of diacyl glyceride and ceramide, and activation of protein kinase C, MAPK, and Ras.[28,29] Proinflammatory and tissue-damaging phenotypic outcomes that follow these signaling events include the proliferation and release of reactive oxygen intermediates, leukotrienes, thromboxane, and platelet-derived growth factor.[32–34] Platelets respond to C5b-9 MAC insertion by degranulation and expression of procoagulant activity.[35] The concept that MAC plays a major role in human disease is further supported by finding that MAC is present at sites of tissue damage in multiple sclerosis, rheumatoid arthritis (RA), and many forms of glomerulonephritis.[32,35] Indeed, deficiency or inactivation of CD59, the complement regulatory protein that restricts MAC formation, seen in paroxysmal nocturnal hemoglobinuria and diabetes, respectively, is associated with thrombosis and vasculopathy.[36]

Because activated complement fragments have the capacity to bind and damage self-tissues, it is imperative that autologous bystander cells be protected from the deleterious effects of complement. To this end, most human and murine cells express molecules that limit the activation of various complement components. C3 is an important site of such complement regulation.[17]

Inhibition of C3 activation blocks the generation of most mediators of inflammation and tissue injury along the complement pathway. A family of membrane-bound proteins regulate the activation of C3 on the surface of host cells.[37,38] Decay accelerating factor (DAF) and membrane cofactor protein (MCP) are expressed on most human cells. Mouse DAF is also ubiquitously expressed, but murine MCP expression is restricted to the testis. However, mouse cells express an additional complement regulatory molecule, Crry, a widely distributed protein with MCP and DAF-like activity.[39,40]

COMPLEMENT AND FETAL TOLERANCE

Although the relationship between pregnancy failure and histologic evidence of inflammation has been convincingly documented, the triggering factors involved in initiating inflammation have remained elusive in most cases of preterm labor and spontaneous miscarriage. Experimental observations suggest that increased complement activation either causes or perpetuates inflammation during pregnancy.[41,42] As fetal tissues are semi-allogeneic and alloantibodies commonly develop in the mother, the placenta is potentially subject to complement-mediated immune attack at the maternal–fetal interface.[41] Although activated complement components are present in normal placentas,[43,44] it appears that in successful pregnancy uncontrolled complement activation is prevented by three regulatory proteins present on the trophoblast membrane: DAF, MCP, and CD59.[45–47] All three proteins are strategically positioned on the trophoblast in contact with maternal blood and cells and provide a mechanism to protect the fetus from damage due to complement pathway activation by alloantibodies. Indeed, based on their distribution patterns, it is likely that these proteins are strategically positioned for this purpose. Studies in mice show that complement regulatory proteins critically determine the sensitivity of host tissues to complement injury in autoimmune, ischemic, and inflammatory disorders.[48,49] The importance of complement regulatory proteins in humans is underscored by recent reports of a strong association between mutations in MCP and factor H (causing ineffective C3 inactivation)

with the hemolytic uremic syndrome and glomerular endothelial injury.[50,51]

Studies in mouse experimental models underscore the importance of complement regulation in fetal control of maternal processes that mediate tissue damage (Figure 27.3). In mice, Crry, a membrane-bound intrinsic complement regulatory protein (like DAF and MCP), blocks C3 and C4 activation on self-membranes[40] and thereby inhibits classical and alternative pathway C3 convertases and blocks C3, C5, and subsequent MAC activation. That appropriate complement inhibition is an absolute requirement for normal pregnancy has been demonstrated by the finding that Crry deficiency *in utero* leads to progressive embryonic lethality.[10] $Crry^{-/-}$ embryos are surrounded by activated C3 fragments and PMNs, primarily around the ectoplacental cone and surrounding trophoectoderm. Importantly, $Crry^{-/-}$ embryos are completely rescued from 100% lethality and live pups are born at a normal Mendelian frequency when C3 deficiency or factor B deficiency is introduced to $Crry^{-/-}$ embryos.[10,52] Defects in placental formation were associated with pregnancy loss and were solely dependent on alternative pathway activation and required maternal C3.[52] These observations emphasize the importance of the alternative pathway in initiating or amplifying complement activation in the placenta and provide genetic proof that $Crry^{-/-}$ embryos die *in utero* due to their inability to suppress complement activation and tissue damage mediated by C3. Overall, these findings support the concept that appropriate complement regulation is necessary to control maternal alloreactivity and placental inflammation and that a local increase in complement activation fragments is highly deleterious to the developing fetus.

COMPLEMENT IN MOUSE MODELS OF PREGNANCY LOSS

Complement activation mediates antiphospholipid antibody-induced pregnancy loss

The antiphospholipid antibody syndrome (APS) is characterized by arterial and venous thrombosis and pregnancy complications, including fetal

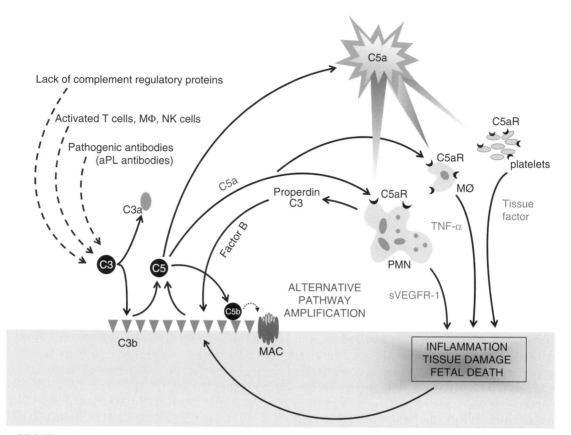

Figure 27.3 The role of complement activation in mouse models of pregnancy complications. The most striking finding is the remarkable similarity of the mechanisms leading to destruction of the feto–placental unit. Whether initiated by pathogenic antibodies (aPL antibodies), activated inflammatory cells, or lack of expression of complement regulatory proteins, there is C3 deposition, inflammatory cell infiltration, and tissue damage, likely products of complement activation. Activation of C5 leads to the generation of potent anaphylatoxins and mediators of effector cell activation, particularly C5a. C5a attracts and activates neutrophils, monocytes, and platelets, and stimulates the release of inflammatory mediators, including reactive oxidants, proteolytic enzymes, chemokines, cytokines, and complement factors C3 and properdin. Secretion of C3 and properdin by neutrophils, as well as the presence of apoptotic and necrotic decidual tissue, may accelerate alternative pathway activation, creating a proinflammatory amplification loop at sites of leukocyte infiltration that enhances C3 activation and deposition and generates additional C5a. This results in further influx of neutrophils, inflammation within the placenta, and ultimately fetal injury. Depending on the extent of damage, either death *in utero* or fetal growth restriction ensues. Adapted from Girardi *et al.* Complement C5a receptors and neutrophils mediate fetal injury in the antiphospholipid syndrome. J Clin Invest 2003; 112(11): 1644–54. With kind permission from the American Society for Clinical Investigation.

death and growth restriction, in association with antiphospholipid (aPL) antibodies. Over the last two decades, APS has emerged as a leading cause of pregnancy loss and pregnancy-related morbidity. Pregnancy loss is a defining criterion for APS and occurs with particularly high frequency in SLE patients bearing this antibody.[53–55] APS is defined as the association of aPL antibodies

(lupus anticoagulant or anticardiolipin antibodies) with one or both of these clinical events. Patients meet criteria for APS if they have three otherwise unexplained embryonic losses (before 10 weeks gestation) or one otherwise unexplained fetal loss (after 10 weeks), with or without placental infarction or fetal growth restriction.[53–55] The *in vivo* mechanisms by which aPL antibodies lead to vascular events, particularly recurrent fetal loss, are largely unknown. Our studies in a murine model of APS indicate that *in vivo* complement activation is necessary for fetal loss and vascular thrombosis caused by aPL antibodies.

Using a mouse model of APS induced by passive transfer of human aPL antibodies, we have shown that complement activation plays an essential and causative role in pregnancy loss and fetal growth restriction.[13] Passive transfer of IgG from women with recurrent miscarriage and aPL antibodies results in a 40% frequency of fetal resorption compared to < 10% in mice treated with IgG from healthy individuals, and a 50% reduction in the average weight of surviving fetuses. In our initial studies, we found that inhibition of the complement cascade *in vivo*, using the C3 convertase inhibitor Crry-Ig, prevented fetal loss and growth restriction and that mice deficient in complement C3 were resistant to fetal injury induced by aPL antibodies.[13]

To define the initiating pathways and critical effectors of aPL-induced pregnancy injury, we used mice deficient in complement elements (C4, factor B, C5, C5a receptor) and inhibitors of complement activation (anti-C5 monoclonal antibodies (mAbs), anti-factor B mAbs, C5a receptor antagonist peptide) in our mouse model of APS.[14] We identified complement component C5, and particularly its cleavage product C5a, as key mediators of fetal injury and showed that antibodies or peptides that block C5a–C5a receptor interactions prevent pregnancy complications. Furthermore, our results indicate that both classical and alternative complement pathway activation contribute to damage (Figure 27.3). Mice deficient in alternative and classical pathway complement components (factor B, C4, C3, and C5) were resistant to fetal injury induced by aPL antibodies. Based on the results of our mouse studies, we proposed a mechanism for pregnancy complications associated with aPL antibodies: aPL antibodies preferentially targeted at decidua and placenta activate complement via the classical pathway (Fc- and C4-dependent), leading to the generation of potent anaphylatoxins (C3a and C5a) and mediators of effector cell activation. Recruitment of inflammatory cells accelerates local alternative pathway activation and creates a proinflammatory amplification loop that enhances C3 activation and deposition, generates additional C3a and C5a, and results in further influx of inflammatory cells into the placenta. Depending on the extent of damage, either death *in utero* or fetal growth restriction ensues.

These studies underscore the importance of inflammation, rather than thrombosis, in fetal injury associated with aPL antibodies. Histopathologic findings in placentas from women with APS also argue that proinflammatory factors may contribute to tissue injury.[56,57] Given that the primary treatment for APS patients is anticoagulation throughout pregnancy, usually with sub-anticoagulant doses of heparin, and evidence that heparin inhibits complement activation *in vitro*, we considered the possibility that heparin prevents pregnancy loss by inhibiting complement activation on trophoblasts and that anticoagulation, in and of itself, is not sufficient to prevent pregnancy complications in APS. We found that treatment with unfractionated heparin or low molecular weight heparin protected pregnancies from aPL antibody-induced damage even at doses that did not cause detectable interference with coagulation.[58] In contrast, treatment with hirudin or fondaparinux (anticoagulants without anti-complement effects) was not protective, demonstrating that anticoagulation is insufficient therapy for APS-associated miscarriage.[58] Furthermore, heparins inhibited both aPL antibody-induced elevations in circulating C3a and increased C3b deposition in decidual tissues (neither was altered by the other anticoagulants) and blocked C3 cleavage *in vitro*. Thus, heparin may prevent pregnancy complications by limiting complement activation and the ensuing inflammatory response at the maternal–fetal interface, rather than by inhibiting thrombosis.

Our experiments indicate that aPL antibodies targeted to decidual tissues damage pregnancies by engagement of the classical pathway of complement activation, followed by amplification through the alternative pathway, and it appears that the heparins prevent obstetric complications caused by aPL antibodies because they block activation of complement. This work also provides a framework for understanding how sub-anticoagulant doses of heparin exert beneficial effects in antibody-mediated tissue injury.

Complement activation is a required intermediary event in antibody-independent mouse models of spontaneous miscarriage and IUGR

Studies in antibody-independent murine models of pregnancy loss strongly indicate a role for complement in fetal injury. Mellor et al.[12] and Munn et al.[59] demonstrated that cells expressing the enzyme indoleamine 2,3-dioxygenase (IDO) protect murine allogeneic concepti from maternal T-cell-mediated immunity and that treatment of pregnant mice with an IDO inhibitor results in a uniform loss of allogeneic, but not syngeneic, fetuses. In this model of murine fetal allograft rejection, maternal T cells specific for paternal antigens trigger complement activation and extensive deposition of C3 at the maternal–fetal interface, despite adequate Crry expression (Figure 27.3).[12,59] It appears that the inhibitory effects of Crry on complement activation are inadequate to prevent complement deposition when, under these pathological conditions, maternal T cells induce the production of large amounts of activated complement. Fetal allogaft rejection and complement activation were evident in T-cell-repleted mothers lacking B cells and pathogenic antibodies, indicating that complement activation is mediated by the antibody-independent alternative pathway.[59] It has been suggested that maternal T cells activated by contact with fetal cells release properdin and provoke activation of the alternative pathway and deposition of complement at the maternal–fetal interface, and cause fetal allograft rejection and death.[60,61] Alternatively, maternal T cells may induce properdin release by myeloid cells. Activated T cells may thus harness the potent inflammatory activities of complement, a constituent of the innate immune system, in a manner similar to antibodies.

We have studied a model of immunologically mediated peri-implantation pregnancy loss that shares features with human recurrent miscarriage: DBA/2-mated female CBA/J mice (CBA/J × DBA/2).[62,63] Embryos derived from mating CBA/J females with DBA/2 males showed 30% frequency of resorption, more than three times greater than that seen within these and other strains or strain combinations. Embryonic lethality

in DBA/2-mated female CBA/J mice is believed to represent rejection of the semi-allogeneic placenta by maternal-derived activated effectors. Resorption is not universal, however, and surviving fetuses show consistent and significant growth restriction.[15] The average weight of fetuses from CBA/J × DBA/2 matings was nearly 30% lower than that of fetuses from the BALB/c-mated female CBA/J mice (the control low-abortion mating combination) at the same gestational age. Pregnancies complicated by miscarriage or growth restriction were characterized by complement C3 deposition and inflammatory infiltrates in placentas and by defective placental development. Inhibition of complement activation in vivo at the level of C3, C5, and C5a–C5a receptor interactions (using Crry-Ig, anti-C5 mAb, or C5a receptor antagonist peptide) rescued pregnancies.[15] As predicted by results of experiments with complement inhibitors, administration of low-dose heparin was also effective in preventing fetal resorptions in DBA/2-mated CBA/J females.[15] These results re-emphasize the importance of complement in fetal damage and provide a framework for understanding how sub-anticoagulant doses of heparin (an empirical treatment administered to some patients with recurrent miscarriage of undefined etiology) exert beneficial effects.

Because immunohistologic analysis of deciduas from CBA/J × DBA/2 mice treated with C5aR antagonist peptide showed minimal C3 deposition surrounding normal-appearing fetuses and no evidence of inflammation, we considered the possibility that recruited inflammatory cells amplify complement activation on trophoblasts and within decidua. Activated myeloid cells have been shown to generate factor B and factor D.[64] Indeed, cognate T-cell–macrophage interactions are accompanied by alternative pathway activation (due to production of C3, factor B, and factor D, and down-regulation of complement regulatory protein expression) leading to generation of C5a and creation of a local amplification loop.[65] Given the extensive infiltration of monocytes and neutrophils observed in deciduas of CBA/J × DBA/2 mice, we hypothesized that alternative pathway activation contributes to fetal injury.

Treatment of CBA/J × DBA/2 and CBA/J × BALB/c mice with an anti-factor B mAb known to inhibit the alternative pathway *in vitro* and *in vivo* by blocking formation of the C3bBb complex[14,66] prevented fetal rejection and growth failure, indicating that the alternative pathway plays a central role in initiating and/or amplifying injury.

THE ALTERNATIVE PATHWAY AS A TARGET FOR ANTI-INFLAMMATORY THERAPIES: PREGNANCY FAILURE AND BEYOND

While the 'traditional' view of the alternative pathway is that it is simply a mechanism to amplify classical and lectin pathway activation, recent studies in pregnancy noted above, and in several other experimental models of human disease have demonstrated that the alternative pathway and its amplification loop play an essential role in disease pathogenesis (Table 27.1). In addition, genetic associations of dysfunctional alleles or mutants of factor H, the major alternative pathway regulatory protein, as well as MCP/CD46, another membrane regulator of alternative pathway activation, have highlighted the role of the alternative pathway in age-related macular degeneration and atypical hemolytic uremic syndrome. The activation and regulatory steps for the alternative pathway amplification loop are illustrated in Figure 27.2.

The evidence that the alternative pathway plays an essential role in the pathogenesis of inflammation first emerged in studies using the K/BxN-derived anti-glucose-6-phosphate isomerase (GPI) passive serum transfer model of rheumatoid arthritis (RA), where inflammatory joint disease was found to be ameliorated in *fB*−/− C57BL/6 mice but not in *C4*−/− or *MBL-A*−/− mice.[67] While the mechanism by which the antigen–antibody complexes were able to activate complement was not clearly defined, the findings challenged the assumption that immune complexes require the classical pathway to be pathogenic *in vivo*. In the collagen-induced arthritis (CIA) mouse model, back-crossing of the *fB*−/− genotype into the DBA1/j strain resulted in substantial disease amelioration, but introduction of the H-2b MHC into DBA1/j (which is H-2q) did not allow the investigators to conclude that factor B itself is responsible for injury rather other H-2 genes.[68] Subsequent studies of the anti-type II collagen (CII) arthritis induced by passive transfer demonstrated that C57BL/6

Table 27.1 Human disease models and complement pathway requirements

Human disease	Mouse model(s)	Complement pathway requirements	
		Classical	Alternative
1. Rheumatoid arthritis	K/BxN serum transfer	No	Yes
	Anti-collagen antibody transfer	No	Yes
2. Antiphospholipid syndrome	Antiphospholipid antibody transfer	Yes	Yes
3. Lupus nephritis	MRL/*lpr* strain	?	Yes
	C4−/−/B6 lpr strain	No	?
4. Asthma	Ova, ragweed immunization/inhalation	No	Yes
5. Ischemia-reperfusion Injury	Intestinal	Yes	Yes
	Renal	No	Yes
6. Type II membrano-proliferative glomerulonephritis	*fH*−/− strain	No	Yes
7. Macular degeneration	Choroid neovascularization	No	Yes
8. Spontaneous fetal loss	*Crry*−/− strain	No	Yes
	CBA/J × DBA/2	?	Yes

Modified from Thurman and Holers, The central role of the alternative complement pathway in human disease. J Immunol 2006; 176(3): 1305–10. With kind permission from the American Association of Immunologists.

mice deficient in factor B were protected from disease, while C4-deficient mice in the same strain were not.[69] Thus, in two models of passive transfer arthritis the alternative pathway was found to be essential, while the classical pathway was dispensable. It must be emphasized that these results do not exclude a role for the classical pathway in arthritis. Rather, they do demonstrate that in wild-type mice it is likely that the classical pathway plays an important role in generating target-fixed C3b that engages the alternative pathway amplification loop, but indeed inflammatory injury can occur in absence of classical pathway activation. In contrast to findings in passive transfer arthritis models, other examples of antibody-mediated tissue injury demonstrate a key role for both the classical and alternative pathways. As described above, fetal loss and growth restriction caused by transfer of aPL antibodies into pregnant mice require the activation of both the classical and alternative pathways, shown in studies using $C4^{-/-}$ mice, $fB^{-/-}$ mice and a specific alternative pathway inhibitory mAb directed to factor B. Taken together, results from experiments in antibody-mediated disease models show that regardless of whether the classical pathway is required, engagement of the alternative pathway appears to be the key pathogenic event.[70]

Other animal models of rheumatic diseases also identify the alternative pathway as a mediator of injury. In the MRL/*lpr* model of SLE, introduction of $fB^{-/-}$[71] or $fD^{-/-}$[72] genotypes results in a substantial decrease in renal disease. In contrast, MRL/*lpr* mice deficient in C3 have extremely high immune complex levels and severe renal disease, like that seen in C3-sufficient mice.[73] These results are not surprising based on studies of C1q- and C4-deficient C57BL/6 mice showing that inhibition of the classical pathway results in disease acceleration due to inadequate clearance of apoptotic bodies and immune complexes,[74] and they highlight the differences in outcomes between therapies that target C3 and the classical pathway compared with those directed at blocking the alternative pathway.

An important role for the alternative pathway has been shown in several antibody-independent models of inflammatory disease, including the CBA/J × DBA/2 model of pregnancy loss described above. In experimental asthma generated by sensitization of mice with ovalbumin or ragweed followed by intrapulmonary challenge with inhaled antigens, $C4^{-/-}$ mice are not protected but both $fB^{-/-}$ mice and mice treated with an inhibitor of factor B do not develop airway disease.[75] In this model, instillation of the alternative pathway inhibitor directly into the lung at doses insufficient to cause a systemic complement inhibition was effective and reconstitution of factor B into the lungs of $fB^{-/-}$ mice resulted in the generation of airway hyper-reactivity, suggesting that pathogenic complement products are generated in the airways where they can stimulate effector cells via C5a and C3a receptors. It should be noted that, as described for antibody-mediated injury, the relative contribution of classical pathway activation varies depending upon the model studied. For example, while ischemia-reperfusion injury of the intestine requires C4, ischemia-reperfusion injury of the kidney occurs in the absence of the classical pathway, and for both target organs alternative pathway activation is necessary for damage.[75]

Finally, as noted above, recent genetic studies have implicated the alternative pathway regulatory protein, factor H, and factor B in susceptibility to age-related macular degeneration in humans.[76] Dysfunctional alleles of factor H (a complement inhibitor) and hyper-functional alleles of factor B (alternative pathway amplifier) are linked to age-related macular degeneration. These results suggest that long-standing dysregulation of the alternative pathway in the eye leads to the formation of drusen and vascular endothelial growth factor (VEFG)-induced neovascularization. Indeed, recent studies using a mouse model of choroidal neovascularization (CNV) that mimics age-related macular degeneration have shown that the alternative pathway, not the classical pathway, is required for the development of CNV and that activation of the complement cascade drives the production of VEGF.[77]

In summary, mouse studies demonstrate that alternative pathway activation is a key mediator in the generation of proinflammatory complement components that lead to pregnancy complications, ischemia-reperfusion injury, arthritis, nephritis, and age-related macular degeneration.

Indeed, experimental models of pregnancy loss were pivotal in elucidating the role of the alternative pathway in immune-mediated injury. They demonstrated that the alternative pathway may be initiated by intrinsic mechanisms, as in the CBA/J × DBA/2 model of miscarriage, or through the classical/lectin pathway-catalyzed amplification loop, as in the model of aPL antibody-mediated fetal loss. Whether these results from human genetic studies and murine models can be translated into a therapeutically effective strategy is not yet known, but the generation of small molecule and mAb inhibitors directed to the three alternative pathway proteins (factor B, factor D, and properdin) will address this possibility in the coming years.

REFERENCES

1. Mills JL, Simpson JL, Driscoll SG et al. Incidence of spontaneous abortion among normal women and insulin-dependent diabetic women whose pregnancies were identified within 21 days of conception. N Engl J Med 1988; 319(25): 1617–23.
2. Hill JA. Immunological contributions to recurrent pregnancy loss. Baillieres Clin Obstet Gynaecol 1992; 6(3): 489–505.
3. Lu GC, Goldenberg RL. Current concepts on the pathogenesis and markers of preterm births. Clin Perinatol 2000; 27(2): 263–83.
4. Challis JRG. Mechanism of parturition and preterm labor. Obstet Gynecol Surv 2000; 55(10): 650–60.
5. Resnik R, Creasy RK. Intrauterine growth restriction. In: Iams JD, ed. Maternal–Fetal Medicine: Principles and Practice, 5th edn. Philadelphia, PA: Saunders, 2003: 495–512.
6. Godfrey KM, Barker DJ. Fetal nutrition and adult disease. Am J Clin Nutr 2000; 71(5 Suppl): 1344S-52S.
7. Mellor AL, Munn DH. Immunology at the maternal–fetal interface: lessons for T cell tolerance and suppression. Annu Rev Immunol 2000; 18: 367–91.
8. Hunt JS, Petroff MG, McIntire RH et al. HLA-G and immune tolerance in pregnancy. FASEB J 2005; 19(7): 681–93.
9. Guleria I, Khosroshahi A, Ansari MJ et al. A critical role for the programmed death ligand 1 in fetomaternal tolerance. J Exp Med 2005; 202(2): 231–7.
10. Xu C, Mao D, Holers VM et al. A critical role for murine complement regulator crry in fetomaternal tolerance. Science 2000; 287(5452): 498–501.
11. Aluvihare VR, Kallikourdis M, Betz AG. Regulatory T cells mediate maternal tolerance to the fetus. Nat Immunol 2004; 5(3): 266–71.
12. Mellor AL, Sivakumar J, Chandler P et al. Prevention of T cell-driven complement activation and inflammation by tryptophan catabolism during pregnancy. Nat Immunol 2001; 2(1): 64–8.
13. Holers VM, Girardi G, Mo L et al. Complement C3 activation is required for antiphospholipid antibody-induced fetal loss. J Exp Med 2002; 195(2): 211–20.
14. Girardi G, Berman J, Redecha P et al. Complement C5a receptors and neutrophils mediate fetal injury in the antiphospholipid syndrome. J Clin Invest 2003; 112(11): 1644–54.
15. Girardi G, Yarilin D, Thurman JM et al. Complement activation induces dysregulation of angiogenic factors and causes fetal rejection and growth restriction. J Exp Med 2006; 203(9): 2165–75.
16. Mao D, Wu X, Deppong C et al. Negligible role of antibodies and C5 in pregnancy loss associated exclusively with C3-dependent mechanisms through complement alternative pathway. Immunity 2003; 19(6): 813–22.
17. Abbas AK, Lichtman AH, Pober JS. Effector mechanisms of humoral immunity. In: Cellular and Molecular Immunology. Philadelphia, PA: WB Saunders, 2000: 316–34.
18. Schmidt BZ, Colten HR. Complement: a critical test of its biological importance. Immunol Rev 2000; 178: 166–76.
19. Weiser MR, Williams JP, Moore FD Jr et al. Reperfusion injury of ischemic skeletal muscle is mediated by natural antibody and complement. J Exp Med 1996; 183(5): 2343–8.
20. Korb LC, Ahearn JM. C1q binds directly and specifically to surface blebs of apoptotic human keratinocytes: complement deficiency and systemic lupus erythematosus revisited. J Immunol 1997; 158(10): 4525–8.
21. Fearon DT, Locksley RM. The instructive role of innate immunity in the acquired immune response. Science 1996; 272(5258): 50–3.
22. Fujita T, Matsushita M, Endo Y. The lectin-complement pathway – its role in innate immunity and evolution. Immunol Rev 2004; 198: 185–202.
23. Hugli TE. Structure and function of C3a anaphylatoxin. Curr Top Microbiol Immunol 1990; 153: 181–208.
24. Brown EJ. Complement receptors and phagocytosis. Curr Opin Immunol 1991; 3(1): 76–82.
25. Holers VM. In: Rich R ed. Complement, Principles and Practices of Clinical Immunology. St Louis, MO: Mosby, 1995: 363.
26. Gerard NP, Gerard C. The chemotactic receptor for human C5a anaphylatoxin. Nature 1991; 349(6310): 614–17.
27. Wetsel RA. Structure, function and cellular expression of complement anaphylatoxin receptors. Curr Opin Immunol 1995; 7(1): 48–53.
28. Shin ML, Rus HG, Nicolescu FI. Membrane attack by complement: assembly and biology of terminal complement complexes. Biomembranes 1996; 4: 123–49.

29. Morgan BP, Meri S. Membrane proteins that protect against complement lysis. Springer Semin Immunopathol 1994; 15(4): 369–96.

30. Carroll MC. The role of complement and complement receptors in induction and regulation of immunity. Annu Rev Immunol 1998; 16: 545–68.

31. Foreman KE, Vaporciyan AA, Bonish BK et al. C5a-induced expression of P-selectin in endothelial cells. J Clin Invest 1994; 94(3): 1147–55.

32. Morgan BP. Effects of the membrane attack complex of complement on nucleated cells. Curr Top Microbiol Immunol 1992; 178: 115–40.

33. Benzaquen LR, Nicholson-Weller A, Halperin JA. Terminal complement proteins C5b-9 release basic fibroblast growth factor and platelet-derived growth factor from endothelial cells. J Exp Med 1994; 179(3): 985–92.

34. Hattori R, Hamilton KK, McEver RP et al. Complement proteins C5b-9 induce secretion of high molecular weight multimers of endothelial von Willebrand factor and translocation of granule membrane protein GMP-140 to the cell surface. J Biol Chem 1989; 264(15): 9053–60.

35. Devine DV. The effects of complement activation on platelets. Curr Top Microbiol Immunol 1992; 178: 101–13.

36. Manzi S, Rairie JE, Carpenter AB et al. Sensitivity and specificity of plasma and urine complement split products as indicators of lupus disease activity. Arthritis Rheum 1996; 39(7): 1178–88.

37. Hourcade D, Holers VM, Atkinson JP. The regulators of complement activation (RCA) gene cluster. Adv Immunol 1989; 45: 381–416.

38. Lublin DM, Atkinson JP. Decay-accelerating factor and membrane cofactor protein. Curr Top Microbiol Immunol 1990; 153: 123–45.

39. Molina H, Wong W, Kinoshita T et al. Distinct receptor and regulatory properties of recombinant mouse complement receptor 1 (CR1) and Crry, the two genetic homologues of human CR1. J Exp Med 1992; 175(1): 121–9.

40. Kim YU, Kinoshita T, Molina H et al. Mouse complement regulatory protein Crry/p65 uses the specific mechanisms of both human decay-accelerating factor and membrane cofactor protein. J Exp Med 1995; 181(1): 151–9.

41. Holmes CH, Simpson KL. Complement and pregnancy: new insights into the immunobiology of the fetomaternal relationship. Baillieres Clin Obstet Gynaecol 1992; 6(3): 439–60.

42. Morgan BP, Holmes CH. Immunology of reproduction: protecting the placenta. Curr Biol 2000; 10(10): R381–3.

43. Weir PE. Immunofluorescent studies of the uteroplacental arteries in normal pregnancy. Br J Obstet Gynaecol 1981; 88(3): 301–7.

44. Wells M, Bennett J, Bulmer JN et al. Complement component deposition in uteroplacental (spiral) arteries in normal human pregnancy. J Reprod Immunol 1987; 12(2): 125–35.

45. Cunningham DS, Tichenor JR Jr. Decay-accelerating factor protects human trophoblast from complement-mediated attack. Clin Immunol Immunopathol 1995; 74(2): 156–61.

46. Tedesco F, Narchi G, Radillo O et al. Susceptibility of human trophoblast to killing by human complement and the role of the complement regulatory proteins. J Immunol 1993; 151(3): 1562–70.

47. Liszewski MK, Farries TC, Lublin DM et al. Control of the complement system. Adv Immunol 1996; 61: 201–83.

48. Song WC. Membrane complement regulatory proteins in autoimmune and inflammatory tissue injury. Curr Dir Autoimmun 2004; 7: 181–99.

49. Yamada K, Miwa T, Liu J et al. Critical protection from renal ischemia reperfusion injury by CD55 and CD59. J Immunol 2004; 172(6): 3869–75.

50. Noris M, Brioschi S, Caprioli J et al. Familial haemolytic uraemic syndrome and an MCP mutation. Lancet 2003; 362(9395): 1542–7.

51. Goodship TH, Liszewski MK, Kemp EJ et al. Mutations in CD46, a complement regulatory protein, predispose to atypical HUS. Trends Mol Med 2004; 10(5): 226–31.

52. Mao D, Xiaobo W, Molina H. A dispensable role for neutrophils, C5, and the classical pathway of complement activation in the abnormal fetomaternal tolerance found in crry-deficient mice. International Immunopharmacology 2002; 2: 1233.

53. Wilson WA, Gharavi AE, Koike T et al. International consensus statement on preliminary classification criteria for definite antiphospholipid syndrome: report of an international workshop. Arthritis Rheum. 1999; 42(7): 1309–11.

54. Lockshin MD, Sammaritano LR, Schwartzman S. Validation of the Sapporo criteria for antiphospholipid syndrome. Arthritis Rheum. 2000; 43(2): 440–3.

55. Levine JS, Branch DW, Rauch J. The antiphospholipid syndrome. N Engl J Med 2002; 346(10): 752–63.

56. Out HJ, Kooijman CD, Bruinse HW et al. Histopathological findings in placentae from patients with intra-uterine fetal death and anti-phospholipid antibodies. Eur J Obstet Gynecol Reprod Biol 1991; 41: 179–86.

57. Magid MS, Kaplan C, Sammaritano LR et al. Placental pathology in systemic lupus erythematosus: a prospective study. Am J Obstet Gynecol 1998; 179(1): 226–34.

58. Girardi G, Redecha P, Salmon JE. Heparin prevents antiphospholipid antibody-induced fetal loss by inhibiting complement activation. Nat Med 2004; 10(11): 1222–6.

59. Munn DH, Zhou M, Attwood JT et al. Prevention of allogeneic fetal rejection by tryptophan catabolism. Science 1998; 281(5380): 1191–3.

60. Schwaeble WJ, Reid KB. Does properdin crosslink the cellular and the humoral immune response? Immunol Today 1999; 20(1): 17–21.

61. Mellor AL, Munn DH. Tryptophan catabolism prevents maternal T cells from activating lethal anti-fetal immune responses. J Reprod Immunol 2001; 52(1–2): 5–13.

62. Clark DA, Chaouat G, Arck PC et al. Cytokine-dependent abortion in CBA × DBA/2 mice is mediated by the procoagulant fgl2 prothrombinase [correction of prothombinase]. J Immunol 1998; 160(2): 545–9.

63. Blois S, Tometten M, Kandil J et al. Intercellular adhesion molecule-1/LFA-1 cross talk is a proximate mediator capable of disrupting immune integration and tolerance mechanism at the feto-maternal interface in murine pregnancies. J Immunol 2005; 174(4): 1820–9.

64. Sundsmo JS, Chin JR, Papin RA et al. Factor B, the complement alternative pathway serine proteinase, is a major constitutive protein synthesized and secreted by resident and elicited mouse macrophages. J Exp Med 1985; 161(2): 306–22.

65. Heeger PS, Lalli PN, Lin F et al. Decay-accelerating factor modulates induction of T cell immunity. J Exp Med 2005; 201(10): 1523–30.

66. Thurman JM, Kraus DM, Girardi G et al. A novel inhibitor of the alternative complement pathway prevents antiphospholipid antibody-induced pregnancy loss in mice. Mol Immunol 2005; 42(1): 87–97.

67. Ji H, Ohmura K, Mahmood U et al. Arthritis critically dependent on innate immune system players. Immunity 2002; 16(2): 157–68.

68. Hietala MA, Jonsson IM, Tarkowski A et al. Complement deficiency ameliorates collagen-induced arthritis in mice. J Immunol 2002; 169(1): 454–9.

69. Banda NK, Thurman JM, Kraus D et al. Alternative complement pathway activation is essential for inflammation and joint destruction in the passive transfer model of collagen-induced arthritis. J Immunol 2006; 177(3): 1904–12.

70. Thurman JM, Holers VM. The central role of the alternative complement pathway in human disease. J Immunol 2006; 176(3): 1305–10.

71. Watanabe H, Garnier G, Circolo A et al. Modulation of renal disease in MRL/lpr mice genetically deficient in the alternative complement pathway factor B. J Immunol 2000; 164(2): 786–94.

72. Elliott MK, Jarmi T, Ruiz P et al. Effects of complement factor D deficiency on the renal disease of MRL/lpr mice. Kidney Int 2004; 65(1): 129–38.

73. Sekine H, Reilly CM, Molano ID et al. Complement component C3 is not required for full expression of immune complex glomerulonephritis in MRL/lpr mice. J Immunol 2001; 166(10): 6444–51.

74. Botto M, Walport MJ. C1q, autoimmunity and apoptosis. Immunobiology 2002; 205(4–5): 395–406.

75. Taube C, Thurman JM, Takeda K et al. Factor B of the alternative complement pathway regulates development of airway hyperresponsiveness and inflammation. Proc Natl Acad Sci U S A 2006; 103(21): 8084–9.

76. Donoso LA, Kim D, Frost A et al. The role of inflammation in the pathogenesis of age-related macular degeneration. Surv Ophthalmol 2006; 51(2): 137–52.

77. Bora NS, Kaliappan S, Jha P et al. Complement activation via alternative pathway is critical in the development of laser-induced choroidal neovascularization: role of factor B and factor H. J Immunol 2006; 177(3): 1872–8.

28

Matrix metalloproteinases

Thomas Pap, Steffen Gay and Georg Schett

Introduction • Structure, nomenclature, and function of matrix metalloproteinases • Regulation • Animal models • Expression of MMPs in RA • MMPs as therapeutic targets • References

INTRODUCTION

Tissue remodeling is a central feature of rheumatoid arthritis (RA). It essentially contributes to a progressive loss of joint function and leads to severe crippling that characterizes the high burden of disease. Tissue remodeling in RA is a complex mechanism and is composed of three major pathophysiological events: (i) growth, spreading, and invasion of inflammatory synovial tissue; (ii) destruction of cartilage; and (iii) bone erosion. All three processes are based on a common underlying mechanism, which is the degradation of extracellular matrix (ECM).

STRUCTURE, NOMENCLATURE, AND FUNCTION OF MATRIX METALLOPROTEINASES

Matrix metalloproteinases (MMPs) are a family of zinc-containing enzymes involved in the degradation and remodeling of ECM proteins. The MMP protein family comprises at least 16 different zinc-dependent endopeptidases.[1] All of these enzymes act extracellularly. The structure of MMPs consists of a catalytic domain containing histidine residues which form a complex with the catalytic zinc atom. The localization of this active site cleft varies among different members of the MMP family and partly influences the substrate specificity of each of the proteins. For example, the fibronectin type II repeats of MMP-2 and -9 allow their binding to denatured collagen.

The regulatory domain is a second essential domain of all MMPs. The regulatory domain locks the catalytic zink site by chelating it to a cysteine residue and thus maintains the MMP in an inactive state. Upon activation of the MMP, this regulatory domain is cleaved from the protease domain, thus uncovering the active catalytic pocket. This cleavage is either autocatalytic or mediated by enzymes such as plasmin, trypsin, furin, or other MMPs, especially membrane-type MMPs (MT-MMPs). Except MMP-7, which is the simplest MMP containing a protease and a regulatory domain, other MMPs contain a variable number of structural domains. These domains partly determine substrate specificity of MMPs and are involved in the binding of matrix proteins and tissue inhibitors of metalloproteinases (TIMPs), the natural inhibitors of MMP activity. Examples of structural domains are the hemopexin domains of collagenases (MMP-1, -8, -13, and -14) allowing the binding to triple-helical collagen and the transmembrane domains of MT-MMPs (MMPs 14–17) serving as anchors to the cell membrane.

The nomenclature of MMPs is now based on an MMP number (MMP-1, MMP-2, etc.). Earlier nomenclatures were based on the assumption that each MMP is highly substrate-specific and MMPs were named according to their capacity to degrade collagen (collagenases), denatured collagen (gelatinases), and elastin (elastases).[2] However, it was recognized that each MMP

Table 28.1 Nomenclature and substrates of MMPs, including the alternative names of MMP family members

Name	Alternative name	Major substrates	MMP substrates
MMP-1	Interstitial collagenase collagenase 1	Collagens (I, II, III, VII, VIII, X), gelatin, aggrecan	MMP-2, -9
MMP-2	Gelatinase A, type IV collagenase	Collagens (I, IV, V, VII, X, XI, XIV), gelatin	MMP-1, -9, -13
MMP-3	Stromelysin-1	Collagens (III, IV, V, IX) gelatin, aggrecan	MMP-1, -2, -7, -8, -9, -13
MMP-7	Matrilysin	Collagens (IV, X) gelatin, aggrecan	MMP-1, -2, -9
MMP-8	Neutrophil collagenase, collagenase 2	Collagens (I, II, III, V, VII, VIII, X) gelatin, aggrecan	–
MMP-9	Gelatinase B, 92 kDa gelatinase	Collagens (IV, V, VII, X, XIV) gelatin, aggrecan	–
MMP-10	Stromelysin-2	Collagens (II, IV, V) gelatin, aggrecan	MMP-1, -8
MMP-11	Stromelysin-3	α_2-Antitrypsin, α_2-macroglobulin	–
MMP-12	Macrophage metalloelastase	Collagen (IV), gelatin, elastin	–
MMP-13	Collagenase-3	Collagens (I, II, III, IV, IX, X, XIV) gelatin, aggrecan	MMP-9
MMP-14	MT1-MMP	Collagens (I, II, III), gelatin, elastin	MMP-2, -13
MMP-15	MT2-MMP	Fibronectin, aggrecan	MMP-2
MMP-16	MT3-MMP	Collagen (III), gelatin	MMP-2
MMP-17	MT4-MMP	–	–
MMP-19	–	Gelatin	–
MMP-20	–	Amelogenin	–

usually degrades multiple substrates and that there is substantial substrate overlap between individual MMPs. Therefore, a numeric nomenclature has become widely accepted (Table 28.1).

The function of MMPs is confined to the extracellular compartment, and MMPs act either in a soluble form outside the cells or anchored to the cell membrane (MT-MMPs). Firstly, members of the MMP family are involved in tissue remodeling under both normal and pathological conditions. Secondly, MMPs are a prerequisite for the migration of normal and malignant cells through the ECM; and, thirdly, they act as regulatory molecules by processing matrix proteins, cytokines, and adhesion molecules. In all these instances, MMP activity underlies a fine balance with the activity of their endogenous inhibitors (TIMPs). Once activated, MMPs are a substrate for TIMPs as well as they are bound and inactivated by plasma proteins such as α2-macroglobulin. To date, four different forms of TIMPs (TIMP 1–4) have been described.[3]

Two types of protein families are structurally related to MMPs: the ADAMs (a desintegrin and a metalloproteinase)[4] and the ADAMTSs (a desintegrin and a metalloproteinase with thrombospondin motifs).[5] Both families are also multidomain proteases and consist of a catalytic and a regulatory domain structurally related to MMPs. However, both families have a desintegrin domain which allows binding to cell surface integrins. Whereas ADAMs are membrane-bound molecules, ADAMTSs lack a transmembrane part, but contain thrombospondin type I motifs, allowing its binding to proteoglycans. The most known ADAM is TACE (ADAM-17, tumor necrosis factor (TNF) converting enzyme), which cleaves membrane-bound TNF-α to a soluble form.[6,7] The most famous ADAMTSs are ADAMTS-4 and -5, which are commonly known as 'aggrecanases' cleaving aggrecan, which is the most important proteoglycan of the cartilage.[8]

REGULATION

With the exception of MMP-2 and the MT-MMPs, which are constitutively expressed, MMP expression is induced (or suppressed) by extracellular signals via transcriptional activation. Three major groups of inducers can be differentiated: (i) proinflammatory cytokines, (ii) growth factors, (iii) matrix molecules, and (iv) advanced glycosylation end products (AGEs). Among proinflammatory cytokines, interleukin (IL)-1 is a central inducer of a variety of MMPs, including MMP-1, -3, -8, -13, and –14.[9–12] The effect of IL-1 on MMP expression highlights the complex nature of MMP induction: the specific effect of an extracellular signal such as IL-1 on MMP expression can be variable and depends on the type of MMP induced, the cell type, and the signal transduction pathway which appears predominantly activated. Thus, for example, IL-1 up-regulates differentially MMP-13, via JNK and p38 protein kinase signaling[9] and MMP-1, via STAT transcription factors,[12] in chondrocytes. Also, additive effects between IL-1 and other cytokines, such as TNF-α or oncostatin M,[12,13] or growth factors, such as fibroblast growth factor (FGF) and platelet-derived growth factor (PDGF), on the induction of MMPs are known.[14] Other cytokines pivotally involved in tissue remodeling of rheumatic diseases which induce MMP expression are TNF-α (MMP 1–3)[15] and IL-17 (MMP-1, -3, -9, and 13)[16,17] and transforming growth factor TGF-β (MMP-13).[18] Among growth factors, FGF and PDGF are known inducers of MMPs, as they potentiate the effect of IL-1 on MMP expression.[14] Vascular endothelial growth factor (VEGF) is an inducer of MMP-13 in chondrocytes,[19] and MIP acts on MMP-9 and –13.[20] The third group of MMP inducers are matrix proteins (collagen, fibronectin), and especially their degradation products activate MMP expression in chondrocytes and fibroblasts, providing the possibility for a site-specific MMP activation at places of matrix breakdown.[21,22] Recently, AGEs have been identified as inducers for MMPs, particularly of articular chondrocytes.[23]

Transcriptional silencers of MMPs are the anti-inflammatory and regulatory cytokines IL-4, IL-10 and IL-13,[24] as well as signaling via the p53 protein.[25] Some interesting data have also come from studies showing that microparticles derived from immune cells can directly stimulate the expression of both inflammatory cytokines and disease-relevant MMPs in synovial cells.[26]

Signaling for transcriptional activation of MMPs is mediated by several pathways. The activator protein-1 (AP-1) binding site is present in the promotor region of all MMPs (except MMP-2), suggesting a central role of jun/fos

transcription factor binding. Indeed, there is abundant experimental evidence that all three mitogen/stress-activated protein kinase (MAPK/SAPK) families, ERK, JNK, and p38 kinase, which integrate extracellular signals upstream from jun/fos, are involved in the regulation of MMP expression. In particular, the induction of MMP-1, -9 and -13 is mediated through MAPK/SAPK signalling.[11,20,27–29] Besides AP-1, the promotor regions of some MMPs contain NF-κB,[27,28] STAT,[30] and ETS[31,32] binding sites. Indeed, activation of these transcription factors has been demonstrated to occur during the induction of MMP-1, -3, and -13, which are thought to be essential for the joint damage in rheumatoid arthritis (RA). Activation of the various MAPK/SAPK and transcription factors, none of which are tissue-specific signaling molecules, occurs at very distinct subcompartments of the rheumatoid joint, thus determining a specific pattern of MMP expression in the synovium.[33,34] On the other hand, tissue-specific transcription factors of MMP do exist. One example is Cbfa-1 (a runx-protein family member) which is essential for MMP-13 expression in cartilage and bone.[35] Recently, regulation of MMPs by the Ets-1 transcription factor has received some interest, because in addition to the well established rolle of Ets-1 in regulating the expresion of MMPs in vascular endothelial cells[36] novel data from the Ets-1 knockout mouse indicate that Ets-1 is also involved in the expression of MMPs in fibroblasts.[37] In this study, it was found that Ets-1 is involved prominently in the fast induction of MMP-2, -3, and -13 by bFGF.

ANIMAL MODELS

MMP activation has been assessed in a variety of animal models of arthritis to gain an insight into the sequence of events leading to degeneration of articular cartilage. The increased catabolism of the cartilage proteoglycan aggrecan is a principal pathological process which leads to the degeneration of articular cartilage in arthritic joint diseases. The consequent loss of sulphated glycosaminoglycans (GAGs), which are intrinsic components of the aggrecan molecule, compromises both the functional and structural integrity of the cartilage matrix and ultimately renders the tissue incapable of resisting the compressive loads applied during joint articulation. Over time, this process leads to irreversible cartilage erosion. *In situ* degradation of aggrecan is a proteolytic process involving cleavage at specific peptide bonds located within the core protein. Studies on collagen-induced arthritis (CIA) and antigen-induced arthritis (AIA) have clearly established that aggrecanases, which belong to the ADAMTS protein family (ADAMTS-4 and -5), are primarily responsible for the catabolism and loss of aggrecan from articular cartilage in the early stages of arthritic joint diseases that precede overt collagen catabolism and disruption of the tissue integrity.[38] Cleavage of aggrecan by aggrecanases leads to the formation of specific neoepitopes (NITEGEs), which are fingerprints for the action of aggrecanase. NITEGE neoepitopes can be stained in the cartilage of arthritic mice, appear early in the course of disease, and indicate a progressive loss of GAGs. The typical morphological result is the inability of articular cartilage to retain dyes like toluidine blue or safranin O, which bind to GAGs. Whereas the loss of GAGs due to aggrecanase cleavage is reversible, later steps of cartilage damage are irreversible. MMPs (especially MMP-1, -3, and -13) govern the cleavage of collagen type II, which is the major matrix constituent of cartilage, and collagen type IX, which provides a link between collagen type II fibrils and GAGs.[39] When the collagen fibrils are lost, the cartilage has no effective way to retain GAGs, thus leading to irreversible damage of cartilage. Furthermore, MMPs also cleave the remaining aggrecan molecules at specific sites, leading to formation of neoepitopes (such as VDIPEN), which differ from that induced by aggrecanases. Studies with MMP-3$^{-/-}$ mice have confirmed these data, showing a lack of cartilage erosion as well as no formation of collagen type II or VDIPEN neoepitopes.[39] However, the loss of GAGs was still evident in MMP-3$^{-/-}$ mice, underlining the action of aggrecanases. Thus, the expression and activation of MMPs seems to be a fateful event in irreversible damage of cartilage. Animal models of arthritis, such as AIA, have also demonstrated an early up-regulation of crucial MMPs, MMP-1, -3, and -13, in the course of disease.[40,41] MMPs are produced from synovial cells invading cartilage and bone (fibroblasts, macrophages, osteoclasts) as well from chondrocytes lying adjacent but not distant from cartilage and bone erosions[42] (G. Schett, unpublished observations) (Figure 28.1). This suggests that cytokines synthesized by synovial cells induce a change of the expression pattern of chondrocyte proteins, shifting it from matrix synthesis to matrix degradation. Furthermore, animal models of arthritis have taught that latent MMP expression is even found in resting phases of disease, thus entailing a more rapid activation of MMPs leading to a faster and more severe cartilage resorption in flares of disease than in its primary onset.[41]

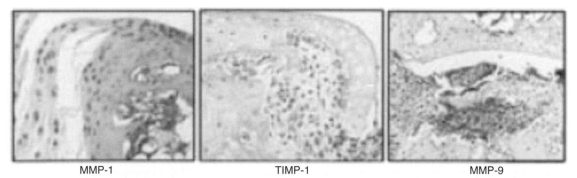

MMP-1   TIMP-1   MMP-9

Figure 28.1 MMPs and TIMPs are expressed by chondrocytes and pannocytes at the site of bone and cartilage destruction. Microphotographs show the junction zone between pannus, cartilage, and bone of paw sections from TNF transgenic mice. Sections were stained for MMP-3, TIMP-1, and MMP-9 (dark colors). MMPs and TIMP are abundantly expressed by cells of the synovial membrane, the invading inflammatory synovial tissue, and adjacent cartilage.

The role of overexpression of MMPs in cartilage resorption is also highlighted by mice transgenic for MMP-13, which develop severe cartilage damage.[43] However, knockout models of MMP have also shown that some MMPs are not crucial for soft tissue remodeling including cartilage resorption (MMP-2$^{-/-}$ mice)[44] and others may even have a key regulatory role, like MT1-MMP (MMP-14), since the knockout mice develop arthritis.[45]

Interesting data have come also from the SCID mouse co-implantation model of RA, where synovial fibroblasts (SFs) are implanted together with normal human articular cartilage into severe combined immunodeficient (SCID) mice (Figure 28.2). Due to their lack of a functional immune system, SCID mice do not reject the human implants and allow the study of the interactions of fibroblasts and cartilage. It has been shown in a number of studies, that in the SCID mouse model, RA synovial fibroblasts (RA-SFs) attach to the co-implanted cartilage and deeply invade the cartilage matrix,[46,47] while normal SFs, osteoarthritis (OA) SFs, or dermal fibroblasts do not show such invasion. Of note, this experimental approach investigates the behavior of RA-SFs in the absence of human inflammatory cells. Therefore, the differences between RA-SFs, OA-SFs, and normal SFs have been taken as evidence for the stable, intrinsic activation of RA-SFs. It has been understood that apart from different proinflammatory cytokines, internal, cytokine-independent pathways contribute to the increased expression of MMPs and that overexpression of MMPs is associated closely with the activated phenotype of RA-SFs.[48] Conversely, inhibition of signaling pathways that are activated in RA-SFs and result in the up-regulation of MMPs can reduce the invasion into the cartilage. Thus, inhibition of MAPK signaling through the delivery of dominant negative mutants of c-Raf-1 decreases the invasiveness of RA-SFs in the SCID mouse model. This is due to reduced phosphorylation of c-Jun and subsequent lower expression of MMP-1 and MMP-13.[49] Unfortunately, there has been no exact estimate as to how individual MMPs contribute to the invasiveness of RA-SFs. This lack of understanding has been one major obstacle to developing specific strategies for the inhibition of MMPs. Although data from the aforementioned MMP knockout mice indicate the particular importance of some MMPs, these models are limited by their purely immunological nature. In addition, they have demonstrated a great overlap between different MMP family members. In this context, the SCID mouse model offers the opportunity to selectively inhibit single MMPs or MMP activation pathways in human RA-SFs and to assess their effects on the invasiveness of these cells. In this context, inhibition of plasmin – one major activator of MMPs – reduces the invasion of RA-SFs by about 30%.[50] Conversely, overexpression of TIMPs in RA-SFs through adenoviral gene transfer resulted in a 50% invasion compared with control fibroblasts.[51] Other studies analyzing the role of individual MMPs in the SCID mouse model are under way and will provide more detailed insights into the concerted action of MMP family members in rheumatoid joint destruction. First data from such analyses indicate that in the SCID mouse model of rheumatoid cartilage destruction, inhibition of a single MMP, such as MMP-1 or MT1-MMP, may reduce the invasion of RA-SFs by about 40%.[52,53]

EXPRESSION OF MMPs IN RA

MMPs are expressed abundantly in the RA synovium, and there have been a number of studies correlating the expression levels of MMPs and their tissue distribution to synovial inflammation and joint destruction. In line with cell culture studies and SCID mouse experiments, RA-SFs in the lining layer constitute the major source of MMPs, underlining their role in the destruction of articular cartilage in RA. Also, there is growing evidence that in addition to the absolute levels of MMPs, the ratio of MMPs to their naturally occurring inhibitors, the TIMPs, is of importance for joint destruction to occur.[54]

MMP-1 (interstitial collagenase, collagenase 1) belongs to the major enzymes in the rheumatoid synovium. It is found in all RA patients but only in about 55–80% of trauma samples.[55] Synovial lining cells produce most MMP-1 in the diseased synovium, and MMP-1 is released from these cells immediately after production.[56] Consequently, the expression of MMP-1 in the synovial fluid

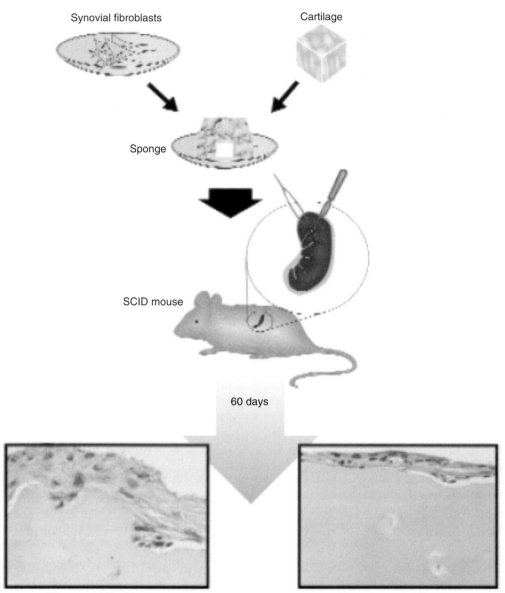

Figure 28.2 SCID mouse co-implantation model of rheumatoid arthritis (RA). Synovial fibroblasts (SFs) were isolated from RA patients (RA-SFs) or non-arthritic patients undergoing leg amputation (normal SFs). Human cartilage was obtained from cardiac surgery (rib cartilage) or non-arthritic amputations (knee cartilage). SFs and cartilage were first inserted into a cavity of inert sterile gel sponge and then co-implanted in a pocket of the surgically opened renal capsule. Sixty days after implantation histological analysis revealed cartilage invasion by RA-SFs (left) but not normal SFs (right).

correlates positively with the degree of synovial inflammation.[57] However, it appears that serum concentrations of MMP-1 do not reflect the levels in the synovial fluids and, therefore, measuring serum MMP-1 has not been proven as a marker for disease activity.

As mentioned before, MMP-2 (gelatinase A) is expressed constitutively in synovial tissues from RA as well as from OA and trauma patients, but several studies have shown increased expression of MMP-2 in the rheumatoid synovium.[55] This is also true for the second member of the gelatinase family, MMP-9 (gelatinase B). MMP-9 can be found at elevated levels in the sera and synovial fluids of RA patients compared with healthy controls,[58,59] and both SFs and macrophages of the RA synovium express MMP-9. Another source of MMP-9 in the synovium is mast cells, which express MMP-9 upon challenge with pro-inflammatory cytokines such as TNF and IL-1.[60] Analyzing the expression of MMP-9 in the synovial fluid of patients with RA, OA, and other inflammatory arthritides, Ahrens et al. found an association between increased levels of MMP-9 and inflammatory arthritis.[59] These data are of interest, because MMP-9 has also been found in osteoclasts and implicated in the resorption of bone.[61] Despite the potential of synovial macrophages to differentiate into bone resorbing, osteoclast-like cells, it is not clear how the expression pattern of MMP-9 correlates with erosions in RA.

Due to its specific properties, MMP-3 plays an important role in the degradation of cartilage matrix, and early reports in the 1980s demonstrated that active MMP-1, -2, and -3 can together destroy a number of structural proteins in the synovium.[62] MMP-3 has been assigned a key role in the destruction of rheumatoid joints because it not only degrades ECM molecules but is also involved in the activation of pro-MMPs into their active forms. It is produced abundantly by RA-SFs when stimulated with macrophage-conditioned medium[63] and again, RA-SFs in the lining layer are the cells that predominantly express MMP-3 in the RA synovium[64] Of interest, there is evidence that the hypoxic environment in the RA synovial membrane increases the expression of MMP-1 and also MMP-3, thus contributing directly to the destructive process.[65] Synovial fluids from patients with RA show about 100-fold higher concentrations of active MMP-3 than control samples.[66] Interestingly, increased levels of MMP-3 are also found in the sera of patients with RA[67–71] and correlate with systemic inflammation at clinical[69,71] and serological[68,70,71] levels. However, the question as to whether increased levels of circulating MMP-3 reflect radiological damage has been discussed controversially. No correlation between serum MMP-3 and radiological or functional scores was seen in the study

by Manicourt et al.[70] So et al. failed to establish differences in the serum levels of MMP-3 between RA patients with long-standing RA (> 5 years) that had low or high erosion scores.[68] In contrast, Yamanaka et al. reported recently that serum MMP-3 was a predictor of joint damage at early stages of disease.[72] At the moment, it can be concluded that the serum levels of MMP-3 at least to a certain degree reflect synovial inflammation and as such may correlate with ongoing joint destruction rather than past damage.

Most other MMPs have also been demonstrated in the RA synovium and particularly in RA-SFs. Among these, MMP-8, which had been described exclusively in polymorphonuclear neutrophils, is also expressed by RA-SFs,[73] and this observation was made not only *in vivo* but also in fibroblast cell cultures under *in vitro* conditions.

MMP-13 (collagenase 3) has been implicated most prominently in cartilage destruction in RA. Using degenerate primers that corresponded to highly conserved regions of the MMP gene family, Wernicke et al. cloned MMP-13 from the synovium of patients with RA,[74] and subsequent studies demonstrated the expression of MMP-13, particularly in SFs but also in macrophages in the lining layer of rheumatoid synovium.[75] Due to this localization and its substrate specificity for collagen type II, MMP-13 plays an important role in joint destruction. Of interest, expression of MMP-13 correlates with elevated levels of systemic inflammation markers[76] but studies in OA demonstrated clearly that the expression of MMP-13 is not specific for RA. Rather, it appears that MMP-13 is associated closely with degeneration of cartilage in different pathologies.

MT-MMPs are also expressed abundantly in cells aggressively destroying cartilage and bone in RA.[77] Although MT1-MMP is expressed constitutively in RA-SFs, elevated levels have been found in RA. This is of importance, because MT1-MMP degrades ECM components and also activates other disease-relevant MMPs such as MMP-2 and MMP-13. In a recent study that compared the expression of MT-MMPs in RA, we suggested that MT1-MMP is of particular relevance to RA.[77] In this analysis, the expression of MT3-MMP mRNA was seen in fibroblasts and some macrophages, particularly in the lining layer, but expression of MT2- and MT4-MMP was characterized by a scattered staining of only a few CD68-negative fibroblasts.

Collectively, all MMPs that have been associated with the remodeling of connective tissue as well as inflammatory processes can be found at elevated levels in the rheumatoid synovium. Although it appears that certain metalloproteinases (MMP-1, -3, -13, together with MT1- and MT3-MMP, and aggrecanases) may contribute most significantly to the destruction of articular cartilage, no specific pattern of MMP expression has been found for RA. Specifically, the relation of disease-induced MMP activity to normal expression in different tissues including the synovium needs to be established. A more detailed understanding of natural MMP inhibitors and metalloproteinase functions that are distinct from matrix degradation will help to develop disease-specific inhibitors for RA.

MMPs AS THERAPEUTIC TARGETS

Based on these data, a number of strategies have been considered to interfere with the expression and activation of MMPs in the rheumatoid joint (Table 28.2).

The understanding that inflammatory stimuli contribute to the up-regulation of MMPs in the rheumatoid synovium has resulted in several studies investigating the potential of anti-inflammatory and disease-modifying therapies to inhibit MMPs in the RA synovium. It was shown that by decreasing synovial inflammation drugs such as methotrexate or leflunomide also affect the production of MMPs and result in decreased levels of MMP-1.[78] Therefore, the retardation of radiological disease progression as seen with some of these disease-modifying anti-rheumatic drugs (DMARDs) may be attributed to decreased levels of MMPs. This notion is also supported by recent advances in the treatment of RA that have come from the use of biologic agents. The use of TNF-α inhibitors such as monoclonal antibodies (mAbs) has not only offered new perspectives to treat inflammation, but first data suggest that they retard at least to a certain degree radiological damage. In this context, Brennan et al. demonstrated that serum levels of MMP-1

Table 28.2 Current strategies to inhibit MMPs in RA

Agents

Anti-inflammatory treatment
    DMARDs (e.g. methotrexate, leflunomide)
    Biologicals (e.g. infliximab, etanercept)

Tetracyclines
    Antimicrobially effective tetracyclins (e.g., doxycycline)
    Chemically modified teracyclines (not antimicrobial)

Specific, pharmacological MMP inhibitors
    Substrate (peptide) inhibitor with alternative chelators
    Non-peptide inhibitors (e.g. sulfone-hydroxamates, biaryl keto-acids)

Gene transfer
    Delivery of naturally occurring inhibitors (TIMP-1, TIMP-3)
    Generation of artificial inhibitors of MMP activation (ATF.BPTI)
    Antisense constructs (αS ODNs, αS expression constructs, ribozymes)

DMARDs, disease-modifying anti-rheumatic drugs; TIMP, tissue inhibitor of metalloproteinases; ODN, oligonucleotide.

and MMP-3 decrease following treatment with anti-TNF-α agents.[79,80]

Among available drugs, tetracyclines have been shown to have anti-collagenolytic effects that are due to different mechanisms, among them inhibition of MMP-1 as well as prevention of MMP activation.[81] Based on this understanding, some clinical trials have been initiated that aimed to use such drugs for the treatment of RA. Nordstrom et al. reported that a 3-month treatment of RA patients with daily 150 mg doxycycline has anti-collagenolytic effects.[82] This effect is not necessarily related to the antimicrobial activity of tetracyclines, as there are a number of modified tetracyclines that are not antimicrobial but still inhibit MMPs. However, their efficacy is far less than what can be achieved with specific inhibitors of MMPs.

Based on our advanced understanding of MMP structures, small molecular weight pharmacological compounds have been developed by nearly all major pharmaceutical companies as well as research institutes (for a comprehensive review of their characteristics, pharmacological properties, and development see Skotnicki et al.[83]). According to their structures, two strategies can be distinguished as follows. Early but continuing efforts have started out from the structure of MMP substrates and resulted in the development of peptide and peptide-like MMP inhibitors that contained alternative chelators such as aminocarboxylates, carboxylic acids, thiol amides, and others. Alternatively, non-peptide inhibitors of MMPs have been synthesized since Novartis disclosed its substance CGS 23161 in.1994 CGS 23161 is rather specific for MMP-3 (K_i 71 nM) and has served as a lead substance for the development of a number of sulfonamide-hydroxamates and derivatives.[83,84] Both peptide and non-peptide inhibitors of MMPs are being developed continuously, and a number of compounds have been used in animal models of arthritis or have even entered early phase clinical studies. Thus, the peptide-type broad-spectrum MMP inhibitors, BB-2516 (marimastat) and BB-94 (batimastat), have been evaluated for arthritis. Batimastat was demonstrated to have favorable effects in adjuvant arthritis[85] but was not followed further due to its poor bioavailability. Marimastat, which that was tested in parallel in patients with advanced cancers,[86–88] had much better pharmacokinetic properties. However, as seen in the cancer studies, marimastat had major musculoskeletal side effects, with muscular pain, stiffness, and even inflammatory polyarthritis.[89,90] Notably, such musculoskeletal symptoms have also been observed with other MMP inhibitors, but their cause remains unclear. Specifically, it has not been clarified whether these side effects are due to MMP inhibition or are caused by common but non-MMP-specific features of MMP inhibitors. It has been suggested that the musculoskeletal side effects are related to the inhibition of MMP-1, but this hypothesis has not been proven so far. Nonetheless, more selective MMP inhibitors have been tested for arthritis, such as RS-130830 (Roche Bioscience),[83] that inhibits MMP-13 much more effectively than MMP-1, and several non-peptide inhibitors with different specificities have been developed. Although the focus appears to shift from inflammatory arthritis to a potential application in OA, nearly all MMP inhibitors are tested for their efficacy in animal or *in vitro* models of RA.

In terms of clinical applications, the Roche compound, Ro 32–3555l (Trocade), has become most advanced.[91,92] Trocade predominantly inhibits collagenases (MMP-1, MMP-3, and MMP-13) and has demonstrated its efficacy in different *in vitro* and *in vivo* models of cartilage degradation. However, no significant effects were seen in animal models of inflammatory arthritis and early clinical data suggest that the progression of joint damage was not prevented.[91] Despite good initial data on tolerability over short periods of time,[92] long term data from clinical trials have been less favorable. So far, no MMP inhibitor has made its way into the clinic, clearly illustrating the problem: although a multitude of pharmacological agents have been developed that inhibit MMPs with even picomolar efficacy, there seem to be conceptual difficulties with their application in RA[93] In this context, it also appears interesting to explore the effect of MMP inhibition on apoptosis in more detail.

Consequently, alternative strategies have been worked out that focus on the specific modulation of MMP activity through interfering with both expression and activation of MMPs. Among them, gene transfer has become one tool that allows blockage of distinct steps of MMP action in a highly selective manner.[94] Specific inhibition of MMPs has been associated mainly with three strategies (Table 28.2): (i) the delivery of naturally occurring inhibitors of MMPs (TIMPs), (ii) the design and delivery of novel inhibitory molecules or modifications of naturally occurring inhibitors, and (iii) targeting the mRNA of MMPs through different antisense strategies.

As mentioned, MMP activity is balanced by natural inhibitors (TIMPs), but in RA the amount of MMPs produced outweighs that of the TIMPs. Therefore, it has been suggested that the delivery of functional genes for TIMPs may 'correct' for this dysbalance and result in a decrease of matrix degradation. Although initial studies by Apparailly et al[95] failed to demonstrate a significant effect of TIMP-1 gene transfer in DBA/1 mice with CIA, most recent studies in both the TNF-α transgenic animal models of RA[33] and the SCID mouse model have shown that delivery of TIMP-1 may have beneficial effects on the destruction of cartilage.[51] Most recently, TIMP-3 has become of particular interest among the TIMPs. This is because in addition to inhibiting MMPs, TIMP-3 has been associated with a number of features that are distinct from other TIMPs. It binds to extracellular matrix, also inhibits MT-MMPs and ADAMs, and has the ability to induce apoptosis in different cell types. With respect to RA, it has been shown that overexpression of TIMP-3 reduces the invasiveness of RA-SFs *in vitro* and *in vivo*.[51] In addition, it was shown recently that TIMP-3 not only induces apoptosis but also modulates the apoptosis-inhibiting effects of TNF-α in RA-SFs.[96]

As an alternative approach, genes for artificial inhibitors of MMP activation can be delivered to the rheumatoid synovium. Thus, it has been proposed that delivery of a gene for a hybrid protein targeting plasmin on the surface of RA-SFs may reduce their invasive potential.[50] This is based on the aforementioned understanding that components of the plasminogen activation system are expressed at significantly higher levels in RA than in osteoarthritic and non-arthritic synovium. Therefore, a protein was constructed that consisted of the plasmin inhibitor, bovine pancreatic trypsin inhibitor (BPTI), linked to the receptor-binding aminoterminal fragment (ATF) of urokinase-type plasminogen activator. Adenoviral delivery of the respective gene into RA-SFs resulted in a significant reduction of cartilage degradation *in vitro* and in the SCID mouse model.[50] Although cartilage destruction was reduced to about 88% *in vitro*, cartilage degradation *in vivo* was reduced by only 30% in the ATF.BTPI transduced fibroblasts. These results indicate a role of plasmin in SF-dependent cartilage degradation and invasion in RA and demonstrate an effective way to inhibit this by gene transfer of a cell surface-targeted plasmin inhibitor. However, these data also demonstrate the limitations of *in vitro* assays for evaluating inhibitors of matrix degradation in favor of humanized animal models (i.e. SCID mice).

Finally, several strategies have been developed that are aimed at modulating the terminal phase of MMP expression by cleaving the mRNA for these enzymes.[94] This can be achieved by different antisense strategies such as antisense oligonucleotides (ODNs), the delivery[53] and expression of antisense expression constructs,

and through ribozymes. Ribozymes are RNA molecules that – like antisense RNA – bind to complementary mRNA but in addition are able to cleave RNA site-specifically. Such ribozymes can be used to destroy messages inside cells. RA-SFs that express ribozymes cleaving collagenase will, therefore, produce no or only limited amounts of this enzyme. The usefulness of this mode to reduce the invasiveness of RA-SFs has been evaluated recently.[52] The failure of numerous MMP inhibitors in the past[97] and the discovery of novel protease substrates, including MMP substrates such as chemokines and cytokines (substrates of MT1-MMP and MMP-2[98]) have resulted in novel strategies to inhibit MMPs. In this regard, for example, the thiirane inhibitors are currently beeing explored.[99] A more complete assessment of future prospects in the field can be found in a recent review by Turk.[100]

REFERENCES

1. Nagase H, Woessner JF. Matrix metalloproteinases. J Biol Chem 1999; 274: 21491–94.
2. Nagase H. Matrix metalloproteinases. In Hooper NM, ed. Zinc Metalloproteases in Health and Disease, London: Taylor and Francis, 1996: 153–204.
3. Brew K, Dinakarpandian D, Nagase H. Tissue inhibitors of metalloproteinases: evolution, stucture and function. Biochim Biophys Acta 2000; 1477: 267–83.
4. Wolfsberg TG, Primakoff P, Myles DG, White JM. ADAM, a novel family of membrane proteins containing a disintegrin and metalloprotease domain: multipotential functions in cell-cell and cell-matrix interactions. J Cell Biol 1995; 131: 275–8.
5. Kaushal GP, Shah SV. The new kids on the block: ADAMTSs, potentially multifunctional metalloproteinases of the ADAM family. J Clin Invest 2000; 105: 1335–7.
6. Black RA, Rauch CT, Kozlosky CJ et al. A metalloproteinase disintegrin that releases tumour-necrosis factor-alpha from cells. Nature 1997; 385: 729–33.
7. Moss ML, Jin SL, Milla ME et al. Cloning of a disintegrin metalloproteinase that processes precursor tumour-necrosis factor-alpha. Nature 1997; 385: 733–6.
8. Tortorella MD, Burn TC, Pratta MA et al. Purification and cloning of aggrecanase-1: a member of the ADAMTS family of proteins. Science 1999; 284: 1664–6.
9. Mengshol JA, Vincenti MP, Brinckerhoff CE. IL-1 induces collagenase-3 (MMP-13) promoter activity in stably transfected chondrocytic cells: requirement for

Runx-2 and activation by p38 MAPK and JNK pathways. Nucleic Acids Res 2001; 29: 4361–72.

10. Gouze JN, Bianchi A, Becuwe P et al. Glucosamine modulates IL-1-induced activation of rat chondrocytes at a receptor level, and by inhibiting the NF-kappaB pathway. FEBS Lett 2002; 510: 166–70.

11. Eberhardt W, Huwiler A, Beck KF et al. Amplification of IL-1 beta-induced matrix metalloproteinase-9 expression by superoxide in rat glomerular mesangial cells is mediated by increased activities of NF-kappa B and activating protein-1 and involves activation of the mitogen-activated protein kinase pathways. J Immunol 2000; 165: 5788–97.

12. Catterall JB, Carrere S, Koshy PJ et al. Synergistic induction of matrix metalloproteinase 1 by interleukin-1alpha and oncostatin M in human chondrocytes involves signal transducer and activator of transcription and activator protein 1 transcription factors via a novel mechanism. Arthritis Rheum 2001; 44(10): 2296–310.

13. Langdon C, Leith J, Smith F, Richards CD. Oncostatin M stimulates monocyte chemoattractant protein-1- and interleukin-1-induced matrix metalloproteinase-1 production by human synovial fibroblasts in vitro. Arthritis Rheum 1997; 40: 2139–46.

14. Bond M, Fabunmi RP, Baker AH, Newby AC. Synergistic upregulation of metalloproteinase-9 by growth factors and inflammatory cytokines: an absolute requirement for transcription factor NF-kappa B. FEBS Lett 1998; 435: 29–34.

15. Han YP, Tuan TL, Wu H, Hughes M, Garner WL. TNF-alpha stimulates activation of pro-MMP2 in human skin through NF-(kappa)B mediated induction ofMT1-MMP. J Cell Sci 2001; 114: 131–9.

16. Jovanovic DV, Martel-Pelletier J, Di Battista JA et al. Stimulation of 92-kd gelatinase (matrix metalloproteinase 9) production by interleukin-17 in human monocyte/macrophages: a possible role in rheumatoid arthritis. Arthritis Rheum 2000; 43: 1134–44.

17. Koenders MI, Kolls JK, Oppers-Walgreen B et al. Interleukin-17 receptor deficiency results in impaired synovial expression of interleukin-1 and matrix metalloproteinases 3, 9, and 13 and prevents cartilage destruction during chronic reactivated streptococcal cell wall-induced arthritis. Arthritis Rheum 2005; 52: 3239–47.

18. Ravanti L, Toriseva M, Penttinen R et al. Expression of human collagenase-3 (MMP-13) by fetal skin fibroblasts is induced by transforming growth factor beta via p38 mitogen-activated protein kinase. FASEB J 2001; 15: 1098–100.

19. Matsubara T, Funahashi K, Umegaki Y et al. Effect of VEGF on the synthesis of metalloproteinase (MMP)-13 by human chondrocytes. Arthritis Rheum 2001; 44 (Suppl 65): A78.

20. Onodera S, Nishihira J, Iwabuchi K et al. Macrophage migration inhibitory factor up-regulates matrix metalloproteinase-9 and -13 in rat osteoblasts. J Biol Chem 2002; 277: 7865–74.

21. Loeser RF, Forsyth CB. Integrin signalingincreases collagenase-3 (MMP-13) production in human articular chondrocytes. Arthritis Rheum 2001; 44 (Suppl 45): A35.

22. Yasuda T, Shimizu M Nakagawa T et al. COOH-terminal heparin-binding fibronectin fragment induces matrix metalloproteinases in human articular cartilage. Arthritis Rheum 2001; 44 (Suppl 63): 63.

23. Yammani RR, Carlson CS, Bresnick AR, Loeser RF. Increase in production of matrix metalloproteinase 13 by human articular chondrocytes due to stimulation with S100A4: role of the receptor for advanced glycation end products Arthritis Rheum 2006; 54: 2901–11.

24. Chabaud M, Garnero P, Dayer JM et al. Contribution of interleukin 17 to synovium matrix destruction in rheumatoid arthritis. Cytokine 2000; 12: 1092–9.

25. Sun Y, Cheung JM, Wenger L et al. Rheumatoid arthritis-derived p53 mutants lose their ability to downregulate the promotors of MMP-1 and MMP-13. Arthritis Rheum 2001; 44 (Suppl 182): 780

26. Distler JH, Jungel A, Huber LC et al. The induction of matrix metalloproteinase and cytokine expression in synovial fibroblasts stimulated with immune cell microparticles. Proc Natl Acad Sci U S A 2005; 102: 2892–7.

27. Mengshol JA, Vincenti MP, Coon CI et al. Interleukin-1 induction of collagenase 3 (matrix metalloproteinase 13) gene expression in chondrocytes requires p38, c-Jun N-terminal kinase, and nuclear factor kappa B: differential regulation of collagenase 1 and collagenase3. Arthritis Rheum 2000; 43: 801–11.

28. Barchowsky A, Frleta D, Vincenti MP. Integration of the NF-kappaB and mitogen-activated protein kinase/AP-1 pathways at the collagenase-1 promoter: divergence of IL-1 and TNF-dependent signal transduction in rabbit primary synovial fibroblasts. Cytokine 2000; 12: 1469–79.

29. Brauchle M, Gluck D, Di Padova F, Han J, Gram H. Independent role of p38 and ERK1/2 mitogen-activated kinases in the upregulation of matrix metalloproteinase-1. Exp Cell Res 2000; 258: 135–44.

30. Li WQ, Dehnade F, Zafarullah M. Oncostatin M-induced matrix metalloproteinase and tissue inhibitor of metalloproteinase-3 genes expression in chondrocytes requires Janus kinase/STAT signaling pathway. J Immunol 2001; 166: 3491–8.

31. Bosc DG, Goueli BS, Janknecht R. HER2/Neu-mediated activation of the ETS transcription factor ER81 and its target gene MMP-1. Oncogene 2001; 20: 6215–24.

32. Westermarck J, Seth A, Kahari VM. Differential regulation of interstitial collagenase (MMP-1) gene

expression by ETS transcription factors. Oncogene 1997; 14: 2651–60.

33. Schett G, Tohidast-Akrad M, Smolen JS et al. Activation, differential localization, and regulation of the stress-activated protein kinases, extracellular signal-regulated kinase, c-JUN N-terminal kinase, and p38 mitogen-activated protein kinase, in synovial tissue and cells in rheumatoid arthritis. Arthritis Rheum 2000; 43: 2501–12.

34. Redlich K, Kiener HP, Schett G et al. Overexpression of transcription factor Ets-1 in rheumatoid arthritis synovial membrane: regulation of expression and activation by interleukin-1 and tumor necrosis factor alpha. Arthritis Rheum 2001; 44: 266–74.

35. Mengshol JA, Vincenti MP, Brinckerhoff CE. IL-1 induces collagenase-3 (MMP-13) promoter activity in stably transfected chondrocytic cells: requirement for Runx-2 and activation by p38 MAPK and JNK pathways. Nucleic Acids Res 2001; 29: 4361–72.

36. Naito S, Shimizu S, Matsuu M et al. Ets-1 upregulates matrix metalloproteinase-1 expression through extracellular matrix adhesion in vascular endothelial cells. Biochem Biophys Res Commun 2002; 291: 130–8.

37. Hahne JC, Fuchs T, El Mustapha H et al. Expression pattern of matrix metalloproteinase and TIMP genes in fibroblasts derived from Ets-1 knock-out mice compared to wild-type mouse fibroblasts. Int J Mol Med 2006; 18: 153–9.

38. van Meurs JB, van Lent PL, Holthuysen AE et al. Kinetics of aggrecanase- and metalloproteinase-induced neoepitopes in various stages of cartilage destruction in murine arthritis. Arthritis Rheum 1999; 42: 1128–39.

39. van Meurs J, van Lent P, Stoop R et al. Cleavage of aggrecan at the Asn341-Phe342 site coincides with the initiation of collagen damage in murine antigen-induced arthritis: a pivotal role for stromelysin 1 in matrix metalloproteinase activity. Arthritis Rheum 1999; 42: 2074–84.

40. Poole AR. Cartilage in health and disease. In: Koopmann WJ, ed. Arthritis and Allied Conditions, 15th edn. Baltimore: Lippincott, Williams & Wilkins, 2005: 223–90.

41. van Meurs JB, van Lent PL, van de Loo AA et al. Increased vulnerability of postarthritic cartilage to a second arthritic insult: accelerated MMP activity in a flare up of arthritis. Ann Rheum Dis 1999; 58: 350–6.

42. Schett G, Hayer S, Tohidast-Akrad M et al. Adenoviral-based overexpression of TIMP-1 reduces tissue damage in the joints of TNF α transgenic mice. Arthritis Rheum 2001; 44: 2888–98.

43. Neuhold LA, Killar L, Zhao W et al. Postnatal expression in hyaline cartilage of constitutively active human collagenase-3 (MMP-13) induces osteoarthritis in mice. J Clin Invest 2001; 107: 35–44.

44. Vaillant B, Chiaramonte MG, Cheever AW et al. Regulation of hepatic fibrosis and extracellular matrix genes by the th response: new insight into the role of tissue inhibitors of matrix metalloproteinases. J Immunol 2001; 167: 7017–26.

45. Holmbeck K, Bianco P, Caterina J et al. MT1-MMP-deficient mice develop dwarfism, osteopenia, arthritis, and connective tissue disease due to inadequate collagen turnover. Cell 1999; 99: 81–92.

46. Müller-Ladner U, Kriegsmann J, Franklin BN et al. Synovial fibroblasts of patients with rheumatoid arthritis attach to and invade normal human cartilage when engrafted into SCID mice. Am J Pathol 1996; 149: 1607–15.

47. Pap T, Aupperle KR, Gay S, Firestein GS, Gay RE. Invasiveness of synovial fibroblasts is regulated by p53 in the SCID mouse in vivo model of cartilage invasion. Arthritis Rheum 2001; 44: 676–81.

48. Pap T, Franz JK, Hummel KM et al. Activation of synovial fibroblasts in rheumatoid arthritis: lack of expression of the tumour suppressor PTEN at sites of invasive growth and destruction. Arthritis Res 1999; 2: 59–64.

49. Pap T, Nawrath M, Heinrich J et al. Cooperation of Ras- and c-Myc-dependent pathways in regulating the growth and invasiveness of synovial fibroblasts in rheumatoid arthritis. Arthritis Rheum 2004; 50: 2794–802.

50. van der Laan WH, Pap T, Ronday HK et al. Cartilage degradation and invasion by rheumatoid synovial fibroblasts is inhibited by gene transfer of a cell surface-targeted plasmin inhibitor. Arthritis Rheum 2000; 43: 1710–18.

51. van der Laan WH, Quax PHA, Seemayer CA et al. Cartilage degradation and invasion by rheumatoid synovial fibroblasts is inhibited by gene transfer of TIMP-1 and TIMP-3. Gene Ther 2003; 10: 234–42.

52. Rutkauskaite E, Zacharias W, Schedel J et al. Ribozymes that inhibit the production of MMP-1 reduce the invasiveness of rheumatoid arthritis synovial fibroblasts. Arthritis Rheum 2004; 50: 1448–56.

53. Rutkauskaite E, Volkmer D, Shigeyama Y et al. Retroviral gene transfer of an antisense construct against membrane-type matrix metalloproteinase 1 (MT1-MMP) reduces the invasiveness of rheumatoid arthritis. Arthritis Rheum 2005; 52: 2010–14.

54. Tchetverikov I, Ronday HK, Van El B et al. MMP profile in paired serum and synovial fluid samples of patients with rheumatoid arthritis. Ann Rheum Dis 2004; 63: 881–3.

55. Konttinen YT, Ainola M, Valleala H et al. Analysis of 16 different matrix metalloproteinases (MMP-1 to MMP-20) in the synovial membrane: different profiles in trauma and rheumatoid arthritis. Ann Rheum Dis 1999; 58: 691–7.

56. Sorsa T, Konttinen YT, Lindy O et al. Collagenase in synovitis of rheumatoid arthritis. Semin Arthritis Rheum 1992; 22: 44–53.

57. Maeda S, Sawai T, Uzuki M et al. Determination of interstitial collagenase (MMP-1) in patients with rheumatoid arthritis. Ann Rheum Dis 1995; 54: 970–5.

58. Gruber BL, Sorbi D, French DL et al. Markedly elevated serum MMP-9 (gelatinase B) levels in rheumatoid arthritis: a potentially useful laboratory marker. Clin Immunol Immunopathol 1996; 78: 161–71.

59. Ahrens D, Koch AE, Pope RM, Stein PM, Niedbala MJ. Expression of matrix metalloproteinase 9 (96-kd gelatinase B) in human rheumatoid arthritis. Arthritis Rheum 1996; 39: 1576–87.

60. Di Girolamo N, Indoh I, Jackson N et al. Human mast cell-derived gelatinase B (matrix metalloproteinase-9) is regulated by inflammatory cytokines: role in cell migration. J Immunol 2006; 177: 2638–50.

61. Okada Y, Naka K, Kawamura K et al. Localization of matrix metalloproteinase 9 (92-kilodalton gelatinase/ type IV collagenase = gelatinase B) in osteoclasts: implications for bone resorption. Lab Invest 1995; 72: 311–22.

62. Okada Y, Nagase H, Harris ED Jr. Matrix metalloproteinases 1, 2, and 3 from rheumatoid synovial cells are sufficient to destroy joints. J Rheumatol 1987; 14 (Spec No): 41–2.

63. Okada Y, Takeuchi N, Tomita K, Nakanishi I, Nagase H. Immunolocalization of matrix metalloproteinase 3 (stromelysin) in rheumatoid synovioblasts (B cells): correlation with rheumatoid arthritis. Ann Rheum Dis 1989; 48: 645–53.

64. Tetlow LC, Lees M, Ogata Y, Nagase H, Woolley DE. Differential expression of gelatinase B (MMP-9) and stromelysin-1 (MMP- 3) by rheumatoid synovial cells in vitro and in vivo. Rheumatol Int 1993; 13: 53–9.

65. Cha HS, Ahn KS, Jeon CH et al. Influence of hypoxia on the expression of matrix metalloproteinase-1, -3 and tissue inhibitor of metalloproteinase-1 in rheumatoid synovial fibroblasts. Clin Exp Rheumatol 2003; 21: 593–8.

66. Beekman B, van El B, Drijfhout JW, Ronday HK, TeKoppele JM. Highly increased levels of active stromelysin in rheumatoid synovial fluid determined by a selective fluorogenic assay. FEBS Lett 1997; 418: 305–9.

67. Taylor DJ, Cheung NT, Dawes PT. Increased serum proMMP-3 in inflammatory arthritides: a potential indicator of synovial inflammatory monokine activity. Ann Rheum Dis 1994; 53: 768–72.

68. So A, Chamot AM, Peclat V, Gerster JC. Serum MMP-3 in rheumatoid arthritis: correlation with systemic inflammation but not with erosive status. Rheumatology (Oxford) 1999; 38: 407–10.

69. Ichikawa Y, Yamada C, Horiki T, Hoshina Y, Uchiyama M. Serum matrix metalloproteinase-3 and fibrin degradation product levels correlate with clinical disease activity in rheumatoid arthritis. Clin Exp Rheumatol 1998; 16: 533–40.

70. Manicourt DH, Fujimoto N, Obata K, Thonar EJ. Levels of circulating collagenase, stromelysin-1, and tissue inhibitor of matrix metalloproteinases 1 in patients with rheumatoid arthritis. Relationship to serum levels of antigenic keratan sulfate and systemic parameters of inflammation. Arthritis Rheum 1995; 38: 1031–9.

71. Yoshihara Y, Obata K, Fujimoto N et al. Increased levels of stromelysin-1 and tissue inhibitor of metalloproteinases-1 in sera from patients with rheumatoid arthritis. Arthritis Rheum 1995; 38: 969–75.

72. Yamanaka H, Matsuda Y, Tanaka M et al. Serum matrix metalloproteinase 3 as a predictor of the degree of joint destruction during the six months after measurement, in patients with early rheumatoid arthritis. Arthritis Rheum 2000; 43: 852–8.

73. Hanemaaijer R, Sorsa T, Konttinen YT et al. Matrix metalloproteinase-8 is expressed in rheumatoid synovial fibroblasts and endothelial cells. Regulation by tumor necrosis factor-alpha and doxycycline. J Biol Chem 1997; 272: 31504–9.

74. Wernicke D, Seyfert C, Hinzmann B, Gromnica-Ihle E. Cloning of collagenase 3 from the synovial membrane and its expression in rheumatoid arthritis and osteoarthritis. J Rheumatol 1996; 23: 590–5.

75. Lindy O, Konttinen YT, Sorsa T et al. Matrix-metalloproteinase 13 (collagenase 3) in human rheumatoid synovium. Arthritis Rheum 1997; 40: 1391–9.

76. Westhoff CS, Freudiger D, Petrow P et al. Characterization of collagenase 3 (matrix metalloproteinase 13) messenger RNA expression in the synovial membrane and synovial fibroblasts of patients with rheumatoid arthritis. Arthritis Rheum 1999; 42: 1517–27.

77. Pap T, Shigeyama Y, Kuchen S et al. Differential expression pattern of membrane-type matrix metalloproteinases in rheumatoid arthritis. Arthritis Rheum 2000; 43: 1226–32.

78. Kraan MC, Reece RJ, Barg EC et al. Modulation of inflammation and metalloproteinase expression in synovial tissue by leflunomide and methotrexate in patients with active rheumatoid arthritis. Findings in a prospective, randomized, double-blind, parallel-design clinical trial in thirty-nine patients at two centers. Arthritis Rheum 2000; 43: 1820–30.

79. Brennan FM, Browne KA, Green PA et al. Reduction of serum matrix metalloproteinase 1 and matrix metalloproteinase 3 in rheumatoid arthritis patients following anti-tumour necrosis factor-alpha (cA2) therapy. Br J Rheumatol 1997; 36: 643–50.

80. Catrina AI, Lampa J, Ernestam S et al. Anti-tumour necrosis factor (TNF)-alpha therapy (etanercept) down-regulates serum matrix metalloproteinase (MMP)-3 and

MMP-1 in rheumatoid arthritis. Rheumatology (Oxford) 2002; 41: 484–9.

81. Greenwald RA, Golub LM, Ramamurthy NS et al. In vitro sensitivity of the three mammalian collagenases to tetracycline inhibition: relationship to bone and cartilage degradation. Bone 1998; 22: 33–8.

82. Nordstrom D, Lindy O, Lauhio A et al. Anticollagenolytic mechanism of action of doxycycline treatment in rheumatoid arthritis. Rheumatol Int 1998; 17: 175–80.

83. Skotnicki JS, Levin JI, Zask A, Killar LM. Matrix metalloproteinase inhibitors. In: Bottomley KMK, Bradshaw D, Nixon JS, eds. Metalloproteinases as targets for anti-inflammatory drugs. Basel: Birkhäuser-Verlag, 1999: 17–57.

84. MacPherson LJ, Bayburt EK, Capparelli MP et al. Discovery of CGS 27023A, a non-peptidic, potent, and orally active stromelysin inhibitor that blocks cartilage degradation in rabbits. J Med Chem 1997; 40: 2525–32.

85. DiMartino MJ, High W, Galloway WA, Crimmin MJ. Preclinical antiarthritic activity of matrix metalloproteinase inhibitors. Ann N Y Acad Sci 1994; 732: 411–13.

86. Nemunaitis J, Poole C, Primrose J et al. Combined analysis of studies of the effects of the matrix metalloproteinase inhibitor marimastat on serum tumor markers in advanced cancer: selection of a biologically active and tolerable dose for longer-term studies. Clin Cancer Res 1998; 4: 1101–9.

87. Primrose JN, Bleiberg H, Daniel F et al. Marimastat in recurrent colorectal cancer: exploratory evaluation of biological activity by measurement of carcinoembryonic antigen. Br J Cancer 1999; 79: 509–14.

88. Tierney GM, Griffin NR, Stuart RC et al. A pilot study of the safety and effects of the matrix metalloproteinase inhibitor marimastat in gastric cancer. Eur J Cancer 1999; 35: 563–8.

89. Drummond AH, Beckett P, Brown PD et al. Preclinical and clinical studies of MMP inhibitors in cancer. Ann N Y Acad Sci 1999; 878: 228–35.

90. Wojtowicz-Praga S, Torri J, Johnson M et al. Phase I trial of Marimastat, a novel matrix metalloproteinase inhibitor, administered orally to patients with advanced lung cancer. J Clin Oncol 1998; 16: 2150–6.

91. Close DR. Matrix metalloproteinase inhibitors in rheumatic diseases. Ann Rheum Dis 2001; 60 (Suppl 3): iii62–iii67.

92. Hemmings FJ, Farhan M, Rowland J, Banken L, Jain R. Tolerability and pharmacokinetics of the collagenase-selective inhibitor Trocade in patients with rheumatoid arthritis. Rheumatology (Oxford) 2001; 40: 537–43.

93. Greenwald RA. Thirty-six years in the clinic without an MMP inhibitor. What hath collagenase wrought? Ann N Y Acad Sci 1999; 878: 413–19.

94. Pap T, Muller-Ladner U, Gay R, Gay S. Gene therapy in rheumatoid arthritis: how to target joint destruction? Arthritis Res 1999; 1: 5–9.

95. Apparailly F, Noel D, Millet V et al. Paradoxical effects of tissue inhibitor of metalloproteinases 1 gene transfer in collagen-induced arthritis. Arthritis Rheum 2001; 44: 1444–54.

96. Drynda A, Quax PHA, Neumann M et al. Gene transfer of TIMP-3 reverses the inhibitory effects of TNF-alpha on Fas-induced apoptosis in rheumatoid arthritis synovial fibroblasts. J Immunol 2005; 174: 6524–31.

97. Coussens LM, Fingleton B, Matrisian LM. Matrix metalloproteinase inhibitors and cancer: trials and tribulations. Science 2002; 295: 2387–92.

98. Tam EM, Morrison CJ, Wu YI, Stack MS, Overall CM. Membrane protease proteomics: isotope-coded affinity tag MS identification of undescribed MT1-matrix metalloproteinase substrates. Proc Natl Acad Sci U S A 2004; 101: 6917–22.

99. Ikejiri M, Bernardo MM, Bonfil RD et al. Potent mechanism-based inhibitors for matrix metalloproteinases. J Biol Chem 2005; 280: 33992–4002.

100. Turk B. Targeting proteases: successes, failures and future prospects. Nat Rev Drug Discov 2006; 5: 785–99.

29

MMPs and ADAMs as targets for therapies in arthritis

Hideaki Nagase, Gillian Murphy and Andrew Parker

Introduction • The MMP family and metzincins • MMPs in arthritis • ADAMTSs • Biological and pathological functions of ADAMTSs • ADAMTSs in arthritis • ADAMs • ADAM gene ablation to determine their role in mammalian physiology • ADAMs in relation to arthritic diseases and inflammation • Synthetic inhibitors and clinical trials • Other therapeutic opportunities • Conclusions • Acknowledgements • References

INTRODUCTION

Degradation of cartilage matrix impairs joint function and is a common feature of rheumatoid arthritis (RA) and osteoarthritis (OA), although the etiology of the two diseases is different. The cartilage consists of a relatively small number of chondrocytes and abundant extracellular matrix (ECM) components, of which about 40–45% are aggregated proteoglycans, aggrecans, and a similar amount of type II collagen. The type II collagen forms a fibrillar network, together with type IX and XI collagens, which provides the tissue with tensile strength. Aggrecans present within this meshwork are highly hydrated due to the anionic property of chondroitin sulfate and keratan sulfate polysaccharide chains attached to the core protein, and this property is important for the tissue to withstand compressive forces. During the progression of RA and OA, degradation of aggrecan occurs initially, followed by the degradation of collagen fibrils. These two events are effected by elevated metalloproteinase activities, which arise primarily from proliferative synovial tissues in RA and from cartilage in OA. The predominant metalloproteinases involved in cartilage degradation are the matrix metalloproteinases (MMPs) and the metalloproteinases with disintegrin and thrombospondin domains (ADAMTSs). In addition, the metalloproteinases with disintegrin domains (ADAMs) that cleave and release cell surface cytokines, growth factors and their receptors also play key roles in inflammation and subsequent tissue destruction. A number of reviews have described the importance of MMPs in arthritis and their inhibitor development as potential therapeutics.[1–3] In this review, we briefly introduce the members of the MMP family, but the main focus is to describe the roles of ADAMTSs and ADAMs in joint destruction and current approaches to intervening in arthritic diseases by developing metalloproteinase inhibitors.

THE MMP FAMILY AND METZINCINS

There are 24 MMP genes in the human genome, but there are 23 MMP proteins, since MMP-23 is coded for by two identical genes on chromosome 1. The MMPs are also collectively called 'matrixins'. All matrixins have a signal peptide and a propeptide domain and a catalytic metalloproteinase domain, and many have a C-terminal hemopexin domain, with the exception of MMP-7, MMP-23, and MMP-26 (Figure 29.1). Gelatinases (MMP-2 and MMP-9) have three

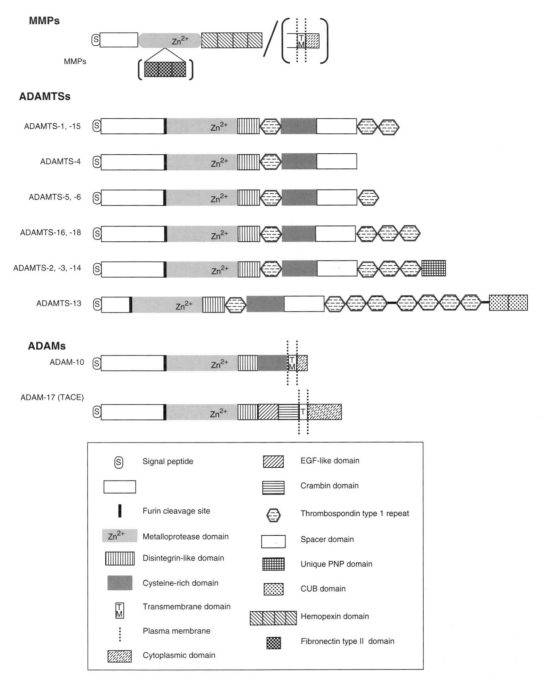

Figure 29.1 Domain arrangements of MMPs, ADAMTSs, and ADAMs. MMPs have secreted forms and membrane-bound forms. MMP-2 and MMP-9 have three repeats of fibronectin type II domains in the catalytic metalloproteinase domain. ADAMTSs have a variable number of TS domains. All ADAMs have a transmembrane and cytoplasmic domains.

repeats of fibronectin type II motifs inserted in the catalytic domain, whose interaction with collagen and other ECM molecules influences enzyme activities. The catalytic domains of MMPs have the zinc binding motif HEXXHXXGXXH where three histidines bind to the catalytic zinc atom. The C-terminal hemopexin (Hpx) domains in MMPs are important for some members to express biological activities, e.g. for collagenases to cleave triple helical collagen,[4] and for MT1-MMP (MMP-14) to assume a dimeric form on the cell surface which is crucial for its biological activities, including the activation of pro-MMP-2, cell migration, and collagenolysis.[5] Most MMPs are secreted from the cell as inactive pro-enzymes, but six are plasma membrane-anchored MT-MMPs (four are type I transmembrane type harboring a cytosolic domain and two have a glycosidic phosphatidyl inositol anchor). Pro-enzymes secreted from the cell need to be activated by tissue or plasma proteinases or by oxidants. Ten pro-MMPs including six MT-MMPs have a pro-protein convertase susceptible sequence at the junction between the pro-peptide and the catalytic domain and they are likely to be activated intracellularly by furin or a related pro-protein convertase. MMPs have been characterized with respect to their abilities to cleave ECM components, but recent studies showed that they can also act on cytokines, chemokines, growth factors, growth factor binding proteins, proteinase inhibitors, cell surface adhesion molecules, and receptors to regulate their biological activities.[6] MMP activities are inhibited by endogenous inhibitors called TIMPs (tissue inhibitors of metalloproteinases). The human genome encodes four TIMPs that can inhibit all MMPs so far tested, with the exception that TIMP-1 is a poor inhibitor of MMP-14 (MTI-MMP), MMP-15 (MT2-MMP), MMP-16 (MT3-MMP), MMP-24 (MT5-MMP), and MMP-19.[7]

ADAMs and ADAMTSs are sometimes mistaken for a subgroup of MMPs, but the primary structures of catalytic domains of MMPs are different from those of ADAMs and ADAMTSs. The latter two are related to snake venom metalloproteinases, reprolysins. The MEROPS database (http:www.merops.sanger.ac.uk/) classifies the MMPs as in the M10 family of metalloproteinases and ADAMs and ADAMTSs in the

M12 family. Crystal structures of MMPs, a crayfish metalloproteinase astacin, snake venom reprolysins, and a bacterial metalloproteinase serralysin all revealed the conserved zinc-binding motif HEXXHXXGXXH and the 'Met-turn' located after the zinc-binding motif. The latter methionine forms a base to create the active site for these metalloproteinases. These enzyme families are collectively called 'metzincins'[8] and all ADAMTSs and ADAMs contain these two motifs. It is notable, however, that amino acid sequences among these metalloproteinase families are not related to each other, but their peptide folds in three dimensions show similarity.[9] All synthetic inhibitors of MMPs are targeted to the active site of the metalloproteinase domain as discussed below.

MMPs IN ARTHRITIS

MMP activities are not readily detected in the normal steady-state tissues, but their production is transcriptionally regulated by cytokines, growth factors, physical stimuli, etc. Thus, MMPs have a functional role regulating both physiological demands and pathological stimuli. Induction of MMPs by interleukin (IL)-1, tumor necrosis factor (TNF)-α, the combination of oncostatin M and IL-1, IL-17, IL-18 in synovial cells or chondrocytes suggests their involvement in inflammation-driven tissue destruction.[3] OA cartilage expresses elevated MMP-1, MMP-3, and MMP-13.[10,11] Injurious mechanical insult to cartilage increases the level of MMP-3 and ADAMTS-5.[12] Proteolytic products of ECM such as fibronectin fragments can also stimulate the production of MMPs.[13–15] As listed in Table 29.1, MMPs are able to cleave a number of ECM components of cartilage. MMPs cleave aggrecan at the Glu[341]-Phe[342] bond in the so-called interglobular domain (IGD) located between the N-terminal G1 and G2 domains. MMP-generated G1-VDIPEN[341] fragments of aggrecan are found in RA and OA cartilage.[16,17] Collagenases degrade type II collagen fibrils and specific collagenase-generated fragments are also detected in RA and OA cartilage.[18] Potential candidate enzymes are MMP-1 and MMP-13 in interterritorial collagenolysis and MMP-2 and MMP-14 in pericellular collagenolysis. Prevention of cartilage and bone destruction

Table 29.1 Matrix metalloproteinases

Enzyme	MMP	Expression	Substrates related to joint destruction
Collagenases			
Collagenase 1	MMP-1	Fibroblasts, synovial cells, chondrocytes, macrophages	Collagen (types I, II, III, VII, VIII, X, and XI) fibronectin, aggrecan, versican, tenascin, link protein, serum amyloid A, IL-1β
Collagenase 2	MMP-8	Neutrophils, chondrocytes	Collagen (types I, II, and III), aggrecan, substance P, bradykinin
Collagenase 3	MMP-13	Chondrocytes, synovial cells, fibroblasts	Collagen (types I, II, III, IX, and X), collagen telopeptides, fibronectin, SPARC, aggrecan, perlecan, tenascin-C
Gelatinases			
Gelatinase A	MMP-2	Fibroblasts, chondrocytes	Collagen (types I, II, III, IV, V, X, and XI), fibronectin, tenascin, SPARC, aggrecan link protein, big endothelin 1, IL-1β, FGFR-1
Gelatinase B	MMP-9	Fibroblasts, chondrocytess, macrophages, neutrophils	Collagen (types IV, V, XI, and XIV), SPARC, aggrecan, link protein, versican, decorin
Stromelysins			
Stromelysin 1	MMP-3	Fibroblasts, chondrocytes	Collagen (types III, IV, V, VII, IX, X, and XI), collagen telopeptides, fibronectin, tenascin, SPARC, IGFBP-3, IL-1β
Stromelysin 2	MMP-10	Epithelial cells	Collagen (types III, IV, and V), fibronectin, aggrecan, link protein
Stromelysin 3	MMP-11	Stromal cells	Weak proteolytic activity. α-Anti-trypsin. IGFBP-1
Matrilysins			
Matrilysin 1	MMP-7	Epithelial cells	Collagen IV, fibronectin, tenascin, aggrecan, link protein, SPARC, decorin, versican, fibulin, pro-α-defensin, FasL, pro-TNF-α, B4 integrin
Matrilysin 2	MMP-26	Epithelial cells	Collagen IV, fibronectin
Membrane-type MMPs			
A) Transmembrane type			
MT1-MMP	MMP-14	Synovial cells, cartilage, placenta, carcinoma	Collagen (types I, II and III), fibronectin, aggrecan, perlecan, CD44, pro-TNF-α, fibrinogen tissue transglutaminase, pro-MMP-2 and pro-MMP-13 activation

MT2-MMP	MMP-15	Endometrium, breast cancer	Fibronectin, tenascin, aggrecan, perlecan, activation of pro-MMP-2, pro-TNF-α, tissue transglutaminase
MT3-MMP	MMP-16	Brain, placenta, breast tumour	Fibronectin, aggrecan, dermatan sulfate proteoglycans, Pro-MMP-2 activation, tissue transglutaminase
MT5-MMP	MMP-24	cerebellum	Gelatin, fibrinogen
B) GPI-anchored			
MT4-MMP	MMP-17	Carcinomas	Collagen IV, fibronectin, chondroitin, sulfate proteoglycan, dermatan sulfate proteoglycan
MT6-MMP	MMP-25	Peripheral blood, leukocytes	
Others			
Macrophage elastase	MMP-12	Macrophages, hypertrophic chondrocytes, osteoclasts	Elastin, fibronectin, osteonectin, aggrecan, fibrinogen, plasminogen
	MMP-19	Synovial cells, lymphocytes (RA), keratinocytes	Collagen IV, fibronectin, tenascin-C, aggrecan, COMP, fibrinogen, fibrin
Enamelysin	MMP-20	Tooth enamel	Amelogenin, aggrecan, COMP
	MMP-21	Various fetal and adult tissues	Gelatin
CA-MMP	MMP-23	Ovary, testis, prostate	Gelatin
	MMP-27	Embryonic fibroblasts (chicken)	Gelatin, casein
Epilysin	MMP-28	Lung, placenta, heart, basal keratinocytes	Casein

in animal models of RA and OA by synthetic MMP inhibitors[19–21] also indicates that MMPs play a key role in joint destruction. However, it is still unclear which MMPs are key enzymes for cartilage destruction in humans.

ADAMTSs

The treatment of cartilage in culture with proinflammatory cytokines such as IL-1 or TNF-α resulted in the cleavage of aggrecan core protein at the Glu[373]-Ala[374] bond in the IGD,[22] which is not normally cleaved by MMPs. The findings of some studies[23,24] suggested that this enzymatic activity was important in aggrecanolysis in arthritis. This enzymic activity was referred to as 'aggrecanases' and the first two enzymes were identified as ADAMTS-4 (aggrecanase 1) and ADAMTS-5 (aggrecanase 2).[25,26]

There are 19 ADAMTS genes in humans and they are all multi-domain proteins.[27] A first ADAMTS was reported in 1997 by Kuno et al.[28] in cachetic carcinoma cells. It is a secreted metalloproteinase whose gene encodes a signal peptide, a large pro-peptide domain, a metalloproteinase domain, a disintegrin domain, a thrombospondin type I (TS) domain, a cysteine-rich domain, a spacer domain, and two additional thrombospondin type I domains (Figure 29.1). The metalloproteinase domain and disintegrin domains are related to those of ADAMs, but TS domains are unique. Thus the name ADAMTS (ADAMs with thrombospondin motif) was coined.

A second enzyme cloned was ADAMTS-2, which processes the N-pro-peptide of pro-collagens I, II, and III.[29] Subsequently, ADAMTS-3[30] and ADAMTS-14[31] have been shown to have pro-collagen N-proteinase activity. Those enzymes have a unique PNP (pro-collagen N-proteinase) domain in the C-terminus (Figure 29.1). The activities of ADAMTS-2 are negatively regulated by the PNP domain but the C-terminal TS domains are required for the full enzyme activity.[32]

Since ADAMTS-4 and -5 were designated as aggrecanase 1 and 2, respectively, ADAMTS-1, -8, -9, -15, -17, and -18[27,33] have been reported to cleave the Glu[373]-Ala[374] bond of aggrecan. Among them, ADAMTS-4 is biochemically the most well characterized. An interesting property is that the metalloproteinase domain alone does not exhibit any aggrecanolytic activity, and full-length ADAMTS-4 is most active on aggrecan, suggesting that non-catalytic domains play an important role in determining aggrecanolytic activity. However, the activity of full-length ADAMTS-4 is primarily on the chondroitin sulfate-rich region of the aggrecan core protein (B, C, D, E sites in Figure 29.2), but not on the Glu[373]-Ala[374] bond.[34] When the C-terminal spacer domain is removed by MT4-MMP on the chondrocyte surface,[35] ADAMTS-4 gains the activity to cleave the Glu[373]-Ala[374] bond in the IGD. This form also can digest non-aggrecan substrates such as fibromodulin, decorin, and biglycan, and a general protein substrate, S-carboxymethylated transferrin.[34] Such changes of activity due to C-terminal processing are accompanied by changes in the extracellular localization of the enzyme. Full-length ADAMTS-4 binds to cell surface proteoglycans and pericellular matrix, but the spacer domain-deleted ADAMTS-4 does not,[34] and can potentially diffuse away from the pericellular region into the interterritorial area of the cartilage. ADAMTS-5 cleaves similar sites of the aggrecan core protein to ADAMTS-4,[36] but ADAMTS-5 is a far more potent aggrecandegrading enzyme than ADAMTS-4 and the ancillary non-catalytic domains also influence its activity greatly (C. Gendron and H. Nagase, unpublished observations). Other ADAMTSs exhibit much lower activities than these two aggrecanases.[33,37]

Another well studied ADAMTS is ADAMTS-13, which cleaves unusually large multimeric forms of von Willebrand factor under shear stress. This activity is crucial for the prevention of unnecessary platelet aggregation in capillaries.[38] ADAMTS-13 has two CUB (complement C1r/C1s-urchin epidermal growth factor-bone morphogenetic protein-1) domains in the C-terminus. The first CUB domain interacts with multimeric von Willebrand factor [39] and the spacer domain is important for the cleavage of the substrate.[40]

TIMPs are not the inhibitors of ADAMTSs in general, but TIMP-3, which is largely an ECM-bound protein, inhibits ADAMTS-1, -4, and -5. ADAMTS-2 is weakly inhibited by TIMP-3 but the affinity is enhanced in the presence of heparin, suggesting that TIMP-3 is a possible regulator of the enzyme in the tissue.[41]

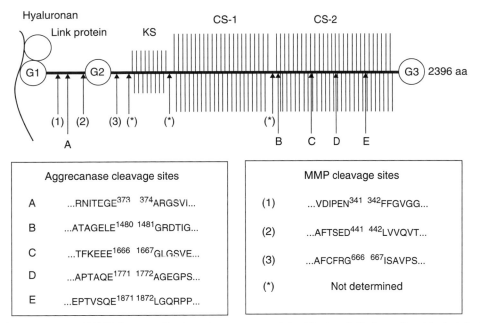

Figure 29.2 Aggrecanase and MMP cleavage sites in aggrecan core protein. Site A and site 1 are the signatorial cleavage sites of aggrecanase and MMP, respectively.

BIOLOGICAL AND PATHOLOGICAL FUNCTIONS OF ADAMTSs

ADAMTS-1 null mice display abnormal morphogenesis of kidney, ureteric ducts, and adrenal glands and defects in ovulation, indicating that the enzyme plays a critical role in development and reproduction.[42] ADAMTS-1 also has anti-angiogenic activity and this activity is derived from binding of the two C-terminal TS domains to vascular endothelial growth factor (VEGF)-165.[43] Although ADAMTS-8 also has anti-angiogenic activity,[44] the mechanism has not been elucidated. Mutations of ADAMTS-2 cause dermatosparaxis in cattle and Ehlers–Danlos syndrome VIIC in humans, an autosomal recessive disorder with skin fragility and joint laxity.[45] ADAMTS-2-null mice, which are essentially normal at birth, developed skin fragility in 1–2 months and the male mice were sterile, although the females are normal in fertility.[46] Reduced activity of ADAMTS-13 due to either mutation or generation of autoantibodies against ADAMTS-13 is a cause of thrombotic thrombocytopenic purpura (TPP), characterized by severe anemia, renal failure, and neurological disorder caused by formation of platelet-rich thrombi in capillaries.[47] There are a number of ADAMTSs whose substrates and biological functions are currently unknown (Table 29.2).

ADAMTSs IN ARTHRITIS

The role of ADAMTSs in arthritis is considered to be their participation in catabolism of aggrecan and possibly other ECM molecules in cartilage. The treatment of human cartilage with IL-1 or TNF-α increases aggrecanase activity, but it has no effect on mRNA levels for ADAMTS-1, -4, and -5.[48] mRNA levels for ADAMTS-4 and ADAMTS-5 in OA cartilage are not significantly elevated compared to that in normal cartilage,[49] but ADAMTS-5 mRNA levels are higher than ADAMTS-4 mRNA.[11] Treatment of human chondrocytes in culture with IL-1β induced ADAMTS-4 mRNA, but did not alter the levels of ADAMTS-5 mRNA.[11] Nonetheless, an increase in the aggrecan fragments generated by aggrecanases is found in RA and OA cartilage and in synovial fluids, suggesting that ADAMTSs are important enzymes in aggrecanolysis. ADAMTS-4-null mice and

Table 29.2 ADAMTSs

	Potential functions	Expression	Substrates
ADAMTS-1	Organ morphogenesis (kidney, adrenal glands, urinary tract, female reproductive organs), anti-angiogenesis	Urinary epithelium, ovary, muscle, kidney, many other tissues	Aggrecan, versican, α2-macroglobulin
ADAMTS-2	Pro-collagen N-pro-peptide processing	Skin, uterus, arteries, fibroblasts	Pro-collagen I, II, and III
ADAMTS-3	Procollagen N-pro-peptide processing	Cartilage, bone and musculotendinous tissue during development	Pro-collagen I and II
ADAMTS-4	Tissue breakdown	Synovium, cartilage, CNS	Aggrecan, versican, brevican, decorin, biglycan, fibromodulin, COMP
ADAMTS-5	Tissue breakdown	Placenta, uterus, cervix, cartilage	Aggrecan, versican, brevican, decorin, biglycan, fibromodulin
ADAMTS-6		Placenta	
ADAMTS-7		Synovium, cartilage	COMP
ADAMTS-8		(Not expressed in cartilage)	Aggrecan
ADAMTS-9		Chondrocytes, fibroblasts, embryonic tissues	Aggrecan, versican
ADAMTS-10		Kidney, liver, heart, placenta	α2-macroglobulin
ADAMTS-12		Cartilage, synovium	COMP
ADAMTS-13	Processing of unusually large von Willebrand factor	Liver, prostate, brain	von Willebrand factor
ADAMTS-14	Pro-collagen N-pro-peptide processing	Prostate, brain, liver, fetal lung	Pro-collagen I and III
ADAMTS-15		Cartilage, fetal kidney, fetal lung	Aggrecan
ADAMTS-16		Cartilage, brain, ovary, fetal lung, fetal kidney	
ADAMTS-17		Ovary, fetal lung	
ADAMTS-18		Brain, submaxillary gland, fetal lung, fetal kidney	
ADAMTS-19		Osteosarcoma, fetal lung	
ADAMTS-20	Neural crest-derived melanoblast migration through dermal mesenchyme or survival and proliferation within the ectoderm	Subectodermal mesenchyme during development	

ADAMTS-5-null mice show no obvious abnormality, but when challenged either via surgically induced joint instability[50,51] or antigen-induced arthritis (AIA),[52] the degradation of aggrecan in the cartilage of ADAMTS-5-null mice was protected, but not that of ADAMTS-4-null mice, indicating that ADAMTS-5 is a major aggrecan-degrading enzyme in cartilage, at least in mice. Whether ADAMTS-5 is a key aggrecanase in the development of human OA will only be determined by further investigation.

While the importance of aggrecanases in aggrecanolysis is well recognized, aggrecan can be degraded by MMPs as well as ADAMTSs (Figure 29.2). Using neoepitope antibodies that detect either MMP-cleaved fragments or ADAMTS-cleaved fragments, Lark et al.[53] showed that both RA and OA cartilages contain aggrecan fragments generated by MMPs (G1-NITEGE[373]) and ADAMTSs (G1-VDIPEN[341]). Recent studies by Struglics et al.[17] confirm these observations in OA cartilage and suggest that MMP-mediated aggrecanolysis is mostly pericellular while ADAMTSs are both pericellular and in the intraterritorial regions. Based on the fact that MT1-MMP-null mice and MMP-9-null mice cause destruction of articular cartilage, impairment of endochondral ossification and fracture repairs, Sandy suggests that some MMPs may be important in cartilage matrix homeostasis.[54] Kevorkian et al.[49] showed that ADAMTS-16 is elevated in late OA cartilage, but its function is not known.

ADAMs

The ADAMs are type I transmembrane proteins with a characteristic domain structure composed of a pro-peptide, a catalytic domain, a disintegrin and cysteine-rich domain, an EGF-like (or other) domain, a transmembrane domain, and a cytoplasmic domain (Figure 29.1).[55] The domains define the ability of these proteins to act as proteinases; 13 of a total of 21 ADAMs in the human genome have a potentially functional catalytic domain with the characteristic zinc-binding motif, and act as adhesion and signaling molecules. The pro-peptide acts as a molecular chaperone during synthesis and interacts with the catalytic cleft, rendering it inactive. Proteolytic cleavage of the pro-peptide by proprotein convertases, such as furin, in the secretory pathway generates a mature active form of the ADAM in many cases. The catalytic domain defines the ability of individual ADAMs to cleave specific cell surface protein substrates, hence acting as up- or down-regulators of their function (Table 29.3).[56,57] A crystal structure that is available for ADAM-17[58] shows that, although the substrate-binding site resembles that of the MMPs, there are several structural features with respect to surface charge and shape that should enable the design of selective inhibitors. The disintegrin and cysteine-rich domain are probably disulfide-bonded[59] to form an adhesive structure interacting with integrins, syndecans, and possibly other ECM or cell surface proteins.[60–62] They also appear to have a role in substrate targeting.[63] The cytoplasmic domain of the ADAMs contains different identifiable signaling motifs and may be involved in the assembly of complexes containing adaptors, and cytoskeletal and signaling

proteins. Regulation of the ADAMs occurs at the level of gene transcription and also by cellular trafficking and activation.[64] Most ADAMs appear to reside in intracellular vesicles and move to the cell surface and are quickly endocytosed. The proteolytic functions of some may be regulated by members of the TIMP family. TIMP-3 seems to play a major role in the control of ADAM-17[65] and has some ability to inhibit ADAM-10, -12, and -33.[56] TIMP-1 is an ADAM-10 inhibitor *in vitro* and in cell-based assays, but its function in this respect *in vivo* has not been addressed.

ADAM GENE ABLATION TO DETERMINE THEIR ROLE IN MAMMALIAN PHYSIOLOGY

The biological role of the ADAMs is a topic of extensive investigation, particularly for those members that have a potential proteolytic function. ADAM-8, -9, -10, -12, -15, -17, -19, and -28 have all been shown to cleave cell surface proteins, such as cytokines, growth factors, growth factor receptors and binding proteins, and cell adhesion molecules, a process referred to as 'shedding' (Table 29.3).[55–57] There are also some references to their activity in the cleavage of ECM components.[57]

The phenotypic outcomes of the generation of mice in which individual ADAM genes have been ablated, as well as combinations of ADAMs, have often given little indication of their function and it is clear that more detailed study involving specific 'challenges' will be necessary.[62,64] ADAM-8$^{-/-}$ mice and ADAM-9$^{-/-}$ mice have no evident phenotype, but ADAM-10$^{-/-}$ mice show early embryonic lethality, probably due to angiogenic defects. ADAM-12$^{-/-}$ mice show 30% embryonic lethality and defects in brown adipose tissue and ADAM-15$^{-/-}$ mice show no phenotype apart from defects in pathological neovascularization. ADAM-17$^{-/-}$ mice show perinatal lethality, probably due to defects in heart development. There are also defects in lung morphogenesis. Significantly, these mice have a phenotype resembling that of EGFR$^{-/-}$ mice, TGF-$\alpha^{-/-}$ mice, HB-EGF$^{-/-}$ mice, or amphiregulin$^{-/-}$ mice. ADAM-19$^{-/-}$ mice have 80% postnatal lethality with defects in cardiovascular morphogenesis. ADAM-28$^{-/-}$ and ADAM-33$^{-/-}$ mice have no overt phenotype. TIMP-3$^{-/-}$ mice

Table 29.3 Human ADAMs: localization and potential function

ADAM	Common name(s)	Potential functions	Expression	Detection in arthritic joint tissues	Substrates related to arthritic disease	Integrin binding
8	MS2, CD156	Sheddase, osteoclast differentiation, brain function	Granulocytes, monocytes, cartilage, bone, lung, CNS	(✓)	TGF-α, TNF-α, TRANCE, IL-RII, CHL1, KL-1, CD16, CD23, CD163, CX3CL1, L-selectin, PSGL-1	NK
9	Meltrin-γ, MDC9	Sheddase, cell migration, osteoclast differentiation	Myeloma, most mesenchymal and epithelial cells, CNS	✓	Pro-HBEGF, TNF-α, epiregulin	α2β1, α3β1, α6β1, α9β1, α6β4, αVβ5
10	Kuz, MADM, SUP-17	Sheddase, cell fate determination, development of angiogenesis	Most mesenchymal and epithelial cells, CNS	✓	Notch, L1, pro-EGF, pro-betacellulin, ephrins, CX3CL1, CX3CL16, IL-6R, CD23, CD44, N-cadherin, E-cadherin	NK
12	Meltrin-α	Sheddase, adipogenesis, myogenesis, bone growth	Most mesenchymal cells, CNS	✓	Pro-HBEGF, epiregulin, IGFBP-3, -5	α4β1, α7β1, α9β1
15	Metargidin, MDC15	Cell/cell binding, neovascularization	Endothelial and epithelial cells	✓	TGF-α, epiregulin	α4β1, α5β1, α9β1, αVβ3
17	TACE	Sheddase, osteoclast recruitment, heart development	Most cells, CNS	✓	CX3CL1, TRANCE, TNF-α, TGF-α, pro-HBEGF, amphiregulin, FasL TNFRII, MUC1 IL-6R TrkA Mucin-1, Notch, CD23, CD30, CD40, L-selectin, VCAM-1, ICAM-1	α5β1
19	Meltrin-β, MADDAM	Sheddase, dendritic cell development, cardiovascular morphogenesis	Mesenchymal cells, dendritic cells, CNS	✓	Neuregulins	α4β1, α5β1
28	MDC-L, eMDC-II	Immune surveillance	Epididymis, lung, lymphocytes	(✓)	CD23	α4β1, α4β7, α9β1
33		Genetically linked to asthma	Mesenchymal cells, lung			α4β1, α5β1, α9β1

For further details see the reference list and the ADAMs website: http://www.people.virginia.edu/%7Ejw7g/Table_of_the_ADAMs.html
NK, not known.

have proved very informative in defining the importance of ADAM-17 in the regulation of TNF-α in systemic inflammation.[66] When AIA was studied in Timp3[-/-] mice, compared with wild-type animals they showed a dramatic increase in the initial inflammatory response to intra-articular antigen injection, and serum TNF-α levels were greatly elevated. However, these differences in clinical features disappeared by days 7–14.[67]

ADAMs IN RELATION TO ARTHRITIC DISEASES AND INFLAMMATION

Specific studies of ADAM expression and potential roles in normal or arthritic joint tissues are still fairly limited. A study by Böhm et al.[68] described the expression of ADAM-15 in RA and OA synovial tissue by immunohistochemistry and *in situ* hybridization. Their results demonstrated high levels of ADAM-15 expression in macrophage-like and fibroblast-like synoviocytes, as well as in plasma cells in RA synovial tissue, compared with normal or OA synovial tissue. This suggests a potential role of ADAM-15 in the pathogenesis of cartilage destruction in inflammatory joint disease. Komiya et al.[69] determined the mRNA expression levels of 10 different ADAMs in synovial tissues of patients with RA or OA and found that ADAM-15 mRNA was more frequently expressed in RA samples. The mRNA and protein were localized to synovial lining cells, endothelial cells, and macrophage-like cells of the sub-lining, with a direct correlation between ADAM-15 mRNA and vascular density. ADAM-15 was up-regulated by VEGF-165. Negligible mRNA for ADAM-8 and ADAM-28 could be found, whilst ADAM-9, -10, and -17 were constitutively expressed in RA and OA tissue. ADAM-12 was higher in RA compared with OA synovium. Böhm et al.[70] have also studied aging ADAM-15[-/-] mice which showed accelerated development of OA lesions compared with wild-type mice. The results were interpreted as showing that ADAM-15 had a protective role in the maintenance of joint integrity. Mice overexpressing soluble ADAM-12 exhibit a pronounced increase in the length of the long bones, due to effects on growth plate chondrocyte proliferation and maturation.[71] An imbalance in pro- and anti-inflammatory cytokines is thought to be a major feature of RA and may have some role to play in OA. The major proinflammatory cytokines, TNF-α and IL-1, are produced by synovial macrophages and ADAM-17 is thought to be responsible for the solubilization of the membrane-bound pro form of TNF-α (hence the alternative name, TNF-α converting enzyme, TACE). A major question concerns the significance of TNF shedding in relation to the inflammatory response.[72] ADAM-17 also releases a number of other key effectors including TRANCE, fractalkine, and various EGF receptor (EGFR) ligands which play roles in the development of arthritic disease. Interestingly ADAM-17 has also been shown to be potentially responsible for the proteolysis of receptors such as TNFR-I and TNFR-II, c-Met, IL-1 receptor-II, trkA, IL-6 receptor (IL-6R), and others (Table 29.3). The generation of soluble forms of receptors, e.g. IL-6R, may be critical for the down-regulation of ligand function.[73] The shedding of cell adhesion molecules such as L-selectin, VCAM-1, ICAM-1, CD30, and CD40 by ADAM-17 also has implications for cell behavior within inflammatory and immune pathways. Other ADAMs can carry out some of these shedding functions (Table 29.3); notably, ADAM-8 cleaves both TNF-α and TGF-α and ADAM-9, -10, and -12 can release EGFR ligands such as HB-EGF from the cell surface. Many ADAMs also regulate chemokines by proteolysis or may in turn be activated by chemokine receptors and by other G protein-coupled receptors to release EGFR ligands from the cell surface in a transactivation mechanism. ADAM-10 may regulate CD44 and E- and N-cadherin levels and function in Notch and Ephrin signalling.[62]

SYNTHETIC INHIBITORS AND CLINICAL TRIALS

As discussed above, a number of MMPs, and more recently ADAMTSs and ADAMs, have been implicated in the progression of RA and OA. Thus, synthetic metalloproteinase inhibitors have been designed and pursued for the last two decades as a therapeutic strategy for arthritis (and also for cancer and cardiovascular disease). Early clinical studies using broad-spectrum peptidic hydroxamate inhibitors such as marimastat (BB-2516, Vernalis), focused on opportunities in oncology. More recently we have seen a number of hydroxamate compounds (e.g. BMS-275921, Bristol-Myers Squib; CGS 27023A, Novartis; BAY 12-9566, Bayer; Ro 32-3555, Roche) with nanomolar K_i values for multiple MMPs progress into clinical studies for arthritis. Whilst all compounds showed good efficacy and tolerability in animal models of arthritis, all have been discontinued citing either lack of efficacy or appearance of musculoskeletal syndrome (MSS) in humans.

Lack of efficacy could be associated with a number of factors including pharmacokinetic properties of the compound in man (e.g. altered pharmacokinetics in patients, ability to achieve adequate concentration in the joint space), limited study design (duration and dosing regime), or a flawed hypothesis. MSS manifests itself as musculoskeletal pain and tendonitis, notably in the small joints of the hands and shoulder. The effects are dose- and time-related and reversible following withdrawal of treatment. The cause of this side effect is not clear but is thought to be a reflection of the lack of selectivity, with MMP-1 inhibition originally hypothesized as a culprit. More recently Pfizer progressed a sulfonamide hydroxamic acid, CP-544439[74] (Table 29.4, compound 1), a potent inhibitor of MMP-13 ($IC_{50} <$ 1 nM) but weak for MMP-1, into a 6-week phase II study in OA patients. A significant reduction was seen in the type II collagen degradation biomarker but MSS was also a feature in 40% of the patients, indicating that avoiding MMP-1 inhibition is not sufficient to mitigate MSS risk. This has led to a focus on identification of more selective MMP inhibitors and a move away from hydroxamic acid compounds. Progress has been enhanced by the use of three-dimensional crystal and/or solution structures with bound inhibitors that have now been described for many MMPs as well as a limited number of ADAMs.

MMP-13, ADAM-17 (TACE), and aggrecanases are three targets where there has been significant recent success in identification of selective, orally bioavailable inhibitors, which demonstrate good efficacy in preclinical models of arthritis. In the MMP-13 area, Wyeth have described a series of carboxylic acids with benzofuran carboxamide groups,[75] which were optimized using homology modeling of MMP S1'

pockets. These compounds have a zinc-binding moiety and demonstrate low nanomolar IC_{50}s against MMP-13, > 10-fold selectivity against MMP-3 and -8, and > 100-fold selectivity against MMP-1, -2, -7, -9, and -14 and ADAMTS-4, and are active in an *in vitro* bovine nasal cartilage degradation assay (Table 29.4, compound 2).[75] Inhibition of MMPs without chelation of the zinc has also recently been exemplified by Pfizer, who described a series of potent, selective non-zinc-binding inhibitors of MMP-13 (Table 29.4, compound 3).[76] Co-crystallization with the MMP-13 catalytic domain demonstrates that the compounds bind deep in the S1' pocket of the enzyme. They are highly potent and selective with picomolar IC_{50} against MMP-13 and > 30 micromolar IC_{50} against MMP-1, -2, -3, -7, -8, -9, -12, -14, and -17.[76] Johnson (Pfizer) presented further data at the 7th World Congress on Inflammation (2005) demonstrating activity in the bovine nasal cartilage *in vitro* assay and efficacy in the rabbit anterior cruciate ligament transection/partial medial meniscectomy model of OA. This profile offers an exciting opportunity for the future with the potential to address MSS concerns and MMP-13-dependent efficacy in man.

Inhibition of aggrecan loss represents an alternative therapeutic strategy for OA. Since the first aggrecanase was cloned and shown to belong to the ADAMTS family, multiple ADAMTS enzymes have now been shown to cleave aggrecan at the disease-associated Glu^{373}-Ala^{374} site, with ADAMTS-4 and ADAMTS-5 believed to be the principal aggrecanases in human disease. Using a pharmacophore model of the P1' site and homology modeling of ADAMTS-4 against the 3-D structure of atrolysin C,[77] Bristol-Myers Squib identified a series of hydroxyl butane diamide derivatives as potent, selective, and orally bioavailable aggrecanase inhibitors (Table 29.4, compound 4).[77] Adopting a similar strategy, Wyeth identified a series of biphenylsulfonamide carboxylate compounds as dual inhibitors of ADAMTS-4 and MMP-13[78] (Table 29.4, compound 5) with limited selectivity against other MMPs. The future development of aggrecanase inhibitors will require a greater understanding of the relative contribution of ADAMTS-4 and ADAMTS-5 to disease as well as the physiological roles of the other ADAMTS family members,

Table 29.4 *In vitro* inhibition profile of selective MMP inhibitors

Compound	Originator	In vitro *profile (IC$_{50}$s – nM)*
1 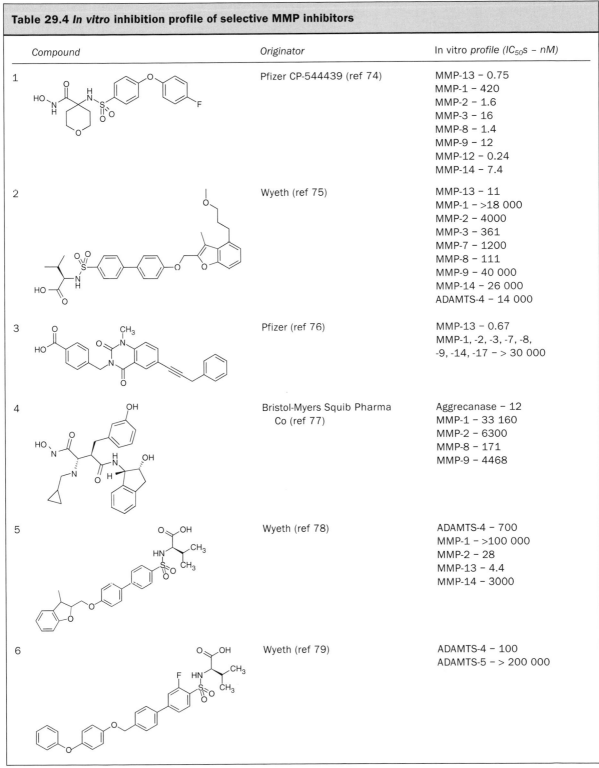	Pfizer CP-544439 (ref 74)	MMP-13 – 0.75 MMP-1 – 420 MMP-2 – 1.6 MMP-3 – 16 MMP-8 – 1.4 MMP-9 – 12 MMP-12 – 0.24 MMP-14 – 7.4
2	Wyeth (ref 75)	MMP-13 – 11 MMP-1 – >18 000 MMP-2 – 4000 MMP-3 – 361 MMP-7 – 1200 MMP-8 – 111 MMP-9 – 40 000 MMP-14 – 26 000 ADAMTS-4 – 14 000
3	Pfizer (ref 76)	MMP-13 – 0.67 MMP-1, -2, -3, -7, -8, -9, -14, -17 – > 30 000
4	Bristol-Myers Squib Pharma Co (ref 77)	Aggrecanase – 12 MMP-1 – 33 160 MMP-2 – 6300 MMP-8 – 171 MMP-9 – 4468
5	Wyeth (ref 78)	ADAMTS-4 – 700 MMP-1 – >100 000 MMP-2 – 28 MMP-13 – 4.4 MMP-14 – 3000
6	Wyeth (ref 79)	ADAMTS-4 – 100 ADAMTS-5 – > 200 000

Continued

Table 29.4 *In vitro* inhibition profile of selective MMP inhibitors—cont'd

Compound	Originator	In vitro profile (IC_{50}s – nM)
7 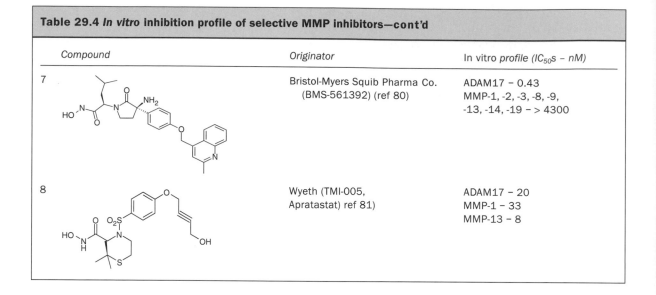	Bristol-Myers Squib Pharma Co. (BMS-561392) (ref 80)	ADAM17 – 0.43 MMP-1, -2, -3, -8, -9, -13, -14, -19 – > 4300
8	Wyeth (TMI-005, Apratastat) ref 81)	ADAM17 – 20 MMP-1 – 33 MMP-13 – 8

including the ability to establish *in vitro* enzyme assays, currently hampered by a lack of substrates for many family members. Nevertheless, prospects for achieving selectivity within closely related ADAMTS family members look promising with the recent description by Wyeth of additional biphenylsulfonamide carboxylate compounds which are potent ADAMTS-4 inhibitors with > 2000-fold selectivity against ADAMTS-5 (Table 29.4, compound 6).[79]

Two examples of hydroxamate-based inhibitors of ADAM-17 have progressed into clinical evaluation for RA. Bristol-Myers Squibb Co. identified BMS-561392 (DPC-333) as a picomolar inhibitor of ADAM-17 which demonstrated > 1000-fold selectivity against MMP-1, -2, -3, -8, -9, -13, -14, and -19, and ADAM-9 and -10[80] (Table 29.4 compound 7). This compound demonstrated efficacy in preclinical models and was progressed into clinical trials for RA. Unfortunately clinical development was put on hold during phase IIa studies, due to a potential hepatotoxicity risk. It is not yet clear whether this is a compound- or mechanism-dependent effect.

Several examples of dual MMP-13 and ADAM-17 inhibitors have also been described.[81,82] Wyeth identified a series of thiomorpholine sulfonamide hydroxamate compounds as dual inhibitors of TACE and MMPs.[81,82] Further optimization led to apratastat (TMI-005) (Table 29.4 compound 8),[81] which has nanomolar IC_{50}s against ADAM-17, MMP-1, and MMP-13 and has demonstrated efficacy in preclinical models of arthritis. Apratastat has progressed through phase I studies in healthy volunteers and RA patients and is currently undergoing phase II evaluation.

OTHER THERAPEUTIC OPPORTUNITIES

In addition to synthetic inhibitors targeted to the catalytic domain of MMPs, Kureha Corp. are evaluating CPA-926, a pro-drug of esculetin, which has been shown to reduce cartilage destruction in a rabbit model of OA.[83] The mechanism of action is not clearly defined, although the compound appears to broadly suppress MMP synthesis and activity. CPA-926 is currently undergoing phase II trials for OA. The chemically modified tetracyclines have been shown to weakly inhibit collagenases and affect secretion of MMPs. Recent data from clinical studies with doxycycline have demonstrated a reduction in the rate of joint space narrowing (JSN) in established OA of the knee, although there was no effect upon pain or JSN in the contralateral knee.[84] Doxycycline has a weak inhibitory activity for MMPs but it is not known whether the clinical effect is due to inhibition of metalloproteinases or to other activities.

Another therapeutic opportunity may come from recent advancement of structural and functional research into TIMPs and generation of selective TIMP mutants. Mutagenesis studies have allowed generation of TIMP mutants selective to specific MMPs[85] by and also converted TIMP-1 and TIMP-2 to inhibit ADAM-17.[86,87] Recent studies of Wei et al. showed that addition of an extra Ala to the N-terminus or mutation of Thr2 to a Gly of TIMP-3 destroyed its ability to inhibit MMPs, but retained the inhibitory activity of ADAM-17.[88] Those studies suggest that there are several key sites in the TIMP molecules that dictate specific interactions with a particular metalloproteinase. The detailed structural analyses of such interaction may provide further clues to design new types of selective inhibitors for ADAMs.

MMPs, ADAMs, and ADAMTSs are multi-domain proteinases and in many cases their activities for the natural ECM substrates are regulated by non-catalytic ancillary domains. Deletion of such domains critically impairs their activity, suggesting that molecules that modify their functions (exosite inhibitors) may specifically affect the enzymatic activity on natural substrates. An example may be seen in autoantibodies found in patients with thrombotic thrombocytopenic purpura that inhibit the activity of ADAMTS-13 to cleave von Willebrand factor. Those antibodies are directed to the non-catalytic domains of the proteinase, not toward the catalytic domain.[40] Specific antibodies and exosite inhibition are ideal for selective inhibition of a target proteinase.

CONCLUSIONS

TNF-α-neutralizing agents such as infliximab (Remicade) and etanercept (Enbrel) are currently used clinically for the treatment of many inflammatory diseases including RA, ankylosing spondylitis, juvenile RA and psoriatic arthritis. An alternative approach to lowering the levels of TNF-α in inflammatory disease is therefore to inhibit ADAM-17. However, a variety of MMPs have been found to be overexpressed in RA synovial tissue and have been implicated in the destruction of cartilage in RA joints, but the optimal ADAM-17 over MMP selectivity profile for a

drug to treat RA is at present unresolved. In the case of OA, it may be necessary to inhibit several metalloproteinases. We will still need to elucidate the physiological and pathological roles of MMPs and ADAMTSs in the progressive degradation of cartilage matrix to design effective therapeutic strategies. Based upon recent success in achieving selectivity and bioavailability with MMP inhibitors targeted at MMP-13, ADAM-17, and ADAMTS-4/-5, the prospects for the next generation of selective metalloproteinase inhibitors look encouraging, although we must now await progression of these compounds to human clinical studies.

ACKNOWLEDGMENTS

We thank Alan Lyons and Ngee Han Lim for drawing the figures and Christine Greig for typing the manuscript. The work is supported by grants from the Arthritis Research Campaign, Wellcome Trust, the Medical Research Council, Cancer Reserch UK, and National Institutes of Health grant AR40994.

REFERENCES

1. Murphy G, Knäuper V, Atkinson S et al. Matrix metalloproteinases in arthritic disease. Arthritis Res 2002; 4 (Suppl 3): S39–S49.

2. Pap T, Gay S, Schett G. Matrix metalloproteinases. In Smolen J, Lipsky P, eds. Targeted Therapies in Rheumatology. London: Martin Dunitz, 2003: 483–97.

3. Milner JM, Cawston TE. Matrix metalloproteinase knock-out studies and the potential use of matrix metalloproteinase inhibitors in the rheumatic diseases. Curr Drug Targets Inflamm Allergy 2005; 4: 363–75.

4. Chung L, Dinakarpandian D, Yoshida N et al. Collagenase unwinds triple-helical collagen prior to peptide bond hydrolysis. EMBO J 2004; 23: 3020–30.

5. Itoh Y, Seiki M. MT1-MMP: a potent modifier of pericellular microenvironment. J Cell Physiol 2006; 206: 1–8.

6. Nagase H, Visse R, Murphy G. Structure and function of matrix metalloproteinases and TIMPs. Cardiovasc Res 2006; 69: 562–73.

7. Baker AH, Edwards DR, Murphy G. Metalloproteinase inhibitors: biological actions and therapeutic opportunities. J Cell Sci 2002; 115: 3719–27.

8. Bode W, Gomis-Rüth FX, Stocker W. Astacins, serralysins, snake venom and matrix metalloproteinases exhibit identical zinc-binding environments (HEXXHXXGXXH and

Met-turn) and topologies and should be grouped into a common family, the 'metzincins'. FEBS Lett 1993; 331: 134–40.

9. Gomis-Rüth FX. Structural aspects of the metzincin clan of metalloendopeptidases. Mol Biotechnol 2003; 24: 157–202.

10. Okada Y, Shinmei M, Tanaka O et al. Localization of matrix metalloproteinase 3 (stromelysin) in osteoarthritic cartilage and synovium. Lab Invest 1992; 66: 680–90.

11. Bau B, Gebhard PM, Haag J et al. Relative messenger RNA expression profiling of collagenases and aggrecanases in human articular chondrocytes in vivo and in vitro. Arthritis Rheum 2002; 46: 2648–57.

12. Lee JH, Fitzgerald JB, DiMicco MA, Grodzinsky AJ. Mechanical injury of cartilage explants causes specific time-dependent changes in chondrocyte gene expression. Arthritis Rheum 2005; 52: 2386–95.

13. Stanton H, Ung L, Fosang AJ. The 45 kDa collagen-binding fragment of fibronectin induces matrix metalloproteinase-13 synthesis by chondrocytes and aggrecan degradation by aggrecanases. Biochem J 2002; 364: 181–90.

14. Yasuda T, Shimizu M, Nakagawa T, Julovi SM, Nakamura T. Matrix metalloproteinase production by COOH-terminal heparin-binding fibronectin fragment in rheumatoid synovial cells. Lab Invest 2003; 83: 153–62.

15. Forsyth CB, Pulai J, Loeser RF. Fibronectin fragments and blocking antibodies to α2β1 and α5β1 integrins stimulate mitogen-activated protein kinase signaling and increase collagenase 3 (matrix metalloproteinase 13) production by human articular chondrocytes. Arthritis Rheum 2002; 46: 2368–76.

16. Lark MW, Bayne EK, Flanagan J et al. Aggrecan degradation in human cartilage – evidence for both matrix metalloproteinase and aggrecanase activity in normal, osteoarthritic, and rheumatoid joints. J Clin Invest 1997; 100: 93–106.

17. Struglics A, Larsson S, Pratta MA et al. Human osteoarthritis synovial fluid and joint cartilage contain both aggrecanase- and matrix metalloproteinase-generated aggrecan fragments. Osteoarthritis Cartilage 2006; 14: 101–13.

18. Dodge GR, Poole AR. Immunohistochemical detection and immunochemical analysis of type II collagen degradation in human normal, rheumatoid, and osteoarthritic articular cartilages and in explants of bovine articular cartilage cultured with interleukin 1. J Clin Invest 1989; 83: 647–61.

19. Conway JG, Wakefield JA, Brown RH et al. Inhibition of cartilage and bone destruction in adjuvant arthritis in the rat by a matrix metalloproteinase inhibitor. J Exp Med 1995; 182: 449–57.

20. Sabatini M, Lesur C, Thomas M et al. Effect of inhibition of matrix metalloproteinases on cartilage loss in vitro and in a guinea pig model of osteoarthritis. Arthritis Rheum 2005; 52: 171–80.

21. Ishikawa T, Nishigaki F, Miyata S et al. Prevention of progressive joint destruction in collagen-induced arthritis in rats by a novel matrix metalloproteinase inhibitor, FR255031. Br J Pharmacol 2005; 144: 133–43.

22. Sandy JD, Neame PJ, Boynton RE, Flannery CR. Catabolism of aggrecan in cartilage explants. Identification of a major cleavage site within the interglobular domain. J Biol Chem 1991; 266: 8683–85.

23. Sandy JD, Flannery CR, Neame PJ, Lohmander LS. The structure of aggrecan fragments in human synovial fluid. Evidence for the involvement in osteoarthritis of a novel proteinase which cleaves the Glu 373-Ala 374 bond of the interglobular domain. J Clin Invest 1992; 89: 1512–16.

24. Lohmander LS, Neame PJ, Sandy JD. The structure of aggrecan fragments in human synovial fluid. Evidence that aggrecanase mediates cartilage degradation in inflammatory joint disease, joint injury, and osteoarthritis. Arthritis Rheum 1993; 36: 1214–22.

25. Tortorella MD, Burn TC, Pratta MA et al. Purification and cloning of aggrecanase-1: a member of the ADAMTS family of proteins. Science 1999; 284: 1664–66.

26. Abbaszade I, Liu RQ, Yang F et al. Cloning and characterization of ADAMTS11, an aggrecanase from the ADAMTS family. J Biol Chem 1999; 274: 23443–50.

27. Porter S, Clark IM, Kevorkian L, Edwards DR. The ADAMTS metalloproteinases. Biochem J 2005; 386: 15–27.

28. Kuno K, Kanada N, Nakashima E et al. Molecular cloning of a gene encoding a new type of metalloproteinase-disintegrin family protein with thrombospondin motifs as an inflammation associated gene. J Biol Chem 1997; 272: 556–62.

29. Colige A, Li SW, Sieron AL et al. cDNA cloning and expression of bovine procollagen I N-proteinase: a new member of the superfamily of zinc-metalloproteinases with binding sites for cells and other matrix components. Proc Natl Acad Sci U S A 1997; 94: 2374–9.

30. Fernandes RJ, Hirohata S, Engle JM et al. Procollagen II amino propeptide processing by ADAMTS-3. Insights on dermatosparaxis. J Biol Chem 2001; 276: 31502–9.

31. Colige A, Vandenberghe I, Thiry M et al. Cloning and characterization of ADAMTS-14, a novel ADAMTS displaying high homology with ADAMTS-2 and ADAMTS-3. J Biol Chem 2002; 277: 5756–66.

32. Colige A, Ruggiero F, Vandenberghe I et al. Domains and maturation processes that regulate the activity of ADAMTS-2, a metalloproteinase cleaving the amino-propeptide of fibrillar procollagens types I-III and V. J Biol Chem 2005; 280: 34397–408.

33. Zeng W, Corcoran C, Collins-Racie LA et al. Glycosaminoglycan-binding properties and aggrecanase activities of truncated ADAMTSs: comparative analyses with ADAMTS-5, -9, -16 and -18. Biochim Biophys Acta 2006; 1760: 517–24.

34. Kashiwagi M, Enghild JJ, Gendron C et al. Altered proteolytic activities of ADAMTS-4 expressed by C-terminal processing. J Biol Chem 2004; 279: 10109–19.

35. Gao G, Plaas A, Thompson VP et al. ADAMTS4 (aggrecanase-1) activation on the cell surface involves C-terminal cleavage by glycosylphosphatidyl inositol-anchored membrane type 4-matrix metalloproteinase and binding of the activated proteinase to chondroitin sulfate and heparan sulfate on syndecan-1. J Biol Chem 2004; 279: 10042–51.

36. Tortorella MD, Liu RQ, Burn T, Newton RC, Arner E. Characterization of human aggrecanase 2 (ADAM-TS5): substrate specificity studies and comparison with aggrecanase 1 (ADAM-TS4). Matrix Biol 2002; 21: 499–511.

37. Collins-Racie LA, Flannery CR, Zeng W et al. ADAMTS-8 exhibits aggrecanase activity and is expressed in human articular cartilage. Matrix Biol 2004; 23: 219–30.

38. Levy GG, Nichols WC, Lian EC et al. Mutations in a member of the ADAMTS gene family cause thrombotic thrombocytopenic purpura. Nature (Lond) 2001; 413: 488–94.

39. Majerus EM, Anderson PJ, Sadler JE. Binding of ADAMTS13 to von Willebrand factor. J Biol Chem 2005; 280: 21773–8.

40. Soejima K, Matsumoto M, Kokame K et al. ADAMTS-13 cysteine-rich/spacer domains are functionally essential for von Willebrand factor cleavage. Blood 2003; 102: 3232–7.

41. Wang WM, Ge G, Lim NH, Nagase H, Greenspan DS. TIMP-3 inhibits the procollagen N-proteinase ADAMTS-2. Biochem J 2006; 398: 515–19.

42. Shindo T, Kurihara H, Kuno K et al. ADAMTS-1: a metalloproteinase-disintegrin essential for normal growth, fertility, and organ morphology and function. J Clin Invest 2000; 105: 1345–52.

43. Luque A, Carpizo DR, Iruela-Arispe ML. ADAMTS1/METH1 inhibits endothelial cell proliferation by direct binding and sequestration of VEGF165. J Biol Chem 2003; 278: 23656–65.

44. Vazquez F, Hastings G, Ortega MA et al. METH-1, a human ortholog of ADAMTS-1, and METH-2 are members of a new family of proteins with angio-inhibitory activity. J Biol Chem 1999; 274: 23349–57.

45. Colige A, Sieron AL, Li SW et al. Human Ehlers-Danlos syndrome type VII C and bovine dermatosparaxis are caused by mutations in the procollagen I N-proteinase gene. Am J Hum Genet 1999; 65: 308–17.

46. Li SW, Arita M, Fertala A et al. Transgenic mice with inactive alleles for procollagen N-proteinase (ADAMTS-2) develop fragile skin and male sterility. Biochem J 2001; 355: 271–8.

47. Terrell DR, Williams LA, Vesely SK et al. The incidence of thrombotic thrombocytopenic purpura-hemolytic uremic syndrome: all patients, idiopathic patients, and patients with severe ADAMTS-13 deficiency. J Thromb Haemost 2005; 3: 1432–6.

48. Flannery CR, Little CB, Hughes CE, Caterson B. Expression of ADAMTS homologues in articular cartilage. Biochem Biophys Res Commun 1999; 260: 318–22.

49. Kevorkian L, Young DA, Darrah C et al. Expression profiling of metalloproteinases and their inhibitors in cartilage. Arthritis Rheum 2004; 50: 131–41.

50. Glasson SS, Askew R, Sheppard B et al. Characterization of and osteoarthritis susceptibility in ADAMTS-4-knockout mice. Arthritis Rheum 2004; 50: 2547–58.

51. Glasson SS, Askew R, Sheppard B et al. Deletion of active ADAMTS5 prevents cartilage degradation in a murine model of osteoarthritis. Nature (Lond) 2005; 434: 644–8.

52. Stanton H, Rogerson FM, East CJ et al. ADAMTS5 is the major aggrecanase in mouse cartilage in vivo and in vitro. Nature (Lond) 2005; 434: 648–52.

53. Lark MW, Bayne EK, Flanagan J et al. Aggrecan degradation in human cartilage. Evidence for both matrix metalloproteinase and aggrecanase activity in normal, osteoarthritic, and rheumatoid joints. J Clin Invest 1997; 100: 93–106.

54. Sandy JD. A contentious issue finds some clarity: on the independent and complementary roles of aggrecanase activity and MMP activity in human joint aggrecanolysis. Osteoarthritis Cartilage 2006; 14: 95–100.

55. White JM. ADAMs: modulators of cell-cell and cell-matrix interactions. Curr Opin Cell Biol 2003; 15: 598–606.

56. Becherer JD, Blobel CP. Biochemical properties and functions of membrane-anchored metalloprotease-disintegrin proteins (ADAMs). Curr Top Dev Biol 2003; 54: 101–23.

57. Seals DF, Courtneidge SA. The ADAMs family of metalloproteases: multidomain proteins with multiple functions. Genes Dev 2003; 17: 7–30.

58. Maskos K, Fernandez-Catalan C, Huber R et al. Crystal structure of the catalytic domain of human tumor necrosis factor-alpha-converting enzyme. Proc Natl Acad Sci U S A 1998; 95: 3408–12.

59. Janes PW, Saha N, Barton WA et al. Adam meets Eph: an ADAM substrate recognition module acts as a molecular switch for ephrin cleavage in trans. Cell 2005; 123: 291–304.

60. Huang J, Bridges LC, White JM. Selective modulation of integrin-mediated cell migration by distinct ADAM family members. Mol Biol Cell 2005; 16: 4982–91.

61. Bridges LC, Bowditch RD. ADAM-integrin interactions: potential integrin regulated ectodomain shedding activity. Curr Pharm Des 2005; 11: 837–47.

62. Huovila AP, Turner AJ, Pelto-Huikko M, Karkkainen I, Ortiz RM. Shedding light on ADAM metalloproteinases. Trends Biochem Sci 2005; 30: 413–22.

63. Smith KM, Gaultier A, Cousin H et al. The cysteine-rich domain regulates ADAM protease function in vivo. J Cell Biol 2002; 159: 893–902.

64. Blobel CP. ADAMs: key components in EGFR signalling and development. Nat Rev Mol Cell Biol 2005; 6: 32–43.

65. Amour A, Slocombe PM, Webster A et al. TNF-alpha converting enzyme (TACE) is inhibited by TIMP-3. FEBS Lett 1998; 435: 39–44.

66. Smookler DS, Mohammed FF, Kassiri Z et al. Tissue inhibitor of metalloproteinase 3 regulates TNF-dependent systemic inflammation. J Immunol 2006; 176: 721–5.

67. Mahmoodi M, Sahebjam S, Smookler D, Khokha R, Mort JS. Lack of tissue inhibitor of metalloproteinases-3 results in an enhanced inflammatory response in antigen-induced arthritis. Am J Pathol 2005; 166: 1733–40.

68. Böhm BB, Aigner T, Blobel CP, Kalden JR, Burkhardt H. Highly enhanced expression of the disintegrin metalloproteinase MDC15 (metargidin) in rheumatoid synovial tissue. Arthritis Rheum 2001; 44: 2046–54.

69. Komiya K, Enomoto H, Inoki I et al. Expression of ADAM15 in rheumatoid synovium: up-regulation by vascular endothelial growth factor and possible implications for angiogenesis. Arthritis Res Ther 2005; 7: R1158–R1173.

70. Böhm BB, Aigner T, Roy B et al. Homeostatic effects of the metalloproteinase disintegrin ADAM15 in degenerative cartilage remodeling. Arthritis Rheum 2005; 52: 1100–9.

71. Kveiborg M, Albrechtsen R, Rudkjarr L et al. ADAM12-S stimulates bone growth in transgenic mice by modulating chondrocyte proliferation and maturation. J Bone Miner Res 2006; 21: 1288–96.

72. Decoster E, Vanhaesebroeck B, Vandenabeele P, Grooten J, Fiers W. Generation and biological characterization of membrane-bound, uncleavable murine tumor necrosis factor. J Biol Chem 1995; 270: 18473–8.

73. Scheller J, Ohnesorge N, Rose-John S. Interleukin-6 trans-signalling in chronic inflammation and cancer. Scand J Immunol 2006; 63: 321–9.

74. Reiter LA, Robinson RP, McClure KF et al. Pyran-containing sulfonamide hydroxamic acids: potent MMP inhibitors that spare MMP-1. Bioorg Med Chem Lett 2004; 14: 3389–95.

75. Wyeth. US Patent Application 2005/0143422 A1. Biaryl sulfonamides and methods for using same (2005).

76. Warner Lambert Company. Patent Application WO02/064080 A2 76 Matrix Metalloproteinase Inhibitors (2002).

77. Yao W, Wasserman ZR, Chao M et al. Design and synthesis of a series of (2R)-N(4)-hydroxy-2-(3-hydroxybenzyl)-N(1)-[(1S,2R)-2-hydroxy-2,3-dihydro-1H-inden-1-yl]butanediamide derivatives as potent, selective, and orally bioavailable aggrecanase inhibitors. J Med Chem 2001; 44: 3347–50.

78. Xiang JS, Hu Y, Rush TS et al. Synthesis and biological evaluation of biphenylsulfonamide. carboxylate aggrecanase-1 inhibitors. Bioorg Med Chem Lett 2006; 16: 311–16.

79. Wyeth. US Patent Application 2006/0004066 A1 79. Methods for treating ADAMTS-5 associated disease (2006).

80. Liu R, Magolda R, Newton R et al. Pharmacological profile of DPC 333, a selective TACE inhibitor. J Inflammat Res Suppl 2002; 2: S125.

81. Levin JI, Chen JM, Laakso LM et al. Acetylenic TACE inhibitors. Part 3: Thiomorpholine sulfonamide hydroxamates. Bioorg Med Chem Lett 2006; 16: 1605–9.

82. Letavic MA, Barberia JT, Carty TJ et al. Synthesis and biological activity of piperazine-based dual MMP-13 and TNF-alpha converting enzyme inhibitors. Bioorg Med Chem Lett 2003; 13: 3243–6.

83. Yamada H, Watanabe K, Saito T et al. Esculetin (dihydroxycoumarin) inhibits the production of matrix metalloproteinases in cartilage explants, and oral administration of its prodrug, CPA-926, suppresses cartilage destruction in rabbit experimental osteoarthritis. J Rheumatol 1999; 26: 654–62.

84. Brandt KD, Mazzuca SA, Katz BP et al. Effects of doxycycline on progression of osteoarthritis: results of a randomized, placebo-controlled, double-blind trial. Arthritis Rheum 2005; 52: 2015–25.

85. Nagase H, Brew K. Designing TIMP (tissue inhibitor of metalloproteinases) variants that are selective metalloproteinase inhibitors. Biochem Soc Symp 2003; (70): 201–12.

86. Lee MH, Rapti M, Knauper V, Murphy G. Threonine 98, the pivotal residue of tissue inhibitor of metalloproteinases (TIMP)-1 in metalloproteinase recognition. J Biol Chem 2004; 279: 17562–9.

87. Lee MH, Rapti M, Murphy G. Delineating the molecular basis of the inactivity of tissue inhibitor of metalloproteinase-2 against tumor necrosis factor-alpha-converting enzyme. J Biol Chem 2004; 279: 45121–9.

88. Wei S, Kashiwagi M, Kota S et al. Reactive site mutations in tissue inhibitor of metalloproteinase-3 disrupt inhibition of matrix metalloproteinases but not tumor necrosis factor-alpha-converting enzyme. J Biol Chem 2005; 280: 32877–82.

30

Update on proinflammatory cytokine blockade in rheumatoid arthritis

Ferdinand C Breedveld

Introduction • Infliximab • Adalimumab • Etanercept • TNF antagonists • Adverse reactions • Summary and conclusions • References

INTRODUCTION

The active search for new treatment modalities for established rheumatoid arthritis (RA) has created a dynamic period for rheumatology. Both innovative application of established disease-modifying anti-rheumatic drugs (DMARDs) and the availability of targeted interventions have improved therapeutic results. The emphasis in RA clinical research has been on measures of inflammatory activity such as joint scores and acute phase response. Control of inflammation is regarded as an effective strategy to improve long-term outcome, although few studies are available to assess how completely inflammation must be controlled. The benefit of early treatment is indisputable, as is tight disease control to detect non-responders in an early phase.[1,2] In the last 5 years the results of many studies have emerged that allow an optimal introduction of tumor necrosis factor (TNF) antagonists in the treatment armamentarium of rheumatologists. Given the availability of three TNF antagonists, the emergence of two new targeted therapies in RA (abatacept and rituximab) and the judgment on clinical efficacy, the usage of recombinant interleukin (IL)-1 receptor antagonist has sharply declined. This chapter will focus on the new insights in efficacy and toxicity of TNF antagonists obtained between 2001 and 2006.

INFLIXIMAB

Infliximab (Remicade) was the first TNF antagonist studied in RA in the Kennedy Institute of Rheumatology. Several placebo-controlled trials showed efficacy of infliximab in combination with methotrexate in patients with advanced RA.[3–5] The efficacy of infliximab in patients with RA of less than 3 years was assessed in a study where 1049 methotrexate-naïve patients were randomized to methotrexate, methotrexate and infliximab 3 mg/kg, or methotrexate and infliximab 6 mg/kg.[6] At 54 weeks the ACR 20% response rates were significantly higher in the methotrexate and infliximab groups (62% and 66%, respectively) when compared with the methotrexate only group (53%). In addition, patients in the infliximab groups showed less radiographic progression (mean Sharp score progression of 0.4) compared with the progression in the methotrexate only group (mean 3.7). Physical function improved significantly more in the infliximab-treated groups, as did employability.[7] The relation between the anti-inflammatory effects of infliximab and the effect on joint destruction was studied in those patients who did not show a clinical response to infliximab and methotrexate therapy.[8] It could be shown that even in these patients treatment with infliximab and methotrexate provided significant benefit with regard to the destructive process, suggesting that in such patients these two aspects of disease are dissociated.

Infliximab was also studied for its potential to induce a state of remission with a temporary intervention. Quinn et al. treated 20 patients with early RA with methotrexate and either placebo or infliximab for 1 year in a controlled study. Intriguingly 7 of the 10 patients who stopped infliximab remained in a state of low disease activity in the second year.[9] In a larger-scale study four treatment strategies were compared as initial therapy in patients with early RA: (1) sequential monotherapy, (2) step-up combination therapy, (3) initial combination therapy with corticosteroids, and (4) initial treatment with methotrexate and corticosteroids. After 1 year the primary outcomes (ACR 20 + HAQ (Health Assessment Questionnaire) + Sharp score) were significantly better in groups 3 and 4 compared with groups 1 and 2.[10] The patients in group 4 who initially started with infliximab and methotrexate (n = 120) discontinued infliximab when they showed low disease activity for 6 consecutive months. Of the 77 patients who discontinued infliximab and entered years 2 and 3 of the study with low disease activity and a mean of 10 mg methotrexate per week, only 14 patients flared and no patient developed radiographic progression.[11] These data provide evidence for the window of opportunity hypothesis in RA. If larger studies confirm these data, this protocol may provide a solution to the economic issues of early therapy with biologics. The approach presented may offer the potential for the drug to be used for a limited period of a time when it has the greatest opportunity to make a difference. Large-scale controlled studies are under way to confirm these findings.

ADALIMUMAB

Adalimumab (Humira) is a fully human anti-TNF monoclonal antibody (mAb) that has shown efficacy as monotherapy or in combination with methotrexate in several randomized, placebo-controlled, phase III trials. In therapy-naïve patients with early aggressive RA (n = 799), subcutaneous administration of adalimumab was significantly more effective than either drug alone in achieving ACR 50 responses, the co-primary efficacy endpoint, from 6 months to 2 years.[12] Adalimumab plus methotrexate was also significantly more effective than either drug alone in slowing the rate of joint destruction, as shown by the significant small increases in the modified Sharp score after 52 weeks of therapy. After 2 years of treatment significantly more patients receiving combination therapy than those receiving monotherapy had a meaningful improvement in physical function. In this trial adalimumab and methotrexate monotherapy had similar effects on clinical outcome but adalimumab was associated with less radiographic progression.

In patients with advanced disease, adalimumab in combination with methotrexate produced more rapid, statistically significant, and sustained improvements in ACR responses compared with the same regimen without adalimumab in several phase III trials of 24–52 weeks. The ACR 20% response at 24 weeks was two to four times more frequent with adalimumab and methotrexate compared with methotrexate and placebo.[13,14] The control of the disease activity achieved with adalimumab and methotrexate in the first 6 months could be maintained for up to 4 years in patients remaining on treatment in open-label extension.[15] Adalimumab plus methotrexate was more effective than placebo plus methotrexate in slowing radiographic progression.[13]

ETANERCEPT

Etanercept (Enbrel) was developed by linking DNA encoding the extracellular portion of the P75 TNF receptor with DNA encoding the Fc portion of human IgG1.[16] Its efficacy as monotherapy or in combination in the treatment of advanced RA has been shown in several phase III trials.[17–19] Etanercept 10 or 25 mg was compared to methotrexate in 632 patients with early RA.[20] At 12 months, 72% of the patients in the group assigned to receive 25 mg etanercept had an ACR 20% response as compared with 65% of those in the methotrexate group. Among the patients who received 25 mg etanercept, 72% had no increase in the erosion score as compared with 60% of the patients in the methotrexate group. Etanercept was also studied in what is now seen as a classical three-arm study comparing etanercept plus methotrexate with etanercept or methotrexate alone[21] in 682 patients with a mean disease duration of 6 years. At week 52 a mean of 85% of patients in the combination group achieved an ACR 20% response compared with 75% and 76% of the methotrexate and etanercept monotherapy groups, respectively. With respect to the radiographic primary outcome the mean Sharp score change for the combination group was lower than for the monotherapy groups at week 52. The mean difference between combination and methotrexate groups was −3.34. Etanercept-treated patients had less change in Sharp scores than did methotrexate-treated patients. The results of the HAQ indicated improvement over baseline values in disability in patients allocated to combination treatment compared with the monotherapies. This improved outcome of etanercept plus methotrexate therapy was sustained during the 2-year extension of the study.[22]

TNF ANTAGONISTS

Adalimumab and etanercept are both approved as monotherapy for RA, while infliximab is approved for use with methotrexate in RA. However, the cumulative weight of evidence from several trials suggests that the combination of a TNF-blocking agent and methotrexate yields superior results. TNF inhibitors have been used with combinations of various background DMARDs without increased toxicity.[23] There is no evidence that any one TNF-blocking agent is more effective than any other. Many uncontrolled observational studies have reported that failure to respond to one TNF inhibitor does not predict response to another. The efficacy of combination therapy of etanercept and anakinra was assessed in a randomized double-blind study including 244 patients. Combination therapy provided no treatment benefit over etanercept alone but was associated with increased safety risk: 0 versus 4% serious infections.

ADVERSE REACTIONS

Data from clinical trials with TNF-inhibiting agents have reported relatively low levels of toxicity of these drugs. An increased susceptibility of tuberculosis (TB) or re-activation of latent TB should be considered as a class characteristic of TNF antagonists. The picture of TB may be atypical in those patients, as has been seen with other immunocompromised patients. There have been more reported cases of TB in patients treated with infliximab and adalimumab than etanercept but no definitive data are available regarding a difference in TB risk between the agents. Screening patients about to start TNF-blocking agents has reduced the risk of activating TB. Other opportunistic infections such as *Listeria* and histoplasmosis are rare but have been reported in the setting of TNF-blocking agents. A systemic literature search conducted through December 2005 on the published trials on infliximab and adalimumab revealed an increased risk of infections requiring antimicrobial therapy and malignancies compared with control patients. The pooled odds ratios were 3.3 for malignancy and 2.0 for infection.[24]

However, several large observational databases including prospective case-control studies did not demonstrate an increased incidence of solid tumors or lymphomas after TNF-blocking therapy. Surprisingly such studies seem to indicate a decreased risk of cardiovascular events during treatment with TNF antagonists compared with control patients. Despite initial warnings there is presently no substantive evidence that TNF antagonists increase the risk of congestive heart failure. Some patients have become pregnant while being treated with TNF blocking therapy and small surveys have not shown that the rates of normal live births, miscarriages, and therapeutic terminations are different from the published rates for the normal population. There are insufficient data to advise continuation or starting of anti-TNF therapy if a patient becomes pregnant. The incidence of pancytopenia, pulmonary fibrosis, and demyelinating-like syndromes is not greater than expected in the general population; however, in rare cases these syndromes have been reported.

SUMMARY AND CONCLUSIONS

The concept of a targeted therapy that could affect one or more specific pathological processes in RA has enormous implications for the future. Heretofore, all the available therapies have been truly non-specific, often borrowed from other disciplines (e.g. oncology, infectious diseases), and having side effect profiles that limit their usefulness. With the new biologic agents, new therapeutic perspectives appear but many questions need to be addressed to further clarify their role. These include the following: (1) do these drugs maintain efficacy with treatments longer than 5 years; (2) do these treatments maintain the integrity of joint structures during long-term therapy; (3) are they safe with long-term therapy; (4) how can we explain non-responders; (5) how can we select patients for different forms of targeted therapies; (6) is it justified to use the, by definition, restricted financial resources in healthcare for long-term RA treatment with biologic agents?

The three TNF antagonists may be used as either first- or second-line options and their first-time use is currently recommended only in exceptional circumstances. Usage of TNF antagonists is generally recommended for patients who have failed DMARD therapy. Whether this will change depends on more studies on the optimal therapeutic strategy in early RA.

RA is a severe disease despite established treatment. The most promising therapies at present include products of biotechnology. These therapies, which have become available for many rheumatologists, may certainly be seen as breakthroughs in the treatment of RA. Methotrexate is presently regarded as the gold standard of traditional DMARD therapy. However, the biologic agents discussed are significantly more effective than methotrexate in slowing radiographic progression of joint destruction. The optimal initial approach for controlling disease activity in RA is now being studied in many centers. The indication is that early introduction of the combination of methotrexate and a TNF antagonist may achieve a sustained remission more frequently than initial monotherapy.[9,11] The optimization of biologic therapies through increasing experience and extended careful surveillance of patients should ensure cytokine-targeted agents a pivotal place in the therapy of RA.

REFERENCES

1. Pincus T, Breedveld FC, Emery P. Does partial control of inflammation prevent long-term joint damage? Clinical rationale for combination therapy with multiple disease-modifying antirheumatic drugs. Clin Exp Rheumatol 1999; 17 (Suppl 18): S2–S7.

2. Grigor C, Capell H, Stirling A et al. Effect of a treatment strategy of tight control for rheumatoid arthritis (the TICORA study): a single-blind randomised controlled trial. Lancet 2004; 364: 263–9.

3. Maini RN, Breedveld FC, Kalden JR et al. Therapeutic efficacy of multiple intravenous infusions of anti-tumor necrosis factor α monoclonal antibody combined with low-dose weekly methotrexate in rheumatoid arthritis. Arthritis Rheum 1998; 41: 1552–63.

4. Maini R, St Clair EW, Breedveld F et al. Infliximab (chimeric anti-tumour necrosis factor α monoclonal antibody) versus placebo in rheumatoid arthritis patients receiving concomitant methotrexate: a randomised phase III trial. Lancet 1999; 354: 1932–9.

5. Lipsky PE, van der Heijde DM, St Clair EW et al. Infliximab and methotrexate in the treatment of rheumatoid arthritis. Anti-tumor necrosis factor trial in rheumatoid arthritis with Concomitant Therapy Group. N Engl J Med 2000; 343: 1594–602.

6. St Clair EW, van der Heijde DMFM, Smolen JS et al. Combination of infliximab and methotrexate therapy for early rheumatoid arthritis: a randomized, controlled trial. Arthritis Rheum 2004; 50: 3432–43.

7. Smolen JS, Han C, van der Heijde D et al. Infliximab treatment maintains employability in patients with early rheumatoid arthritis. Arthritis Rheum 2006; 54: 716–22.

8. Smolen JS, Han C, Bala M et al. Evidence of radiographic benefit of treatment with infliximab plus methotrexate in rheumatoid arthritis patients who had no clinical improvement: a detailed subanalysis of data from the anti-tumor necrosis factor trial in rheumatoid arthritis with concomitant therapy study. Arthritis Rheum 2005; 52: 1020–30.

9. Quinn MA, Conaghan PhG, O'Connor PhJ et al. Very early treatment with infliximab in addition to methotrexate in early, poor-prognosis rheumatoid arthritis reduces magnetic resonance imaging evidence of synovitis and damage, with sustained benefit after infliximab withdrawal: results from a twelve-month randomized, double-blind, placebo-controlled trial. Arthritis Rheum 2005; 52: 27–35.

10. Goekoop-Ruiterman YPM, de Vries-Bouwstra JK, Allaart CF et al. Clinical and radiographic outcomes of four different treatment strategies in patients with early rheumatoid arthritis (the BeSt study). Arthritis Rheum 2005; 52: 3381–90.

11. Bijl AE, van der Kooij SM, Goekoop-Ruiterman YP et al. Persistent good clinical response after tapering and discontinuation of initial infliximab therapy in patients with early rheumatoid arthritis: 3-year results from the Best trial. Ann Rheum Dis 2006; 65 (Suppl II): 109 (abstract).

12. Breedveld FC, Weisman MH, Kavanaugh AF et al. The PREMIER study. A multicenter, randomized, double-blind clinical trial of combination therapy with adalimumab plus methotrexate versus methotrexate alone or adalimumab alone in patients with early, aggressive rheumatoid arthritis who had not had previous methotrexate treatment. Arthritis Rheum 2006; 54: 26–37.

13. Keystone EC, Kavanaugh AF, Sharp JT et al. Radiographic, clinical, and functional outcomes of treatment with adalimumab (a human anti-tumor necrosis factor monoclonal antibody) in patients with active rheumatoid arthritis receiving concomitant methotrexate therapy: a randomized, placebo-controlled, 52-week trial. Arthritis Rheum 2004; 50: 1400–11.

14. Furst DE, Schiff MH, Fleischman RM et al. Adalimumab, a fully human anti tumor necrosis factor-alpha monoclonal antibody, and concomitant standard antirheumatic therapy for the treatment of rheumatoid arthritis: results of STAR (Safety Trial of Adalimumab in Rheumatoid Arthritis). J Rheumatol 2003; 30: 2563–71.

15. Weinblatt ME, Keystone EC, Furst DE et al. Long term efficacy and safety of adalimumab plus methotrexate in patients with rheumatoid arthritis: ARMADA 4 year extended study. Ann Rheum Dis 2006; 65: 753–9.

16. Mohler KM, Torrance DS, Smith CA et al. Soluble tumor necrosis factor (TNF) receptors are effective therapeutic agents in lethal endotoxemia and function simultaneously as both TNF carriers and TNF antagonists. J Immunol 1993; 151: 1548–61.

17. Moreland LW, Margolies G, Heck LW Jr et al. Recombinant soluble tumor necrosis factor receptor (p80) fusion protein: toxicity and dose finding trial in refractory rheumatoid arthritis. J Rheumatol 1996; 23: 1849–55.

18. Moreland LW, Baumgartner SW, Schiff MH et al. Treatment of rheumatoid arthritis with recombinant human tumor necrosis factor receptor (p75)-FC fusion protein. N Engl J Med 1997; 337: 141–7.

19. Moreland LW, Schiff MH, Baumgartner SW et al. Etanercept therapy in rheumatoid arthritis: a randomized, controlled study. Ann Intern Med 1999; 130: 478–86.

20. Bathon JM, Martin RW, Fleischmann RM et al. A comparison of etanercept and methotrexate in patients with early rheumatoid arthritis. N Engl J Med 2000; 343: 1586–93.

21. Klareskog L, van der Heijde D, de Jager JP et al. Therapeutic effect of the combination of etanercept and methotrexate compared with each treatment alone in patients with rheumatoid arthritis: double-blind randomised controlled trial. Lancet 2004; 363: 675–81.

22. Gomez-Reino JJ, Pavelka K, Kekow J et al. The effect of adding etanercept to methotrexate and methotrexate to etanercept monotherapies on physical function and patient-reported outcomes in RA patients: TEMPO trial extension results. Ann Rheum Dis 2006; 65 (Suppl II): 319 (abstract).

23. Furst DE, Schiff MH, Fleischman RM et al. Adalimumab, a fully human anti tumor necrosis factor-alpha monoclonal antibody, and concomitant standard antirheumatic therapy for the treatment of rheumatoid arthritis: results of STAR (Safety Trial of Adalimumab in Rheumatoid Arthritis). J Rheumatol 2003; 30: 2563–71.

24. Bongartz T, Sutton AJ, Sweeting MJ et al. Anti-TNF antibody therapy in rheumatoid arthritis and the risk of serious infections and malignancies: systematic review and meta-analysis of rare harmful effects in randomized controlled trials. JAMA 2006; 295: 2275–85.

31

Targeting interleukin-1 in rheumatic diseases

Cem Gabay and William P Arend

Introduction • Nomenclature and structure of the IL-1 family of cytokines and receptors • Toll/IL-1R signaling pathways • Endogenous inhibitors of Toll/IL-1R signaling • IL-1 receptor antagonist • Administration of IL-1Ra in rheumatic diseases • Administration of IL-1Ra in periodic fever syndromes • Potential biologic function of novel IL-1 and IL-1R homologs • Conclusion • References

INTRODUCTION

The first identified members of the interleukin (IL)-1 family of cytokines include two agonist forms of IL-1, IL-1α and IL-1β, and a natural inhibitor IL-1 receptor antagonist (IL-1Ra). Excess or unopposed production of IL-1 may lead to inflammation and tissue damage. The IL-1 family of cytokines also extends to other members that are related to IL-1 by their amino acid sequence and structural homologies. This family includes IL-18 and six novel cytokines, IL-1F5 to IL-1F10. IL-1 and IL-18 use different receptors but both cytokines induce similar intracellular signals through a receptor complex including a ligand binding chain and an accessory protein. IL-1F6, IL-1F8, and IL-1F9 bind to IL-1Rrp2 and use the IL-1R accessory protein. Several endogenous inhibitors regulate IL-1 and IL-18 signals, some of which are used in therapy or are currently being tested in clinical trials.

NOMENCLATURE AND STRUCTURE OF THE IL-1 FAMILY OF CYTOKINES AND RECEPTORS

IL-1 cytokines

The IL-1 family of cytokines includes 10 different ligands which share some amino acid sequence homology (Table 31.1). The biological activity of IL-1 resides in two cytokines derived from two different genes, IL-1α and IL-1β, which bind to the same receptors.[1] The interactions of IL-1α and IL-1β with IL-1 receptor I (IL-1RI) lead to the recruitment of the IL-1R homolog, IL-1R accessory protein (IL-1RAcP), and of subsequent intracellular signaling.[2] IL-1Ra competes with IL-1 for its interaction with cell surface IL-1RI and acts as an endogenous IL-1 inhibitor. These three members of the IL-1 family are highly homologous to each other and are tightly conserved across species. The genes for IL-1α, IL-1β, and IL-1Ra are located close to each other in the human chromosome 2q14 region.[3,4]

Both IL-1α and IL-1β are synthesized as 31 kDa precursor peptides (pre-IL-1α and pre- IL-1β) and are cleaved to generate 17 kDa mature IL-1α and IL-1β. IL-1β is primarily produced by macrophages and is secreted after cleavage of its proform by the cystein protease caspase-1.[5] Pre-IL-1α is cleaved by calpain proteases to release mature carboxy-terminal IL-1α. Most IL-1α is placed on the plasma membrane and can exert its function by stimulating cells by direct cell–cell interaction.[6] In addition, pre-IL-1α contains a nuclear localization sequence in its amino terminal domain allowing the nuclear translocation of pre-IL-1α and its amino-terminal 16 kDa propiece,[7] where they exert different

Table 31.1 IL-1 family of cytokines and receptors

Ligands	Receptors	Characterized and postulated functions
IL-1α (IL-1F1)	IL-1RI, IL-1RII, IL-1RAcP	Proinflammatory Promotes tissue damage Unique intracellular functions
IL-1β (IL-1F2)	IL-1RI, IL-1RII, IL-1RAcP	Proinflammatory Promotes tissue damage
IL-1Ra (IL-1F3)	IL-1RI, IL-1RII (weakly)	Anti-inflammatory
IL-18 (IL-1F4)	IL-18Rα, IL-18Rβ	Promotes Th1 responses Proinflammatory
IL-1F5	IL-1Rrp2?	IL-1Rrp2 antagonist?
IL-1F6	IL-1Rrp2, IL-1RAcP	Weak IL-1 agonist activities
IL-1F7	IL-18Ra, IL-18BP	IL-18 inhibitor? Antitumoral activity?
IL-1F8	IL-1Rrp2, IL-1RAcP	Weak IL-1 agonist activities
IL-1F9	IL-1Rrp2, IL-1RAcP	Weak IL-1 agonist activities
IL-1F10	IL-1RI (weakly)	Not characterized
IL-33	T1/ST2, IL-1RAcP	Promotes Th2 responses IL-1R, IL-18, TLR4 signaling inhibition
Not characterized	SIGIRR	IL-1R, IL-18, TLR4 signaling inhibition
Not characterized	APL	Not characterized
Not characterized	TIGIRR	Not characterized

effects on cell growth, tumor transformation, apoptosis, pro-collagen-I and cytokine production, and NF-κB activation.[8–11]

Like IL-1β, IL-18 is produced as a pro-peptide, which is cleaved by caspase-1 to generate mature and active IL-18.[12] Six new members of the IL-1 family have been identified primarily through use of DNA database searches for homologs of IL-1, and termed IL-1F5 to IL-1F10.[13,14] The genes encoding for IL-1α, IL-1β, IL-1Ra, and the six novel members form a cluster on the long arm of chromosome 2. In humans, all of the genes encoding for IL-1F5 to IL-1F10 map to less than 300 kb of chromosome 2, where they are flanked by IL-1α, IL-1β, and IL-1Ra. Reported similarities between the amino acid sequences of human IL-1 homologs range from 52% (between IL-1F5 and IL-1Ra) to 13% (between IL-1F5 and IL-18). As opposed to the human, IL-1F7 gene is not present in the mouse. Different splice variants for IL-1F5, F7, F8, F9, and F10 have been reported. IL-33, a novel member of the IL-1 family was recently shown to bind to ST2 and to use IL-1RAcP as a co-receptor for cell signaling. IL-33 is a potent inducer of Th2 activities in vitro and in vivo.[14a] In addition, IL-33 stimulates the production of pro-inflammatory cytokines by mast cells via a mechanism independent of cell degranulation (personal communication).

IL-1 receptors

The first member of the IL-1 receptor family (IL-1RI) was cloned in 1988 but findings in recent years have expanded our knowledge on IL-1 receptor homologs, which now include 10 members (IL-1RI, IL-1RII, IL-1RAcP, IL-18Rα, IL-18Rβ, IL-1Rrp2, APL, T1/ST2, SIGIRR, and TIGIRR) (Table 31.1). These receptors are defined as membrane-spanning proteins that possess at least one but usually three immunoglobulin-like extracellular domains and, with the exception of IL-1RII, a cytoplasmic domain related to the Toll-like receptor (TLR) superfamily, the Toll-like/IL-1R (TIR) domain. Many of the genes of receptors (IL-1RI, IL-1RII, IL-18Rα, IL-18Rβ, T1/ST2, IL-1Rrp2) are located in a 530 kb cluster on human chromosome 2q12.[15] IL-1RAcP gene is on chromosome 3q28,[16] SIGIRR lies on chromosome 11p15,[17] and TIGIRR and APL map on the X chromosome.[18] IL-1RII has a short cytoplasmic domain (29 amino acids) and may exist only as a decoy receptor.[19]

T1/ST2 and IL-1Rrp2 resemble IL-1RI in structure. Although T1/ST2 activates MAP kinases, it is not able to stimulate NF-κB activation.[20] T1/ST2 is expressed on T-helper type 2 (Th2) lymphocytes and some evidence indicates that T1/ST2 plays an important role in Th2 responses (IL-4, IL-5, IgE production).[21] The cytoplasmic domains of APL, SIGGIR, and TIGGIR have an additional 100 amino acid carboxy-terminal tail in their TIR domains. SIGGIR has a single extracellular immunoglobulin domain. Ligands for APL, SIGIRR, and TIGIRR have not been clearly characterized so far, and thus, are considered as orphan receptors.

TOLL/IL-1R SIGNALING PATHWAYS

TIR domain-containing superfamily members can be divided into three groups. The first contains extracellular immunoglobulin domains and includes IL-1R family members. The second possesses extracellular leucine-rich repeats and includes TLRs. The third consists of intracellular adapter peptides such as MyD88, MyD88 adaptor-like (MAL), TIR domain-containing adaptor inducing interferon (IFN)-β (Trif), and TLR4 adaptor TRAM. MyD88 is an essential component for IL-1 and IL-18 signaling.[22] It interacts with TIR domain of IL-1R and recruits IL-1R-associated kinase (IRAK)-4 and IRAK-1 through death domain interactions and TNF receptor associated factor (TRAF)6.[23–25] Phosphorylation of IRAK leads to the formation of a larger complex with transforming growth factor (TGF)-β activated kinase (TAK)1-TGF-β and activated protein kinase 1 binding protein (TAB)1-TAB2.[26] Activation of TAK1 leads to the phosphorylation of IKK,[27] and subsequent NF-κB activation. Activated TAK1 is also thought to participate in activation of p38 MAP kinase, JNK, and ERK1/2 pathways.[28] Mitogen-activated extracellular signal regulated kinase activating kinase (MEKK)3 has also been implicated in NF-κB activation through interaction with TRAF6.[29]

ENDOGENOUS INHIBITORS OF TOLL/IL-1R SIGNALING

The activity of the IL-1R family is tightly regulated at different levels by different endogenous inhibitors, including soluble receptors, receptor antagonists, inhibitory receptors, and intracellular

signaling inhibitors. Soluble IL-1RII binds IL-1 with higher affinity than IL-1Ra, thus further increasing the inhibitory effect of IL-1Ra.[30] Upon IL-1 binding, cell surface IL-1RII can also recruit IL-1RAcP, thus preventing IL-1RAcP from forming a receptor complex with IL-1RI.[31] A soluble form of IL-1RAcP exerts inhibitory actions on IL-1 signaling.[32,33]

IL-1Ra is currently the only receptor antagonist recognized in the IL-1 family. IL-1F5 has been reported to inhibit the stimulatory effects of IL-1F9, supposedly by interfering with the binding of IL-1F9 to IL-1Rrp2.[34] However, this effect was not confirmed in a recent study by using other *in vitro* systems and stimulation with IL-1F6, IL-1F8, and IL-1F9.[35]

Recently, it has been shown that membrane-bound T1/ST2 negatively regulates cell signals induced by IL-1, IL-18, and lipopolysaccharide (LPS) by sequestrating the adapters MyD88 and Mal. Consistently, ST2-deficient mice are unable to develop tolerance to LPS stimulation.[36] SIGIRR inhibits NF-κB activation by members of the IL-1R/TLR family by trapping of signaling molecules TRAF6 and IRAK1.[37] SIGIRR-deficient mice were found to be more susceptible to LPS-induced lethality[37] and to exhibit a more severe form of experimental colitis.[38] An alternatively spliced short MyD88 variant lacking the intermediate domain inhibits IL-1R/TLR-triggered signals by preventing IRAK-1 phosphorylation.[39] IRAK-M, a member of the IRAK family without kinase activity, prevents the formation of IRAK-TRAF6 complexes and down-regulates downstream signals induced by IL-1 and some TLR ligands.[40]

IL-1 RECEPTOR ANTAGONIST

A description of the characterization, cloning, and expression of the IL-1Ra molecule is summarized in Chapter 12 in the previous edition of this monograph[41] and in a recent comprehensive review on IL-1Ra.[42] Four members of the IL-1Ra family have now been described: (1) sIL-1Ra, the original secreted 17 kDa isoform; (2) icIL-1Ra1, an 18 kDa intracellular isoform; (3) icIL-1Ra2, another intracellular isoform found only as mRNA; and (4) icIL-1Ra3, a 16 kDa intracellular isoform. Both sIL-1Ra and icIL-1Ra1 bind avidly to IL-1 receptors and readily inhibit the binding of IL-1α and IL-1β *in vitro* and *in vivo*. The major intracellular isoform of IL-1Ra, icIL-1Ra1, is released from keratinocytes and macrophages under certain conditions but may also carry out unique biological functions within cells. icIL-1Ra1 was described to inhibit IL-1-induced IL-6 and IL-8 production in Caco-2 intestinal epithelial cells through inhibition of p38 mitogen-activated protein kinase (MAPK) and NF-κB pathways.[43] In addition, icIL-1Ra1 was shown to inhibit IL-1-induced IL-6 and IL-8 production in keratinocytes through binding to the third component of the COP9 signalosome with subsequent inhibition of the p38 MAPK pathway.[44] Thus, the major intracellular isoform of IL-1Ra may exert anti-inflammatory activities inside the cell as well as in the pericellular micro-environment after release.

Balance between IL-1 and IL-1Ra

The balance between IL-1 and IL-1Ra is important in natural host defense against inflammatory diseases and in the treatment of human diseases.[45] The role of a physiologic balance between IL-1 and IL-1Ra was dramatically illustrated by the observations that particular inbred strains of mice genetically lacking all isoforms of IL-1Ra spontaneously developed arterial inflammation[46] or a chronic inflammatory arthritis.[47] Subsequent studies indicated that the absence of IL-1Ra led to the development of arthritis by enhancing IL-1-induced T-cell-dependent antibody production through augmenting CD40 ligand and OX40 expression on T cells.[48] However, arthritis did not occur in IL-1Ra-deficient mice in the absence of IL-17, with excess IL-17 production in these mice being secondary to OX40 induction by IL-1.[49] The arteritis observed in IL-1Ra-deficient mice also appeared to be mediated by effector T cells.[50] Thus, endogenous IL-1Ra may serve an important role in preventing or limiting organ damage in IL-1-mediated inflammatory diseases through controlling T-cell stimulation of antibody production or reducing effector T-cell function.

IL-1Ra gene polymorphisms and disease

The importance of endogenous IL-1Ra in regulating disease processes is further illustrated by studies on IL-1Ra gene polymorphisms.[45,51,52]

An allelic polymorphism exists in intron 2 of the IL-1Ra gene, caused by the presence of two to six copies of an 86 bp tandem repeat. The allele containing two repeats (IL-1RN*2) is found in 21.4% of the normal Caucasian population and is present in increased frequencies in a variety of human diseases primarily of epithelial or endothelial cell origin (Table 31.2). The possible mechanism of disease associations with IL-1RN*2 has been best characterized through studies on endothelial cells and coronary artery disease. icIL-1Ra1 is the only isoform found in human umbilical vein endothelial cells and human coronary artery endothelial cells, with lower levels of icIL-1Ra1 produced by cells from individuals carrying IL-1RN*2.[53] In addition, the presence of IL-1RN*2 predisposes endothelial cells to a decrease in growth and an increase in senescence, characteristics thought to lead to accelerated atherosclerosis.[54] Local production of IL-1 in coronary artery endothelial cells is found in patients with dilated cardiomyopathy[55] and in atherosclerotic plaques of patients with coronary artery disease.[56] The carriage of IL-1RN*2 is associated with a higher rate of

---

Table 31.2 Human diseases associated with IL-1Ra gene allele 2 (IL-1RN*2)

Systemic lupus erythematosus, particularly skin lesions
Sjögren's syndrome
Juvenile chronic arthritis
Rheumatoid arthritis in certain population groups
Ankylosing spondylitis
Osteoarthritis
Ulcerative colitis in certain population groups
Severity of alopecia areata
Lichen sclerosis
Early-onset psoriasis
Multiple sclerosis in certain population groups
Hypochlorhydria and gastric cancer
Diabetic nephropathy
Susceptibility to sepsis
Henoch–Schönlein purpura
IgA nephropathy
Early-onset periodontitis
Bronchial asthma
Fibrosing alveolitis
Silicosis
Severity of acute graft-versus-host disease in bone
    marrow transplant patients
Idiopathic recurrent miscarriage
Peptic ulcer disease

single-vessel coronary artery disease[56] as well as with protection from restenosis after coronary angioplasty.[57,58] In addition, the carriage of IL-1RN*2 predisposes to increased serum levels of soluble markers of endothelial inflammation in patients with non-ST-elevation acute coronary syndromes.[59] Lastly, IL-1RN*2 is also a susceptibility factor in the development of carotid atherosclerosis.[60] These data suggest that individuals carrying IL-1RN*2 demonstrate an alteration in the balance between IL-1 and IL-1Ra in endothelial cells with a relative lack of icIL-1Ra1 production. This imbalance may predispose to accelerated atherosclerosis in both coronary and carotid arteries with an increased risk of clinical disease.

IL-1Ra in animal models of arthritis

The administration of IL-1Ra and other inhibitors of IL-1 in animal models of arthritis was reviewed in Chapter 12 in the first edition of this monograph.[41] The major benefit of therapeutic delivery of IL-1Ra by gene therapy over administration of recombinant protein was in the maintenance of high protein levels in local tissues.[61] Technical advances have been made in gene therapy systems to enhance expression of IL-1Ra in the synovium in experimental animal models of inflammatory arthritis. An inducible expression system was described for the local production of IL-1Ra in the joints of mice with collagen-induced arthritis (CIA).[62] Lentiviral-mediated gene delivery of IL-1Ra to the synovium led to stable integration with amplification of IL-1Ra protein production through inflammation-induced proliferation of the transduced cells.[63] Intramuscular gene therapy with plasmid DNA containing the IL-1Ra cDNA was also successful in preventing the development of CIA.[64] Local intra-articular gene expression of IL-1Ra through *ex vivo* gene therapy ameliorated arthritis in contralateral joints through modulating the function of resident antigen-presenting cells that traffic to distant regional lymph nodes.[65] Thus, intra-articular gene therapy of inflammatory arthritis with IL-1Ra may lead to prolonged suppression of disease in multiple joints, possibly rendering this treatment more feasible for human disease. Experimental animal models of osteoarthritis have also been successfully treated with IL-1Ra administered either alone by intra-articular injection,[66] or in combination with IL-10,[67] or with insulin-like growth factor to enhance chondrocyte synthesis of matrix.[68]

A soluble form of the IL-1 receptor accessory protein (sIL-1RAcP) has also been employed as a therapeutic agent in CIA. sIL-1RAcP increases the affinity of binding of IL-1α or IL-1β to the soluble type II IL-1 receptor by 100-fold, while leaving unaltered the low binding affinity of IL-1Ra.[32] Local production of sIL-1RAcP by injection of transduced fibroblasts into knee joints led to a marked reduction in inflammation and in cartilage and bone destruction.[69] Systemic delivery of either IL-1Ra or sIL-1RAcP using adenoviral vectors prevented the development of CIA; in contrast to IL-1Ra, IL-1RAcP ameliorated the arthritis without affecting T-cell immunity.[33] A form of the sIL-1RAcP is currently being evaluated in clinical trials in patients with RA.

ADMINISTRATION OF IL-1Ra IN RHEUMATIC DISEASES

The results of early clinical trials of IL-1Ra in the treatment of RA were reviewed in Chapter 12 in the first edition of this monograph.[41] New information has been provided by the results of additional clinical trials, as reviewed in two monographs[70,71] and four editorials.[72–75] In a 48-week extension of an earlier 24-week trial, IL-1Ra (anakinra) alone gave a sustained clinical response with excellent tolerance and no increased number of withdrawals or clinical complications.[76] In addition, a significantly greater retardation of radiologic joint damage was observed at 48 weeks in comparison with 24 weeks in patients treated with IL-1Ra alone.[77] In two further trials in RA, anakinra was administered in combination with methotrexate and exhibited significantly greater responses than did methotrexate alone.[78,79] Anakinra also improved the functional status of responding RA patients[80] and led to greater improvements in patient-reported than physician-reported outcomes.[81] The safety profile of anakinra was high even in patients with multiple comorbid condition.[82–84] Patients who failed anti-TNF-α therapy exhibited a poor response to anakinra[85] and combination therapy with etanercept and anakinra in methotrexate failures provided no increased efficacy and exhibited increased toxicity compared with etanercept alone.[86] The first clinical trial of gene transfer with IL-1Ra in RA was reported[87] and discussed in a review.[88]

IL-1Ra treatment was reported to be dramatically successful in patients with Still's disease, of either juvenile or adult onset.[89,90] These patients had failed treatment with numerous other agents including steroids, methotrexate, and TNF-α inhibitors. Anakinra treatment was safe and efficacious in 4 patients with severe lupus arthritis[91] and in 13 patients with osteoarthritis, the latter after intra-articular injection.[92] In contrast, anakinra treatment was only modestly successful in a subset of patients with ankylosing spondylitis.[93,94] Administration of anakinra had a favorable effect on the course of acute gout in a recent open-label study.[94a]

ADMINISTRATION OF IL-1Ra IN PERIODIC FEVER SYNDROMES

Periodic fever syndromes are a subset of hereditary autoinflammatory disorders characterized by recurrent and severe attacks of fever, arthritis, and skin lesions. Mutations in members of a new family of genes, the PYRINs, lead to familial Mediterranean fever and to other clinical disorders through overproduction of caspase-1 with unregulated release of active IL-1β.[95–103] Patients with three of these clinical syndromes all responded dramatically to treatment with IL-1Ra: Muckle-Wells syndrome,[104,105] neonatal-onset multisystem inflammatory disorder (NOMID),[106,107] and familial cold autoinflammatory syndrome (FCAS).[108] It is highly likely that other described clinical syndromes in this family may also be due to overproduction of IL-1β and will exhibit a similar response to treatment with IL-1Ra.

POTENTIAL BIOLOGIC FUNCTION OF NOVEL IL-1 AND IL-1R HOMOLOGS

Little is known regarding the biologic function of novel IL-1 homologs and our knowledge derives mostly from *in vitro* studies. IL-1F7 binds to IL-18BP and enhances its ability to inhibit IL-18 activities.[109] IL-1F6, IL-1F8, and IL-1F9

bind to IL-1Rrp2 and IL-1RAcP and induce similar signals to IL-1, but at much higher concentrations (100–1000-fold).[35] Recently, we have observed that recombinant IL-1F8 induces the production of IL-6 by human synovial fibroblasts and articular chondrocytes in culture. However, these stimulatory effects were present when using at least 100-fold higher concentrations of IL-1F6 and IL-1F8 than of IL-1β (personal data). Differential splicing of mouse T1/ST2 generates two mRNA of 2.7 and 5.2 kb encoding for a shorter soluble ST2 and a longer membrane-bound variant.[110,111] A soluble ST2-human IgG fusion protein decreased the production of proinflammatory cytokines TNF-α, IL-6, and IL-12 by LPS-stimulated mouse macrophages, the LPS-induced lethality in mice,[112] and the severity of collagen-induced arthritis.[113]

CONCLUSION

IL-1 plays a major role in inflammatory conditions such as RA and other rheumatic diseases. In addition, recent findings have demonstrated that some periodic fever syndromes are associated with IL-1β overproduction. The use of IL-1Ra-deficient mice has demonstrated that uncontrolled IL-1 activities may lead to various inflammatory conditions. The administration of IL-1Ra was successful in treating RA patients and other inflammatory conditions such systemic onset juvenile idiopathic arthritis, adult Still's disease, and periodic fever syndromes. In addition to IL-1 and IL-1R, many other members of this family of cytokines and receptors have been characterized. Their functions are starting to be elucidated. Some of them control Th1 and Th2 responses or possess weak IL-1 agonist activity, whereas others exhibit inhibitory functions on TIR signaling.

REFERENCES

1. Dinarello CA. Biologic basis for interleukin-1 in disease. Blood 1996; 87: 2095–147.
2. Huang J, Gao X, Li S, Cao Z. Recruitment of IRAK to the interleukin 1 receptor complex requires interleukin 1 receptor accessory protein. Proc Natl Acad Sci U S A 1997; 94: 12829–32.
3. Steinkasserer A, Spurr NK, Cox S et al. The human IL-1 receptor antagonist gene (IL1RN) maps to chromosome

2q14-q21, in the region of the IL-1 alpha and IL-1 beta loci. Genomics 1992; 13: 654–7.

4. Patterson D, Jones C, Hart I et al. The human interleukin-1 receptor antagonist (IL1RN) gene is located in the chromosome 2q14 region. Genomics 1993; 15: 173–6.

5. Black RA, Kronheim SR, Cantrell M et al. Generation of biologically active interleukin-1 beta by proteolytic cleavage of the inactive precursor. J Biol Chem 1988; 263: 9437–42.

6. Niki Y, Yamada H, Kikuchi T et al. Membrane-associated IL-1 contributes to chronic synovitis and cartilage destruction in human IL-1 alpha transgenic mice. J Immunol 2004; 172: 577–84.

7. Wessendorf JH, Garfinkel S, Zhan X et al. Identification of a nuclear localization sequence within the structure of the human interleukin-1 alpha precursor. J Biol Chem 1993; 268: 22100–4.

8. Stevenson FT, Turck J, Locksley RM et al. The N-terminal propiece of interleukin 1 alpha is a transforming nuclear oncoprotein. Proc Natl Acad Sci U S A 1997; 94: 508–13.

9. Pollock AS, Turck J, Lovett DH. The prodomain of interleukin 1alpha interacts with elements of the RNA processing apparatus and induces apoptosis in malignant cells. FASEB J 2003; 17: 203–13.

10. Hu B, Wang S, Zhang Y et al. A nuclear target for interleukin-1alpha: interaction with the growth suppressor necdin modulates proliferation and collagen expression. Proc Natl Acad Sci U S A 2003; 100: 10008–13.

11. Werman A, Werman-Venkert R, White R et al. The precursor form of IL-1alpha is an intracrine proinflammatory activator of transcription. Proc Natl Acad Sci U S A 2004; 101: 2434–9.

12. Ghayur T, Banerjee S, Hugunin M et al. Caspase-1 processes IFN-gamma-inducing factor and regulates LPS-induced IFN-gamma production. Nature 1997; 386: 619–23.

13. Sims JE, Nicklin MJ, Bazan JF et al. A new nomenclature for IL-1-family genes. Trends Immunol 2001; 22: 536–7.

14. Dunn E, Sims JE, Nicklin MJ et al. Annotating genes with potential roles in the immune system: six new members of the IL-1 family. Trends Immunol 2001; 22: 533–6.

14a. Schmitz J, Owyang A, Ololham E, et al. IL-33, an interleukin-1-like cytokine that signals via the IL-1 receptor-related protein ST2 and induces T helper type 2- associated cytokines. Immunity 2005; 23: 479–90.

15. Dale M, Nicklin MJ. Interleukin-1 receptor cluster: gene organization of IL1R2, IL1R1, IL1RL2 (IL-1Rrp2), IL1RL1 (T1/ST2), and IL18R1 (IL-1Rrp) on human chromosome 2q. Genomics 1999; 57: 177–9.

16. Dale M, Hammond DW, Cox A et al. The human gene encoding the interleukin-1 receptor accessory protein (IL1RAP) maps to chromosome 3q28 by fluorescence in situ hybridization and radiation hybrid mapping. Genomics 1998; 47: 325–6.

17. Thomassen E, Renshaw BR, Sims JE. Identification and characterization of SIGIRR, a molecule representing a novel subtype of the IL-1R superfamily. Cytokine 1999; 11: 389–99.

18. Born TL, Smith DE, Garka KE et al. Identification and characterization of two members of a novel class of the interleukin-1 receptor (IL-1R) family. Delineation of a new class of IL-1R-related proteins based on signaling. J Biol Chem 2000; 275: 29946–54.

19. Colotta F, Dower SK, Sims JE et al. The type II 'decoy' receptor: a novel regulatory pathway for interleukin 1. Immunol Today 1994; 15: 562–6.

20. Brint EK, Fitzgerald KA, Smith P et al. Characterization of signaling pathways activated by the interleukin 1 (IL-1) receptor homologue T1/ST2. A role for Jun N-terminal kinase in IL-4 induction. J Biol Chem 2002; 277: 49205–11.

21. Coyle AJ, Lloyd C, Tian J et al. Crucial role of the interleukin 1 receptor family member T1/ST2 in T helper cell type 2-mediated lung mucosal immune responses. J Exp Med 1999; 190: 895–902.

22. Adachi O, Kawai T, Takeda K et al. Targeted disruption of the MyD88 gene results in loss of IL-1- and IL-18-mediated function. Immunity 1998; 9: 143–50.

23. Wesche H, Henzel WJ, Shillinglaw W et al. MyD88: an adapter that recruits IRAK to the IL-1 receptor complex. Immunity 1997; 7: 837–47.

24. Suzuki N, Suzuki S, Duncan GS et al. Severe impairment of interleukin-1 and Toll-like receptor signalling in mice lacking IRAK-4. Nature 2002; 416: 750–6.

25. Cao Z, Xiong J, Takeuchi M et al. TRAF6 is a signal transducer for interleukin-1. Nature 1996; 383: 443–6.

26. Jiang Z, Ninomiya-Tsuji J, Qian Y et al. Interleukin-1 (IL-1) receptor-associated kinase-dependent IL-1-induced signaling complexes phosphorylate TAK1 and TAB2 at the plasma membrane and activate TAK1 in the cytosol. Mol Cell Biol 2002; 22: 7158–67.

27. Zandi E, Rothwarf DM, Delhase M et al. The IkappaB kinase complex (IKK) contains two kinase subunits, IKKalpha and IKKbeta, necessary for IkappaB phosphorylation and NF-kappaB activation. Cell 1997; 91: 243–52.

28. Ninomiya-Tsuji J, Kishimoto K, Hiyama A et al. The kinase TAK1 can activate the NIK-I kappaB as well as the MAP kinase cascade in the IL-1 signalling pathway. Nature 1999; 398: 252–6.

29. Huang Q, Yang J, Lin Y et al. Differential regulation of interleukin 1 receptor and Toll-like receptor signaling by MEKK3. Nat Immunol 2004; 5: 98–103.

30. Burger D, Chicheportiche R, Giri JG et al. The inhibitory activity of human interleukin-1 receptor antagonist is enhanced by type II interleukin-1 soluble receptor and

hindered by type I interleukin-1 soluble receptor. J Clin Invest 1995; 96: 38–41.

31. Lang D, Knop J, Wesche H et al. The type II IL-1 receptor interacts with the IL-1 receptor accessory protein: a novel mechanism of regulation of IL-1 responsiveness. J Immunol 1998; 161: 6871–7.

32. Smith DE, Hanna R, Della F et al. The soluble form of IL-1 receptor accessory protein enhances the ability of soluble type II IL-1 receptor to inhibit IL-1 action. Immunity 2003; 18: 87–96.

33. Smeets RL, Joosten LA, Arntz OJ et al. Soluble interleukin-1 receptor accessory protein ameliorates collagen-induced arthritis by a different mode of action from that of interleukin-1 receptor antagonist. Arthritis Rheum 2005; 52: 2202–11.

34. Debets R, Timans JC, Homey B et al. Two novel IL-1 family members, IL-1 delta and IL-1 epsilon, function as an antagonist and agonist of NF-kappa B activation through the orphan IL-1 receptor-related protein 2. J Immunol 2001; 167: 1440–6.

35. Towne JE, Garka KE, Renshaw BR et al. Interleukin (IL)-1F6, IL-1F8, and IL-1F9 signal through IL-1Rrp2 and IL-1RAcP to activate the pathway leading to NF-kappaB and MAPKs. J Biol Chem 2004; 279: 13677–88.

36. Brint EK, Xu D, Liu H et al. ST2 is an inhibitor of interleukin 1 receptor and Toll-like receptor 4 signaling and maintains endotoxin tolerance. Nat Immunol 2004; 5: 373–9.

37. Wald D, Qin J, Zhao Z et al. SIGIRR, a negative regulator of Toll-like receptor-interleukin 1 receptor signaling. Nat Immunol 2003; 4: 920–7.

38. Garlanda C, Riva F, Polentarutti N et al. Intestinal inflammation in mice deficient in Tir8, an inhibitory member of the IL-1 receptor family. Proc Natl Acad Sci U S A 2004; 101: 3522–6.

39. Burns K, Janssens S, Brissoni B et al. Inhibition of interleukin 1 receptor/Toll-like receptor signaling through the alternatively spliced, short form of MyD88 is due to its failure to recruit IRAK-4. J Exp Med 2003; 197: 263–8.

40. Kobayashi K, Hernandez LD, Galan JE et al. IRAK-M is a negative regulator of Toll-like receptor signaling. Cell 2002; 110: 191–202.

41. Gabay C, Arend WP. Interleukin 1. In: Smolen JS, Lipsky PE, eds. Targeted Therapies in Rheumatology. London: Martin Dunitz, 2003: 213–29.

42. Arend WP. Interleukin-1 receptor antagonist. Adv Immunol 1993; 54: 167–227.

43. Garat C, Arend WP. Intracellular IL-1Ra type 1 inhibits IL-1-induced IL-6 and IL-8 production in Caco-2 intestinal epithelial cells through inhibition of p38 mitogen-activated protein kinase and NF-kappaB pathways. Cytokine 2003; 23: 31–40.

44. Banda NK, Guthridge C, Sheppard D et al. Intracellular IL-1 receptor antagonist type 1 inhibits IL-1-induced cytokine production in keratinocytes through binding to the third component of the COP9 signalosome. J Immunol 2005; 174: 3608–16.

45. Arend WP. The balance between IL-1 and IL-1Ra in disease. Cytokine Growth Factor Rev 2002; 13: 323–40.

46. Nicklin MJ, Hughes DE, Barton JL et al. Arterial inflammation in mice lacking the interleukin 1 receptor antagonist gene. J Exp Med 2000; 191: 303–12.

47. Horai R, Saijo S, Tanioka H et al. Development of chronic inflammatory arthropathy resembling rheumatoid arthritis in interleukin 1 receptor antagonist-deficient mice. J Exp Med 2000; 191: 313–20.

48. Nakae S, Asano M, Horai R et al. IL-1 enhances T cell-dependent antibody production through induction of CD40 ligand and OX40 on T cells. J Immunol 2001; 167: 90–7.

49. Nakae S, Saijo S, Horai R et al. IL-17 production from activated T cells is required for the spontaneous development of destructive arthritis in mice deficient in IL-1 receptor antagonist. Proc Natl Acad Sci U S A 2003; 100: 5986–90.

50. Shepherd J, Nicklin MJ. Elastic-vessel arteritis in interleukin-1 receptor antagonist-deficient mice involves effector Th1 cells and requires interleukin-1 receptor. Circulation 2005; 111: 3135–40.

51. Arend WP, Evans CH. Interleukin-1 receptor antagonist. In: Thomson AW, Lotze MT, eds. The Cytokine Handbook, 4th edn. London: Elsevier; 2003: 669–708.

52. Arend WP. The role of interleukin-1 receptor antagonist in the prevention and treatment of disease. Mod Rheumatol 2003; 13: 1–6.

53. Dewberry R, Holden H, Crossman D et al. Interleukin-1 receptor antagonist expression in human endothelial cells and atherosclerosis. Arterioscler Thromb Vasc Biol 2000; 20: 2394–400.

54. Dewberry RM, Crossman DC, Francis SE. Interleukin-1 receptor antagonist (IL-1RN) genotype modulates the replicative capacity of human endothelial cells. Circ Res 2003; 92: 1285–7.

55. Francis SE, Holden H, Holt CM et al. Interleukin-1 in myocardium and coronary arteries of patients with dilated cardiomyopathy. J Mol Cell Cardiol 1998; 30: 215–23.

56. Francis SE, Camp NJ, Dewberry RM et al. Interleukin-1 receptor antagonist gene polymorphism and coronary artery disease. Circulation 1999; 99: 861–6.

57. Francis SE, Camp NJ, Burton AJ et al. Interleukin 1 receptor antagonist gene polymorphism and restenosis after coronary angioplasty. Heart 2001; 86: 336–40.

58. Marculescu R, Mlekusch W, Exner M et al. Interleukin-1 cluster combined genotype and restenosis after balloon angioplasty. Thromb Haemost 2003; 90: 491–500.

59. Ray KK, Camp NJ, Bennett CE et al. Genetic variation at the interleukin-1 locus is a determinant of changes in soluble endothelial factors in patients with acute coronary syndromes. Clin Sci (Lond) 2002; 103: 303–10.

60. Worrall BB, Azhar S, Nyquist PA et al. Interleukin-1 receptor antagonist gene polymorphisms in carotid atherosclerosis. Stroke 2003; 34: 790–3.

61. Gouze JN, Gouze E, Palmer GD et al. A comparative study of the inhibitory effects of interleukin-1 receptor antagonist following administration as a recombinant protein or by gene transfer. Arthritis Res Ther 2003; 5: R301–9.

62. Bakker AC, van de Loo FA, Joosten LA et al. C3-Tat/ HIV-regulated intraarticular human interleukin-1 receptor antagonist gene therapy results in efficient inhibition of collagen-induced arthritis superior to cytomegalovirus-regulated expression of the same transgene. Arthritis Rheum 2002; 46: 1661–70.

63. Gouze E, Pawliuk R, Gouze JN et al. Lentiviral-mediated gene delivery to synovium: potent intra-articular expression with amplification by inflammation. Mol Ther 2003; 7: 460–6.

64. Kim JM, Jeong JG, Ho SH et al. Protection against collagen-induced arthritis by intramuscular gene therapy with an expression plasmid for the interleukin-1 receptor antagonist. Gene Ther 2003; 10: 1543–50.

65. Kim SH, Lechman ER, Kim S et al. Ex vivo gene delivery of IL-1Ra and soluble TNF receptor confers a distal synergistic therapeutic effect in antigen-induced arthritis. Mol Ther 2002; 6: 591–600.

66. Frisbie DD, Ghivizzani SC, Robbins PD et al. Treatment of experimental equine osteoarthritis by in vivo delivery of the equine interleukin-1 receptor antagonist gene. Gene Ther 2002; 9: 12–20.

67. Zhang X, Mao Z, Yu C. Suppression of early experimental osteoarthritis by gene transfer of interleukin-1 receptor antagonist and interleukin-10. J Orthop Res 2004; 22: 742–50.

68. Nixon AJ, Haupt JL, Frisbie DD et al. Gene-mediated restoration of cartilage matrix by combination insulin-like growth factor-I/interleukin-1 receptor antagonist therapy. Gene Ther 2005; 12: 177–86.

69. Smeets RL, van de Loo FA, Joosten LA et al. Effectiveness of the soluble form of the interleukin-1 receptor accessory protein as an inhibitor of interleukin-1 in collagen-induced arthritis. Arthritis Rheum 2003; 48: 2949–58.

70. Targeting IL-1 – a new approach to the management of rheumatoid arthritis. Rheumatology (Oxford) 2003; 42: ii1-ii43.

71. The role of interleukin-1 in rheumatoid arthritis. Rheumatology (Oxford) 2004; 43: ii1-ii23.

72. Dayer JM, Bresnihan B. Targeting interleukin-1 in the treatment of rheumatoid arthritis. Arthritis Rheum 2002; 46: 574–8.

73. Hoffman HM, Patel DD. Genomic-based therapy: targeting interleukin-1 for autoinflammatory diseases. Arthritis Rheum 2004; 50: 345–9.

74. Dinarello CA. Blocking IL-1 in systemic inflammation. J Exp Med 2005; 201: 1355–9.

75. Dinarello CA. The many worlds of reducing interleukin-1. Arthritis Rheum 2005; 52: 1960–7.

76. Nuki G, Bresnihan B, Bear MB et al. Long-term safety and maintenance of clinical improvement following treatment with anakinra (recombinant human interleukin-1 receptor antagonist) in patients with rheumatoid arthritis: extension phase of a randomized, double-blind, placebo-controlled trial. Arthritis Rheum 2002; 46: 2838–46.

77. Bresnihan B, Newmark R, Robbins S et al. Effects of anakinra monotherapy on joint damage in patients with rheumatoid arthritis. Extension of a 24-week randomized, placebo-controlled trial. J Rheumatol 2004; 31: 1103–11.

78. Cohen S, Hurd E, Cush J et al. Treatment of rheumatoid arthritis with anakinra, a recombinant human interleukin-1 receptor antagonist, in combination with methotrexate: results of a twenty-four-week, multicenter, randomized, double-blind, placebo-controlled trial. Arthritis Rheum 2002; 46: 614–24.

79. Cohen SB, Moreland LW, Cush JJ et al. A multicentre, double blind, randomised, placebo controlled trial of anakinra (Kineret), a recombinant interleukin 1 receptor antagonist, in patients with rheumatoid arthritis treated with background methotrexate. Ann Rheum Dis 2004; 63: 1062–8.

80. Cohen SB, Woolley JM, Chan W. Interleukin 1 receptor antagonist anakinra improves functional status in patients with rheumatoid arthritis. J Rheumatol 2003; 30: 225–31.

81. Cohen SB, Strand V, Aguilar D et al. Patient- versus physician-reported outcomes in rheumatoid arthritis patients treated with recombinant interleukin-1 receptor antagonist (anakinra) therapy. Rheumatology (Oxford) 2004; 43: 704–11.

82. Fleischmann RM, Schechtman J, Bennett R et al. Anakinra, a recombinant human interleukin-1 receptor antagonist (r-metIIuIL-1ra), in patients with rheumatoid arthritis: a large, international, multicenter, placebo-controlled trial. Arthritis Rheum 2003; 48: 927–34.

83. Schiff MH, DiVittorio G, Tesser J et al. The safety of anakinra in high-risk patients with active rheumatoid arthritis: six-month observations of patients with comorbid conditions. Arthritis Rheum 2004; 50: 1752–60.

84. Tesser J, Fleischmann R, Dore R et al. Concomitant medication use in a large, international, multicenter, placebo controlled trial of anakinra, a recombinant interleukin 1 receptor antagonist, in patients with rheumatoid arthritis. J Rheumatol 2004; 31: 649–54.

85. Buch MH, Bingham SJ, Seto Y et al. Lack of response to anakinra in rheumatoid arthritis following failure of tumor necrosis factor alpha blockade. Arthritis Rheum 2004; 50: 725–8.

86. Genovese MC, Cohen S, Moreland L et al. Combination therapy with etanercept and anakinra in the treatment of patients with rheumatoid arthritis who have been

treated unsuccessfully with methotrexate. Arthritis Rheum 2004; 50: 1412–19.

87. Evans CH, Robbins PD, Ghivizzani SC et al. Gene transfer to human joints: progress toward a gene therapy of arthritis. Proc Natl Acad Sci U S A 2005; 102: 8698–703.

88. van de Loo FA, Smeets RL, van den Berg WB. Gene therapy in animal models of rheumatoid arthritis: are we ready for the patients? Arthritis Res Ther 2004; 6: 183–96.

89. Pascual V, Allantaz F, Arce E et al. Role of interleukin-1 (IL-1) in the pathogenesis of systemic onset juvenile idiopathic arthritis and clinical response to IL-1 blockade. J Exp Med 2005; 201: 1479–86.

90. Fitzgerald AA, Leclercq SA, Yan A et al. Rapid responses to anakinra in patients with refractory adult-onset Still's disease. Arthritis Rheum 2005; 52: 1794–803.

91. Ostendorf B, Iking-Konert C, Kurz K et al. Preliminary results of safety and efficacy of the interleukin 1 receptor antagonist anakinra in patients with severe lupus arthritis. Ann Rheum Dis 2005; 64: 630–3.

92. Chevalier X, Giraudeau B, Conrozier T et al. Safety study of intraarticular injection of interleukin 1 receptor antagonist in patients with painful knee osteoarthritis: a multicenter study. J Rheumatol 2005; 32: 1317–23.

93. Tan AL, Marzo-Ortega H, O'Connor P et al. Efficacy of anakinra in active ankylosing spondylitis: a clinical and magnetic resonance imaging study. Ann Rheum Dis 2004; 63: 1041–5.

94. Haibel H, Rudwaleit M, Listing J et al. Open label trial of anakinra in active ankylosing spondylitis over 24 weeks. Ann Rheum Dis 2005; 64: 296–8.

94a. So A, De Smedt T, Revaz S, et al. A pilot study on IL-1 inhibition by anakinra in acute gout. Arthritis Res & Ther 2007; 12:R28.

95. Hoffman HM, Mueller JL, Broide DH et al. Mutation of a new gene encoding a putative pyrin-like protein causes familial cold autoinflammatory syndrome and Muckle-Wells syndrome. Nat Genet 2001; 29: 301–5.

96. Aganna E, Martinon F, Hawkins PN et al. Association of mutations in the NALP3/CIAS1/PYPAF1 gene with a broad phenotype including recurrent fever, cold sensitivity, sensorineural deafness, and AA amyloidosis. Arthritis Rheum 2002; 46: 2445–52.

97. Hull KM, Shoham N, Chae JJ et al. The expanding spectrum of systemic autoinflammatory disorders and their rheumatic manifestations. Curr Opin Rheumatol 2003; 15: 61–9.

98. Shoham NG, Centola M, Mansfield E et al. Pyrin binds the PSTPIP1/CD2BP1 protein, defining familial Mediterranean fever and PAPA syndrome as disorders in the same pathway. Proc Natl Acad Sci U S A 2003; 100: 13501–6.

99. Agostini L, Martinon F, Burns K et al. NALP3 forms an IL-1beta-processing inflammasome with increased activity in Muckle-Wells autoinflammatory disorder. Immunity 2004; 20: 319–25.

100. Neven B, Callebaut I, Prieur AM et al. Molecular basis of the spectral expression of CIAS1 mutations associated with phagocytic cell-mediated autoinflammatory disorders CINCA/NOMID, MWS, and FCU. Blood 2004; 103: 2809–15.

101. Martinon F, Tschopp J. Inflammatory caspases: linking an intracellular innate immune system to autoinflammatory diseases. Cell 2004; 117: 561–74.

102. Stehlik C, Reed JC. The PYRIN connection: novel players in innate immunity and inflammation. J Exp Med 2004; 200: 551–8.

103. Arostegui JI, Aldea A, Modesto C et al. Clinical and genetic heterogeneity among Spanish patients with recurrent autoinflammatory syndromes associated with the CIAS1/PYPAF1/NALP3 gene. Arthritis Rheum 2004; 50: 4045–50.

104. Hawkins PN, Lachmann HJ, McDermott MF. Interleukin-1-receptor antagonist in the Muckle-Wells syndrome. N Engl J Med 2003; 348: 2583–4.

105. Hawkins PN, Lachmann HJ, Aganna E et al. Spectrum of clinical features in Muckle-Wells syndrome and response to anakinra. Arthritis Rheum 2004; 50: 607–12.

106. Hawkins PN, Bybee A, Aganna E et al. Response to anakinra in a de novo case of neonatal-onset multisystem inflammatory disease. Arthritis Rheum 2004; 50: 2708–9.

107. Lovell DJ, Bowyer SL, Solinger AM. Interleukin-1 blockade by anakinra improves clinical symptoms in patients with neonatal-onset multisystem inflammatory disease. Arthritis Rheum 2005; 52: 1283–6.

108. Hoffman HM, Rosengren S, Boyle DL et al. Prevention of cold-associated acute inflammation in familial cold autoinflammatory syndrome by interleukin-1 receptor antagonist. Lancet 2004; 364: 1779–85.

109. Bufler P, Azam T, Gamboni-Robertson F et al. A complex of the IL-1 homologue IL-1F7b and IL-18-binding protein reduces IL-18 activity. Proc Natl Acad Sci U S A 2002; 99: 13723–8.

110. Gachter T, Werenskiold AK, Klemenz R. Transcription of the interleukin-1 receptor-related T1 gene is initiated at different promoters in mast cells and fibroblasts. J Biol Chem 1996; 271: 124–9.

111. Iwahana H, Yanagisawa K, Ito-Kosaka A et al. Different promoter usage and multiple transcription initiation sites of the interleukin-1 receptor-related human ST2 gene in UT-7 and TM12 cells. Eur J Biochem 1999; 264: 397–406.

112. Sweet MJ, Leung BP, Kang D et al. A novel pathway regulating lipopolysaccharide-induced shock by ST2/T1 via inhibition of Toll-like receptor 4 expression. J Immunol 2001; 166: 6633–9.

113. Leung BP, Xu D, Culshaw S et al. A novel therapy of murine collagen-induced arthritis with soluble T1/ST2. J Immunol 2004; 173: 145–50.

32

Update on targeted therapy in psoriatic arthritis

Philip Mease

Introduction • **Classification and epidemiology** • **Immunopathogenesis of PsA** • **Outcome measures** • **Update on conventional therapies** • **Update on biologic agents for PsA** • **Other biologic agents** • **Other potential treatments** • **Conclusion** • **References**

INTRODUCTION

Psoriatic arthritis (PsA) is a chronic, progressive form of inflammatory arthritis that occurs in individuals with psoriasis. It affects at least 0.3% of the population, although estimates of its prevalence vary widely, and is generally considered an autoimmune disease with unknown antigenic determinants. There currently is no predictive marker indicating which psoriasis patients will develop arthritis.[1] PsA often is classified as a subtype of spondyloarthropathy, due to shared HLA associations among those with spinal involvement, and characteristic inflammatory clinical and immunopathologic features.[2] Although it is heterogeneous in presentation, this disease often results in significant functional impairment and reduced quality of life.[3] Since the previous edition of this textbook, a number of developments have occurred including development of a new classification criteria for PsA, deepening understanding of pathophysiology, further validation of outcome measures for clinical trials, new observations on more prolonged use of targeted therapy agents reviewed in the previous edition of this textbook, and data from trials of newly emerging agents.

CLASSIFICATION AND EPIDEMIOLOGY

Historically the Moll and Wright criteria have been used for the classification of PsA,[4] according to which, PsA is an inflammatory arthropathy in patients with psoriasis, usually with negative rheumatoid factor, and five distinct clinical subsets: (1) oligoarticular (< 5 tender and swollen joints) asymmetric arthritis, (2) polyarticular arthritis, (3) distal interphalangeal joint (DIP) predominant, (4) spondylitis predominant, and (5) arthritis mutilans. Although several classification criteria for PsA have been proposed since the initial Moll and Wright criteria,[5,6] the Classification of Psoriatic Arthritis study group (CASPAR), based on the results of an international study involving extensive analysis of over 500 patients with PsA and 500 patients with another inflammatory arthritis serving as controls, has developed new classification criteria for PsA to improve classification sensitivity and specificity utilizing elements of history, exam, laboratory and X-ray (Table 32.1).[7,8]

It is known that psoriasis affects approximately 2–3% of the general population and the prevalence of PsA in psoriasis patients is between 6% and 39%.[9,10] Telephone surveys

Table 32.1 Diagnostic criteria for PsA (CASPAR)[7,8]

Established inflammatory articular disease (joint, spine, or entheseal) with 3 or more of the following

1. Psoriasis	(a) Current*	Psoriatic skin or scalp disease present today as judged by a qualified health professional
	(b) History	A history of psoriasis that may be obtained from patient, or qualified health professional
	(c) Family history	A history of psoriasis in a first or second degree relative according to patient report
2. Nail changes		Typical psoriatic nail dystrophy including onycholysis, pitting, and hyperkeratosis observed on current physical examination
3. A negative test for RF		By any method except latex but preferably by ELISA or nephelometry, according to the local laboratory reference range
4. Dactylitis	(a) Current	Swelling of an entire digit
	(b) History	A history of dactylitis recorded by a qualified health professional
5. Radiological evidence of juxta-articular new bone formation		Ill-defined ossification near joint margins (but excluding osteophyte formation) on plain X-rays of hand or foot

*Current psoriasis awarded 2 points
Specificity 98.7%, sensitivity 91.4%

recently conducted in Europe and in the US, respectively, suggest a prevalence of 30%[11] and 11%.[12] This range is partly related to the lesser severity of psoriasis in the US population studied, which may be correlated with difference in PsA prevalence.[12,13] It is also likely that the condition remains generally underdiagnosed, related to lack of awareness by both the patient and physician and subclinical presentation.[14]

Genetic epidemiology

The relative risk for PsA amongst first-degree relatives is second only to ankylosing spondylitis among rheumatic diseases, indicating a strong genetic association.[4,15] Current research evidence points to a multifactorial pattern of inheritance[15] with a possible parent-of-origin effect (paternal).[16] The concordance of PsA in identical twins is 30–40%.[17]

PsA is associated with human leukocyte antigen (HLA) class 1 alleles. Linkage with the short arm of chromosome 6 has been shown, demonstrating associations with HLA-B13, B-17, B-27, B-38, B-39, HLA-Cw6, and HLA-DRB1*07.[18,19]

IMMUNOPATHOGENESIS OF PsA

Synovial biopsy studies have documented the similarity of immunohistology of various spondyloarthropathy (SpA) subsets, including PsA and ankylosing spondylitis (AS), and distinction of these from rheumatoid arthritis (RA), by such features as increased vascularity, infiltration with polymorphonuclear cells (PMNs) and CD163+ macrophages, and up-regulation of Toll-like receptors 2 and 4.[20-23] These findings support the construct of SpA at least partly being related to activation of the innate immune system and presentation of 'arthritogenic' peptides to T cells, including infectious antigens. Angiogenesis is prominent in both the synovium and psoriatic skin lesions, driven by a number of angiogenic growth factors such as vascular endothelial growth factor (VEGF), transforming growth factor (TGF)-β, and angiopoietins.[22,24-27]

Ample evidence now exists documenting the central role of tumor necrosis factor (TNF)-α in both PsA and psoriasis.[22,28] High levels of TNF-α are found in psoriatic skin lesions and in the synovial fluid, serum, and synovial tissue of patients with PsA. TNF-α inhibition continues to gain much attention, since biologic agents that block its activity demonstrate significant benefit in PsA. Studies of these agents re-confirm the central role of TNF-α in the inflammation of PsA and psoriasis. TNF-α is produced by macrophages, keratinocytes, mast cells, monocytes, dendritic cells, and activated T cells. It up-regulates nuclear transcription factors, including NF-kB, resulting in enhanced expression of many molecules central to the inflammatory response, including other cytokines (e.g. IL-1, IL-6) and chemokines. In the joints, TNF-α mediates other biological processes that can result in cartilage and bone damage, including expression of metalloproteinases by fibroblasts and chondrocytes, maturation and activation of osteoclasts from monocytic stem cells, and angiogenesis. In relation to both the joints and the skin, TNF-α induces the expression of endothelial, keratinocyte, and dendritic cell surface adhesion molecules such as intercellular adhesion molecule (ICAM)-1 and E-selectin (CD62E). In addition to stimulating proinflammatory cells and cytokines in the skin, a key role played by TNF-α is promotion of keratinocyte hyperproliferation and survival, which is important in the psoriatic lesion.[22,28,29]

Other potential targets for therapy include inhibition of cytokines IL-1, IL-6, IL-12, IL-15, and IL-18, all of which are pathogenic through pleiotropic cellular and cytokine mechanisms as well as direct inhibition of cellular targets such as T cells via blockade of 'second signal' pathways. Results of early work with agents which target these cytokines and pathways will be reviewed below. To date, inhibition of TNF continues to demonstrate the most comprehensive effect in PsA, so most of these agents are being tried in patients who have not responded adequately to or have had adverse effects from anti-TNF therapy.

Recently, a Viennese group has developed an animal model for psoriasis and PsA. Inducible epidermal deletion of the gene JunB and its functional companion c-Jun in adult mice led to the histologic and immunohistochemical hallmarks of psoriasis and arthritis. In humans, JunB is a component of the activator protein 1 (AP-1) transcription factor, localized in the psoriasis susceptibility region *PSORS6*, and has diminished expression in human psoriatic skin lesions. They further showed that development of arthritis, but not psoriasis, required the presence of T and B cells and signaling through tumor necrosis factor 1 (TNFR1). Their conclusion was that deletion, or at least diminishment, of JunB/AP-1 in keratinocytes induces chemokine/cytokine expression, which in turn recruits

PMNs and macrophages to the epidermis, leading to both skin and joint lesions.[30]

OUTCOME MEASURES

For the most part, outcome measures have been adapted from similar measures used in assessment of RA and psoriasis. These are used both in longitudinal studies of the natural history of PsA and in clinical trials. These measures have been shown to effectively assess peripheral joint and skin inflammation, function, quality of life, fatigue, and structural damage determined by X-ray, and distinguish treatment from placebo (Table 32.2). Approaches to assessment of enthesitis, dactylitis, and spine involvement are still in development. Studies performed by members of the Group for Research and Assessment of Psoriasis and Psoriatic Arthritis (GRAPPA), an international research consortia of rheumatologists and dermatologists, have begun the process of validation of some of these measures in PsA.[31-34] A detailed review of these measures is given elsewhere.[35-37] An exercise to evaluate the performance quality of composite measures of disease activity and change, including the ACR scoring system, the Disease Activity Score (DAS)

Table 32.2 Examples of outcome measures used in PsA clinical trials[35,36]

- **Arthritis response**
  - ACR Response Criteria (including DIP and CMC joints)
  - Psoriatic Arthritis Response Criteria (PsARC)
  - Disease Activity Score (DAS)
- **Radiographic assessment**
  - Modified Sharp
  - Modified van der Heijde/Sharp
- **Skin response**
  - Psoriasis Area and Severity Index (PASI)
  - Dermatologist Static Global
  - Physician Global Assessment (PGA) of Psoriasis
- **QOL/function improvement**
  - Short-Form 36 Health Survey (SF-36®)
  - Health Assessment Questionnaire (HAQ) Disability Index
  - Dermatology Life Quality Index (DLQI)
  - Fatigue (FACIT)

*Current psoriasis = 2 points

as employed in the EULAR Response Criteria (both used in RA), and the Psoriatic Arthritis Response Criteria (PsARC) was performed utilizing the data from two phase 2 trials of anti-TNF-α drugs in PsA. This demonstrated that various modifications of the DAS scoring system were the most sensitive and accurate measures of disease activity and discrimination of change between treatment and placebo groups, although the ACR and PsARC systems performed adequately.[31]

Several studies have documented the effectiveness of ultrasound[38-43] and MRI[43-45] in detecting inflammation in the joints and enthesium of PsA patients, as well as the extent of structural damage. As these tools become more refined, they also will enhance our ability to assess the effectiveness of new therapies on the progression of joint damage in PsA.

PsA was the subject of a workshop at the seventh and module at the eighth biannual meeting of the Outcome Measures in Rheumatology (OMERACT) group. A core set of domains of the disease to be included in PsA trials was agreed upon and key outcome measures to assess these domains were reviewed.[46,46b]

UPDATE ON CONVENTIONAL THERAPIES

Conventional disease-modifying anti-rheumatic drugs (DMARDs) used in PsA such as methotrexate and sulfasalazine, are not considered as 'targeted' as the more highly specifically targeted biologic therapies, because of their more non-specific immunomodulatory effects and thus are not comprehensively reviewed here. These agents were reviewed in the previous edition of this textbook[47] and in a recent comprehensive review.[48] Two studies conducted since the previous textbook should be noted. The agent leflunomide, a pyrimidine antagonist approved in RA at a dose of 20 mg per day, was assessed in 188 PsA patients. PsARC response, the primary endpoint, was met by 59% of leflunomide-treated patients compared with 29.7% of placebo-treated patients ($p < 0.0001$). ACR 20 response was achieved by 36.3% and 20%, respectively ($p = 0.0138$), and PASI 75 response by 17.4% and 7.8%, respectively ($p = 0.048$).[49] As with methotrexate, liver function test

abnormalities may be noted and need to be monitored, an issue more paramount in patients who are overweight and may have co-existent hepatic steatosis (fatty liver).

In a separate study, 72 patients with incomplete response to methotrexate were randomized to placebo or addition of cyclosporine.[50] At 48 weeks, significant improvements in tender and swollen joint count, CRP, PASI, and synovial ultrasound score occurred in the combination group, but statistical differentiation between the combination and methotrexate alone group occurred just in PASI and ultrasound score.

UPDATE ON BIOLOGIC AGENTS FOR PsA

Biologic agents currently approved for treatment of PsA, based on controlled phase 2 and 3 trials and the safety database from these trials and the RA database, include the anti-TNF-α compounds, etanercept (Enbrel®),[51] infliximab (Remicade®),[52] and adalimumab (Humira®).[53] Controlled phase 2 trials have been completed with the costimulatory blockade agents alefacept and efalizumab. Pilot trials with other biologics in development have been completed. Several agents either approved or in development for RA and psoriasis, will likely be assessed in PsA.

TNF-α Inhibitors

The anti-TNF-α agents approved for use in PsA and psoriasis include etanercept, infliximab, and adalimumab. Etanercept and infliximab continue to be studied in patients, as originally described in the first edition of this textbook.[54]

In the placebo-controlled portion of the phase 3 etanercept trial ($n = 205$), utilizing 25 mg administered subcutaneously twice a week, ACR 20 response was achieved by 59% of etanercept-treated patients vs 15% in the placebo group (42% and 41% on background methotrexate respectively) ($p < 0.0001$) (Figure 32.1a).[55] Skin response, as measured by the PASI score which was considered evaluable (BSA >3%) in 66 of the etanercept and 62 of the placebo patients, showed a 75% improvement in 23% and 3%, respectively, at 24 weeks ($p = 0.001$) (Figure 32.1b). A sub-study of this trial

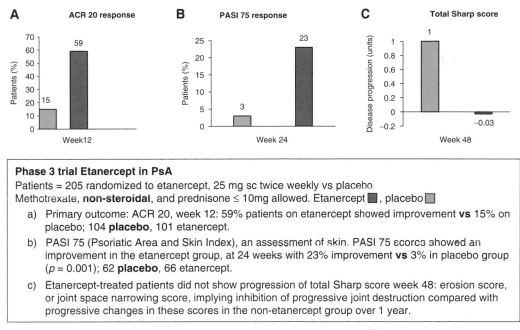

Figure 32.1 Phase 3 trial of etanercept in PsA.[55]

established the minimal clinically important difference (MCID) of the HAQ score in PsA (judged to be 0.22 in RA).[56] Two different methodologies were used: patient-derived to characterize within-treatment group change and standard error of measurement (SEM)-derived to characterize within-subject change. The former established a change of 0.3 units of HAQ score and the latter 0.4 as clinically important differences.[57] A change of 0.51 was noted in the etanercept group, significantly superior to the placebo group. Improvement in quality of life (SF-36) was also demonstrated in the treatment group. Inhibition of progression of joint space narrowing and erosions was shown, with 1 unit of modified total Sharp score (mTSS) progression in the placebo group and none (–0.03 units) in the etanercept group ($p = 0.001$) (Figure 32.1c). A total of 169 patients participated in open-label follow-up use of etanercept for between 1 and 2 years. At the end of this time period, 64% and 63% of the originally etanercept-treated and placebo patients, respectively, demonstrated an ACR 20 response; 38% of all patients achieved a PASI 75 response by 12 weeks, indicating an enduring clinical response in joints and skin.

The mTSS, evaluable in 141 patients at 2 years, showed a change of –0.38 and –0.22 units in the original etanercept and placebo groups, respectively, indicating continued inhibition of structural damage.[58,59] The drug was well tolerated and no new safety issues emerged apart from those seen in clinical trial and general clinical experience with etanercept.

A phase 3 study of infliximab in 200 PsA patients (IMPACT II) has been completed.[60] Baseline demographic and disease activity characteristics were similar to those of the etanercept phase 3 trial. At week 14, 58% of infliximab patients and 11% of placebo patients achieved an ACR 20 response ($p < 0.001$) (Figure 32.2a). Presence of dactylitis decreased in the infliximab group (41% to 18%), compared with the placebo group (40% to 30%) ($p = 0.025$). Likewise, incidence of enthesitis, assessed by palpation of the Achilles tendon and plantar fascia insertions, decreased in the infliximab group (42% to 22%) compared with the placebo group (35% to 34%) ($p = 0.016$).[61] At 24 weeks, PASI 75 was achieved by 64% of the treatment group and 2% of the placebo group ($p < 0.001$) (Figure 32.2b). The median PASI response was

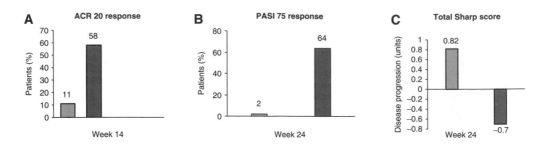

Figure 32.2 Phase 3 trial of infliximab in Ps/PsA.[60]

87% in ACR 20 responders and 74% in ACR 20 non-responders, suggesting that infliximab may be effective in treating skin symptoms, even when joints do not improve significantly.[62] Utilizing the van der Heijde-Sharp scoring method (hands and feet), modified for PsA, infliximab-treated patients showed inhibition of radiographic disease progression at 24 weeks, compared with placebo patients, although PsA-specific radiographic features, including pencil-in-cup deformities and gross osteolysis, did not differ between the treatment groups, as has been observed in other anti-TNF-α trials, presumably due to the more fixed nature of theses changes (Figure 32.2c).[61] HAQ score improved for 59% of infliximab patients, compared with 19% of placebo patients, while both the physical and mental components of SF-36 scores improved for patients receiving infliximab. The observed benefits obtained with infliximab were sustained at 1 year in those originally on infliximab and when the placebo group went on infliximab at 24 weeks, it too achieved a similar degree of benefit.[60]

Adalimumab is a fully human anti-TNF-α monoclonal antibody (mAb) administered subcutaneously, 40 mg, every other week or weekly. It is approved for treatment of RA[63-65] and was shown to be effective for PsA in an open-label trial ($n = 15$).[66] Safety and efficacy of the 40 mg every other week dose was studied in a large ($n = 313$) phase 3 study, the Adalimumab Effectiveness in Psoriatic Arthritis Trial (ADEPT).[67] At 12 weeks, 58% of patients receiving adalimumab achieved ACR 20 compared with 14% of patients receiving placebo ($p < 0.001$) (Figure 32.3a). This response rate did not differ between patients taking adalimumab in combination with methotrexate (50% of patients) and those taking adalimumab alone, similar to observations made in the etanercept and infliximab trials. Mean improvement in enthesitis and dactylitis was greater for patients receiving adalimumab, but this result did not achieve statistical significance. In all, 138 patients were evaluable for PASI response; PASI 75 was achieved by 59% in the adalimumab-treated group and 1% in the placebo group ($p < 0.001$) (Figure 32.3b). Radiographic progression of disease was significantly inhibited by adalimumab, as evaluated by X-rays of hands and feet, using a modified Sharp score

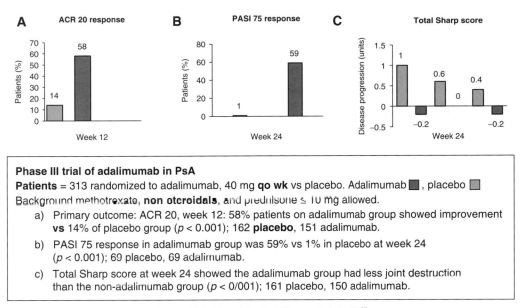

Figure 32.3 Phase 3 of adalimumab in PsA.[67]

(Figure 32.3c).[67] Mean change in TSS was –0.2 for patients receiving adalimumab and 1.0 for patients receiving placebo ($p < 0.001$). Mean change in HAQ was –0.4 for adalimumab patients and –0.1 for placebo patients ($p < 0.001$). Mean change in the physical component of the SF-36 was 9.3 for the treatment group and 1.4 for the placebo group ($p < 0.001$). A second, smaller phase 3 study was performed and also showed significant efficacy in the adalimumab-treated group in clinical measures.[68]

In summary, the anti-TNF-α medications have shown the greatest efficacy of any treatment to date in the various clinical aspects of PsA. Their efficacy in joint disease activity, inhibition of structural damage, function, and quality of life is similar. There may be some differentiation in efficacy in the skin and enthesium, but all have excellent effects in these domains. These agents tend to be well tolerated and patients generally acclimate to their parenteral administration, especially when they experience significant efficacy. Safety concerns are present, such as risk for infection, but no new concerns have arisen in the PsA population compared to the more extensively studied RA patient experience.

Biologic medicines are much costlier to develop and produce than conventional pharmaceutical agents. Therefore, proper pharmacoeconomic assessment of their utility must take into account not only their cost but also the cost of the disease on both the individual and society in direct medical costs, including caring for adverse effects, but also the cost of lost work capacity and disability, diminished family and social participation, and ability to perform activities of daily living. A highly effective medicine may be shown to be as cost-effective or more so than less expensive therapies if it can be shown to significantly lessen the cost of a worsening rheumatic disease. Recent studies have demonstrated the cost-effectiveness of anti-TNF-α therapy in PsA.[69–71]

New anti-TNF-α agents are being developed for use in PsA, including cimzia and golimumab, each with advantages of infrequent subcutaneous administration. Experience in management of RA suggests that when a clinician switches from one of these agents to another, if the first has not had or has lost efficacy, or caused side effects, a substantial percentage of patients will respond to another medication in this class.[72–74] Anecdotally, a similar experience has been noted in the management of PsA patients.

OTHER BIOLOGIC AGENTS

Alefacept is a fully human fusion protein that blocks interaction between leukocyte function-associated antigen (LFA)-3 on the antigen-presenting cell and CD2 on the T cell, or by attracting natural killer (NK) lymphocytes to interact with CD2 to yield apoptosis of particular T-cell clones.[75] It is approved for treatment of psoriasis[76,77] and is administered weekly as a 15 mg intramuscular injection, in a 12 weeks on, 12 weeks off regimen in order to allow return of depleted CD4 cells. An open-label trial ($n = 11$) of this compound in PsA showed that more than one-half of patients achieved an ACR 20 response and a decrease of CD4, CD8, and CD68 cells in the synovial lining.[75] A controlled trial ($n = 185$) showed that 54% of patients given a combination of alefacept and methotrexate had an ACR 20 response as compared with 23% in the methotrexate alone group ($p < 0.001$) at week 24. PASI 75 results were 28% and 24%, respectively.[78,79]

Efalizumab is a humanized mAb to the CD11 subunit of LFA-1 on T cells which inteferes with its coupling with ICAM-1 on antigen-presenting and endothelial cells. It interferes with activation of T lymphocytes and migration of cells to the site of inflammation. It is administered subcutaneously, once per week and is approved for use in psoriasis.[80] In a 12-week trial of efalizumab in patients with PsA, 28% of patients achieved an ACR 20 response versus 19% in the placebo group ($p = 0.2717$). Since this response was not statistically significant, it cannot be clearly recommended for treatment of arthritis.[81]

Abatacept (CTLA4-Ig) is a recombinant human fusion protein that binds to the CD80/86 receptor on an antigen-presenting cell, thus blocking the second signal activation of the CD28 receptor on the T cell. It is administered intravenously once per month and has been approved for use in RA.[82] A phase II trial for use in psoriasis has been conducted.[83] It is anticipated that further assessment of this drug will be conducted for psoriasis and for PsA.

OTHER POTENTIAL TREATMENTS

A pilot trial of anti-IL-15 compound has shown efficacy in PsA.[84] A trial is currently under way to assess the efficacy and safety of an IL-1 antagonist, anakinra, in PsA (IL-1 antagonist, anakinra, in PsA). A mAb to the IL-6 receptor (MRA) is in phase III development for the treatment of RA, and will likely be tested in PsA.[85,85a]

A humanized antibody to the α-subunit (CD25) of the IL-2 receptor has been tried for psoriasis, but with some loss of efficacy noted over time.[86,87] Several inhibitors of IL-12 are being evaluated in psoriasis, with good success (C Leonardi, personal communication), and will likely be assessed in PsA. It is anticipated that inhibitors of IL-18 also will be studied.

Pioglitazone is a ligand for PPAR-γ originally developed to treat diabetes and extended to PsA because of the observation that it could inhibit angiogenesis and down-regulate proinflammatory cytokines.[88] In an uncontrolled trial of pioglitazone administered orally, 50% achieved an ACR 20 response after 12 weeks.[89] This agent may be beneficial for treating PsA, but its efficacy must be evaluated in a controlled study.

A recombinant IL-10 agent demonstrated preliminary benefit in psoriasis;[87,90] a controlled study of this agent in PsA showed benefit in the skin, but not in joints.[91] Recombinant human IL-11 has been utilized in psoriasis, with preliminary clinical and histological benefit noted.[92] A mAb to CD3 has also demonstrated some benefit in PsA, although issues such as transient T-cell depletion and mild cytokine release symptoms have been noted.[93]

CONCLUSION

Numerous studies have increased our understanding of the basic pathophysiology of PsA, providing support for the clinical effects of targeted therapy, e.g. inhibition of TNF-α. The consequent emerging treatments for PsA have demonstrated significant benefit for clinical signs and symptoms in the joints, enthesium, and skin, inhibition of joint damage as assessed by radiographic progression, and improved quality of life and functional status. Agents that block the cell–cell interactions required to activate T cells are effective in the skin and may benefit the joints as well. Observation of the effectiveness of these agents has helped to elucidate the pathogenesis of PsA and psoriasis which, in turn, may lead to more novel and effective interventions.

Development of these targeted therapies has also increased interest in the accurate diagnosis and classification of PsA, which would facilitate the institution of appropriate therapy in a timely fashion. Significant efforts are under way to further develop and validate outcome measures that accurately assess the effect of therapies and determine the natural history of these diseases. This effort, along with the development of evidence-based treatment guidelines and general educational initiatives, is being led by international research consortia such GRAPPA and other groups.

The benefits of biologic agents must be weighed against their cost: patient improvement and inhibition of disease progression on one hand, versus allocating limited resources on the other. Comprehensive health economic analyses are being developed to aid our ability to see the full impact of these more effective treatments on patient function, productivity, and quality of life in the context of society as a whole.

REFERENCES

1. Mease P. Targeting therapy in psoriatic arthritis. Drug Discovery Today 2004; 1(3): 389–96.
2. Kruithof E, Baeten D, De Rycke L et al. Synovial histopathology of psoriatic arthritis, both oligo- and polyarticular, resembles spondyloarthropathy more than it does rheumatoid arthritis. Arthritis Res Ther 2005; 7(3): R569–80.
3. Husted JA, Gladman DD, Farewell VT, Cook RJ. Health-related quality of life of patients with psoriatic arthritis: a comparison with patients with rheumatoid arthritis. Arthritis Rheum 2001; 45(2): 151–8.
4. Moll J, Wright V. Psoriatic arthritis. Semin Arthritis Rheum 1973; 3: 55–78.
5. Helliwell P, Taylor W. Classification and diagnostic criteria for psoriatic arthritis. Ann Rheum Dis 2005; 64 (Suppl 2): ii3–ii8.
6. Taylor W, Marchesoni A, Arreghini M, Sokol K, Helliwell P. A comparison of the performance characteristics of classification criteria for the diagnosis of psoriatic arthritis. Semin Arthritis Rheum 2004; 34(3): 575–84.
7. Taylor W, Helliwell P, Gladman D et al. A validation of current classification criteria for the diagnosis of psoriatic arthritis–preliminary results of the CASPAR Study. Ann Rheum Dis 2005; 64 (Suppl 3): 107.
8. Taylor W, Gladman D, Helliwell P et al. Classification criteria for psoriatic arthritis: development of new criteria from a large international study. Arthritis Rheum 2006; 54: 2665–73.
9. Leonard DG, O'Duffy JD, Rogers RS. Prospective analysis of psoriatic arthritis in patients hospitalized for psoriasis. Mayo Clin Proc 1978; 53(8): 511–18.
10. Shbeeb M, Uramoto KM, Gibson LE, O'Fallon WM, Gabriel SE. The epidemiology of psoriatic arthritis in Olmsted County, Minnesota, USA, 1982–1991. J Rheumatol 2000; 27(5): 1247–50.
11. Salonen S. The EUROPSO psoriasis patient study: treatment history and satisfaction reported by 17,900 members of European psoriasis patients associations (poster). In: Spring Symposium of the European Academy of Dermatology and Venereology, Malta, 2003.
12. Gelfand J, Gladman D, Mease P et al. Epidemiology of psoriatic arthritis in the population of the United States. J Am Acad Dermatol 2005; 53: 573.
13. Gladman D, Antoni C, Mease P, Clegg DO, Nash P. Psoriatic arthritis: epidemiology, clinical features, course, and outcome. Ann Rheum Dis 2005; 64 (Suppl 2): ii14–ii17.
14. Offidani A, Cellini A, Valeri G, Giovagnoni A. Subclinical joint involvement in psoriasis: magnetic resonance imaging and X-ray findings. Acta Derm Venereol 1998; 78(6): 463–5.
15. Rahman P, Elder J. Genetic epidemiology of psoriasis and psoriatic arthritis. Ann Rheum Dis 2005; 64 (Suppl 2): ii37–ii9.
16. Rahman P, Gladman D, Schentag C, Petronis A. Excessive paternal transmission in psoriatic arthritis. Arthritis Rheum 1999; 42: 1228–31.
17. Sege-Peterson K, Winchester R. Psoriatic arthritis. In: Freedberg IM, Eisen AZ, Wolff K et al. eds. Fitzpatrick's Dermatology in General Medicine, 5 edn. New York: McGraw Hill, 1999: 522–3.
18. Gladman DD, Farewell VT, Pellett F, Schentag C, Rahman P. HLA is a candidate region for psoriatic arthritis. evidence for excessive HLA sharing in sibling pairs. Hum Immunol 2003; 64(9): 887–9.
19. Gladman DD, Anhorn KA, Schachter RK, Mervart H. HLA antigens in psoriatic arthritis. J Rheumatol 1986; 13(3): 586–92.
20. Baeten D, Kruithof E, De Rycke L et al. Infiltration of the synovial membrane with macrophage subsets and polymorphonuclear cells reflects global disease activity in spondyloarthropathy. Arthritis Res Ther 2005; 7(2): R359–69.
21. De Rycke L, Vandooren B, Kruithof E et al. Tumor necrosis factor alpha blockade treatment downmodulates the increased systemic and local expression of Toll-like receptor 2 and Toll-like receptor 4 in spondylarthropathy. Arthritis Rheum 2005; 52(7): 2146–58.

22. Veale D, Ritchlin C, FitzGerald O. Immunopathology of psoriasis and psoriatic arthritis. Ann Rheum Dis 2005; 65 (Suppl 2): ii26–ii29.

23. Kruithof E, Baeten D, De Rycke L et al. Synovial histopathology of psoriatic arthritis, either oligo- or polyarticular, resembles more spondyloarthropathy than rheumatoid arthritis [abstract]. Arthritis Rheum 2004; 50 (Suppl 431): S209.

24. Kuroda K, Sapadin A, Shoji T, Fleischmajer R, Lebwohl M. Altered expression of angiopoietins and Tie2 endothelium receptor in psoriasis. J Invest Dermatol 2001; 116(5): 713–20.

25. Markham T, Fearon U, Mullan R et al. Anti-TNF alpha therapy in psoriasis: clinical and angiogenic responses. Br J Dermatol 2003; 143 (Suppl 59): 40.

26. Fearon U, Griosios K, Fraser A et al. Angiopoietins, growth factors, and vascular morphology in early arthritis. J Rheumatol 2003; 30(2): 260–8.

27. Creamer D, Sullivan D, Bicknell R, Barker J. Angiogenesis in psoriasis. Angiogenesis 2002; 5(4): 231–6.

28. Mease P. TNFalpha therapy in psoriatic arthritis and psoriasis. Ann Rheum Dis 2004; 63(7): 755–8.

29. Krueger J, Bowcock A. Psoriasis pathophysiology: current concepts of pathogenesis. Ann Rheum Dis 2005; 64 (Suppl 2): ii30–ii36.

30. Zenz R, Eferl R, Kenner L et al. Psoriasis-like skin disease and arthritis caused by inducible epidermal deletion of Jun proteins. Nature 2005; 437(7057): 369–75.

31. Fransen J, Antoni C, Mease P et al. Performance of response criteria for assessing peripheral arthritis in patients with psoriatic arthritis: analysis of data from randomized, controlled trials of two tumor necrosis factor inhibitors. Ann Rheum Dis 2006; 65:1373–8.

32. Husted JA, Gladman DD, Cook RJ, Farewell VT. Responsiveness of health status instruments to changes in articular status and perceived health in patients with psoriatic arthritis. J Rheumatol 1998; 25(11): 2146–55.

33. Husted JA, Gladman DD, Farewell VT, Long JA, Cook RJ. Validating the SF-36 health survey questionnaire in patients with psoriatic arthritis. J Rheumatol 1997; 24(3): 511–17.

34. Singh A, Mease P, Yu E et al. Health Assessment Questionnaire has similar psychometric properties in psoriatic arthritis and rheumatoid arthritis. Arthritis Rheum 2005; 52 (Suppl 9): S402.

35. Mease P, Antoni C, Gladman DD, Taylor W. Psoriatic arthritis assessment tools in clinical trials. Ann Rheum Dis 2005; 64 (Suppl 2): ii49–ii54.

36. Gladman DD, Helliwell P, Mease PJ et al. Assessment of patients with psoriatic arthritis: a review of currently available measures. Arthritis Rheum 2004; 50(1): 24–35.

37. van der Heijde D, Sharp J, Wassenberg S et al. Psoriatic arthritis imaging: a review of scoring methods. Ann Rheum Dis 2005; 64 (Suppl 2): ii61–ii64.

38. Wakefield RJ, Balint PV, Szkudlarek M et al. Musculoskeletal ultrasound including definitions for ultrasonographic pathology. J Rheumatol 2005; 32(12): 2485–7.

39. D'Agostino MA, Said-Nahal R, Hacquard-Bouder C et al. Assessment of peripheral enthesitis in the spondylarthropathies by ultrasonography combined with power Doppler: a cross-sectional study. Arthritis Rheum 2003; 48(2): 523–33.

40. De Simone C, Guerriero C, Giampetruzzi AR et al. Achilles tendinitis in psoriasis: clinical and sonographic findings. J Am Acad Dermatol 2003; 49(2): 217–22.

41. Kane D, Greaney T, Bresnihan B, Gibney R, FitzGerald O. Ultrasonography in the diagnosis and management of psoriatic dactylitis. J Rheumatol 1999; 26(8): 1746–51.

42. Klauser A, Halpern EJ, Frauscher F et al. Inflammatory low back pain: high negative predictive value of contrast-enhanced color Doppler ultrasound in the detection of inflamed sacroiliac joints. Arthritis Rheum 2005; 53(3): 440–4.

43. Ory P, Gladman DD, Mease P. Psoriatic arthritis and imaging. Ann Rheum Dis 2005; 64 (Suppl 2): ii55–ii57.

44. Baraliakos X, Braun J. Magnetic resonance imaging in spondyloarthropathies. Joint Bone Spine 2006; 73(1): 1–3.

45. McGonagle D, Gibbon W, O'Connor P et al. Characteristic magnetic resonance imaging entheseal changes of knee synovitis in spondylarthropathy. Arthritis Rheum 1998; 41(4): 694–700.

46. Gladman DD, Mease PJ, Krueger G, et al. Outcome measures in psoriatic arthritis. J Rheumatol. 32(11): 2262-9, 2005.

46a. Gladman D, Mease P, Strand V, et al. Consensus on a core set of domains for psoriatic arthritis. J Rheum. 2007;34:1167-70.

46b. Gladman D, Mease P, Healy P, et al. Outcome measures in psoriatic arthritis. J Rheum. 2007;34:1159-66.

47. Mease PJ. Psoriatic arthritis/psoriasis. In: Smolen JS, Lipsky PE, eds. Targeted Therapies in Rheumatology. London: Martin Dunitz, 2003: 525–48.

48. Nash P, Clegg DO. Psoriatic arthritis therapy: NSAIDs and traditional DMARDs. Ann Rheum Dis 2005; 64 (Suppl 2): ii74–ii77.

49. Kaltwasser JP, Nash P, Gladman D et al. Efficacy and safety of leflunomide in the treatment of psoriatic arthritis and psoriasis. Arthritis Rheum 2004; 50(6): 1939–50.

50. Fraser AD, van Kuijk AW, Westhovens R et al. A randomised, double blind, placebo controlled, multicentre trial of combination therapy with methotrexate plus ciclosporin in patients with active psoriatic arthritis. Ann Rheum Dis 2005; 64(6): 859–64.

51. Enbrel® (Etanercept) prescribing information. Thousand Oaks, CA: Immunex Corporation, 2003.

52. Remicade (infliximab) prescribing information. Malvern, PA: Centocor Inc., 2003.

53. Humira™ (adalimumab) prescribing information. North Chicago, IL: Abbott Laboratories., 2003.

54. Mease PJ. Psoriatic arthritis/psoriasis. In: Smolen JS, Lipsky PE, eds. Targeted Therapies in Rheumatology. London: Martin Dunitz, 2003: 525–48.

55. Mease P, Kivitz A, Burch F et al. Etanercept treatment of psoriatic arthritis: safety, efficacy, and effect on disease progression. Arthritis Rheum 2004; 50(7): 2264–72.

56. Wells GA, Tugwell P, Kraag GR et al. Minimum important difference between patients with rheumatoid arthritis: the patient's perspective. J Rheumatol 1993; 20(3): 557–60.

57. Mease P, Ganguly L, Wanke E, Yu E, Singh A. How much improvement in functional status is considered important by patients with active psoriatic arthritis: applying the outcome measures in rheumatoid arthritis clinical trials (OMERACT) group guidelines. Ann Rheum Dis 2004; 63 (Suppl 1): 391 (abstract).

58. Mease P, Kivitz AJ, Burch FX et al. Continued inhibition of radiographic progression in patients with psoriatic arthritis following 2 years of treatment with etanercept. J Rheumatol 2006; 33: 712–21.

59. Mease P, Ruderman EM, Ritchlin C, Ory P, Tsuji W. Etanercept in psoriatic arthritis: sustained improvement in joint and skin disease and inhibition of radiographic progression at 2 years. Ann Rheum Dis 2004; 63 (Suppl 1) (OP0136): 99 (abstract).

60. Antoni C, Krueger GG, de Vlam K et al. Infliximab improves signs and symptoms of psoriatic arthritis: results of the IMPACT 2 trial. Ann Rheum Dis 2005; 64(8): 1150–7.

61. Van der Heidje D, Gladman D, Kavanaugh A et al. Infliximab inhibits progression of radiographic damage in patients with active psoriatic arthritis: 54 week results from IMPACT 2. Arthritis Rheum 2005; 52 (Suppl 9): S281.

62. Mease P, Kavanaugh A, Krueger G et al. Infliximab improves psoriasis regardless of arthritis response in patients with active psoriatic arthritis: results from IMPACT 2 Trial. Arthritis Rheum 2004; 50 (Suppl 9): S616 (abstract).

63. Weinblatt ME, Keystone EC, Furst DE et al. Adalimumab, a fully human anti-tumor necrosis factor alpha monoclonal antibody, for the treatment of rheumatoid arthritis in patients taking concomitant methotrexate: the ARMADA trial. Arthritis Rheum 2003; 48(1): 35–45.

64. van de Putte LB, Atkins C, Malaise M et al. Efficacy and safety of adalimumab as monotherapy in patients with rheumatoid arthritis for whom previous disease modifying antirheumatic drug treatment has failed. Ann Rheum Dis 2004; 63(5): 508–16.

65. Furst DE, Schiff MH, Fleischmann RM et al. Adalimumab, a fully human anti tumor necrosis factor-alpha monoclonal antibody, and concomitant standard antirheumatic therapy for the treatment of rheumatoid arthritis: results of STAR (Safety Trial of Adalimumab in Rheumatoid Arthritis). J Rheumatol 2003; 30(12): 2563–71.

66. Ritchlin C, Anandarajaha A, Totterman S et al. Preliminary data from a study of adalimumab in the treatment of psoriatic arthritis. Ann Rheum Dis 2004; 63 (Suppl 1): 403 (abstract).

67. Mease P, Gladman D, Ritchlin C. Adalimumab in the treatment of patients with moderately to severely active psoriatic arthritis: results of ADEPT. Arthritis Rheum 2005; 58: 3279–89.

68. Genovese M, Mease P, Thomson G et al. Adalimumab efficacy in patients with psoriatic arthritis who failed prior DMARD therapy. Ann Rheum Dis 2005; 64 (Suppl 3): 313.

69. Marra CA. Valuing health states and preferences of patients. Ann Rheum Dis 2005; 64 (Suppl 3): 36.

70. Guh D, Bansback N, Nosyk B, Melilli L, Anis A. Improvement in health utility in patients with psoriatic arthritis treated with adalimumab (Humira). Ann Rheum Dis 2005; 64 (Suppl 3): 401.

71. Bansback N, Barkham N, Ara R et al. The economic implications of TNF-inhibitors in the treatment of psoriatic arthritis. Arthritis Rheum 2004; 50 (Suppl 9): S509.

72. Hansen KE, Hildebrand JP, Genovese MC et al. The efficacy of switching from etanercept to infliximab in patients with rheumatoid arthritis. J Rheumatol 2004; 31(6): 1098–102.

73. Haraoui B, Keystone EC, Thorne JC et al. Clinical outcomes of patients with rheumatoid arthritis after switching from infliximab to etanercept. J Rheumatol 2004; 31(12): 2356–9.

74. Bombardieri S, Tzioufas AG, McKenna F et al. Efficacy evaluation of adalimumab (Humira) in patients with single and multiple prior biologics in the ReAct trial. Arthritis Rheum 2004; 50 (Suppl 9): S187 (abstract).

75. Kraan MC, van Kuijk AW, Dinant HJ et al. Alefacept treatment in psoriatic arthritis: reduction of the effector T cell population in peripheral blood and synovial tissue is associated with improvement of clinical signs of arthritis. Arthritis Rheum 2002; 46(10): 2776–84.

76. Krueger GG, Papp KA, Stough DB et al. A randomized, double-blind, placebo-controlled phase III study evaluating efficacy and tolerability of 2 courses of alefacept in patients with chronic plaque psoriasis. J Am Acad Dermatol 2002; 47(6): 821–33.

77. Lebwohl M, Christophers E, Langley R et al. An international, randomized, double-blind, placebo-controlled phase 3 trial of intramuscular alefacept in patients with chronic plaque psoriasis. Arch Dermatol 2003; 139(6): 719–27.

78. Mease P, Gladman D, Keystone E. Efficacy of alefacept in combination with methotrexate in the treatment of psoriatic arthritis. Ann Rheum Dis 2005; 64 (Suppl 3): 324 (abstract).

79. Mease P, Gladman D, Keystone E. Alefacept in combination with methotrexate for the treatment of psoriatic arthritis: results of a randomized, double-blind, placebo-controlled study. Arthritis Rheum 2006; 54: 1638–45.

80. Lebwohl M, Tyring SK, Hamilton TK et al. A novel targeted T-cell modulator, efalizumab, for plaque psoriasis. N Engl J Med 2003; 349(21): 2004–13.

81. Papp K, Mease P, Garovoy M et al. Efalizumab in patients with psoriatic arthritis: results of a phase II randomized double-blind placebo controlled study. In: International Psoriasis Symposium, Toronto; 10 June 2004.

82. Kremer JM, Westhovens R, Leon M et al. Treatment of rheumatoid arthritis by selective inhibition of T-cell activation with fusion protein CTLA4Ig. N Engl J Med 2003; 349(20): 1907–15.

83. Abrams JR, Lebwohl M, Guzzo C. CTLA4Ig-mediated blockade of T cell co-stimulation in patients with psoriasis vulgaris. J Clin Invest 1999; 103: 1243–52.

84. McInnes IB, Gracie JA. Interleukin-15: a new cytokine target for the treatment of inflammatory diseases. Curr Opin Pharmacol 2004; 4(4): 392–7.

85. Nishimoto N YK, Miyasaka N et al. Long-term safety and efficacy of anti-interleukin 6 receptor antibody (MRA) in patients with rheumatoid arthritis. Arthritis Rheum 2003; 48 (Suppl 9): S126.

85a. Gibbs A, Gogarty M, Bresnihan B, et al. Moderate clinical response and absence of MRI or immunohistological change suggests that anakinra is ineffective in psoriatic arthritis. Arth Rheum. 2006; 54(Suppl 9):S719

86. Krueger JG, Walters IB, Miyazawa M et al. Successful in vivo blockade of CD25 (high-affinity interleukin 2 receptor) on T cells by administration of humanized anti-Tac antibody to patients with psoriasis. J Am Acad Dermatol 2000; 43: 448–58.

87. Jung JH ZT, Kavanaugh A. Other biologic therapy. Heidelberg: Springer-Verlag, 2005.

88. Mease PJ. Recent advances in the management of psoriatic arthritis. Curr Opin Rheumatol 2004; 16(4): 366–70.

89. Bongartz T, Coras B, Vogt T, Scholmerich J, Muller-Ladner U. Treatment of active psoriatic arthritis with the PPARgamma ligand pioglitazone: an open-label pilot study. Rheumatology (Oxford) 2005; 44(1): 126–9.

90. Reich K, Garbe C, Blaschke V et al. Response of psoriasis to interleukin-10 is associated with suppression of cutaneous type 1 inflammation, downregulation of the epidermal interleukin-8/CXCR2 pathway and normalization of keratinocyte maturation. J Invest Dermatol 2001; 116(2): 319–29.

91. McInnes IB, Illei GG, Danning CL et al. IL-10 improves skin disease and modulates endothelial activation and leukocyte effector function in patients with psoriatic arthritis. J Immunol 2001; 167(7): 4075–82.

92. Trepicchio WL, Ozawa M, Walters IB et al. Interleukin-11 therapy selectively downregulates type I cytokine proinflammatory pathways in psoriasis lesions. J Clin Invest 1999; 104(11): 1527–37.

93. Utset TO, Auger JA, Peace D et al. Modified anti-CD3 therapy in psoriatic arthritis: a phase I/II clinical trial. J Rheumatol 2002; 29(9): 1907–13.

33

Spondyloarthritides

Joachim Sieper and Jürgen Braun

Introduction • Treatment of AS with NSAIDs • Treatment with DMARDs • Treatment with TNF blockers • References

INTRODUCTION

This chapter is an update of the chapter in the previous edition on targeted therapies in spondyloarthritides (SpA) and will only discuss studies that have been published since then. Recent years have confirmed the unique position of the tumor necrosis factor (TNF) blocking agents for the treatment of patients with SpA, especially in active ankylosing spondylitis (AS), while data on other forms of SpA are still quite limited.

Most recently recommendations for the management of AS have been published for the first time, which were developed by an international group of experts inside the 'ASsessment in Ankylosing Spondylitis' (ASAS) working group and as part of the EULAR recommendations for various rheumatic diseases.[1] These recommendations summarize in 10 bullet points the most important points for the treatment of AS.

Non-steroidal anti-inflammatory drugs (NSAIDs) and TNF blockers are regarded in these recommendations as the most important and only effective part of drug treatment which has to be combined during the entire course of the disease with non-pharmacologic treatments. NSAIDs are recommended as first-line drug therapy for AS patients with pain and stiffness. Corticosteroid injections directed to the local site of musculoskeletal inflammation are useful in experienced centers but the use of systemic corticosteroids for axial disease is not supported by evidence. Similarly, there is no evidence for the usefulness of disease-modifying anti-rheumatic drugs (DMARDs), including sulfasalazine and methotrexate, to treat axial disease, but sulfasalazine may be useful in patients with peripheral arthritis. Anti-TNF therapy should be given to patients with persistently high disease activity and failure of other treatments according to the ASAS recommendations.[2]

TREATMENT OF AS WITH NSAIDs

The Cox-II selective drug etericoxib given in a doses of 90 mg/day was shown to be not more effective than 120 mg but more effective than 1000 mg/day naproxen in a 1 year treatment study of AS.[3] A recent study allocated a total of 215 patients to receive either continuous treatment with NSAIDs or only on demand for a period of 2 years.[4] Most interestingly, there was significantly less radiographic progression in the continuous treatment group in comparison with the on-demand treatment group, suggesting that NSAIDs may have disease-controlling properties. In this study there was no increased toxicity in the continuous treatment group. However, the fact that the overall level of clinical disease activity was not clearly different between the groups during the 2-year treatment period raises the question whether such a possible disease-controlling effect is due to the anti-inflammatory action of these drugs or whether there are additional independent effects. More data are needed in the future to confirm these exciting findings and to address these questions.

TREATMENT WITH DMARDs

The use of DMARDS for the treatment of axial disease in SpA has been rather disappointing, which is also reflected in the ASAS/EULAR recommendations. In a meta-analysis sulfasalazine has been shown to improve SpA-associated peripheral arthritis, but not spinal pain.[5] In a recent multicenter randomized controlled trial of sulfasalazine in undifferentiated SpA and early AS a small efficacy on spinal pain was noted, since patients with inflammatory back pain (IBP) but no peripheral arthritis had a significantly larger improvement in disease activity than the placebo group despite using less NSAIDs.[6] However, since all groups improved and since other subgroups were not different from placebo it is difficult to draw definite conclusions from this study.

Methotrexate is commonly used in rheumatoid arthritis (RA) with good results, improving symptoms and slowing the progression of erosive disease. This is clearly different in AS, suggesting different pathomechanisms of these diseases. In a recent systematic review on the use of methotrexate in AS, the conclusion was that there is no evidence for an effect on IBP and inconclusive evidence of efficacy for peripheral joint disease.[7] The only randomized controlled trial of methotrexate in AS has failed to show a significant effect of 7.5 mg oral methotrexate weekly on spondylitis, while some improvement of peripheral arthritis was reported in that study.[8] A recent open-label trial treating 20 active AS patients with 20 mg methotrexate s.c. for 16 weeks also did not detect an effect on axial symptoms, with some limited effect on peripheral arthritis.[9] Thus, methotrexate should not be used for the treatment of axial manifestations but (similar to other DMARDs) might have some role in the therapy of peripheral arthritis. Similarly, leflunomide is effective in treating the symptoms and slowing radiographic change in RA. However, recent studies in AS suggest that it is not effective for the axial manifestations of AS,[10,11] while patients with peripheral arthritis may have had some benefit from this agent.[10] Leflunomide is effective in the treatment of psoriatic arthritis.[12]

There are only two open studies with conflicting results addressing the efficacy of the interleukin (IL)-1 receptor antagonist anakinra in AS. In the first study, nine patients with active AS were treated with 100 mg anakinra given as a daily subcutaneous injection for 3 months. Significant improvement was observed both in clinical parameters and in acute inflammatory lesions determined by MRI.[13] This efficacy could not be confirmed in another open study treating 20 AS patients with the same dosage over 6 months. There was no change in the disease activity index or other clinical parameters, but also no change in bony inflammation, as detected by MRI.[14]

TREATMENT WITH TNF BLOCKERS

The introduction of TNF blockers has been the most substantial development in the treatment of AS and other SpA in the last few years. All three such agents – infliximab, etanercept, and adalimumab – have now been approved for the treatment of active AS. This success of anti-TNF treatment is likely to be a class effect because there is no major difference in their efficacy regarding the rheumatic manifestations. There is even some evidence that this therapy works better in AS and other SpA than in RA.[15]

Large randomized controlled trials of infliximab[16,17] and etanercept[18,19] have shown impressive short-term improvements in spinal pain, function, and inflammatory markers as compared with placebo. Uniformly, at least 50% of patients reach a 50% improvement of their disease activity as judged by the BASDAI 50 or the ASAS 40 improvement criteria, while this level of improvement is only achieved in about 10% of the placebo patients. Furthermore, about 25% of patients can be expected to achieve partial remission despite previous failure of NSAID treatment. Recently, one open-label[20] and one placebo-controlled double-blind study[21] showed very similar results for adalimumab in the treatment of AS.

Long-term follow-up data have been published for treatment with both infliximab and etanercept. The survival rate for infliximab treatment after 3 years was 69%;[22,23] efficacy has been seen to persist over this time. However, if treatment with infliximab was stopped patients relapsed between week 7 and 45, and by week 52 all except one patient out of 41 (97.6%) became active again. When treatment with inflixmab was commenced again all except one patient responded similarly to the first time and the drug was well tolerated.[22]

The good efficacy of infliximab on signs and symptoms is paralleled by a clear reduction of active spinal inflammation as detected by MRI.[24,25] When AS patients were followed over 2 years of treatment with infliximab there was even a further reduction of inflammation over this time.[26] However, the value of this drug as a disease modifier has not been clarified. No significant radiologic progression of disease as assessed by the modified SASSS (Stoke Ankylosing Spondylitis Spine Score), validated for use in scoring X-rays in AS,[27] was seen in a small number of AS patients.[28] However, more data are needed.

The efficacy of etanercept in AS has also been demonstrated[29] and recently reconfirmed in two large multicenter randomized placebo-controlled trials.[18,19] In contrast to other studies, the patients were allowed to continue DMARD and corticosteroid medication, and this occurred in about 30% of the patients. Patients from one of these randomized controlled studies[29] were enrolled in an open extension trial, after several months without therapy.[30] These patients have now been followed for 2 years after restart of treatment with etanercept.[31] This study design allowed two important conclusions to be made: the beneficial effect of therapy with etanercept does not persist after cessation of active drug; and response to therapy on re-introduction of etanercept shows a similar efficacy and safety profile to that in treatment-naïve patients. In another study 277 patients were enrolled in 1 of the randomized controlled trials over 24 weeks and subsequently all treated with etanercept and followed up in an open-label extension trial for a further 72 weeks.[32] After 2 years, 200 of the patients (72%) were still being treated with the drug; 50% of patients showed an ASAS

50% response at week 48 and 54% of the patients reached this level of response at week 96.

MRI results during treatment were also reported from the same two studies. From the larger study MRI of the spine was available at baseline, week 12, week 24, and week 48.[33] After 12 weeks spinal inflammation regressed by 54% in the etanercept group but worsened by 13% in the placebo group. In the second study, MRI of the spine and/or the sacroiliac joint was performed at baseline ($n = 25$), after 6 weeks (end of placebo-controlled phase, $n = 20$), and after 24 weeks of continuous treatment with etanercept ($n = 12$). Significant regression of spinal inflammation was already seen after 6 weeks in patients treated with etanercept but not in patients with placebo. Continuous treatment with etanercept for 24 weeks resulted in a further decrease of inflammation.[34]

A reduction of acute inflammation in spine and sacroiliac joint was also found in the small open-label trial with adlimumab over 1 year of treatment.[20]

Infliximab[35] and etanercept[36] were also effective in small studies in undifferentiated SpA. Similar to infliximab,[37] etanercept[38] has been shown to be effective for peripheral joint and skin symptoms in patients with psoriatic arthritis. Etanercept is effective for SpA associated with inflammatory bowel disease (IBD) regarding joint and spine but not gut symptoms.[39] In line with that, etanercept has no effect on IBD.[40] This is in contrast to infliximab, which has been approved for Crohn's disease[41] and ulcerative colitis.[42] Thus, etanercept is not recommended for the comparatively small SpA subgroup with concomitant IBD.

Most recently data from four placebo-controlled trials with TNF blockers for the treatment of AS (two with etanercept and two with infliximab) were analyzed for the incidence of reported flares of anterior uveitis during treatment.[43] The calculated frequency of flares of anterior uveitis in the placebo group was 15.6 per 100 patient-years, while patients treated with TNF blockers had significantly less flares (mean of 6.8 flares per 100 patient-years). Flares occurred less frequently in patients treated with infliximab (3.4 per 100 patient-years) than in those treated with etanercept (7.9 per 100 patient-years), although this difference was not significant. However, while treatment with TNF blockers can reduce the frequency of anterior uveitis, the exact role of TNF blocker in the treatment of severe treatment refractory cases of anterior uveitis has still to be defined.

Recommendations on which AS patients should be treated with TNF blockers were published in 2003[44] and confirmed in 2006[2] after 3 years of experience with the treatment of AS with TNF blockers: patients should have a definite diagnosis of AS, should be active despite an adequate treatment with NSAIDs, should have a disease activity as measured by the BASDAI of at least 4 (on a scale between 0 and 10) or higher and should have other objective signs of inflammation, as judged by an expert, normally a rheumatologist. Treatment should only be continued after 6–12 weeks if there is at least 50% improvement of the BASDAI or an absolute improvement of 2 points on the BASDAI scale between 0 and 10. A prediction of response to anti-TNF therapy is difficult, patients with shorter disease duration, elevated C-reactive protein (CRP), and, possibly, positive MRI findings may have better benefit from this treatment.[45]

Cost-effectiveness is always an issue when expensive therapies such as the TNF blockers are discussed. Despite the relative expense of infliximab compared with more traditional therapies for musculoskeletal disease, it was recently demonstrated that the significant clinical benefits[16] and improvement in quality of life with infliximab result in lower disease-associated costs than standard care, resulting in an approximate short-term cost of approximately £35 000 per quality-adjusted life year (QALY) gained,[46] an amount of money societies might be willing to pay. In another analysis of two of the randomized placebo-controlled studies, one with infliximab[16] and one with etanercept,[29] these calculated costs were higher.[47] When modeling for long-term therapy, using annual disease progression of 0.07 on BASFI in the sensitivity analysis, the cost per QALY gained is reduced to £9600.[46]

REFERENCES

1. Zochling J, van der Heijde D, Burgos-Vargas R et al. ASAS/EULAR recommendations for the management of ankylosing spondylitis. Ann Rheum Dis 2006; 65(4): 442–52.

2. Braun J, Davis J, Dougados M et al. First update of the international ASAS consensus statement for the use of anti-TNF agents in patients with ankylosing spondylitis. Ann Rheum Dis 2006; 65(3): 316–20.

3. van der Heijde D, Baraf HS, Ramos-Remus C et al. Evaluation of the efficacy of etoricoxib in ankylosing spondylitis: results of a fifty-two-week, randomized, controlled study. Arthritis Rheum 2005; 52(4): 1205–15.

4. Wanders A, Heijde D, Landewe R et al. Nonsteroidal antiinflammatory drugs reduce radiographic progression in patients with ankylosing spondylitis: a randomized clinical trial. Arthritis Rheum 2005; 52(6): 1756–65.

5. Chen J, Liu C. Sulfasalazine for ankylosing spondylitis. Cochrane Database Syst Rev 2005(2): CD004800.

6. Braun J, Zochling J, Baraliakos X et al. Efficacy of sulfasalazine in patients with inflammatory back pain due to undifferentiated spondyloarthritis and early ankylosing spondylitis: a multicentre randomised controlled trial. Ann Rheum Dis 2006; 65: 1147–53.

7. Chen J, Liu C. Methotrexate for ankylosing spondylitis. Cochrane Database Syst Rev 2004(3): CD004524.

8. Gonzalez-Lopez L, Garcia-Gonzalez A, Vazquez-Del-Mercado M, Munoz-Valle JF, Gamez-Nava JI. Efficacy of methotrexate in ankylosing spondylitis: a randomized, double blind, placebo controlled trial. J Rheumatol 2004; 31(8): 1568–74.

9. Haibel H, Brandt HC, Song IH et al. Results of an open label pilot study with 20mg methotrexate parenterally for the treatment of active anklyosing spondylitis. Ann Rheum Dis 2006; in press.

10. Haibel H, Rudwaleit M, Braun J, Sieper J. Six months open label trial of leflunomide in active ankylosing spondylitis. Ann Rheum Dis 2005; 64(1): 124–6.

11. Van Denderen JC, Van der Paardt M, Nurmohamed MT et al. Double blind, randomised, placebo controlled study of leflunomide in the treatment of active ankylosing spondylitis. Ann Rheum Dis 2005; 64: 1761–4.

12. Kaltwasser JP, Nash P, Gladman D et al. Efficacy and safety of leflunomide in the treatment of psoriatic arthritis and psoriasis: a multinational, double-blind, randomized, placebo-controlled clinical trial. Arthritis Rheum 2004; 50(6): 1939–50.

13. Tan AL, Marzo-Ortega H, O'Connor P et al. Efficacy of anakinra in active ankylosing spondylitis: a clinical and magnetic resonance imaging study. Ann Rheum Dis 2004; 63(9): 1041–5.

14. Haibel H, Rudwaleit M, Listing J, Sieper J. Open label trial of anakinra in active ankylosing spondylitis over 24 weeks. Ann Rheum Dis 2005; 64(2): 296–8.

15. Heiberg MS, Nordvag BY, Mikkelsen K et al. The comparative effectiveness of tumor necrosis factor-blocking agents in patients with rheumatoid arthritis and

patients with ankylosing spondylitis: a six-month, longitudinal, observational, multicenter study. Arthritis Rheum 2005; 52(8): 2506–12.

16. Braun J, Brandt J, Listing J et al. Treatment of active ankylosing spondylitis with infliximab: a randomised controlled multicentre trial. Lancet 2002; 359(9313): 1187–93.

17. van der Heijde D, Dijkmans B, Geusens P et al. Efficacy and safety of infliximab in patients with ankylosing spondylitis: results of a randomized, placebo-controlled trial (ASSERT). Arthritis Rheum 2005; 52(2): 582–91.

18. Davis JC Jr, Van Der Heijde D, Braun J et al. Recombinant human tumor necrosis factor receptor (etanercept) for treating ankylosing spondylitis: a randomized, controlled trial. Arthritis Rheum 2003; 48(11): 3230–6.

19. Calin A, Dijkmans BA, Emery P et al. Outcomes of a multicentre randomised clinical trial of etanercept to treat ankylosing spondylitis. Ann Rheum Dis 2004; 63(12): 1594–600.

20. Haibel H, Rudwaleit M, Brandt HC et al. Adalimumab reduces spinal symptoms in active ankylosing spondylitis – clinical and magnetic resonance imaging results of a fifty-two week open label trial. Arthritis Rheum 2006; 54: 678–81.

21. van der Heijde D, Kivitz A, Schiff M et al. Adalimumab therapy results in significant reduction of signs and symptoms in subjects with ankylosing spondylitis: the ATLAS trial. Arthritis Rheum 2006; 54: 2136–46.

22. Baraliakos X, Listing J, Brandt J et al. Clinical response to discontinuation of anti-TNF therapy in patients with ankylosing spondylitis after 3 years of continuous treatment with infliximab. Arthritis Res Ther 2005; 7(3): R439–44.

23. Braun J, Baraliakos X, Brandt J et al. Persistent clinical response to the anti-TNF-alpha antibody infliximab in patients with ankylosing spondylitis over 3 years. Rheumatology (Oxford) 2005; 44(5): 670–6.

24. Braun J, Baraliakos X, Golder W et al. Magnetic resonance imaging examinations of the spine in patients with ankylosing spondylitis, before and after successful therapy with infliximab: evaluation of a new scoring system. Arthritis Rheum 2003; 48(4): 1126–36.

25. Braun J, Landewe R, Hermann KG et al. Major reduction in spinal inflammation in patients with ankylosing spondylitis after treatment with infliximab: results of a multicenter, randomized, double-blind, placebo-controlled magnetic resonance imaging study. Arthritis Rheum 2006; 54(5): 1646–52.

26. Sieper J, Baraliakos X, Listing J et al. Persistent reduction of spinal inflammation as assessed by magnetic resonance imaging in patients with ankylosing spondylitis after 2 yrs of treatment with the anti-tumour necrosis factor agent infliximab. Rheumatology (Oxford) 2005; 44: 1525–30.

27. Creemers MC, Franssen MJ, van't Hof MA et al. Assessment of outcome in ankylosing spondylitis: an extended radiographic scoring system. Ann Rheum Dis 2005; 64(1): 127–9.

28. Baraliakos X, Listing J, Rudwaleit M et al. Radiographic progression in patients with ankylosing spondylitis after 2 years of treatment with the tumour necrosis factor alpha antibody infliximab. Ann Rheum Dis 2005; 64(10): 1462–6.

29. Brandt J, Khariouzov A, Listing J et al. Six-month results of a double-blind, placebo-controlled trial of etanercept treatment in patients with active ankylosing spondylitis. Arthritis Rheum 2003; 48(6): 1667–75.

30. Brandt J, Listing J, Haibel H et al. Long-term efficacy and safety of etanercept after readministration in patients with active ankylosing spondylitis. Rheumatology (Oxford) 2005; 44(3): 342–8.

31. Baraliakos X, Brandt J, Listing J et al. Outcome of patients with active anklyosing spondylitis after 2 years of therapy with etanercept – clinical and magnetic resonance imaging data. Arthritis Res Ther 2005; in press.

32. Davis JC, van der Heijde DM, Braun J et al. Sustained durability and tolerability of etanercept in ankylosing spondylitis for 96 weeks. Ann Rheum Dis 2005; 64: 1557–62.

33. Baraliakos X, Davis J, Tsuji W, Braun J. Magnetic resonance imaging examinations of the spine in patients with ankylosing spondylitis before and after therapy with the tumor necrosis factor alpha receptor fusion protein etanercept. Arthritis Rheum 2005; 52(4): 1216–23.

34. Rudwaleit M, Baraliakos X, Listing J et al. Magnetic resonance imaging of the spine and the sacroiliac joints in ankylosing spondylitis and undifferentiated spondyloarthritis during treatment with etanercept. Ann Rheum Dis 2005; 64(9): 1305–10.

35. Brandt J, Haibel H, Reddig J, Sieper J, Braun J. Successful short term treatment of severe undifferentiated spondyloarthropathy with the anti-tumor necrosis factor-alpha monoclonal antibody infliximab. J Rheumatol 2002; 29(1): 118–22.

36. Brandt J, Khariouzov A, Listing J et al. Successful short term treatment of patients with severe undifferentiated spondyloarthritis with the anti-tumor necrosis factor-alpha fusion receptor protein etanercept. J Rheumatol 2004; 31(3): 531–8.

37. Antoni CE, Kavanaugh A, Kirkham B et al. Sustained benefits of infliximab therapy for dermatologic and articular manifestations of psoriatic arthritis: results from the infliximab multinational psoriatic arthritis controlled trial (IMPACT). Arthritis Rheum 2005; 52(4): 1227–36.

38. Mease PJ, Kivitz AJ, Burch FX et al. Etanercept treatment of psoriatic arthritis: safety, efficacy, and effect on

disease progression. Arthritis Rheum 2004; 50(7): 2264–72.

39. Marzo-Ortega H, McGonagle D, O'Connor P, Emery P. Efficacy of etanercept for treatment of Crohn's related spondyloarthritis but not colitis. Ann Rheum Dis 2003; 62(1): 74–6.

40. Sandborn WJ, Hanauer SB, Katz S et al. Etanercept for active Crohn's disease: a randomized, double-blind, placebo-controlled trial. Gastroenterology 2001; 121(5): 1088–94.

41. Hanauer SB, Feagan BG, Lichtenstein GR et al. Maintenance infliximab for Crohn's disease: the ACCENT I randomised trial. Lancet 2002; 359(9317): 1541–9.

42. Rutgeerts P, Sandborn WJ, Feagan BG et al. Infliximab for induction and maintenance therapy for ulcerative colitis. N Engl J Med 2005; 353(23): 2462–76.

43. Braun J, Baraliakos X, Listing J, Sieper J. Decreased incidence of anterior uveitis in patients with ankylosing spondylitis treated with the anti-tumor necrosis factor agents infliximab and etanercept. Arthritis Rheum 2005; 52(8): 2447–51.

44. Braun J, Pham T, Sieper J, et al. International ASAS consensus statement for the use of anti-tumour necrosis factor agents in patients with ankylosing spondylitis. Ann Rheum Dis 2003; 62(9): 817–24.

45. Rudwaleit M, Listing J, Brandt J, Braun J, Sieper J. Prediction of a major clinical response (BASDAI 50) to tumour necrosis factor alpha blockers in ankylosing spondylitis. Ann Rheum Dis 2004; 63(6): 665–70.

46. Kobelt G, Andlin-Sobocki P, Brophy S et al. The burden of ankylosing spondylitis and the cost-effectiveness of treatment with infliximab (Remicade). Rheumatology (Oxford) 2004; 43(9): 1158–66.

47. Boonen A, van der Heijde D, Severens JL et al. Markov model into the cost-utility over five years of etanercept and infliximab compared with usual care in patients with active ankylosing spondylitis. Ann Rheum Dis 2006; 65(2): 201–8.

34

Early Arthritis

Paul Emery and Sally Cox

Early disease • Biological therapy • High-dose anti-TNF as potential remission-induction therapy • Summary • References

EARLY DISEASE

In recent years, treatment of rheumatoid arthritis (RA) has changed beyond recognition. Advances in the identification, linked with an understanding of the prognosis of patients with inflammatory arthritis, has enabled early initiation of effective therapies. It is recognized that suppression of inflammation should be as rapid as possible.[1-3] Persistent inflammation leads to damage, with substantial irreversible damage occurring within the first 2 years of symptoms.[2] This rate of damage occurrence appears to be greater in the earlier phase of the disease, rather than being simply cumulative. Permanent damage leads to disability, which in turn leads to costs, both to the individual and society. Treatment strategies have developed based on principles taking account of the above.

'Early' disease has often been defined as symptom duration of less than 2 years (although in earlier studies this was conventionally defined as less than 5 years).[4] The concept of a 'window of opportunity' suggests that there may be a time-frame early in the disease process in which there may be a disproportionate response to therapy that results in long-term sustained benefits.[5] Currently it is not clear whether this may occur during the first 1 or 2 years of disease onset, or may be just limited to a few months.

Objective measures of damage include bone erosions on radiographs,[6] but ultrasound (US)[7] and magnetic resonance imaging (MRI)[8] have also been increasingly used to detect early erosions not yet detectable by conventional radiography. Local osteoporosis assessed by dual-energy X-ray absorptiometry (DEXA) has been used as a measure of the impact of inflammation on bone, and shows that rapid bone loss occurs early in the disease process. It is accepted that the degree of damage is associated with the amount of inflammation present.[9] Loss of function, which correlates with the level of inflammation, also occurs early.[10] It is recognized that there is a 'therapeutic window of opportunity' in which early treatment provides better outcomes than treatment later in the disease.[1] This stage may represent a time of potentially transient reversibility of damage. With early treatment, it has been shown there is a reversal of functional loss,[10] less erosive change, and improvements in bone density measurements with DEXA.[9]

BIOLOGICAL THERAPY

Anti-tumor necrosis factor (TNF) therapy was first assessed in patients' refractory to traditional disease-modifying anti-rheumatic drug (DMARD) therapy.[11] Studies of anti-TNF agents confirmed their effectiveness in treating established disease in patients with ongoing inflammation and joint destruction, despite DMARD therapy. The biologics had a good safety profile, with few adverse events. What was not clear was whether anti-TNF would be as successful in treating early patients compared to conventional DMARDs given earlier.

Etanercept in early RA

The Early Rheumatoid Arthritis (ERA) study was designed to determine whether TNF monotherapy was superior to traditional DMARD therapy used early in the disease.[12] A total of 632 patients with early erosive disease (< 3 years) received etanercept or methotrexate monotherapy. Those patients receiving anti-TNF therapy had a faster clinical response (with more patients achieving an ACR 20/50/70) at 6 months and these differences were apparent within the first 2 weeks of therapy. Both groups had good clinical outcomes at 12 months and a profound reduction in the rates of progression of radiographic damage.[12] Etanercept halted erosions in 72% of patients compared with 60% of those receiving methotrexate. There was a good correlation between clinical improvement and the reduction in radiographic progression. Interestingly, this study did not demonstrate superiority of a biologic agent over methotrexate in methotrexate-naïve patients with early disease (at the primary endpoint of 12 months). Two issues may explain these somewhat unexpected results. Firstly, the methotrexate regimen was more aggressive than traditionally used regimes, both with earlier initiation of therapy and more rapid escalation (0 to 20 mg in 8 weeks). Secondly, the patient population had a high number of responders to methotrexate. The patient population was naïve to methotrexate, and generally patients respond better to their first therapy than subsequent treatments. As regards symptoms and signs within the responder population, patients did as well on methotrexate as etanercept, and thus the effective difference between the two therapies was confined to the higher number of methotrexate non-responders. This represents a much smaller proportion of the total population than would have been predicted.

What was clear from this study was that early aggressive treatment is imperative to providing better outcomes. An open-label extension study showed some advantages of etanercept over methotrexate in reducing disease activity and structural damage at 2 years.[13] ACR response rates were maintained for the duration of the study. Etanercept was also more effective in improving quality of life (QoL) during this time.

Infliximab in early RA

ATTRACT was one of the key studies in the efficacy of biologic therapy in RA.[14] In patients with long-standing disease with active inflammation despite methotrexate, combination therapy halted joint progression and improved QoL, as would be expected with the reduction in disease burden achieved with adequate suppression of inflammation. Control of inflammation was rapid with infliximab. Over half of responders had achieved this response within a fortnight and 90% within 6 weeks.[11] A subgroup of the ATTRACT patient population[14] had disease duration of less than 3 years. The patients in this cohort had been given one of five dosing regimens including methotrexate monotherapy or combination with various regimens of infliximab. As in all infliximab studies (after phase III) it was used with methotrexate, so the relative benefits of monotherapy versus methotrexate could not be tested. Combination infliximab and methotrexate inhibited structural damage in patients with early disease during the 2 years of treatment, and worked equally well in early and late disease. This sub-analysis was retrospective, had small numbers, and was not adequately powered to draw firm conclusions. However, it did support the early use of TNF to prevent initial damage.

A large multicenter trial, ASPIRE, evaluated efficacy of infliximab in combination with methotrexate versus methotrexate alone in methotrexate-naïve, early RA patients.[15] In all, 1049 patients were enrolled into one of three treatment arms: methotrexate/placebo or methotrexate/infliximab (3 mg/kg or 6 mg/kg). Superior clinical, functional, and radiological outcomes were seen at 1 year in the combination group. DAS 28 remission rates were significantly higher, with 31.0% of patients in the combination infliximab (6 mg/kg) group achieving remission compared with 15.0% of those receiving monotherapy. This trial confirmed that erosive joint disease occurs early and supported the need for early, aggressive therapy. It demonstrated that the combination of methotrexate and anti-TNF was superior to methotrexate alone in preventing progression of joint destruction,[16] improving clinical responses, and reducing disability.[17]

Adalimumab in early RA

The PREMIER study allowed the assessment of the impact of the combination by comparing the two monotherapies, adalimumab and methotrexate, with the combination of the two.[18] Importantly PREMIER showed that at 2 years 50% of the patients treated with the combination were in clinical remission, providing a gold standard outcome for new poor prognosis patients (they were selected for likelihood of developing erosions). In all, 799 patients in the PREMIER study had disease duration of less than 3 years (mean 0.7 years). The co-primary endpoint of ACR 50 response was achieved in 61% of combination patients, but in only 46% and 42% of those patients receiving monotherapy (with methotrexate and adalimumab, respectively). Change in total Sharp score was significantly lower in the combination group, indicating significantly less radiological progression. ACR 20/50/70 responses were significantly better by week 2 in the combination group, and this result was sustained over the 2-year period. Although adalimumab and methotrexate monotherapy had equivalent clinical outcomes at 2 years, there was twice as much radiographic damage in the methotrexate group.[19] Again, use in combination with methotrexate in early disease showed superior clinical outcomes and inhibition of structural damage when compared with either agent as monotherapy. Combination therapy was superior to methotrexate monotherapy in improvement of health-related QoL, physical function, and structure, reducing radiologic progress by 80% compared with methotrexate.[20] Overall rates of adverse events were comparable among treatment groups. ERA and PREMIER demonstrated that anti-TNF monotherapy was equivalent to methotrexate for managing symptoms and signs, but TNF blockade was superior for damage prevention.

The findings in PREMIER and ASPIRE support early aggressive intervention in RA. Both studies confirm that combination therapy with anti-TNF-α and methotrexate has rapid onset of effect and superior long-term clinical and radiologic outcomes. However, these studies had 'sacrificed' the earliness of disease duration for poor prognostic factors (patients were selected for either the presence of erosions or factors predicting erosions).

HIGH DOSE ANTI-TNF AS POTENTIAL REMISSION-INDUCTION THERAPY

We have aimed for remission for some time;[21] for the first time it has become an attainable goal. A small pilot study[22] was performed to determine whether a high dose induction TNF therapy regimen could induce sustained imaging remission. Five patients with poor prognosis RA were given high dose infliximab (10 mg/kg) at weeks 0, 2, 6, and 14. These patients all had early disease with minimal X-ray damage – MRI was used as both selection and outcome measures. By selection, using the presence of synovitis on MRI, the study population has increased homogeneity and increased the power of the study. After the first induction phase, one patient had clinical remission but no patients achieved imaging remission (MRI and US) according to the protocol. Patients were re-induced; however, there were no further improvements in response to the re-induction. Furthermore, all patients relapsed on ceasing infliximab. This study concluded that any variability in response to infliximab was not due to insufficient drug and that short-term treatment did not lead to drug-free remission.

Remission-induction with 12 months infliximab treatment

Quinn et al.[23] performed a 12-month double-blind randomized placebo-controlled trial with the aim of remission-induction in patients with early poor prognosis RA. Twenty patients received methotrexate and induction infliximab/placebo, then 8 weekly infusions through to 46 weeks. The primary endpoint was synovitis as measured by MRI. However, there was the opportunity to look at the long-term impact of 12 months of infliximab. At 1 year, all MRI scores were significantly better in the infliximab group, with no new erosions. Improvement in joint counts was rapid and seen within 2 weeks in the active group and significant differences were seen in functional and QoL measures. Importantly, in the cohort that received early infliximab therapy, response was sustained 12 months after therapy was ceased, with a median disease activity score in 28 joints (DAS 28) of 2.05 (remission range) at 2 years, with median HAQ (Health Assessment Questionnaire) and QoL also normal. Functional benefits and QoL were also maintained at 24 months. This was one of the first studies to demonstrate the feasibility of sustained remission following a course of infliximab therapy. The question was whether this was a 'one-off' in a selected population or a genuine reproducible event. The answer was provided by BeSt.

BeSt study

The BeSt trial was a multi-center, single-blind study.[24,25] A total of 508 patients with < 2 years of symptoms were randomized to 1 of 4 treatment arms: sequential monotherapy starting with methotrexate, step-up therapy from methotrexate, step-down (including initial high dose oral prednisolone), or combination methotrexate/infliximab. Adjustments in doses were made at 3 monthly intervals with the goal of achieving DAS 44 ≤ 2.4. Co-primary endpoints were functional ability (measured by HAQ) and radiographic damage (measured by modified Sharp/Van der Heijde score [SHS]). A significantly greater and more rapid improvement in function (as measured by HAQ) was seen with the initial combination treatment and initial treatment with infliximab and methotrexate. Mean HAQ scores at 3 months were 0.6 on groups 3 and 4, compared with 1.0 in groups 1 and 2. At 12 months, there was still a clinically detectable difference between the groups (0.5 [groups 3 and 4] versus 0.7 [groups 1 and 2]). There was also significantly less radiologic damage than with sequential monotherapy or step-up therapy. In the group receiving infliximab, 46% showed no radiologic progression at

1 year (versus 29% and 37% in the monotherapy or step-up patients, respectively). Also, 53%, 64%, 71%, and 74% of patients in groups 1–4, respectively, achieved DAS44 ≤ 2.4 at 12 months. Only the differences between group 1 versus groups 3 and 4 were significant. After 6 months in remission, four patients stopped infliximab and in the second year, approximately 50% of patients were able to stop their infliximab yet remain in remission. This provided further support that combination anti-TNF-α blocker and methotrexate was optimal in the treatment of early RA.

SUMMARY

It is recognized that there is a 'therapeutic window of opportunity' in which early treatment provides better outcomes than treatment later in the disease.[5] The ultimate goal of treatment is prevention of arthritis by modification of the underlying disease process. Although a proportion of early patients will have good responses to traditional DMARDs, anti-TNF therapies provide more rapid control of inflammation and better long-term outcomes (in combination with methotrexate). However, they are substantially more expensive than standard DMARDs. This raises the question that if you treat aggressively later, rather than early, can you ever 'catch up' with respect to disease suppression? A further question is whether biologic therapy can induce a sustainable remission. Early trials have shown positive results; however, numbers were small and as yet there are no longer-term data. In this era of exciting new developments, further research is needed to determine optimal use of these resources, with the ultimate aim of arthritis remission and eventual prevention of the disease.

REFERENCES

1. Nell VPK, Machold KP, Eberl G et al. Benefit of very early referral and very early therapy with disease modifying anti-rheumatic drugs in patients with early rheumatoid arthritis. Rheumatology 2004; 43: 906–14.
2. Van der Heide A, Jacobs JWG, Bijlsma JWJ et al. The effectiveness of early treatment with anti-rheumatic drugs: a randomised controlled trial. Ann Intern Med 1996: 124; 699–707.

3. Emery P. Early arthritis. In: Smolen JS, Lipsky PE, eds. Targeted Therapies in Rheumatology. London: Martin Dunitz, 2003: 509–13.

4. Quinn MA, Conaghan PG, Emery P The therapeutic approach of early intervention for rheumatoid arthritis: what is the evidence? Rheumatology 2001; 40: 1211–20.

5. Quinn M, Emery P. Window of opportunity in ERA: possibility of altering disease process with early intervention. Clin Exp Rheumatol 2003; 21 (Suppl.31): S154–7.

6. Abu-Shakra M, Toker R, Flusser D et al. Clinical and radiographic outcomes of rheumatoid arthritis in patients not treated with disease modifying drugs. Arthritis Rheum 1998; 41: 1190–5.

7. Wakefield RJ, Gibbon W, Conaghan P et al. The value of sonography in the detection of cortical bone erosions: a comparative study with conventional radiography Arthritis Rheum 2000; 43(12): 2762–70.

8. McGonagle D, Conaghan P, O'Connor P et al. The relationship between synovitis and bone changes in early untreated RA – a controlled MRI study. Arthritis Rheum 1999; 42: 1706–11.

9. Gough AK, Lilley J, Eyre S et al. Generalised bone loss in patients with early rheumatoid arthritis occurs early and relates to disease activity. Lancet 1994; 344: 23–7.

10. Devlin J, Gough A, Huissoon A et al. The acute phase and function in early rheumatoid arthritis. CRP levels correlate with functional outcome. J Rheumatol 1997; 24: 9–13.

11. Maini R, St Clair EW, Breedveld F et al. Infliximab (chimeric anti-tumour necrosis factor α monoclonal antibody) versus placebo in rheumatoid arthritis patients receiving concomitant methotrexate: a randomised phase III trial. Lancet 1999; 354: 1932–9.

12. Bathon, JM, Martin RW, Fleischman RM et al. A comparison of etanercept and methotrexate in patients with early rheumatoid arthritis. N Engl J Med 2000; 343(22): 1586–93.

13. Genovese MC, Bathon JM, Martin RW et al Etanercept versus methotrexate in patients with early rheumatoid arthritis – two year radiographic and clinical outcomes. Arthritis Rheum 2002; 46 (6): 1443–50.

14. Breedveld FC, Emery P, Keystone E et al. Infliximab in active early rheumatoid arthritis. Ann Rheum Dis 2004; 63: 149–55.

15. St Clair EW, van der Heijde MFM, Smolen JS et al. Combination of infliximab and methotrexate therapy for early rheumatoid arthritis. Arthritis Rheum 2004; 50(11): 3432–43.

16. Van der Heijde D, Emery P, Bathon J et al. Reduction in radiographic progression in the hands and feet of patients with early rheumatoid arthritis after receiving infliximab in combination with methotrexate. Arthritis Rheum 2005; 52 (Suppl): S739.

17. Smolen J, Han C, Bala M et al. Patients with early rheumatoid arthritis achieved a clinically meaningful and sustained improvement in physical function after treatment with infliximab. Arthritis Rheum 2005; 52 (Suppl): S37.

18. Breedveld FC, Weissman MH, Kavanaugh AF et al. The efficacy and safety of adalimumab plus MTX vs adalimumab or MTX alone in the early treatment of RA: 1 and 2 year results of the PREMIER Study. Ann Rheum Dis 2005; 64 (Suppl III): 60.

19. Van der Heijde D Landewe R, Keystone EC et al. Adalimumab (HUMIRA) plus MTX prevents nearly all Severe radiographic progression observed with methotrexate monotherapy in early, aggressive rheumatoid arthritis. Arthritis Rheum 2005; 52 (Suppl): S110.

20. Weisman M, Strand V, Cifaldi MA et al. Adalimumab (HUMIRA) plus methotrexate is superior to MTX alone in improving physical function, as measured by the SF-36, in patients with early rheumatoid arthritis. Arthritis Rheum 2005; 52 (Suppl): S395.

21. Emery P, Salmon M. Early rheumatoid arthritis: time to aim for remission Ann Rheum Dis 1995; 54(12): 944–7.

22. Conaghan P, Quinn M, O'Connor P et al. The impact of a very high dose TNF blockade on new rheumatoid arthritis patients: a clinical and imaging pilot study. Arthritis Rheum 2002; 46(7): 1971–2.

23. Quinn M, Conaghan PG, O'Connor PJ et al. Very early treatment with infliximab in addition to methotrexate in early, poor-prognosis rheumatoid arthritis reduces magnetic resonance imaging evidence of synovitis and damage with sustained benefit after infliximab withdrawal. Arthritis Rheum 2005; 52(1): 27–35.

24. Vries-Bouwstra JK, Goekoop-Ruiterman YPM, Van Zeben D et al. A comparison of clinical and radiological outcomes of four treatment strategies for early rheumatoid arthritis: results of the BeSt Trial. Ann Rheum Dis 2004; 50(Suppl): 4096.

25. Goekoop-Ruiterman YPM, Vries-Bouwstra JK, Allaart CF et al. Clinical and radiographic outcomes of four different treatment strategies in patients with early rheumatoid arthritis (the BeSt Study). Arthritis Rheum 2005; 52(11): 3381–90.

35

Juvenile arthritis

Patricia Woo

Introduction • Impact of juvenile idiopathic arthritis • Types of juvenile idiopathic arthritis • Imbalances in cellular and cytokine networks • Genetic influences and possible targets • Therapeutic cytokine modulation • TNF-α blockade • Potential risks from TNF blockade • Other immunomodulation • Trial design and ethical considerations • Practical management of new therapies • Conclusion • References

INTRODUCTION

For children and young people with severe juvenile idiopathic arthritis (JIA), whose disease is uncontrolled by conventional disease-modifying drugs and steroids, a new group of therapies with exciting potential has emerged. Research examining cellular and cytokine control of inflammation in JIA has provided some of the scientific rationale for therapeutic agents targeting biological pathways. These biological agents include antagonists to cytokines such as tumor necrosis factor (TNF)-α, and blockade of cytokine signaling (e.g. interleukin (IL)-1 and IL-6), which have shown early promise by producing dramatic clinical benefit in many children with JIA and other autoimmune diseases. However, despite targeting specific molecules, the therapeutic actions of these new agents remain non-specific, producing variable clinical responses that raise additional ethical and administrative considerations.

IMPACT OF JUVENILE IDIOPATHIC ARTHRITIS

JIA affects 1 in 1000 children.[1] For the majority of children with polyarticular disease, methotrexate and other second-line agents[2,3] have improved the prognosis of this group of diseases. However, significant numbers (approximately 30%) of children with JIA are refractory to conventional management, and suffer in addition the cumulative side effects of long-term immunosuppressive medication. Such disease activity results in joint damage, which often necessitates joint replacement, severe growth retardation, chronic pain, and functional disability. There is also a significant impact on emotional and psychological development, lifestyle, and employment.[4,5] It is to this group of patients that biological therapy is currently targeted.

TYPES OF JUVENILE IDIOPATHIC ARTHRITIS

The classification of chronic arthritis in children has been a clinical one, attempting to separate the heterogeneous spectrum of disease into more homogeneous subgroups according to clinical features at presentation and their prognosis. There were two systems of classification in use from the 1970s, which were not identical (Table 35.1). An international taskforce convened by the International League of Associations of Rheumatology (ILAR) proposed and subsequently revised a unifying classification which aimed to produce clinically homogeneous subgroups that are mutually exclusive, so as to aid research into pathogenesis and therapeutic studies.[6] The discussions in this chapter will use this ILAR classification.

Table 35.1 Comparison of the classifications of arthritis in children

ARA: Juvenile Rheumatoid Arthritis (1977)	EULAR: Juvenile chronic Arthritis (1977)	ILAR: Juvenile Idiopathic Arthritis(1977)
Pauciarticular (four or less joints affected, includes RF+, extended, some psoriatic and ERA as defined in ILAR)	**Pauciarticular** (four or less joints affected, includes RF+, extended, some ERA and psoriatics as defined in ILAR)	**Oligoarticular** (four or less joints affected, RF− only)
		Extended oligoarticular (RF− only)
Polyarticular (includes RF+ and RF−, some psoriatics and ERA as defined in ILAR)	**Polyticular** (includes RF+ and RF−, some ERA and psoriatics as defined in ILAR)	**Polyarticular, RF−**
		Polyarticular RF+
Systemic	**Systemic**	**Systemic**
Juvenile ankylosing Spondyloarthritis excluded	**Probable and definite juvenile ankylosing spondylitis**	**Enthesitis-related arthritis** (not all would fit juvenile ankylosing spondylitis as in EULAR)
Psoriatics included in pauci/poly	Psoriatics included in pauci/poly	**Psoriatic arthritis**
		Unclassified

The categories are in bold type.
ERA, enthesis-related arthritis; RF, rheumatoid factor.

Since there are no obvious infectious triggers or reproducible observations of seasonality in any of these diseases, they are regarded at present as autoimmune diseases. The persistent inflammatory response is perceived by current researchers to depend on the balance of the immune and inflammatory mediators, which can be reactive to foreign antigens or self-antigens, but are also controlled genetically. Imbalances in cellular functions and interactions, and in pro- and anti-inflammatory cytokines, have been found in JIA. Modulation of these imbalances is the rationale for the development of newer biological therapies, as is the case for other rheumatic diseases. In addition, the case can be strengthened in JIA, where there are genetic variations that are proinflammatory.

IMBALANCES IN CELLULAR AND CYTOKINE NETWORKS

A type 1 T-cell response (predominance of interferon (IFN)-γ-producing cells) is found in the synovial fluid and membranes of children with oligoarticular, polyarticular, and enthesitis-related arthritis, but not in the peripheral blood mononuclear cells, indicating sequestration and/or *in situ* differentiation and polarization of T cells.[7,8] Currently, there are no data on the type of synovial T-cell response in systemic arthritis, but there is one report of a mixed type 1 and 2 response in the peripheral blood mononuclear cells.[9] Differences between rheumatoid arthritis (RA) and JIA include:

1. the lack of IgM rheumatoid factor (RF), except for the subgroup of RF-positive arthritis, which constitutes about 1% of all JIA
2. the presence of IFN-γ and interleukin (IL)-4-producing cells in the synovial fluid and synovium of JIA
3. the variable levels of TNF-α and its soluble receptor (sTNFR) in subgroups.
4. the multisystem inflammation seen in systemic JIA.

Evidence that the pathological processes in JIA are cytokine-dependent includes the positive correlation of serum and synovial concentrations of various cytokines with disease activity.[10–12] The effects of proinflammatory cytokines on synovial cells and osteoclasts are well described, and it is clear that the general principle of using antagonists of proinflammatory cytokines is applicable to JIA as well. The issue is whether there is a 'master cytokine' to target.

Research so far in JIA suggests that there are different cytokine imbalances in at least three areas. Systemic JIA is characterized by quotidian fevers, transient rash, enlargement of the reticuloendothelial system, serositis, and systemic vasculitis, in addition to arthritis. These patients have a vigorous acute phase response and their serum cytokine profiles reflect excess production of IL-6 and its agonist sIL-6R,[13,14] although other proinflammatory cytokines are also present.[11,15] The ratio of TNF and its natural inhibitor, sTNFR, is higher in the synovial fluid of polyarticular JIA as compared with enthesitis-related arthritis, consistent with a more aggressively erosive disease in the former.[16] The difference between oligoarticular and polyarticular JIA is that IL-4 is detected only in the synovium and fluid in oligoarticular JIA,[7,8] even though both showed type 1 T-cell responses. An additional important consideration is the genetic component of the imbalance.

GENETIC INFLUENCES AND POSSIBLE TARGETS

It is clear that HLA association studies have identified class II antigens in case-control as well as family association studies. HLA-DR*0801 has been identified as being the genetic background of early-onset JIA, particularly oligoarticular JIA.[17] The exception is systemic JIA. How these class II antigens present peptides in JIA versus controls is an active area of research, and could yield novel therapeutic approaches.

The cytokine milieu is influential in the process of antigen presentation, cellular polarization, and apoptosis. Thus, the balance of pro- and anti-inflammatory cytokines is important in the outcome of inflammation. Studies of genetic associations with variants of pro- and anti-inflammatory cytokines have shown interesting results in JIA. Our case-control study of the IL-10 gene has shown that the low IL-10-producing variant is significantly associated with extended oligoarticular JIA, suggesting a genetic effect on disease severity.[18,19] This genetic variant was also shown to be a severity factor for asthma.[20] More recently we have also found association of this allele with

sJIA in a case-control study.[21] Thus the role of regulatory T and possibly B cells that secrete IL-10 in these diseases merits further research. Recent studies of the TNF-α gene suggest that the −308 variant is associated with severity in a sample of Turks,[22] and a Japanese sample population.[23] This variant has been shown to influence transcription of the TNF-α gene.[24] A more comprehensive analysis of all the nucleotide variants in the regulatory region of the TNF-α gene has been reported recently for oligoarticular JIA, using a family study.[25] The function of the haplotypes remains to be characterized. Other associations include the macrophage inhibitory factor (MIF) and IL-6. MIF was found to have a genetic variant in the regulatory region which is significantly associated with all types of JIA, but its functional significance awaits further characterization.[26] The IL-6 gene has several variants in its regulatory region, and the −174 gene variant has a dominant effect on gene expression, and has been shown to be associated with systemic JIA in case-control as well as in family studies.[27,28] Its biological significance is illustrated by its association with type I and II insulin-dependent diabetes, peak bone mass in adolescent young men, increased bone turnover in postmenopausal women, and survival after coronary bypass graft. Confirmation of these studies as well as analysis of the interaction of these genetic influences would provide the scientific basis for new biological therapies in each of these types of arthritis in children.

THERAPEUTIC CYTOKINE MODULATION

Cytokine modulation aims to restore homeostasis by influencing a perceived imbalance of cytokines or by promoting a particular cellular response. Established therapies have been shown to alter production of cytokines at the level of transcription and translation. Corticosteroids and cyclosporin A inhibit nuclear factors important for gene expression,[29–31] thalidomide enhances TNF-α mRNA degradation,[32] and leflunamide inhibits signal transduction pathways by blocking tyrosine phosphorylation.[33] In contrast, the principal means of TNF blockade, and of current new biologicals, is to block the molecule itself from interacting with cells, using monoclonal neutralizing antibodies or recombinant soluble cytokine receptors. Receptor interference is achieved by using naturally derived cytokine antagonists (e.g. recombinant IL-1ra) and by using monoclonal antibodies (mAbs, e.g. anti-IL-6R).

TNF-α BLOCKADE

Etanercept is licensed for use in children in the USA and Europe. It is a recombinant protein consisting of the binding portion of the human soluble TNF-α receptor attached to the Fc portion of human IgG. It neutralizes TNF by binding with an affinity 50–1000 times that of the naturally occurring TNF receptors, and has a longer half-life. It may also exert its effect by binding other cytokines, such as lymphotoxin. It has a UK licence for use in children aged 4–17 years who show an inadequate response to, or are intolerant of, methotrexate. Early safety and efficacy data in children less than 4 years of age are encouraging.[34] It is administered by subcutaneous injection twice weekly, for an indefinite period, and may be used with or without methotrexate.

The most detailed trial to date enrolled 69 patients with chronic polyarthritis of variable etiology and unresponsive to maximum conventional treatment.[35] The duration of the study was 1 year, although 5-year follow-up data are now available.[36] The initial study had a novel design, in that all patients received etanercept for the first 3 months, while all other medications, except low dose steroids and non-steroidal anti-inflammatory drugs (NSAIDs), were stopped. Figure 35.1 shows the structure of the trial and the patient responses. Non-responders in the first 3 months were withdrawn from stage 2 of the study, as they required additional therapy. The definition of improvement was as described by Giannini et al.[37] Seventy-four per cent of all patients benefited over the first 3 months. A secondary endpoint was the time to flare of disease: during the 7 months after randomization, 77% of those receiving placebo flared at a median of 28 days, whereas only 24% of those still receiving etanercept flared at a median of 116 days. During the final, open-label phase, 74% of all patients benefited, 64% of patients improving by 50% and 36% improving by 70% (Figure 35.1). There are limitations to the interpretation of this

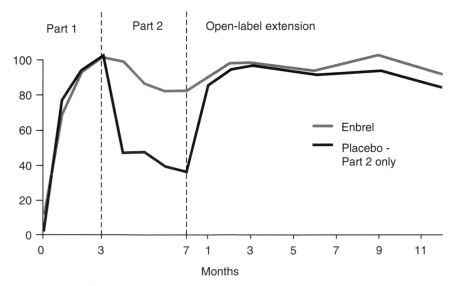

Figure 35.1 The three phases of the trial of etanercept in children with polyarticular JIA. In part 1, both groups received etanercept. In part 2, patients were blinded and randomized to receive etanercept or placebo. Part 3 was again open-label, with all patients receiving the active agent.[35,36]

study, but given that the patient population represents the more severe end of the disease spectrum, this is a remarkable response to treatment. At a median 2.3 years of subsequent treatment, 67% of all patients had a 70% improvement in disease activity. Other smaller studies have found similar improvements in polyarticular JIA,[38] and juvenile anklylosing spondylitis,[39] and there are reports of benefit from the simultaneous use of methotrexate.[40]

Infliximab is a chimeric human–murine mAb that binds both soluble and cell-bound TNF-α. Infliximab is given by intravenous infusions, and combination treatment with methotrexate is recommended to avoid the development of tachyphylaxis to the murine component of the agent. There is a licence for its use in adults with RA, and although there is no current license for its use in children, there are anecdotal reports of its success in JIA.[41–43] High dose anti-TNF therapy is now being piloted, showing early success in systemic JIA.[43] Table 35.2 shows a comparison of the two agents used in JIA. Finally, Humira is another humanized recombinant antibody that is licensed for adult use, but may be applicable to larger children with JIA.

POTENTIAL RISKS FROM TNF BLOCKADE

Etanercept appears to be well tolerated by children. Although headache, nausea, abdominal pain, and vomiting were more common in children than were reported by adults treated with etanercept for RA, this did not result in discontinuation of treatment. Reports of skin rashes, some at the site of injection, and some vasculitic, have not led to discontinuation of the drug. There are no reports of increased risk from infection, but this remains a theoretical possibility.

There have been isolated case reports of aplastic anemia, severe leukopenia, and pancytopenia, and a possible association with demyelinating diseases of the central nervous system in adults receiving TNF blockade. The theoretical increased risk of malignancy, over that of the disease itself, has not been reflected clinically,[45] but 10 years of follow-up is still insufficient to determine the long-term risk. The risk of infection, including tuberculosis reactivation, is thought to be higher with the use of anti-TNF agents, particularly infliximab.[46] In a recent double-blind placebo-controlled trial of infliximab in children with JIA, the incidence of infusion reaction and development of antibody to the drug were four times as high in the 3 mg/kg dose range when given every 8 weeks, but dropped to approximately 7% at 6 mg/kg equivalent to the incidence obtained in adult trials. There are reports that adult patients receiving both types of TNF antagonist may develop antibodies to anti-nuclear antigen and dsDNA, and precipitate the clinical development of systemic lupus erythematosus (SLE) or a lupus-like syndrome.[47,48] There have been no reports of dsDNA or lupus so far in children.

Table 35.2 Comparison of etanercept and infliximab

	Etanercept	Infliximab
Licensed indications	Polyarticular JIA failing to respond to, or intolerant of, methotrexate	Not licensed
Half-life	70 h	200 h
Dose	0.4 mg/kg (maximum 25 mg) twice weekly	3 mg/kg at week zero, 2, 6, 8, and 14 weekly thereafter
Route of administration	Subcutaneous injection	Intravenous infusion
Side effects	Risk of sepsis	Risk of sepsis, tachyphylaxis
Cost of vials	Four 25 mg vials – £325	100 mg vial – £451
Cost per year[a]	£4225	£4059

[a]Costs based on 30-kg child and using same vial of etanercept for both weekly doses.

OTHER IMMUNOMODULATION

IL-1 receptor antagonist (IL-1ra)

This is a non-signaling peptide of the IL-1 family, which exerts its actions by blocking the proinflammatory actions of both IL-1a and IL-1b. Despite considerable natural regulation of IL-1 activity, studies have shown benefit from supra-physiological doses of recombinant IL-1ra. IL-1ra is now licensed for use in the USA and parts of Europe. Early trials in JIA have yet to complete. The rationale would be that IL-1 is more active in cartilage and bone erosions in animal models of arthritis, and should have a place in the more erosive forms of JIA. Of interest is the recent anecdotal report of its efficacy in systemic JIA.[49]

Recombinant IL-10

This has been infused systemically to inhibit the synthesis of proinflammatory cytokines and alter cellular differentiation and polarization. It too has a short half-life that results in poor clinical efficacy, and high systemic doses have not been well tolerated.[50] These results have led to exploration of the alternative approaches of local therapy and gene therapy.[51–53]

IL-6

This is a possible target for the treatment of systemic JIA, as discussed above. Overproduction of the cytokine promotes proinflammatory cellular activity, although it also stimulates cytokine antagonists such as IL-1ra, sTNFR, and TIMP (Figure 35.2). A recombinant anti-human

IL-6R mAb of the IgG1 subclass has undergone successful phase II studies in RA and a phase III multicenter study in Europe has been concluded with good efficacy. Phase II therapeutic trials in Japan and Europe have shown dramatic changes in disease activity in systemic JIA.[53,54]

Modulation of T- and B-cell ontogeny

Inconsistent results and the observation of prolonged $CD4^+$ T-cell depletion have been reported, thus raising anxieties about the longer-term consequences of such manipulations. Antibody targeted against CD20 markers expressed by B cells is undergoing phase II trials in RA. The rationale for its use in RA depends on the hypothesis of a clone of rheumatoid factor (RF)-producing B cells,[56] and this is unlikely to be applicable since most JIA subtypes are RF-negative.

Future developments are likely to include targeting of other cytokines such as IFN-γ, combination therapy, and the use of cytokines to either divert the immune response towards tolerance or to control apoptosis. Genetic research will also continue, not only in terms of gene therapy, but also in the identification of genetic populations most likely to respond to treatment.

TRIAL DESIGN AND ETHICAL CONSIDERATIONS

The use of anti-TNF therapy in children with chronic diseases highlights important technical and ethical considerations. The use of a novel drug in children with severe JIA must address questions of safety and efficacy in the context of a patient group previously receiving complex long-term medication. A placebo-controlled study is not ethical or appropriate in this context. Lovell et al. needed to stop other disease-modifying drugs to demonstrate that beneficial effects were attributable to etanercept alone, and therefore treated all recruits with the trial medication before randomization (it being unethical to stop all disease-modifying medication in children with severe disease).[35] Other concerns included the management of

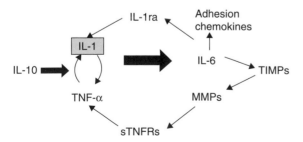

Figure 35.2 Positive and negative cytokine feedback. MMP, matrix metalloproteinase.

non-responders, the period of follow-up, and the interpretation of results thereafter, especially in a chronic disease characterized by relapses and remission. The open-label extension of the study addressed the problem of what to do at the end of a trial before the results were available and license obtained.[35]

Owing to concerns about long-term safety of this new group of drugs, and to identify long-term benefit, clear guidelines and a central registry to monitor responses and side effects are critical. This has now been established in the UK and in other European countries. The pediatric rule of the FDA in the USA has made early trials of new therapies possible in children, but other parts of the world still need to subscribe to such a policy. The pharmacokinetics and the dosages that would be efficacious are different in children and need to be adequately assessed. It is important to acknowledge, first, that JIA comprises a group of diseases which differ from RA and should be examined separately, and second, that children require treatment during unique periods of physiological and psychological change.

PRACTICAL MANAGEMENT OF NEW THERAPIES

In addition to resources being available for supervision nationally, the success of these new drugs requires appropriate local provision. The pediatric rheumatology nurse specialist's role is to provide effective practical, educational, and emotional support for the child and family. Guidance on administration, blood test monitoring, management of side effects (which may include injection site reactions), and appropriate response to infection are important aspects of continuing care. Effective education for both the patient and parents ensures understanding, appropriate expectations, and adherence to the new drug following many years of 'ineffective' treatment and uncontrolled disease activity. Cooperation will depend on a balance between their belief that this time 'it may work', and excessive faith in a new wonder drug.

CONCLUSION

The impact of etanercept on many children and their families has been dramatic, despite uncertainty about the long-term side effects and efficacy. Refinement of the use of TNF blockade, combination therapies, and alternative biologicals are being investigated, and in due course biologicals may be used to treat a wider cohort of children with less severe disease. To this end, vigilance and appropriate assessment of potential risks are paramount. Ultimately, these therapeutic developments may fundamentally alter our therapeutic approach to all chronic autoimmune diseases.

REFERENCES

1. Gare BA. Epidemiology. Baillieres Clin Rheumatol 1998; 12: 191–208.
2. Wallace CA. The use of methotrexate in childhood rheumatic diseases. Arthritis Rheum 1998; 41: 381–91.
3. Wallace CA. On beyond methotrexate: treatment of severe juvenile rheumatoid arthritis. Clin Exp Rheum 1999; 17: 499–504.
4. Martin K, Woo P. Outcome in JCA. Rev Rheum 1997; 64: 5242.
5. David J, Cooper C, Hickey L et al. The functional and psychological outcomes of juvenile chronic arthritis in young adulthood. Br J Rheumatol 1994; 33: 876–81.
6. Petty RE, Southwood TR, Baum J et al. Revision of the proposed classification criteria for juvenile idiopathic arthritis: Durban, 1997. J Rheumatol 1998; 25: 1991–4.
7. Wedderburn LR, Robinson N, Patel A et al. Selective recruitment of polarized T cells expressing CCR5 and CXCR3 to the inflamed joints of children with juvenile idiopathic arthritis. Arthritis Rheum 2000; 43: 765–74.
8. Murray KJ, Grom AA, Thompson SD et al. Contrasting cytokine profiles in the synovium of different forms of juvenile rheumatoid arthritis and juvenile spondyloarthropathy: prominence of interleukin 4 in restricted disease. J Rheumatol 1998; 25: 1388–98.
9. Raziuddin S, Bahabri S, Al-Dalaan A et al. A mixed Th1/Th2 cell cytokine response predominates in systemic onset juvenile rheumatoid arthritis: immunoregulatory IL-10 function. Clin Immunol Immunopathol 1998; 86: 192–8.
10. De Benedetti F, Ravelli A, Martini A. Cytokines in juvenile rheumatoid arthritis. Curr Opin Rheumatol 1997; 9: 428–33.
11. Rooney M, David J, Symons J et al. Inflammatory cytokine responses in juvenile chronic arthritis. Br J Rheumatol 1995; 34: 454–60.
12. Grom AA, Murray KJ, Luyrink L et al. Patterns of expression of tumor necrosis factor alpha, tumor necrosis factor beta and their receptors in synovia of

patients with juvenile rheumatoid arthritis and juvenile spondyloarthropathy. Arthritis Rheum 1996; 39: 1703–10.

13. De Benedetti F, Massa M, Pignatti P et al. Serum soluble interleukin-6 (IL-6) receptor and IL-6/soluble IL-6 receptor complex in systemic juvenile rheumatoid arthritis. J Clin Invest 1994; 93: 2114–9.

14. Keul R, Heinrich PC, Muller-Newen G et al. A possible role for soluble IL-6 receptor in the pathogenesis of systemic onset juvenile chronic arthritis. Cytokine 1998; 10: 729–34.

15. Prieur AM, Roux-Lombard P, Dayer JM. Dynamics of fever and the cytokine network in systemic juvenile arthritis. Rev Rhum Engl Ed 1996; 63: 163–70.

16. Rooney M, Varsani H, Martin K et al. Tumour necrosis factor alpha and its soluble receptors in juvenile chronic arthritis. Rheumatology 2000; 39: 432–8.

17. Prahalad S, Ryan MH, Shear ES et al. Juvenile rheumatoid arthritis: linkage to HLA demonstrated by allele sharing in affected sibpairs. Arthritis Rheum 2000; 43: 2335–8.

18. Crawley E, Kon S, Woo P. Hereditary predisposition to low interleukin-10 production in children with extended oligoarticular juvenile idiopathic arthritis. Rheumatology 2001; 40: 574–8.

19. Crawley E, Kay R, Sillibourne J et al. Polymorphic haplotypes of the interleukin-10 5′ flanking region determine variable interleukin-10 transcription and are associated with particular phenotypes of juvenile rheumatoid arthritis. Arthritis Rheum 1999; 42: 1101–8.

20. Lim S, Crawley E, Woo P, Barnes PJ. Haplotype associated with low interleukin-10 production in patients with severe asthma. Lancet 1998; 352: 113.

21. Fife MS, Gutierrez A, Ogilvie EM et al. Novel IL-10 gene family associations with systemic juventile idiopathic arthritis. Arthritis Res Ther (2006); 8: R148.

22. Ozen S, Alikasifoglu M, Bakkaloglu A et al. Tumour necrosis factor alpha G→A −238 and G→A −308 polymorphisms in juvenile idiopathic arthritis. Rheumatology 2002; 41(2): 223–7.

23. Date Y, Seki N, Kamizono S et al. Identification of a genetic risk factor for systemic juvenile rheumatoid arthritis in the 5′-flanking region of the TNF alpha gene and HLA genes. Arthritis Rheum 1999; 42: 2577–82.

24. Abraham LJ, Kroeger KM. Impact of the −308 TNF promoter polymorphism on the transcriptional regulation of the TNF gene: relevance to disease. J Leukoc Biol 1999; 66(4): 562–6.

25. Zeggini E, Thomson W, Kwiatkowski D et al. Linkage and association studies of single nucleotide polymorphism-tagged tumor necrosis factor haplotypes in juvenile oligoarthritis. Arthritis Rheum 2002; 46: 3304–11.

26. Donn R, Alourfi Z, De Benedetti F et al. Mutation screening of the macrophage migration inhibitory factor gene: positive association of a functional polymorphism of macrophage migration inhibitory factor with juvenile idiopathic arthritis. Arthritis Rheum 2002; 46: 2402–9.

27. Fishman D, Faulds G, Jeffery R et al. The effect of novel polymorphisms in the interleukin-6 (IL-6) gene on IL-6 transcription and plasma IL-6 levels, and an association with systemic onset juvenile chronic arthritis. J Clin Invest 1998; 102: 1369–76.

28. Ogilvie EM, Fife MS, Thompson SD et al. The -174G allele of the interleukin-6 gene confers susceptibility to systemic arthritis in children: a multicenter study using simplex and multiplex juvenile idiopathic arthritis families. Arthritis Rheum 2003 Nov; 48(11): 3202–6.

29. Auphan N, DiDonato JA, Rosette C et al. Immunosuppression by glucocorticoids: inhibition of NF-kappa B activity through induction of I kappa B synthesis. Science 1995; 270: 286–90.

30. Almawi WY, Beyhum HN, Rahme AA, Rieder MJ. Regulation of cytokine and cytokine receptor expression by glucocorticoids. J Leukoc Biol 1996; 60: 563–72.

31. Matsuda S, Koyasu S. Mechanisms of action of cyclosporine. Immunopharmacology 2000; 47(2–3): 119–25.

32. Sampaio EP, Sarno EN, Galilly R et al. Thalidomide selectively inhibits tumor necrosis factor α production by stimulating human monocytes. J Exp Med 1991; 173: 699–703.

33. Xu X, Williams JW, Bremer EG et al. Inhibition of protein tyrosine phosphorylation in T cells by a novel immunosuppressive agent, leflunomide. J Biol Chem 1995; 270: 12398–403.

34. Rothman D, Smith K, Kimura Y. Safety and efficacy of etanercept in children with JRA less than 4 years of age. Arthritis Rheum 2001; 44: S292 (abstract 1435).

35. Lovell DJ, Reiff A, Jones OY et al. Long-term and efficacy of etanercept in children with polyarticular-course juvenile rheumatoid arthritis. Arthritis Rheum 2006; 54: 1987–94.

36. Lovell DJ, Giannini EH, Passo M et al. Long-term efficacy of etanercept (ENBREL) in children with polyarticular-course juvenile rheumatoid arthritis. PRES 2001; 60 (Suppl 2): II17–II52.

37. Giannini EH, Ruperto N, Ravelli A et al. Preliminary definition of improvement in juvenile arthritis. Arthritis Rheum 1997; 40: 1202–9.

38. Kietz DA, Pepmueller PH, Moore TL. Clinical response to etanercept in polyarticular course juvenile rheumatoid arthritis. J Rheumatol 2001; 28: 360–2.

39. Reiff A, Henrickson M. Prolonged efficacy of etanercept in refractory juvenile ankylosing spondylitis. Arthritis Rheum 2001; 44: S292 (abstract 1434).

40. Brunner HI, Tomasi AL, Sherrard TM et al. Effectiveness and safety of etanercept for the treatment of juvenile rheumatoid arthritis (JRA) in clinical practice. Arthritis Rheum 2001; 44: S292 (abstract 1436).

41. Vinje E, Obiora O, Forre O. Juvenile chronic polyarthritis treated with infliximab. Ann Rheum Dis 2000; 59: 745 (abstract).

42. Billiau AD, Wouters C. Improved articular and systemic disease in a boy treated with anti-TNFα monoclonal antibody (Remicade) for refractory JIA. Ann Rheum Dis 2000; 59: 744 (abstract 11.20).

43. Gerloni V, Pontikaki I, Desiati F et al. Infliximab in the treatment of persistently active refractory juvenile idiopathic chronic arthritis. Ann Rheum Dis 2000; 59: 740 (abstract 1.4).

44. Kimura Y, Imundo LF, Li SC. High dose infliximab in the treatment of resistant systemic juvenile rheumatoid arthritis. Arthritis Rheum 2001; 44: S272 (abstract 1316).

45. Klareskog L, Moreland LM, Cohen SB et al. Global safety and efficacy of up to five years of etanercept (Enbrel) therapy. Arthritis Rheum 2001; 44: S77 (abstract 150).

46. De Rosa FG, Bonora S, Di Perri G. Tuberculosis and treatment with infliximab. N Engl J Med 2002; 346(8): 623–6.

47. Shakoor N, Michalska M, Harris CA, Block JA. Drug-induced systemic lupus erythematosus associated with etanercept therapy. Lancet 2002; 359: 579–80.

48. Jones RE, Moreland LW. Tumor necrosis factor inhibitors for rheumatoid arthritis. Bull Rheum Dis 1999; 48: 1–3.

49. Pascual V, Allantaz F, Arce E, Punaro M, Banchereau J. Role of interleukin-1 (IL-1) in the pathogenesis of systemic onset juvenile idiopathic arthritis and clinical response to IL-1 blockade. J Exp Med 2005; 201(9): 1479–86.

50. van Roon JA, Lafeber FP, Bijlsma JW. Synergistic activity of interleukin-4 and interleukin-10 in suppression of inflammation and joint destruction in rheumatoid arthritis. Arthritis Rheum. 2001; 44: 3–12.

51. Fellowes R, Etheridge CJ, Coade S et al. Amelioration of established collagen induced arthritis by systemic IL-10 gene delivery. Gene Ther 2000; 7: 967–77.

52. Lechman ER, Jaffurs D, Ghivizzani SC et al. Direct adenoviral gene transfer of viral IL-10 to rabbit knees with experimental arthritis ameliorates disease in both injected and contralateral control knees. J Immunol 1999; 163: 2202–8.

53. Minter RM, Ferry MA, Murday ME et al. Adenoviral delivery of human and viral IL-10 in murine sepsis. J Immunol 2001; 167: 1053–9.

54. Yokota S, Miyamae T, Imagawa T et al. Therapeutic efficacy of humanized recombinant anti-interleukin-6 receptor antibody in children with systemic-onset juvenile idiopathic arthritis. Arthritis Rheum. 2005; 52: 818–25.

55. Woo P, Wilkinson N, Prieur A M et al. Open label phase II trial of single, ascending doses of MRA in Caucasian children with severe systemic juvenile idiopathic arthritis: proof of principle of the efficacy of IL-6 receptor blockade in this type of arthritis and demonstration of prolonged clinical improvement. Arthritis Res Ther 2005; 7: R1281.

56. Edwards JC, Cambridge G, Abrahams VM. Do self-perpetuating B lymphocytes drive human autoimmune disease? Immunology 1999; 97: 188–96.

36

Update – systemic lupus erythematosus

Bevra H Hahn and Sonwoo Lee

Introduction • **Conventional therapies** • **Targeting B cells in SLE** • **Inhibition of costimulatory signals** • **Anti-cytokine therapy** • **Induction of regulatory/suppressive T cells** • **Autologous hematopoietic stem cell transplant (HSCT)** • **Complement therapy with anti-C5b** • **References**

INTRODUCTION

Systemic lupus erythematosus (SLE) is a multi-system autoimmune disorder with organ damage from autoantibodies and immune complexes, which activate complement, which causes infiltration of inflammatory cells. Clinical manifestations include polyarthritis, dermatitis, nephritis, cytopenias, vasculitis, pulmonitis, myocarditis, endocarditis, pleural and pericardial effusions, damage to central and peripheral nerves, and, particularly in patients with antibodies to phospholipids, fetal loss and clotting. Diagnosis requires one or more autoantibodies (including anti-nuclear antibody – ANA) and ≥ 1 typical organ manifestation. Criteria for classification as SLE for studies require ≥ 4 of 11 manifestations.[1,2] The mortality rate is approximately 10% over 10 years; nephritis and infections are the main causes of death.

Prognosis has improved in recent decades[3,4] with earlier detection and improved therapies, dialysis and renal transplantation, new vaccines, and improved antihypertensive and antimicrobial drugs. However, non-selective immunosuppressive drugs, mainstays of therapy, are associated with marked toxicity.[5] Recently identification of immunopathogenic mechanisms in lupus has allowed development of novel therapeutic agents. These new therapies are expected to be at least as effective as conventional therapies, and less toxic. An overview of novel therapeutic modalities for SLE is presented in Figure 36.1.

CONVENTIONAL THERAPIES

Until recently, clinical trials in SLE were avoided because of lack of financial support for treatments that are generic (e.g. corticosteroids and cyclophosphamide), relatively small numbers of patients, heterogeneity in clinical and laboratory manifestations, lack of a single biomarker or surrogate marker for disease activity that applies to all patients, and the natural disease course of flares alternating with improvement. Recently, several valid measures of disease activity, flares, and damage have been developed and used in drug trials.[6–8] Because universal measures of activity and progression of nephritis are available, effective therapies have been established in lupus nephritis. The 'gold standard' therapy for lupus proliferative glomerulonephritis (the 'NIH regimen') is a combination of high dose corticosteroids (1000 mg intravenous (i.v.) pulse of SoluMedrol followed by 60 mg daily doses of prednisone or equivalent for a few weeks, then tapered to as low a dose as possible) plus 6 monthly pulses of i.v. cyclophosphamide, 750 mg/m² of body surface area, followed by

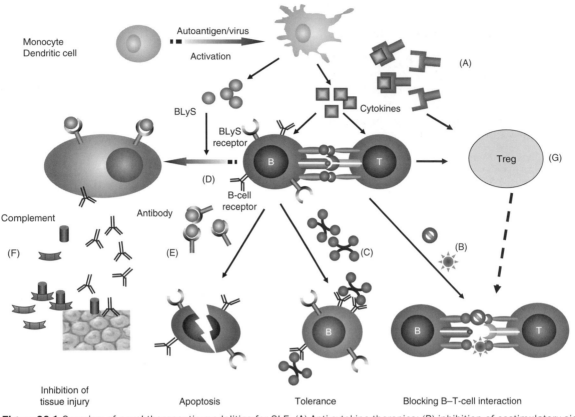

Figure 36.1 Overview of novel therapeutic modalities for SLE. (A) Anti-cytokine therapies; (B) inhibition of costimulatory signals using anti-CD40L or CTLA-4-Ig; (C) induction of B-cell tolerance using LJP-394; (D) eliminating B cells with anti-CD20, anti-CD22; (E) blocking survival signal for B cell by anti-BLyS; (F) inhibition of tissue injury by antibody against terminal complements; (G) induction of regulatory/inhibitory CD4+ and CD8+ T cells.

quarterly i.v. cyclophosphamide for an additional 2 years.[9–13] Although this treatment is effective in approximately 80% of patients and improves survival, relapse rates are high and toxicity is considerable. Adverse effects of corticosteroids include life-threatening infections, disfiguring weight gain, hypertension, diabetes, edema, cataract, ischemic necrosis of bone, osteoporosis, poor wound healing, emotional lability, acne, stretch marks, psychosis, and difficulty sleeping. Adverse effects of cyclophosphamide include life-threatening infections, cytopenias, malignancies, infertility, nausea, diarrhea, hair loss, hemorrhagic cystitis, and fatigue.

Variations in conventional therapies for severe SLE

Alterations in the NIH regimen have been tested to attain better response rates in shorter times and/or to miminize exposure to prolonged corticosteroid/immunosuppressive therapies. A prospective, blinded, controlled trial of high dose i.v. cyclophosphamide (50 mg/kg/day for 4 days), added to corticosteroids, with no subsequent cyclophosphamide was ultimately somewhat more effective for nephritis (but not for other SLE manifestations), but not less toxic than the NIH regimen.[14–17] The Euro-Lupus Nephritis Trial Group study[18,19] of lower doses of cyclophosphamide in a prospective, randomized trial comparing the NIH regimen to 500 mg of cyclophosphamide i.v. every 2 weeks for six doses, followed by daily azathioprine, showed similar efficacy to the higher doses of cyclophosphamide in the NIH regimen; side effects were somewhat, although not significantly, less. The patients in this trial were almost all Caucasian; results may not apply to other ethnic groups.

Substitution of mycophenolate mofetil for cyclophosphamide in conventional therapies.

Substituting a safer cytotoxic drug for cyclophosphamide has been successful in some patients. A randomized, prospective controlled trial in Hong Kong of MMF (mycophenolate mofetil) in lupus patients with proliferative nephritis showed comparable efficacy at 12 months between daily oral MMF and daily oral cyclophosphamide given for 6 months, then followed by azathioprine maintenance. The low cyclophosphamide group had less drug-related toxicity.[20] In fact, after a median follow-up of 5 years, the groups had similar outcomes, but serious infections were lower in the MMF group.[21] Doses of mycophenolate were gradually reduced after the initial year of therapy, but when doses were low, the relapse rate was higher in MMF than in the cyclophosphamide/ azathioprine group, suggesting the necessity of long-term therapy in this patient subset. Later, a randomized controlled study[22] looking at efficacy of MMF or azathioprine or quarterly i.v. cyclophosphamide as maintenance therapies, following induction of improvement with six doses of cyclophosphamide monthly i.v. (500–750 mg/m²), demonstrated that the 72-month event-free survival rate and relapse-free survival rate were better in groups maintained with MMF or azathioprine than with quarterly i.v. cyclophosphamide. Adverse effects were also lower in MMF or azathioprine groups. Finally, a recent study[23] randomizing patients with severe proliferative lupus nephritis into initial therapy with the NIH cyclophosphamide regimen or MMF 3 g per day as induction therapy showed that by 6 months higher proportions of patients were improved in the MMF group. Improvement occurred in 52% of MMF-treated patients compared with 30% of cyclophosphamide patients. Furthermore, the rate of life-threatening infections was lower in MMF, although that of diarrhea was higher.

In summary, MMF is a reasonable and safer choice than cyclophosphamide for inducing or maintaining improvement in severe lupus nephritis, and either MMF or azathioprine may be superior to cyclophosphamide in maintaining improvement once it is achieved. There are no controlled trials to say that MMF is as effective as or better than cyclophosphamide in any life-threatening aspect of SLE other than nephritis. Furthermore, in the authors' experience, some patients with lupus nephritis respond better to cyclophosphamide than to MMF (and vice versa), so it is premature to say that MMF should replace cyclophosphamide in the management of severe nephritis or other life-threatening manifestations of SLE. With MMF, duration of therapy, tapering schedules, and management of refractory or relapsing disease (seen with all regimens) are yet to be established.

TARGETING B CELLS IN SLE

B lymphocytes play important roles in initiation, propagation, and amplification of autoimmunity.[24] They are precursors to plasma cells that secrete pathogenic autoantibodies, and serve as antigen-presenting cells that activate helper T cells. Therapies that deplete/inactivate B cells or subsets are under intense study.

Anti-CD20

CD20 is a surface antigen expressed on all B cells from pre-B through mature B; it is not expressed on plasma cells.[25] Rituximab (IDEC-C2B8, MabThera, Rituxan) is a chimeric humanized monoclonal antibody (mAb) to CD20 composed of a human IgG1 kappa constant region and a variable region of murine anti-CD20. It mediates complement and antibody-dependent cell-mediated cytotoxicity with direct antiproliferative effects against B-cell lines *in vitro*,[26] depletes peripheral B cells, and down-regulates costimulatory molecule.[27,28] Rituximab has been FDA-approved for treatment of low grade B-cell lymphoma and for rheumatoid arthritis (RA)[29,30] (http://arthritis.about.com/od/mabtherarituxan 2006). In open trials in autoimmune diseases, it has been acceptably safe (adverse effects include infusion reactions, arrhythmias, and possibly increased infection rates), and it has been efficacious in approximately 50% of patients with chronic idiopathic thrombocytopenic purpura (ITP),[31] and autoimmune hemolytic anemia.[32] In seropositive RA, a controlled prospective randomized trial demonstrated efficacy.[33,34] Open trials in SLE patients[35–38] have been promising. In one trial,[36] 17 of 24 patients (failing standard treatments) improved. Reduction of anti-dsDNA antibodies was modest. B-cell depletion persisted for 3–6 months on average (for years in one patient) and clinical improvement lasted for 12 months in most.[35–39–41] Some patients relapsed when the B cells started to repopulate the immune system; others did not. Rituximab doses that depleted B cells were more likely to suppress disease activity than smaller doses. Four weekly doses of 375 mg/m^2, two weekly doses of 1000 mg (full dose), or two weekly doses of 500 mg (half dose) were effective in some patients and showed more sustained reduction in global disease activity (BILAG or SLAM) and improvement in serological and renal parameters than did lower doses.[37,39] Some investigators give rituximab concomitantly with 750 mg i.v. cyclophosphamide; all give high dose i.v. corticosteroids with each infusion, which probably reduces infusion reactions. The frequency of human antichimeric antibody (HACA) production in SLE patients is significantly higher than in lymphoma patients.[39,42] HACA may abolish efficacy of rituximab.[43] Its production is associated with lower doses of rituximab, less depletion of B cells, higher baseline SLAM scores, African–American ancestry, and repeated treatments.[37] Large multicenter double-blind placebo-controlled clinical trials with rituximab in SLE are in progress. However, questions regarding optimal dose, durability of response, need to give therapy for one round and then as needed, or on a regular basis, escape from response related to HACA, appropriate combination therapies, and long-term side effects will probably require additional studies.

Other mAbs against B-cell surface markers are available for study, including fully humanized anti-CD20[41,44] and anti-CD22.[45] The humanized anti-CD20 might be less likely to induce HACA. Anti-CD22 should be similar in action to anti-CD20, but has the theoretical advantage of delivery of toxins to B cells via antibody conjugates, since CD22 is internalized upon ligation.[46]

LJP-394

LJP-394 (abetimus sodium, Riquent) is a synthetic B-cell tolerogen composed of four oligonucleotide epitopes attached to a nonimmunogenic polyethylene glycol platform. Acting as antigen, it cross-links anti-dsDNA antibodies on the surface of autoreactive B cells, theoretically leading to their anergy or deletion.

It is possible that it works by binding antibody, thus forming immune complexes that can be eliminated from the body. In a prospective, randomized double-blind trial (16 weekly i.v. doses of 100 mg) in lupus nephritis, serum levels of anti-dsDNA fell and C3 rose in the LJP-394 treated group, but time to renal flare was not significantly different compared to controls.[47,48] Further analysis of a subgroup of patients with high affinity antibodies to LJP-394 and higher serum creatinine levels (Cr $\geq$ 1.5 mg/dl), showed significant reduction in time to renal flare, time to increased immunosuppressive treatment, and improved HRQOL (health-related quality of life).[49] LJP-394 was well tolerated. At present, LJP-394 is a novel B-cell 'tolerogen', probably effective in nephritis patients with high affinity antibody. Additional studies are planned to clarify its clinical application for either induction or maintenance therapy.

INHIBITION OF COSTIMULATORY SIGNALS

Anti-CD40

CD40 ligand (CD40L, CD154) on activated immune cells (mainly T cells) or platelets binds with CD40 on the surface of B cells, APCs (antigen-presenting cells), or vascular endothelial cells.[50–53] This interaction provides costimulatory signals that activate B cells, APCs, and vascular endothelial cells.[54–58]

Increased expression of CD40L on multiple cells in SLE patients promotes pathogenic autoantibody production and glomerulonephritis.[59–62] Blockade of the CD40–CD40L pathway has been effective in animal models of lupus.[63–66] Two humanized anti-CD40L mAbs (IDEC-131 and BG9588) were tested in SLE patients. Treatment with IDEC-131 failed to demonstrate clinical efficacy over placebo in a double-blind, placebo-controlled study.[67] Although BG9588 therapy in patients with proliferative glomerulonephritis reduced anti-dsDNA antibodies, increased C3 levels, and decreased hematuria, the study was terminated prematurely due to unexpected thromboembolic complications.[68] While blocking CD40–CD40L interaction retards atherogenesis, CD40L is necessary to maintain stability in thrombi; blocking CD40L on platelets might permit instability in thrombi resulting in thromboembolism. This problem might discourage additional human trials in the near future.

CTLA-4 –Ig

Surface expression of CTLA-4 is restricted to activated and memory T cells.[69] CTLA-4 binds B7 molecules with much higher avidity than CD28 (which provides costimulatory signals for T cells).[70–72] Therefore, ligation between CTLA-4 and B7 molecules (a) suppresses CD28-mediated T-cell activation, and (b) induces anergy or apoptosis by blocking survival signals or by inducing release of tolerogenic IDO (indoleamine 2,3-dioxygenase) from dendritic cells.[73–76] CTLA-4 ligation inhibits T-cell-dependent antibody production by B cells.[77–80] CTLA-4-Ig (abatacept, belatacept), a fusion protein of the extracellular domain of CTLA-4 and the Fc portion of human IgG1, was engineered to block CD28–B7 interaction. Prospective, double-blind, randomized studies of abatacept demonstrated clinical efficacy in patients with RA (the US FDA has approved its use in RA), psoriasis, and allogenic bone marrow transplantation.[73,81–84] Combination therapy with CTLA-4-Ig and cyclophosphamide dramatically reduced proteinuria, autoantibody production, and mortality in a murine model of active lupus nephritis.[85,86] Clinical trials in SLE patients have been designed and are expected to begin soon.

Anti-BLyS

B-lymphocyte stimulator (BLyS; BAFF, TALL-1, THANK, and zTNF4) is a member of the tumor necrosis factor (TNF) ligand superfamily; it is expressed on the surface membrane of myeloid cells and released as a soluble protein.[87] Its expression is regulated by interferon (IFN)-γ, IFN-α, interleukin (IL)-10, and CD40L.[87–89] Interactions of BLyS with its receptors (TACI, BCMA, and BAFF-R) on B cells support maturation, differentiation, and survival of B cells by activation of NF-κB via TRAF and up-regulation of anti-apoptotic bcl-2 family proteins.[90] Experiments using receptor knockout mice show that ligation of each receptor results in different biologic functions. In B cells, BAFF-R mediates a survival signal, whereas TACI ligation transmits a negative signal.[91,92] Excessive BLyS/BAFF expression occurs in some patients with SLE, RA, and Sjögren's syndrome.[93] Elevated levels in blood are generally correlated with disease activity and autoantibody titers (RF and anti-dsDNA).[94] Moreover, treatment with soluble BLyS decoy receptors (TACI-Ig or BAFFR-Ig) in lupus-prone mice resulted in decreased disease progression and improved survival.[95–97] Human anti-BLyS mAb (LymphoStat-B) showed adequate safety in phase I human trials.[98] In one phase II trial, the impact on the SLEDAI measure of disease activity was not significantly different from placebo, although levels of anti-DNA were reduced (Human Genome Sciences, press release 10/05/05). Additional phase II/III studies in SLE of LymphoStat-B, TACI-Ig (which is effective in murine lupus[96]) or BAFF inhibitors are awaited.

ANTI-CYTOKINE THERAPY

Up-regulation of IL-10, IL-6, IL-18, type 1 IFNs, IFN-γ, IL-1, and TNF-α has been found in murine and human SLE. In humans, levels of expression tend to correlate with disease activity.[99–105] Anti-dsDNA and immune complexes stimulate release of these proinflammatory cytokines from dendritic, mononuclear, T, and endothelial cells.[106,107] Other inflammatory cytokines involved in pathogenesis (IL-18, IFN-γ) also up-regulate IL-6, IL-1, and TNF-α.[101] Therefore, these cytokines are reasonable targets for lupus therapy.

Anti-IL10

IL-10 regulates apoptosis of lymphoid cells and potentiates autoantibody production in lupus.[108,109] Serum levels and secretion by peripheral blood mononuclear cells are increased in SLE patients; in some studies high levels correlate with disease activity.[102,108] Administration of IL-10 accelerated renal disease; anti IL-10 mAb delayed its onset in a murine lupus model.[110] In a small open-label study,[111] anti-IL-10 murine mAb was administered for 3 weeks to steroid-dependent lupus patients. Observation for 6 months showed improvement of dermatitis, arthritis, MEX-SLEDAI scores (Mexican version of the Systemic Lupus Disease Activity Index), and daily steroid dose, with reduction of serum IL-10 levels. However, all six patients developed antibodies against the murine mAb, making it unlikely that this particular mAb can be used. Development of a humanized mAb might permit additional trials.

Anti-IL-6R mAb

Secretion of serum and urinary IL-6 is increased in active lupus.[112,113] IL-6 promotes B-lymphocyte maturation and mesangial cell proliferation, and blocks suppression by $CD4^+CD25^+$ regulatory T cells.[114,115] Exogenous IL-6 accelerated progression of glomerulonephritis; anti-IL-6 receptor (anti-IL-6R) suppressed anti-DNA production, delayed proteinuria, and improved survival in murine SLE.[116,117] Treatment with humanized anti-IL-6R (MRA, Tocilizumab, containing CDR from mouse anti-human IL6R fused with human IgG) was well tolerated and reduced disease activity in a multicenter, double-blind, placebo-controlled trial of RA and in smaller, open trials in juvenile inflammatory arthritis (JIA), adult-onset Still's disease, Crohn's disease, and Castleman's disease.[118–120] A clinical trial in SLE is in progress.

Anti-TNF-α

The role of TNF-α in the pathogenesis of lupus remains unclear. As a proinflammatory cytokine, it activates immune cells and endothelial cells, and induces adhesion molecules and other proinflammatory cytokines such as IL-1 and IL-6. While it participates in the pathophysiology of some autoimmune disease like RA, Crohn's disease, or spondyloarthropathy, its blocking may promote autoimmunity. Clinical trials showed that anti-TNF therapy in patients with other autoimmune disease may develop lupus-like

syndromes with anti-nuclear antibodies, anti-dsDNA (IgM isotype in about 7–16% in RA), and anti-cardiolipin antibodies; discontinuance of TNF blockade ameliorated symptoms and titers of autoantibodies.[121,122] In contrast, TNF-α was detected in the serum and renal tissues in lupus patients and its levels were correlated with disease activity.[123,124] In an open-label pilot study in six refractory lupus patients, four doses of infliximab induced reduction of proteinuria and disease activity with resolution of arthritis.[125] Arthritis relapsed 2 or 3 months after the last dose of infliximab, but decreased proteinuria lasted for several months. Although titers of anti-dsDNA antibody (IgG isotypes) and anti-cardiolipin antibody were increased with infliximab administration, it was transient and not associated with flare of disease. Double-blind, placebo-controlled multicenter trials are anticipated to evaluate safety and clinical efficacy for SLE patients.

Anti-IL-1

Increased levels of IL-1 were detected in the spinal fluid of CNS lupus patients and in the kidneys of human and murine SLE (MRL/lpr and NZB/W F1 mice).[126–128] Stimulating normal human mononuclear cells with anti-dsDNA resulted in release of IL-1.[106] Administration of low doses of IL-1 accelerated glomerulonephritis in the NZB/W F1 mice, but administration of its soluble receptor antagonist (IL-1Ra, Kineret) did not improve established nephritis in MRL/lpr mice.[126,129] Two small open-label studies in lupus patients with refractory arthritis showed transient benefit and acceptable safety.[130,131] IL-1Ra has not yet been investigated in lupus nephritis patients.

Type 1 interferons (IFN-α, IFN-β)

Recently several laboratories have reported that a characteristic 'signature' of gene expression in the peripheral blood leukocytes of SLE patients is elevated expression of IFN-inducible genes.[99,100,103] Some genes are up-regulated primarily by type 1 IFNs, although IFN-γ also regulates many of them. Furthermore, lupus-prone mice with the receptors for type1 IFN knocked out are protected from disease.[132] There is great interest in developing inhibitors of type 1 IFN binding for potential clinical trials.

INDUCTION OF REGULATORY/SUPPRESSIVE T CELLS

A strategy of recent interest is to control clinical autoimmunity by inducing T cells that can down-regulate it. Several T-cell subsets have this capability. Among CD4+CD25+ T cells in the periphery are cells that express CTLA-4 and also up-regulate expression of Foxp3.[133,134] Those cells suppress autoantibody formation – some by inhibiting proliferation of helper CD4+ T cells, and others by direct suppression of B-cell production of Ig. In addition, there are subsets of CD8+ T cells which can also suppress proliferation in CD4+ helper T-cells.[135] With regard to SLE, two strategies have been successful in inducing several of these CD4+ and CD8+ regulatory/inhibitory T-cell subsets. One has been to educate peripheral lymphocytes by incubation with IL-2 and transforming growth factor (TGF)-β, which generates regulatory cells;[133,136] such educated cells could then be re-infused. This strategy should be adaptable to human use in the near future. The second method is to inject on a regular basis short, soluble peptides from autoantigens which induce regulatory/inhibitory T cells powerful enough to suppress autoreactive cells and disease in murine lupus models. Peptides which have been clinically successful in these models have been derived from Ig of antibodies to DNA,[134,135,137,138] histones in nucleosomal antigen,[139] the D1 peptide of Sm,[140] and the 70 K protein of U1RNP.[141] One of the Ig-derived peptides, edratide,[138] which is injected subcutaneously once a week, seemed safe in a phase I clinical trial in patients with SLE, and is currently in phase II trials to assess efficacy.

AUTOLOGOUS HEMATOPOIETIC STEM CELL TRANSPLANT (HSCT)

Multiple case reports record improvement of coincidental autoimmune diseases (RA, SSc, SLE, JIA, or MS, etc.) in patients receiving HSCT for other disorders, and there have been excellent results in animal models of autoimmune disease with experimental stem cell transplantation. These reports suggested that HSCT is a viable option for severe autoimmune disease that is refractory to conventional therapy.[142,143]

Data from the European Group for Blood and Marrow Transplantation (EMBT) showed a remission rate of 66% in SLE patients, with partial remission in an additional 14% following autologous HSCT. Remission was defined as SLEDAI ≤ 3 and dose of prednisolone ≤ 10 mg/day.[144,145] Relapse occurred in 32% of those patients within 40 months. Unfortunately, 16% of patients died within 6 months after HSCT. These data must be interpreted with the realization that patients included in all the trials were refractory to standard therapies for SLE. In the most recent US study[146,147] the probability of disease-free survival was 50% at 5 years, and overall survival was 86%. Most of the deaths were from recurrent active SLE, and several were from infections. It is likely that careful patient selection and standardized techniques will be useful in future studies. Autologous HSCT is safer than allogeneic HSCT because it avoids complications related to graft-versus-host responses, but allogeneic HSCT might be more effective to eradicate autoantigen-reactive progenitor cells. A phase II HSCT trial has been designed in the USA to compare efficacy of HSCT to current standard care in patients refractory to usual therapeutic approaches.

COMPLEMENT THERAPY WITH ANTI-C5b

Pathophysiologic roles of the complement system are complex in lupus. While complement activation is a marker of active SLE as it correlates with disease activity, deficiency of its early components predisposes or accelerates lupus nephritis.[148] Early components of the classical pathway like C1q protect from emerging autoimmunity via clearance of immune complexes or apoptotic cell debris, but the late components (C5b-9) formed after activation of C3 to C3a are involved in renal injury.[149–151] Classical, alternative, and lectin complement pathways are activated in human and murine lupus. In particular, self-perpetuating activation of the alternative pathway plays a major role in lupus nephritis after the classical pathway initiates activation of the alternative pathway. Reduced disease activity in lupus-prone mice with deficient alternative components (factor B or D) supports the role of that pathway.[149] Blocking C3 or C5 activation has been a goal for complement-targeted therapy, because activation of both pathways results in cleaving of those components and produces MAC (membrane attack complex C5b-9). Anti-C5 mAb was effective in murine SLE; thus humanized chimeric mAb to complement 5 (eculizumab, h5G1.1-mAb:the CDR from mouse anti-human C5 fused with human IgG2 F(ab)' region and with a human IgG4 Fc region) was designed. A multicenter randomized placebo-controlled phase II trial of eculizumab in 122 patients with idiopathic membranous glomerulonephritis did not show differences in outcomes between the treatment and placebo groups.[152] However, this result may have been influenced by the short duration of therapy – perhaps insufficient for biologic effects to result in disease improvement. Eculizumab therapy had acceptable safety, and further studies are awaited.

In summary, advanced understanding of the immuno-pathogenesis of lupus has translated into several novel therapeutic strategies which target specific immunologic reactions. As more biologic agents are tested, the effective therapeutic regimens will emerge. It is likely that greater benefits will occur when effective biologics are combined with some of the standard, current, less targeted therapies, and/or that combinations of biologics will be more effective than single agents. We look forward to developing treatments that are safer and better targeted for each patient with SLE.

REFERENCES

1. Tan EM, Cohen AS, Fries JF et al. The 1982 revised criteria for the classification of systemic lupus erythematosus. Arthritis Rheum 1982; 25(11): 1271–7.

2. Hochberg MC. Updating the American College of Rheumatology revised criteria for the classification of systemic lupus erythematosus. Arthritis Rheum 1997; 40(9): 1725.

3. Korbet SM, Lewis EJ, Schwartz MM et al. Factors predictive of outcome in severe lupus nephritis. Lupus Nephritis Collaborative Study Group. Am J Kidney Dis 2000; 35(5): 904–14.

4. Bongu A, Chang E, Ramsey-Goldman R. Can morbidity and mortality of SLE be improved? Best Pract Res Clin Rheumatol 2002; 16(2): 313–32.

5. Pryor BD, Bologna SG, Kahl LE. Risk factors for serious infection during treatment with cyclophosphamide and high-dose corticosteroids for systemic lupus erythematosus. Arthritis Rheum 1996; 39(9): 1475–82.

6. Griffiths B, Mosca M, Gordon C. Assessment of patients with systemic lupus erythematosus and the use of lupus disease activity indices. Best Pract Res Clin Rheumatol 2005; 19(5): 685–708.

7. Buyon JP, Petri MA, Kim MY et al. The effect of combined estrogen and progesterone hormone replacement therapy on disease activity in systemic lupus erythematosus: a randomized trial. Ann Intern Med 2005; 142(12 Pt 1): 953–62.

8. Petri M, Kim MY, Kalunian KC et al. Combined oral contraceptives in women with systemic lupus erythematosus. N Engl J Med 2005; 353(24): 2550–8.

9. Takada K, Illei GG, Boumpas DT. Cyclophosphamide for the treatment of systemic lupus erythematosus. Lupus 2001; 10(3): 154–61.

10. Bansal VK, Beto JA. Treatment of lupus nephritis: a meta-analysis of clinical trials. Am J Kidney Dis 1997; 29(2): 193–9.

11. Illei GG, Austin HA, Crane M et al. Combination therapy with pulse cyclophosphamide plus pulse methylprednisolone improves long-term renal outcome without adding toxicity in patients with lupus nephritis. Ann Intern Med 2001; 135(4): 248–57.

12. Gourley MF, Austin HA, III, Scott D et al. Methylprednisolone and cyclophosphamide, alone or in combination, in patients with lupus nephritis. A randomized, controlled trial. Ann Intern Med 1996; 125(7): 549–57.

13. Austin HA III, Klippel JH, Balow JE et al. Therapy of lupus nephritis. Controlled trial of prednisone and cytotoxic drugs. N Engl J Med 1986; 314(10): 614–19.

14. Brodsky RA, Petri M, Smith BD et al. Immunoablative high-dose cyclophosphamide without stem-cell rescue for refractory, severe autoimmune disease. Ann Intern Med 1998; 129(12): 1031–5.

15. Petri M, Jones RJ, Brodsky RA. High-dose cyclophosphamide without stem cell transplantation in systemic lupus erythematosus. Arthritis Rheum 2003; 48(1): 166–73.

16. Petri M, Brodsky R. High-dose cyclophosphamide and stem cell transplantation for refractory systemic lupus erythematosus. JAMA 2006; 295(5): 559–60.

17. Petri M, Brodsky R, Jones R, Brodsky I, Magder L. High-dose cyclophosphamide vs monthly cyclophosphamde: eighteen month results. Arthritis Rheum 2005; 52: 539–40.

18. Houssiau FA, Vasconcelos C, D'Cruz D et al. Immunosuppressive therapy in lupus nephritis: the Euro-Lupus Nephritis Trial, a randomized trial of

low-dose versus high-dose intravenous cyclophosphamide. Arthritis Rheum 2002; 46(8): 2121–31.

19. Houssiau FA, Vasconcelos C, D'Cruz D et al. Early response to immunosuppressive therapy predicts good renal outcome in lupus nephritis: lessons from long-term followup of patients in the Euro-Lupus Nephritis Trial. Arthritis Rheum 2004; 50(12): 3934–40.

20. Chan TM, Li FK, Tang CS et al. Efficacy of mycophenolate mofetil in patients with diffuse proliferative lupus nephritis. Hong Kong-Guangzhou Nephrology Study Group. N Engl J Med 2000; 343(16): 1156–62.

21. Chan TM, Tse KC, Tang CS, Mok MY, Li FK. Long-term study of mycophenolate mofetil as continuous induction and maintenance treatment for diffuse proliferative lupus nephritis. J Am Soc Nephrol 2005; 16(4): 1076–84.

22. Contreras G, Pardo V, Leclercq B et al. Sequential therapies for proliferative lupus nephritis. N Engl J Med 2004; 350(10): 971–80.

23. Ginzler EM, Dooley MA, Aranow C et al. Mycophenolate mofetil or intravenous cyclophosphamide for lupus nephritis. N Engl J Med 2005; 353(21): 2219–28.

24. Lipsky PE. Systemic lupus erythematosus: an autoimmune disease of B cell hyperactivity. Nat Immunol 2001; 2(9): 764–6.

25. Stashenko P, Nadler LM, Hardy R, Schlossman SF. Characterization of a human B lymphocyte-specific antigen. J Immunol 1980; 125(4): 1678–85.

26. Alas S, Ng CP, Bonavida B. Rituximab modifies the cisplatin-mitochondrial signaling pathway, resulting in apoptosis in cisplatin-resistant non-Hodgkin's lymphoma. Clin Cancer Res 2002; 8(3): 836–45.

27. Reff ME, Carner K, Chambers KS et al. Depletion of B cells in vivo by a chimeric mouse human monoclonal antibody to CD20. Blood 1994; 83(2): 435–45.

28. Tokunaga M, Fujii K, Saito K et al. Down-regulation of CD40 and CD80 on B cells in patients with life-threatening systemic lupus erythematosus after successful treatment with rituximab. Rheumatology (Oxford) 2005; 44(2): 176–82.

29. Grillo-Lopez AJ, White CA, Varns C et al. Overview of the clinical development of rituximab: first monoclonal antibody approved for the treatment of lymphoma. Semin Oncol 1999; 26(5 Suppl 14): 66–73.

30. Hainsworth JD, Burris HA III, Morrissey LH et al. Rituximab monoclonal antibody as initial systemic therapy for patients with low-grade non-Hodgkin lymphoma. Blood 2000; 95(10): 3052–6.

31. Stasi R, Pagano A, Stipa E, Amadori S. Rituximab chimeric anti-CD20 monoclonal antibody treatment for adults with chronic idiopathic thrombocytopenic purpura. Blood 2001; 98(4): 952–7.

32. Perrotta S, Locatelli F, La MA et al. Anti-CD20 monoclonal antibody (Rituximab) for life-threatening autoimmune haemolytic anaemia in a patient with

systemic lupus erythematosus. Br J Haematol 2002; 116(2): 465–7.

33. Edwards JC, Leandro MJ, Cambridge G. B lymphocyte depletion therapy with rituximab in rheumatoid arthritis. Rheum Dis Clin North Am 2004; 30(2): 393–403, viii.

34. Edwards JC, Szczepanski L, Szechinski J et al. Efficacy of B-cell-targeted therapy with rituximab in patients with rheumatoid arthritis. N Engl J Med 2004; 350(25): 2572–81.

35. Leandro MJ, Edwards JC, Cambridge G, Ehrenstein MR, Isenberg DA. An open study of B lymphocyte depletion in systemic lupus erythematosus. Arthritis Rheum 2002; 46(10): 2673–7.

36. Leandro MJ, Cambridge G, Edwards JC, Ehrenstein MR, Isenberg DA. B-cell depletion in the treatment of patients with systemic lupus erythematosus: a longitudinal analysis of 24 patients. Rheumatology (Oxford) 2005; 44(12): 1542–5.

37. Looney RJ, Anolik JH, Campbell D et al. B cell depletion as a novel treatment for systemic lupus erythematosus: a phase I/II dose-escalation trial of rituximab. Arthritis Rheum 2004; 50(8): 2580–9.

38. Sfikakis PP, Boletis JN, Lionaki S et al. Remission of proliferative lupus nephritis following B cell depletion therapy is preceded by down-regulation of the T cell costimulatory molecule CD40 ligand: an open-label trial. Arthritis Rheum 2005; 52(2): 501–13.

39. Looney RJ, Anolik J, Sanz I. B lymphocytes in systemic lupus erythematosus: lessons from therapy targeting B cells. Lupus 2004; 13(5): 381–90.

40. Ng KP, Leandro MJ, Edwards JC et al. Repeated B cell depletion in treatment of refractory systemic lupus erythematosus. Ann Rheum Dis 2006; 65: 942–5.

41. Tahir H, Isenberg DA. Novel therapies in lupus nephritis. Lupus 2005; 14(1): 77–82.

42. McLaughlin P, Grillo Lopez AJ, Link BK et al. Rituximab chimeric anti-CD20 monoclonal antibody therapy for relapsed indolent lymphoma: half of patients respond to a four-dose treatment program. J Clin Oncol 1998; 16(8): 2825–33.

43. Saito K, Nawata M, Iwata S, Tokunaga M, Tanaka Y. Extremely high titer of anti-human chimeric antibody following re-treatment with rituximab in a patient with active systemic lupus erythematosus. Rheumatology (Oxford) 2005; 44(11): 1462–4.

44. Stein R, Qu Z, Chen S et al. Characterization of a new humanized anti-CD20 monoclonal antibody, IMMU-106, and its use in combination with the humanized anti-CD22 antibody, epratuzumab, for the therapy of non-Hodgkin's lymphoma. Clin Cancer Res 2004; 10(8): 2868–78.

45. Leonard JP, Coleman M, Ketas J et al. Combination antibody therapy with epratuzumab and rituximab in

relapsed or refractory non-Hodgkin's lymphoma. J Clin Oncol 2005; 23(22): 5044–51.

46. Carnahan J, Wang P, Kendall R et al. Epratuzumab, a humanized monoclonal antibody targeting CD22: characterization of in vitro properties. Clin Cancer Res 2003; 9(10 Pt 2): 3982S–3990S.

47. Furie RA, Cash JM, Cronin ME et al. Treatment of systemic lupus erythematosus with LJP 394. J Rheumatol 2001; 28(2): 257–65.

48. Alarcon-Segovia D, Tumlin JA, Furie RA et al. LJP 394 for the prevention of renal flare in patients with systemic lupus erythematosus: results from a randomized, double-blind, placebo-controlled study. Arthritis Rheum 2003; 48(2): 442–54.

49. Strand V, Aranow C, Cardiel MH et al. Improvement in health-related quality of life in systemic lupus erythematosus patients enrolled in a randomized clinical trial comparing LJP 394 treatment with placebo. Lupus 2003; 12(9): 677–86.

50. Toubi E, Shoenfeld Y. The role of CD40-CD154 interactions in autoimmunity and the benefit of disrupting this pathway. Autoimmunity 2004; 37: 457–64.

51. Yellin MJ, Brett J, Baum D et al. Functional interactions of T cells with endothelial cells: the role of CD40L-CD40-mediated signals. J Exp Med 1995; 182(6): 1857–64.

52. Hollenbaugh D, Mischel-Petty N, Edwards CP et al. Expression of functional CD40 by vascular endothelial cells. J Exp Med 1995; 182(1): 33–40.

53. Sidiropoulos PI, Boumpas DT. Lessons learned from anti-CD40L treatment in systemic lupus erythematosus patients. Lupus 2004; 13(5): 391–7.

54. Lederman S, Yellin MJ, Cleary AM et al. T-BAM/CD40-L on helper T lymphocytes augments lymphokine-induced B cell Ig isotype switch recombination and rescues B cells from programmed cell death. J Immunol 1994; 152(5): 2163–71.

55. Renshaw BR, Fanslow WC III, Armitage RJ et al. Humoral immune responses in CD40 ligand-deficient mice. J Exp Med 1994; 180(5): 1889–900.

56. Barrett TB, Shu G, Clark EA. CD40 signaling activates CD11a/CD18 (LFA-1)-mediated adhesion in B cells. J Immunol 1991; 146(6): 1722–9.

57. Grammer AC, Lipsky PE. CD154-CD40 interactions mediate differentiation to plasma cells in healthy individuals and persons with systemic lupus erythematosus. Arthritis Rheum 2002; 46(6): 1417–29.

58. Mach F, Schonbeck U, Sukhova GK et al. Functional CD40 ligand is expressed on human vascular endothelial cells, smooth muscle cells, and macrophages: implications for CD40-CD40 ligand signaling in atherosclerosis. Proc Natl Acad Sci U S A 1997; 94(5): 1931–6.

59. Koshy M, Berger D, Crow MK. Increased expression of CD40 ligand on systemic lupus erythematosus lymphocytes. J Clin Invest 1996; 98(3): 826–37.

60. Desai-Mehta A, Lu L, Ramsey-Goldman R, Datta SK. Hyperexpression of CD40 ligand by B and T cells in human lupus and its role in pathogenic autoantibody production. J Clin Invest 1996; 97(9): 2063–73.

61. Devi BS, Van NS, Krausz T, Davies KA. Peripheral blood lymphocytes in SLE—hyperexpression of CD154 on T and B lymphocytes and increased number of double negative T cells. J Autoimmun 1998; 11(5): 471–5.

62. Yellin MJ, D'Agati V, Parkinson G et al. Immunohistologic analysis of renal CD40 and CD40L expression in lupus nephritis and other glomerulonephritides. Arthritis Rheum 1997; 40(1): 124–34.

63. Kalled SL, Cutler AH, Datta SK, Thomas DW. Anti-CD40 ligand antibody treatment of SNF1 mice with established nephritis: preservation of kidney function. J Immunol 1998; 160(5): 2158–65.

64. Quezada SA, Eckert M, Adeyi OA et al. Distinct mechanisms of action of anti-CD154 in early versus late treatment of murine lupus nephritis. Arthritis Rheum 2003; 48(9): 2541–54.

65. Wang X, Huang W, Schiffer LE et al. Effects of anti-CD154 treatment on B cells in murine systemic lupus erythematosus. Arthritis Rheum 2003; 48(2): 495–506.

66. Wang X, Huang W, Mihara M, Sinha J, Davidson A. Mechanism of action of combined short-term CTLA4Ig and anti-CD40 ligand in murine systemic lupus erythematosus. J Immunol 2002; 168(4): 2046–53.

67. Kalunian KC, Davis JC Jr, Merrill JT, Totoritis MC, Wofsy D. Treatment of systemic lupus erythematosus by inhibition of T cell costimulation with anti-CD154: a randomized, double-blind, placebo-controlled trial. Arthritis Rheum 2002; 46(12): 3251–8.

68. Boumpas DT, Furie R, Manzi S et al. A short course of BG9588 (anti-CD40 ligand antibody) improves serologic activity and decreases hematuria in patients with proliferative lupus glomerulonephritis. Arthritis Rheum 2003; 48(3): 719–27.

69. Rudd CE, Schneider H. Unifying concepts in CD28, ICOS and CTLA4 co-receptor signalling. Nat Rev Immunol 2003; 3(7): 544–56.

70. Scheipers P, Reiser H. Role of the CTLA-4 receptor in T cell activation and immunity. Physiologic function of the CTLA-4 receptor. Immunol Res 1998; 18(2): 103–15.

71. Reiser H, Stadecker MJ. Costimulatory B7 molecules in the pathogenesis of infectious and autoimmune diseases. N Engl J Med 1996; 335(18): 1369–77.

72. Brunet JF, Denizot F, Luciani MF et al. A new member of the immunoglobulin superfamily – CTLA-4. Nature 1987; 328(6127): 267–70.

73. Guinan EC, Boussiotis VA, Neuberg D et al. Transplantation of anergic histoincompatible bone marrow allografts. N Engl J Med 1999; 340(22): 1704–14.

74. Walunas TL, Lenschow DJ, Bakker CY et al. CTLA-4 can function as a negative regulator of T cell activation. Immunity 1994; 1(5): 405–13.

75. Gribben JG, Freeman GJ, Boussiotis VA et al. CTLA4 mediates antigen-specific apoptosis of human T cells. Proc Natl Acad Sci U S A 1995; 92(3): 811–15.

76. Greenwald RJ, Boussiotis VA, Lorsbach RB, Abbas AK, Sharpe AH. CTLA-4 regulates induction of anergy in vivo. Immunity 2001; 14(2): 145–55.

77. Judge TA, Tang A, Spain LM et al. The in vivo mechanism of action of CTLA4Ig. J Immunol 1996; 156(6): 2294–9.

78. Linsley PS, Wallace PM, Johnson J et al. Immunosuppression in vivo by a soluble form of the CTLA-4 T cell activation molecule. Science 1992; 257(5071): 792–5.

79. Mellor AL, Chandler P, Baban B et al. Specific subsets of murine dendritic cells acquire potent T cell regulatory functions following CTLA4-mediated induction of indoleamine 2,3 dioxygenase. Int Immunol 2004; 16(10): 1391–401.

80. Munn DH, Sharma MD, Mellor AL. Ligation of B7-1/B7-2 by human CD4+ T cells triggers indoleamine 2,3-dioxygenase activity in dendritic cells. J Immunol 2004; 172(7): 4100–10.

81. Abrams JR, Kelley SL, Hayes E et al. Blockade of T lymphocyte costimulation with cytotoxic T lymphocyte-associated antigen 4-immunoglobulin (CTLA4Ig) reverses the cellular pathology of psoriatic plaques, including the activation of keratinocytes, dendritic cells, and endothelial cells. J Exp Med 2000; 192(5): 681–94.

82. Abrams JR, Lebwohl MG, Guzzo CA et al. CTLA4Ig-mediated blockade of T-cell costimulation in patients with psoriasis vulgaris. J Clin Invest 1999; 103(9): 1243–52.

83. Teng GG, Turkiewicz AM, Moreland LW. Abatacept: a costimulatory inhibitor for treatment of rheumatoid arthritis. Expert Opin Biol Ther 2005; 5(9): 1245–54.

84. Kremer JM, Westhovens R, Leon M et al. Treatment of rheumatoid arthritis by selective inhibition of T-cell activation with fusion protein CTLA4Ig. N Engl J Med 2003; 349(20): 1907–15.

85 Daikh DI, Wofsy D. Cutting edge: reversal of murine lupus nephritis with CTLA4Ig and cyclophosphamide. J Immunol 2001; 166(5): 2913–16.

86. Finck BK, Linsley PS, Wofsy D. Treatment of murine lupus with CTLA4Ig. Science 1994; 265(5176): 1225–7.

87. Nardelli B, Belvedere O, Roschke V et al. Synthesis and release of B-lymphocyte stimulator from myeloid cells. Blood 2001; 97(1): 198–204.

88. Moore PA, Belvedere O, Orr A et al. BLyS: member of the tumor necrosis factor family and B lymphocyte stimulator. Science 1999; 285(5425): 260–3.

89. Litinskiy MB, Nardelli B, Hilbert DM et al. DCs induce CD40-independent immunoglobulin class switching through BLyS and APRIL. Nat Immunol 2002; 3(9): 822–9.

90. Tardivel A, Tinel A, Lens S et al. The anti-apoptotic factor Bcl-2 can functionally substitute for the B cell survival but not for the marginal zone B cell differentiation activity of BAFF. Eur J Immunol 2004; 34(2): 509–18.

91. Yan M, Wang H, Chan B et al. Activation and accumulation of B cells in TACI-deficient mice. Nat Immunol 2001; 2(7): 638–43.

92. Shulga-Morskaya S, Dobles M, Walsh ME et al. B cell-activating factor belonging to the TNF family acts through separate receptors to support B cell survival and T cell-independent antibody formation. J Immunol 2004; 173(4): 2331–41.

93. Stohl W, Metyas S, Tan SM et al. B lymphocyte stimulator overexpression in patients with systemic lupus erythematosus: longitudinal observations. Arthritis Rheum 2003; 48(12): 3475–86.

94. Cheema GS, Roschke V, Hilbert DM, Stohl W. Elevated serum B lymphocyte stimulator levels in patients with systemic immune-based rheumatic diseases. Arthritis Rheum 2001; 44(6): 1313–19.

95. Stohl W. A therapeutic role for BLyS antagonists. Lupus 2004; 13(5): 317–22.

96. Ramanujam M, Wang X, Huang W et al. Mechanism of action of transmembrane activator and calcium modulator ligand interactor-Ig in murine systemic lupus erythematosus. J Immunol 2004; 173(5): 3524–34.

97. Gross JA, Johnston J, Mudri S et al. TACI and BCMA are receptors for a TNF homologue implicated in B-cell autoimmune disease. Nature 2000; 404(6781): 995–9.

98. Stohl W. BlySfulness does not equal blissfulness in systemic lupus erythematosus: a therapeutic role for BLyS antagonists. Curr Dir Autoimmun 2005; 8: 289–304.

99. Baechler EC, Batliwalla FM, Karypis G et al. Interferon-inducible gene expression signature in peripheral blood cells of patients with severe lupus. Proc Natl Acad Sci U S A 2003; 100(5): 2610–15.

100. Bennett L, Palucka AK, Arce E et al. Interferon and granulopoiesis signatures in systemic lupus erythematosus blood. J Exp Med 2003; 197(6): 711–23.

101. Grondal G, Gunnarsson I, Ronnelid J et al. Cytokine production, serum levels and disease activity in systemic lupus erythematosus. Clin Exp Rheumatol 2000; 18(5): 565–70.

102. Kalsi JK, Grossman J, Kim J et al. Peptides from antibodies to DNA elicit cytokine release from peripheral blood mononuclear cells of patients with systemic lupus erythematosus: relation of cytokine pattern to disease duration. Lupus 2004; 13(7): 490–500.

103. Kirou KA, Lee C, George S et al. Activation of the interferon-alpha pathway identifies a subgroup of systemic

lupus erythematosus patients with distinct serologic features and active disease. Arthritis Rheum 2005; 52(5): 1491–503.

104. Linker-Israeli M, Deans RJ, Wallace DJ et al. Elevated levels of endogenous IL-6 in systemic lupus erythematosus. A putative role in pathogenesis. J Immunol 1991; 147(1): 117–23.

105. Merrill JT, Buyon JP. The role of biomarkers in the assessment of lupus. Best Pract Res Clin Rheumatol 2005; 19(5): 709–26.

106. Sun KH, Yu CL, Tang SJ, Sun GH. Monoclonal anti-double-stranded DNA autoantibody stimulates the expression and release of IL-1beta, IL-6, IL-8, IL-10 and TNF-alpha from normal human mononuclear cells involving in the lupus pathogenesis. Immunology 2000; 99(3): 352–60.

107. al-Janadi M, al-Dalaan A, al-Balla S, al-Humaidi M, Raziuddin S. Interleukin-10 (IL-10) secretion in systemic lupus erythematosus and rheumatoid arthritis: IL-10-dependent CD4+CD45RO+ T cell-B cell antibody synthesis. J Clin Immunol 1996; 16(4): 198–207.

108. Park YB, Lee SK, Kim DS et al. Elevated interleukin-10 levels correlated with disease activity in systemic lupus erythematosus. Clin Exp Rheumatol 1998; 16(3): 283–8.

109. Smolen JS, Steiner G, Aringer M. Anti-cytokine therapy in systemic lupus erythematosus. Lupus 2005; 14(3): 189–91.

110. Ishida H, Muchamuel T, Sakaguchi S et al. Continuous administration of anti-interleukin 10 antibodies delays onset of autoimmunity in NZB/W F1 mice. J Exp Med 1994; 179(1): 305–10.

111. Llorente L, Richaud-Patin Y, Garcia-Padilla C et al. Clinical and biologic effects of anti-interleukin-10 monoclonal antibody administration in systemic lupus erythematosus. Arthritis Rheum 2000; 43(8): 1790–800.

112. Iwano M, Dohi K, Hirata E et al. Urinary levels of IL-6 in patients with active lupus nephritis. Clin Nephrol 1993; 40(1): 16–21.

113. Tsai CY, Wu TH, Yu CL, Lu JY, Tsai YY. Increased excretions of beta2-microglobulin, IL-6, and IL-8 and decreased excretion of Tamm-Horsfall glycoprotein in urine of patients with active lupus nephritis. Nephron 2000; 85(3): 207–14.

114. Pasare C, Medzhitov R. Toll pathway-dependent blockade of CD4+CD25+ T cell-mediated suppression by dendritic cells. Science 2003; 299(5609): 1033–6.

115. Horii Y, Iwano M, Hirata E et al. Role of interleukin-6 in the progression of mesangial proliferative glomerulonephritis. Kidney Int Suppl 1993; 39: S71–S75.

116. Mihara M, Takagi N, Takeda Y, Ohsugi Y. IL-6 receptor blockage inhibits the onset of autoimmune kidney disease in NZB/W F1 mice. Clin Exp Immunol 1998; 112(3): 397–402.

117. Ryffel B, Car BD, Gunn H, Roman D, Hiestand P, Mihatsch MJ. Interleukin-6 exacerbates glomerulonephritis in (NZB x NZW)F1 mice. Am J Pathol 1994; 144(5): 927–37.

118. Nishimoto N, Yoshizaki K, Miyasaka N et al. Treatment of rheumatoid arthritis with humanized anti-interleukin-6 receptor antibody: a multicenter, double-blind, placebo-controlled trial. Arthritis Rheum 2004; 50(6): 1761–9.

119. Mihara M, Nishimoto N, Ohsugi Y. The therapy of autoimmune diseases by anti-interleukin-6 receptor antibody. Expert Opin Biol Ther 2005; 5(5): 683–90.

120. Yokota S, Miyamae T, Imagawa T et al. Therapeutic efficacy of humanized recombinant anti-interleukin-6 receptor antibody in children with systemic-onset juvenile idiopathic arthritis. Arthritis Rheum 2005; 52(3): 818–25.

121. Charles PJ, Smeenk RJ, De JJ, Feldmann M, Maini RN. Assessment of antibodies to double-stranded DNA induced in rheumatoid arthritis patients following treatment with infliximab, a monoclonal antibody to tumor necrosis factor alpha: findings in open-label and randomized placebo-controlled trials. Arthritis Rheum 2000; 43(11): 2383–90.

122. Mohan AK, Edwards ET, Cote TR, Siegel JN, Braun MM. Drug-induced systemic lupus erythematosus and TNF-alpha blockers. Lancet 2002; 360(9333): 646.

123. Studnicka-Benke A, Steiner G, Petera P, Smolen JS. Tumour necrosis factor alpha and its soluble receptors parallel clinical disease and autoimmune activity in systemic lupus erythematosus. Br J Rheumatol 1996; 35(11): 1067–74.

124. Gabay C, Cakir N, Moral F et al. Circulating levels of tumor necrosis factor soluble receptors in systemic lupus erythematosus are significantly higher than in other rheumatic diseases and correlate with disease activity. J Rheumatol 1997; 24(2): 303–8.

125. Aringer M, Graninger WB, Steiner G, Smolen JS. Safety and efficacy of tumor necrosis factor alpha blockade in systemic lupus erythematosus: an open-label study. Arthritis Rheum 2004; 50(10): 3161–9.

126. Brennan DC, Yui MA, Wuthrich RP, Kelley VE. Tumor necrosis factor and IL-1 in New Zealand Black/White mice. Enhanced gene expression and acceleration of renal injury. J Immunol 1989; 143(11): 3470–5.

127. Boswell JM, Yui MA, Burt DW, Kelley VE. Increased tumor necrosis factor and IL-1 beta gene expression in the kidneys of mice with lupus nephritis. J Immunol 1988; 141(9): 3050–4.

128. Alcocer-Varela J, Aleman-Hoey D, Alarcon-Segovia D. Interleukin-1 and interleukin-6 activities are increased in the cerebrospinal fluid of patients with CNS lupus erythematosus and correlate with local late T-cell activation markers. Lupus 1992; 1(2): 111–17.

129. Kiberd BA, Stadnyk AW. Established murine lupus nephritis does not respond to exogenous interleukin-1 receptor antagonist; a role for the endogenous molecule? Immunopharmacology 1995; 30(2): 131–7.

130. Moosig F, Zeuner R, Renk C, Schroder JO. IL-1RA in refractory systemic lupus erythematosus. Lupus 2004; 13(8): 605–6.

131. Ostendorf B, Iking-Konert C, Kurz K et al. Preliminary results of safety and efficacy of the interleukin 1 receptor antagonist anakinra in patients with severe lupus arthritis. Ann Rheum Dis 2005; 64(4): 630–3.

132. Santiago-Raber ML, Baccala R, Haraldsson KM et al. Type-I interferon receptor deficiency reduces lupus-like disease in NZB mice. J Exp Med 2003; 197(6): 777–88.

133. Horwitz DA, Zheng SG, Gray JD et al. Regulatory T cells generated ex vivo as an approach for the therapy of autoimmune disease. Semin Immunol 2004; 16: 135–43.

134. Hahn BH, Ebling F, Singh RR et al. Cellular and molecular mechanisms of regulation of autoantiobdy production in lupus. Ann N Y Acad Sci 2005; 1051: 433–41.

135. Hahn BH, Singh RP, La Cava A, Ebling FM. Tolerogenic treatment of lupus mice with consensus peptide induces Foxp3-expressing, apoptosis-resistant, TGFbeta-secreting CD8+ T cell suppressors. J Immunol 2005; 175: 7728–37.

136. Zheng SG, Wang JH, Stohl W et al. TGF-beta requires CTLA-4 early after T cell activation to induce Foxp3 and generate adaptive CD4+CD25+ regulatory cells. J Immunol 2006; 176: 3321–9.

137. Zinger H, Eilat E, Meshorer A, Mozes E. Peptides based on the complementarity-determining regions of a pathogenic autoantibody mitigate lupus manifestations of (NZBxNZW)F1 mice via active suppression. Int Immunol 2003; 15: 205–14.

138. Mauremann N, Sthoeger Z, Zinger H, Mozes E. Amelioration of lupus manifestations by a peptide based on the complementarity determining region 1 of an autoantibody in severe combined immunodeficient (SCID) mice engrafted with peripheral blood lymphocytes of SLE patients. Clin Exp Immunol 2004; 137: 513–20.

139. Kang HK, Michaels MA, Berner BR, Datta SK. Very low-dose tolerance with nucleosomal peptides controls lupus and induces potent regulatory T cell subsets. J Immunol 2005; 174: 3247–55.

140. Riemekasten G, Langnickel D, Enghard P et al. Intravenous injection of a D1 protein of the Smith proteins postpones murine lupus and induces type 1 regulatory T cells. J Immunol 2004; 173: 5835–42.

141. Monneaux F, Hoebeke J, Sordet C et al. Selective modulation of CD4+ T cells from lupus patients by a promiscuous, protective peptide analog. J Immunol 2005; 175: 5839–47.

142. Marmont AM. Stem cell transplantation for autoimmune disorders. Coincidental autoimmune disease in patients transplanted for conventional indications. Best Pract Res Clin Haematol 2004; 17(2): 223–32.

143. Hough RE, Snowden JA, Wulffraat NM. Haemopoietic stem cell transplantation in autoimmune diseases: a European perspective. Br J Haematol 2005; 128(4): 432–59.

144. Jayne D, Passweg J, Marmont A et al. Autologous stem cell transplantation for systemic lupus erythematosus. Lupus 2004; 13(3): 168–76.

145. Tyndall A, Gratwohl A. Blood and marrow stem cell transplants in autoimmune disease. A consensus report written on behalf of the European League Against Rheumatism (EULAR) and the European Group for Blood and Marrow Transplantation (EBMT). Br J Rheumatol 1997; 36(3): 390–2.

146. Burt RK, Traynor A, Statkute L et al. Nonmyeloablative hematopoietic stem cell transplantation for systemic lupus erythematosus. JAMA 2006; 295(5): 527–35.

147. Traynor AE, Corbridge TC, Eagan AE et al. Prevalence and reversibility of pulmonary dysfunction in refractory systemic lupus: improvement correlates with disease remission following hematopoietic stem cell transplantation. Chest 2005; 127(5): 1680–9.

148. Manderson AP, Botto M, Walport MJ. The role of complement in the development of systemic lupus erythematosus. Annu Rev Immunol 2004; 22:431–56.

149. Boackle SA, Holers VM. Role of complement in the development of autoimmunity. Curr Dir Autoimmun 2003; 6: 154–68.

150. Nangaku M, Pippin J, Couser WG. Complement membrane attack complex (C5b-9) mediates interstitial disease in experimental nephrotic syndrome. J Am Soc Nephrol 1999; 10(11): 2323–31.

151. Pickering MC, Walport MJ. Links between complement abnormalities and systemic lupus erythematosus. Rheumatology (Oxford) 2000; 39(2): 133–41.

152. Javaid B, Quigg RJ. Treatment of glomerulonephritis: will we ever have options other than steroids and cytotoxics? Kidney Int 2005; 67(5): 1692–703.

37

Vasculitis

Gary S Hoffman, Leonard H Calabrese and Carol A Langford

Introduction • Giant cell (temporal) arteritis • Takayasu's arteritis • Wegener's granulomatosis and microscopic polyangiitis • Churg–Strauss syndrome • Vasculitis associated with chronic viral infection • References

INTRODUCTION

The systemic vasculitides are heterogeneous in regard to clinical phenotype, prognosis, and etiology. In only a few instances is the cause of a specific form of vasculitis well established. For severe forms of disease, treatment has been frustratingly familiar, incorporating corticosteroids (CS), and, in some cases, cytotoxic therapies. It is important for the practitioner to not become prematurely jaded about these broad-based immunosuppressive/anti-inflammatory agents, as when used judiciously they reduce disease morbidity and may be life-saving. The provision of more disease-specific treatments will emerge as our understanding of pathogenesis improves. This, in fact, is being addressed in randomized controlled trials of biologic agents. In this chapter, we will focus primarily on new insights into the pathogenesis of certain vasculitides and how those insights are changing approaches to patient care.

GIANT CELL (TEMPORAL) ARTERITIS

Giant cell arteritis (GCA) is a disease of unknown cause, affecting large and medium-sized arteries, in patients generally older than 50 years. Women are affected at least twice as often as men.[1,2] In the USA, the annual incidence is approximately 2.5/100 000 population, and 18/100 000 among persons > 50 years old. The prevalence of GCA in this age group has been estimated to be 223/100 000 population[1–4] and the approximate total number of prevalent cases in the USA alone is 162 340.

Characteristic features of GCA are provided in Table 37.1.[3–9] Morbidity from GCA itself is substantial. In the era preceding the availability of CS, 30–60% of patients experienced visual loss, compared with 5–25% of CS-treated patients in more recent series.[10–15] In one population-based study, 17% of GCA patients developed aortic aneurysms that were sometimes associated with dissection or vessel rupture.[16] Aortic branch vessel stenoses may cause extremity (upper > lower) claudication (~15%).[17,18] Patients may also experience polymyalgia rheumatica (PMR) (~50%), constitutional symptoms (~50%), and stroke (0–5%).[3–9,19–22]

Conventional medical therapy for giant cell arteritis

There is general agreement that once a convincing diagnosis of GCA is assumed, treatment with CS should begin immediately. This sense of urgency is conveyed because of the knowledge that in the pre-CS era, GCA was frequently complicated by blindness.

How much prednisone?

How long should the initial dose be maintained before it is tapered? How long should one expect

Table 37.1 Giant cell arteritis: clinical features (% frequency)

Author (no. of cases)	Hunder (94)	Liozan (147)	Gonzalez-Gay (239)	Chevalet (164)	Hoffman (98)[a]
Headache	77	NS	83	67	93
Abnormal temporal artery	53	55	72	21	NS
Jaw claudication/pain	51	38	39	16	60
Constitutional symptoms	48	65	70	NS	NS
Polymyalgia rheumatica	34	27	47	49	55
Fever	27	NS	11	46	5
Diplopia	12	NS	7	NS	NS
Amaurosis	5	NS	17	NS	NS
Blindness	13	13	14	NS	18
Stroke	NS	NS	3.5	NS	0
Mean age (years)	75	75	73	73	74
Percentage female	74	63	56	71	71

[a]At presentation; NS, not stated.

to treat a patient with GCA? The answers to such questions are as numerous as the authorities who have studied GCA. Comparative studies have not been performed that would clearly recommend any one approach above others.

Whereas some early reports of GCA suggested that treatment may only be necessary for 6–12 months, in 1973 Beevers et al.[23] recognized the chronic nature of this illness and noted that in many cases CS therapy may be required for several years. Indeed, this is now a widely accepted perception. Relapse rates in the course of CS tapering have been reportedly ~30% to > 80% over 1–4 years of follow-up.[20–27]

It is apparent that GCA is not readily controlled in many patients once CS therapy is reduced to low or moderate doses (i.e. prednisone 5–15 mg/day). Even after 2–3 years of therapy, about 50% of patients remain CS-dependent, a situation that has led to substantial morbidity in an already fragile elderly population. The risks of fractures and cataracts are five and three times greater, respectively, in patients with GCA compared with age-matched controls not treated with CS.[19] Nesher et al.[28,29] found that among 43 patients followed for a mean period of 3 years, 35% had fractures and 21% had severe infections, which in two-thirds of cases led to death. An important role for CS

could be implicated in 37% of all deaths. The need for prolonged CS therapy to control GCA, and the goal of reducing disease- and treatment-related morbidity and mortality, have led investigators to explore the use of adjunctive agents to improve outcomes.

Adjunctive therapy to corticosteroids in giant cell arteritis

Conventional immunosuppressive agents

Numerous studies have explored the utility of either methotrexate (MTX) or azathioprine (AZA) as a means of achieving improved disease control and less dependence on CS therapy. Two recent randomized, double-blind, placebo-controlled studies of weekly MTX have been completed. In both, the rate of CS taper was rapid, so that in the absence of relapse, CS withdrawal could be accomplished in 4 months[24] or 6 months.[9] In both studies, relapses were frequent, and the first relapse occurred with equal frequency in the CS-only and CS + MTX groups. However, the frequency of more than one relapse differed between groups in one study and not in the other. The reason for these differences is uncertain. Consequently, the role that MTX or other adjunctive therapies may play in GCA remains unsettled.

New insights into pathogenesis, new opportunities for treatment

Our inability to control GCA, without producing CS-related morbidity, may not be at an impasse. Although the pathogenesis of GCA has not been completely elucidated, our understanding of the disease has grown substantially. Biopsy specimens obtained at different stages in the evolution of vascular lesions have revealed that inflammatory cells are initially concentrated in the adventitia and are absent or sparse in the intima, with an intermediate presence in the media. Mononuclear cells migrate into the vessel wall from the adventitia[30–36] (Figure 37.1). CD4+ T cells are prevalent in this infiltrate, and may play a key role in driving the inflammatory attack. Production of interleukin (IL)-2, tumor necrosis factor (TNF)-α and interferon (IFN)-γ by CD4+ T cells indicates a predominant Th1 response.[30,33–36] Products of activated macrophages include IL-1 and TNF-α (Figure 37.2),[33] which are proinflammatory cytokines that further stimulate the Th1 response. Granuloma formation depends on Th1 cytokines and, in animal models, anti-TNF-α therapy has been shown to block granuloma formation. Blockade of these cytokines could theoretically play an important role in selective interference with disease progression.

TNF-α inhibitors such as infliximab and etanercept, and IL-1 receptor antagonist (IL-1ra), have been shown to abrogate inflammatory responses and limit tissue damage in patients with rheumatoid arthritis (RA), and are being studied in other illnesses in which macrophage- and Th1-mediated responses may be important. Our new understanding of the pathogenesis of GCA suggests that interfering with vascular injury due to the products of activated macrophages and Th1 lymphocytes would be worthy of investigation.

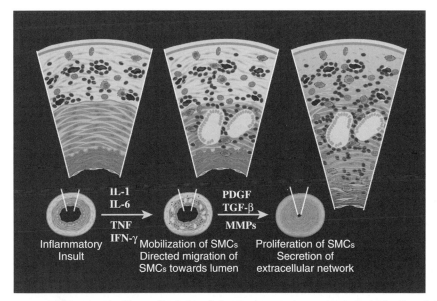

Figure 37.1 GCA: proposed pathogenesis. The earliest sign of disease in vessels appears to be activation of dendritic cells and Th1 lymphocytes (that produce TNF and IFN-γ). About 2–5% of these cells are clonally expanded in the adventitia of vessels, but not in the circulation, suggesting that antigen presentation may occur in the vascular adventitia. In turn, macrophages are activated (and produce IL-1, IL-6, TNF). As macrophages migrate into the media, they assume a different phenotype, producing matrix metalloproteinases (MMPs), toxic oxygen radicals, and toxic nitration of proteins that damages the media. Subsequently, synthetic products include growth factors [platelet-derived growth factor (PDGF), transforming growth factor-β (TGF-β)] and vascular endothelial growth factor (VEGF), that leads to microvascular neoangiogenesis within the vessel wall. Eventually myointimal proliferation, including smooth muscle cells (SMCs), leads to vascular stenosis and ischemia. (Adapted from Weyand and Goronzy.[30,34–36])

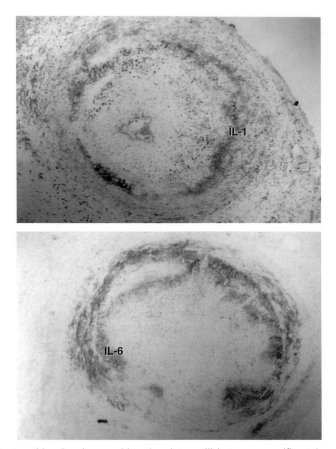

Figure 37.2 GCA: temporal artery biopsies. Immunohistochemistry, utilizing monospecific stains, demonstrates IL-1, IL-6 TNF and IFN-γ in the vessel wall. (Courtesy of Dr Maria Cid and Jose Hernandez-Rodriguez, Barcelona.)

The first use of a biologic agent in a randomized trial was recently reported by Hoffman and colleagues.[37] The authors evaluated the efficacy of adding placebo or the monoclonal antibody (mAb) to TNF, infliximab, to standard of care (CS) in patients with newly diagnosed GCA. Addition of anti-TNF-α therapy did not improve the durability of remissions or reduce cumulative CS requirements.[37] A similar study designed for polymyalgia rheumatica[38] also failed to demonstrate efficacy. These observations raise the question of whether other pathways and mediators play more important or pivotal roles in GCA and PMR disease pathogenesis.

Aspirin – targeted therapy of a different kind

Two recent retrospective studies have noted that low dose aspirin antiplatelet or anticoagulant therapy may reduce the risk of ischemic events in patients with GCA by a factor of 3–5-fold. An increased risk of bleeding complications was not observed.[39,40]

TAKAYASU'S ARTERITIS

Takayasu's arteritis (TA) is an idiopathic systemic inflammatory disease that may lead to segmental stenosis, occlusion, dilatation and/or aneurysm formation of the aorta and/or its main branches. Coronary and/or pulmonary arteries may also be affected. A significant number of patients fail to achieve and sustain remission despite prolonged treatment with CS and cytotoxic agents.

As is true for GCA, granuloma formation is a characteristic feature in the inflammatory lesions of TA. Granuloma formation is in part

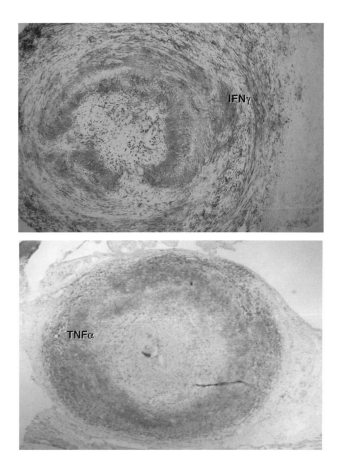

Figure 37.2, cont'd

dependent on TNF-α. TNF-α production occurs primarily in macrophages, T cells, and natural killer (NK) cells. TNF-α induces macrophage production of IL-12 and IL-18, which are potent cytokines that bias CD4 T cells to differentiate as Th1 cells, and activate NK cells. IL-18-influenced Th1 lymphocyte production of IFN-γ leads to enhanced recruitment and activation of macrophages, a critical feature of granuloma formation. The pathogenesis of TA includes vessel injury due to activated T cells, NK cells, γδ cells, and macrophages. Therefore, it is logical to consider that TNF-α inhibition, as was noted for GCA, might enhance control of the inflammatory process in TA. Although one might anticipate a similar result to that noted for GCA, it is important to recall that immunologic function and disease susceptibility differ in many ways in youth and in the elderly.

Preliminary data from an open-label trial of 15 patients with treatment-refractory TA has demonstrated encouraging results that will hopefully lead to a randomized controlled study.[41] TA patients had previously failed to maintain remission on tapering courses of CS and concurrent therapy with cyclophosphamide (CP), MTX, AZA, cyclosporin, mycophenolate mofetil, and/or tacrolimus. Median duration of disease prior to anti-TNF therapy was 6 years. Patients had previously experienced multiple relapses. Prior to trials of anti-TNF therapy, relapses had occurred when the median prednisone dose was less than 20 mg of prednisone a day. At lower doses, relapses occurred that led to starting anti-TNF therapy. Ten patients were able to discontinue prednisone during the period of follow up (1–3.3 years) after starting anti-TNF therapy, and an additional four patients achieved sustained remissions while taking < 10 mg prednisone daily (> 50% reduction in prior CS requirements). One patient did not achieve remission and died of complications of myocardial infarction. Although these results must be regarded as preliminary, they do suggest that anti-TNF therapy is a useful adjunct to CS in the treatment of TA. Anti-TNF therapy for TA should be evaluated in a larger study to determine its potential utility in producing remission, while minimizing the use of CS.

WEGENER'S GRANULOMATOSIS AND MICROSCOPIC POLYANGIITIS

Wegener's granulomatosis (WG) is a systemic inflammatory disease of unknown etiology characterized by necrotizing granulomatous inflammation of the upper and lower airways, necrotizing crescentic glomerulonephritis, and systemic vasculitis of small and medium vessels. Manifestations may be limited to the respiratory tract, or may be more generalized.[42,43]

Microscopic polyangiitis (MPA) is also a form of small and medium-sized vessel vasculitis, and is distinguished histologically from WG by not having granuloma formation. MPA manifests most often as necrotizing crescentic glomerulonephritis, pulmonary hemorrhage, constitutional symptoms, and skin and peripheral nervous system involvement. Like WG, it can present as a pulmonary–renal syndrome.[44] If granulomas are not found on a biopsy, because either they are truly not present or the biopsy sample was inadequate for detection, the vasculitic component of WG may not be histologically distinguishable from MPA. In the absence of destructive upper airway disease, these two syndromes may also be clinically indistinguishable.

Before the introduction of CS plus CP, WG and MPA were usually fatal diseases with mortality occurring from pulmonary or renal failure. Although this regimen has been proven to prolong survival and induce remission in a majority of patients, long-term CP use is associated with substantial toxicity.[42] Recent therapeutic approaches have utilized regimens that reduce the duration of CP exposure by switching to MTX or AZA after 3–6 months,[45,46] or avoid the use of CP altogether by the use of MTX for remission induction of non-severe disease.[47–49] Unfortunately, even with the ability to successfully induce remission and limit CP exposure, relapse of disease and drug-related adverse events still impact a substantial proportion of patients, underscoring the need for better therapy. As pathogenic mechanisms of WG and MPA become understood, it may be possible to selectively target critical pathways and, hopefully, establish more effective, less toxic treatment approaches.

Evolving concepts in pathogenesis

Histologic features of affected tissues, genetic influences, and the presence of circulating anti-neutrophil cytoplasmic antibodies (ANCA) have provided important avenues of investigation in the pathophysiology of WG and MPA.

Granuloma formation

Classical histopathologic features of tissues from the upper and lower airways in WG consist of multifocal lesions that include a mixed inflammatory infiltrate, areas of dense polymorphonuclear neutrophil (PMN) accumulations (microabcesses), geographic necrosis surrounded by palisading histiocytes and giant cells, granuloma formation, and vasculitis.[50–52] The renal lesion seen in WG and MPA consists of a focal, segmental necrotizing glomerulonephritis in which there are few to no immune complexes. Collectively, these findings have suggested dominance of cell-mediated immune responses in the pathogenesis of WG.

Granuloma formation may result from an inability or reduced capabilities of activated macrophages to eradicate an antigen, be it exogenous (e.g. mycobacteria, or non-infectious, particulate materials, such as silica) or endogenous (e.g. self-antigens, elastic fibers).[53,54] A typical granuloma consists of a focal accumulation of macrophages, macrophage-derived epithelioid cells, multinucleate giant cells, and lymphocytes. Other cells that may also be present include B cells, plasma cells, NK cells, fibroblasts, and neutrophils. As noted in discussions of GCA and TA (see above), TNF-α and IFN-γ have been shown to be important in the process of giant cell and granuloma formation.[55,56]

In active WG, macrophages are activated, as reflected by increased expression of surface markers and production of neopterin, a monocyte-specific protein.[57,58] Peripheral blood monocytes from WG patients produce increased IL-12 and IL-18, thereby favoring a Th1 pattern of cytokine secretion (Figure 37.3).[59] TNF-α, INF-γ, IL-12, and IL-18 have been identified in diseased tissues, consistent with a Th1-mediated process.[59–61] Based upon these data, it has been hypothesized that dysregulated secretion of Th1 cytokines may be important in the granulomatous inflammation seen in WG.

Genetic influences

The role of genetic influences in WG and MPA has remained an area of intense interest and investigation.[62] Although there have been limited data thus far to suggest clear genetic associations with these diseases, one of the most intriguing areas of study has focused on genetic polymorphisms of costimulatory molecules in the pathogenesis of WG. Cytotoxic T-lymphocyte antigen 4 (CTLA-4) has been found to play an important role in regulation of T-cell immune responses through inhibition of the costimulatory signal required for complete T-cell activation.[63,64]

Polymorphisms in the CTLA-4 gene have been identified and are associated with various autoimmune diseases, including WG.[65] In both Swedish and American cohorts, significant differences were found to exist in a microsatellite polymorphism, (AT)n, located in the 3'-untranslated region of exon 3 in WG patients and normal controls. The shortest microsatellite allele (86 AT base pairs) was markedly underrepresented in WG patients compared with normal controls.[65,66] The shorter CTLA-4 alleles are associated with a more stable form of messenger RNA and, consequently, greater CTLA-4 protein production. Under-representation of these alleles in WG patients could then result in less cell surface CTLA-4 expression, with the end result being enhanced T-cell activation (Figure 37.4). In another study, CD4+ T-cell surface expression of CTLA-4 was found to be increased in WG,[67] reflecting an activated state. However, upon stimulation by mitogen, these T cells failed to up-regulate CTLA-4, again suggesting an impairment of T-cell function in WG. Collectively, these data raise further questions about the role of cellular immunity and T-cell activation in WG and whether this represents a potential avenue for therapeutic exploration.

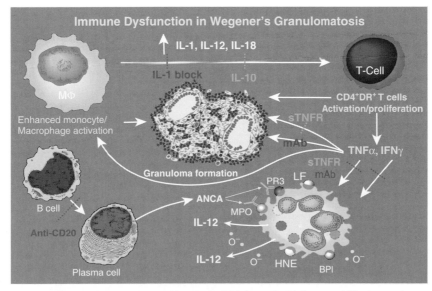

Figure 37.3 Immune dysfunction in Wegener's granulomatosis. BPI, bacteriocidal permeability increasing protein; HNE, human neutrophil elastase; LF, lactoferrin; MF, macrophage; MPO, myeloperoxidase.

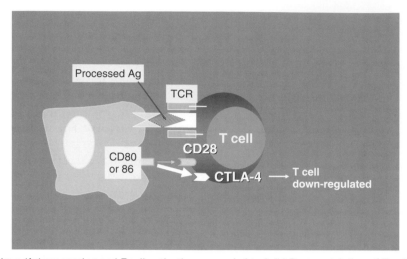

Figure 37.4 (a) Antigen (Ag) processing and T-cell activation: second signal. (b) Down-regulation of T cells by CTLA-4. CTLA-4 resembles CD28 and binds CD80 and CD86 more avidly than CD28, but CTLA-4 provides an inhibitory signal.

Role of ANCA

The high degree of association between ANCA and the small vessel vasculitides of WG and MPA has raised important questions regarding their role in disease pathogenesis. Arguing against a primary pathogenic role for ANCA has been the existence of patients with well characterized disease who lack ANCA, the absence of a tight association between ANCA and disease activity, the ability for patients to have high levels of ANCA yet remain in clinical remission, and the inability of this model to account for selection of targeted organs in these diseases.

Despite these questions, there has been a growing body of evidence from *in vitro* and *in vivo* murine studies to support a pathogenic role for ANCA. ANCA are directed against enzymes located within the cytoplasm or cytoplasmic granules of neutrophils and the lysosomes of monocytes.[68] In WG patients, specificity of ANCA is usually to proteinase 3 (PR3) (~80%), and less often to myeloperoxidase (MPO) (~20%), whereas in MPA, ANCA most often target MPO. ANCA can be detected in the majority of patients with active generalized WG and MPA. Substantial *in vitro* evidence points to a pathogenic role for these antibodies.[68–71] One proposed sequence of events leading to vessel injury suggests an interaction between activated endothelial cells, PMNs, and monocytes that have been attracted by chemokines and are bound by adhesion molecules. When primed by inflammatory stimuli, PMNs and monocytes express PR3 and MPO on their surface.[72,73] ANCA can bind to PR3 or MPO, and fully activate the PMNs, with resultant degranulation and enhanced respiratory burst.[68,74] When they are in proximity to endothelial cells, cytotoxity from proteolytic enzymes and reactive oxygen intermediates (ROI) may result.[74] In addition, free PR3 may also become bound to endothelial cells. *In vitro*, ANCA binding to PR3 present on endothelial surface have been shown to induce neutrophil-mediated antibody-dependent cell cytotoxicity (ADCC).[75] Thus, vessel damage may result from the combined effects of proteolytic enzymes, ROI, and ADCC. Adding to this experience have been data gained from the investigation of ANCA utilizing an innovative MPO knockout (KO) mouse model.[76] In these studies, MPO KO mice were immunized with mouse MPO. Splenocytes from these mice and control mice were injected into mice lacking functional T or B lymphocytes. Only mice that received anti-MPO splenocytes developed severe necrotizing and crescentic glomerulonephritis. Purified anti-MPO IgG was then obtained from the MPO KO mice and injected into healthy wild-type mice and mice lacking functional T or B lymphocytes. The introduction of anti-MPO IgG was able to cause pauci-immune glomerular necrosis and crescent formation in both populations of mice regardless of whether there was a deficient or intact immune system. While this series of experiments provides compelling evidence of a direct pathogenic role for ANCA IgG in the animal model, its direct applicability to human disease remains unclear.

Developing new therapies from new insights

The introduction of agents capable of blocking TNF together with the strong body of evidence linking this cytokine with tissue injury in WG made TNF inhibitory therapies an attractive choice for therapeutic investigation in this disease. In a pilot study aimed at evaluating the safety of etanercept in WG, 20 patients received the drug at a dose of 25 mg subcutaneously, twice a week, together with conventional therapy.[77] During the 6-month period of the trial, a favorable safety profile was observed and 16 patients (80%) achieved remission at some point, although mild-to-moderate flares were reported in 12 patients.

These encouraging results led to the WG Etanercept Trial (WGET), a multicenter, double-blind, placebo-controlled, randomized trial in which the objective was to test the efficacy of etanercept in maintaining disease remission when added to conventional therapies.[78] In this trial of 180 patients, there were no significant differences between etanercept and placebo in rate of sustained remission, sustained periods of low levels of disease activity, time to sustained remission, or number of disease flares. These results therefore, did not provide support for the use of etanercept in either the induction or the maintenance of remission in WG. Of particular concern was the observation that six patients in the etanercept arm developed solid malignancies, all of whom were also treated with CP during the trial.[79] These findings suggest that the combination of TNF inhibition and CP may heighten the risk of cancer beyond that observed with CP alone.

A question that has been raised is whether there could be therapeutic differences between anti-TNF agents in WG, as was observed in Crohn's disease. To date, there have been no randomized controlled trials examining infliximab or adalimumab in WG. Outside of several small series involving less than 10 patients,[80,81] the largest published experience comes from the use of infliximab that was given to 32 patients with WG or MPA.[82] Patients reported in this study fell into two groups, 16 patients with acute disease or relapse where infliximab was added to standard induction therapies and 16 patients with persistent disease where infliximab was added to the patients' existing treatment regimen. Although 88% of patients experienced remission, severe infections occurred in 21% of patients and two patients (7%) died. These data raise further concern regarding the safety and utility of anti-TNF therapies in WG. Unless further information emerges, TNF modulatory therapies are not recommended for use in WG.

The exploration of B-cell-depleting therapies was initially prompted by the question as to whether removal of the cellular precursor to ANCA-producing plasma cells could be of benefit in reducing disease activity. B-cell depletion can be achieved with rituximab, a humanized mAb directed against CD20, a B-cell-restricted differentiation antigen. In a study of one patient who suffered from a chronic relapsing course of WG associated with PR3-ANCA, the administration of rituximab and solumedrol brought about a reduction of ANCA and improvement in disease activity.[83] This favorable experience prompted further study of rituximab through compassionate and open-label trials.[84,85] These studies collectively demonstrated that following rituximab treatment all patients achieved swift B-lymphocyte depletion, and complete clinical remission. Remission was maintained while B cells were absent, with relapse occurring in some patients following reconstitution of B lymphocytes. Overall, rituximab had a favorable side effect profile consisting of mild infusion-related events and non-serious infections primarily affecting the upper respiratory tract. Of interest was that although modulation of ANCA had been the initial rationale for studying rituximab in WG, ANCA levels did not become negative in all patients, particularly on retreatment in the absence of CS. This has raised important questions regarding the pathways through which rituximab may be acting in WG and in turn how these pathways may reflect the pathophysiologic mechanisms taking place in WG.[86] These questions are currently being explored through an ongoing randomized, double-blind trial, that will compare the efficacy of rituximab to CP for remission induction in WG and MPA.

The role of T-cell activation together with the data regarding CTLA-4 polymorphisms in WG has made costimulation blockage an interesting area for therapeutic investigation. Abatacept (CTLA-4–Ig) is a soluble fusion protein consisting of CTLA-4 linked to the Fc portion of a human IgG1 antibody that was approved by the FDA in 2006 for the treatment of RA. The utility of this agent in WG remains unknown.

CHURG–STRAUSS SYNDROME

Churg–Strauss syndrome (CSS) is a rare vasculitic disorder, occurring in 2.4 patients/million population.[87] The full-blown vasculitic syndrome is typically preceded by a prodromal phase of asthma, allergic rhinitis, and eosinophilia. Peripheral neuropathy, cutaneous purpura, gastrointestinal symptoms, cardiomyopathy, non-cavitating pulmonary infiltrates, and glomerulonephritis are the characteristic vasculitic manifestations of CSS.[87–89] CS used as the sole agent may be able to achieve remission for patients without critical organ- or life-threatening disease.[90] For more serious or refractory disease, another immunosuppressive agent, usually CP, is added and can be changed to a less toxic drug as the disease enters remission.[87–89,91]

Evolving concepts in pathogenesis

ANCA positivity has been reported with variable frequency, ranging from approximately one-third to two-thirds of patients.[92] Given the large proportion of patients with CSS who are ANCA-negative, it appears unlikely that ANCA play a major or essential role in pathogenesis. Evidence suggests that CSS is predominantly a T-cell-mediated process.[93] Activated T cells (CD4+ and CD8+) are present in diseased tissues and in peripheral blood.[94,95] T-cell lines in CSS are characterized by both a Th1 and Th2 response.[93] However, the cytokine profile in peripheral blood (IL-13, IL-4, and IL-10) suggests that a Th2 process predominates in CSS.[93]

The prominent eosinophilia and eosinophil-rich infiltrates that are found in CSS, as well as the observation that disease activity is closely linked to eosinophil counts, suggest that eosinophils play a central role in CSS. However, the factors that bring about the increased activation and numbers of eosinophils in CSS are unknown. One hypothesis regarding the origin of eosinophilia in CSS is that this results from a hypersensitivity reaction to an exogenous antigen, as disease onset has been linked to prior vaccination, desensitization, drugs,[96] and inhalation of allergens.[97] Proteins stored within the eosinophils' granules may be responsible for the tissue damage seen in CSS. In the idiopathic hypereosinophilic syndrome, eosinophil cationic protein is thought to be responsible for the observed cardiotoxicity and could also be important in CSS.[98] Another protein, eosinophil-derived neurotoxin, could participate in causing neuropathy. Eotaxin, a chemokine specific for eosinophils,[99] has been shown to induce the expression of the adhesion molecules intercellular adhesion molecule-1 (ICAM-1) and vascular cellular adhesion molecule-1 (VCAM-1) on endothelial cells.[100]

CSS: developing new therapies from new insights

To the extent that eosinophils may be prominent factors in CSS, novel therapies that block their recruitment and activation may be useful avenues for investigation as these become available. IFN-α, an inhibitor of eosinophilopoiesis and degranulation,[99] has been studied in CSS.[89] In a small, open-label trial four patients with CSS partially responsive to high doses of CS and cytotoxic agents were treated with varying doses of IFN-α.[101] Improvement was dose-dependent and correlated with a decrease in eosinophil counts. Rapid improvements in pulmonary function and skin lesions in one patient were also reported in another publication.[102] However, a recent report has described the development of leucoencephalopathy in 2 of 12 patients with CSS who had received IFN-α.[103] Although a strict causal relationship cannot be determined, leucoencephalopathy has been described in patients treated with IFN-α for other diseases and these two cases suggested that IFN-α may also cause cerebral cytotoxicity in CSS. This experience suggests that the use of IFN-α should be avoided except in instances where patients have been unresponsive to other forms of treatment and are closely monitored by cerebral MRI to detect asymptomatic leucoencephalopathy at an early stage.

VASCULITIS ASSOCIATED WITH CHRONIC VIRAL INFECTION

There is perhaps no area of vascular inflammatory disease where the rationale for a biological approach is more inviting than for those vasculitic syndromes associated with chronic viral infections.

Traditional therapies for vasculitis rely on broad-based immunosuppression, which is clearly not appealing from the perspective of controlling underlying infectious diseases, and thus a more selective approach to controlling both infection and inflammation is highly desirable. Advances in our understanding of viral pathogenesis, including the role of cytokines, and the development of new and more effective antiviral agents offer new therapeutic approaches to many of these disorders.

The pathogenesis of virus-associated vasculitis is heterogeneous. At least two major mechanisms are involved. First, viral replication within the vessel itself may induce direct injury (e.g. equine viral arteritis). Second, vascular inflammation and damage might result from immune mechanisms, humoral and/or cellular, directed against the virus itself. While numerous viral pathogens have been implicated in the pathogenesis of vasculitis, the evidence for causality is most robust for hepatitis B virus (HBV) and hepatitis C virus (HCV).[104]

Hepatitis B virus

There are two types of vasculitic syndromes associated with HBV infection. A self-limiting small-vessel vasculitis affecting mainly the skin has been described in the early stages of the infection. This condition is generally self-limiting and subsides with the appearance of jaundice. Circulating immune complexes (ICs) appear to play a critical role in this syndrome, having been detected in the circulation, synovium, and vessel wall.[105]

The other form of vascular inflammatory disease, namely a polyarteritis nodosa-like vasculitis, is far more serious. The term 'polyarteritis nodosa (PAN)-like' is used because primary PAN is not associated with a known infectious agent. HBV with a medium-sized vessel arteritis is characterized by multisystem involvement. It usually occurs in the early stages of chronic HBV infection,[106] generally the first 6–12 months following acute HBV infection. The clinical manifestations are similar to those of the idiopathic form of the disease. Despite its explosive nature, HBV arteritis usually lasts for only a few months. In successfully treated patients, relapses are rare.

Conventional therapy of HBV-associated vasculitis

The standard therapy of idiopathic PAN with high dose CS and CP is also effective in controlling the vascular inflammatory phase of HBV-associated arteritis in the short term, but long-term results demonstrate near-universal viral persistence, virus-associated complications, and relapse.[107,108] More recent strategies for HBV-associated arteritis have focused on control of both vascular inflammation and viral infection.

New insights into pathogenesis, new opportunities for therapy

The pathogenesis of this syndrome appears to involve both viral and host elements, with the formation and deposition of viral-specific ICs.[108] A number of studies have provided evidence for a role of ICs in both the early occurring small-vessel vasculitis form of disease and the more severe systemic arteritis phenotype.[109] Evidence includes the presence of circulating ICs containing HBV-specific antibody and complement, hypocomplementemia, and vascular deposition of virus and host-derived immune products. It is not clear whether the pathogenic antigen is actually HbsAg, as originally thought, or HbeAg.[108]

Despite the lack of controlled data, Guillevin and Trepo have demonstrated the efficacy of a combination of therapies for HBV-associated systemic arteritis.[108] Each of their trials has applied four principles: (1) initial use of CS to rapidly control vascular inflammation; (2) discontinuation of CS after about 2 weeks, so as not to compromise immunologic clearance of HBV; (3) concurrent best available antiviral therapy; and (4) plasma exchange to facilitate clearance of ICs. This strategy has appeared to improve outcomes and favor HbeAg to HbeAb seroconversion.

The antiviral therapy approach was initially employed with the relatively weak antiviral agent vidarabin, subsequently with IFN-α, and most recently with the antiviral nucleoside analog lamivudine. Response rates have improved to 90%, with HbeAg to HbeAb seroconversion noted in 70% of patients. Because the vascular inflammation is linked to HBV replication, prospects for improved therapy for vasculitis are tied to new and more effective antiviral drugs. In the past few years several new agents have been approved for HBV treatment including PEG-IFN-α, adefovir dipivoxil, and most recently entecavir. To date there are no reports of their use in this setting, although both adefovir and especially entecavir have strong therapeutic advantages, which make them attractive alternatives to lamivudine.

Unresolved questions include the following. What is the relative importance of CS therapy and plasmapheresis in this treatment regimen? Is it possible that only antiviral therapy may be adequate for certain patients with milder forms of HBV-associated arteritis? What is the ideal or optimal antiviral agent or agents? It is unlikely that large-scale controlled trials of this rare complication of HBV infection will ever be performed.

Hepatitis C virus

HCV has most frequently been associated with small-vessel vasculitis resulting from deposition of IC-containing cryoglobulins in the vessel wall (HCV-associated mixed cryoglobulinemia or HCV-MC). Small studies and scattered case reports have indicated the occasional association

Table 37.2 Clinical findings in hepatitis C-associated mixed cryoglobulinemia

Finding	Prevalence (%)
Purpura	90–100
Arthralgias	50–90
Weakness	70–100
Peripheral neuropathy	3–70
Renal involvement	10–55
Hepatic involvement	60–70
Splenomegaly	50
Lymphadenopathy	Rare–15
Lung involvement	Rare
Sjögren's syndrome	20–40
Raynaud's phenomenon	10–35
Skin ulcers	10–30

of HCV with medium-sized (PAN-like) or large-vessel vasculitides.

In the more common form of HCV vasculitis, HCV-MC, the clinical findings can range from a pure cutaneous leukocytoclastic vasculitis to a multisystem disorder including neuropathies and membranoproliferative glomerulonephritis. The clinical features of HCV-MC are outlined in Table 37.2.[110] The clinical features of the PAN-like disorder associated with HCV are more reminiscent of idiopathic PAN with larger-caliber vessel involvement.[111] It should be emphasized that such cases of PAN-like HCV are quite rare.

Conventional therapy of HCV-associated vasculitis

Prior to the molecular discovery of HCV in 1989 the standard therapy of 'essential' MC was a combination of CS, CP, and plasmapheresis.[112] Such therapy appeared to be effective in the short term but for the most part was palliative and rarely led to long-term remission. In addition, past literature about 'essential' cryoglobulinemia described an increased incidence of lymphomas among CS/CP-treated patients. This gave further pause to the chronic use of alkylating agents in the treatment of HCV vasculitis. Given that > 90% of 'essential MC' cases have been found to be associated with chronic HCV infection, treatment strategies have been reconsidered.

New insights into pathogenesis, new opportunities for therapy

The pathogenesis of this disorder also appears to involve both viral and host-associated factors. Clear evidence of both virus and specific antibody deposition in ICs has been found in skin lesions.[113] Similar evidence in other organs such as nerve and kidney has been less compelling. A role for virus-specific ICs is also supported by the high concentration of virus and specific antibodies within the cryoprecipitates.[110] A clear correlation exists between the effectiveness of antiviral therapy, reductions in cryoglobulin concentrations, and improvements in vasculitis, all of which supports a direct role of HCV as a cause of small-vessel vasculitis in certain predisposed individuals.[110] In the far less common, medium-sized artery form of illness, data on pathogenesis are quite limited. Viral-associated ICs are also presumed to play a critical role in this phenotype, but the reasons for differences in selection of vessel types and the more fulminating course of illness remain unknown.

In addition to IC-mediated vasculitis, HCV infection is associated with a spectrum of lymphoproliferative disorders. These range from monoclonal gammopathies of undetermined origin (MGUS), generally of the IgG class, to low-grade lymphoproliferative disorders resulting in the elaboration of monoclonal immunoglobulins of the IgM class that have rheumatoid factor (RF) activity.[114] Rarely, patients may also develop *de novo* high grade lymphomas of the non-Hodgkin's disease type.[114] The RF produced in the setting of chronic HCV infection appears to arise from a limited set of genes of germ-line origin. The precise stimuli for these monoclonal RFs are still ill-defined. They may arise as a polyspecific response to an HCV-related stimulus and gradually evolve into a monoclonal response, in a stepwise fashion. Alternatively, they may arise clonally in a *de novo* fashion. There is evidence that limited somatic mutations may then lead to the acquisition of RF activity, suggesting that some element of antibody formation is HCV antigen-driven. At this stage, the disorder becomes less dependent on viral stimulation and may pose a further challenge for designing therapy.

The current therapeutic approach to vasculitis in the setting of chronic HCV infection is directed at both the vascular inflammatory state and the underlying viral infection. Data are limited. There have been three controlled trials of IFN-a in the setting of HCV-associated MC. Each study has demonstrated transient benefit in those patients who have had a good antiviral response;[115] unfortunately, the rate of relapse was nearly 100% following discontinuation of therapy. This high relapse rate reflects the recognized ineffectiveness of IFN-α monotherapy for treating chronic HCV infection. More recently, newer therapies, including combinations of IFN-α and the nucleoside analog ribavirin, have significantly increased the enduring viral response rate in HCV infection. Newer versions of IFN-α incorporating polyethylene glycol (PEG) also appear to have improved pharmacokinetic properties of this agent as well as the viral response rate. There are only limited reports, which are uncontrolled, of combination therapy (i.e. standard IFN-α and ribavirin). They describe encouraging results in small numbers of patients with HCV-MC.[116] Even more limited are reports of successful therapy of HCV-MC with PEG-IFN. In a recent pilot study[117] PEG-IFN plus ribavirin achieved a higher rate of complete clinical response in a shorter treatment period (14 months) than those previously reported with IFN-α and ribavirin.

Unfortunately, even with an improved antiviral armamentarium, there appears to be a need for concomitant immunosuppressive therapy in HCV-MC and HCV arteritis patients.[115] This is especially true of those patients with more severe forms of disease, e.g. severe skin involvement, motor neuropathies, and progressive renal disease. The use of antiviral agents alone, in such patients, is often inadequate and has led to exacerbations and even death in rare cases. Although there are no controlled studies of different therapeutic regimens for such patients, a stepwise algorithm has been recently proposed[115] and is summarized in Table 37.3.

There are increasing numbers of reports in the form of case studies and small series describing the efficacy of anti-CD20 mAb (rituximab) in patients with HCV-MC vasculitis who are resistant or intolerant to IFN-α monotherapy.[118–121]

Table 37.3 Treatment approach to vasculitis in the setting of HCV infection[115]

Mild disease
Isolated purpura without ulceration, mild sensory neuropathy
Best antiviral regimen, i.e. INF-α plus ribavirin, or PEG-INF-α plus ribavirin, no glucocorticoids or cytotoxic agents

Moderate to severe disease
Severe skin disease, motor neuropathy, glomerulonephritis
Initial therapy with glucocorticoids to control inflammatory phase with or without cyclophosphamide followed by best antiviral therapy

Catastrophic disease
Ischemic necrosis of extremities, rapidly progressive glomerulonephritis or neuropathy
Same regimen as for moderate to severe disease combined with plasmapheresis

Such an approach involves the use of mAbs directed to CD20 antigen, a transmembrane protein expressed on pre-B lymphocytes and mature lymphocytes but not stem cells or mature plasma cells. Rituximab proved most effective on cutaneous vasculitis, subjective symptoms of peripheral neuropathy, arthralgia, and low grade B-cell lymphoma. Results of such therapy on HCV-associated renal disease are more limited. Most clinical responders had decreases in serum cryoglobulin levels and increases in C4 serum levels, although not to normal levels. In one study a rise in HCV viral load of 0.3 logs was noted at the end of the study, although the clinical significance of this is yet unknown. Such studies should be considered preliminary at present and B-cell targeted therapy should be reserved for those failing or intolerant of standard treatments awaiting further data.

Non-HCV-associated cryoglobulinemia

Cryoglobulins containing a monoclonal immunoglobulin component (types I and II) may arise in a variety of settings aside from chronic HCV infection. These include lymphoproliferative disorders such as Waldenstrom's macroglobulinemia, non-Hodgkin's lymphoma and, rarely,

'autoimmune' diseases, especially Sjögren's syndrome.[122] The clinical manifestations of cryoglobulinemic vasculitis in these settings may be particularly severe. In addition to visceral target organ involvement, cold-induced ischemic changes in the extremities may lead to occlusive vasculopathy and gangrene. Traditional therapy of non-HCV-associated cryoglobulinemia has generally been directed at the underlying condition. Idiopathic or 'essential cases' have been treated with combinations of plasmapheresis, high-dose CS and CP, and other cytotoxic agents.[122] The knowledge that all type I and type II cryoglobulins are associated *de facto* with clonal B-cell expansions provides a theoretical basis for treatment with more specific therapies such as the anti-CD20 chimeric mAb (rituximab). Rituximab has recently been reported to be successful in treating several other autoimmune disorders, including immune-mediated thrombocytopenia.[123] To date, there are only anecdotal reports of efficacy in such settings.[124]

REFERENCES

1. Salvarani C, Gabriel SE, O'Fallon WM, Hunder GG. The incidence of giant cell arteritis in Olmsted County, Minnesota: apparent fluctuations in a cyclic pattern. Ann Intern Med 1995; 123: 192–4.
2. Matteson EL, Gold KN, Block DA, Hunder GG. Long-term survival of patients with giant cell arteritis in the American College of Rheumatology giant cell arteritis classification criteria cohort. Am J Med 1996; 100: 193–6.
3. Hunder GG. Giant cell (temporal) arteritis. Rheum Dis Clin North Am 1990; 16: 399–409.
4. Hunder GG, Valente RM, Hoffman GS, Weyand CM. Giant cell arteritis: clinical aspects. In: Hoffman GS, Weyand CM, eds. Inflammatory Diseases of Blood Vessels. New York: Marcel Dekker; 2002: 425–41.
5. Liozon E, Herrmann F, Ly K et al. Risk factors for visual loss in giant cell (temporal) arteritis: a prospective study of 174 patients. Am J Med 2001; 111: 211–17.
6. Gonzáles-Gay MA, García-Porrúa C, Vázquez-Caruncho M et al. The spectrum of polymyalgia rheumatica in northwestern Spain: incidence and analysis of variables associated with relapse in a 10 year study. J Rheumatol 1999; 26: 1326–32.
7. Gonzalez-Gay MA, Blanco R, Rodriguez-Valverde V et al. Permanent visual loss and cerebrovascular accidents in giant cell arteritis – predictors and response to treatment. Arthritis Rheum 1998; 41: 1497–504.

8. Chevalet P, Barrier JH, Pottier P et al. A randomized, multicenter, controlled trial using intravenous pulses of methylprednisolone in the initial treatment of simple forms of giant cell arteritis: a one year followup study of 164 patients. J Rheumatol 2000; 27: 1484–91.

9. Hoffman GS, Cid MC, Hellmann DB et al. A multicenter, randomized, double-blind, placebo-controlled trial of adjuvant methotrexate treatment for giant cell arteritis. Arthritis Rheum 2002; 46: 1309–18.

10. Gordon LK, Levin LA. Visual loss in giant cell arteritis. JAMA 1998; 280: 385–6.

11. Myklebust G, Gran JT. A prospective study of 287 patients with polymyalgia rheumatica and temporal arteritis: clinical and laboratory manifestations at onset of disease and at the time of diagnosis. Br J Rheumatol 1996; 35: 1161–8.

12. Bengtsson B A, Malmvall B-E. The epidemiology of giant cell arteritis including temporal arteritis and polymyalgia rheumatica. Arthritis Rheum 1981; 24: 899–904.

13. Font C, Cid MC, Coll-Vincent B, Lopez-Soto A, Grau JM. Clinical features in patients with permanent visual loss due to biopsy-proven giant cell arteritis. Br J Rheumatol 1997; 36: 251–4.

14. Cid MC, Font C, Oristrell J et al. Association between strong inflammatory response and low risk of developing visual loss and other cranial ischemic complications in giant cell (temporal) arteritis. Arthritis Rheum 1998; 41: 26–32.

15. Aillo PD, Trantmann JC, McPhee TJ et al. Visual prognosis in giant cell arteritis. Ophthalmology 1993; 100: 550–5.

16. Evans JM, O'Fallen WM, Hunder GG. Increased incidence of aortic aneurysm and dissection in giant cell (temporal) arteritis. Ann Intern Med 1995; 122: 502–7.

17. Greene GM, Lain D, Sherwin RM et al. Giant cell arteritis of the legs. Am J Med 1986; 81: 727–33.

18. Ninet JP, Bachet P, Dumontet CM et al. Subclavian and axillary involvement in temporal arteritis and polymyalgia rheumatica. Am J Med 1990; 88: 13–20.

19. Rob-Nicholson C, Chang RW, Anderson S et al. Diagnostic value of the history and examination in giant cell arteritis: a clinical pathological study of 81 temporal artery biopsies. J Rheumatol 1988; 15: 1793–6.

20. Delecoeuillerie G, Joly P, DeLara AC, Paolaggi JB. Polymyalgia rheumatica and temporal arteritis: a retrospective analysis of prognostic features and different corticosteroid regimens (11 year survey of 210 patients). Ann Rheum Dis 1988; 47: 733–9.

21. Graham E, Holland A, Avery A, Russel RWR. Prognosis in giant cell arteritis. BMJ 1981; 282: 269–71.

22. Hachulla E, Boivin V, Pasturel-Michon U et al. Prognosis factors and long term evolution in a cohort of 133 patients with giant cell arteritis. Clin Exp Rheumatol 2001; 19: 171–6.

23. Beevers DG, Harpur JE, Turk KAD. Giant cell arteritis – the need for prolonged treatment. J Chronic Dis 1973; 26: 571–84.

24. Jover JA, Hernández-García C, Morado IC et al. Combined treatment of giant-cell arteritis with methotrexate and prednisone. A randomized, double-blind, placebo-controlled trial. Ann Intern Med 2001; 134: 106–14.

25. Kyle V, Hazleman BL. Treatment of polymyalgia rheumatica and giant cell arteritis. I. Steroid regimens in the first two months. Ann Rheum Dis 1989; 48: 658–61.

26. Kyle V, Hazleman BL. Treatment of polymyalgia rheumatica and giant cell arteritis. II. Relation between steroid dose and steroid associated diseases. Ann Rheum Dis 1989; 48: 662–6.

27. Lundberg I, Hedfors E. Restricted dose and duration of corticosteroid treatment in patients with polymyalgia rheumatica and temporal arteritis. J Rheumatol 1990; 17: 1340–5.

28. Nesher G, Sonnenblick M, Friedlander Y. Analysis of steroid related complications and mortality in temporal arteritis: a 15-year survey of 43 patients. J Rheumatol 1994; 21: 1283–6.

29. Nesher G, Rubinow A, Sonnenblick M. Efficacy and adverse effects of different corticosteroid dose regimens in temporal arteritis: a retrospective study. Clin Exp Rheumatol 1997; 15: 303–6.

30. Weyand CM. The pathogenesis of giant cell arteritis. J Rheumatol. 2000; 27: 517–22.

31. Nordborg E, Nordborg C. The inflammatory reaction in giant cell arteritis: an immunohistochemical investigation. Clin Exp Rheumatol 1998; 16: 165–8.

32. Nordborg C, Nordborg E, Petursdottir V. The pathogenesis of giant cell arteritis: morphological aspects. Clin Exp Rheumatol. 2000; 18 (Suppl. 20): 18–21.

33. Cid MC, Hernandez-Rodriguez J, Sanchez M et al. Tissue expression of pro-inflammatory cytokines (IL-1b, IL-6, TNF-a) in giant cell arteritis patients. Correlation with intensity of systemic inflammatory response. Arthritis Rheum 2001; 44(S): 341.

34. Brack A, Geisler A, Martinez-Taboada VM et al. Giant cell arteritis is a T cell-dependent disease. Mol Med 1997; 3: 530–43.

35. Weyand CM, Goronzy JJ. Arterial wall injury in giant cell arteritis. Arthritis Rheum 1999; 42: 844–53.

36. Weyand CM, Wagner AD, Bjornsson J, Goronzy JJ. Correlation of topographical arrangement and functional pattern of tissue-infiltrating macrophages in giant cell arteritis. J Clin Invest 1996; 98: 1642–9.

37. Hoffman GS, Cid MC, Rendt KE, Merkel PA, Weyand CM, Stone JH, Salvarani C, Xu W, Visvanathan S,

Rahman MU, *for the Infliximab-GCA study group*. Infliximab for maintenance of glucocorticosteroid-induced remission of giant cell arteritis: A placebo-controlled randomized trial. Ann Intern Med. 2007; 146: 621-30

38. Salvarani C, Macchioni PL, Manzini C, Polazzi G, Trotta A, Manganelli P, Cimmino M, Gerli R, Cantanosa MG, Boiardi L, Cantini F, Klersy C, Hunder GG. Infliximab plus prednisone or placebo plus prednisone for initial treatment of polymyalgia rheumatica. Ann Intern Med. 2007; 146: 631-39.

39. Nesher G, Berkun Y, Mates M et al. Low-dose aspirin and prevention of cranial ischemic complications in giant cell arteritis. Arthritis Rheum 2004; 50: 1332–7.

40. Lee MS, Smith SD, Galor A, Hoffman GS. Antiplatelet and anticoagulant therapy in patients with giant cell arteritis. Arthritis Rheum 2006; 54: 3071–4.

41. Hoffman GS, Merkel PA, Brasington RD et al. Anti-tumor necrosis factor therapy in patients with difficult to treat Takayasu arteritis. Arthritis Rheum 2004; 50: 2296–304.

42. Hoffman GS, Kerr GS, Leavitt RY et al. Wegener granulomatosis: an analysis of 158 patients. Ann Intern Med 1992; 116: 488–98.

43. Reinhold-Keller E, Beuge N, Latza U et al. An interdisciplinary approach to the care of patients with Wegener's granulomatosis. Long term outcome in 155 patients. Arthritis Rheum 2000; 43: 1021–32.

44. Guillevin L, Durand-Gasselin B, Cevallos R et al. Microscopic polyangiitis. Clinical and laboratory findings in eighty-five patients. Arthritis Rheum 1999; 42: 421–30.

45. Jayne D, Rasmussen N, Andrassy K et al. A randomized trial of maintenance therapy for vasculitis associated with antineutrophil cytoplasmic autoantibodies. N Engl J Med 2003; 349: 36–44.

46. Langford CA, Talar-Williams C, Barron KS et al. Use of a cyclophosphamide-induction methotrexate-maintenance regimen for the treatment of Wegener's granulomatosis: extended follow-up and rate of relapse. Am J Med 2003; 114: 463–9.

47. Hoffman GS, Leavitt RY, Kerr GS, Fauci AS. The treatment of Wegener's granulomatosis with glucocorticoids and methotrexate. Arthritis Rheum 1992; 35: 1322–9.

48. Sneller MC, Hoffman GS, Talar-Williams C et al. An analysis of forty-two Wegener's granulomatosis patients treated with methotrexate and prednisone. Arthritis Rheum 1995; 38: 608–13.

49. De Groot K, Rasmussen N, Bacon PA et al. Randomized trial of cyclophosphamide versus methotrexate for induction of remission in early systemic antineutrophil cytoplasmic antibody-associated vasculitis. Arthritis Rheum 2005; 52: 2461–9.

50. Devaney KO, Travis WD, Hoffman G et al. Interpretation of head and neck biopsies in Wegener's granulomatosis. A pathologic study of 126 biopsies in 70 patients. Am J Surg Pathol 1990; 14: 555–64.

51. Jennette JC. Antineutrophil cytoplasmic autoantibody-associated diseases; a pathologist's perspective. Am J Kidney Dis 1991; 18: 164–70.

52. Travis WD, Hoffman GS, Leavitt RY et al. Surgical pathology of the lung in Wegener's granulomatosis. Review of 87 open lung biopsies from 67 patients. Am J Surg Pathol 1991; 15: 315–33.

53. Williams GT, Williams WJ. Granulomatous inflammation – a review. J Clin Pathol 1983; 36: 723–33.

54. Sneller MC. Granuloma formation, implications for the pathogenesis of vasculitis. Cleve Clin J Med 2002; 69 (Suppl 2): SII40–3.

55. Kindler V, Sappino AP, Grau GE et al. The inducing role of tumor necrosis factor in the development of bactericidal granulomas during BCG infection. Cell 1989; 56: 731–40.

56. Vignery A. Osteoclasts and giant cells: macrophage–macrophage fusion mechanism. Int J Exp Pathol 2000; 81: 291–304.

57. Nassonov E, Samsonov M, Beketova T et al. Serum neopterin concentrations in Wegener's granulomatosis correlate with vasculitis activity. Clin Exp Rheum 1995; 13: 353–6.

58. Muller Kobold AC, Kallenberg CGM, Cohen Tervaert JW. Monocyte activation in patients with Wegener's granulomatosis. Ann Rheum Dis 1999; 58: 237–45.

59. Ludviksson BR, Sneller MC, Chua KS et al. Active Wegener's granulomatosis is associated with HLA-DR+ CD4+ T cells exhibiting an unbalanced Th1-type T cell cytokine pattern: reversal with IL-10. J Immunol 1998; 160: 3602–9.

60. Csernok E, Trabandt A, Müller A et al. Cytokine profile in Wegener's granulomatosis. Predominance of type 1 (Th1) in the granulomatous inflammation. Arthritis Rheum 1999; 42: 742–50.

61. Müller A, Trabandt A, Gloeckner-Hofmann K et al. Localized Wegener's granulomatosis: predominance of CD26 and IFN-γ expression. J Pathol 2000; 192: 113–20.

62. Huang D, Zhou Y, Hoffman GS. Pathogenesis: immuno-genetic factors. Best Pract Res Clin Rheum 2001; 15: 239–58.

63. Bluestone JA, St Clair EW, Turka LA. CTLA4Ig: bridging the basic immunology with clinical application. Immunity 2006; 24: 233–8.

64. Cron RQ. A signal achievement in the treatment of arthritis. Arthritis Rheum 2005; 52: 2229–32.

65. Huang D, Giscombe R, Zhou Y, Lefvert AK. Polymorphisms in CTLA-4 but not tumor necrosis factor-α or interleukin 1β genes are associated with Wegener's granulomatosis. J Rheumatol 2000; 27: 397–401.

66. Zhou Y, Huang D, Hoffman GS. Genetic polymorphisms in the TNF, IL-1, IL-6 and cytotoxic lympho-cyte-associated antigen 4 (CTLA-4) in Wegener's granulomatosis (WG). Arthritis Rheum 2001; 44 (Suppl): S344.

67. Steiner K, Moosig F, Csernok E et al. Increased expression of CTLA-4 (CD152) by T and B lymphocytes in Wegener's granulomatosis. Clin Exp Immunol 2001; 126: 143–50.

68. Jennette JC, Xiao H Falk RJ. Pathogenesis of vascular inflammation by anti-neutrophil cytoplasmic antoibodies. J Am Soc Nephrol 2006; 17: 1235–42.

69. Russel KA, Specks U. Are antineutrophil cytoplasmic antibodies pathogenic? Experimental approaches to understand the antineutrophil cytoplasmic antibody phenomenon. Rheum Dis Clin North Am 2001; 27: 815–32.

70. Harper L, Savage CO. Pathogenesis of ANCA-associated systemic vasculitis. J Pathol 2000; 190: 349–59.

71. Heeringa P, Jennette JC, Falk RJ. Microscopic polyangiitis: pathogenesis. In: Hoffman GS, Weyand CM, eds. Inflammatory Diseases of Blood Vessels. New York: Marcel Dekker, 2001: 339–53.

72. Harper L, Cockwell P, Dwoma A, Savage COS. Neutrophil priming and apoptosis in anti-neutrophil cytoplasmic autoantibody-associated vasculitis. Kidney Int 2001; 59: 1729–38.

73. Csernok E, Ernst M, Schmitt W et al. Activated neutrophils express proteinase 3 on their plasma membrane in vitro and in vivo. Clin Exp Immunol 1994; 95: 244–50.

74. Savage COS, Pottinger BE, Gaskin G et al. Autoantibodies developing to myeloperoxidase and proteinase 3 in systemic vasculitis stimulate neutrophil cytotoxicity toward cultured endothelial cells. Am J Pathol 1992; 141: 335–42.

75. Mayet WJ, Schwarting A, Meyer Zum Büschenfelde KH. Cytotoxic effects of antibodies to proteinase 3 (C-ANCA) on human endothelial cells. Clin Exp Immunol 1994; 97: 458–65.

76. Xiao H, Heeringa P, Hu P et al. Antineutrophil cytoplasmic autoantibodies specific for myeloperoxidase cause glomerulonephritis and vasculitis in mice. J Clin Invest 2002; 110: 955–63.

77. Stone JH, Uhlfelder ML, Hellman DB et al. Etanercept combined with conventional treatment in Wegener's granulomatosis. A six-month open-label trial to evaluate safety. Arthritis Rheum 2001; 44: 1149–54.

78. WGET Research Group. Etanercept plus standard therapy for Wegener's granulomatosis. N Engl J Med 2005; 352: 351–61.

79. Stone JH, Holbrook JT, Marriott MA et al. Solid malignancies among the patients in the Wegener's granulomatosis etanercept trial. Arthritis Rheum 2006; 54: 1608–18.

80. Lamprecht P, Voswinkel J, Lilienthal T et al. Effectiveness of TNFα blockade with infliximab in refractory Wegener's granulomatmosis. Rheumatology 2002; 41: 1303–7.

81. Bartolucci P, Ramanoelina J, Cohen P et al. Efficacy of the anti-TNF-α antibody infliximab against refractory systemic vasculitides: an open pilot study on 10 patients. Rheumatology 2002; 41: 1126–32.

82. Booth A, Harper L, Hammad T et al. Prospective study of TNFα blockade with infliximab in anti-neutrophil cytoplasmic antibody-associated systemic vasculitis. J Am Soc Nephrol 2004; 15: 717–21.

83. Specks U, Fervenza FC, McDonald TJ, Hogan MCE. Response of Wegener's granulomatosis to anti-CD20 chimeric monoclonal antibody therapy. Arthritis Rheum 2001; 44: 2836–40.

84. Keogh KA, Wylam ME, Stone JH, Specks U. Induction of remission by B-lymphocyte depletion in eleven patients with refractory antineutrophil cytoplasmic antibody-associated vasculitis. Arthritis Rheum 2005; 52: 262–8.

85. Keogh KA, Ytterberg SR, Fervenza FC et al. Rituximab for refractory Wegener's granulomatosis: report of a prospective, open-label pilot trial. Am J Respir Crit Care Med 2006; 173: 180–7.

86. Sneller MC. Rituximab and Wegener's granulomatosis: are B cells a target in vasculitis treatment? Arthritis Rheum 2005; 52: 1–5.

87. Guillevin L, Cohen P, Gayraud M et al. Churg–Strauss syndrome. Clinical study and long-term follow-up of 96 patients. Medicine 1999; 78: 26–37.

88. Keogh KA, Specks U. Churg-Strauss syndrome. Semin Respir Crit Care Med 2006; 27: 148–57.

89. Hellmich B, Gross WL. Recent progress in the pharmacotherapy of Churg-Strauss syndrome. Expert Opin Pharmacother 2004; 5: 25–35.

90. Cohen P, Mouthon L, Godmer P et al. Corticosteroids (CS) alone for Churg–Strauss syndrome (CSS) without initial poor prognostic factor (Five factor score (FFS) = 0): preliminary results at 4 years of a French multicenter prospective study. Arthritis Rheum 2001; 44 (Suppl): S56.

91. Guillevin L, Cohen P, Mahr A et al. Treatment of polyarteritis nodosa and microscopic polyangiitis with poor prognosis factors: a prospective trial comparing glucocorticoids and six or twelve cyclophosphamide pulses in sixty-five patients. Arthritis Rheum 2003; 49: 93–100.

92. Sable-Fourtassou R, Cohen P, Mahr A et al. Antineutrophil cytoplasmic antibodies and the Churg-Strauss syndrome. Ann Intern Med 2005; 143: 632–8.

93. Kiene M, Csernok E, Muller A et al. Predominant Th2 cytokine profile in Churg–Strauss syndrome. Clin Exp Immunol 2000; 120 (Suppl 1): 49.

94. Hattori N, Ichimura M, Nagamatsu M et al. Clinicopathological features of Churg–Strauss syndrome-associated neuropathy. Brain 1999; 122: 427–39.

95. Schmitt WH, Csernok E, Kobayashi S et al. Churg–Strauss syndrome. Serum markers of lymphocyte activation and endothelial damage. Arthritis Rheum 1998; 41: 445–52.

96. D'Cruz DP, Barnes NC, Lockwood CM. Difficult asthma or Churg–Strauss syndrome? BMJ 1999; 318: 475–6.

97. Mouthon L, Khaled M, Cohen P et al. Antigen inhalation as triggering factor in systemic small-sized-vessel vasculitis. Ann Med Interne 2001; 152: 152–6.

98. Eustace JA, Nadasdy T, Choi M. The Churg Strauss syndrome. J Am Soc Nephrol 1999; 10: 2048–55.

99. Rothenberg ME. Eosinophilia. N Engl J Med 1998; 338: 1592–600.

100. Hohki G, Terada N, Hamano N et al. The effects of eotaxin on the surface adhesion molecules of endothelial cells and on eosinophil adhesion to microvascular endothelial cells. Biochem Biophys Res Commun 1997; 241: 136–41.

101. Tatsis E, Schnabel A, Gross W. Interferon-α treatment of four patients with the Churg–Strauss syndrome. Ann Intern Med 1998; 129: 370–4.

102. Termeer CC, Simon J, Schopf E. Low-dose interferon alfa-2b for the treatment of Churg–Strauss syndrome with prominent skin involvement. Arch Dermatol 2001; 137: 136–8.

103. Metzler C, Lamprecht P, Hellmich B et al. Leucoencephalopathy after treatment of Churg-Strauss syndrome with interferon α. Ann Rheum Dis 2005; 64: 1242–3.

104. Vassilopoulos D, Calabrese LH. Viral associated vasculitides: clinical aspects. In: Hoffman GS, Weyand CM, eds. Inflammatory Diseases of the Blood Vessels. New York: Marcel Dekker, 2002: 553–64.

105. Dienstag JL. Immunopathogenesis of the extrahepatic manifestations of hepatitis B virus infection. Springer Semin Immunopathol 1981; 3: 461–72.

106. Guillevin L, Lhote F, Cohen P et al. Polyarteritis nodosa related to hepatitis B virus. A prospective study with long-term observation of 41 patients. Medicine (Baltimore) 1995; 74: 238–53.

107. McMahon BJ, Heyward WL, Templin DW et al. Hepatitis B-associated polyarteritis nodosa in Alaskan Eskimos: clinical and epidemiologic features and long-term follow-up. Hepatology 1989; 9: 97–101.

108. Trepo C, Guillevin L. Polyarteritis nodosa and extrahepatic manifestations of HBV I infection: the case against autoimmune intervention. J Autoimmun 2001; 16: 269–74.

109. Misiani R. Viral associated vasculitides: basic aspects. In: Hoffman GS, Weyand CM, eds. Inflammatory Diseases of the Blood Vessels. New York: Marcel Dekker, 2002: 553–64.

110. Agnello V. The etiology and pathophysiology of mixed cryoglobulinemia secondary to hepatitis C virus infection. Springer Semin Immunopathol 1997; 19: 111–29.

111. Cacoub P, Maisonobe T, Thibault V et al. Systemic vasculitis in patients with hepatitis C. J Rheumatol 2001; 28: 109–18.

112. Gorevic PD, Kassab HJ, Levo Y et al. Mixed cryoglobulinemia: clinical aspects and long-term follow-up of 40 patients. Am J Med 1980; 69: 287–308.

113. Agnello V, Abel G. Localization of hepatitis C virus in cutaneous vasculitic lesions in patients with type II cryoglobulinemia. Arthritis Rheum 1997; 40: 2007–15.

114. Dammacco F, Sansonno D, Piccoli C et al. The lymphoid system in HCV infection: autoimmunity, mixed cryoglobulinemia and overt B-cell malignancy. Semin Liver Dis 2000; 20: 143–57.

115. Vassilopoulos D, Calabrese LH. Hepatitis C virus infection and vasculitis: implications of antiviral and immunosuppressive therapies. Arthritis Rheum 2002; 46: 585–97.

116. Zuckerman E, Keren D, Slobodin G et al. Treatment of refractory, symptomatic, hepatitis C virus related mixed cryoglobulinemia with ribavirin and interferon-alpha. J Rheumatol 2000; 27: 2172–8.

117. Cacoub P, Saadoun D, Limal N et al. PEGylated interferon alfa-2b and ribavirin treatment in patients with hepatitis C virus-related systemic vasculitis. Arthritis Rheum 2005; 52(3): 911–15.

118. Sansonno D, De Re V, Lauletta G et al. Monoclonal antibody treatment of mixed cryoglobulinemia resistant to interferon alpha with an anti-CD20. Blood 2003; 101: 3818–26.

119 Zaja F, Vianelli N, Sperotto A et al. Anti-CD20 therapy for chronic lymphocytic leukemia-associated autoimmune diseases. Leuk Lymphoma 2003; 44(11): 1951–5.

120. Roccatello D, Baldovino S, Rossi D et al. Long-term effects of anti-CD20 monoclonal antibody treatment of cryoglobulinaemic glomerulonephritis. Nephrol Dial Transplant 2004; 19(12): 3054–61.

121. Quartuccio L, Soardo G, Romano G et al. Rituximab treatment for glomerulonephritis in HCV-associated mixed cryoglobulinaemia: efficacy and safety in the absence of steroids. Rheumatology (Oxford) 2006; 45: 842–6.

122. Lamprecht P, Gause A, Gross W. Cryoglobulinemic vasculitis. Arthritis Rheum 1999; 42: 2507–16.

123. Ratanatharathorn V, Carson E, Reynolds C et al. Anti D20 monoclonal antibody treatment of immune mediated thrombocytopenia in a patient with chronic graft-versus-host disease. Ann Intern Med 2000; 133: 275–9.

124. Ghijseis E, Lerut E, Vanrenterghem Y, Kuypers D. Anti-CD20 antibody (Rituximab) therapy for HCV negative therapy resistant essential mixed cryoglobulinemia with renal and cardiac failure. Am J Kidney Dis 2004; 43: E24.

Myositis

Frederick W Miller

INTRODUCTION

The myositis syndromes, or idiopathic inflammatory myopathies (IIMs), are a diverse group of rare, acquired, systemic disorders, which share the primary feature of chronic muscle inflammation of unknown cause.[1] The main clinicopathologic forms of these juvenile and adult onset diseases are polymyositis (PM), dermatomyositis (DM), and inclusion body myositis (IBM), but less common variants include cancer-associated forms and those in which myositis is seen as an overlap syndrome with other disorders such as lupus or scleroderma. Given that the pathogeneses are unknown, but that inflammation in affected tissues is the primary pathologic finding associated with muscle weakness and other symptoms, the treatment of these conditions has been directed at inhibiting immune responses via immunosuppressive agents and at strengthening remaining muscles via exercise and physical therapy. In the past, most immunosuppressive therapies have been non-specific in terms of cellular targets, but recently, clinical trials have attempted to utilize new information, which suggests possible immune-mediated pathogenetic mechanisms, to more finely focus therapy to the relevant molecular targets. This chapter summarizes current evidence supporting this more targeted molecular biologic approach in myositis and the preliminary clinical findings that have resulted from them.

PATHOLOGY AND IMMUNE ABNORMALITIES

Whatever mechanisms are hypothesized to result in the IIM must be consistent with the pathology that is seen.[2] The pathology in the muscle, skin, and other affected tissues is characterized by collections of mononuclear cells.[3] This inflammation is often focal and inhomogeneous. Thus, essentially normal tissue can be present next to active inflammatory lesions, which can juxtapose areas characterized by nearly complete fibrosis from prior inflammation. In skeletal muscle, the muscle cells (myocytes) show evidence of focal necrosis with degeneration and regeneration and there is often increased connective tissue or fibrosis in the interstitial areas around the myocytes.

Immunohistochemical and other investigations implicate different pathogeneses in the various forms of myositis.[1,4,5] In PM and IBM, the weight of evidence suggests a predominant cytotoxic T-lymphocyte-mediated process with CD8+ T cells surrounding and invading otherwise normal appearing myocytes in endomysial areas. In DM, on the other hand, the infiltrate is mainly B lymphocytes and CD4+ helper T cells in perimysial areas around the muscle fascicles and small blood vessels. Blood vessel pathology with endothelial cell damage from complement deposition and atrophy of the myofibers at the periphery of the fascicle due to the more tenuous blood supply in this area – called perifascicular atrophy – is also characteristic of DM, as well as a decrease in the overall vasculature in muscle.[6] Of interest, the same cellular infiltrates and vasculopathy found in muscle are also present in the skin and other target organs in DM.[1,7] IBM differs pathologically from PM and DM by the presence of myocytes with characteristic reddish inclusions and vacuoles rimmed by purple granules on trichrome staining, as well as by amyloid beta protein deposition and nuclear or cytoplasmic 15–18 nm tubulofilamentous inclusions as demonstrated by electron microscopy.[8]

The immunopathology in the IIMs consists of a wide variety of cellular and humoral abnormalities (Table 38.1). Cellular findings include T and B lymphocyte activation in circulation and infiltrating target tissues. A variety of lines of other evidence are consistent with the working hypothesis that cell-mediated myotoxicity is operative, especially in PM and IBM.[9] Humoral abnormalities include autoantibodies, which are found in over 90% of PM and DM patients.[10] Although it remains unclear what role, if any, autoantibodies play in IIM pathogenesis, they inhibit the function of their targets, serum levels of autoantibodies do correlate highly with myositis disease activity, and they can become negative after prolonged remission.[11–14] The most frequent autoantibodies in IIMs are antinuclear antibodies (ANAs), but many others are commonly seen, including rheumatoid factor (RF), anti-La, anti-Ro, and those known as myositis-associated autoantibodies (anti-U1RNP, anti-PM/Scl, anti-Ku, and anti-p155 autoantibodies).[15] None of these are diagnostic for PM or DM, but if present, they do assist in distinguishing the IIM from other non-inflammatory forms of myopathy. About a third of IIM patients have autoantibodies that are diagnostic for IIM, known as myositis-specific autoantibodies.[16] The most common of these are anti-synthetase (including anti-Jo-1) autoantibodies, anti-signal recognition particle (SRP) autoantibodies, and anti-Mi-2 autoantibodies. Each of these autoantibodies is strongly associated with a distinct clinical presentation, immunogenetic risk factor, response to therapy, and prognosis, suggesting that each may represent a truly different myositis syndrome.[17, 18]

POSSIBLE PATHOGENIC MECHANISMS

The inflammatory pathology, the frequent finding of autoantibodies and other immune abnormalities, the overlap of myositis with

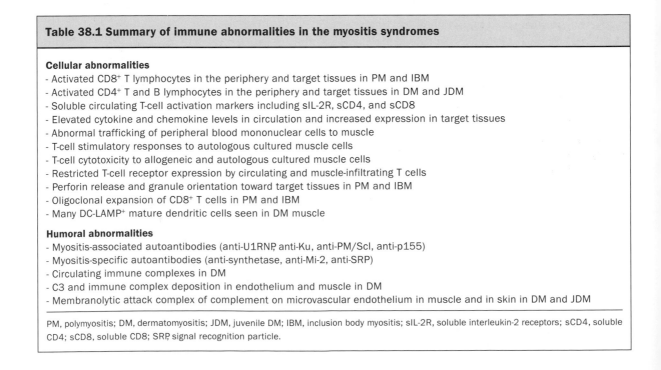

Table 38.1 Summary of immune abnormalities in the myositis syndromes

Cellular abnormalities
- Activated CD8+ T lymphocytes in the periphery and target tissues in PM and IBM
- Activated CD4+ T and B lymphocytes in the periphery and target tissues in DM and JDM
- Soluble circulating T-cell activation markers including sIL-2R, sCD4, and sCD8
- Elevated cytokine and chemokine levels in circulation and increased expression in target tissues
- Abnormal trafficking of peripheral blood mononuclear cells to muscle
- T-cell stimulatory responses to autologous cultured muscle cells
- T-cell cytotoxicity to allogeneic and autologous cultured muscle cells
- Restricted T-cell receptor expression by circulating and muscle-infiltrating T cells
- Perforin release and granule orientation toward target tissues in PM and IBM
- Oligoclonal expansion of CD8+ T cells in PM and IBM
- Many DC-LAMP+ mature dendritic cells seen in DM muscle

Humoral abnormalities
- Myositis-associated autoantibodies (anti-U1RNP, anti-Ku, anti-PM/Scl, anti-p155)
- Myositis-specific autoantibodies (anti-synthetase, anti-Mi-2, anti-SRP)
- Circulating immune complexes in DM
- C3 and immune complex deposition in endothelium and muscle in DM
- Membranolytic attack complex of complement on microvascular endothelium in muscle and in skin in DM and JDM

PM, polymyositis; DM, dermatomyositis; JDM, juvenile DM; IBM, inclusion body myositis; sIL-2R, soluble interleukin-2 receptors; sCD4, soluble CD4; sCD8, soluble CD8; SRP, signal recognition particle.

autoimmune diseases such as systemic lupus erythematosus (SLE) and rheumatoid arthritis (RA) in some patients, the immunogenetic risk factors, and the clinical response to anti-inflammatory agents – all suggest an immune-mediated component to the pathogenesis of the myositis syndromes.[1] As is the case with other autoimmune conditions, however, the IIMs are likely complex disorders resulting from chronic immune activation and dysregulation following selected environmental exposures in genetically susceptible individuals.[19] As summarized above, many lines of current evidence suggest that the mechanisms differ for different forms of myositis and possibly differ at different stages of disease.[4,18,20,21]

Therefore, although the cause of IIM is unknown, immune-mediated mechanisms certainly play a role in disease pathogenesis. Yet, possibly due to different methodologies and the assessment of relatively small numbers of patients from different populations, prior studies have sometimes been contradictory and the exact mechanisms that result in the myositis syndromes remain unclear. Some immunopathogenetic mechanisms appear to be common to different phenotypes, while in other cases the mechanisms may differ.

Immune-mediated mechanisms

Given the pathology seen in the IIMs, a number of investigations have focused on understanding possible immunoregulatory control mechanisms that could account for the inflammation seen. A variety of lines of evidence have shown abnormalities in the expression of immunological synapse components, cytokines, chemokines and their receptors, costimulatory molecules, cell migration regulators, matrix metalloproteinases (MMPs), complement factors, and endoplasmic reticulum (ER) stress response components in association with immune effector and/or target cells in IIMs (Table 38.2). Further evidence for the linkage of many of these findings to the disease process comes from investigations that suggest strong correlations between the

Table 38.2 Possible targets for biologic therapy of idiopathic inflammatory myopathies (IIMs)

Target	Increased expression in IIM	Comments	References
Immunological synapse components			
HLA class I	PM, DM, JDM, IBM	Classical HLA A, B, and C antigens on myocytes	96, 97
HLA-G	PM, DM, IBM	Non-classical HLA class I protein co-expressed on all HLA class I+ myocytes	98
HLA class II	PM, DM, JDM, IBM	Increased expression by PBLs and myocytes	99, 100
TCR	PM, IBM, anti-Jo-1 autoantibody+	Restricted a/b families found in the periphery and muscle-infiltrating T cells	101–104
ICAM-1	PM, DM, JDM, IBM	Expressed on muscle microvessel (arteriole, capillary, and venule) endothelium (more prominent in JDM) and myofibers (more prominent in PM and DM)	105–109
LFA-1a	PM, DM	Expressed on muscle-infiltrating T cells	108, 110
ICOS, ICOS-L	PM, DM, IBM	Supports role of CD8+ T cells in pathogenesis	111
Cytokines			
IL-1a	PM, DM, JDM, IBM	Expressed by endothelial cells > inflammatory cells, may be directly myotoxic	96, 112
IL-1Ra	PM, DM, JDM	Increased circulating levels, polymorphisms in gene a risk factor for JDM	113–115
IL-1b	PM, DM, IBM	Expressed on inflammatory cells	110, 112
IL-6	Possibly in PM, DM, IBM	Constitutive expression by myoblasts	116
TNF-α	PM, DM, JDM, IBM	Expressed on CD8+ T cells and myocytes and increased in serum; may be directly myotoxic	117–119
sTNF-R	PM, DM, JDM	Elevated in serum	113, 120

Continued

Table 38.2 Possible targets for biologic therapy of idiopathic inflammatory myopathies (IIMs)—cont'd

Target	Increased expression in IIM	Comments	References
TGF-β1-3	PM, DM, IBM	Antigen and mRNA both up-regulated in muscle	110, 112
IFN-α/β	DM	IFN signatures distinguished DM from PM and IBM	60
Chemokines/receptors			
MIP-1a (CCL3)	PM, DM, IBM	Both message and protein increased	112, 121
MIP-1b (CCL4)	PM, DM, IBM	Both message and protein increased	121
RANTES (CCL5)	PM, DM, IBM	Expressed on inflammatory cells	121
MCP-1 (CCL2)	DM > PM, IBM	Expressed on myocytes, binds to CCR2	122
CCR2	PM and IBM > DM	Expressed on vessel walls and mononuclear cells, the primary receptor for MCP-1	122
Co-stimulators			
BB-1 (CD 80, B7 family)		Expressed on MHC-I⁺ cells and makes contact with CD28 or CTLA-4	123
CD40	PM, DM	Expressed on myocytes	124
CD40L	PM, DM	Expressed on muscle-infiltrating T cells	124
CTLA-4	PM, DM	Expressed on muscle and infiltrating T cells	125
CD28	PM, DM	Expressed on muscle cells	125
Cell migration regulators			
VCAM-1	PM, DM, IBM	Studies suggest different expression in different groups	105–107, 109
VLA-4	PM, DM, IBM	Up-regulated on infiltrating leukocytes; interacts with VCAM-1 expressed on endothelial cells	126
CD142 and CD31	DM	Both molecules facilitate dendritic cell transmigration	23
Metalloproteinases			
MMP-9/MMP-2	PM, IBM	MMP-9 and -2 on non-necrotic and MHC-1-expressing myofibers; MMP-9 on CD8⁺ T cells	127
Complement factors			
C3, C5b-9 membrane attack complex	DM, JDM	C3 and the membranolytic attack complex on capillary endothelium and myocytes	35, 128
ER stress response			
Protein 78 pathway and NF-κB	PM, DM, IBM	Up-regulated compared with controls suggesting a possible non-immune pathogenetic mechanism	43, 56

PM, polymyositis; DM, dermatomyositis; JDM, juvenile DM; IBM, inclusion body myositis; CD, complementary determining; MNC, mononuclear cell; ICAM-1, intercellular adhesion molecule-1; VCAM-1, vascular cellular adhesion molecule-1; LFA-1, leukocyte function-associated antigen 1; VLA-4, very late antigen-4; TCR, T-cell receptor; HLA, human leukocyte antigen; IL-1, interleukin-1; IL-1Ra, IL-1 receptor antagonist; PBL, peripheral blood lymphocytes; TNF-α, tumor necrosis factor-α; TGF-β, transforming growth factor-β; MIP-1, macrophage inflammatory protein-1; RANTES, regulated on activation, normal T-cell expressed and secreted; MCP-1, monocyte chemoattractant protein-1; CCR2, chemokines receptor-2; CTLA-4, cytotoxic T-lymphocyte antigen-4; MMP, matrix metalloproteinases; C3, third component of complement; ICOS, inducible costimulatory molecule; ICOS-L, ICOS-ligand.

immune abnormalities noted and the severity of disease.[1] Some of these studies also suggest that myocytes, myoblasts, or endothelial cells themselves may serve as antigen-presenting cells (APCs), but the finding of CD86/CD40 and CD86/MHC class II antigens and cells with dendritic cell (DC) morphologies in myositis muscle biopsies implies that some professional APCs may also be present in the inflamed muscle tissue.[22,23]

Recent findings suggest that the autoantigenic aminoacyl-tRNA synthetases may perpetuate the development of myositis by recruiting mononuclear cells that induce innate and adaptive immune responses. For example, several amino acid domains of the Jo-1 autoantigen (histidyl-tRNA synthetase) can induce CD4[+] and CD8[+] lymphocytes, interleukin (IL)-2-activated monocytes, and immature DCs (iDCs) to migrate and are chemotactic for lymphocytes and activated monocytes.[24] Another autoantigen, asparaginyl-tRNA synthetase, induced migration of lymphocytes, activated monocytes, iDCs, and CCR3-transfected HEK-293 cells; however, the non-autoantigenic aspartyl-tRNA and lysyl-tRNA synthetases were not chemotactic. Therefore, the selection of a self-molecule as a target for an autoantibody response may be a consequence of the proinflammatory properties of the molecule itself.

These findings, taken together, strongly suggest intimate cell–cell interactions, cell–cell communication, and immune activation as necessary, but likely not sufficient, activities prior to cell migration and other effector functions in IIMs. Despite the impressive pathologic differences in the various forms of IIMs, it is somewhat surprising that many studies suggest that the same molecular abnormalities may be found in all forms of myositis.[20,25] Nonetheless, it remains unclear as to whether these are primary events or possibly secondary non-specific changes induced by whatever primary events are actually triggering these diseases.

Complement

Complement has been hypothesized to play a role in the pathogenesis of myositis in a number of possible ways. The first evidence for this came from early studies demonstrating deposition of immunoglobulin and complement (C3) in the microvasculature, particularly in DM and juvenile DM (JDM).[26] Since that time, others have confirmed these findings and suggested the possible role of infectious agents,[27,28] cryoglobulins,[29] or other mechanisms to explain these deposits.[30] Circulating immune complexes or abnormal complement levels have also been found in DM[31] and PM[32] cases and in a spontaneous familial canine dermatomyositis syndrome that closely mimics human DM.[33,34] The C5b–C9 membrane attack complex has been implicated in the pathology of DM vessels and myocytes.[35]

Hypoxia or oxidative stress

Primary processes – which could be myotrophic infections, myotoxic or immune-activating environmental exposures – may result in secondary inflammatory responses or altered physiology in muscle, skin or other target organs.[1,36,37] These or other changes could affect blood supply to muscles and induce subsequent hypoxia. This has been hypothesized in DM, in which decreased capillary density and increased markers of hypoxia, including IL-1 and transforming growth factor-β (TGF-β) are prominently found,[20] and one study has actually documented hypoxia in the muscle tissue of myositis patients.[38] Hypoxia may also alter endothelial cell function by increasing IL-1 and intercellular adhesion molecule-1 (ICAM-1) expression.[39] Another pathologic finding in IIM is that of occasional ragged red fibers and cytochrome c oxidase (COX)-negative fibers in muscle biopsies.[40] This may be further evidence for ischemic changes in IIM, since animal models show similar ischemia-induced mitochondrial changes and ragged red fibers in skeletal muscle.[41] Alternatively, oxidative stress may also play a role in IIM, as has been specifically suggested in IBM based upon the finding of excess intracellular nitric oxide, which can combine with superoxide to produce highly toxic peroxynitrite that can nitrate tyrosines of proteins and possibly result in the misfolding of proteins.[8,42,43] Additional evidence for metabolic disturbances in myositis comes from magnetic resonance spectroscopy studies, suggesting decreased energy production[44] and altered choline/lipid and creatine/lipid ratios,[45] and from a Coxsackie B virus-induced animal model in which muscle lactate and CO_2 are significantly elevated.[46] Again, the major uncertainty regarding the implications of these metabolic studies is whether they represent primary etiopathogenic events or secondary processes resulting from the complex physiological changes that accompany chronic inflammatory changes in muscle and other target tissues.

Direct myotoxic effects from cytokines

The cytokines present in the muscle and endothelium of myositis biopsies may be involved in the regulation of immune responses, but may also have diverse direct effects on muscle and other target tissues.[20] This is true for tumor necrosis factor (TNF)-α, which has been shown to directly induce a wide array of changes in muscle from accelerated catabolism to contractile dysfunction to inhibition of myogenic differentiation through nuclear factor kappaB (NF-κB).[47,48] IL-1a also may play a role in direct myotoxicity via its influence on insulin-like growth factor, leading to metabolic disturbances in nutrition supply[49] and by suppressing myoblast proliferation as well as myoblast fusion, leading to poor muscle regeneration.[50]

Inhibitors of apoptosis

Although apoptosis of multinucleated muscle fibers could be an expected outcome – given the muscle pathology, the many inflammatory processes described above, and the fact that Fas/FasL are expressed in some muscle tissue – evidence for myocyte apoptosis has not been convincingly produced in IIM.[22] This somewhat surprising finding has resulted in a number of investigations that have attempted to define the mechanisms that may block muscle cell apoptosis. Using laser capture microscopy, it has been shown that Fas-associated death domain-like IL-1-converting enzyme-inhibitory protein (FLIP) is expressed in the muscle fibers and on infiltrating lymphocytes of myositis biopsies.[51] Other apoptotic inhibitors also appear to be expressed in myositis biopsies, including an inhibitor of apoptosis (IAP)-like protein (hILP),[52] as well as Bcl-2 on Fas+ muscle fibers and Bcl-XL and cyclin-dependent kinase inhibitory proteins p16 and p57 on Fas+ inflammatory cells.[53] Therefore, both the effector cells and the target cells in the muscle of IIM patients may have separate mechanisms for inhibiting apoptotic events. Nevertheless, recent findings suggest that myocyte apoptosis might still be induced under certain conditions. The expression of MRP8 and MRP14 by muscle-infiltrating activated macrophages was found to associate with degeneration of myofibers in biopsies, and further, purified MRP8/MRP14 complex inhibited proliferation and differentiation of C2C12 myoblasts and it induced apoptosis via

activation of caspase-3 in a time- and dose-dependent manner.[54]

MHC and the endoplasmic reticulum stress response

Although muscle fibers do not normally express major histocompatibility complex (MHC) class I antigens, in PM, DM, and IBM, MHC class I antigens are expressed in many myocytes regardless of whether they are invaded by T cells or contain vacuoles. This observation, as well as the finding that transgenic overexpression of MHC class I can also induce inflammatory myopathies in mice,[55] suggested that combined immune and non-immune processes involving metabolic stress due to up-regulation of MHC class I antigen expression may be at work in the IIM. The assembly and folding of MHC class I molecules occurs in the ER and involves a complex process wherein chaperones bind to proteins to assure their proper folding and to prevent accumulation of unfolded proteins. Studies provide evidence that the ER chaperones calnexin, calreticulin, GRP94, BiP/GRP78, and ERp72 physically associate with AβPP in s-IBM muscle, suggesting their role in AβPP folding and processing.[43] In DM the pathways of ER stress response, the unfolded protein response (glucose-regulated protein 78 pathway), and the ER overload response (NF-κB pathway) were significantly activated in muscle tissue of human myositis patients and in the mouse model.[56] Taken together, these findings suggest that secondary effects of up-regulation of MHC molecules may induce both immune and non-immune processes, both of which may play a role in IIM pathogenesis via activation of NF-κB, resulting in the induction of a number of cytokines, chemokines, adhesion molecules, and further MHC up-regulation, thus initiating a self-sustaining positive-feedback loop.

Lessons from gene expression studies

In support of other lines of evidence listed above, findings from recent gene expression array investigations in muscle biopsies were that genes encoding a variety of MHC, immunoglobulin, complement (factor B, C7, factor I, C1S, factor H, and C4), adhesion (cathepsin B (CTSB), Endo 1-associated antigen (CD146), anosmin-1), angiogenesis (CX3CL1, CCR1, CD47, VCAM-1, ICAM-1, PECAM1, and ICAM2), chemokine (CCL2, CCL3, and the CXC-chemokine ligands (CXCL) 9 and 10) and cytokine (IL-1, IL-2, IL-5, IL-10, TNF, and TGF-β) molecules were up-regulated in IIM.[23,25,57–60] These studies also demonstrated up-regulation of interferon (IFN) signatures as one of the major features differentiating DM from PM and IBM, calling into question the theory of ischemia as the cause of muscle damage, as IFN signatures are not a feature of ischemic tissue. One investigation of serial muscle biopsies from three DM and four IBM patients, before and after treatment with intravenous immunoglobulin, suggested decreases in selected chemokine and ICAM genes in those DM patients who responded to therapy.[61]

BIOLOGICAL THERAPY OF MYOSITIS

The rarity and heterogeneity of the IIMs have limited therapeutic studies in these diseases. Additionally, it has been difficult to interpret or compare the results of the few studies that have been performed due to the lack of validated outcome measures, little consistency in the use of classification criteria and no prior consistency in clinical trial designs. Only recently have worldwide, multidisciplinary consortia of experts been organized (the International Myositis Assessment and Clinical Studies group, IMACS, https://dir-apps.niehs.nih.gov/imacs/) to define and validate outcome measures and standardize the conduct of clinical trials in juvenile and adult myositis.[62,63]

No proven treatments exist for myositis and those in use often result in serious toxic and other complications. Standard therapy has focused on inhibiting immune responses with immunosuppressive agents and on strengthening muscles through exercise and physical therapy.[64] The usual therapeutic approach is to begin treatment with corticosteroids alone in less severe cases with good prognostic factors, or corticosteroids in addition to azathioprine, methotrexate or similar non-specific immunomodulatory drugs in severe cases with poor prognostic factors, using

drug doses proportionate to the degree of disease activity present.[1] Although many patients respond to such therapies to some extent, the IIMs remain serious diseases, with high morbidity and mortality, in need of safer and more effective therapies. The molecular immunopathologic findings described above have generated interest in developing targeted therapies for IIMs using similar approaches as have been successfully employed in other rheumatic diseases (see other chapters). Possible common pathogenetic mechanisms in all forms of IIMs suggest additional specific targets that may have more general applicability. Over the last decade, a variety of biologic agents have been reported to possibly benefit IIM patients on the basis of case reports, case series, or controlled trials (Table 38.3). For the most part these data represent preliminary, and sometimes conflicting, clinical observations, often not controlled, without validated endpoints, and from which conclusions are unable to be firmly drawn. Thus, compared with some other rheumatic diseases, the biologic therapy of myositis is in its infancy.

Intravenous immunoglobulin

Intravenous immunoglobulin (IVIG) is the best studied biologic agent in the treatment of myositis.[65] Based upon empiric IVIG therapy in a patient with X-linked agammaglobulinemia who developed echovirus meningoencephalitis and myositis-fasciitis that resulted in dramatic clinical response[66] and anecdotal responses in other immune-mediated diseases, controlled and uncontrolled trials have been reported in PM, DM, and IBM, and uncontrolled studies have been performed in JDM and retrovirus-associated PM (Table 38.3).

The strongest evidence for the effectiveness of IVIG in IIMs comes from a double-blind, placebo-controlled, crossover protocol of 1 g/kg/day for 2 consecutive days each month in DM, which demonstrated an improvement in strength in 11 of 12 patients who received IVIG compared with 3 of 11 in the placebo group.[67] These patients also had significant improvements in a neuromuscular symptoms score and in their skin rashes. These clinical changes were accompanied by significant histologic improvements

Table 38.3 Published studies of biologic therapies in myositis

Agent	Clinical experience	Subgroup	Outcome	Reference
IVIG	Open-label trial (n = 6)	DM	5 of 6 patients improved in strength on 2 g/kg/month for 4 months	129
IVIG	Double-blind, placebo-controlled crossover trial (n = 12)	DM	Significant clinical, laboratory, and muscle biopsy improvement after 3 months of 2 g/kg/month treatment	130
IVIG	Open-label trial (n = 19)	DM	7 of 19 patients (with severe skin disease, no cancer or antibodies) improved in strength and rash	131
IVIG	Open-label trial (n = 5)	JDM	5 of 5 refractory patients improved in strength and rash	132
IVIG	Retrospective clinic review (n = 9)	JDM	9 of 9 patients showed evidence of clinical improvement, but most were on other therapies	133
IVIG	Open-label trial (n = 7)	JDM	6 of 7 patients showed evidence of clinical strength improvement, but few maintained responses	70
IVIG	Retrospective chart review (n = 18)	JDM	12 of 18 patients showed evidence of clinical strength improvement, but many were on other immunosuppressive therapies	71
IVIG	Open-label trial (n = 14 PM of 20 IIM)	PM	10 of 14 patients improved in strength on 2 g/kg/month for 4 months	129
IVIG	Open-label trial (n = 35)	PM	Clinical and laboratory improvement in 25 of 35 patients after 6 months of 2 g/kg/month treatment, 7 relapsed in 4–23 months, but the rest were stable	73
IVIG	Open-label case series (n = 3)	HIV-1+ or HTLV-1+ PM	No improvement seen	74
IVIG	Open-label (n = 4)	IBM	Improvement in 3 of 4 patients after 2 g/kg/month for 2 months	134
IVIG	Double-blind, placebo-controlled, crossover trial (n = 19)	IBM	No significant improvement in strength in 9 patients on 2 g/kg/month treatment	76
IVIG	Double-blind, placebo-controlled trial (n = 36)	IBM	No significant improvement in strength in 19 patients on 2 g/kg/month treatment with prednisone vs 17 on placebo and prednisone for 3 months	77

Agent	Study design	Disease	Comments	Reference
Anti-C5 mAb	Randomized, double-blind, placebo-controlled phase 1 trial (n = 12)	DM	Little toxicity noted, study completed	Personal communication, Dr Chris Mojcik
Etanercept	Open-label (n = 4)	JDM	Little response, little toxicity	82
Etanercept	Open-label (n = 4)	PM, DM, JDM	Improvements in all patients; all had been refractory to prior therapies	135
Etanercept	Open-label, retrospective (n = 9)	IBM	No improvement over baseline or IBM patients in other studies	136
Infliximab	Open-label (n = 2)	PM, DM	Clinical, laboratory, and pathologic improvement in both patients	84
Infliximab	Double-blind, placebo-controlled, phase 2 (n = 28)	PM, DM	Single-center trial, ongoing	http://www.clinicaltrials.gov/ct/show/NCT00338891?order=8
Anti-T-cell globulin	Open-label, randomized trial with or without MTX (n = 11)	IBM	6 subjects randomized to anti-T-cell globulin plus MTX had improved myometry compared with 5 with MTX alone after 12 months	93
IFN-β1a	Phase 1 randomized, placebo-controlled trial (n = 30)	IBM	Little toxicity, little evidence of improvement	92
IFN-β1a	Phase 2 randomized, placebo-controlled trial (n = 30)	IBM	Little toxicity, little evidence of improvement	137
Rituximab (anti-CD20)	Phase 1, open-label, trial (n = 6)	DM	Initial improvements in all 6/6 evaluable DM patients – 2 JDM patients treated out of protocol also improved	87
Stem cell therapy	Case reports (n = 2)	Anti-Jo-1[+] PM	Improved myositis and pulmonary disease, but toxicity in both patients; experience accumulating in ongoing European and US studies	138, 139

IVIG, intravenous immunoglobulin; anti-Jo-1, autoantibodies to Jo-1 antigen (histidyl-tRNA synthetase) present; CK, creatine kinase; mAb, monoclonal antibody; MTX, methotrexate; see also footnote to Table 38.2.

in muscle biopsies, including decreases in the expression of MHC class I and ICAM-1, and significant increases in muscle fiber diameter and capillary density. The limitations of this study include the fact that many patients were also receiving corticosteroids and other immunomodulatory agents that may have influenced these responses and that each treatment period was only 3 months long, with little follow-up after the end of the protocol to assess adverse events and response durability.

Juvenile-onset DM, which shares many clinical, immunologic, and pathologic features with adult-onset DM,[68] has also been reported to be responsive to IVIG therapy in uncontrolled studies.[69] In several small open-label or retrospective case series, the majority of patients had some response; however, often it was short-lived and, because most patients were also taking other immunosuppressive therapy, it remains unclear what role the IVIG truly played in the responses.[70,71]

Studies of IVIG therapy in PM and IBM, which are thought to be cytotoxic T-cell-mediated diseases rather than involving complement activation and immunoglobulin deposition in the case of DM, have been inconclusive (Table 38.3). An attempt to use IVIG as first-line therapy in PM and DM, as proposed by some investigators, failed to show any benefit.[72] Although open-label studies in which PM patients received IVIG with other immunosuppressive therapy suggest short- and long-term responses in some patients,[73] results from an ongoing controlled trial have not been reported.[74] And, despite encouraging responses from an open-label study in IBM patients,[75] two subsequent double-blind, placebo-controlled trials in IBM have failed to demonstrate significant benefit from IVIG.[76,77]

The mechanism of action of IVIG in most diseases for which it is prescribed remains unknown and it is likely that different mechanisms may be at work in different diseases. Possible effects of IVIG include Fc receptor blockade, inactivation of complement effector functions, inhibition of lymphocyte activation and cytokine release, increased catabolism of IgG, immunomodulation by anti-idiotype antibodies, or diverse immunologic effects from the non-IgG components present in IVIG.[65,78] In both DM and animal model (experimental autoimmune myositis) studies, however, it appears that IVIG may exert its positive effects via blocking complement activation and inhibiting the deposition of the membranolytic attack complex of complement on myocytes and vascular endothelium.[79,80]

The problems associated with IVIG are numerous and include: high cost, as measured by both the cost of preparations and extensive time commitments of patients and health care providers; intermittent product shortages; variable composition and effectiveness from manufacturer to manufacturer and from lot to lot; few data on frequencies, risk factors, and rates of adverse events at the doses being used for myositis; uncertain long-term risks; the need for repeated administration; and, of greatest importance, the lack of response or tachyphylaxis in most patients.[81] Other difficulties with IVIG are: anaphylaxis, especially as a result of preformed IgE anti-IgA antibodies in IgA-deficient persons; infusion-related back pain, nausea, vomiting, abdominal pain, myalgias, and fevers; possible interference with responses to live vaccines (measles, mumps, rubella) resulting in the recommendation that vaccinations should be deferred for 6 months after IVIG if possible; aseptic meningitis, in which a risk factor in DM appears to be history of migraine headaches; false positive lab tests for hepatitis B and C and other assays relating to the presence of infused immunoglobulin; occasional transmission of infectious agents, including hepatitis C in the past; thromboembolic events in patients with high serum viscosity; and rare hemolysis, wheezing, pulmonary edema, congestive heart failure, arthralgias, rashes, and renal and immune complex disease in patients with high titer rheumatoid factors.[81]

In summary, despite numerous studies of IVIG in IIMs, there remains inadequate information as regards the optimal dose or schedule to use for treatment, and which groups of myositis patients, under what circumstances, and for how long, respond to IVIG. At present, given the many limitations of the product and its questionable cost-effectiveness, it would seem reasonable to reserve IVIG treatment for short-term therapy in those patients, especially with DM and JDM, who have failed methotrexate and/or azathioprine, are severely ill, or are so immunocompromised or infected that other agents would not be advisable.

Anti-TNF agents

As outlined above, data from a number of studies suggest the central role of TNF-α in the pathogenesis of myositis (Table 38.2). Therefore, attempts to block TNF-α effects by use of etanercept (a dimeric fusion protein consisting of the extracellular ligand-binding portion of the soluble human 75 kDa TNF-α receptor linked to the Fc portion of human IgG1) or infliximab (a chimeric IgG1k monoclonal antibody (mAb) composed of human constant and murine variable regions directed against TNF-α) have been clinically assessed. Anti-TNF-α therapy in phase 1 studies or case series has been reported to result in improvements in strength and the capacity to taper other medications in some patients with IIM (Table 38.3). An open-label trial of etanercept in JDM has not resulted in improvements to date.[82] Other reports, however, claim substantial clinical, laboratory, and pathologic improvement from open-label experience with etanercept and infliximab in PM or DM patients who were particularly difficult to manage and had failed multiple prior agents.[83–86] Several phase 1/2 studies in children and adults are ongoing and should give a more complete understanding of the benefit/risk ratios when they are completed (Table 38.4).

Other biologic therapies

Several other biologic therapies have been studied in small numbers of IIM patients. Based on the hypothesized important role of complement in the pathogenesis of DM, a randomized, double-blind, placebo-controlled pilot study of the effect of h5G1.1-mAb (a monoclonal antibody which binds C5, the fifth component of complement, preventing cleavage into C5a and C5b) has undergone a multicenter phase 1/2 trial in DM patients. Another mAb, rituximab, which is directed against the B-lymphocyte marker CD20 and is approved for use in B-cell lymphoma and RA, has resulted in clinical improvements in six of seven DM patients in an open-label trial[87] and is undergoing further study in the largest multicenter study ever performed in myositis. This phase 2 international trial in PM, DM, and JDM will also utilize the new proposed IMACS outcome criteria and clinical trial design elements (Table 38.4).

Although treatment of malignancies and infections with IFN-α has been associated with the development of myositis in case reports,[88–91] the positive response in multiple sclerosis to IFN-β1a has prompted a phase 1, randomized,

Agent	Study design	IIM subgroup	Website
Etanercept	Phase 1 double-blind, placebo-controlled, single-center trial ($n = 40$)	DM	http://www.clinicaltrials.gov/ct/show/NCT00112385?order=12
Infliximab	Phase 2, double-blind, placebo-controlled, single-center trial ($n = 28$)	PM, DM	http://www.clinicaltrials.gov/ct/show/NCT00033891?order=8
Rituximab (anti-CD20)	Phase 2, double-blind, placebo phase design, multicenter, international trial ($n = 76$ PM, 76 DM, and 50 JDM)	PM, DM, JDM	http://www.clinicaltrials.gov/ct/show/NCT00106184?order=5
Stem cell therapy	Phase 1 open-label, single-center study in multiple autoimmune diseases	DM	http://www.clinicaltrials.gov/ct/show/NCT00010335?order=11

Table 38.4 Ongoing clinical trials of biologic therapies in myositis

Abbreviations: see footnotes to Tables 38.2 and 38.3.

placebo-controlled trial of 30 IBM patients.[92] This was a 24-week, multicenter, clinical trial of 30 μg of IFN-β1a administered intramuscularly once a week. Twenty-nine of the 30 subjects enrolled completed the study; however, two subjects (one in the placebo group, one in the IFN-β1a group) experienced severe adverse events. No subjects required dosage reductions, and the adverse event profile was similar for the placebo and IFN-β1a groups. Unfortunately, there were no significant differences in the changes in muscle strength and muscle mass between the placebo and IFN-β1a groups at 6 months. Nonetheless, this study demonstrated little evidence of toxicity, resulting in a phase 2 trial that also showed little evidence of efficacy.

In an open-label, randomized study, six IBM subjects, who received anti-T-cell globulin plus methotrexate, had improved myometry compared to the five with metrotrexate alone after 12 months, suggesting a possible beneficial effect of anti-T-cell therapy in IBM.[93] Another agent, alemtuzumab (Campath, directed against CD52) is being explored as a possible therapy for IBM in an open-label trial of 20 IBM patients.

The intriguing concept that one might be able to reset the 'immunostat' by depleting a patient's current immune system of activated cells and replenishing them with autologous stem cells, which would be expected to undergo differentiation to different effector cells in a new environment, has resulted in a wide range of investigations of stem cell therapy (SCT) in many pediatric and adult autoimmune diseases.[94,95] Case reports of muscle and lung improvement in two PM subjects with the anti-synthetase syndrome (interstitial lung disease with anti-Jo-1 autoantibodies) have supported the basis for the several ongoing SCT investigations in adult and juvenile IIM.

SYNTHESIS

Dramatic strides in understanding the molecular immunopathologic abnormalities in the myositis syndromes have been achieved in the last decade. The up-regulation of a number of cell surface or soluble proteins – critical to the function of the immunological synapse, the activation, recruitment and trafficking of effector cells into target tissues, the complement system, and the breakdown of extracellular matrix components via MMPs – have now been documented and confirmed. While it remains unclear if these abnormal expressions are primary or secondary events, they have served as the basis for the initiation of a number of clinical observations and trials of novel biologic agents that specifically inhibit or block the action of these proteins. Although we must temper the early optimism that often accompanies positive case reports and other uncontrolled experiences when a new agent is introduced, it is likely that one or more biologic therapies directed against targets summarized in this review will find a role in the armamentarium of physicians who treat myositis in the future. Novel biologic and cellular therapies – coupled with the recent establishment of international multidisciplinary consortia that have developed consensus on outcome measures and clinical trial design issues in IIM to increase the efficiency and reliability of trials – will likely play an increasing role in understanding the best management of myositis disease activity and damage and will hopefully result in safer and more effective treatments in the near future.

ACKNOWLEDGMENTS

The author thanks Dr Lisa Rider for constructive comments on the manuscript and useful discussions.

REFERENCES

1. Miller FW. Inflammatory myopathies: polymyositis, dermatomyositis, and related conditions. In: Koopman W, Moreland L, eds. Arthritis and Allied Conditions, A Textbook of Rheumatology. Philadelphia: Lippincott, Williams and Wilkins, 2004: 1593–620.
2. Dalakas MC. Muscle biopsy findings in inflammatory myopathies. Rheum Dis Clin North Am 2002; 28: 779–98, vi.
3. Engel AG, Hohlfeld R. The polymyositis and dermatomyositis syndromes. In: Engel AG, Franzini-Armstrong C, eds. Myology. New York: McGraw-Hill, 2004: 1321–66.
4. Engel AG, Arahata K, Emslie-Smith A. Immune effector mechanisms in inflammatory myopathies. Res Publ Assoc Res Nerv Ment Dis 1990; 68: 141–57.

5. Dalakas MC, Hohlfeld R. Polymyositis and dermatomyositis. Lancet 2003; 362: 971–82.

6. Emslie-Smith AM, Engel AG. Microvascular changes in early and advanced dermatomyositis: a quantitative study. Ann Neurol 1997; 27: 343–56.

7. Crowson AN, Magro CM. The role of microvascular injury in the pathogenesis of cutaneous lesions of dermatomyositis. Hum Pathol 1996; 27: 15–19.

8. Askanas V, Engel WK. Sporadic inclusion-body myositis and hereditary inclusion-body myopathies: current concepts of diagnosis and pathogenesis. Curr Opin Rheumatol 1998; 10: 530–42.

9. Dalakas MC. Inflammatory, immune, and viral aspects of inclusion-body myositis. Neurology 2006; 66: S33–S38.

10. Sarkar K, Miller FW. Autoantibodies as predictive and diagnostic markers of idiopathic inflammatory myopathies. Autoimmunity 2004; 37: 291–4.

11. Miller FW. Humoral immunity and immunogenetics in the idiopathic inflammatory myopathies. Curr Opin Rheumatol 1991; 3: 902–10.

12. Miller FW, Waite KA, Biswas T, Plotz PH. The role of an autoantigen, histidyl-tRNA synthetase, in the induction and maintenance of autoimmunity. Proc Natl Acad Sci U S A 1990; 87: 9933–7.

13. Miller FW, Twitty SA, Biswas T, Plotz PH. Origin and regulation of a disease-specific autoantibody response. Antigenic epitopes, spectrotype stability, and isotype restriction of anti-Jo-1 autoantibodies. J Clin Invest 1990; 85: 468–75.

14. Romisch K, Miller FW, Dobberstein B, High S. Human autoantibodies against the 54 kDa protein of the signal recognition particle block function at multiple stages. Arthritis Res Ther 2006; 8: R39.

15. Targoff IN. Immune manifestations of inflammatory muscle disease. Rheum Dis Clin North Am 1994; 20: 857–80.

16. Love LA, Leff RL, Fraser DD et al. A new approach to the classification of idiopathic inflammatory myopathy: myositis-specific autoantibodies define useful homogeneous patient groups. Medicine (Baltimore) 1991; 70: 360–74.

17. Miller FW. Myositis-specific autoantibodies. Touchstones for understanding the inflammatory myopathies. JAMA 1993; 270: 1846–9.

18. O'Hanlon TP, Carrick DM, Targoff IN et al. Immunogenetic risk and protective factors for the idiopathic inflammatory myopathies: distinct HLA-A, -B, -Cw, -DRB1, and -DQA1 allelic profiles distinguish European American patients with different myositis autoantibodies. Medicine (Baltimore) 2006; 85: 111–27.

19. Shamim EA, Miller FW. Familial autoimmunity and the idiopathic inflammatory myopathies. Curr Rheumatol Rep 2000; 2: 201–11.

20. Lundberg IE. The physiology of inflammatory myopathies: an overview. Acta Physiol Scand 2001; 171: 207–13.

21. Miller FW. Polymyositis and dermatomyositis. In: Goldman L, Ausiello D, eds. Cecil Textbook of Medicine. Philadelphia: Saunders, 2004: 1680–4.

22. Nagaraju K. Update on immunopathogenesis in inflammatory myopathies. Curr Opin Rheumatol 2001; 13: 461–8.

23. Nagaraju K, Rider LG, Fan C et al. Endothelial cell activation and neovascularization are prominent in dermatomyositis. J Autoimmune Dis 2006; 3: 2.

24. Howard OM, Dong HF, Yang D et al. Histidyl-tRNA synthetase and asparaginyl-tRNA synthetase, autoantigens in myositis, activate chemokine receptors on T lymphocytes and immature dendritic cells. J Exp Med 2002; 196: 781–91.

25. Zhou X, Dimachkie MM, Xiong M, Tan FK, Arnett FC. cDNA microarrays reveal distinct gene expression clusters in idiopathic inflammatory myopathies. Med Sci Monit 2004; 10: BR191–BR197.

26. Whitaker JN, Engel WK. Vascular deposits of immunoglobulin and complement in idiopathic inflammatory myopathy. N Engl J Med 1972; 286: 333–8.

27. Roig QM, Damjanov I. Dermatomyositis as an immunologic complication of toxoplasmosis. Acta Neuropathol (Berl) 1982; 58: 183–6.

28. Damjanov I, Moser RL, Katz SM, Lyons P. Immune complex myositis associated with viral hepatitis. Hum Pathol 1980; 11: 478–81.

29. Lambie PB, Quismorio FP Jr. Interstitial lung disease and cryoglobulinemia in polymyositis. J Rheumatol 1991; 18: 468–9.

30. Shimada K, Koh CS, Tsukada N, Shoji S, Yanagisawa N. [Detection of immune complexes in the sera and around the muscle fibers in a case of myasthenia gravis and polymyositis.] Rinsho Shinkeigaku 1989; 29: 432–5.

31. Solling J, Solling K, Jacobsen KU. Circulating immune complexes in lupus erythematosus, scleroderma and dermatomyositis. Acta Derm Venereol 1979; 59: 421–6.

32. Behan WM, Barkas T, Behan PO. Detection of immune complexes in polymyositis. Acta Neurol Scand 1982; 65: 320–34.

33. Hargis AM, Winkelstein JA, Moore MP, Weidner JP, Prieur DJ. Complement levels in dogs with familial canine dermatomyositis. Vet Immunol Immunopathol 1988; 20: 95–100.

34. Hargis AM, Prieur DJ, Haupt KH, McDonald TL, Moore MP. Prospective study of familial canine dermatomyositis. Correlation of the severity of dermatomyositis and circulating immune complex levels. Am J Pathol 1986; 123: 465–79.

35. Kissel JT, Mendell JR, Rammohan KW. Microvascular deposition of complement membrane attack complex in dermatomyositis. N Engl J Med 1986; 314: 329–34.

36. Love LA, Miller FW. Noninfectious environmental agents associated with myopathies. Curr Opin Rheumatol 1993; 5: 712–18.

37. Reed AM, Ytterberg SR. Genetic and environmental risk factors for idiopathic inflammatory myopathies. Rheum Dis Clin North Am 2002; 28: 891–916.

38. Niinikoski J, Paljarvi L, Laato M, Lang H, Panelius M. Muscle hypoxia in myositis. J Neurol Neurosurg Psychiatry 1986; 49: 1455.

39. Shreeniwas R, Koga S, Karakurum M et al. Hypoxia-mediated induction of endothelial cell interleukin-1 alpha. An autocrine mechanism promoting expression of leukocyte adhesion molecules on the vessel surface. J Clin Invest 1992; 90: 2333–9.

40. Chariot P, Ruet E, Authier FJ et al. Cytochrome c oxidase deficiencies in the muscle of patients with inflammatory myopathies. Acta Neuropathol (Berl) 1996; 91: 530–6.

41. Heffner RR, Barron SA. The early effects of ischemia upon skeletal muscle mitochondria. J Neurol Sci 1978; 38: 295–315.

42. Yang CC, Alvarez RB, Engel WK, Heller SL, Askanas V. Nitric oxide-induced oxidative stress in autosomal recessive and dominant inclusion-body myopathies. Brain 1998; 121(Pt 6): 1089–97.

43. Askanas V, Engel WK. Sporadic inclusion-body myositis: a proposed key pathogenetic role of the abnormalities of the ubiquitin-proteasome system, and protein misfolding and aggregation. Acta Myol 2005; 24: 17–24.

44. Park JH, Vital TL, Ryder NM et al. Magnetic resonance imaging and P-31 magnetic resonance spectroscopy provide unique quantitative data useful in the longitudinal management of patients with dermatomyositis. Arthritis Rheum 1994; 37: 736–46.

45. Chung YL, Smith EC, Williams SC et al. In vivo proton magnetic resonance spectroscopy in polymyositis and dermatomyositis: a preliminary study. Eur J Med Res 1997; 2: 483–7.

46. Chowdhury SA, Ytterberg SR, Wortmann RL. Abnormal energy metabolism in murine polymyositis. Arthritis Rheum 1989; 32: S125 (abstract).

47. Li YP, Reid MB. Effect of tumor necrosis factor-alpha on skeletal muscle metabolism. Curr Opin Rheumatol 2001; 13: 483–7.

48. Langen RC, Schols AM, Kelders MC, Wouters EF, Janssen-Heininger YM. Inflammatory cytokines inhibit myogenic differentiation through activation of nuclear factor-kappaB. FASEB J 2001; 15: 1169–80.

49. Fang CH, Li BG, James JH, Fischer JE, Hasselgren PO. Cytokines block the effects of insulin-like growth factor-I (IGF-I) on glucose uptake and lactate production in skeletal muscle but do not influence IGF-I-induced changes in protein turnover. Shock 1997; 8: 362–7.

50. Ji SQ, Neustrom S, Willis GM, Spurlock ME. Proinflammatory cytokines regulate myogenic cell proliferation and fusion but have no impact on myotube protein metabolism or stress protein expression. J Interferon Cytokine Res 1998; 18: 879–88.

51. Nagaraju K, Casciola-Rosen L, Rosen A et al. The inhibition of apoptosis in myositis and in normal muscle cells. J Immunol 2000; 164: 5459–65.

52. Li M, Dalakas MC. Expression of human IAP-like protein in skeletal muscle: a possible explanation for the rare incidence of muscle fiber apoptosis in T-cell mediated inflammatory myopathies. J Neuroimmunol 2000; 106: 1–5.

53. Vattemi G, Tonin P, Filosto M et al. T-cell anti-apoptotic mechanisms in inflammatory myopathies. J Neuroimmunol 2000; 111: 146–51.

54. Seeliger S, Vogl T, Engels IH et al. Expression of calcium-binding proteins MRP8 and MRP14 in inflammatory muscle diseases. Am J Pathol 2003; 163: 947–56.

55. Nagaraju K, Raben N, Loeffler L et al. From the cover: conditional up-regulation of MHC class I in skeletal muscle leads to self-sustaining autoimmune myositis and myositis-specific autoantibodies [see comments]. Proc Natl Acad Sci U S A 2000; 97: 9209–14.

56. Nagaraju K, Casciola-Rosen L, Lundberg I et al. Activation of the endoplasmic reticulum stress response in autoimmune myositis: potential role in muscle fiber damage and dysfunction. Arthritis Rheum 2005; 52: 1824–35.

57. Tezak Z, Hoffman EP, Lutz JL et al. Gene expression profiling in DQA1*0501+ children with untreated dermatomyositis: a novel model of pathogenesis. J Immunol 2002; 168: 4154–63.

58. Greenberg SA, Sanoudou D, Haslett JN et al. Molecular profiles of inflammatory myopathies. Neurology 2002; 59: 1170–82.

59. Tian L, Greenberg SA, Kong SW et al. Discovering statistically significant pathways in expression profiling studies. Proc Natl Acad Sci U S A 2005; 102: 13544–9.

60. Greenberg SA, Pinkus JL, Pinkus GS et al. Interferon-alpha/beta-mediated innate immune mechanisms in dermatomyositis. Ann Neurol 2005; 57: 664–78.

61. Raju R, Dalakas MC. Gene expression profile in the muscles of patients with inflammatory myopathies: effect of therapy with IVIg and biological validation of clinically relevant genes. Brain 2005; 128: 1887–96.

62. Rider LG, Giannini EH, Brunner HI et al. International consensus on preliminary definitions of improvement in adult and juvenile myositis. Arthritis Rheum 2004; 50: 2281–90.

63. Oddis CV, Rider LG, Reed AM et al. International consensus guidelines for trials of therapies in the idiopathic

inflammatory myopathies. Arthritis Rheum 2005; 52: 2607–15.

64. Baer AN. Advances in the therapy of idiopathic inflammatory myopathies. Curr Opin Rheumatol 2006; 18: 236–41.

65. Patel SY, Kumararatne DS. From black magic to science: understanding the rationale for the use of intravenous immunoglobulin to treat inflammatory myopathies. Clin Exp Immunol 2001; 124: 169–71.

66. Mease PJ, Ochs HD, Wedgwood RJ. Successful treatment of echovirus meningoencephalitis and myositis-fasciitis with intravenous immune globulin therapy in a patient with X-linked agammaglobulinemia. N Engl J Med 1981; 304: 1278–81.

67. Dalakas MC, Illa I, Dambrosia JM et al. A controlled trial of high-dose intravenous immune globulin infusions as treatment for dermatomyositis. N Engl J Med 1993; 329: 1993–2000.

68. Rider LG, Miller FW. Idiopathic inflammatory muscle disease: clinical aspects. Baillieres Best Pract Res Clin Rheumatol 2000; 14: 37–54.

69. Rider LG, Miller FW. Classification and treatment of the juvenile idiopathic inflammatory myopathies. Rheum Dis Clin North Am 1997; 23: 619–55.

70. Tsai MJ, Lai CC, Lin SC et al. Intravenous immunoglobulin therapy in juvenile dermatomyositis. Zhonghua Min Guo Xiao Er Ke Yi Xue Hui Za Zhi 1997; 38: 111–15.

71. Al Mayouf SM, Laxer RM, Schneider R, Silverman ED, Feldman BM. Intravenous immunoglobulin therapy for juvenile dermatomyositis: efficacy and safety. J Rheumatol 2000; 27: 2498–503.

72. Cherin P, Piette JC, Wechsler B et al. Intravenous gamma globulin as first line therapy in polymyositis and dermatomyositis: an open study in 11 adult patients [see comments]. J Rheumatol 1994; 21: 1092–7.

73. Cherin P, Pelletier S, Teixeira A et al. Results and long-term followup of intravenous immunoglobulin infusions in chronic, refractory polymyositis: an open study with thirty-five adult patients. Arthritis Rheum 2002; 46: 467–74.

74. Dalakas MC. Controlled studies with high-dose intravenous immunoglobulin in the treatment of dermatomyositis, inclusion body myositis, and polymyositis. Neurology 1998; 51: S37–S45.

75. Soueidan SA, Dalakas MC. Treatment of inclusion-body myositis with high-dose intravenous immunoglobulin. Neurology 1993; 43: 876–9.

76. Dalakas MC, Sonies B, Dambrosia J et al. Treatment of inclusion-body myositis with IVIg: a double-blind, placebo-controlled study [see comments]. Neurology 1997; 48: 712–16.

77. Dalakas MC, Koffman B, Fujii M et al. A controlled study of intravenous immunoglobulin combined with prednisone in the treatment of IBM. Neurology 2001; 56: 323–7.

78. Miller FW. Polymyositis, dermatomyositis and related conditions. In: Koopman W, ed. Arthritis and allied conditions. Baltimore: Williams and Wilkins, 1996.

79. Basta M, Dalakas MC. High-dose intravenous immunoglobulin exerts its beneficial effect in patients with dermatomyositis by blocking endomysial deposition of activated complement fragments. J Clin Invest 1994; 94: 1729–35.

80. Wada J, Shintani N, Kikutani K et al. Intravenous immunoglobulin prevents experimental autoimmune myositis in SJL mice by reducing anti-myosin antibody and by blocking complement deposition. Clin Exp Immunol 2001; 124: 282–9.

81. Miller FW. Intravenous immunoglobulin in polymyositis/dermatomyositis. In: Strand V, ed. Proceedings: Early Decisions in DMARD Development IV. Biologic Agents in Autoimmune Disease. Atlanta: Arthritis Foundation, 1996: 205–12.

82. Miller ML, Mendez E, Klein-Gitelman M, Pachman LM. Experience with Etanercept in chronic juvenile dermatomyositis: preliminary results. Arthritis Rheum 2000; (Suppl): Vol 43(9): S380 (abstract).

83. Saadeh CK. Etanercept is effective in the treatment of polymyositis/dermatomyositis which is refractory to conventional therapy. Arthritis Rheumatism 2001; 43 9 (Suppl): S193 (abstract).

84. Hengstman GJ, van den Hoogen FH, van Engelen BG, Barrera P, Netea M, van de Putte LB. Anti-TNF-blockade with infliximab (Remicade) in polymyositis and dermatomyositis. Arthritis Rheum 2000; 43 9 (Suppl): S193 (abstract).

85. Hengstman GJ, van den Hoogen FH, Barrera P et al. Successful treatment of dermatomyositis and polymyositis with anti-tumor-necrosis-factor-alpha: preliminary observations. Eur Neurol 2003; 50: 10–15.

86. Nzeusseau A, Durez P, Houssiau FA, Devogelaer JP. Successful use of infliximab in a case of refractory juvenile dermatomyositis. Arthritis Rheum 2001; 39 (Suppl): (abstract).

87. Levine TD. Rituximab in the treatment of dermatomyositis: an open-label pilot study. Arthritis Rheum 2005; 52: 601–7.

88. Matsuya M, Abe T, Tosaka M et al. The first case of polymyositis associated with interferon therapy. Intern Med 1994; 33: 806–8.

89. Cirigliano G, Della RA, Tavoni A, Viacava P, Bombardieri S. Polymyositis occurring during alpha-interferon treatment for malignant melanoma: a case report and review of the literature. Rheumatol Int 1999; 19: 65–7.

90. Hengstman GJ, Vogels OJ, ter Laak HJ, de Witte T, van Engelen BG. Myositis during long-term interferon-alpha treatment. Neurology 2000; 54: 2186.

91. Dietrich LL, Bridges AJ, Albertini MR. Dermatomyositis after interferon alpha treatment. Med Oncol 2000; 17: 64–9.

92. Muscle Study Group. Randomized pilot trial of betaINF1a (Avonex) in patients with inclusion body myositis. Neurology 2001; 57: 1566–70.

93. Lindberg C, Trysberg E, Tarkowski A, Oldfors A. Anti-T-lymphocyte globulin treatment in inclusion body myositis: a randomized pilot study. Neurology 2003; 61: 260–2.

94. Barron KS, Wallace C, Woolfrey CEA et al. Autologous stem cell transplantation for pediatric rheumatic diseases. J Rheumatol 2001; 28: 2337–58.

95. Furst DE. The status of stem cell transplantation for rheumatoid arthritis: a rheumatologist's view. J Rheumatol 2001; 28 (Suppl 64): 60–1.

96. Nyberg P, Wikman AL, Nennesmo I, Lundberg I. Increased expression of interleukin 1alpha and MHC class I in muscle tissue of patients with chronic, inactive polymyositis and dermatomyositis. J Rheumatol 2000; 27: 940–8.

97. Zhou X, Filemon KT, Xion M, Dimachkie MM, Arnett FC Jr. Gene expression profile of muscle biopsies from patients with inflammatory myopathies. Arthritis Rheum 2000; (Suppl): 1254 (abstract).

98. Wiendl H, Behrens L, Maier S et al. Muscle fibers in inflammatory myopathies and cultured myoblasts express the nonclassical major histocompatibility antigen HLA-G. Ann Neurol 2000; 48: 679–84.

99. Inukai A, Kuru S, Liang Y et al. Expression of HLA-DR and its enhancing molecules in muscle fibers in polymyositis. Muscle Nerve 2000; 23: 385–92.

100. Miller FW, Love LA, Barbieri SA, Balow JE, Plotz PH. Lymphocyte activation markers in idiopathic myositis: changes with disease activity and differences among clinical and autoantibody subgroups. Clin Exp Immunol 1990; 81: 373–9.

101. O'Hanlon T, Miller FW. T cell-mediated immune mechanisms in myositis. Curr Opin Rheumatol 1995; 503–9.

102. Fyhr IM, Moslemi AR, Tarkowski A, Lindberg C, Oldfors A. Limited T-cell receptor V gene usage in inclusion body myositis. Scand J Immunol 1996; 43: 109–14.

103. Lindberg C, Oldfors A, Tarkowski A. Restricted use of T cell receptor V genes in endomysial infiltrates of patients with inflammatory myopathies. Eur J Immunol 1994; 24: 2659–63.

104. Amemiya K, Granger RP, Dalakas MC. Clonal restriction of T-cell receptor expression by infiltrating lymphocytes in inclusion body myositis persists over time: Studies in repeated muscle biopsies. Brain 2000; 123: 2030–9.

105. De Bleecker JL, Engel AG. Expression of cell adhesion molecules in inflammatory myopathies and Duchenne dystrophy. J Neuropathol Exp Neurol 1994; 53: 369–76.

106. Tews DS, Goebel HH. Expression of cell adhesion molecules in inflammatory myopathies. J Neuroimmunol 1995; 59: 185–94.

107. Lundberg IE. The role of cytokines, chemokines, and adhesion molecules in the pathogenesis of idiopathic inflammatory myopathies. Curr Rheumatol Rep 2000; 2: 216–24.

108. Iannone F, Cauli A, Yanni G et al. T-lymphocyte immunophenotyping in polymyositis and dermatomyositis. Br J Rheumatol 1996; 35: 839–45.

109. Sallum AM, Kiss MH, Silva CA et al. Difference in adhesion molecule expression (ICAM-1 and VCAM-1) in juvenile and adult dermatomyositis, polymyositis and inclusion body myositis. Autoimmun Rev 2006; 5: 93–100.

110. Lundberg I, Ulfgren AK, Nyberg P, Andersson U, Klareskog L. Cytokine production in muscle tissue of patients with idiopathic inflammatory myopathies. Arthritis Rheum 1997; 40: 865–74.

111. Wiendl H, Mitsdoerffer M, Schneider D et al. Muscle fibres and cultured muscle cells express the B7.1/2-related inducible co-stimulatory molecule, ICOSL: implications for the pathogenesis of inflammatory myopathies. Brain 2003; 126: 1026–35.

112. Lundberg IE, Nyberg P. New developments in the role of cytokines and chemokines in inflammatory myopathies. Curr Opin Rheumatol 1998; 10: 521–9.

113. Rider L, Ahmed A, Beausang L et al. Elevations of interleukin-1 receptor antagonist (IL-1RA), sTNFR, sIL2R, and IL-10 in juvenile idiopathic inflammatory myopathies suggest a role for monocyte/macrophage and B lymphocyte activation. Arthritis Rheum 1998; 41 (Suppl): S265.

114. Son K, Tomita Y, Shimizu T et al. Abnormal IL-1 receptor antagonist production in patients with polymyositis and dermatomyositis. Intern Med 2000; 39: 128–35.

115. Rider LG, Artlett CM, Foster CB et al. Polymorphisms in the IL-1 receptor antagonist gene VNTR are possible risk factors for juvenile idiopathic inflammatory myopathies. Clin Exp Immunol 2000; 121: 47–52.

116. De Rossi M, Bernasconi P, Baggi F, de Waal MR, Mantegazza R. Cytokines and chemokines are both expressed by human myoblasts: possible relevance for the immune pathogenesis of muscle inflammation. Int Immunol 2000; 12: 1329–35.

117. Kuru S, Inukai A, Liang Y et al. Tumor necrosis factor-alpha expression in muscles of polymyositis and dermatomyositis. Acta Neuropathol (Berl) 2000; 99: 585–8.

118. Fedczyna TO, Lutz J, Pachman LM. Expression of TNF alpha by muscle fibers in biopsies from children with untreated juvenile dermatomyositis: association with the TNFalpha-308A allele. Clin Immunol 2001; 100: 236–9.

119. De Bleecker JL, Meire VI, Declercq W, Van Aken EH. Immunolocalization of tumor necrosis factor-alpha and its receptors in inflammatory myopathies. Neuromuscul Disord 1999; 9: 239–46.

120. Shimizu T, Tomita Y, Son K et al. Elevation of serum soluble tumour necrosis factor receptors in patients with polymyositis and dermatomyositis. Clin Rheumatol 2000; 19: 352–9.

121. Adams EM, Kirkley J, Eidelman G, Dohlman J, Plotz PH. The predominance of beta (CC) chemokine transcripts in idiopathic inflammatory muscle diseases. Proc Assoc Am Physicians 1997; 109: 275–85.

122. Bartoli C, Civatte M, Pellissier JF, Figarella Branger D. CCR2A and CCR2B, the two isoforms of the monocyte chemoattractant protein-1 receptor are up-regulated and expressed by different cell subsets in idiopathic inflammatory myopathies. Acta Neuropathol (Berl) 2001; 102: 385–92.

123. Murata K, Dalakas MC. Expression of the costimulatory molecule BB-1, the ligands CTLA-4 and CD28, and their mRNA in inflammatory myopathies. Am J Pathol 1999; 155: 453–60.

124. Sugiura T, Kawaguchi Y, Harigai M et al. Increased CD40 expression on muscle cells of polymyositis and dermatomyositis: role of CD40-CD40 ligand interaction in IL-6, IL-8, IL-15, and monocyte chemoattractant protein-1 production. J Immunol 2000; 164: 6593–600.

125. Nagaraju K, Raben N, Villalba ML et al. Costimulatory markers in muscle of patients with idiopathic inflammatory myopathies and in cultured muscle cells. Clin Immunol 1999; 92: 161–9.

126. Cid MC, Grau JM, Casademont J et al. Leucocyte/endothelial cell adhesion receptors in muscle biopsies from patients with idiopathic inflammatory myopathies (IIM). Clin Exp Immunol 1996; 104: 467–73.

127. Choi YC, Dalakas MC. Expression of matrix metalloproteinases in the muscle of patients with inflammatory myopathies. Neurology 2000; 54: 65–71.

128. Whitaker JN, Engel WK. Vascular deposits of immunoglobulin and complement in inflammatory myopathy. Trans Am Neurol Assoc 1971; 96: 24–8.

129. Cherin P, Herson S, Wechsler B et al. Efficacy of intravenous gammaglobulin therapy in chronic refractory polymyositis and dermatomyositis: an open study with 20 adult patients. Am J Med 1991; 91: 162–8.

130. Dalakas MC, Illa I, Dambrosia JM et al. A controlled trial of high-dose intravenous immune globulin infusions as treatment for dermatomyositis. N Engl J Med 1993; 329: 1993–2000.

131. Gottfried I, Seeber A, Anegg B et al. High dose intravenous immunoglobulin (IVIG) in dermatomyositis: clinical responses and effect on sIL-2R levels. Eur J Dermatol 2000; 10: 29 35.

132. Lang BA, Laxer RM, Murphy G, Silverman ED, Roifman CM. Treatment of dermatomyositis with intravenous gammaglobulin. Am J Med 1991; 91: 169–72.

133. Sansome A, Dubowitz V. Intravenous immunoglobulin in juvenile dermatomyositis—four year review of nine cases. Arch Dis Child 1995; 72: 25–8.

134. Soueidan SA, Dalakas MC. Treatment of inclusion-body myositis with high-dose intravenous immunoglobulin. Neurology 1993; 43: 876–9.

135. Saadeh CK. Etanercept is effective in the treatment of polymyositis/dermatomyositis which is refractory to conventional therapy including steroids and other disease modifying agents. Arthritis Rheum 2000; (Suppl): 757 (abstract).

136. Barohn RJ, Herbelin L, Kissel JT et al. Pilot trial of etanercept in the treatment of inclusion-body myositis. Neurology 2006; 66: S123–S124.

137. Muscle Study Group. Randomized pilot trial of high-dose betaINF-1a in patients with inclusion body myositis. Neurology 2004; 63: 718–20.

138. Bingham S, Griffiths B, McGonagle D et al. Autologous stem cell transplantation for rapidly progressive Jo 1 positive polymyositis with long-term follow-up. Br J Haematol 2001; 113: 840–41.

139. Baron F, Ribbens C, Kaye O et al. Effective treatment of Jo-1-associated polymyositis with T-cell-depleted autologous peripheral blood stem cell transplantation. Br J Haematol 2000; 110: 339–42.

39

TNF blockade in orphan rheumatic diseases

Michael Voulgarelis and Haralampos M Moutsopoulos

Introduction • Primary Sjögren's syndrome • Adult Still's disease • Sarcoidosis • Polymyositis/ dermatomyositis • Vasculitis • Behcet's disease • Conclusion • References

INTRODUCTION

Tumor necrosis factor (TNF)-α is a pleiotropic proinflammatory cytokine that has been implicated in the pathogenesis of a variety of autoimmune disorders. Its presence instigates the production and secretion of a cascade of several inflammatory mediators resulting in altered tissue remodeling, epithelial barrier permeability, macrophage activation, up-regulation of adhesion molecules, and recruitment of inflammatory infiltrates, all of which play a significant role in the pathogenesis of inflammation and immune response.[1,2] In this context, the application of specific TNF-α blockers has paved the way for innovative therapeutic options in the treatment of autoimmune diseases.

Three predominant biological agents capable of inhibiting TNF-α currently prevail: infliximab, etanercept, and adalimumab. Infliximab is a recombinant chimeric IgG1 anti-TNF-α specific antibody (whether the TNF-α be membrane-bound or secreted in the extracellular area) which, as anticipated, impedes TNF-α binding to its membranous and soluble receptors, i.e. TNF-R1/p55 or TNF-R2/p75. Further advancement in biotechnology saw the advent of adalimumab, a fully human monoclonal antibody (mAb) with TNF-α-blocking properties. Finally, etanercept as a fusion protein combines the ligand-binding portion of human TNF-R2 with sequences of the human Fc portion of IgG1. Whereas TNF-R1 is a constitutive membrane receptor, TNF-R2 is stimuli-induced and can be found on virtually every cell surface. Bearing greater affinity to its ligand (TNF-α), TNF-R2 is more effective than TNF-R1 in compromising the cytokine.

The successful application of TNF-α blockade in several disorders including rheumatoid arthritis (RA), psoriatic arthritis, ankylosing spondylitis, and Crohn's disease has been well documented.[3–6] However, there are indications that the use of TNF-α blockade could potentially be extended to treat other rheumatic diseases. Preliminary evidence from open-label trials and case reports, for instance, suggest that these TNF-α inhibitors may be effective in the treatment of Behcet's disease, Wegener's granulomatosis, and sarcoidosis. The purpose of this chapter is to review and discuss recent data concerning the scope of TNF-α inbitors in a number of other orphan rheumatic disorders including primary Sjögren's syndrome, adult Still's disease, polymyositis, vasculitis, sarcoidosis, and Behcet's disease.

PRIMARY SJÖGREN'S SYNDROME

Sjögren's syndrome (SS) is an autoimmune disease characterized by broad organ-specific and systemic manifestations, the most common being diminished lacrimal and salivary gland function, xerostomia, keratoconjunctivitis sicca, and parotid gland enlargement. The etiology of

SS has not yet been clarified. While lymphoid infiltrates are a characteristic histopathological finding in SS, there is evidence suggesting that proinflammatory cytokines such as TNF-α may also play an important role in the pathogenesis of the disease. TNF-α can be secreted not only by mononuclear cells infiltrating the glands, but also by ductal epithelial cells.[7,8] In addition, infiltrating mononuclear inflammatory cells, vascular endothelial cells, ductal epithelial cells, and fibroblasts all co-express TNF-α and TNF-R.[9] This inter-related localization of TNF-R and its ligand TNF-α in inflammatory and epithelial cells may suggest a proinflammatory role of TNF-α in SS. The increased presence of TNF-α in the lacrimal glands of MRL/lpr mice compared with control glands further indicates that TNF-α is a potential mediator of lacrimal gland damage in these murine models of SS.[10] Finally, in NOD mice, TNF-α inhibition has been shown to be effective in suppressing tissue destruction in lacrimal glands and preventing sicca symptoms.[11]

On the basis of recent evidence concerning the efficacy of TNF-α blockers in RA, a pilot open-label study was conducted involving 16 patients with active primary SS treated with 3 mg/kg of infliximab at weeks 0, 2, and 6.[12] The treatment yielded impressive results over a 3-month follow-up period in the reduction of fatigue, joint pain, symptoms of sicca, salivary flow rate, and Shirmer I test. In addition, infusion was well-tolerated and no serious adverse effects were reported. Interestingly, no lupus-like syndrome was observed and no anti-double-stranded DNA antibodies were detected in any SS patients included in the study. The successful results of this study prompted the same authors to extend the protocol by administering additional infusions of infliximab (3–5 mg/kg) every 12 weeks for 1 year.[13] This follow-up study included 10 of the 16 SS patients who had originally participated in the previous pilot study. All 10 patients reported a recurrence of SS symptoms at a median of 9 weeks after receiving the third of the 3 initial infusions. A statistically significant decrease in systemic and local disease manifestations was noted after 1 year of treatment in all 10 patients. Albeit these data suggest that sustained improvement of active SS may be

achieved with infliximab treatment, it would be imprudent to draw any conclusion based on such a small subgroup of patients.

A multicenter, randomized, double-blind, placebo-controlled trial randomly assigned 103 patients with primary SS to receive infliximab 5 mg/kg or placebo in weeks 0, 2, and 6.[14] The patients were then followed up for 22 weeks. All patients had active disease as assessed by values > 50 mm on two of three visual analog scales (VAS: 0–100 mm) that evaluated joint pain, fatigue, and buccal, ocular, skin, vaginal or bronchial dryness. Secondary endpoints included values on each VAS separately, the number of tender and swollen joints, the basal salivary flow rate, results of the Shirmer I test for lacrimal gland function, the focus score on labial salivary gland biopsy, the level of C-reactive protein (CRP), and the erythrocyte sedimentation rate (ESR) evaluated at weeks 0, 10, and 22. At week 10, 26.5% of patients receiving placebo and 27.8% of patients treated with infliximab showed an overall favorable response ($p = 0.89$), while 20.4% of the placebo group and 16.7% of the infliximab group still showed a similar response ($p = 0.62$) at week 22. Consequently, this study failed to prove the efficacy of infliximab in primary SS. Although discrepancies between these two studies[12,14] may be explained by their different designs or different inclusion criteria, results of another recent open study of etanercept in 15 patients with primary SS[15] again did not report any improvement of lacrimal and salivary function or salivary histological features.

Although the lack of change in sicca symptoms and signs following use of TNF inhibitors could be explained by the pre-existence of significant glandular tissue destruction, TNF inhibitors were also found to be ineffective in the subgroup of recently diagnosed patients.[14] The lack of improvement in fatigue, number of tender and swollen joints, ESR, and CRP levels is more surprising, considering that the mechanisms of arthritis may differ in primary SS from RA. The role of TNF-α in the pathogenesis of SS is therefore seriously in question, emphasizing the need for future therapies to focus on other molecular targets.

ADULT STILL'S DISEASE

Still's disease is a systemic rheumatic childhood disease which may persist into adulthood or may develop *de novo* in the adult population. Adult Still's disease (ASD) is traditionally treated with non-steroidal anti-inflammatory drugs and corticosteroids. Those who do not respond or who display serious steroid side effects may alternatively be treated with disease-modifying anti-rheumatic drugs (DMARDs, e.g. gold salts, hydroxychloroquine, methotrexate, D-penicillamine, sulfasalazine), but failures of the latter approach are common.

TNF is elevated in both the serum and the synovial fluid of children with juvenile rheumatoid arthritis (JRA).[16] Serum levels of soluble TNF-R are also elevated in these patients and are correlated with disease activity.[17] Further evidence that TNF may amplify local inflammation and lead to joint destruction was provided in a study in which both TNF-α and lymphotoxin were detected in the majority of synovial tissues obtained from patients with JRA.[18]

To the best of our knowledge, only one randomized, multicenter, double-blind trial of etanercept has been reported for the treatment of polyarticular JRA in children who did not tolerate or who had an inadequate response to methotrexate.[19] In the first part of this study (open-label), 69 children with active JRA received etanercept (0.4 mg/kg twice weekly) for 3 months. The second part of the study comprised a placebo-controlled study in which 51 of the 69 children with clinical response were randomized to continue etanercept or receive placebo for an additional 4 months. Only 28% of those who continued to receive etanercept experienced disease flare, as compared with 88% of the children who were receiving placebo ($p = 0.003$). The results of this study suggest that TNF, lymphotoxin, or both, have a role in JRA and that inhibition of these substances is a valid therapeutic intervention.

On the other hand, limited experience with TNF blockade in ASD has been recorded. Apart from reports of a few isolated cases, the results of only three observation studies have been published.[20–22] Etanercept at 25 mg two or three times per week was used in ASD patients in an uncontrolled trial.[20] Twelve adult patients who met criteria for ASD and had active arthritis were enrolled in a 6-month open-label trial of etanercept. All these patients had previously been treated unsuccessfully with other DMARDs. Seven patients achieved an ACR 20% response, one of three patients with systemic features of ASD (fever and rash) showed improvement, and two patients withdrew because of disease flare. In the second study,[21] six patients with active and severe disease despite conventional immunosuppressive therapy received infliximab at 3–5 mg/kg (at weeks 0, 2, and 6, continuing with intervals of 6–8 weeks depending on the patient's disease activity), resulting in improvements in fever, joint manifestations, myalgias, splenomegaly, rash, and serologic abnormalities. Finally, a French trial[22] involving 20 ASD patients (previously unresponsive to the conventional DMARDs) treated 10 patients with infliximab, 5 with etanercept, and 5 with both drugs consecutively. A partial response was observed in 16 cases: 7 receiving etanercept and 9 infliximab. At a mean follow-up of 13 months, complete remission had occurred in only five cases: one receiving etanercept and four infliximab. No deaths or serious adverse events were reported during the course of these three studies.

This initial investigation indicates that TNF-α blockade treatment may be beneficial to some ASD patients who are unresponsive to conventional treatment. However, most patients achieve only partial remission, indicating that this therapy does not seem to be as effective in ASD as in RA or spondylarthropathies. To conclude, the risk-benefit ratio of TNF-α blockade in refractory ASD patients cannot be accurately evaluated without further studies taking place.

SARCOIDOSIS

Sarcoidosis is a systemic disorder characterized by the presence of non-caseating granulomas. The natural process of pulmonary sarcoidosis ranges from spontaneous remission to chronic disease, resulting in the insidious loss of lung function. Corticosteroids are the mainstay of treatment, although their use frequently incurs serious side effects.

Sarcoidosis has been described as an inflammatory response disorder accompanied by increased proinflammatory cytokine production with alveolar macrophage-derived TNF-α being involved in the induction and maintenance of granulomas.[23] It has been shown that in response to TNF-α, intracellular adhesion molecule-1 (ICAM-1) surface expression on alveolar macrophages is increased in pulmonary sarcoidosis, supporting the role of TNF-α in mediating aggregation of macrophages and inflammatory granuloma formation.[24] High levels of TNF-α released from alveolar macrophages seem to correlate with disease progression.[25] It has also been shown that levels of soluble TNF-R, which are known to inhibit TNF-α activity, are initially increased in the lungs of patients with sarcoidosis at stage I of the disease, decreasing as the disease progresses to stage II/III.[26] Consequently, TNF-α bioactivity is reduced in the lungs of subjects with stage I sarcoidosis compared with patients with stage II/III disease and healthy controls, indicating potential for TNF-α blockade in the therapy of sarcoidosis. It should also be mentioned that previous usage of thalidomide and pentoxifylline as TNF-α inhibitors has been shown to equally benefit patients with sarcoidosis.[27,28]

In this context, a prospective open-label study[29] of etanercept was undertaken in 17 patients with stage II/III progressive pulmonary sarcoidosis. Patients displaying extrapulmonary organ involvement or treated with other immunosuppressive agents were excluded from the study. The dose of etanercept tested was equal to the standard dose (25 mg twice weekly) used to achieve remission in patients with RA. The study was terminated at 15 months due to an excessive number of patients experiencing disease progression while taking etanercept. More specifically, 5 patients displayed no improvement, deterioration was recorded in 11, and 1 patient withdrew from the study. Moreover, TNF-α activity in serum and bronchioalveolar lavage failed to provide response predictor markers. Finally, serious adverse events included one localized intestinal lymphoma and one nasopharyngeal extramedullary plasmacytoma.

Infliximab has been evaluated in several case series with multi-organ sarcoidosis refractory to conventional therapy.[30–35] Patients were treated with 5 mg/kg and followed up every 6 weeks for 25 months of continuous therapy. Infliximab induced rapid resolution of the disease, with relapse occurring on discontinuation. When the case series reporting the use of infliximab in refractory sarcoidosis were reviewed to evaluate its potential role as a treatment option, the following conclusion was reached: although there is insufficient evidence to support infliximab as an appropriate alternative to conventional treatment options as first-line therapy for sarcoidosis, the preliminary outlook on its use in treatment-refractory cases is promising. Infliximab has been shown to improve the clinical picture and reduce the need for corticosteroids in a small number of refractory patients. Furthermore, the data suggest that sarcoidosis is responsive to infliximab but not to etanercept. The results are consistent with the different effect of these two TNF-α antagonists, principally that only infliximab binds and lyses TNF-α-producing cells.

POLYMYOSITIS/DERMATOMYOSITIS

Polymyositis (PM) and dermatomyositis (DM) are inflammatory muscle diseases characterized by systemic proximal muscle weakness, cutaneous lesions (in DM), and systemic manifestations in other organs. Although little is known about the etiology of these diseases, evidence suggests that both cellular and humoral autoimmune mechanisms are involved in their pathogenesis and progression. Levels of circulating soluble p55 and p75 TNFR are increased[36] and TNF-α and other proinflammatory cytokines are expressed in inflammatory lesions in PM and DM,[37] as well as in areas of muscle fiber regeneration.[38] In addition, TNF-α-positive cells infiltrate the endomysium in PM and the perimysium in DM.[39] Despite the potentially pivotal role of TNF-α in PM and DM, corroborating clinical evidence remains insubstantial.

Four female patients, aged 9–35 years, with PM or DM refractory to corticosteroids and various disease-modifying therapies were treated with etanercept.[40] All patients displayed a rapid response to etanercept, three showing complete response and one a partial response, allowing three patients to discontinue all treatment.

In another study,[41] two patients with previously untreated DM/PM were treated with infliximab 10 mg/kg every other week for 6 weeks. The response in both patients was remarkable from the first infusion but PM was not fully controlled by the end of the study at 12 weeks. The authors of both studies claimed that anti-TNF treatment had caused no side effects. One other patient with PM refractory to several lines of treatment (intravenous immunoglobulin, high dose of steroids, methotrexate, azathioprine), responded dramatically to five courses of infliximab (10 mg/kg) infused over 2 weeks, with normalization of creatine phosphokinase (CPK) and impressive improvement in muscle strength.[42] At the same time electromyographic (EMG) studies and pulmonary changes consistently improved, allowing immunosuppressive agents to be considerably reduced or stopped.

In a retrospective study[43] during the period 1998–2004, eight DM/PM patients who were refractory to corticosteroids and immunosuppressive therapy were treated with anti-TNF inhibitors. Six patients were treated with etanercept alone, one with infliximab, and one sequentially with both agents. A favorable response with improved motor strength and decreased fatigue was observed in six patients as well as a significant decrease in the level of serum CPK.

These results provide evidence that TNF-α blockade may incite rapid and dramatic control of DM/PM symptoms, even in the most refractory cases. However, controlled studies are required to determine the appropriate dose and magnitude of response to anti-TNF-α agents in the setting of refractory DM and PM.

VASCULITIS

Anti-neutrophil cytoplasmic antibodies-associated systemic vasculitis (AASV)

AASV includes a group of systemic vasculitides, predominantly characterized by inflammation of microscopic vessels. The pathogenetic mechanisms of systemic vasculitides, particularly those associated with anti-neutrophil cytoplasmic antibodies (ANCAs), may be susceptible to anti-TNF-α inhibitors, in light of the implication of TNF-α in the cytokine cascade responsible for vascular damage and granuloma formation. Evidence suggests that TNF-α plays a central role in the pathogenesis of AASV in which ANCAs are capable of activating neutrophils primed by TNF-α *in vitro*, possibly emulating the induction of the vascular inflammation observed *in vivo*.[44,45] In more detail, the TNF-α-induced enhancement of the neutrophil activation may lead to their secretion of proteins with subsequent binding of these antigens to the endothelial cell surface. Eventually, ANCAs can bind to these antigens, giving rise to enhanced neutrophil adhesion, neutrophil activation, and endothelial cell damage. Interestingly, there are both increased expression of TNF-α at sites of vascular injury[46] and increased serum levels of TNF-α and TNF-R during disease activity.[47] Furthermore, the potential role of TNF-α as a therapeutic target in AASV has been investigated in a rat model of AASV using the anti-rat TNF-α monoclonal antibody (CNTO 1081).[48] Treatment with CNTO 1081 significantly reduced albuminuria, crescent formation, and lung hemorrhage, suggesting that TNF-α plays an important role in the pathogenesis of experimental autoimmune vasculitis.

The first report[49] of etanercept therapy in Wegener's granulomatosis (WG) was a 6-month open-label trial of 20 patients with persistently active disease or with new flares of previously established WG in whom etanercept (25 mg subcutaneously twice weekly) was added to standard therapies (glucocorticoids, methotrexate, cyclophosphamide, azathioprine, cyclosporine). Etanercept was the initial therapy in 14 patients. The mean Birmingham Vasculitis Activity Score for WG (BVAS/WG) improved from 3.6 at entry to 0.6 at 6 months. Among the 14 patients in whom etanercept was the initial treatment, the mean daily prednisone dose decreased from 12.9 at entry to 6.4 mg at 6 months. However, in 15 patients the BVAS at consecutive visits was increased from baseline with severe flares occurring in 3 patients.

Furthermore, a total of 13 patients (in two separate reports)[50,51] with WG refractory to standard treatment were treated with 3–5 mg/kg infliximab mainly in addition to other immunosuppressive therapy. Complete or partial remission for 6–24 months was achieved in most patients, with substantial reduction of the BVAS.

In an open-label, multi-center, prospective trial[52] enrolling 32 patients with WG or microscopic polyangiitis (MPA), infliximab was effective in inducing remission in 88% of patients at a mean time of 6.4 weeks, thereby permitting reduction of steroid therapy. In this study, infliximab was found to be effective as adjuvant therapy for vasculitis both as a component of initial therapy and in management of refractory disease. Interestingly, the incidence of serious infections in this study was higher than that reported for infliximab in RA patients.

In another study, six patients with relapsing WG or MPA refractory to corticosteroids and immunosuppressive medication were treated with infliximab monthly for 3 months.[53] Improvement was demonstrated by reduction of BVAS and corticosteroid doses.

In a cohort of 14 patients[54] with AASV, both disease activity (BVAS) and measures of systemic inflammation were associated with the degree of endothelial dysfunction. Induction of remission through the use of infliximab resulted in a reduction in inflammation and normalization of endothelium-dependent vasomotor responses. In this study, the treatment with anti-TNF-α antibody did not result in any changes in serum TNF-α levels, despite improving endothelial function, suggesting that tissue levels of cytokine are more important in the disease process.

Although much evidence has accumulated concerning the role of TNF-α in inflammatory processes in AASV, there are insufficient published data and experience of TNF-α inhibitors as a treatment in these diseases. However, the potential role of infliximab cannot be discounted. Therefore, further randomized, placebo-controlled studies should be initiated to address the efficacy and safety of TNF-α inhibitors in the treatment of WG or MPA

Takayasu's arteritis

Takayasu's arteritis (TA) is an idiopathic systemic granulomatous disease of the large and medium-sized vessels characterized by segmental stenosis, occlusion, dilatation, and aneurysm formation in the aorta and its main branches. The main pathologic findings of TA include circulating activated T cells bearing restricted T-cell receptor repertoire[55] and predominance of T cells in the vascular lesions.[56] The involvement of these cells in the pathogenesis of TA may be responsible for the production of different inflammatory cytokines such as TNF-α, IL-2 and interferon (IFN)-γ.[57] TNF-α, a key mediator of granulomatous inflammation, has multiple effects on vasculature including adhesion and trans-endothelial migration of inflammatory cells and damage of the vascular wall. In this regard, a recent study has shown the presence of an increased number of TNF-α-positive and IL-2-negative T cells in active TA, connoting the significance of their role in the pathogenesis of the disease.[58]

An open-label trial[59] of 15 patients with active relapsing TA, resistant to conventional therapy, was carried out with 7 patients being treated with etanercept (3 of whom later switched to infliximab) and 8 with infliximab. Ten of the 15 achieved complete remission, sustained for 1–3.3 years without developing new lesions on magnetic resonance imaging (MRI) despite discontinuation of glucocorticoid therapy. Four patients achieved partial remission and were able to discontinue glucocorticoid requirement. In 9 of the 14 responders, an increase in the anti-TNF-α dosage was necessary to sustain remission.

In a report of four patients[60] with TA (three were resistant to previous cytotoxic therapies), three showed improvement treated with infliximab at an initial dose of 3 mg/kg at weeks 0, 2, 6, and 8. However, a higher dose regimen (5 mg/kg) was eventually warranted for two of the responders.

The small number of patients and the design of these studies do not allow further conclusions to be drawn in relation to the efficacy and the role of the two TNF-α inhibitors in TA. However, these data justify the need for an adequately randomized controlled trial to determine whether anti-TNF-α treatment can reduce the morbidity and mortality rate as well as shorten the duration of conventional steroid use in TA.

Giant cell arteritis

Giant cell arteritis (GCA) is characterized by infiltration of the vessel wall by macrophages, giant cells, and T lymphocytes associated with the production of several cytokines that are responsible for the acute phase response. Vasculitic lesions in GCA samples may be characterized by *in situ* production of cytokines indicative of macrophages and T-cell activation.[61] Using immunohistochemical techniques, TNF-α was demonstrated in up to 60% of the cells in all areas of inflamed arteries.[62] In GCA, TNF-α is localized to giant cells and macrophages,[63] suggesting that its predominant source is the monocyte lineage, although occasionally TNF-α is found in areas infiltrated by T cells.[64] Furthermore, the TNF-R1 (p55) was detected on endothelial cells and infiltrating mononuclear cells adjacent to the internal elastic lamina.[65] Given the close proximity of TNF-R and TNF-α to the internal elastic lamina, it has been hypothesized that TNF-α could be involved in the leukocyte infiltration and arterial wall destruction typifying GCA.

Several case reports suggest that GCA may be successfully treated with anti-TNF-α inhibitors. The recent use of infliximab in three of four patients with long-standing corticosteroid-resistant active GCA[66] produced encouraging results. In another report,[67] two patients provided with infliximab as the initial and sole therapy displayed an initial response, but relapse occurred during follow-up. Etanercept was also shown to be beneficial as a steroid-sparing agent in a patient with corticosteroid-resistant GCA.[68] However, the limited number of patients included in these studies does not allow definite conclusions to be drawn.

BEHCET'S DISEASE

Behcet's disease (BD) is a chronic multisystemic vasculitis capable of affecting any human organ or system. Recurrent oral ulcers are a very significant clinical sign. BD is a worldwide pathology, whose prevalence varies according to the population and geographic location. Although BD has been long known, its etiology remains an enigma. Genetic and microbiological factors, immune dysregulation, inflammatory mediators, heat-shock proteins, oxidative stress, lipid peroxidation, and environmental factors have been previously correlated with the pathogenesis of the disease.[69] Th1 phenotype lymphocytes that produce proinflammatory mediators, such as IL-2, IL-6, IL-8, IL-12, IL-18, TNF-α, and IFN-γ are increased in patients with BD.[70] Similarly, the percentages of peripheral γδ+ T lymphocytes that are known to secrete IFN-γ and TNF-α have also been found to be elevated and related to mucocutaneous lesions in such patients, suggesting a direct role of Th1 phenotype lymphocytes in the pathogenesis of BD lesions.[71] Concentration of circulating TNF-α and soluble TNF receptors are increased in the serum of patients with active BD.[72] Following treatment, these patients display reduced levels of Th1 phenotype cytokines,[73] whereas the levels of IL-1 receptor antagonist found at low levels in ocular BD patients were found to be elevated in these treated patients, further supporting the implication of proinflammatory cytokines such as TNF-α in the pathophysiology of the disease.[74]

Patients with relapsing panuveitis were given a single infusion of infliximab whilst receiving their immunosuppressive therapy, which resulted in rapid and effective suppression of acute ocular inflammation and extraocular manifestations. In an open trial[75] of five such patients, treatment with a single dose of infliximab at the onset of a relapse of panuveitis resulted in remission of ocular inflammation within 24 hours and complete suppression of the flare within 7 days in all five patients. According to published data,[76–81] several patients have received anti-TNF treatment. These data strongly suggest that infliximab is remarkably effective in inducing short-term remission of almost all manifestations of the disease, including acute, sight-threatening panuveitis. It is plausible that the efficacy of infliximab is superior to etanercept in BD, but this has yet to be confirmed. Moreover, whether such treatment is superior to the conventional protocol in preventing relapse and progression of the disease remains unknown.

CONCLUSION

TNF-α is a proinflammatory cytokine that plays an important role in the pathophysiology of several inflammatory diseases. TNF inhibition may prove effective in patients with severe, therapy-resistant chronic inflammatory disorders including BD, vasculitis, PM/DM, and sarcoidosis but as yet published data are incomplete. Further studies are currently under way and should provide useful information in defining the more responsive types of inflammatory diseases, patient characteristics, and the proper dosing regimen. There is still much debate but the prospects for the future are intriguing. The logical outcome should be the increased prescription of anti-TNF-α biotherapy. However, we have to be watchful of short or mid-term adverse events, widely described in the literature. Infrequent adverse events such as infections, particularly tuberculosis and less commonly fungal infections, added to the possible increase in risk of lymphoma, all require continued pharmacovigilance. Ongoing surveillance of these and other serious adverse events is necessary to determine the true incidence rates, and the overall risk-benefit of TNF-α antagonists. Last but not least, the high economical cost of these agents should also be taken into the equation.

REFERENCES

1. Suryaprasad AG, Prindiville T. The biology of TNF blockade. Autoimmun Rev 2003; 2: 346–57.
2. Malek NP, Pluempe J, Kubicka S et al. Molecular mechanisms of TNF receptor-mediated signaling. Recent Results Cancer Res 1998; 147: 97–106.
3. Nepom GT. Therapy of autoimmune diseases: clinical trials and new biologics. Curr Opin Immunol 2002; 14: 812–15.
4. Comerford LW, Bickston SJ. Treatment of luminal and fistulizing Crohn's disease with infliximab. Gastroenterol Clin North Am 2004; 33: 387–406.
5. Maini R, St Clair EW, Breedveld F et al. Infliximab (chimeric anti-tumour necrosis factor alpha monoclonal antibody) versus placebo in rheumatoid arthritis patients receiving concomitant methotrexate: a randomised phase III trial. ATTRACT Study Group. Lancet 1999; 354: 1932–9.
6. Braun J, Brandt J, Listing J et al. Long-term efficacy and safety of infliximab in the treatment of ankylosing spondylitis: an open, observational, extension study of a three-month, randomized, placebo-controlled trial. Arthritis Rheum 2003; 48: 2224–33.
7. Boumba D, Skopouli FN, Moutsopoulos HM. Cytokine mRNA expression in the labial salivary gland tissues from patients with primary Sjogren's syndrome. Br J Rheumatol 1995; 34: 326–33.
8. Fox RI, Kang HI, Ando D et al. Cytokine mRNA expression in salivary gland biopsies of Sjogren's syndrome. J Immunol 1994; 152: 5532–9.
9. Koski H, Janin A, Humphreys-Beher MG et al. Tumor necrosis factor-alpha and receptors for it in labial salivary glands in Sjogren's syndrome. Clin Exp Rheumatol 2001; 19: 131–7.
10. Jabs DA, Gerard HC, Wei Y et al. Inflammatory mediators in autoimmune lacrimal gland disease in MRL/Mpj mice. Invest Ophthalmol Vis Sci 2004; 45: 2293–8.
11. Tornwall J, Fox H, Edwards C et al. Treatment with pegylated recombinant methionyl human soluble tumor necrosis factor-type 1 receptor prevents development of Sjögren's syndrome and diabetes in the NOD mouse model. Arthritis Rheum 1999; 42 (Suppl 9): S403.
12. Steinfeld SD, Demols P Salmon I et al. Infliximab in patients with primary Sjogren's syndrome: a pilot study. Arthritis Rheum 2001; 44: 2371–5.
13. Steinfeld SD, Demols P, Appelboom T. Infliximab in primary Sjogren's syndrome: one-year followup. Arthritis Rheum 2002; 46: 3301–3.
14. Mariette X, Ravaud P, Steinfeld S et al. Inefficacy of infliximab in primary Sjogren's syndrome: results of the randomized, controlled Trial of Remicade in Primary Sjogren's Syndrome (TRIPSS). Arthritis Rheum 2004; 50: 1270–6.
15. Sankar V, Brennan MT, Kok MR et al. Etanercept in Sjogren's syndrome: a twelve-week randomized, double-blind, placebo-controlled pilot clinical trial. Arthritis Rheum 2004; 50: 2240–5.
16. Eberhard BA, Laxer RM, Andersson U et al. Local synthesis of both macrophage and T cell cytokines by synovial fluid cells from children with juvenile rheumatoid arthritis. Clin Exp Immunol 1994; 96: 260–6.
17. Mangge H, Kenzian H, Gallistl S et al. Serum cytokines in juvenile rheumatoid arthritis. Correlation with conventional inflammation parameters and clinical subtypes. Arthritis Rheum 1995; 38: 211–20.
18. Grom AA, Murray KJ, Luyrink L et al. Patterns of expression of tumor necrosis factor alpha, tumor necrosis factor beta, and their receptors in synovia of patients

with juvenile rheumatoid arthritis and juvenile spondy-larthropathy. Arthritis Rheum 1996; 39: 1703–10.

19. Lovell DJ, Giannini EH, Reiff A et al. Etanercept in children with polyarticular juvenile rheumatoid arthritis. Pediatric Rheumatology Collaborative Study Group. N Engl J Med 2000; 342: 763–9.

20. Husni ME, Maier AL, Mease PJ et al. Etanercept in the treatment of adult patients with Still's disease. Arthritis Rheum 2002; 46: 1171–6.

21. Kraetsch HG, Antoni C, Kalden JR et al. Successful treatment of a small cohort of patients with adult onset of Still's disease with infliximab: first experiences. Ann Rheum Dis 2001; 60 (Suppl 3): iii55–7.

22. Fautrel B, Sibilia J, Mariette X et al. Tumour necrosis factor alpha blocking agents in refractory adult Still's disease: an observational study of 20 cases. Ann Rheum Dis 2005; 64: 262–6.

23. Baughman RP, Strohofer SA, Buchsbaum J et al. Release of tumor necrosis factor by alveolar macrophages of patients with sarcoidosis. J Lab Clin Med 1990; 115: 36–42.

24. Sasaki M, Namioka Y, Ito T et al. Role of ICAM-1 in the aggregation and adhesion of human alveolar macrophages in response to TNF-alpha and INF-gamma. Mediators Inflamm 2001; 10: 309–13.

25. Ziegenhagen MW, Benner UK, Zissel G et al. Sarcoidosis: TNF-alpha release from alveolar macrophages and serum level of sIL-2R are prognostic markers. Am J Respir Crit Care Med 1997; 156: 1586–92.

26. Armstrong L, Foley NM, Millar AB. Inter-relationship between tumour necrosis factor-alpha (TNF-alpha) and TNF soluble receptors in pulmonary sarcoidosis. Thorax 1999; 54: 524–30.

27. Marques LJ, Zheng L, Poulakis N et al. Pentoxifylline inhibits TNF-alpha production from human alveolar macrophages. Am J Respir Crit Care Med 1999; 159: 508–11.

28. Zabel P, Entzian P, Dalhoff K et al. Pentoxifylline in treatment of sarcoidosis. Am J Respir Crit Care Med 1997; 155: 1665–9.

29. Utz JP, Limper AH, Kalra S et al. Etanercept for the treatment of stage II and III progressive pulmonary sarcoidosis. Chest 2003; 124: 177–85.

30. Ulbricht KU, Stoll M, Bierwirth J et al. Successful tumor necrosis factor alpha blockade treatment in therapy-resistant sarcoidosis. Arthritis Rheum 2003; 48: 3542–3.

31. Yee AM, Pochapin MB. Treatment of complicated sarcoidosis with infliximab anti-tumor necrosis factor-alpha therapy. Ann Intern Med 2001; 135: 27–31.

32. Roberts SD, Wilkes DS, Burgett RA et al. Refractory sarcoidosis responding to infliximab. Chest 2003; 124: 2028–31.

33. Baughman RP, Lower EE. Infliximab for refractory sarcoidosis. Sarcoidosis Vasc Diffuse Lung Dis 2001; 18: 70–4.

34. Pettersen JA, Zochodne DW, Bell RB et al. Refractory neurosarcoidosis responding to infliximab. Neurology 2002; 59: 1660–1.

35. Mallbris L, Ljungberg A, Hedblad MA et al. Progressive cutaneous sarcoidosis responding to anti-tumor necrosis factor-alpha therapy. J Am Acad Dermatol 2003; 48: 290–3.

36. Shimizu T, Tomita Y, Son K et al. Elevation of serum soluble tumour necrosis factor receptors in patients with polymyositis and dermatomyositis. Clin Rheumatol 2000; 19: 352–9.

37. Kuru S, Inukai A, Liang Y et al. Tumor necrosis factor-alpha expression in muscles of polymyositis and dermatomyositis. Acta Neuropathol (Berl) 2000; 99: 585–8.

38. Kuru S, Inukai A, Kato T et al. Expression of tumor necrosis factor-alpha in regenerating muscle fibers in inflammatory and non-inflammatory myopathies. Acta Neuropathol (Berl) 2003; 105: 217–24.

39. Tateyama M, Nagano I, Yoshioka M et al. Expression of tumor necrosis factor-alpha in muscles of polymyositis. J Neurol Sci 1997; 146: 45–51.

40. Saadeh CK. Etanercept is effective in the treatment of polymyositis/dermatomyositis which is refractory to conventional therapy including steroid and other disease modifying agents. Arthritis Rheum 2000; 43: S193.

41. Hengstman GJ, van den Hoogen FH, Barrera P et al. Successful treatment of dermatomyositis and polymyositis with anti-tumor-necrosis-factor-alpha: preliminary observations. Eur Neurol 2003; 50: 10–15.

42. Labioche I, Liozon E, Weschler B et al. Refractory polymyositis responding to infliximab: extended follow-up. Rheumatology (Oxford) 2004; 43: 531–2.

43. Efthimiou P, Schwartzman S, Kagen L. Possible role for tumor necrosis factor inhibitors in the treatment of resistant dermatomyositis and polymyositis. Ann Rheum Dis 2006; 65: 1233–6.

44. Falk RJ, Terrell RS, Charles LA et al. Anti-neutrophil cytoplasmic autoantibodies induce neutrophils to degranulate and produce oxygen radicals in vitro. Proc Natl Acad Sci U S A 1990; 87: 4115–19.

45. Reumaux D, Vossebeld PJ, Roos D et al. Effect of tumor necrosis factor-induced integrin activation on Fc gamma receptor II-mediated signal transduction: relevance for activation of neutrophils by anti-proteinase 3 or anti-myeloperoxidase antibodies. Blood 1995; 86: 3189–95.

46. Noronha IL, Kruger C, Andrassy K et al. In situ production of TNF-alpha, IL-1 beta and IL-2R in ANCA-positive glomerulonephritis. Kidney Int 1993; 43: 682–92.

47. Jonasdottir O, Petersen J, Bendtzen K. Tumour necrosis factor-alpha (TNF), lymphotoxin and TNF receptor levels in serum from patients with Wegener's granulomatosis. APMIS 2001; 109: 781–6.

48. Little MA, Bhangal G, Smyth CL et al. Therapeutic effect of anti-TNF-alpha antibodies in an experimental model of anti-neutrophil cytoplasm antibody-associated systemic vasculitis. J Am Soc Nephrol 2006; 17: 160–9.

49. Stone JH, Uhlfelder ML, Hellmann DB et al. Etanercept combined with conventional treatment in Wegener's granulomatosis: a six-month open-label trial to evaluate safety. Arthritis Rheum 2001; 44: 1149–54.

50. Lamprecht P, Voswinkel J, Lilienthal T et al. Effectiveness of TNF-alpha blockade with infliximab in refractory Wegener's granulomatosis. Rheumatology (Oxford) 2002; 41: 1303–7.

51. Bartolucci P, Ramanoelina J, Cohen P et al. Efficacy of the anti-TNF-alpha antibody infliximab against refractory systemic vasculitides: an open pilot study on 10 patients. Rheumatology (Oxford) 2002; 41: 1126–32.

52. Booth A, Harper L, Hammad T et al. Prospective study of TNFalpha blockade with infliximab in anti-neutrophil cytoplasmic antibody-associated systemic vasculitis. J Am Soc Nephrol 2004; 15: 717–21.

53. Booth AD, Jefferson HJ, Ayliffe W et al. Safety and efficacy of TNFalpha blockade in relapsing vasculitis. Ann Rheum Dis 2002; 61: 559.

54. Booth AD, Jayne DR, Kharbanda RK et al. Infliximab improves endothelial dysfunction in systemic vasculitis: a model of vascular inflammation. Circulation 2004; 109: 1718–23.

55. Nityanand S, Giscombe R, Srivastava S et al. A bias in the alphabeta T cell receptor variable region gene usage in Takayasu's arteritis. Clin Exp Immunol 1997; 107: 261–8.

56. Seko Y, Minota S, Kawasaki A et al. Perforin-secreting killer cell infiltration and expression of a 65-kD heat-shock protein in aortic tissue of patients with Takayasu's arteritis. J Clin Invest 1994; 93: 750–8.

57. Seko Y. Takayasu arteritis. In: Hoffman GS, Weyand C, eds. Inflammatory Diseases of the Blood Vessels. New York: Marcel Dekker, 2002: 443–53.

58. Tripathy NK, Gupta PC, Nityanand S. High TNF-alpha and low IL-2 producing T cells characterize active disease in Takayasu's arteritis. Clin Immunol 2006; 118: 154–8.

59. Hoffman GS, Merkel PA, Brasington RD et al. Anti-tumor necrosis factor therapy in patients with difficult to treat Takayasu arteritis. Arthritis Rheum 2004; 50: 2296–304.

60. Karageorgaki ZT, Mavragani CP, Papathanasiou MA, Skopouli FN. Infliximab in Takayasu arteritis: a safe alternative? Clin Rheumatol 2006 [Epub ahead of print].

61. Blain H, Abdelmouttaleb I, Belmin J et al. Arterial wall production of cytokines in giant cell arteritis: results of a pilot study using human temporal artery cultures. J Gerontol A Biol Sci Med Sci 2002; 57: M241–5.

62. Weyand CM, Hicok KC, Hunder GG et al. Tissue cytokine patterns in patients with polymyalgia rheumatica and giant cell arteritis. Ann Intern Med 1994; 121: 484–91.

63. Wagner AD, Wittkop U, Prahst A et al. Dendritic cells co-localize with activated CD4+ T cells in giant cell arteritis. Clin Exp Rheumatol 2003; 21: 185–92.

64. Baumann H, Gauldie J. The acute phase response. Immunol Today 1994; 15: 74–80.

65. Field M, Cook A, Gallagher G. Immuno-localisation of tumour necrosis factor and its receptors in temporal arteritis. Rheumatol Int 1997; 17: 113–18.

66. Cantini F, Niccoli L, Salvarani C et al. Treatment of longstanding active giant cell arteritis with infliximab: report of four cases. Arthritis Rheum 2001; 44: 2933–5.

67. Andonopoulos AP, Meimaris N, Daoussis D et al. Experience with infliximab (anti-TNF alpha monoclonal antibody) as monotherapy for giant cell arteritis. Ann Rheum Dis 2003; 62: 1116.

68. Tan AL, Holdsworth J, Pease C et al. Successful treatment of resistant giant cell arteritis with etanercept. Ann Rheum Dis 2003; 62: 373–4.

69. Gul A. Behcet's disease: an update on the pathogenesis. Clin Exp Rheumatol 2001; 19 (5 Suppl 24): S6–S12.

70. Mege JL, Dilsen N, Sanguedolce V et al. Overproduction of monocyte derived tumor necrosis factor alpha, interleukin (IL) 6, IL-8 and increased neutrophil superoxide generation in Behcet's disease. A comparative study with familial Mediterranean fever and healthy subjects. J Rheumatol 1993; 20: 1544–9.

71. Yamashita N, Kaneoka H, Kaneko S et al. Role of gammadelta T lymphocytes in the development of Behcet's disease. Clin Exp Immunol 1997; 107: 241–7.

72. Turan B, Gallati H, Erdi H et al. Systemic levels of the T cell regulatory cytokines IL-10 and IL-12 in Bechcet's disease; soluble TNFR-75 as a biological marker of disease activity. J Rheumatol 1997; 24: 128–32.

73. Hamzaoui K, Hamzaoui A, Guemira F et al. Cytokine profile in Behcet's disease patients. Relationship with disease activity. Scand J Rheumatol 2002; 3: 205–10.

74. Yosipovitch G, Shohat B, Bshara J et al. Elevated serum interleukin 1 receptors and interleukin 1B in patients with Behcet's disease: correlations with disease activity and severity. Isr J Med Sci 1995; 31: 345–8.

75. Sfikakis PP, Theodossiadis PG, Katsiari CG et al. Effect of infliximab on sight-threatening panuveitis in Behcet's disease. Lancet 2001; 358: 295–6.

76. Saulsbury FT, Mann JA. Treatment with infliximab for a child with Behcet's disease. Arthritis Rheum 2003; 49: 599–600.

77. Hassard PV, Binder SW, Nelson V et al. Anti-tumor necrosis factor monoclonal antibody therapy for gastrointestinal Behcet's disease: a case report. Gastroenterology 2001; 120: 995–9.

78. Licata G, Pinto A, Tuttolomondo A et al. Anti-tumour necrosis factor alpha monoclonal antibody therapy for recalcitrant cerebral vasculitis in a patient with Behcet's syndrome. Ann Rheum Dis 2003; 62: 280–1.

79. Rozenbaum M, Rosner I, Portnoy E. Remission of Behcet's syndrome with TNFalpha blocking treatment. Ann Rheum Dis 2002; 61: 283–4.

80. Gulli S, Arrigo C, Bocchino L et al. Remission of Behcet's disease with anti-tumor necrosis factor monoclonal antibody therapy: a case report. BMC Musculoskelet Disord 2003; 4: 19.

81. Ribi C, Sztajzel R, Delavelle J et al. Efficacy of TNF {alpha} blockade in cyclophosphamide resistant neuro-Behcet disease. J Neurol Neurosurg Psychiatry 2005; 76: 1733–5.

40

Overview of the safety of TNF inhibitors

Arthur Kavanaugh and John J Cush

Introduction • Assessment of safety data • Target-related reactions: Immunosuppression with TNF inhibitors • Target-related reactions: specific consequences of TNF inhibition • TNF inhibitors: agent-related reactions • Other factors affecting risks for adverse effects • Other considerations • Conclusion • References

INTRODUCTION

Among the most dramatic therapeutic advances in medicine in recent years has been the development of novel biologic therapeutics. In autoimmune disease, the introduction of biologic therapeutics, particularly recombinant proteins and monoclonal antibodies (mAbs), has been driven largely by three factors: (1) a growing recognition of the unmet clinical need for potent therapeutic agents in various disease states; (2) a clearer delineation of the molecular pathogenesis of diverse autoimmune conditions, allowing the identification of specific components of the dysregulated immune response that could serve as relevant therapeutic targets; and (3) advances in biopharmaceutical development, allowing the creation of agents capable of altering the function of specific targets. While a number of biologic agents targeting diverse components of the immune system have been introduced for several autoimmune conditions, the greatest clinical success to date has been achieved with inhibitors of the key proinflammatory cytokine tumor necrosis factor (TNF)-α.[1] Through 2006, more than 1.2 million patients worldwide have received therapy with one of the three approved recombinant macromolecule TNF inhibitors. The three are infliximab, a chimeric IgG1 mAb specific for TNF-α; etanercept, a dimeric soluble type-II TNF receptor (CD120b)–IgG Fc fusion protein that binds

TNF-α as well as lymphotoxin (TNF-β); and adalimumab, a human IgG1 mAb specific for TNF-α. Based on impressive results from a number of controlled clinical trials, these agents have been approved for use in rheumatoid arthritis (RA), Crohn's disease, psoriasis, psoriatic arthritis (PsA), ankylosing spondylitis, juvenile idiopathic arthritis, and ulcerative colitis. They are under study in a variety of other diseases as well. As reviewed elsewhere, the TNF inhibitors have achieved remarkable clinical efficacy, both in terms of substantially improving the signs and symptoms of disease, and in improving quality of life and maintaining or improving functional status, a key outcome for arthritis patients. Moreover, TNF inhibitors have been shown to prevent the progression of structural damage in RA and other conditions, including PsA.

Accompanying appreciation of the tremendous clinical benefit of TNF inhibitors has been the awareness that such potent immunomodulatory agents may also cause untoward reactions and adverse events.[2,3] Adverse reactions related to the use of biologic agents, including TNF inhibitors, may be broadly considered as target-related or agent-related (Table 40.1). Target-related issues derive from inhibition of targets, such as TNF, that are not only important contributors to the immune-driven inflammation central to the etiopathogenesis of autoimmune diseases,

Table 40.1 Potential safety issues with TNF inhibitors
Target-related
Infections
Serious infections
Opportunistic infections
Malignancies
Lymphomas
Solid organ cancers
Autoantibody development
Lupus-like syndromes
Hepatotoxicity
Demyelinating conditions
Hematologic abnormalities
Congestive heart failure
Agent-related
Administration reactions

but also serve key functions in physiologic processes, such as normal inflammatory responses and immunosurveillance. By altering the composition and functional integrity of the normal immune response, TNF inhibitors may predispose patients to certain side effects, such as infections and an increased risk of malignancy. These types of untoward outcomes may theoretically be a concern with any potent immunomodulatory therapy, certainly with any that are strong enough to be clinically effective in autoimmune diseases. In addition, certain types of infections, such as *Mycobacterium tuberculosis*, occur more commonly with TNF-directed therapies than with other agents, suggesting a specific effect of TNF in host defense for particular pathogens. Some target-related adverse events derive not necessarily from potentially wide-ranging immunosuppression, but rather from a unique aspect of the target. In the case of TNF inhibitors, the development of autoantibodies is an adverse effect commonly seen with agents in this class that is not associated with other immunomodulatory therapies. Finally, some adverse events, such as administration reactions, are agent-related. The three available TNF inhibitors are large, peptide-based molecules that are potentially immunogenic. Adverse reactions such as allergic and hypersensitivity reactions and idiosyncratic reactions relate to

characteristics of each specific agent rather than to their common target.

ASSESSMENT OF SAFETY DATA

Pertinent to consideration of safety issues surrounding the TNF inhibitors is a general consideration of the sources of safety data, which relates directly to the interpretation of such information.[4] Data concerning the safety of any therapy come from various sources (Table 40.2). Before a drug's approval, all safety information comes from clinical trials. Because of key attributes that affect its reliability, safety data from randomized clinical trials are often considered the 'gold standard'. Some strengths of data from clinical trials include the presence of controls. Among other benefits, this allows accounting for toxicities that relate to the disease being studied and other medications used, rather than to the treating agent under study. This is crucial for autoimmune diseases, where the disease itself can predispose to certain outcomes that would be considered toxicities. A clear example is the greater proclivity of RA patients to develop infections, as compared with age- and sex-matched controls.[5,6] Controlled trials also provide a complete reporting of all relevant data, including exact times and doses of medications used

Table 40.2 Sources of safety information
Sources
Double-blind, placebo-controlled, randomized clinical trials (DBPCRCTs)
Long-term follow-up of patients from DBPCRCTs
Cohort studies
Patient registries
Mandatory post marketing surveillance
Voluntary/spontaneous post marketing surveillance
Case-control studies
Individual cases/anecdotes
Considerations
Completeness of data
Presence of controls
Attribution of causality
Generalizability of data
Heterogeneity/numbers of patients
Duration of treatment

and other potentially confounding factors. This allows more reliable attribution of causality. However, there are some limitations that affect the interpretation of safety data derived from controlled trials. The primary outcome of clinical studies is efficacy, not safety, and hence studies are powered to appropriately define efficacy outcomes. Therefore, the studies in general are neither large enough in size nor long enough in duration to capture important yet uncommon adverse effects. Moreover, the population of patients typically enrolled in clinical trials may not be generally representative of the overall population of patients for whom the therapy under study may be used in the clinic. Thus, clinical trials patients tend to have less comorbidity and fewer pre-existing conditions that might affect the occurrence of important adverse events. Therefore, safety data derived from other sources are crucial to ascertainment of the overall safety profile of a medication. Collection of safety data from various sources after a drug has been approved is referred to as pharmacovigilance. Various sources of data have different strengths and weaknesses. Some, such as registries, offer some of the benefits of controlled studies, yet provide larger numbers of patients. Even anecdotal reports can have value in highlighting particular safety issues. A particular strength of case reports is that they provide assessment of the drug among patients with certain comorbidities or who are using other medications that would have been excluded from entry into clinical trials. These factors may contribute to certain adverse effects, but would not have been identified from clinical trial data alone. However, pharmacovigilance data are often incomplete, and a comparison group is often not included, precluding estimation of the incidence of the event and causality. Therefore, safety issues identified from pharmacovigilance often are said to provide a 'signal', the true significance of which needs to be delineated from more controlled sources of data.

Host factors can contribute importantly to toxicity, and are relevant to discussions of the safety issues surrounding TNF inhibitors (Table 40.3). To date, the greatest exposure to TNF inhibitors has been in patients with RA and Crohn's disease.

Table 40.3 Host factors relevant to safety data
Disease being treated
Severity/activity of disease
Comorbidity
Age of patients
Concomitant medications

Because the treatment paradigms are more often chronic in RA, the largest exposure to TNF inhibitors in patient-years has been in that disease. As noted, patients with RA have a greater prevalence of certain adverse outcomes, such as infection.[5,6] Compared with an age- and sex-matched general population, RA patients also have a greater prevalence of certain malignancies, specifically lymphoma.[7] Among RA patients, factors associated with a proclivity for infection include advancing age, severity of RA, comorbid conditions (e.g. diabetes mellitus, chronic obstructive pulmonary disease), and the use of concomitant medications such as corticosteroids.[6] For lymphoma, the level of disease activity and advancing age were the most important associated factors. It is important to note that to date, the subset of RA patients most commonly considered appropriate candidates for treatment with TNF inhibitors has been those patients with severe, long-standing, refractory disease. Any consideration of the risks associated with a particular therapeutic intervention needs to take into account the specific population exposed. In recent years, based upon their established success in patients with refractory disease, TNF inhibitors have been increasingly tested in patients with early RA. In such patients, who tend to be younger and suffer less comorbidity, adverse effects have tended to occur less commonly as compared with patients with long-standing refractory disease.[8] The use of TNF inhibitors in diseases other than RA continues to expand.[9,10] In order to be able to attribute the excess risk of adverse events to use of TNF inhibitors in these conditions, there needs to be delineation of the baseline risks of important outcomes and consideration of comorbid conditions and other factors that may predispose to certain adverse effects.

TARGET-RELATED REACTIONS: IMMUNOSUPPRESSION WITH TNF INHIBITORS

Infections and serious infections

In nearly all clinical trials of TNF inhibitors, there has been a greater incidence of infections noted among treated patients as compared with controls. The most common sites of infection have typically been the same types of infection observed in the general population and in RA patients overall, namely the upper and lower respiratory tracts, the skin, and the urinary tract.[11] It is important to note that an increased risk of infection has also been observed in the treatment group of virtually all effective therapies in RA. Moreover, in the clinic, therapy with traditional disease-modifying anti-rheumatic drugs (DMARDs) such as methotrexate has also been shown to be associated with an increased risk for infections.[12]

Serious infections, defined by regulatory agencies as those infections requiring hospitalization or treatment with intravenous antibiotics, were observed in clinical trials of TNF inhibitors in RA. In the majority of trials, the incidence of serious infections in patients treated with TNF inhibitors was small, and did not exceed that observed in the control group.[13] However, the primary outcome of all of these studies was safety, and the trials were not powered to define differences in relatively uncommon safety outcomes. A systematic analysis that combined the results from nine clinical trials of TNF inhibitors has been performed.[14] That analysis did find an increased risk of serious infection among TNF inhibitors compared with controls (3.6% versus 1.7%); however, it should be noted that in that analysis, a non-standard definition of serious infection was used, and no attempt was made to control for the time of exposure, which was nearly always greater in those clinical trials for patients receiving TNF inhibitors.[14] In that same analysis, there was a non-significant trend towards a greater incidence of serious infections with higher doses of TNF inhibitor. In one of the only clinical trials having a primary outcome of safety, the use of high doses of a TNF inhibitor was associated with a greater incidence of serious infections compared with a lower dose, and

the lower dose was not different from placebo in that regard.[15] In pharmacovigilance, serious infections have certainly been observed among patients receiving TNF inhibitors.[13] From those reports, the relative impact of potentially confounding factors such as comorbidities and concomitant medications on the rate of serious infections remains incompletely defined. This important question has also been addressed using registries of RA patients.[16,17] In a German registry, the rate of infections and serious infections among 858 RA patients receiving treatment with TNF inhibitors was compared with that among 601 patients receiving only DMARDs.[16] The relative risk for infections (3.3–4.1) as well as serious infections (2.7–2.8) was significantly higher among patients receiving TNF inhibitors. However, those patients also had more severe and more active RA, thereby placing them at a greater *a priori* risk of infections. When the investigators used propensity scoring methods to control for severity of disease as a confounder, the relative risks were reduced. The risk of infection decreased to 2.3–3.0, and that for serious infection became a non-significant trend of 2.1. In data from the British registry, 7644 RA patients treated with TNF inhibitors were compared to 1354 RA patients on DMARDs alone.[17] In this analysis, the crude rate of serious infections was higher among TNF-treated patients (1.28; 95% confidence interval (CI) 0.94–1.76), although this did not reach statistical significance. Further, when the rates were adjusted for age, sex, severity of RA, use of corticosteroids, and comorbidity, there was no difference between the groups (relative risk 1.03; 95% CI 0.68–1.57).

As a bottom line, it perhaps can be stated that treatment with TNF inhibitors can result in an increased risk of infections and serious infections, but that other factors such as the severity of RA, the use of other medications such as corticosteroids, and the presence of comorbidities are important contributors to these outcomes.

Opportunistic infections

In addition to common infections, various opportunistic infections such as *Pneumocystis carinii*, listeriosis, legionella, atypical mycobacteria, coccidioidomycosis, histoplasmosis, and aspergillosis have been reported in patients receiving therapy with TNF inhibitors.[13] The development of these infections in many cases reflects the overall incidence within the local community. For example, coccidioidomycosis has been noted particularly in the desert southwestern United States, and histoplasmosis in the Ohio and Mississippi river valleys. Overall, while the numbers of cases of these types of opportunistic infections are small, it does appear that treatment with TNF inhibitors contributes to the risk for these infections.[18] Other factors, such as the use of corticosteroids, also play a role. Host factors are also important, as a history of opportunistic infection is a risk factor for the development of subsequent additional opportunistic infections.

Tuberculosis

Data from numerous animal studies has shown that TNF-α plays a critical role in defense against tuberculosis (TB) infection. Thus, inhibition of TNF by various methods has been shown to result in increased susceptibility to TB infection, poor granuloma formation, greater rates of TB reactivation, and higher mortality.[18–22] Although there were few cases of TB during clinical trials with TNF inhibitors, post marketing surveillance revealed a substantial number of cases.[23,24] Through the last quarter of 2002, there were 172 cases of TB seen with infliximab and 38 cases seen with etanercept, with a denominator for both of roughly 230 000 patient-years of exposure. A greater risk was noted initially with the mAb infliximab as compared with the soluble receptor etanercept. Differences in risk could be related to factors including mechanistic differences between the agents, pharmacokinetic/pharmacodynamic differences, alternate avidity for TNF, or factors related to the populations treated. Most cases appear to be reactivation of latent TB, with an onset usually within the first few months of therapy. Importantly, the incidence has decreased substantially with the widespread adoption of screening for latent TB before commencing TNF inhibitors. Interestingly, with all three agents about half of the presentations of TB were extrapulmonary or disseminated. This is in contrast to the general population, where approximately 85% of cases of TB present

with pneumonia. This suggests a class effect among TNF inhibitors. Although screening for latent TB has been very effective, vigilance is still required, as cutaneous anergy is not uncommon among the populations of patients treated with TNF inhibitors. Also, while screening can be effective for discovering latent TB, acquisition of new cases of TB during therapy is always a possibility, particularly in endemic areas.

Malignancies

Initial analyses, after the TNF inhibitors had been available in the clinic for half a decade, suggested that TNF inhibitor therapy was not associated with any greater risk of solid organ tumors, but a question arose regarding lymphoproliferative malignancies, especially non-Hodgkin's lymphoma (NHL).[25] For NHL, a standardized incidence ratio (SIR) of approximately 2 to 6 or more had been observed among RA patients receiving TNF inhibitors, compared with an age- and sex-matched population.[25–28] However, this rate may approximate the baseline risk of the exposed RA population. Thus, it has been shown that RA patients are at a higher risk for developing lymphoma, particularly those with the most severe and active disease.[7] As this is the population of RA patients most likely to receive TNF inhibitor therapy, a larger number of cases of lymphoma would be expected among treated patients. More data with longer follow-up time are necessary to fully define any potential association between lymphoma and these agents. Indeed, given that TNF inhibitors can be highly effective in controlling systemic inflammation and decreasing disease activity in RA, it might be hypothesized that treatment should lead to a reduction in lymphoma patients with sufficient treatment early in the disease course.

Several observations have caused the potential effect of TNF inhibitors on solid tumors to be re-examined. The systematic analysis of data from clinical trials of TNF inhibitors suggested an increased risk of cancer among patients receiving TNF inhibitors (odds ratio 3.3; 95% CI 1.2–9.1).[14] This study also suggested a dose effect with a greater risk for cancer at higher doses. There are several methodologic limitations that affect the interpretation of this analysis, including the lack of accounting for exposure time, an important point for an outcome such as malignancy among patients in clinical trials. However, several studies in conditions other than RA have also raised this issue. In a study of patients with Wegener's granulomatosis, 6 solid tumors developed among 89 patients receiving treatment with a TNF inhibitor compared with none among 91 control patients.[29] It is notable that all of these patients had previously received treatment with cyclophosphamide, an alkylating agent known to be associated with development of malignancies. In a trial of patients with chronic obstructive pulmonary disease (COPD), 1 cancer developed among 77 control patients, whereas 9 were observed among 157 patients treated with a TNF inhibitor.[30] Most of the cancers were lung and laryngeal, cancers known to occur at higher incidence among heavy smokers, and most of the patients included in this study had extensive smoking histories. Thus, it is possible that treatment with TNF inhibitors may alter the risk for development of solid tumors, particularly among patients at higher baseline risk due to other factors. Clinicians need to be vigilant for overall risk of cancer among treated patients, based upon their age, sex, family history, comorbidities, and other factors that affect the incidence of cancer.

TARGET-RELATED REACTIONS: SPECIFIC CONSEQUENCES OF TNF INHIBITION

Pharmacovigilance data have also revealed cases of multiple sclerosis (MS) and other demyelinating conditions among patients treated with TNF inhibitors.[31,32] Animal data have been uninformative in this regard, as inhibition of TNF appears to be effective in experimental allergic encephalomyelitis (EAE), an animal model with semblance to human MS. In humans, inhibition of TNF may modify peripheral T-cell autoreactivity, which in turn may initiate release of proinflammatory cytokines in the CNS.[32] Although the relationship between MS and TNF inhibitor therapy is still not clear, it is worrisome that two studies of TNF inhibitors in patients with MS showed worsening of MRI lesions with treatment. It has been hypothesized that TNF plays a critical role in remyelination and inhibition may

impair this process, or that TNF inhibitors might unmask unidentified latent infections leading to MS. While the true impact of TNF inhibitors on the development of MS remains undefined, most clinicians avoid these agents or use them cautiously in patients with MS or other demyelinating conditions.

An interesting observation among patients treated with TNF inhibitors has been the development of certain autoantibodies that are more typically associated with systemic lupus erythematosus (SLE).[33,34] While positive anti-nuclear antibodies (ANAs) are not uncommon among RA patients, the prevalence increases to 50% or more among those treated with TNF inhibitors. More importantly, approximately 10–15% of RA patients treated with TNF inhibitors also develop autoantibodies against double-stranded DNA (anti-dsDNA); such autoantibodies are much less common in RA, and are more specific for SLE than the generic ANAs. Of note, while some patients have developed what appears to be drug-induced lupus related to TNF inhibitors, this seems to be quite uncommon.[33,34] Therefore, the development of ANAs and anti-dsDNA seems to be of no consequence in the vast majority of treated patients. In addition to ANAs and anti-dsDNA, anticardiolipin antibodies have also been observed in relation to TNF inhibition. However, other antibodies commonly seen in SLE patients have not been observed, suggesting that TNF inhibition is not replicating SLE. Data from animal models have been contradictory as regards SLE and TNF inhibition. In some models, TNF potentiates inflammation and TNF inhibition is therapeutic, whereas in others TNF inhibition results in enhanced autoantibody production and more severe disease.

In many patients with chronic heart failure (CHF), TNF levels are elevated, and there may even be a correlation with disease activity. In animal models of induced ischemic cardiomyopathy, TNF effects various changes that are detrimental to myocardial function and overall survival, and TNF inhibition is dramatically effective. These data provided a seemingly sound rationale for testing TNF inhibitors in patients with CHF. However, multiple clinical trials assessing the efficacy of TNF inhibitors on CHF have failed to show any benefit and, in some, have resulted in increased morbidity and mortality.[35–37] TNF may actually be an adaptive cytokine that induces vasodilation, decreases beta-adrenergic stimulation, and prevents myocyte apoptosis. Importantly, in RA patients, there seems to be no association between the development or worsening of CHF and the use of TNF inhibitors. Nevertheless, caution is indicated when considering the use of TNF inhibitors for patients with autoimmune disease who have concomitant cardiac dysfunction. Other adverse effects that have been infrequently observed among RA patients treated with TNF inhibitors include hematologic cytopenias, especially leukopenia, and hepatic dysfunction, manifest usually as an increase in liver function tests (LFTs).[30,38,39] Attribution of these toxicities to TNF inhibitors among RA patients has been somewhat difficult as patients not uncommonly take other medications that can also be associated with these toxicities. Also, the mechanism by which TNF inhibitors cause these reactions is uncertain. Nevertheless, it does appear that such events do rarely occur among treated patients, and clinicians need to be aware of them.

TNF INHIBITORS: AGENT-RELATED REACTIONS

Various types of adverse reactions specific to each of the different TNF inhibitors have been observed. Antibodies to the individual agents have been noted in treated patients, and may underlie various hypersensitivity reactions. Development of antibodies to biological agents depends on several factors, including the foreignness of the protein (e.g. mouse versus human), route of administration (e.g. subcutaneous versus intravenous), treatment paradigms (e.g. continuous versus intermittent) and, perhaps most importantly, the concomitant use of immunosuppressive medications. Antibodies to infliximab, which appear to be largely anti-idiotypic in specificity, have been associated with type I, type II, and type III hypersensitivity reactions.[2,40,41] These reactions have occurred most commonly during the third and fourth infusions and have ranged from mild urticaria and pruritus to hypotension and even anaphylaxis. Intermittent usage of infliximab, which is more commonly employed in the treatment of Crohn's

disease, has been associated with a greater propensity for the development of antibodies to infliximab.[42,43] Those patients with a higher concentration of antibodies against infliximab were more likely to experience infusion reactions than patients who did not develop these antibodies. The development of these antibodies is attenuated by the concomitant use of immunosuppressives such as corticosteroids, azathioprine, methotrexate, and 6-mercaptopurine.[42,43] By far the most common agent-related reactions to etanercept and adalimumab, which are given subcutaneously, are injection site reactions (ISRs). Histologically, these ISRs have been shown to resemble delayed-type hypersensitivity reaction.[44] Leukocytoclastic vasculitis, which has been hypothesized to relate to the deposition of immune complexes of TNF inhibitor and antibodies to the inhibitor, has also been described with all three TNF inhibitors.[45] In general, reactions related to one TNF inhibitor have not developed with the subsequent use of other TNF inhibitors; thus switching from one agent to another is a feasible option in such cases.

OTHER FACTORS AFFECTING RISKS FOR ADVERSE EFFECTS

TNF certainly has a central role in the inflammatory cascade and has the potential to affect various components of the immune response. Therefore, it could be hypothesized that interference with some aspects of normal immunity might be demonstrated *in vitro* and may be associated with predisposition to certain adverse effects. However, in the several studies that have addressed this, TNF inhibitor therapy has not been shown to have any demonstrable effect on various measures of humoral immunity, cell-mediated immunity, and innate immune responses.[2] Of note, this includes responses to vaccination with both peptide and carbohydrate antigens that are no different than those observed among RA patients in general. Investigators have begun to assess whether any genetic polymorphisms in factors relevant to host defense may contribute to the risk of adverse effects, such as infection among patients treated with TNF inhibitors. It has been suggested that polymorphisms in the genes encoding one of the

Table 40.4 Potential mechanisms of action of TNF inhibitors

Down-regulate other inflammatory mediators
  - other cytokines (IL-1, IL-6, etc.)
  - chemokines (IL-8, etc.)
  - other mediators (e.g. prostaglandins, metalloproteinases)
Alter vascular function
  - alter adhesion molecule expression/function
  - inhibit angiogenesis
Alter innate immune system function
Modulate the function of immunocompetent cells
  - T cells
  - macrophages

Fc gamma receptors (FcγRIII) may correlate with efficacy outcomes among arthritis patients treated with TNF inhibitors.[46] To date, there have been preliminary results that suggest that polymorphisms in genes encoding TNF, lymphotoxin, and FcγRIII may be associated with an increased risk of certain infections.[47] Further work is needed to confirm and expand these results before they can be applied to the clinic.

TNF is a potent central cytokine that effects myriad activities. While inhibition of TNF has certainly proven effective, it is not absolutely clear what the proximate mechanism of action is for various facets of its efficacy. A number of potential mechanisms of action for TNF inhibitors have been described (Table 40.4). Similarly, when considering adverse effects related to the use of TNF inhibitors, the specific mechanisms underlying various toxicities have not been fully defined. It is possible that there may be various dose dependencies for different mechanisms, and that this might allow refinement of therapy so as to maximize efficacy while minimizing toxicity.

OTHER CONSIDERATIONS

The success of TNF inhibition has driven additional research into novel therapies and treatment paradigms for RA and other immune conditions. One question that has arisen regards therapeutic options for patients who do not achieve the desired level of clinical efficacy when treated with TNF inhibitors. Hypothetically, the idea of combining inhibitors of TNF with other cytokine inhibitors has appeal, as it could be reasoned that such an approach might offer synergy. This concept has had support from certain animal models of arthritis, where combinations of therapies inhibiting TNF and IL-1, another important proinflammatory cytokine, achieved clinical results superior to either therapy used alone. Unfortunately, when this approach was tried in RA patients, there was no added clinical efficacy.[48] There was, however, a biologic effect in terms of increased adverse effects, specifically a greater incidence of infections and serious infections with combination therapy. Preliminary results from a study assessing the combination of a TNF inhibitor in conjunction with an inhibitor of T-cell activity similarly revealed no substantial improvement in clinical efficacy but also showed a greater risk of infectious adverse events, serious infections, and cancers among patients receiving the combination of biologic agents.[49] Therefore, while the idea of combining biologic agents with distinct mechanisms of action has theoretical appeal, concern about additive toxicities requires careful planning and very close monitoring for any future studies of this approach.

The notable success of TNF inhibitors in established refractory RA has resulted increasingly in the assessment of these drugs in patients with early RA. Compared with patients with long-standing RA, patients with early disease have even better clinical outcomes. Moreover, adverse events tend to occur less commonly among early RA patients, presumably related to factors such as their less frequent comorbidity and their overall better general health. Thus, from a safety perspective, the use of TNF inhibitors in patients with early RA would seem desirable. However, because such patients are generally younger, the consequences of adverse events, should they occur, may be distinct and possibly have a greater deleterious impact than among older persons. In addition, there may be risks for patients with a long life expectancy that might not be seen among older persons, such as increasing risks for infectious agents that then may eventuate a greater risk of malignancy. This is relevant for considerations of treating juvenile patients with autoimmune disease as well.

As a large number of patients receiving therapy with TNF inhibitors are women of reproductive age, pregnancy is an important issue.[50] All of the TNF inhibitors currently approved are considered category 'B' for pregnancy according to the United States Food and Drug Administration (FDA), as untoward effects have not been noted in animal models, but there is a paucity of human data. To date, in anecdotal reports, it appears that the outcome of pregnancies among patients treated with TNF inhibitors is not different from that among similar persons unexposed to this type of therapy. It is worth noting that other therapeutic choices for RA, such as the DMARDs methotrexate and leflunomide, are contraindicated as regards pregnancy.

CONCLUSION

The introduction of TNF inhibitors has dramatically improved the clinical status of many patients with RA and other autoimmune diseases. The success of the agents already introduced almost guarantees continued development, and the introduction of many more therapeutic agents in this class can be anticipated. Despite their tremendous clinical utility, TNF inhibitors can be associated with adverse reactions. Some adverse reactions are target-related, and derive from inhibition of such a key proinflammatory cytokine. This includes an increased risk of infections and perhaps certain types of cancer, particularly among persons already at increased risk for these outcomes. Other adverse reactions to TNF inhibition relate to the agents themselves rather than the target, such as various hypersensitivity reactions. Although clinical trials provide crucial information on the efficacy and initial tolerability of new drugs, they are an incomplete source of safety information. This is particularly true as regards longer-term safety data on larger numbers of more heterogeneous patients. Therefore, clinicians must be aware of the potential complications of biological therapies, and should report these reactions so that we all might learn more about these important agents. During treatments, assiduous observation for any signs or symptoms suggestive of adverse effects such as infection and malignancy is required during therapy with the TNF inhibitors.

REFERENCES

1. Kavanaugh A, Cohen S, Cush J. The evolving use of tumor necrosis factor inhibitors in rheumatoid arthritis. J Rheumatol 2004; 31: 1881–4.
2. Lee SJ, Yedla P, Kavanaugh A. Secondary immune deficiencies associated with biological therapeutics. Curr Allergy Asthma Rep 2003; 3: 389–95.
3. Weisman MH. What are the risks of biologic therapy in rheumatoid arthritis? An update on safety. J Rheumatol 2002; 29 (Suppl 65): 33–8.
4. Kavanaugh A, Cush JJ, Antoni C. Long term monitoring of novel therapies. In: Smolen JS, Lipsky PE, eds. Targeted Therapies in Rheumatology. London: Martin Dunitz, 2003: 679–90.
5. Doran MF, Crowson CS, Pond GR, O'Fallon WN, Gabriel SE. Frequency of infection in patients with rheumatoid arthritis compared with controls: a population based study. Arthritis Rheum 2002; 46: 2287–93
6. Doran MF, Crowson CS, Pond GR, O'Fallon WN, Gabriel SE. Predictors of infection in rheumatoid arthritis. Arthritis Rheum 2002; 46: 2294–300.
7. Baecklund E, Iliadou A, Askling J et al. Association of chronic inflammation, not its treatment, with increased lymphoma risk in rheumatoid arthritis. Arthritis Rheum 2006; 54: 692–701.
8. Kavanaugh A, Keystone EC. The safety of biologic agents in early rheumatoid arthritis. Clin Exp Rheumatol 2003; 21 (Suppl 31): S203–S208.
9. Colombel JF, Loftus EV, Tremaine WJ et al. The safety profile of infliximab in patients with Crohn's disease: the Mayo Clinic experience in 500 patients. Gastroenterology 2004; 126: 19–31.
10. Kavanaugh A, Tutuncu Z, Catalan-Sanchez T. Update on anti-tumor necrosis factor therapy in the spondyloarthropathies, including psoriatic arthritis. Curr Opin Rheumatol 2006; 18: 347–53.
11. Scott DL, Kingsley GH. Tumor necrosis factor inhibitors for rheumatoid arthritis. N Engl J Med 2006; 355: 704–12.
12. Hernandez-Cruz B, Cardiel MH, Villa AR, Alcocer-Varela J. Development, recurrence and severity of infections in Mexican patients with rheumatoid arthritis: a nested case-control study. J Rheumatol 1998; 25: 1900–7.
13. Cush J, Kavanaugh A. ACR Hotline. FDA meeting March 2003: Update on the safety of new drugs for Rheumatoid Arthritis. Part II: CHF, infections and other safety issues. Available at: http://www.rheumatology.org/research/hotline [Accessed 8/20/03.]

14. Bongartz T, Sutton A, Sweeting MJ et al. Anti-TNF antibody therapy in rheumatoid arthritis and the risk of serious infections and malignancies: systematic review of rare harmful effects in randomized controlled trials. JAMA 2006; 295: 2275–85.

15. Westhovens R, Yocum D, Han J et al. The safety of infliximab, combined with background treatments, among patients with rheumatoid arthritis and various comorbidities: a large, randomized, placebo-controlled trial. Arthritis Rheum 2006; 54: 1075–86.

16. Listing J, Strangfeld A, Kary S et al. Infections in patient with rheumatoid arthritis treated with biologic agents. Arthritis Rheum 2005; 52: 3403–12.

17. Dixon WG, Watson K, Lunt M et al. Rates of serious infection, including site-specific and bacterial intracellular infection, in rheumatoid arthritis patients receiving anti-tumor necrosis factor therapy: results from the British Society for Rheumatology Biologics Register. Arthritis Rheum 2006; 54: 2368–76.

18. Benini J, Ehlers EM, Ehlers S. Different types of pulmonary granuloma necrosis in immunocompetent vs. TNFRp55-gene-deficient mice aerogenically infected with highly virulent *Mycobacterium avium*. J Pathol 1999; 189: 127–37.

19. Kaneko H, Yamada H, Mizuno S et al. Role of tumor necrosis factor-alpha in *Mycobacterium*-induced granuloma formation tumor necrosis factor-alpha-deficient mice. Lab Invest 1999; 79: 379–86.

20. Senaldi G, Yin S, Shaklee CL et al. *Corynebacterium parvum*- and *Mycobacterium bovis* bacillus Calmette-Guerin-induced granuloma formation is inhibited in TNF receptor I (TNF-RI) knockout mice and by treatment with soluble TNF-RI. J Immunol 1996; 1571: 5022–6.

21. Rojas M, Oliverier M, Gros P et al. TNF-α and IL-10 modulate the induction of apoptosis by virulent *Mycobacterium tuberculosis* in murine macrophages. J Immunol 1999; 162: 6122–31.

22. Mohan VP, Scanga CA, Yu K et al. Effects of tumor necrosis factor alpha on host immune response in chronic persistent tuberculosis: possible role for limiting pathology. Infect Immun 2001; 69: 1847–55.

23. Bieber J, Kavanaugh A. Consideration of the risk and treatment of TB in patients with rheumatoid arthritis receiving biologic treatments. Rheum Dis Clin North Am 2004; 30: 257–70.

24. Keane J, Gershon S, Wise RP et al. Tuberculosis associated with infliximab, a tumor necrosis factor α-neutralizing agent. N Engl J Med 2001; 345: 1098–104.

25. Cush J, Kavanaugh A. ACR Hotline. FDA meeting March 2003: Update on the safety of new drugs for Rheumatoid Arthritis. Part I: The risk of lymphoma with RA and TNF Inhibitors. Available at: http://www.rheumatology.org/research/hotline/0303TNFL. htm [Accessed 3/31/03].

26. van Vollenhoven RF. Benefits and risks of biological agents: lymphomas. Clin Exp Rheumatol 2004; 22 (Suppl 35): S122–S125.

27. Symmons DPM, Silman AJ. Anti-tumor necrosis factor α therapy and the risk of lymphoma in rheumatoid arthritis: no clear answer. Arthritis Rheum 2004; 50: 1703–6.

28. Wolfe F, Michaud K. Lymphoma in rheumatoid arthritis. The effect of methotrexate and anti-tumor necrosis factor therapy in 18,572 patients. Arthritis Rheum 2004; 50: 1740–51.

29. Wegener's Granulomatosis Etanercept Trial (WGET) research group. Etanercept plus standard therapy for Wegener's granulomatosis. N Engl J Med 2005; 352: 351–61.

30. Remicade (infliximab) package insert. May 2006.

31. Robinson WH, Genovese MC, Moreland LW. Demyelinating and neurologic events reported in association with tumor necrosis factor α antagonism. Arthritis Rheum 2001; 44: 1977–83.

32. Mohan N, Edwards ET, Cupps TR et al. Demyelination occurring during anti-tumor necrosis factor α therapy for inflammatory arthritides. Arthritis Rheum 2001; 44: 2862–9.

33. Shakoor N, Michalska M, Harris CA et al. Drug-induced systemic lupus erythematosus associated with etanercept therapy. Lancet 2002; 359: 579–80.

34. Debandt M, Vittecoq O, Descamps V et al. Anti-TNF-α-induced systemic lupus syndrome. Clin Rheumatol 2003; 22: 56–61.

35. Anker SD, Coats AJS. How to RECOVER from RENAISSANCE? The significance of the results of RECOVER, RENAISSANCE, RENEWAL and ATTACH. Int J Cardiol 2002; 85: 12–30.

36. Mann DL, McMurray JJV, Packer M et al. Targeted anticytokine therapy in patients with chronic heart failure. Results of the Randomized Etanercept Worldwide Evaluation (RENEWAL). Circulation 2004; 109: 1594–602.

37. Chung ES, Packer M, Lo KH et al. Randomized, double-blind, placebo-controlled, pilot trial of infliximab, a chimeric monoclonal antibody to tumor necrosis factor-α, in patients with moderate-to-severe heart failure. Results of the Anti-TNF Therapy Against Congestive Heart failure (ATTACH) trial. Circulation 2003; 107: 3133–40.

38. Etanercept package insert. May 2006.

39. Humira (adalimumab) package insert. June 2006.

40. Kugathasan S, Levy MB, Saeian K et al. Infliximab retreatment in adults and children with Crohn's disease: risk factors for the development of delayed severe systemic reaction. Am J Gastroenterol 2002; 97: 1408–14.

41. Soykan I, Ertan C, Ozden A et al. Severe anaphylactic reaction to infliximab: report of a case. Am J Gastroenterol 2000; 95: 2395–6.

42. Baert F, Noman M, Verneire S et al. Influence of immunogenicity on the long-term efficacy of infliximab in Crohn's disease. N Engl J Med 2003; 348: 601–8.

43. Sands BE, Anderson FH, Bernstein CH et al. Infliximab maintenance therapy for fistulizing Crohn's Disease. N Engl J Med 2004; 350: 876–85.

44. Zeltser R, Vaale L, Tanck C et al. Clinical, histological, and immunophenotypic characteristics of injection site reactions associated with etanercept. Arch Dermatol 2001; 137: 893–9.

45. Mohan N, Edwards E, Cupps T et al. Leukocytoclastic vasculitis associated with tumor necrosis factor-alpha blocking agents. J Rheumatol 2004; 31: 1955–8.

46. Tutuncu Z, Kavanaugh A, Zvaifler N et al. FcrIIIA polymorphisms influence treatment outcomes in patients with inflammatory arthritis treated with TNF-α blocking agents. Arthritis Rheum 2005; 52: 2693–6.

47. Hughes LB, Criswell LA, Beasley TM et al. Genetic risk factors for infections in patients with early rheumatoid arthritis. Genes Immun 2004; 5: 641–7.

48. Genovese M, Cohen S, Moreland L et al. Combination therapy with etanercept and anakinra in the treatment of patients with rheumatoid arthritis who have been treated unsuccesfully with methotrexate. Arthritis Rheum 2004; 50: 1412–19.

49. Combe B, Weinblatt M, Birbara C et al. Safety and patient-reported outcomes associated with abatacept in the treatment of rheumatoid arthritis patients receiving background disease modifying anti-rheumatic frugs (DMARDs): the ASSURE trial. Arthritis Rheum 2005; 52 (suppl): S709–S710.

50. Salmon JE, Alpert D. Are we coming to terms with tumor necrosis factor inhibition in pregnancy? Arthritis Rheum 2006; 54: 2353–5.

41

Anti-CD20 to further targeted therapies in rheumatology

Kristine P Ng and David A Isenberg

Introduction • B-cell depletion • Inhibition of costimulatory molecules • Immunoablation • Tolerizing T cells • Tolerizing B cells • Anti-cytokine therapies • Complement blockade • Conclusion• Acknowledgments • References

INTRODUCTION

The management of most autoimmune rheumatic diseases (ARDs) has improved with major advances in drug development and our understanding of disease pathogenesis. ARDs share some clinical and serological characteristics and there is considerable overlap of immunosuppressive drugs used in their treatment. The overall goals in the management of these often complex conditions are reducing autoimmunity, suppressing inflammation, arresting disease progression, and achieving remission.

Rheumatoid arthritis (RA) and systemic lupus erythematosus (SLE) are two rheumatological conditions that can share clinical and serological features. About 4% of patients with SLE can have erosive disease resembling RA. The management of RA has changed dramatically since the discovery of anti-tumor necrosis factor (anti-TNF)-α therapy. Several new approaches (some in clinical trials) offer promising additional therapeutic agents for both RA and SLE.

These approaches are based on an improved understanding of the pathogenesis of RA and SLE, leading to the development of specific targeted therapeutic agents which modify the disease process and prevent further damage. This chapter reviews some of these exciting advances.

B-CELL DEPLETION

Rituximab

Rheumatoid arthritis

RA was regarded as largely a T-cell-mediated autoimmune disease in the 1980s to 1990s. This was in part due to the association of HLA-DR allotype and the presence of T cells in the RA synovium.[1] Activated T lymphocytes initiated by arthritogenic antigens stimulate macrophages, monocytes, and synovial fibroblasts. These in turn generate proinflammatory cytokines interleukin (IL)-1, IL-6, and TNF-α, believed to be important in the pathogenesis of RA. Biological therapy with anti-TNF-α drugs is now regarded as standard treatment for RA patients who have failed classic disease-modifying antirheumatic drugs (DMARDs). However, about 30% of RA patients fail to respond to anti-TNF-α therapy, with ongoing disease activity leading to irreversible long-term joint damage.

A renewed interest in the role of B cells in the pathogenesis of RA was raised when Edwards and colleagues proposed the concept of self-perpetuating B lymphocytes driving the disease process.[2] An example of this concept is the generation of IgG rheumatoid factor (RF) immune complexes providing a positive feedback cycle through complex signal interactions between T and B cells. This promotes the production of cytokines and cell surface ligands, creating a vicious cycle. Furthermore, T-cell activation was disrupted when human RA synovium implanted in severe combined immune deficient (SCID) mice treated with anti-CD20 antibodies, demonstrating that T-cell activation is B-cell-dependent.[3] The potential roles of B cells in RA include production of autoantibodies resulting in complement fixation and immune complex deposition, generation of proinflammatory cytokines like TNF-α and IL-1, and serving as antigen-presenting cells (APCs).

CD20 is a specific marker for B cells expressed on the surface of pre-B lymphocytes to the pre-plasma cell stage. It is not expressed on the hematopoietic pro-B cells and plasma cells. Rituximab is a chimeric monoclonal antibody (mAb) that targets CD20. It comprises the variable regions of a murine anti-CD20 B-cell hybridoma fused with human IgG constant regions. The killing of B cells by rituximab is thought to be mediated by induction of complement-mediated activities, activation of antibody-dependent cytotoxic activity (ADCC), and apoptosis.[4] Interestingly, the killing mechanism of rituximab has been shown to be different in different tissue environments.[5] Rituximab was approved by the Food and Drug Administration (FDA) in 1997 for the treatment of patients with non-Hodgkin's lymphoma. The safety profile of rituximab in this population is well defined, with experience in more than 900 000 patients and close to a decade of post marketing surveillance.

In an open study of five refractory seropositive RA patients treated with rituximab, cyclophosphamide, and prednisolone, all achieved major improvement (ACR 50 or 70) for at least 6 months.[6] An extension study involving 22 patients with RA treated with varying rituximab doses and cyclophosphamide with or without steroids demonstrated major improvement in patients who were treated with a rituximab dose

of at least 600 mg/m.[2] All patients tolerated treatment well with no major side effects.[7] These encouraging results led to a phase IIa controlled study in 2004, which confirmed the efficacy of B-cell depletion in RA.[8] In this study, 161 patients with active seropositive RA despite methotrexate of at least 10 mg/week were randomized to four different treatment arms. The treatment regimes were methotrexate 10 mg/week only (control group), rituximab alone (1000 mg on days 1 and 15), rituximab with cyclophosphamide (750 mg intravenously on days 3 and 17), and rituximab with methotrexate. All groups received a 17-day course of corticosteroid which included 100 mg intravenous (i.v.) methylprednisolone prior to rituximab and cyclophosphamide infusions. The primary outcome was ACR 50 response at 24 weeks. At 24 weeks, the ACR 50 response rate was significantly better at 33–43% in the rituximab groups compared with 13% in the control groups. Clinical benefit was maintained at 48 weeks in the rituximab groups. All rituximab regimens were generally safe and well tolerated. Most of the adverse events observed were due to first rituximab infusion reactions (36% vs 30% in the placebo group). This occurred less frequently during the second infusion (17% vs 15% in the placebo group). Total immunoglobulin levels were generally preserved and the incidence of human anti-chimeric antibodies (HACAs) was 4.3%.

Subsequently, a phase IIb (DANCER) study assessed whether a lower dose of rituximab in combination with methotrexate was just as effective and if corticosteroids were necessary in all treatment regimes.[9] The study design was complex with a 3 by 3 multifactorial design resulting in patients randomized to nine different treatment arms. The primary endpoint was the proportion of RA patients who had failed previous DMARD or biological therapy achieving an ACR 20 response rate. In the rituximab groups, patients were randomized to placebo versus 500 mg rituximab (two infusions, 2 weeks apart) vs 1000 mg rituximab (two infusions, 2 weeks apart). The corticosteroid groups were placebo vs 100 mg i.v methylprednisolone (days 1 and 15 before rituximab) vs 100 mg i.v methylprednisolone plus 60 mg oral prednisolone (days 2–7) and 30 mg oral prednisolone (days 8–14). A third of patients in the rituximab groups had failed previous anti-TNF-α therapy. At 24 weeks, patients treated with rituximab had significantly higher ACR 20, ACR 50, and ACR 70 responses compared with placebo groups (Figure 41.1). There was no difference in ACR response rates in the low and high dose rituximab groups except for a higher number of patients achieving ACR 70 in the high dose group, although this was not statistically significant. Corticosteroids did not contribute to clinical efficacy at 24 weeks but i.v corticos teroids reduced the incidence of first rituximab infusion events. Clinically significant infections were uncommon, although there were a few more observed in the high dose rituximab group (2%) compared with placebo (1%) and the low dose group (0%). Rituximab also showed prolonged efficacy at 48 weeks, with ACR 50 responses of 38% in the high dose rituximab, group, 42% in the low dose rituximab, and 20% in the placebo group.[10]

The FDA has now approved rituximab for RA in patients who have failed one or more anti-TNF-α agents. This decision was based in part on the phase III (REFLEX) study.[11] Patients were randomized to receive placebo or two infusions of 1000 mg rituximab (days 1 and 15) with 100 mg i.v. methylprednisolone and a short course of oral steroids between the two rituximab infusions. Rituximab showed ACR 20, ACR 50, and ACR 70 responses of 51%, 27%, and 12% compared with placebo of 18%, 5%, and 1%, respectively, at 24 weeks. Rituximab was well tolerated with serious adverse events occurring in 7% and 10% in the rituximab and placebo groups, respectively.

The REFLEX trial also showed that at week 56 there was a significant difference in mean change of total Sharp/Genant score (measuring radiographic changes) in the rituximab group compared with placebo, suggesting that rituximab can inhibit joint structural damage.[12] The current recommended dose of rituximab in RA is 1000 mg given as two infusions 2 weeks apart.

There are still many unanswered aspects of rituximab treatment in RA, including the role of re-treatment. Edwards and colleagues recently reported a 5-year follow-up on a cohort of 36 RA patients treated with up to 4 cycles of rituximab for persistent disease activity. The mean time to re-treatment was 18 months and each cycle was effective (maintaining ≥ ACR 20) for a mean period of 15 months. Re-treatment was well tolerated but total serum immunoglobulin levels fell below the normal range, particularly serum IgM.[13] Preliminary reports from additional open-label extension of the REFLEX and DANCER studies looking at re-treatment suggest that repeated cycles of rituximab produce

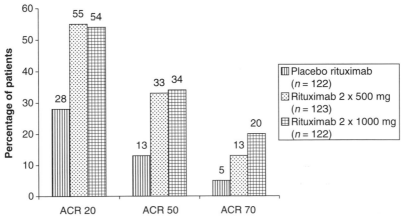

Figure 41.1 Patients who experienced responses according to American College of Rheumatology 20% (ACR 20), 50% (ACR 50), and 70% (ACR 70) improvement criteria at 24 weeks. ACR 20 and ACR 50 (placebo rituximab vs 2 × 500 mg rituximab vs 2 × 1000 mg rituximab, $p \leq 0.001$), ACR 70 (placebo rituximab vs 2 × 500 mg rituximab, $p = 0.029$; placebo vs 2 × 1000 mg rituximab, $p \leq 0.001$). Adapted from Arthritis Rheum 2006; 54: 1394, Emery P et al (with permission from Wiley).

an ACR response rate comparable to baseline, with no added toxicity.[14,15] Although the incidence of the HACA response related to rituximab appears to be relatively low in the RA population, its significance remains uncertain. As a result, the safety and efficacy of a humanized mAb against CD20 (Hu-Max CD20) in RA is being explored in a phase I/II controlled trial.

Systemic lupus erythematosus

The immunopathogenesis of SLE is complex but involves genetic, hormonal, and environmental factors leading to loss of B-cell tolerance, which is central to the development of the disease. B cells play a key role in the immunopathogenesis of SLE.[16] It is postulated that anti-dsDNA antibodies have pathogenic properties, especially in lupus nephritis.[17] However, murine SLE models have shown that B cells are critical to the development of the disease even if they are unable to secrete autoantibodies,[18] suggesting that the mechanisms involved are far more complex than

pathogenic autoantibody production. B cells also present autoantigens to T cells and initiate inflammatory responses through T cells and dendritic cells with the production of proinflammatory cytokines TNF-α, IL-12, IL-6, and interferon (IFN)-γ. This inflammatory response is further enhanced by T- and B-cell interaction via costimulatory molecules resulting in subsequent immune complex deposition and organ damage.

In addition to B-cell hyperactivity, numerous studies have found abnormalities in peripheral B-cell homeostasis in patients with active SLE. These include lymphopenia and expansion of certain B-cell subsets (CD27[high] plasma cells) in peripheral blood.[19] The frequency and number of CD27[high] plasma cells are found to be significantly correlated with SLE disease activity and anti-dsDNA antibody levels.[20] The concept of targeting B cells in SLE is thus a rational therapeutic strategy.

Rituximab has already shown great promise in the treatment of refractory SLE in a number of published uncontrolled observational studies (Figure 41.2 – target 1). Leandro and colleagues

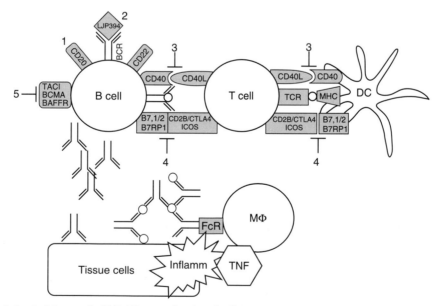

Figure 41.2 B-cell-directed therapy in SLE. (1) monoclonal antibodies against B-cell surface antigen CD20 and CD22. (2) B-cell tolerogen (e.g. LJP 394). (3) Inhibition of costimulatory molecule (e.g. CD40L mAb). (4) Inhibition of costimulatory molecule (e.g. CTLA-4-Ig). (5) Inhibition of B-cell survival (e.g. anti-BLyS or TACI-Ig). DC, dendritic cell; MΦ, macrophage; IL, interleukin; CTLA-4, cytotoxic T-lymphocyte antigen 4; Ig, immunoglobulin; mAb, monoclonal antibody; BLyS, B-lymphocyte stimulator protein; TACI, transmembrane activator and calcium modulating cyclophilin ligand interactor. Reprinted from Best Pract Res Clin Rheumatol, 19, Anolik JH, Aringer M, New treatments for SLE: cell-depleting and anti-cytokine therapies, page 861, copyright (2005), with permission from Elsevier.

published the first trial of six severely active SLE patients who had failed routine immunosuppressives including cyclophosphamide.[21] A combination protocol of two infusions of 500 mg rituximab plus 750 mg cyclophosphamide (given 2 weeks apart) and high dose oral corticosteroid course was used. All patients (except one who was lost to follow-up) had significant improvement with a decrease of mean British Isles Lupus Assessment Group (BILAG) scores from 14 to 6 at 6 months. There was particular benefit in lupus-related fatigue, arthritis/arthralgia, skin vasculitis, and serositis. The mean duration of B-cell depletion was 4.4 months with no significant adverse events noted. An extension of the original study involving 24 refractory SLE patients from the same group confirmed similar benefit using the same protocol but with a higher dose of 1 g rituximab.[22] There was corresponding serologic improvement with a decrease of anti-dsDNA antibodies and increase in serum C3 levels at 6 months. B-cell depletion was achieved by all patients except one. A significant advantage of this protocol is that all immunosuppressives were stopped in all but two patients. Thirteen patients remained well without the need for further immunosuppressives at mean follow-up of 23 months. Furthermore, the addition of cyclophosphamide may provide a higher level of B-cell depletion by directly inducing plasma cell death.

Ongoing long-term follow-up of up to 6 years in 30 patients with SLE treated with combination rituximab and cyclophosphamide at University College London (UCL) suggests that the treatment is relatively safe with infrequent treatment-related toxicity. Of the 30 patients, 2 of the 3 serious adverse events observed are thought to be related to rituximab. One patient developed pneumococcal septicemia 5 months after treatment, whilst B cells remained depleted, and another had a serum sickness-like reaction which resolved with i.v. steroids. A further patient died from complications related to severely active lupus 5 months after treatment with repopulation of B cells at 4 months (KP Ng, DA Isenberg, unpublished observations). Ten patients (seven previously reported[23]) in the UCL cohort have been re-treated with at least another cycle of rituximab on relapse of disease.

Clinical benefit was observed in at least half of the patients. Interestingly, the mean duration of benefit on subsequent cycle was longer than the initial cycle, suggesting additional benefit of re-treatment (13 months vs 7 months). The HACA response appears to be more frequent in lupus individuals compared with lymphoma or RA patients. One patient who developed HACAs on re-treatment was treated successfully with a humanized anti-CD20.[24]

These studies suggest that B-cell depletion is generally harder to achieve in the lupus population compared with RA patients. This may be due to complement dysfunction or different rituximab pharmacokinetics in lupus individuals. In one study, the extent of B-cell depletion was also found to be dependent on the FcγRIIIa genotype, suggesting the importance of ADCC and apoptosis in the mechanism of B-cell lysis.[25]

A phase I/II dose escalation trial of rituximab monotherapy in 18 patients with mild to moderate lupus activity (Systemic Lupus Activity Measure, SLAM > 5) was conducted by Looney and colleagues.[26] Patients who were previously on cyclophosphamide were excluded from the study. All other immunosuppressives were permitted as long as doses were stable for a month before study entry. Patients were allocated to low (100 mg/m^2), intermediate (375 mg/m^2), or high (4 weekly infusions of 375 mg/m^2) rituximab dose regimes. There was a significant improvement of SLAM global scores for up to 12 months in patients with profound B-cell depletion. Only half of these patients had raised anti-dsDNA antibody levels at the outset, making an analysis of the effect of B-cell depletion hard to judge. Six patients developed high titer HACA levels and this response was associated with African–American ancestry, reduced B-cell depletion, high disease activity, and lower doses of rituximab. Serum IgM decreased below the normal range in seven patients whilst IgG and IgA levels remained within the normal limits. Protective anti-tetanus and anti-pneumococcal IgG antibodies remained unchanged. Antibodies to ENA also show little change after B-cell depletion in most cases.[27] Besides clinical improvement, abnormalities of B-cell homeostasis and tolerance in SLE patients also improve after B-cell depletion.[28]

A study of Greek patients with active WHO class III/IV class lupus nephritis treated with a lymphoma dosing regime of 4 weekly rituximab infusions of 375 mg/m[2] demonstrated clinical benefit.[29] Although patient numbers were small, 5 of the 10 patients achieved complete remission defined as normal levels of serum creatinine and albumin, inactive urine sediment, and 24-hour urinary protein < 500 mg. Response was sustained in four patients at 12 months. Interestingly, the authors found down-regulation of expression of costimulatory CD40 ligand (CD40L) on T-helper cells preceding renal remission. This observation lends further support to the additional role of B cells in the mechanisms underlying immunopathogenesis of SLE. Anti-dsDNA antibody titers were decreased in all patients and treatment was well tolerated, with only one patient developing a hypersensitivity reaction which resolved with hydrocortisone. A recent study has shown histologic improvement on repeat renal biopsies of patients with severe lupus nephritis after combination rituximab and cyclophosphamide therapy.[30]

Anti-CD22

Systemic lupus erythematosus

CD22 is a B-cell-specific transmembrane protein of the IgG superfamily that is associated with B-cell receptor signaling and B-cell homing. It is expressed from the late pro-B cell stage until the differentiation of plasma cell phase (Figure 41.2 – target 1). The outcome of an open-label study of an anti-CD22 mAb (epratuzumab) in 14 moderately active SLE patients was recently reported.[31] All patients improved with a decrease in total BILAG scores of ≥ 50% at some point during the 6-month study. No significant change in autoantibody levels was noted and the drug was well tolerated. Moderate B-cell depletion was observed and this may be partially related to the agonist activity of CD22, which contains an immunoreceptor tyrosine-based inhibitory motif.[32] Two phase III clinical trials of epratuzumab in active SLE are currently in progress.

Inhibiting B-cell survival

The survival and maturation of B cells requires the presence of survival and trophic factors like vascular cell adhesion molecule-1 (VCAM-1) and B-cell-activating factor (BAFF), also known as B-lymphocyte stimulator protein (BLyS). BLyS is a member of the TNF superfamily of cytokines. It binds to three receptors, transmembrane activator and calcium modulating cyclophilin ligand interactor (TACI), BAFF-receptor (BAFFR), also called BR3 (BLyS receptor 3) and B-cell maturation protein (BCMA) to form a complex with multiple mode of actions.[33] These actions include differentiation and activation of B cells leading to autoreactivity from antibody production, rescuing B cells from death and inducing a costimulatory response in T cells.[34] A second growth factor with B-cell-stimulating properties, APRIL (A proliferation-inducing ligand) has also been identified.[35] APRIL binds BCMA and TACI receptors but not to BAFFR. Animal models have demonstrated that dysregulation of BAFF expression can lead to autoimmunity.[36] Furthermore, peripheral blood serum BLyS is high and correlated positively with anti-dsDNA antibody in patients with SLE and RF antibodies in patients with RA.[37] Thus, the inhibition of B-cell survival factors BAFF/BLyS is another novel way to deplete B cells. Other targets available include fusion proteins with a BAFF receptor, TACI-Ig (atacicept) or BAFF-receptor 3 (BR3). Circulating levels of BLyS are found to be markedly elevated after B-cell depletion with rituximab in patients with RA. The repopulation of peripheral B cells was associated with a decline in BLyS levels, just before clinical relapse.[38] This observation suggests that combining B-cell survival inhibitor agents and anti-CD20 mAb therapy may act synergistically to achieve a longer duration of clinical remission.

Rheumatoid arthritis

Belimumab/lymphostat-B is a human mAb directed against BLyS. Results of a phase II study with this agent in 283 RA patients demonstrated a modest effect with an ACR 20 response rate of 29% compared with 16% in the placebo group (p = 0.02).[39] No significant adverse events were reported and there was moderate

B-cell depletion with a significant reduction of RF titers.

The pharmacokinetic profile of TACI-Ig was investigated in an initial phase Ib trial of moderate to severe RA patients. The frequency and severity of adverse events were comparable to the placebo group and interestingly, the drug was also found to be present in inflamed joints.[40]

Systemic lupus erythematosus

A phase I dose escalation trial of belimumab in 57 stable SLE patients showed a significant reduction of peripheral B cells but no effect on disease activity[41] (Figure 41.2 – target 5). Outcome from the phase II trial of belimumab in 449 patients with SLE was recently presented.[42] Although there was only a significant improvement of lupus activity measured using the SELENA-SLE Disease Activity Index (SLEDAI) score in serologically active (HEp ANA > 1:80 and/or anti-dsDNA $\geq$ 30 IU) patients, B-cell depletion and improvement of immunological parameters were achieved in most patients at 52 weeks with no notable side effects. However, this study was unusual with > 20% of the patients said to have SLE being ANA-negative. The further evaluation of this drug in a phase III trial is currently planned. A phase Ib trial of TACI-Ig in SLE patients is under way and due to complete soon (Figure 41.2 – target 5).

INHIBITION OF COSTIMULATORY MOLECULES

Abatacept (Orencia)

Rheumatoid arthritis

As discussed, targeting T cells can be a potentially novel strategy for the treatment of RA. This approach has been evaluated in the past with targeting sites like the T-cell surface antigenic determinants (CD4, CD5), T-cell receptors, modulating CD4$^+$ T-cell function via CD4$^+$ mAb and antagonizing the major histocompatibility complex (MHC).[43] Unfortunately, none of these approaches has been very successful.

Another novel method to target T cells is by inhibiting costimulatory molecules. The activation of T cells requires two signaling mechanisms.

The first signal is antigen-specific with the binding of a major histocompatibility peptide–antigen complex to a T-cell receptor. The second costimulatory signal binds an APC surface ligand to a surface protein on the T cell. One of the major costimulatory signals is the interaction of CD28 on T cells with CD80/CD86 on APC. Cytotoxic T-lymphocyte-associated antigen 4 (CTLA-4) is expressed on activated T cells and competes with CD28 for binding to CD80/CD86, generating a negative signal to T cells. The importance of activating CD28 has been highlighted recently in a tragic trial at Northwick Park Hospital in London. Six healthy volunteers given a stimulating CD28 mAb experienced a 'cytokine release' storm leading to severe headaches and later, profound vasoconstriction.

Abatacept (CTLA-4-Ig) is a fusion protein consisting of the external domain human CTLA-4 receptor protein and the Fc domain of human IgG1. It binds to the CD80/CD86 ligand on APCs, which prevents the costimulatory binding of CD28 on T cells. As a consequence, there is down-regulation of T-cell activity resulting in decreased proinflammatory cytokine production and subsequent reduction of B-cell autoantibody production.

Kremer and colleagues conducted a phase II study of 339 active RA patients despite methotrexate, assigned to receive placebo or abatacept 2 mg/kg or abatacept 10 mg/kg plus methotrexate.[44] The optimal dose of abatacept was 10 mg/kg with significantly higher ACR 20, ACR 50, and ACR 70 response rates of 60%, 36.5%, and 16.5% compared with placebo 35.3%, 11.8%, and 1.7%, respectively, at 6 months. CTLA-4-Ig was well tolerated with no deaths. Clinical benefit was sustained for up to 1 year with corresponding improvement in the modified Health Assessment Questionnaire (HAQ) scores in patients treated with 10 mg/kg abatacept.[45] To confirm the phase II study findings, a phase III 1-year Abatacept in Inadequate Responders to Methotrexate (AIM) study was performed.[46] At 1 year, the group receiving abatacept 10 mg/kg had a significantly higher ACR 20, ACR 50, and ACR 70 response rate than the placebo group (73.1%, 48.3%, 28.8% versus 39.7%, 18.2%, 6.1%, respectively). In addition, patients treated with abatacept had a significant slowing of radiographic progression (approximately 50% reduction in change of Genant-modified Sharp scores from baseline) compared with placebo. Improvement of structural joint damage was also sustained at 2 years.[47]

A large phase III randomized placebo-controlled abatacept trial in treatment of anti-TNF-α inadequate responders (ATTAIN) established that abatacept is also efficacious in RA patients who have failed anti-TNF-α therapy.[48] In December 2005, the FDA approved abatacept for use in RA patients who had failed methotrexate or anti-TNF-α antagonists based on the findings of the AIM and ATTAIN trials.

Patients recruited in the ATTAIN trial consisted of current and previous users of anti-TNF-α therapy (washout period of 28 days for etanercept and 60 days for infliximab). No patients had prior adalimunab. Patients continued their stable dose of traditional DMARD or anakinra throughout the trial. The majority of patients were on methotrexate. At 6 months, there was a higher proportion of patients achieving ACR 20 (50.4% vs 19.5%, $p < 0.001$), ACR 50 (20.3% vs 3.8%, $p < 0.001$), and ACR 70 (10.2% vs 1.5%, $p = 0.003$) responses compared with placebo. Although acute infusion reactions were more frequent in the abatacept group, the reactions were mild to moderate intensity and rates of serious adverse events were similar in both groups. Abatacept was administered intravenously over 30 minutes. After the initial infusion, another dose was given 2 weeks and 4 weeks later followed by monthly infusions thereafter.

The ASSURE (Safety and Patient-reported Outcomes Associated with Abatacept in the Treatment of Rheumatoid Arthritis Patients Receiving Background DMARDs) trial was designed to assess the safety of abatacept in combination with traditional DMARDs and other biologics.[49] Patients were randomized to monthly infusion of abatacept 10 mg/kg or placebo for 1 year. Of the 1441 patients recruited in the study, the majority were on combination treatment with non-biologic agents. Only 103 patients were in the abatacept/biologic group compared with the abatacept/non-biologic ($n = 856$), placebo/non-biologic ($n = 418$), and placebo/biologic ($n = 64$) groups. There was a higher frequency of infections in the abatacept/biologic group compared with the other three groups (19.4% vs 6.3–8.8%). This suggests that combination treatment with two biologic therapies of different mode of actions is not advisable. In addition, there were more neoplasms observed in the abatacept/biologic group (6.8% vs 1.6–3.8%). It is important to note that patient numbers in each group were relatively small and a direct association with malignancy is difficult to ascertain.

Systemic lupus erythematosus

In the NZB/NZW mouse model, production of autoantibody was blocked with prolongation of life when mice were treated with murine CTLA-4-Ig.[50] A number of studies have looked at the therapeutic effects of CTLA-4-Ig in lupus-prone mice with nephritis. One study found that combination CTLA4-Ig and cyclophosphamide was needed to treat mice with late stage renal disease.[51] In another study, CTLA-4-Ig monotherapy was beneficial in lupus mouse models with renal disease but combined treatment with cyclophosphamide was more effective.[52] A phase IIb controlled study looking at the potential of CTLA-4 in treating acute flares in patients with SLE has started (Figure 41.2 – target 4). The safety and efficacy of another costimulatory agent, RG2077, in SLE patients treated with cyclophosphamide is currently being assessed in a phase I/II clinical trial.

Anti-CD40L

Systemic lupus erythematosus

The interaction of costimulatory molecule CD40L and CD40 has been studied as another immune pathway to target (Figure 41.2 – target 3). CD40L, expressed on activated T cells, binds avidly to CD40 on B cells facilitating B-cell autoantibody production. Unfortunately, encouraging results from the blockade of CD40L/CD40 in animal studies have not translated to human studies. The two humanized anti-CD40L mAbs involved in therapeutic trials are BG9588 and IDEC-131. IDEC-131 targets a different epitope to BG9588. Although a phase I trial of IDEC-131 was safe and well tolerated in patients with SLE,[53] it was no better compared to placebo in the treatment of active lupus in a phase II controlled trial.[54] Another phase II trial of BG9588 in lupus nephritis was halted because of increased incidence of thromboembolic events in treated subjects.[55]

IMMUNOABLATION

Systemic lupus erythematosus

Immunoablation with or without hematopoietic stem cell transplant (HSCT) has been used in patients with severe refractory lupus who have failed conventional immunosuppressive treatment. This concept, derived from hematologists, aims to 'reset' the immune system by ablating abnormal cells with high dose chemotherapy followed by repopulation of healthy hematopoietic stem cells. This non-specific method of cellular depletion can be associated with significant morbidity and mortality.

A retrospective review from the European Blood and Marrow Registry identified 53 patients with SLE treated with autologous HSCT using a conditioning regime of cyclophosphamide, anti-thymocyte globulin, or lymphoid irradiation.[56] Remission (SLEDAI < 3) was achieved in 66% of patients at 6 months. However, relapse rate was high, with 32% of patients relapsing after 6 months. Treatment-related mortality was high at 12%.

The results of a study involving 48 severe lupus subjects with life-threatening organ involvement treated with autologous non-myeloablative HSCT were recently published.[57] Mortality rate was 4% with two deaths, one from a fungal infection and the other from active lupus after a delayed period to transplant. At follow-up of 29 months, there was improvement of disease activity and lupus serological profile, and stabilization of organ dysfunction.

Petri and colleagues used immunoablation without HSCT in 14 SLE patients based on the rationale that autoreactive effector cells may be reinfused with HSCT.[58] Patients were treated with 50 mg/kg cyclophosphamide for 4 days followed by granulocyte colony stimulating factor (G-CSF). All patients improved, with no deaths

or fungal infection observed. Another group also confirmed similar benefit and safety using immunoablation without HSCT in four SLE patients.[59] At present, immunoblation should be reserved for severe refractory SLE patients with life-threatening organ dysfunction.

Rheumatoid arthritis

Since 1996, most published reports on the use of autologous HSCT in RA have been individual cases or case series. Clinical benefit is often modest and short-lived, with most patients relapsing after 6 months.[60] This treatment may also have a favorable effect on the rate of radiographic joint damage.[61] An analysis of 76 severe RA patients from the European bone marrow and transplant registry showed an ACR 50 response rate of 67% at 12 months.[62] The majority of these patients had a high dose treatment regime of cyclophosphamide 200 mg/kg with autologous HSCT. There was one death related to sepsis but most patients relapsed, with 74% of patients needing to restart a DMARD after 1 year post HSCT. Recently, with the advent of new technology, new conditioning regimes have been used to lower the incidence of acute graft versus host disease, resulting in microchimerism.[63] The first non-myeloablative allogeneic HSCT was performed in a patient with severe refractory RA on this background.[64] Results were encouraging, with remission of disease 1 year post HSCT without further requirement of immunosuppressive drugs. A phase 1 trial looking at induction of tolerance with mixed microchimerism from allogeneic HSCT in RA is currently recruiting.

TOLERIZING T CELLS

Edratide

Systemic lupus erythematosus

Edratide (TV-4710) is a synthetic peptide which has been developed to modulate the immune system by tolerizing T cells. The peptide has 19 amino acid residues based on the complementarity determining region 1 (CDR 1) of a pathogenic human anti-DNA mAb bearing the 16/6 idiotype (Id).[65] Edratide has demonstrated its ability to down-regulate autoreactive T-cell responses of peripheral blood lymphocytes in SLE patients.[66] Two placebo-controlled phase 1 trials of edratide in patients with SLE were completed in 2004. A phase II trial is in progress.

TOLERIZING B CELLS

LJP 394

Systemic lupus erythematosus

LJP 394 (abetimus sodium) is a conjugate tetravalent oligonucleotide attached to an inert polyethylene glycol platform. It acts as a B-cell tolerizing agent by binding to anti-dsDNA receptors and modulates B-cell responses to induce anergy or apoptosis[67] (Figure 41.2 – target 2). It has been used to treat patients with lupus nephritis since the 1990s. LJP 394 has been shown to reduce anti-dsDNA antibody titers in lupus subjects.[68] A phase II/III trial was conducted in 230 lupus subjects with a past history of nephritis to investigate if this compound could prevent future renal flares.[69] The study was stopped prematurely because no difference in time to renal flare and number of flares between the abetimus and placebo groups was found. However, a sub-analysis showed that patients with high affinity antibodies to abetimus had a longer time to renal flare, experienced fewer flares, and restarted cyclophosphamide much later compared with the placebo group. Serious adverse events were comparable for both groups. In addition, patients in the treated group showed a significant improvement of health-related quality of life measured by the SF-36.[70] A subsequent randomized placebo-controlled phase III trial of 298 high affinity lupus patients did not confirm the phase II/III study findings, with 12% and 16% of patients flaring in the high affinity group and placebo group, respectively.[71] However, patients treated with LJP 394 had a statistically significant decrease of greater than 50% 24-hour urinary protein compared with placebo when the two studies were analyzed (44% LJP 394 group vs 18% placebo group – phase II/III study, $p = 0.002$ and 41% LJP 394 group vs 28% placebo group – phase III study, $p = 0.047$).[72] Because of these contradictory results, another phase III controlled trial is in progress.

ANTI-CYTOKINE THERAPIES

Anti-TNF-α

Rheumatoid arthritis

The use of anti-TNF-α agents is well established in the management of RA. The three anti-TNF-α agents approved for use in RA are infliximab, etanercept, and adalimumab. Several randomized controlled trials have confirmed the significant clinical efficacy of these three agents in combination with methotrexate or monotherapy in achieving remission for patients with early and long-standing RA.[73–75] In addition, anti-TNF-α therapy can slow progression of radiographic structural joint damage. Whilst it is clear that patients treated with anti-TNF-α agents are at risk of infections,[76] long-term complications are still unknown. The British Society of Rheumatology's Biologics Register is nearing full recruitment of 4000 patients each on these three drugs. The analysis of infections and other complications (including cancer rates) in these 12 000 patients compared to 4000 controls (with active RA but not on any of the TNF-α blockers) over a 5-year period should provide definitive answers as to how effective and safe these drugs are. The use of pegylated anti-TNF-α agents (certolizumab pegol [CDP-870] and CNTO 148) is currently being investigated.

Systemic lupus erythematosus

The role of anti-TNF-α therapy in lupus is yet to be determined. The mixed results from experimental mouse models have pointed towards a somewhat unclear role of TNF-α in the pathogenesis of SLE.[77] Furthermore, the development of ANAs has been observed amongst patients receiving anti-TNF-α therapy, although the incidence of clinical lupus is rare.[78] Aringer and colleagues controversially treated six lupus patients with arthritis and nephritis of low to moderate disease activity on a background of low dose corticosteroids and azathioprine or methotrexate with infliximab[79] (Figure 41.3 – target 6). Patients received four infusions of 300 mg infliximab (~ 5 mg/kg) on day 0, and week 2, 6, and 10. All patients completed the study at 52 weeks and no infusion reactions were noted. There was a significant reduction of proteinuria in all four patients with lupus nephritis and benefit was sustained for more than 6 months after the last infusion. Three patients with arthritis only had short-lived benefit and one of these patients was treated on relapse with another infusion of infliximab at week 20. Half of the patients had urinary tract infections, highlighting the risk of infections with anti-TNF-α therapy. Not surprisingly, two-thirds of the patients had transient elevated anti-dsDNA antibodies after the infusions but without any increase in disease activity. More studies are needed before anti-TNF-α therapy can be recommended for patients with SLE.

IL-6

Rheumatoid arthritis

IL-6 is a pleiotropic cytokine with proinflammatory and anti-inflammatory properties. It is produced by a variety of cells including fibroblasts, synoviocytes, lymphocytes, monocytes, and endothelial cells. In addition, it aids the production of autoantibodies by stimulating B cells. IL-6 is a key proinflammatory cytokine in the pathogenesis of RA. Levels of IL-6 are higher in the serum and synovial fluid of patients with RA compared with controls and correlated with disease activity.[80]

An open-label study of murine anti IL-6 mAb in five RA patients showed encouraging results, although benefit was short-lived.[81] IL-6 may also be targeted via blocking its receptor IL-6R. MRA (tocilizumab) is a humanized mAb that blocks the IL-6R. In a phase I/II placebo-controlled randomized study of 45 active RA patients who failed at least one DMARD, a single dose of 5 mg/kg MRA produced a significantly higher ACR 20 response rate of 55.6% compared with placebo at 2 weeks.[82] Clinical benefit was maintained at 8 weeks. Inflammatory markers were normalized

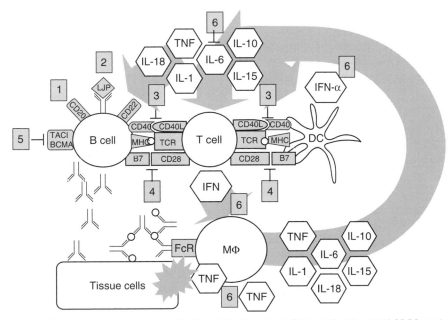

Figure 41.3 Overview of targeted therapies in SLE. (1) Antibodies to surface molecules (anti-CD20 and anti-CD22 mAb). (2) B-cell tolerogen (LJP 394). (3) Inhibition costimulatory molecule (CD40L). (4) Inhibition costimulatory molecule (CTLA-4-Ig). (5) Inhibition B-cell-directed cytokines. (6) Inhibition proinflammatory/immunoregulatory cytokines derived from monocytes/macrophages (MΦ), dendritic cells (DC) such as TNF, IL-6, IL-10, IL-15, IL-18. IL, interleukin; CTLA-4, cytotoxic T-lymphocyte antigen 4; Ig, immunoglobulin; mAb, monoclonal antibody; TNF, tumor necrosis factor; IFN, interferon. Reprinted from Best Pract Res Clin Rheumatol, 19, Anolik JH, Aringer M, New treatments for SLE: cell-depleting and anti-cytokine therapies, page 866, copyright (2005) with permission from Elsevier.

and diarrhea was the most common side effect reported (8% of patients).

Another phase II trial confirmed similar benefit and optimal efficacy with a 4 weekly infusions MRA dose of 8 mg/kg in combination with methotrexate.[83] This dose benefit was confirmed in a 3-month study of 164 RA patients randomized to receive MRA 8 mg/kg, 4 mg/kg, or placebo administered every 4 weeks.[84] The ACR 20 responses were 78%, 57%, and 11% in the respective groups, indicating a dose-dependent response. The ACR 50 and ACR 70 responses were also significantly better than placebo in the 8 mg/kg group. Five serious adverse events were observed, with three in the MRA groups and the remaining two in the placebo group. One patient died from Epstein–Barr virus infection and hemophagocytosis syndrome 61 days after receiving a single dose of 8 mg/kg MRA. Of concern, 44% of patients in the MRA groups had an elevated cholesterol level. Although the authors commented that no cardiovascular complications were observed, the duration of this study was too short to determine this. The results of a recent phase III trial of 125 RA patients on low dose methotrexate treated with 8 mg/kg MRA were recently presented.[85] At 24 weeks, ACR 20 responses were higher in the MRA group compared with placebo (80.3% vs 25%, $p < 0.001$). Lipid levels were also elevated but stabilized at upper limit of normal in the MRA group. Long-term trials are needed to establish the significance of this aspect, RA patients are already at increased risk of developing cardiovascular events.[86].

Systemic lupus erythematosus

Evidence from animal models and SLE patients suggest that IL-6 may play a role in the pathogenesis of SLE. Anti-dsDNA antibodies can promote expression of IL-6 in animal models.[87] Lupus-prone mice injected with an anti-IL6 mAb resulted in decreased renal proteinuria and anti-dsDNA antibody production.[88] High serum IL-6 levels are present in patients with SLE and found to be associated with active disease activity in the hematological organ system but not other organ systems using the BILAG activity index.[89] The outcome of a phase I

open-label trial of MRA in SLE is awaited (Figure 41.3 – target 6).

IL-1

Rheumatoid arthritis

IL-1 is a proinflammatory cytokine that is believed to play an important role in the pathogenesis of RA. Anakinra is a recombinant human IL-1 receptor antagonist that is approved in Europe and United States for use in RA. Anakinra is efficacious as monotherapy and when combined with methotrexate in treating active RA.[90] It is capable of slowing radiographic progression.[91] Although there are no head to head trials comparing these agents, its effects are perceived to be modest when compared to the commercially available anti-TNF-α agents. A higher incidence of infections was observed with combination anakinra and anti-TNF-α therapy,[92] highlighting the concern of combination biologic therapy. Unfortunately, anakinra has not been shown to be effective in patients who have failed anti-TNF-α therapy.[93] The outcome of a study with a high affinity IL-1 receptor antagonist (IL-1 TRAP) was also disappointing.[94]

IL-10

Systemic lupus erythematosus

Targeting IL-10 has been explored as a therapeutic agent for patients with SLE (Figure 41.3 – target 6). Serum IL-10 is elevated and correlated with disease activity in lupus subjects.[95] A murine IgG1 anti-IL-10 mAb demonstrated reduction of disease activity in an open-label study.[96] Treatment was well tolerated. Phase I trials are anticipated with a human anti-IL-10 mAb.

COMPLEMENT BLOCKADE

Rheumatoid arthritis and systemic lupus erythematosus

The complement system plays an important role in the pathogenesis of SLE. Patients with SLE have decreased levels of circulating complement related to systemic consumption. In the MRL/lpr murine SLE model, development of experimental lupus can be blocked with a mAb to C5.[97] The immunomodulatory effect of a humanized C5 mAb (eculizumab) is currently being investigated in phase I and II trials of patients with SLE and RA.

CONCLUSION

The next few years will be an exciting time in the treatment of patients with RA and SLE. It is realistic to anticipate that some of the novel therapeutic agents reviewed here will be translated to effective treatments and add to the growing number of biological therapies available. Research into newer pharmacological agents in RA and SLE is ongoing (Tables 41.1 and 41.2).

Future challenges include tailoring therapy for the individual patient with minimal side effects and developing cheaper novel therapies using the advances in biotechnology. It is also important to ascertain if these new therapies will improve morbidity and mortality. The design of future clinical trials will need to explore the efficacy of combination biological therapies and comparative trials between the various drugs. Although the ultimate goal of cure in RA and SLE seems unrealistic at present, it is hoped that achieving remission is a realistic goal with improved understanding of pathogenic pathways and availability of new and better treatments.

ACKNOWLEDGMENTS

Dr Kristine Ng is a recipient of the New Zealand Rose Hellaby Medical Scholarship.

Table 41.1 New targeted therapies for rheumatoid arthritis

Class of therapy	Agent	Mechanism of action/target	Clinical stage
Cytokines			
TNF inhibitors	Certolizumab pegol (CDP-870)	Human anti-TNF-α antibody fragment	Phase III
	Golimumab (CNTO 148)	Human anti-TNF-α antibody	Phase III
	Pegsunercept	PEGylated soluble TNF receptor type 1	Phase II
	ISIS 104838	TNF-α antisense oligonucleotide	Phase II
Interleukin-based therapies	HuMax-IL-15	IL-15 mAb	Phase II
	ABT-874	IL-12 mAb	Phase II
	IL-18bp (Tadekinig-α)	Recombinant IL-18 binding protein	Phase II
	MRA (tocilizumab)	IL-6 mAb	Phase III
Interferon cytokines	Fontolizumab	IFN-γ mAb	Phase II
B-cell depletion	Rituximab	Anti-CD20 chimeric mAb	FDA approved
	Hu-Max CD20	Anti-CD20 humanized mAb	Phase II
	Belimumab	Anti-BLyS mAb	Phase II
	TACI-Ig (atacicept)	BAFF receptor	Phase Ib
Costimulatory molecules	Abatacept	CTLA-4-Ig fusion protein	FDA approved
Complement	Eculizumab	C5 mAb	Phase II
Bone remodeling	Zoledronic acid	Bisphosphonate	Phase II
	AMG 162	RANKL mAb	Phase II
Small molecules	SB-681323	p38 MAPK inhibitor	Phase II
	p38 inh (4)	p38 MAPK inhibitor	Phase II
	TASKI-1	Syk kinase inhibitor	Phase II
Allogeneic HSCT			Phase I

TNF, tumor necrosis factor; MAPK, mitogen-activated protein kinase; MAb, monoclonal antibody; IL, interleukin; HSCT, hematopoietic stem cell transplant; RANKL, receptor activator of NF-κB ligand; Syk, spleen tyrosine kinase; CTLA, cytotoxic T-lymphocyte antigen 4; BAFF, B-cell-activating factor; Ig, immunoglobulin.

Table 41.2 New targeted therapies for systemic lupus erythematosus

Class of therapy	Agent	Mechanism of action/ target	Clinical stage
Cytokines			
Interleukin-based therapies	MRA (tocilizumab)	IL-6 mAb	Phase I
		IL-10 mAb	Phase I
Interferon cytokines	MEDI-545	IFN-α	Phase I
B-cell-depletion	Rituximab	Anti-CD20 mAb	Phase II/III
	Epratuzumab	Anti-CD22 mAb	Phase III
	Belimumab	Anti-BLyS mAb	Phase II (completed)
	TACI-Ig	TACI receptor fusion protein	Phase 1b
Costimulatory molecules	Abatacept	CTLA-4-Ig	Phase IIb
	RG2077	CTLA-4-IgG4m	Phase I/II
	Alemtuzumab	CD52 humanized mAb	Phase I
Antigen-targeted therapies	Edratide (TV4710)	T-cell tolerogen	Phase II
	Abetimus sodium (LJP 394)	B-cell tolerogen	Phase III
	Recombinant human DNase	Degradation of DNA	Phase I
Complement	Eculizumab	C5 mAb	Phase II
Allogeneic HSCT			Phase I
Autologous HSCT			Phase II

mAb, monoclonal antibody; IL, interleukin; HSCT, Hematopoietic stem cell transplant; CTLA, cytotoxic T-lymphocyte antigen 4; TACI, transmembrane activator and calcium modulating cyclophilin ligand interactor; IFN, interferon, BLyS, B-lymphocyte stimulator protein; DNA, deoxyribonucleic acid, Ig, immunoglobulin.

REFERENCES

1. Van Boxel JA, Paget SA. Predominantly T-cell infiltrate in rheumatoid synovial membranes. N Engl J Med 1975; 293: 517–20.

2. Edwards JC, Cambridge G, Abrahams VM. Do self-perpetuating B lymphocytes drive human autoimmune disease? Immunology 1999; 97: 188–96.

3. Takemura S, Klimiuk PA, Braun A et al. T cell activation in rheumatoid synovium is B cell dependent. J Immunol 2001; 167: 4710–18.

4. Edwards JC, Cambridge G, Leandro MJ. B cell depletion in rheumatic disease. Best Pract Res Clin Rheumatol 2006; 20: 915–28.

5. Gong Q, Ou Q, Ye S et al. Importance of cellular microenvironment and circulatory dynamics in B cell immunotherapy. J Immunol 2005; 174: 817–26.

6. Edwards JC, Cambridge G. Sustained improvement in rheumatoid arthritis following a protocol designed to deplete B lymphocytes. Rheumatology (Oxford) 2001; 40: 205–11.

7. Leandro MJ, Edwards JC, Cambridge G. Clinical outcome in 22 patients with rheumatoid arthritis treated with B lymphocyte depletion. Ann Rheum Dis 2002; 61: 883–8.

8. Edwards JC, Szczepanski L, Szechinski J et al. Efficacy of B-cell-targeted therapy with rituximab in patients with rheumatoid arthritis. N Engl J Med 2004; 350: 2572–81.

9. Emery P, Fleischmann R, Filipowicz-Sosnowska A et al. The efficacy and safety of rituximab in patients with active rheumatoid arthritis despite methotrexate treatment: results of a phase IIB randomized, double-blind, placebo-controlled, dose-ranging trial. Arthritis Rheum 2006; 54: 1390–400.

10. Emery P, Fleischmann R, Martin-Mola E et al. Prolonged efficacy of rituximab in rheumatoid arthritis patients with an inadequate response to methotrexate: 1 year follow up of a subset of patients receiving a single course in a controlled trial (DANCER trial). Ann Rheum Dis 2006; 65: 190.

11. Cohen S, Greenwald M, Dougados MR et al. Efficacy and safety of rituximab in active rheumatoid arthritis patients who experienced an inadequate response to one or more anti-TNFα therapies (REFLEX). Arthritis Rheum 2005; 52: S677.

12. Keystone E, Emery P, Peterfy CG et al. Prevention of joint structural damage at 1 year with rituximab in rheumatoid arthritis patients with an inadequate response to one or more TNF inhibitors (REFLEX study). Ann Rheum Dis 2006; 65: 58.

13. Edwards JC, Leandro MJ, Cambridge G. Repeated B lymphocyte depletion therapy in rheumatoid arthritis: 5 year follow-up. Arthritis Rheum 2005; 52: S133.

14. Keystone E, Fleischmann R, Emery P et al. Long term efficacy and safety of a repeat treatment course of rituximab in rheumatoid arthritis patients with an inadequate response to one or more TNF inhibitors. Ann Rheum Dis 2006; 65: 323.

15. Van Vollenhoven RF, Cohen S, Pavelka K et al. Response to rituximab in patients with rheumatoid arthritis is maintained by repeat therapy: results of an open label trial. Ann Rheum Dis 2006; 65: 510.

16. Chan OT, Madaio MP, Shlomchik MJ. The central and multiple roles of B cells in lupus pathogenesis. Immunol Rev 1999; 169: 107–21.

17. Okamura M, Kanayama Y, Amastu K et al. Significance of enzyme linked immunosorbent assay (ELISA) for antibodies to double stranded and single stranded DNA in patients with lupus nephritis: correlation with severity of renal histology. Ann Rheum Dis 1993; 52: 14–20.

18. Chan OT, Hannum LG, Haberman AM. A novel mouse with B cells but lacking serum antibody reveals an antibody-independent role for B cells in murine lupus. J Exp Med 1999; 189: 1639–48.

19. Odendahl M, Jacobi A, Hansen A et al. Disturbed peripheral B lymphocyte homeostasis in systemic lupus erythematosus. J Immunol 2000; 165: 5970–9.

20. Jacobi AM, Odendahl M, Reiter K et al. Correlation between circulating CD27high plasma cells and disease activity in patients with systemic lupus erythematosus. Arthritis Rheum 2003; 48: 1332–42.

21. Leandro MJ, Edwards JC, Cambridge G et al. An open study of B lymphocyte depletion in systemic lupus erythematosus. Arthritis Rheum 2002; 46: 2673–7.

22. Leandro MJ, Cambridge G, Edwards JC et al. B-cell depletion in the treatment of patients with systemic lupus erythematosus: a longitudinal analysis of 24 patients. Rheumatology (Oxford) 2005; 44: 1542–5.

23. Ng KP, Leandro MJ, Edwards JC et al. Repeated B cell depletion in treatment of refractory systemic lupus erythematosus. Ann Rheum Dis 2006; 65: 942–5.

24. Tahir H, Rohrer J, Bhatia A et al. Humanized anti-CD20 monoclonal antibody in the treatment of severe resistant systemic lupus erythematosus in a patient with antibodies against rituximab. Rheumatology (Oxford) 2005; 44: 561–2.

25. Anolik JH, Campbell D, Felgar RE et al. The relationship of FcgammaRIIIa genotype to degree of B cell depletion by rituximab in the treatment of systemic lupus erythematosus. Arthritis Rheum 2003: 48: 455–9.

26. Looney RJ, Anolik JH, Campbell D et al. B cell depletion as a novel treatment for systemic lupus erythematosus: a phase I/II dose-escalation trial of rituximab. Arthritis Rheum 2004; 50: 2580–9.

27. Cambridge G, Leandro M, Teodorescu M et al. B cell depletion therapy in systemic lupus erythematosus: effect on autoantibody and antimicrobial antibody profiles. Arthritis Rheum 2006; 54: 3612–22.

28. Anolik JH, Barnard J, Cappione A et al. Rituximab improves peripheral B cell abnormalities in human systemic lupus erythematosus. Arthritis Rheum 2004; 50: 3580–90.

29. Sfikakis PP, Boletis JN, Lionaki S et al. Remission of proliferative lupus nephritis following B cell depletion therapy is preceded by down-regulation of the T cell costimulatory molecule CD40 ligand: an open-label trial. Arthritis Rheum 2005; 52: 501–13.

30. Gunnarsson I, Sundelin B, Jonsdottir T et al. Histopathological and clinical changes in patients with severe lupus nephritis treated with rituximab plus cyclophosphamide: a rebiopsy in 7 patients. Ann Rheum Dis 2006; 65: 64.

31. Dorner T, Kaufmann J, Wegener WA et al. Initial clinical trial of epratuzumab (humanized anti-CD22 antibody) for immunotherapy of systemic lupus erythematosus. Arthritis Res Ther 2006; 8: R74.

32. Otipoby KL, Draves KE, Clark EA. CD22 regulates B cell receptor-mediated signals via two domains that independently recruit Grb2 and SHP-1. J Biol Chem 2001; 276: 44315–22.

33. Thompson JS, Bixler SA, Qian F et al. BAFF-R, a novel TNF receptor that specifically interacts with BAFF. Science 2001; 293: 2108–11.

34. Huard B, Schneider P, Mauri D et al. T cell costimulation by the TNF ligand BAFF. J Immunol 2001; 167: 6225–31.

35. Roschke V, Sosnovtseva S, Ward CD et al. BLyS and APRIL form biologically active heterotrimers that are expressed in patients with systemic immune-based rheumatic diseases. J Immunol 2002; 169: 4314–21.

36. Mackay F, Woodcock SA, Lawton P et al Mice transgenic for BAFF develop lymphocytic disorders along with autoimmune manifestations. J Exp Med 1999; 190: 1697–71.

37. Cheema GS, Roschke V, Hilbert DM. Elevated serum B lymphocyte stimulator levels in patients with systemic immune-based rheumatic diseases. Arthritis Rheum 2001; 44: 1313–19.

38. Cambridge G, Stohl W, Leandro M et al. Circulating levels of B lymphocyte stimulator in patients with rheumatoid arthritis following rituximab treatment. Arthritis Rheum 2006; 54: 723–32.

39. McKay J, Chwalinska-Sadowska H, Boling E et al. Belimumab, a fully human monoclonal antibody to BLyS, combined with standard of care therapy reduces the signs and symptoms of rheumatoid arthritis in a heterogenous subject population. Arthritis Rheum 2005; 52: S710.

40. Munafo A, Rossier C, Peter N et al. TACI-Ig in patients with RA: an exploratory, multi-centre, double-blind,

placebo-controlled, dose-escalating, single and repeat dose phase study. Ann Rheum Dis 2006; 65: 108.

41. Furie R, Stohl W, Ginzler E at al. Safety, pharmacokinetic and pharmacodynamic results of a phase 1 single and double dose escalation study of lymphostat-B (human monoclonal antibody to BLyS) in SLE patients. Arthritis Rheum 2003; 48: S377.

42. Wallace D, Lisse J, Stohl W et al. Belimumab, a fully human monoclonal antibody to B-lymphocyte stimulator (BLyS), shows bioactivity and reduces SLE disease activity. Ann Rheum Dis 2006; 65: 62.

43. Moreland LW, Pratt PW, Mayes MD et al. Double-blind, placebo-controlled multicenter trial using chimeric monoclonal anti-CD4 antibody, cM-T412, in rheumatoid arthritis patients receiving concomitant methotrexate. Arthritis Rheum 1995; 38: 1581–8.

44. Kremer JM, Westhovens R, Leon M et al. Treatment of rheumatoid arthritis by selective inhibition of T-cell activation with fusion protein CTLA4Ig. N Engl J Med 2003; 349: 1907–15.

45. Kremer JM, Dougados M, Emery P et al. Treatment of rheumatoid arthritis with the selective costimulation modulator abatacept: twelve-month results of a phase iib, double-blind, randomized, placebo-controlled trial. Arthritis Rheum 2005; 52: 2263–71.

46. Kremer JM, Genant HK, Moreland LW et al. Effects of abatacept in patients with methotrexate-resistant active rheumatoid arthritis: a randomized trial. Ann Intern Med 2006; 144: 865–76.

47. Genant HK, Peterfy C, Westhovens R et al. Abatacept sustains inhibition of radiographic progression over 2 years in RA patients with an inadequate response to methotrexate: results from the long term extension of the AIM trial. Ann Rheum Dis 2006; 65: 57.

48. Genovese MC, Becker JC, Schiff M et al Abatacept for rheumatoid arthritis refractory to tumor necrosis factor alpha inhibition. N Engl J Med 2005; 353: 1114–23.

49. Combe B, Weinblatt M, Birbara C et al. Safety and patient-reported outcomes associated with abatacept in the treatment of rheumatoid arthritis patients receiving background DMARDs: the ASSURE trial. Arthritis Rheum 2005; 52; S709.

50. Finck BK, Linsley PS, Wofsy D. Treatment of murine lupus with CTLA4Ig. Science 1994; 265: 1225–7.

51. Daikh DI, Wofsy D. Cutting edge: reversal of murine lupus nephritis with CTLA4Ig and cyclophosphamide. J Immunol 2001; 166: 2913–16.

52. Cunnane G, Chan OT, Cassafer G et al. Prevention of renal damage in murine lupus nephritis by CTLA-4Ig and cyclophosphamide. Arthritis Rheum 2004; 50: 1539–48.

53. Davis JC Jr, Totoritis MC, Rosenberg J et al. Phase I clinical trial of a monoclonal antibody against CD40-ligand (IDEC-131) in patients with systemic lupus erythematosus. J Rheumatol 2001; 28: 95–101.

54. Kalunian KC, Davis JC Jr, Merrill JT et al. Treatment of systemic lupus erythematosus by inhibition of T cell costimulation with anti-CD154: a randomized, double-blind, placebo-controlled trial. Arthritis Rheum 2002; 46: 3251–8.

55. Boumpas DT, Furie R, Manzi S et al. A short course of BG9588 (anti-CD40 ligand antibody) improves serologic activity and decreases hematuria in patients with proliferative lupus glomerulonephritis. Arthritis Rheum 2003; 48: 719–27.

56. Jayne D, Passweg J, Marmont A et al. Autologous stem cell transplantation for systemic lupus erythematosus. Lupus 2004; 13: 168–76.

57. Burt RK, Traynor A, Statkute L et al. Nonmyeloablative hematopoietic stem cell transplantation for systemic lupus erythematosus. JAMA 2006; 295: 527–35.

58. Petri M, Jones RJ, Brodsky RA. High-dose cyclophosphamide without stem cell transplantation in systemic lupus erythematosus. Arthritis Rheum 2003; 48: 166–73.

59. Gladstone DE, Prestrud AA, Pradhan A et al. High-dose cyclophosphamide for severe systemic lupus erythematosus. Lupus 2002; 11: 405–10.

60. Snowden JA, Biggs JC, Milliken ST et al. A phase I/II dose escalation study of intensified cyclophosphamide and autologous blood stem cell rescue in severe, active rheumatoid arthritis. Arthritis Rheum 1999; 42: 2286–92.

61. Verburg RJ, Sont JK, van Laar JM. Reduction of joint damage in severe rheumatoid arthritis by high-dose chemotherapy and autologous stem cell transplantation. Arthritis Rheum 2005; 52: 421–4.

62. Snowden JA, Passweg J, Moore JJ et al. Autologous hemopoietic stem cell transplantation in severe rheumatoid arthritis: a report from the EBMT and ABMTR. J Rheumatol 2004; 31: 482–8.

63. Lowsky R, Takahashi T, Liu YP et al. Protective conditioning for acute graft-versus-host disease. N Engl J Med 2005; 353: 1321–31.

64. Burt RK, Oyama Y, Verda L et al. Induction of remission of severe and refractory rheumatoid arthritis by allogeneic mixed chimerism. Arthritis Rheum 2004; 50: 2466–70.

65. Dayan M, Segal R, Sthoeger Z et al. Immune response of SLE patients to peptides based on the complementarity determining regions of a pathogenic anti-DNA monoclonal antibody. J Clin Immunol 2000; 20: 187–94.

66. Sthoeger ZM, Dayan M, Tcherniack A et al. Modulation of autoreactive responses of peripheral blood lymphocytes of patients with systemic lupus erythematosus by peptides based on human and murine anti-DNA autoantibodies. Clin Exp Immunol 2003; 131: 385–92.

67. Jones DS, Barstad PA, Feild MJ et al. Immunospecific reduction of antioligonucleotide antibody-forming cells with a tetrakis-oligonucleotide conjugate (LJP 394), a

therapeutic candidate for the treatment of lupus nephritis. J Med Chem 1995; 38: 2138–44.

68. Weisman MH, Bluestein HG, Berner CM et al. Reduction in circulating dsDNA antibody titre after administration of LJP 394. J Rheumatol 1997; 24: 314–18.

69. Alarcon-Segovia D, Tumlin JA, Furie RA et al. LJP 394 for the prevention of renal flare in patients with systemic lupus erythematosus: results from a randomized, double-blind, placebo-controlled study. Arthritis Rheum 2003; 48: 442–54.

70. Strand V, Aranow C, Cardiel MH et al. Improvement in health-related quality of life in systemic lupus erythematosus patients enrolled in a randomized clinical trial comparing LJP 394 treatment with placebo. Lupus 2003; 12: 677–86.

71. Linnik MD, Hu JZ, Heilbrunn KR et al. Relationship between anti-double-stranded DNA antibodies and exacerbation of renal disease in patients with systemic lupus erythematosus. Arthritis Rheum 2005; 52: 1129–37.

72. Tumlin JA, Hura C, Joh T et al. Reduction in 24 hour urine protein levels associated with treatment of SLE patients with LJP 394 in two randomised, placebo controlled clinical trials. Presented at the American Society of Nephrology Annual Scientific Meeting, 2004.

73. Blumenauer B, Judd M, Cranney A et al. Etanercept for the treatment of rheumatoid arthritis. Cochrane Database Syst Rev 2003; (4): CD004525.

74. Lipsky PE, van der Heijde DM, St Clair EW et al. Infliximab and methotrexate in the treatment of rheumatoid arthritis. Anti-Tumor Necrosis Factor Trial in Rheumatoid Arthritis with Concomitant Therapy Study Group. N Engl J Med 2000; 343: 1594–602.

75. Weinblatt ME, Keystone EC, Furst DE et al. Adalimumab, a fully human anti-tumor necrosis factor alpha monoclonal antibody, for the treatment of rheumatoid arthritis in patients taking concomitant methotrexate: the ARMADA trial. Arthritis Rheum 2003; 48: 35–45.

76. Listing J, Strangfeld A, Kary S et al. Infections in patients with rheumatoid arthritis treated with biologic agents. Arthritis Rheum 2005; 52: 3403–12.

77. Jacob CO, McDevitt HO. Tumour necrosis factor-alpha in murine autoimmune 'lupus' nephritis. Nature 1988; 331: 356–8.

78. De Rycke L, Baeten D, Kruithof E et al. Infliximab, but not etanercept, induces IgM anti-double-stranded DNA autoantibodies as main antinuclear reactivity: biologic and clinical implications in autoimmune arthritis. Arthritis Rheum 2005; 52: 2192–201.

79. Aringer M, Graninger WB, Steiner G et al. Safety and efficacy of tumor necrosis factor alpha blockade in systemic lupus erythematosus: an open-label study. Arthritis Rheum 2004; 50: 3161–9.

80. Houssiau FA, Devogelaer JP, Van Damme J et al. Interleukin-6 in synovial fluid and serum of patients with rheumatoid arthritis and other inflammatory arthritides. Arthritis Rheum 1988; 31: 784–8.

81. Wendling D, Racadot E, Wijdenes J. Treatment of severe rheumatoid arthritis by anti-interleukin 6 monoclonal antibody. J Rheumatol 1993; 20: 259–62.

82. Choy EH, Isenberg DA, Garrood T et al. Therapeutic benefit of blocking interleukin-6 activity with an anti-interleukin-6 receptor monoclonal antibody in rheumatoid arthritis: a randomized, double-blind, placebo-controlled, dose-escalation trial. Arthritis Rheum 2002; 46: 3143–50.

83. Maini RN, Taylor PC, Pavelka K et al. Efficacy of IL6 receptor antogonist MRA in rheumatoid arthritis patients with an incomplete response to methotrexate (CHARISMA). Arthritis Rheum 2003; 48: S652.

84. Nishimoto N, Yoshizaki K, Miyasaka N et al. Treatment of rheumatoid arthritis with humanized anti-interleukin-6 receptor antibody: a multicenter, double-blind, placebo-controlled trial. Arthritis Rheum 2004; 50: 1761–9.

85. Nishimoto N, Miyasaka N, Yamamoto K et al. Efficacy and safety of tocilizumab in monotherapy, an anti IL-6 receptor monoclonal antibody, in patients with active rheumatoid arthritis: results from a 24 week double-blind phase III study. Ann Rheum Dis 2006; 65: 59.

86. del Rincon ID, Williams K, Stern MP et al. High incidence of cardiovascular events in a rheumatoid arthritis cohort not explained by traditional cardiac risk factors. Arthritis Rheum 2001; 44: 2737–45.

87. Yu CL, Sun KH, Tsai CY et al. Anti-dsDNA antibody up-regulates interleukin 6, but not cyclo-oxygenase, gene expression in glomerular mesangial cells: a marker of immune-mediated renal damage? Inflamm Res 2001; 50: 12–18.

88. Finck BK, Chan B, Wofsy D et al. Interleukin 6 promotes murine lupus in NZB/NZW F1 mice. J Clin Invest 1994; 94: 585–91.

89. Ripley BJ, Goncalves B, Isenberg DA et al. Raised levels of interleukin 6 in systemic lupus erythematosus correlate with anaemia. Ann Rheum Dis 2005; 64: 849–53.

90. Cohen S, Hurd E, Cush J et al. Treatment of rheumatoid arthritis with anakinra, a recombinant human interleukin-1 receptor antagonist, in combination with methotrexate: results of a twenty-four-week, multicenter, randomized, double-blind, placebo-controlled trial. Arthritis Rheum 2002; 46: 614–24.

91. Jiang Y, Genant HK, Watt I et al. A multicenter, double-blind, dose-ranging, randomized, placebo-controlled study of recombinant human interleukin-1 receptor antagonist in patients with rheumatoid arthritis: radiologic progression and correlation of Genant and Larsen scores. Arthritis Rheum 2000; 43: 1001–9.

92. Weisman MH. What are the risks of biologic therapy in rheumatoid arthritis? An update on safety. J Rheumatol Suppl 2002; 65: 33–8.

93. Buch MH, Bingham SJ, Seto Y et al. Lack of response to anakinra in rheumatoid arthritis following failure of tumor necrosis factor alpha blockade. Arthritis Rheum 2004; 50: 725–8.

94. Bingham C, Genovese M, Moreland L et al. Results of a phase II study of interleukin-1 (IL1)-Trap in moderate to severe rheumatoid arthritis. Arthritis Rheum 2004; 50 (Suppl): S237.

95. Park YB, Lee SK, Kim DS et al. Elevated interleukin-10 levels correlated with disease activity in systemic lupus erythematosus. Clin Exp Rheumatol 1998; 16: 283–8.

96. Llorente L, Richaud-Patin Y, Garcia-Padilla C et al. Clinical and biologic effects of anti-interleukin-10 monoclonal antibody administration in systemic lupus erythematosus. Arthritis Rheum 2000; 43: 1790–800.

97. Bao L, Osawe I, Puri T et al. C5a promotes development of experimental lupus nephritis which can be blocked with a specific receptor antagonist. Eur J Immunol 2005; 35: 2496–506.

42

Targeting B-lymphocyte stimulator (BLyS) in immune-based rheumatic diseases: a therapeutic promise waiting to be fulfilled

William Stohl

Introduction • **General biology of BLyS** • **BLyS receptors** • **Biologic consequences of BLyS/BLyS receptor interactions** • ***In vivo*** **consequences of BLyS overexpression** • ***In vivo*** **consequences of BLyS/BLyS receptor deficiency** • **Elimination/neutralization of BLyS in murine disease** • **Contributory/confounding role for a proliferation-inducing ligand (APRIL)** • **BLyS overexpression in human rheumatic diseases** • **Therapeutic neutralization of BLyS in human disease** • **BLyS antagonism as part of combination therapy** • **Concluding remarks** • **References**

INTRODUCTION

Rheumatologists need no reminder that current treatment options for patients with systemic immune-based rheumatic diseases are inadequate and fraught with serious toxicities. Although many of our patients do respond clinically to corticosteroids, cytotoxic drugs, and/or tumor necrosis factor (TNF)-α antagonists, the responses are almost always sub-total, and complications from the medications are too often more pernicious than the underlying disease itself.

In the summer of 1999, this author was perusing a recent issue of *Science* and came across an article that literally made him jump from his seat. This article focused on a molecule dubbed BLyS (B-lymphocyte stimulator), a soluble factor derived from non-T cells (monocytes), and its potent ability to costimulate B-cell proliferation *in vitro* and promote hypergammaglobulinemia *in vivo*.[1] The exquisite specificity of BLyS binding to B cells suggested that neutralization of BLyS might selectively affect B-cell function without perturbing the function of other cell types (lymphoid and non-lymphoid). That is, BLyS antagonists could be highly safe, yet biologically potent, weapons in combating the many human disorders associated with B-cell hyperactivity. Since publication of that seminal paper in 1999, considerable (albeit still very incomplete) insight and knowledge has been gained into the biology of BLyS, its role in systemic immune-based diseases in both mouse and man, and its striking therapeutic efficacy in murine disease but perceived dearth of same in human disease.

GENERAL BIOLOGY OF BLyS

BLyS (also known as BAFF, TALL-1, THANK, TNFSF13B, and zTNF4) is a 285-amino acid member of the TNF ligand superfamily and is expressed as a type II transmembrane protein.[1-6]

Cleavage of BLyS by a furin protease from the cell surface results in release of a soluble, biologically active 17-kDa molecule.[3,7] Like other members of the TNF ligand superfamily, soluble BLyS circulates in trimeric form.[3,8] What still remains uncertain is whether the membrane-bound form has biological activity, and what remains highly controversial is whether higher-order multimers of BLyS exist under physiologic conditions. Some laboratories have induced BLyS to assemble into virus-like clusters of 60 monomers under appropriate *in vitro* conditions,[9–11] but other laboratories have been unsuccessful in coaxing BLyS to assume a multimeric configuration.[12,13] It has been suggested that multimeric self-assembly of BLyS is an artifactual consequence of the manner in which BLyS is 'tagged' for *in vitro* experimentation,[14] although this notion has itself been challenged.[15] Even if virus-like clusters of BLyS are present systemically in the circulation or locally in tissues, the issue of their *in vivo* biologic activity, if any, remains an open one.

At least two isoforms of BLyS are expressed. The full-length BLyS mRNA isoform codes for the biologically active full-length protein, and the alternatively spliced ΔBLyS mRNA isoform codes for a protein with a small peptide deletion.[16] ΔBLyS does not bind to cells expressing BLyS receptors and, therefore, has no agonistic activity. Moreover, ΔBLyS can form biologically inactive heterotrimers with full-length BLyS, thereby functioning as a dominant-negative antagonist of BLyS activity. Indeed, selective over-expression of the ΔBLyS isoform can result in functional BLyS neutralization *in vivo*.[17] How ΔBLyS expression is normally regulated and whether ΔBLyS expression is dysregulated in the rheumatic diseases are largely unknown.

Our knowledge regarding the regulation of full-length BLyS expression is only modestly greater. A polymorphism in the BLyS promoter region exists at position -871. Monocyte BLyS mRNA levels are greater in individuals bearing the -871T polymorphism than in those bearing the -871C polymorphism,[18] and transfectants with reporter constructs containing the -871T polymorphism had > 2-fold more luciferase activity than did transfectants with reporter constructs containing the -871C polymorphism.[19]

The ramifications for this observations with regard to the rheumatic diseases is uncertain, inasmuch as no association between systemic lupus erythematosus (SLE) or rheumatoid arthritis (RA) with either polymorphism was appreciated in a Japanese cohort.[18]

Systemic expression of BLyS is largely restricted to myeloid lineage cells (monocytes, dendritic cells, macrophages, neutrophils)[1–3,5,7,20] and to bone marrow-derived radiation-resistant stromal cells.[21] In myeloid lineage cells, BLyS mRNA and protein levels are up-regulated by interferon (IFN)-γ, interleukin (IL)-10, IFN-α, CD40 ligand, RANTES, and SDF-1α.[7,20,22,23] BLyS is also expressed to some degree by T cells.[3] Although purified SLE peripheral blood T cells stimulated *in vitro* with an anti-CD3 monoclonal antibody (mAb) produce substantial amounts of BLyS,[24] it remains unknown whether T-cell engagement *in vivo* can also trigger BLyS production by T cells.

BLyS is not expressed by peripheral blood B cells, but its expression can be detected in several tonsillar B-cell subsets.[25] Nuclear CD40 may be playing an important contributory role in driving BLyS expression in these cells.[26] Although any pathogenic ramifications for CD40-driven BLyS production in systemic rheumatic diseases remain purely speculative, the ability of certain B cells to produce BLyS has already been suggested as an autocrine pathway of survival in neoplastic B cells.[27–30]

In addition to systemic BLyS expression, BLyS is expressed locally in a tissue-specific manner. This includes expression of BLyS by astrocytes in the central nervous system,[31] which may be crucial to survival of virus-specific antibody-secreting cells that control viral persistence.[32] BLyS is also locally expressed by fibroblast-like synoviocytes in synovial tissue,[33] an observation which may be especially germane to patients with RA undergoing B-cell-depleting therapy with the anti-CD20 mAb rituximab. BLyS produced by fibroblast-like synoviocytes can blunt the B-cell-depleting effects of rituximab in the joint and, thereby, limit the clinical effectiveness of rituximab therapy.[34] Of note, reactive oxygen species can augment BLyS expression.[35] Thus, in the context of inflammatory diseases in which B cells contribute to the pathogenic outcome, anti-inflammatory therapies may not only primarily attenuate ongoing inflammation but may also secondarily attenuate BLyS-driven pathology.

BLyS RECEPTORS

The ability of BLyS to exert biological effects on B cells perforce demonstrates that B cells express receptors for BLyS. Indeed, three BLyS receptors (BCMA, TACI, and BAFFR [also called BR3]) have been identified, and their expression is largely (but not exclusively) limited to B cells.[36–39] BLyS binds strongly to B cells and weakly to T cells, but not to natural killer (NK) cells or monocytes.[1,40] The vast majority, if not all, of the BLyS that binds to human peripheral blood B cells does so via surface BAFFR and/or TACI, with little, if any, BLyS binding via BCMA.[28] Nevertheless, levels of BCMA mRNA in terminally differentiated plasma cells are much greater than those in mature B cells,[41,42] and *in vitro*-generated human plasmablasts up-regulate surface BCMA and down-regulate surface BAFFR and TACI.[43] The numbers of antigen-specific long-lived Ig-secreting cells in the bone marrow are greatly reduced in BCMA-deficient mice in comparison with those in BCMA-intact mice,[44] strongly suggesting that engagement of BCMA by BLyS is biologically consequential.

BIOLOGIC CONSEQUENCES OF BLyS/BLyS RECEPTOR INTERACTIONS

A complex intracellular signaling scheme is triggered following engagement by BLyS of its receptors. Several TNF receptor-associated factors (TRAFs), including TRAF1, TRAF2, TRAF3, TRAF5, and TRAF6, interact with one or more of the three BLyS receptors.[40,45–47] Phospholipase C-γ2, NF-κB1, and NF-κB2 are all activated,[48–51] HSH2 expression is up-regulated,[52] nuclear accumulation of PKCδ is prevented,[53] CD19 surface expression is enhanced,[54,55] and B-cell survival is increased.[43,51,56–60] Up-regulation of cyclooxygenase-2, production of prostaglandin E$_2$, and increased expression of Mcl-1 may be especially important in BlyS-driven viability and continued cell cycling of recently stimulated B cells.[61] Enhanced survival may also, at least in part, be secondary to BLyS-induced down-regulation of Bim.[62] Indeed, BLyS has little effect on survival of Bim-deficient B cells.[63] Moreover, BLyS-driven B-cell survival may, in part, be related to up-regulation of Bcl-2 and/or Bcl-x$_L$,[57] given that B cells with enforced overexpression of Bcl-x$_L$ are protected from the premature death that ensues in the absence of BLyS signaling.[64] Moreover, the canonical NF-κB pathway (NF-κB1) may be especially vital in that its constitutive activation in B cells obviates the need for BLyS/BAFFR interactions in normal B cell development.[65]

In addition to its role as a B-cell survival factor, BLyS also serves as a B-cell differentiation factor, promoting the differentiation of immature B cells to mature B cells, including marginal zone (MZ) B cells.[66,67] Moreover, BLyS promotes Ig class switching and Ig production by B cells via engagement of TACI and BAFFR.[22,68,69] Accordingly, protracted neutralization of BLyS could, in principle, adversely affect global humoral immunity. Whether this concern actually becomes clinically meaningful remains to be empirically established.

The effects of BLyS are not limited to 'conventional' B2 B cells. Peritoneal B1 (CD5$^+$) B cells treated in culture with BLyS demonstrate up-regulation of surface CD21, activation of the non-canonical NF-κB pathway (NF-κB2), and enhanced survival. Moreover, in B1 B cells triggered by engagement of Toll-like receptors, BLyS has a costimulatory effect in terms of expression of activation markers, proliferation, and cytokine production.[70]

IN VIVO CONSEQUENCES OF BLyS OVEREXPRESSION

Given the ability of BLyS to promote B-cell survival and differentiation, it is not surprising that overexpression of BLyS, either through exogenous administration of BLyS or endogenous overproduction, has profound consequences. Administration of exogenous BLyS to mice at the time of immunization with antigen enhances *in vivo* antigen-specific antibody production.[57] Moreover, repeated administration of BLyS to mice without specific antigenic immunization results in B-cell expansion and polyclonal hypergammaglobulinemia.[1] Increased levels of BLyS may relax the selection stringency as B cells mature through the transitional stages, thereby dampening the elimination of autoreactive B cells.[71] Thus, not only is some of the increased Ig production in BLyS-overexpressing mice likely directed to ambient environmental (foreign) antigens, but some of the increased Ig production is likely directed to self-antigens. Indeed, constitutive overexpression of BLyS in BLyS-transgenic (Tg) mice bearing a non-autoimmune-prone genetic background (largely derived from C57BL/6 [B6] mice) often leads to SLE-like features (elevated circulating titers of multiple autoantibodies and renal pathology), with clinical disease (increased proteinuria) being manifest by 8 months (but not 5 months) of age.[6,72,73] Although BLyS overexpression may rescue autoreactive B cells only when the proportion of competing (non-autoreactive) B cells is small,[74] the development of autoimmunity in BLyS-Tg mice (bearing a full Ig repertoire) may reflect BLyS-driven expansion of autoreactive B cells that escape tolerance even without BLyS overexpression rather than BLyS-driven selection of otherwise tolerant autoreactive B-cell populations.

In any case, BLyS overexpression also has striking effects on hosts with an underlying diathesis to autoimmunity. Congenic autoimmune-prone B6 mice were generated by introgressing into B6 mice the *Sle1* or *Nba2* loci on mouse chromosome 1 (derived from NZW and NZB mice, respectively), each locus being strongly implicated in the loss of tolerance to nucleosomal autoantigens.[75,76] Accordingly, B6.Sle1 mice and B6.Nba2 mice each have an incomplete genetic predisposition to development of SLE in that they spontaneously develop elevated circulating titers of IgG anti-chromatin autoantibodies but rarely develop renal disease.[76–78] Introduction of a BLyS Tg into these mice dramatically accelerated development of target organ (kidney) pathology.[79] Of note, acceleration of clinical disease (increased proteinuria and/or death) was not observed, suggesting that even in an autoimmune-prone host, factors beyond just BLyS overexpression are required for development of clinical disease.

Even without 'artificial' Tg-driven BLyS overexpression, BLyS overexpression is a feature of murine SLE, in that circulating BLyS levels are elevated in (NZB × NZW)F1 and MRL-*lpr/lpr* mice at the time of disease onset.[6] It may be that BLyS facilitates phenotypic expression of a latent SLE diathesis, with greater cumulative BLyS exposure leading to greater penetrance of the autoimmune phenotype (Figure 42.1).

Importantly, SLE is not the only phenotype associated with BLyS overexpression. Although many BLyS-Tg mice succumb to SLE nephritis by ~12 months of age, not all do. Of those that do not, many develop a phenotype resembling Sjögren's syndrome, with enlarged salivary glands, periductal infiltrates, acinar destruction, and reduced production of saliva.[80] BLyS overexpression is also a feature of inflammatory arthritis, as evidenced by the up-regulation of BLyS during the development of collagen-induced arthritis (CIA).[81]

IN VIVO CONSEQUENCES OF BLyS/BLyS RECEPTOR DEFICIENCY

Just as excessive BLyS production leads to profound immune perturbations, so too does BLyS deficiency. Mice that are genetically BLyS-deficient display considerable global reductions in B cells beyond the transitional type 1 (T1) stage. This includes virtually all mature B2 B cells (although numbers of peritoneal B1 B cells and immature bone marrow B cells remain nearly intact) and leads to marked reductions in baseline serum Ig levels and Ig responses to T-cell-dependent and T-cell-independent antigens.[82,83]

Of note, the phenotypes of mice genetically deficient in individual BLyS receptors are highly disparate. In two of the cases, the phenotypes do not resemble that of BLyS-deficient mice at all, highlighting the non-overlapping functions subserved by each BLyS receptor. Immunized BCMA-deficient mice do not harbor as many antigen-specific long-lived Ig-secreting cells in their bone marrow as do BCMA-intact mice,[44] although BCMA-deficient mice otherwise exhibit no discernible phenotypic or functional abnormalities.[83,84]

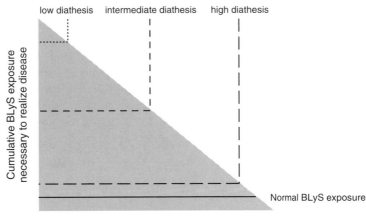

Figure 42.1 Hypothetical relationship between underlying SLE diathesis and cumulative BLyS exposure. A persistent up-regulation in endogenous BLyS expression may not necessarily lead to clinical disease (SLE). For example, circulating BLyS levels are elevated in a large percentage of HIV-infected individuals,[147,148] but these subjects do not manifest features of SLE or related autoimmune disorders. The ability of BLyS overexpression to promote SLE-like disease is likely dependent upon the host's underlying diathesis to SLE, which includes both genetic constitution and environmental exposures. In a host with a high SLE diathesis (long-dashed line), relatively little BLyS overexpression is necessary to 'push' the host over the disease threshold. Such an individual is at very high risk for developing SLE during her/his lifetime. In a host with a low SLE diathesis (dotted line), the cumulative BLyS expression required to cross the disease threshold is so high that it is most unlikely ever to be achieved during the host's lifetime. In a host with an intermediate SLE diathesis (short-dashed line), an intermediate degree of cumulative BLyS exposure is needed to develop disease.

These BCMA-deficient mice all bore a non-autoimmune-prone genetic background, demonstrating that in a normal (non-autoimmune) environment, surface expression of BLyS receptors other than BCMA is sufficient to transmit the requisite BLyS-triggered signals for 'normal' B-cell survival and function (at least until terminal differentiation into plasma cells). Nevertheless, this by no means excludes a potential pathogenic role for BLyS/BCMA interactions in the context of autoimmunity or autoimmune disease. Engagement of BCMA can trigger B cells to up-regulate surface expression of costimulatory molecules which, in turn, enhances the ability of the B cells to serve as antigen-presenting cells (APCs).[85] The APC function of B cells may be as important, if not more important, than their autoantibody-producing capacities in promoting autoimmune disease, as has compellingly been shown in SLE-prone MRL-*lpr/lpr* mice.[86–88] Thus, it is entirely plausible that BLyS overexpression in an autoimmune-prone host drives increased signaling via BCMA which, in turn,

leads to increased B-cell expression of costimulatory molecules and APC function. By therapeutically blocking BLyS/BCMA interactions, development of disease may be abrogated (ameliorated) even in the context of BLyS overexpression and even in the context of increased total numbers of B cells and circulating Ig (autoantibody) levels.

The phenotype of mice genetically deficient in TACI, a second BAFF receptor, strikingly differs from those of either BLyS-deficient or BCMA-deficient mice. The latter is not surprising, since in contrast to the up-regulation of B-cell costimulatory molecules and APC function upon engagement of BCMA, engagement of TACI has no such effects.[85] Strikingly, TACI-deficient mice harbor increased numbers of B cells rather than the decreased or normal numbers of B cells observed in BLyS-deficient or BCMA-deficient mice, respectively.[89,90] As TACI-deficient mice age, they develop elevated circulating titers of autoantibodies, Ig deposition in their kidneys with concomitant glomerulonephritis, and premature death.[91] *In vitro* treatment of normal B cells with anti-TACI mAb blocks B-cell responses to agonists,[91] strongly suggesting that TACI transmits a negative signal to B cells.

Nevertheless, the physiologic function of TACI cannot be limited to simply transmitting a negative signal to B cells. TACI-deficient mice, despite their B-cell expansion and serological and clinical autoimmunity, manifest impaired Ig responses to T-cell-independent antigens.[89,90] In humans, mutations of the *Taci* gene are associated with common varied immunodeficiency and IgA deficiency,[92,93] strongly suggesting that the intact (wild-type) TACI molecule plays a vital role in normal Ig class switching and Ig production. Subtle differences in the manner by which TACI is engaged may trigger different intracellular signaling pathways and result in divergent phenotypes.

In contrast to BCMA- or TACI-deficient mice, A/WySnJ mice (which bear a mutated *Baffr* gene) and BAFFR-deficient mice display deficiencies in mature B-cell number and antibody responses qualitatively similar to those of BLyS-deficient mice.[38,39,94,95] When injected with exogenous BLyS, A/WySnJ and BAFFR-deficient mice do not undergo splenic B lymphocytosis, whereas similarly treated A/J and BLyS-deficient control mice do.[59,95] Moreover, in bone marrow chimeric mice harboring B cells that bear the mutated *Baffr* gene and B cells that bear the wild-type *Baffr* gene, the B cells bearing the mutated *Baffr* gene have decreased *in vivo* survival.[59] Taken together, these observations strongly point to BLyS/BAFFR interactions as essential for the pro-survival effects of BLyS on peripheral B cells.

ELIMINATION/NEUTRALIZATION OF BLyS IN MURINE DISEASE

Of great importance, the reductions in B-cell number and function even in BLyS-deficient mice (and even within the B2 subset) are not total, and the magnitude of these reductions has previously been overstated due to concomitant effects of BLyS deficiency on surface expression of CD21 and CD23 (markers typically used to delineate discrete maturational subsets of B cells).[96] This incomplete B-cell depletion points

to some BLyS-independent means of B-cell survival and function. Although studies in hen egg lysozyme (HEL)/anti-HEL double-Tg mice had suggested that survival of autoreactive B cells is more dependent upon BLyS than is survival of non-autoreactive B cells,[97,98] considerable levels of IgG autoantibodies did develop with age in BLyS-deficient SLE-prone NZM 2328 mice despite the life-long total absence of BLyS.[99] This indicated that at least some autoreactive B cells survived and differentiated into autoantibody-secreting cells via an as yet undefined BLyS-independent pathway. Ig deposition and proliferative glomerulonephritis developed in many of these mice. Nevertheless, clinical autoimmunity (severe proteinuria, premature death) was markedly attenuated, suggesting that in hosts with a strong diathesis to autoimmune disease, elimination of BLyS may have a disproportionately greater effect on clinical features of disease than on serological or pathological features of the disease.

The clinical response observed in NZM 2328 mice by genetic ablation of BLyS is paralleled by more standard therapeutic interventions. Both (NZB × NZW)F1 and MRL-*lpr/lpr* mice manifest dramatic clinical responses (decreased disease progression and improved survival) to treatment with BLyS antagonists.[6,50,100,101] In addition, the BLyS antagonist TACI-Ig has both preventive and therapeutic effects in the CIA model of RA.[82,102] Furthermore, the BLyS antagonists BCMA-Ig and BAFFR-Ig therapeutically ameliorate established hyperthyroidism in a murine model of Graves' disease.[103] Thus, BLyS antagonism in the mouse is beneficial in multiple rheumatic and autoimmune disease states, suggesting that the clinical potential of BLyS antagonism in the human arena may extend to multiple rheumatic and autoimmune disorders as well.

CONTRIBUTORY/CONFOUNDING ROLE FOR A PROLIFERATION-INDUCING LIGAND (APRIL)

A close 'relative' of BLyS within the TNF ligand superfamily is APRIL (also known as TALL-2, TRDL-1, and TNFSF13A), a 250-amino acid protein that binds to two of the three BLyS receptors (BCMA and TACI)[104–109] but does not bind to BAFFR.[38] Perhaps related to its differential ability to bind to BLyS receptors, APRIL can costimulate B cells *in vitro* and *in vivo*,[22,106,107] although it does so with considerably less potency than that of BLyS.[110] In addition to its binding to BCMA and TACI, APRIL also binds to heparan sulfate proteoglycans, whereas BLyS does not.[111,112] What ramifications, if any, this last observation has for B-cell function or, by extension, for the rheumatic diseases remain to be established.

Neither complete deficiency of APRIL nor its constitutive overexpression have dramatic effects on *in vivo* biology. APRIL-deficient mice bearing a non-autoimmune-prone genetic background have been described as being phenotypically normal[113] or to have selective deficiencies in circulating IgA levels and IgA responses to mucosal challenges.[114] Similarly, APRIL-Tg mice, which constitutively overexpress APRIL, manifest only subtle immunologic abnormalities.[115] Most noteworthy, no serologic or clinical autoimmune features have been appreciated in such APRIL-overexpressing mice.

Nevertheless, APRIL may play an important role in modifying the net biologic effects of BLyS. BLyS and APRIL can form heterotrimers which are present in the circulation.[116] Although such heterotrimers have BLyS-like biologic activity *in vitro*, what, if any, biologic activity these heterotrimers have *in vivo* remains uncertain. In principle, the biologic activity of BLyS/APRIL heterotrimers may be greater than, less than, or equal to that of BLyS homotrimers. Thus, therapeutic neutralization of APRIL concomitant with neutralization of BLyS might be beneficial, harmful, or neutral in the context of autoimmunity. This can potentially have profound ramifications for the types of BLyS antagonists chosen for use in the clinic. Indeed, differences in various immunologic parameters were appreciated among SLE-prone (NZB × NZW)F1 mice depending on whether they were treated with TACI-Ig or with BAFFR-Ig.[101] Since TACI binds not only to BLyS and APRIL but to certain syndecans as well,[117] some of the immunologic differences between TACI-Ig-treated mice and BAFFR-Ig-treated mice may relate to syndecan-mediated effects.

Although no information is yet available in humans with regard to any differential effects of BLyS-specific antagonists compared to those of agents which antagonize both BLyS and APRIL, there is reason to believe that differences between the two types of antagonists will emerge. In an observational study of SLE patients, serum APRIL levels modestly, but significantly, inversely correlated with disease activity and modestly, but significantly, inversely correlated with serum anti-dsDNA titers in anti-dsDNA-positive patients. Changes in serum levels of BLyS and APRIL over time were usually discordant.[118] Although other interpretations are plausible, one interpretation is that APRIL is a down-regulator of disease activity, at least in human SLE, and perhaps effects such downregulation by complexing to BLyS as heterotrimers. Empiric experience will ultimately determine the relative clinical efficacies of antagonists specific for BLyS and those able to antagonize both BLyS and APRIL.

BLyS OVEREXPRESSION IN HUMAN RHEUMATIC DISEASES

Overexpression of BLyS in association with autoimmune disease is not limited to mice but is also a feature of several human rheumatic diseases. An association between elevated circulating BLyS levels and human rheumatic disease was first noted in SLE, with circulating BLyS levels being increased in as many as 50% of SLE patients.[119–121] Somewhat surprisingly, a large longitudinal study showed only modest correlation between circulating BLyS protein levels and clinical disease activity.[122] However, a separate study (containing both cross-sectional and longitudinal elements), despite being considerably smaller in size than the first, demonstrated substantially stronger correlation between disease activity and BLyS mRNA levels in blood leukocytes.[123] This association between BLyS overexpression and disease activity in human SLE supports the premise that BLyS overexpression not only promotes development of disease but also actively contributes to the ongoing maintenance of disease in SLE patients.

The dichotomy between the relatively strong association between disease activity and BLyS overexpression as measured by blood leukocyte mRNA levels and the weak association between disease activity and BLyS overexpression as measured by circulating protein levels likely reflects the inability of circulating BLyS protein levels in human SLE to faithfully reflect excessive endogenous BLyS production. There are several reasons for this. First, some SLE patients harbor circulating anti-BLyS autoantibodies.[123] It is not yet known whether any of these anti-BLyS autoantibodies are functionally neutralizing, but regardless, such autoantibodies could enhance the clearance of BLyS and/or interfere with *in vitro* detection of BLyS, thereby masking endogenous BLyS overproduction. Second, increased urinary excretion of BLyS has been reported in SLE patients, especially among those with clinically overt renal involvement,[124] so urinary loss of BLyS could lead to spurious reductions in circulating BLyS levels. Third, freshly isolated SLE B cells, despite intact surface expression of BLyS receptors, bind less biotinylated BLyS *ex vivo* than do freshly isolated normal B cells.[125] The most likely explanation for this disparity is that BLyS receptors on B cells in SLE patients are occupied by soluble BLyS *in vivo*. Accordingly, it is likely that BLyS receptors expressed by SLE B cells bind BLyS *in vivo* and remove it from the circulation, resulting in a homeostatic pathway which modulates the effects of BLyS overproduction on circulating BLyS levels.

Elevated circulating BLyS levels are observed not just in SLE patients but in patients with other rheumatic diseases as well. Early reports described elevated circulating BLyS levels in a substantial fraction of RA patients.[119,120] However, it subsequently became apparent that rheumatoid factor (RF) in the samples could lead to spurious elevations in the BLyS determinations. Reassuringly, more recent reports using an assay that minimizes (eliminates) the potential confounding effects of RF have confirmed elevated circulating BLyS levels in RA, albeit not to the extent initially believed.[123,126] In any case, BLyS levels in synovial fluid (SF) from RA patients (and from patients with other inflammatory arthritides) are routinely greater than those in corresponding serum,[127] consistent with local production of BLyS in the inflamed joints.[128]

Several reports have focused on BLyS expression in other rheumatic diseases. Circulating BLyS levels may be especially high in patients with Sjögren's syndrome.[55,80,129–131] Elevated salivary BLyS levels may importantly contribute to the periodontal disease that often plagues these patients,[132] and local overexpression of BLyS in the salivary glands likely contribute to the pathologic changes.[133–135] Salivary gland biopsies have revealed that the predominant phenotypes of the B cells in the ectopic germinal centers are those of T2 and MZ B cells,[136] precisely those B cells expected to expand in response to BLyS overstimulation. Consistent with this notion is the strong expression of BLyS localized to the T2 B-cell area.

Elevated circulating BLyS levels are also found in patients with scleroderma, dermatomyositis, Wegener's granulomatosis, or antineutrophil cytoplasmic antibody (ANCA)-associated vasculitis.[137–139] In scleroderma patients, skin thickness correlates with serum BLyS levels, and local BLyS expression is increased in the skin of patients with early diffuse cutaneous scleroderma. Moreover, declining serum BLyS levels over time correlate with regression of skin sclerosis, whereas increasing serum BLyS levels over time correlate with new onset or worsening of organ involvement.[137] These intriguing correlations notwithstanding, the precise pathogenetic connection between circulating BLyS levels and clinical features in these disorders remains to be fully elucidated.

THERAPEUTIC NEUTRALIZATION OF BLyS IN HUMAN DISEASE

Although no BLyS antagonist has yet been approved by the FDA for use in any rheumatic or non-rheumatic disease, several BLyS antagonists have been developed for human use and have been tested in the context of clinical trials. Based on the very encouraging experience in murine SLE and arthritis models, it was (unrealistically) anticipated by some that therapeutic targeting of BLyS in human rheumatic diseases would have earth-shaking effects on disease activity. To date, this dream has not been realized, but it would be far too premature and very unwise at this point in time to delete BLyS antagonists from the future armamentarium of the practicing rheumatologist.

The greatest experience to date with BLyS antagonists has accrued with belimumab, a fully human anti-BLyS IgG1λ mAb.[140] Belimumab binds and neutralizes BLyS but has no such activity against APRIL. In a randomized, double-blind, placebo-controlled phase I trial in SLE, belimumab was shown to be safe in that the prevalence of adverse events was no different in patients treated with belimumab at any tested dose (1, 4, 10, or 20 mg/kg) than in placebo-treated patients. Moreover, belimumab was demonstrated to be biologically active by virtue of reduction in peripheral blood B-cell counts in belimumab-treated patients but not in placebo-treated patients.[141] No clinical efficacy was demonstrated, although the small number of patients ($n = 70$) and very short treatment schedules (single infusion or two infusions 3 weeks apart) and follow-up period (12 weeks after final infusion) likely precluded demonstration of clinical benefit.

Recently, belimumab was shown to have statistically significant clinical efficacy in a 24-week, randomized, double-blind, placebo-controlled phase II trial in RA.[142] In this trial, patients with active RA ($n = 283$) were treated with one of three doses of belimumab (1, 4, or 10 mg/kg) or placebo at weeks 0, 2, 4, and every 4 weeks thereafter through 24 weeks. Belimumab or placebo was added to standard-of-care therapy, with a major caveat being that the subjects could not concurrently be receiving biologic therapy (e.g. TNF antagonists, rituximab). No dose-dependent clinical response was observed, suggesting that the lowest dose tested exerted the maximal effect. Among all belimumab-treated patients, 29% experienced a clinical response (defined as an ACR 20 response), whereas only 16% of the placebo-treated patients had an ACR 20 response. Among the belimumab-treated patients, peripheral blood B-cell counts declined by ~20%, and serum RF levels declined by ~30% (compared with no change in placebo-treated patients for either).[143] At face value, the low response rate among belimumab-treated patients was disappointing, but it must be viewed in the context of the very low response rate among the placebo-treated patients.

A near-doubling of the clinical response in the drug-treated group compared with the rate in the placebo-treated group is similar to that reported in a recent rituximab-based trial in RA patients.[144] In the matter of belimumab therapy for RA, the jury must be considered to still be out.

More recently, a 52-week, randomized, double-blind, placebo-controlled phase II trial of belimumab in SLE was concluded.[145] In this trial, patients with active SLE ($n = 449$) were treated with belimumab or placebo as in the phase II RA trial, except that the double-blind treatment lasted for 52 weeks rather than for only 24 weeks. The trial failed to meet its co-primary endpoints (disease activity at 24 weeks and time to first flare during the 52 weeks) when considering the entire SLE cohort. However, reduced disease activity was demonstrable at 52 weeks (but not at 24 weeks) in the 71.5% of patients who were 'seropositive' (anti-nuclear antibody (ANA) titer ≥ 1:80 and/or positive for anti-dsDNA antibodies) at entry, raising the hope that belimumab may be clinically efficacious in a substantial subset of SLE patients. The slow onset of clinical efficacy may be related to the persistently increased occupancy by BLyS of BAFFR on SLE B cells, even at times when circulating levels of soluble BLyS are not high.[125] For clinical efficacy, BLyS antagonists may not only have to neutralize circulating BLyS but may also have overcome the extended tight binding of BLyS to its receptors. For this reason, BLyS antagonists may not be ideal agents during the 'induction' phase of treatment but may be better suited for 'maintenance' therapy.

Other BLyS antagonists currently undergoing clinical trials in RA and/or SLE include the fusion proteins TACI-Ig and BR3-Fc and the 'peptibody' AMG 623. TACI-Ig, in contrast to belimumab or BR3-Fc, binds and neutralizes both BLyS and APRIL. Thus, its biologic and clinical effects may substantially differ from those of belimumab (and BR3-Fc). Results from a randomized, double-blind, placebo-controlled phase Ib trial with TACI-Ig in RA ($n = 73$) have not yet been presented in a peer-reviewed forum but were recently reported by press release (http://www.zymogenetics.com/ir/newsItem. php?id=802373). According to the press release,

TACI-Ig was safe and well tolerated. Schedule- and dose-dependent reductions in circulating IgM, IgG, IgA, and RF were observed. In the cohort of 19 patients that received 7 doses of TACI-Ig over a 3-month period, positive trends on some disease activity measures (e.g. ACR 20, DAS 28) were noted.

No clinical trial results are yet available for BR3-Fc, which specifically binds and neutralizes BLyS but not APRIL. A phase I trial in RA with BR3-Fc completed enrollment in the third quarter of 2005.

Clinical trial results are also not yet available for AMG 623, a fusion between the Fc portion of IgG and a peptide sequence selected for its ability to bind with high affinity to BLyS. Phase I trials with AMG 623 in RA and SLE are ongoing.

BLyS ANTAGONISM AS PART OF COMBINATION THERAPY

Although current clinical trials are evaluating BLyS antagonists as single agents (superimposed upon 'standard-of-care' therapy), the most rational utilization of BLyS antagonists may lie in their combination with other B-cell-depleting agents (e.g. rituximab). Circulating BLyS levels are markedly elevated without comparable elevation in BLyS mRNA levels in mice genetically devoid of B cells,[97] suggesting that a physical reduction in B cells (which are the predominant cells that express BLyS receptors) eliminates a major clearance pathway for circulating BLyS. If so, then therapeutic depletion of B cells should lead to increases in circulating BLyS levels, and B-cell repletion should be associated with reductions in circulating BLyS levels.

Recent observations in rituximab-treated RA patients support this notion.[126] Following rituximab-induced B-cell depletion, circulating BLyS levels rise and remain elevated during the entire duration of peripheral blood B-cell depletion. With return of B cells to the peripheral blood, circulating BLyS levels decline, and circulating BLyS levels routinely return to pre-rituximab baseline levels by the onset of clinical relapse. The period during which circulating BLyS levels remain elevated may play a key role in promoting re-emergence of pathogenic autoreactive

B cells. Accordingly, neutralization of BLyS following rituximab-based therapy could delay the re-emergence of such pathogenic autoreactive B cells and prolong the period of clinical remission.

Alternatively, initial treatment of patients with the combination of rituximab and a BLyS antagonist may lead to a more complete global B-cell depletion which, in turn, may result in a more long-lasting clinical remission. Although anti-CD20 mAb treatment of mice leads to profound depletion of peripheral blood B cells, substantial B-cell populations remain intact in lymphoid tissues. However, administration of a BLyS antagonist along with anti-CD20 mAb results in near-total B-cell depletion, even in the lymphoid tissues.[146] If the combination of anti-CD20 mAb and a BLyS antagonist has similar effects in humans, then the more complete global B-cell depletion may translate into more complete and longer-lasting clinical remissions.

CONCLUDING REMARKS

Despite the great excitement generated by BLyS antagonism in murine models of SLE and RA, no widespread excitement has yet been generated from the experience to date with BLyS antagonism in human SLE and RA. Since mice are not simply small furry humans with tails, it is not surprising that differences would emerge between responses to therapy in murine disease and human disease. Although there may yet be several bumps along the road, it remains the contention of this author that BLyS antagonism will be proven to have an important role in the management of patients with SLE, RA, and/or other related rheumatic diseases. With apologies to William Shakespeare, I come not to bury BLyS but to praise it.

REFERENCES

1. Moore PA, Belvedere O, Orr A, et al. BLyS. member of the tumor necrosis factor family and B lymphocyte stimulator. Science 1999; 285: 260–3.
2. Shu H-B, Hu W-H, Johnson H. TALL-1 is a novel member of the TNF family that is down-regulated by mitogens. J Leukoc Biol 1999; 65: 680–3.

3. Schneider P, MacKay F, Steiner V et al. BAFF, a novel ligand of the tumor necrosis factor family, stimulates B cell growth. J Exp Med 1999; 189: 1747–56.

4. Mukhopadhyay A, Ni J, Zhai Y, Yu G-L, Aggarwal BB. Identification and characterization of a novel cytokine, THANK, a TNF homologue that activates apoptosis, nuclear factor-κB, and c-Jun NH_2-terminal kinase. J Biol Chem 1999; 274: 15978–81.

5. Tribouley C, Wallroth M, Chan V et al. Characterization of a new member of the TNF family expressed on antigen presenting cells. Biol Chem 1999; 380: 1443–7.

6. Gross JA, Johnston J, Mudri S et al. TACI and BCMA are receptors for a TNF homologue implicated in B-cell autoimmune disease. Nature 2000; 404: 995–9.

7. Nardelli B, Belvedere O, Roschke V et al. Synthesis and release of B-lymphocyte stimulator from myeloid cells. Blood 2001; 97: 198–204.

8. Kanakaraj P, Migone T-S, Nardelli B et al. BLyS binds to B cells with high affinity and induces activation of the transcription factors NF-κB and ELF-1. Cytokine 2001; 13: 25–31.

9. Liu Y, Xu L, Opalka N et al. Crystal structure of sTALL-1 reveals a virus-like assembly of TNF family ligands. Cell 2002; 108: 383–94.

10. Kim HM, Yu KS, Lee ME et al. Crystal structure of the BAFF-BAFF-R complex and its implications for receptor activation. Nat Struct Biol 2003; 10: 342–8.

11. Liu Y, Hong X, Kappler J et al. Ligand-receptor binding revealed by the TNF family member TALL-1. Nature 2003; 423: 49–56.

12. Karpusas M, Cachero TG, Qian F et al. Crystal structure of extracellular human BAFF, a TNF family member that stimulates B lymphocytes. J Mol Biol 2002; 315: 1145–54.

13. Oren DA, Li Y, Volovik Y et al. Structural basis of BLyS receptor recognition. Nat Struct Biol 2002; 9: 288–92.

14. Zhukovsky EA, Lee J-O, Villegas M, Chan C, Chu S, Mroske C. Is TALL-1 a trimer of a virus-like cluster? Nature 2004; 427: 413–14.

15. Cachero TG, Schwartz IM, Qian F et al. Formation of virus-like clusters is an intrinsic property of the tumor necrosis factor family member BAFF (B cell activating factor). Biochemistry 2006; 45: 2006–13.

16. Gavin AL, Aït-Azzouzene D, Ware CF, Nemazee D. ΔBAFF, an alternate splice isoform that regulates receptor binding and biopresentation of the B cell survival cytokine, BAFF. J Biol Chem 2003; 278: 38220–8.

17. Gavin AL, Duong B, Skog P et al. ΔBAFF, a splice isoform of BAFF, opposes full length BAFF activity *in vivo* in transgenic mouse models. J Immunol 2005; 175: 319–28.

18. Kawasaki A, Tsuchiya N, Fukazawa T, Hashimoto H, Tokunaga K. Analysis on the association of human BLYS (BAFF, TNFSF13B) polymorphisms with systemic lupus erythematosus and rheumatoid arthritis. Genes Immun 2002; 3: 424–9.

19. Novak AJ, Grote DM, Ziesmer SC et al. Elevated serum B-lymphocyte stimulator levels in patients with familial lymphoproliferative disorders. J Clin Oncol 2006; 6: 983–7.

20. Scapini P, Nardelli B, Nadali G et al. G-CSF-stimulated neutrophils are a prominent source of functional BLyS. J Exp Med 2003; 197: 297–302.

21. Gorelik L, Gilbride K, Dobles M et al. Normal B cell homeostasis requires B cell activation factor production by radiation-resistant cells. J Exp Med 2003; 198: 937–45.

22. Litinskiy MB, Nardelli B, Hilbert DM et al. DCs induce CD40-independent immunoglobulin class switching through BLyS and APRIL. Nat Immunol 2002; 3: 822–9.

23. He B, Qiao X, Klasse PJ et al. HIV-1 envelope triggers polyclonal Ig class switch recombination through a CD40-independent mechanism involving BAFF and C-type lectin receptors. J Immunol 2006; 176: 3931–41.

24. Yoshimoto K, Takahashi Y, Ogasawara M et al. Aberrant expression of BAFF in T cells of systemic lupus erythematosus, which is recapitulated by a human T cell line, Loucy. Int Immunol 2006; 18: 1189–96.

25. He B, Chadburn A, Jou E et al. Lymphoma B cells evade apoptosis through the TNF family members BAFF/BLyS and APRIL. J Immunol 2004; 172: 3268–79.

26. Lin-Lee Y-C, Pham LV, Tamayo AT et al. Nuclear localization in the biology of the CD40 receptor in normal and neoplastic human B lymphocytes. J Biol Chem 2006; 281: 18878–87.

27. Novak AJ, Bram RJ, Kay NE, Jelinek DF. Aberrant expression of B-lymphocyte stimulator by B chronic lymphocytic leukemia cells: a mechanism for survival. Blood 2002; 100: 2973–9.

28. Novak AJ, Darce JR, Arendt BK et al. Expression of BCMA, TACI, and BAFF-R in multiple myeloma: a mechanism for growth and survival. Blood 2004; 103: 689–94.

29. Novak AJ, Grote DM, Stenson M et al. Expression of BLyS and its receptors in B-cell non-Hodgkin lymphoma: correlation with disease activity and patient outcome. Blood 2004; 104: 2247–53.

30. Elsawa SF, Novak AJ, Grote DM et al. B-lymphocyte stimulator (BLyS) stimulates immunoglobulin production and malignant B-cell growth in Waldenström macroglobulinemia. Blood 2006; 107: 2882–8.

31. Krumbholz M, Theil D, Derfuss T et al. BAFF is produced by astrocytes and up-regulated in multiple sclerosis lesions and primary central nervous system lymphoma. J Exp Med 2005; 201: 195–200.

32. Tschen S-I, Stohlman SA, Ramakrishna C et al. CNS viral infection diverts homing of antibody-secreting

cells from lymphoid organs to the CNS. Eur J Immunol 2006; 36: 603–12.

33. Ohata J, Zvaifler NJ, Nishio M et al. Fibroblast-like synoviocytes of mesenchymal orgin express functional B cell-activating factor of the TNF family in response to proinflammatory cytokines. J Immunol 2005; 174: 864–70.

34. Goodyear CS, Boyle DL, Silverman GJ. Secretion of BAFF by fibroblast-like synoviocytes from rheumatoid arthritis biopsies attenuates B-cell depletion by rituximab. Arthritis Rheum 2005; 52: S290.

35. Moon E-Y, Lee J-H, Oh S-Y et al. Reactive oxygen species augment B-cell-activating factor expression. Free Radic Biol Med 2006; 40: 2103–11.

36. Laabi Y, Gras M-P, Brouet J-C et al. The BCMA gene, preferentially expressed during B lymphoid maturation, is bidirectionally transcribed. Nucleic Acids Res 1994; 22: 1147–54.

37. von Bülow G-U, Bram RJ. NF-AT activation induced by a CAML-interacting member of the tumor necrosis factor receptor superfamily. Science 1997; 278: 138–41.

38. Thompson JS, Bixler SA, Qian F et al. BAFF-R, a novel TNF receptor that specifically interacts with BAFF. Science 2001; 293: 2108–11.

39. Yan M, Brady JR, Chan B et al. Identification of a novel receptor for B lymphocyte stimulator that is mutated in a mouse strain with severe B cell deficiency. Curr Biol 2001; 11: 1547–52.

40. Xia X-Z, Treanor J, Senaldi G et al. TACI is a TRAF-interacting receptor for TALL-1, a tumor necrosis factor family member involved in B cell regulation. J Exp Med 2000; 192: 137–43.

41. Underhill GH, George D, Bremer EG, Kansas GS. Gene expression profiling reveals a highly specialized genetic program of plasma cells. Blood 2003; 101: 4013–21.

42. Tarte K, Zhan F, De Vos J, Klein B, Shaughnessy J Jr. Gene expression profiling of plasma cells and plasmablasts: toward a better understanding of the late stages of B-cell differentiation. Blood 2003; 102: 592–600.

43. Avery DT, Kalled SL, Ellyard JI et al. BAFF selectively enhances the survival of plasmablasts generated from human memory B cells. J Clin Invest 2003; 112: 286–97.

44. O'Connor BP, Raman VS, Erickson LD et al. BCMA is essential for the survival of long-lived bone marrow plasma cells. J Exp Med 2004; 199: 91–7.

45. Shu H-B, Johnson H. B cell maturation protein is a receptor for the tumor necrosis factor family member TALL-1. Proc Natl Acad Sci U S A 2000; 97: 9156–61.

46. Hatzoglou A, Roussel J, Bourgeade M-F et al. TNF receptor family member BCMA (B cell maturation) associates with TNF receptor-associated factor (TRAF) 1, TRAF2, and TRAF3 and activates NF-κB, Elk-1, c-Jun N-terminal kinase, and p38 mitogen-activated protein kinase. J Immunol 2000; 165: 1322–30.

47. Xu L-G, Shu H-B. TNFR-associated factor-3 is associated with BAFF-R and negatively regulates BAFF-R-mediated NF-κB activation and IL-10 production. J Immunol 2002; 169: 6883–9.

48. Hikida M, Johmura S, Hashimoto A, Takezaki M, Kurosaki T. Coupling between B cell receptor and phospholipase C-γ2 is essential for mature B cell development. J Exp Med 2003; 198: 581–9.

49. Claudio E, Brown K, Park S, Wang H, Siebenlist U. BAFF-induced NEMO-independent processing of NK-κB2 in maturing B cells. Nat Immunol 2002; 3: 958–65.

50. Kayagaki N, Yan M, Seshasayee D et al. BAFF/BLyS receptor 3 binds the B cell survival factor BAFF ligand through a discrete surface loop and promotes processing of NF-κB2. Immunity 2002; 10: 515–24.

51. Hatada EN, Do RKG, Orlofsky A et al. NF-κB1 p50 is required for BLyS attenuation of apoptosis but dispensible for processing of NF-κB2 p100 to p52 in quiescent mature B cells. J Immunol 2003; 171: 761–8.

52. Herrin BR, Justement LB. Expression of the adaptor protein hematopoietic Src homology 2 is up-regulated in response to stimuli that promote survival and differentiation of B cells. J Immunol 2006; 176: 4163–72.

53. Mecklenbräuker I, Kalled SL, Leitges M, Mackay F, Tarakhovsky A. Regulation of B-cell survival by BAFF-dependent PKCδ-mediated nuclear signalling. Nature 2004; 431: 456–61.

54. Hase H, Kanno Y, Kojima M et al. BAFF/BLyS can potentiate B-cell selection with the B-cell co-receptor complex. Blood 2004; 103: 2257–65.

55. d'Arbonneau F, Pers J-O, Devauchelle V et al. BAFF-induced changes in B cell antigen receptor-containing lipid rafts in Sjögren's syndrome. Arthritis Rheum 2006; 54: 115–26.

56. Thompson JS, Schneider P, Kalled SL et al. BAFF binds to the tumor necrosis factor receptor-like molecule B cell maturation antigen and is important for maintaining the peripheral B cell population. J Exp Med 2000; 192: 129–35.

57. Do RKG, Hatada E, Lee H et al. Attenuation of apoptosis underlies B lymphocyte stimulator enhancement of humoral immune response. J Exp Med 2000; 192: 953–64.

58. Batten M, Groom J, Cachero TG et al. BAFF mediates survival of peripheral immature B lymphocytes. J Exp Med 2000; 192: 1453–65.

59. Harless SM, Lentz VM, Sah AP et al. Competition for BLyS-mediated signaling through Bcmd/BR3 regulates peripheral B lymphocyte numbers. Curr Biol 2001; 11: 1986–9.

60. Hsu BL, Harless SM, Lindsley RC, Hilbert DM, Cancro MP. Cutting edge: BLyS enables survival of transitional and mature B cells through distinct mediators. J Immunol 2002; 168: 5993–6.

61. Mongini PKA, Inman JK, Han H et al. APRIL and BAFF promote increased viability of replicating human B2 cells via mechanism involving cyclooxygenase 2. J Immunol 2006; 176: 6736–51.

62. Craxton A, Draves KE, Gruppi A, Clark EA. BAFF regulates B cell survival by downregulating the BH3-only family member Bim via the ERK pathway. J Exp Med 2005; 202: 1363–74.

63. Oliver PM, Vass T, Kappler J, Marrack P. Loss of the proapoptotic protein, Bim, breaks B cell anergy. J Exp Med 2006; 203: 731–41.

64. Amanna IJ, Dingwall JP, Hayes CE. Enforced bcl-x$_L$ gene expression restored splenic B lymphocyte development in BAFF-R mutant mice. J Immunol 2003; 170: 4593–600.

65. Sasaki Y, Derudder E, Hobeika E et al. Canonical NF-κB activity, dispensable for B cell development, replaces BAFF-receptor signals and promotes B cell proliferation upon activation. Immunity 2006; 24: 729–39.

66. Rolink AG, Tschopp J, Schneider P, Melchers F. BAFF is a survival and maturation factor for mouse B cells. Eur J Immunol 2002; 32: 2004–10.

67. Tardivel A, Tinel A, Lens S et al. The anti-apoptotic factor Bcl-2 can functionally substitute for the B cell survival but not for the marginal zone B cell differentiation activity of BAFF. Eur J Immunol 2004; 34: 509–18.

68. Yamada T, Zhang K, Yamada A, Zhu D, Saxon A. B lymphocyte stimulator activates p38 mitogen-activated protein kinase in human Ig class switch recombination. Am J Respir Cell Mol Biol 2005; 32: 388–94.

69. Castigli E, Wilson SA, Scott S et al. TACI and BAFF-R mediate isotype switching in B cells. J Exp Med 2005; 201: 35–9.

70. Ng LG, Ng C-H, Woehl B et al. BAFF costimulation of Toll-like receptor-activated B-1 cells. Eur J Immunol 2006; 36: 1837–46.

71. Miller JP, Stadanlick JE, Cancro MP. Space, selection, and surveillance: setting boundaries with BLyS. J Immunol 2006; 176: 6405–10.

72. Mackay F, Woodcock SA, Lawton P et al. Mice transgenic for BAFF develop lymphocytic disorders along with autoimmune manifestations. J Exp Med 1999; 190: 1697–710.

73. Khare SD, Sarosi I, Xia X-Z et al. Severe B cell hyperplasia and autoimmune disease in TALL-1 transgenic mice. Proc Natl Acad Sci U S A 2000; 97: 3370–5.

74. Aït-Azzouzene D, Gavin AL, Skog P, Duong B, Nemazee D. Effect of cell: cell competition and BAFF expression on peripheral B cell tolerance and B-1 cell survival in transgenic mice expressing a low level of Igκ-reactive macroself antigen. Eur J Immunol 2006; 36: 985–96.

75. Morel L, Rudofsky UH, Longmate JA, Schiffenbauer J, Wakeland EK. Polygenic control of susceptibility to murine systemic lupus erythematosus. Immunity 1994; 1: 219–29.

76. Rozzo SJ, Allard JD, Choubey D et al. Evidence for an interferon-inducible gene, Ifi202, in the susceptibility to systemic lupus. Immunity 2001; 15: 435–43.

77. Morel L, Mohan C, Yu Y et al. Functional dissection of systemic lupus erythematosus using congenic mouse strains. J Immunol 1997; 158: 6019–28.

78. Mohan C, Alas E, Morel L, Yang P, Wakeland EK. Genetic dissection of SLE pathogenesis: Sle1 on murine chromosome 1 leads to a selective loss of tolerance to H2A/H2B/DNA subnucleosomes. J Clin Invest 1998; 101: 1362–72.

79. Stohl W, Xu D, Kim KS et al. BAFF overexpression and accelerated glomerular disease in mice with an incomplete genetic predisposition to systemic lupus erythematosus. Arthritis Rheum 2005; 52: 2080–91.

80. Groom J, Kalled SL, Cutler AH et al. Association of BAFF/BLyS overexpression and altered B cell differentiation with Sjögren's syndrome. J Clin Invest 2002; 109: 59–68.

81. Zhang M, Ko K-H, Lam QLK et al. Expression and function of TNF family member B cell-activating factor in the development of autoimmune arthritis. Int Immunol 2005; 17: 1081–92.

82. Gross JA, Dillon SR, Mudri S et al. TACI-Ig neutralizes molecules critical for B cell development and autoimmune disease: impaired B cell maturation in mice lacking BLyS. Immunity 2001; 15: 289–302.

83. Schiemann B, Gommerman JL, Vora K et al. An essential role for BAFF in the normal development of B cells through a BCMA-independent pathway. Science 2001; 293: 2111–14.

84. Xu S, Lam D-P. B-cell maturation protein, which binds the tumor necrosis factor family members BAFF and APRIL, is dispensible for humoral immune responses. Mol Cell Biol 2001; 21: 4067–74.

85. Yang M, Hase H, Legarda-Addison D et al. BCMA, the receptor for APRIL and BAFF, induces antigen presentation in B cells. J Immunol 2005; 175: 2814–24.

86. Shlomchik MJ, Madaio MP, Ni D, Trounstein M, Huszar D. The role of B cells in lpr/lpr-induced autoimmunity. J Exp Med 1994; 180: 1295–306.

87. Chan O, Shlomchik MJ. A new role for B cells in systemic autoimmunity: B cells promote spontaneous T cell activation in MRL-lpr/lpr mice. J Immunol 1998; 160: 51–9.

88. Chan OTM, Hannum LG, Haberman AM, Madaio MP, Shlomchik MJ. A novel mouse with B cells but lacking serum antibody reveals an antibody-independent role for B cells in murine lupus. J Exp Med 1999; 189: 1639–47.

89. von Bülow G-U, van Deursen JM, Bram RJ. Regulation of the T-independent humoral response by TACI. Immunity 2001; 14: 573–82.

90. Yan M, Wang H, Chan B et al. Activation and accumulation of B cells in TACI-deficient mice. Nat Immunol 2001; 2: 638–43.

91. Seshasayee D, Valdez P, Yan M et al. Loss of TACI causes fatal lymphoproliferation and autoimmunity, establishing TACI as an inhibitory BLyS receptor. Immunity 2003; 18: 279–88.

92. Salzer U, Chapel HM, Webster ADB et al. Mutations in *TNFRSF13B* encoding TACI are associated with common variable immunodeficiency in humans. Nat Genet 2005; 37: 820–8.

93. Castigli E, Wilson SA, Garibyan L et al. TACI is mutant in common variable immunodeficiency and IgA deficiency. Nat Genet 2005; 37: 829–34.

94. Sasaki Y, Casola S, Kutok JL, Rajewski K, Schmidt-Supprian M. TNF family member B cell-activating factor (BAFF) receptor-dependent and -independent roles for BAFF in B cell physiology. J Immunol 2004; 173: 2245–52.

95. Shulga-Morskaya S, Dobles M, Walsh ME et al. B cell-activating factor belonging to the TNF family acts through separate receptors to support B cell survival and T cell-independent antibody formation. J Immunol 2004; 173: 2331–41.

96. Gorelik L, Cutler AH, Thill G et al. Cutting edge: BAFF regulates CD21/35 and CD23 expression independent of its B cell survival function. J Immunol 2004; 172: 762–6.

97. Lesley R, Xu Y, Kalled SL et al. Reduced competitiveness of autoantigen-engaged B cells due to increased dependence on BAFF. Immunity 2004; 20: 441–53.

98. Thien M, Phan TG, Gardam S et al. Excess BAFF rescues self-reactive B cells from peripheral deletion and allows them to enter forbidden follicular and marginal zone niches. Immunity 2004; 20: 785–98.

99. Jacob CO, Pricop L, Putterman C et al. Paucity of clinical disease despite serological autoimmunity and kidney pathology in lupus-prone New Zealand Mixed 2328 mice deficient in BAFF. J Immunol 2006; 177: 2671–80.

100. Ramanujam M, Wang X, Huang W et al. Mechanism of action of transmembrane activator and calcium modulator ligand interactor-Ig in murine systemic lupus erythematosus. J Immunol 2004; 173: 3524–34.

101. Ramanujam M, Wang X, Huang W et al. Similarities and differences between selective and nonselective BAFF blockade in murine SLE. J Clin Invest 2006; 116: 724–34.

102. Wang H, Marsters SA, Baker T et al. TACI-ligand interactions are required for T cell activation and collagen-induced arthritis in mice. Nat Immunol 2001; 2: 632–7.

103. Gilbert JA, Kalled SL, Moorhead H et al. Treatment of autoimmune hyperthyroidism in a murine model of Graves' disease with tumor necrosis factor-family

104. Hahne M, Kataoka T, Schröter M et al. APRIL, a new ligand of the tumor necrosis factor family, stimulates tumor cell growth. J Exp Med 1998; 188: 1185–90.

105. Kelly K, Manos E, Jensen G, Nadauld L, Jones DA. APRIL/TRDL-1, a tumor necrosis factor-like ligand, stimulates cell death. Cancer Res 2000; 60: 1021–7.

106. Marsters SA, Yan M, Pitti RM et al. Interaction of the TNF homologues BLyS and APRIL with the receptor homologues BCMA and TACI. Curr Biol 2000; 10: 785–8.

107. Yu G, Boone T, Delaney J et al. APRIL and TALL-1 and receptors BCMA and TACI: system for regulating humoral immunity. Nat Immunol 2000; 1: 252–6.

108. Wu Y, Bressette D, Carrell JA et al. Tumor necrosis factor (TNF) receptor superfamily member TACI is a high affinity receptor for TNF family members APRIL and BLyS. J Biol Chem 2000; 275: 35478–85.

109. Rennert P, Schneider P, Cachero TG et al. A soluble form of B cell maturation antigen, a receptor for the tumor necrosis factor family member APRIL, inhibits tumor cell growth. J Exp Med 2000; 192: 1677–83.

110. Craxton A, Magaletti D, Ryan EJ, Clark EA. Macrophage- and dendritic cell-dependent regulation of human B-cell proliferation requires the TNF family ligand BAFF. Blood 2003; 101: 4464–71.

111. Hendriks J, Planelles L, de Jong-Odding J et al. Heparan sulfate proteoglycan binding promotes APRIL-induced tumor cell proliferation. Cell Death Differ 2005; 12: 637–48.

112. Ingold K, Zumsteg A Tardivel A et al. Identification of proteoglycans as the APRIL-specific binding partners. J Exp Med 2005; 201: 1375–83.

113. Varfolomeev E, Kischkel F, Martin F et al. APRIL-deficient mice have normal immune system development. Mol Cell Biol 2004; 24: 997–1006.

114. Castigli E, Scott S, Dedeoglu F et al. Impaired IgA class switching in APRIL-deficient mice. Proc Natl Acad Sci U S A 2004; 101: 3903–8.

115. Stein JV, López-Fraga M, Elustondo FA et al. APRIL modulates B and T cell immunity. J Clin Invest 2002; 109: 1587–98.

116. Roschke V, Sosnovtseva S, Ward CD et al. BLyS and APRIL form biologically active heterotrimers that are expressed in patients with systemic immune-based rheumatic diseases. J Immunol 2002; 169: 4314–21.

117. Bischof D, Elsawa SF, Mantchev G et al. Selective activation of TACI by syndecan-2. Blood 2006; 107: 3235–42.

118. Stohl W, Metyas S, Tan S-M et al. Inverse association between circulating APRIL levels and serologic and

clinical disease activity in patients with systemic lupus erythematosus. Ann Rheum Dis 2004; 63: 1096–103.

119. Zhang J, Roschke V, Baker KP et al. Cutting edge: a role for B lymphocyte stimulator in systemic lupus erythematosus. J Immunol 2001; 166: 6–10.

120. Cheema GS, Roschke V, Hilbert DM, Stohl W. Elevated serum B lymphocyte stimulator levels in patients with systemic immune-based rheumatic diseases. Arthritis Rheum 2001; 44: 1313–19.

121. Stohl W, Metyas S, Tan S-M et al. B lymphocyte stimulator overexpression in patients with systemic lupus erythematosus: longitudinal observations. Arthritis Rheum 2003; 48: 3475–86.

122. Petri M, Stohl W, Chatham W et al. Association of BLyS™ with measures of disease activity in a prospective SLE observational study. Arthritis Rheum 2004; 50: S603.

123. Collins CE, Gavin AL, Migone T-S et al. B lymphocyte stimulator (BLyS) isoforms in systemic lupus erythematosus: disease activity correlates better with blood leukocyte BLyS mRNA levels than with plasma BLyS protein levels. Arthritis Res Ther 2006; 8: R6.

124. Davis JC Jr, Gross J, Gescuk B, Harder B, Wofsy D. zTNF4 and soluble TACI receptor levels in serum and urine may reflect disease activity in patients with SLE. Arthritis Rheum 2001; 44: S99.

125. Carter RH, Zhao H, Liu X et al. Expression and occupancy of BAFF-R on B cells in systemic lupus erythematosus. Arthritis Rheum 2005; 52: 3943–54.

126. Cambridge G, Stohl W, Leandro MJ et al. Circulating levels of B lymphocyte stimulator in patients with rheumatoid arthritis following rituximab treatment: relationships with B cell depletion, circulating antibodies, and clinical relapse. Arthritis Rheum 2006; 54: 723–32.

127. Tan S-M, Xu D, Roschke V et al. Local production of B lymphocyte stimulator protein and APRIL in arthritic joints of patients with inflammatory arthritis. Arthritis Rheum 2003; 48: 982–92.

128. Seyler TM, Park YW, Takemura S et al. BLyS and APRIL in rheumatoid arthritis. J Clin Invest 2005; 115: 3083–92.

129. Mariette X, Roux S, Zhang J et al. The level of BLyS (BAFF) correlates with the titre of autoantibodies in human Sjögren's syndrome. Ann Rheum Dis 2003; 62: 168–71.

130. Jonsson MV, Szodoray P, Jellestad S, Jonsson R, Skarstein K. Association between circulating levels of the novel TNF family members APRIL and BAFF and lymphoid organization in primary Sjögren's syndrome. J Clin Immunol 2005; 25: 189–201.

131. Pers J-O, Daridon C, Devauchelle V et al. BAFF overexpression is associated with autoantibody production in autoimmune diseases. Ann N Y Acad Sci 2005; 1050: 34–9.

132. Pers J-O, d'Arbonneau F, Devauchelle-Pensec V et al. Is periodontal disease mediated by salivary BAFF in Sjögren's syndrome? Arthritis Rheum 2005; 52: 2411–14.

133. Szodoray P, Jellestad S, Teague MO, Jonsson R. Attenuated apoptosis of B cell activating factor-expressing cells in primary Sjögren's syndrome. Lab Invest 2003; 83: 357–65.

134. Lavie F, Miceli-Richard C, Quillard J et al. Expression of BAFF (BLyS) in T cells infiltrating labial salivary glands from patients with Sjögren's syndrome. J Pathol 2004; 202: 496–502.

135. Ittah M, Miceli-Richard C, Gottenberg J-E et al. B cell-activating factor of the tumor necrosis factor family (BAFF) is expressed under stimulation by interferon in salivary gland epithelial cells in primary Sjögren's syndrome. Arthritis Res Ther 2006; 8: R51.

136. Daridon C, Pers J-O, Devauchelle V et al. Identification of transitional type II B cells in the salivary glands of patients with Sjögren's syndrome. Arthritis Rheum 2006; 54: 2280–8.

137. Matsushita T, Hasegawa M, Yanaba K et al. Elevated serum BAFF levels in patients with systemic sclerosis: enhanced BAFF signaling in systemic sclerosis B lymphocytes. Arthritis Rheum 2006; 54: 192–201.

138. Krumbholz M, Specks U, Wick M et al. BAFF is elevated in serum of patients with Wegener's granulomatosis. J Autoimmun 2005; 25: 298–302.

139. Sanders JS, Huitma MG, Kallenberg CGM, Stegeman CA. Plasma levels of soluble interleukin 2 receptor, soluble CD30, interleukin 10, and B cell activator of the tumor necrosis factor family during follow-up in vasculitis associated with proteinase-3-antineutrophil cytoplasmic antibodies: associations with disease activity and relapse. Ann Rheum Dis 2006; 65: 1484–9.

140. Baker KP, Edwards BM, Main SH et al. Generation and characterization of LymphoStat-B, a human monoclonal antibody that antagonizes the bioactivities of B lymphocyte stimulator. Arthritis Rheum 2003; 48: 3253–65.

141. Furie R, Stohl W, Ginzler E et al. Safety, pharmacokinetic and pharmacodynamic results of a phase 1 single and double dose-escalation study of Lymphostat-B (human monoclonal antibody to BLyS) in SLE patients. Arthritis Rheum 2003; 48: S377.

142. McKay J, Chwalinska-Sadowska H, Boling E et al. Belimumab (BmAb), a fully human monoclonal antibody to B-lymphocyte stimulator (BLyS), combined with standard of care therapy reduces the signs and symptoms of rheumatoid arthritis in a heterogeneous subject population. Arthritis Rheum 2005; 52: S710–S711.

143. Stohl W, Chatham W, Weisman M et al. Belimumab (BmAb), a novel fully human monoclonal antibody to B-lymphocyte stimulator (BLyS), selectively modulates B-cell sub-populations and immunoglobulins in a

heterogeneous rheumatoid arthritis subject population. Arthritis Rheum 2005; 52: S444.

144. Emery P, Fleischmann RM, Filipowicz-Sosnowska A et al. Rituximab in rheumatoid arthritis: a double-blind, placebo-controlled, dose-ranging trial. Arthritis Rheum 2005; 52: S709.

145. Wallace DJ, Lisse J, Stohl W et al. Belimumab (BMAB), a fully human monoclonal antibody to B-lymphocyte stimulator (BLYS), shows bioactivity and reduces systemic lupus erythematosus disease activity. EULAR Abstracts Online 2006.

146. Gong Q, Ou Q, Ye S et al. Importance of cellular microenvironment and circulatory dynamics in B cell immunotherapy. J Immunol 2005; 174: 817–26.

147. Stohl W, Cheema GS, Briggs W et al. B lymphocyte stimulator protein-associated increase in circulating autoantibody levels may require CD4+ T cells: lessons from HIV-infected patients. Clin Immunol 2002; 104: 115–22.

148. Rodriguez B, Valdez H, Freimuth W et al. Plasma levels of B-lymphocyte stimulator increase with HIV disease progression. AIDS 2003; 17: 1983–5.

43

Anti-CD3 antibody – a history of successful immune interventions

Damien Bresson and Matthias von Herrath

Introduction • Pharmacology of anti-CD3 antibodies • Anti-CD3 antibody in organ transplantation • Tolerogenic capacity of anti-CD3 antibodies in autoimmune diseases • Anti-CD3 therapy in rheumatology • Concluding remarks • Acknowledgments • References

INTRODUCTION

The immune system controls a variety of physiologic but also pathologic mechanisms. Consequently, all autoimmune processes have to be tightly controlled to maintain a healthy balance in the body. In order to counteract any immunological disorders or pathologic events, a plethora of immune interventions have been validated in preclinical studies. Although a majority showed great promise in animal models, the data observed in human clinical trials were more contrasted. The first most promising drugs were highly unspecific and induced strong immune suppression.[1-3] Immuno-suppressive agents available until 1978 included the alkylating agent, cyclophosphomide, the folic acid antagonist, methotrexate, and in addition azothioprine and corticosteroids. They block cellular division non-specifically. All these methods produce severe side effects due to their general cytotoxicity or their inherent lack of pharmacological specificity. Then, cyclosporin A was the first of a new generation of immuno-suppressive agents with a specific site of action within the immune system.[4] Its action is directed specifically towards the lymphocyte, at an early stage of its activation. It has a very low degree of myelotoxicity, which has made its use in clinical transplantation attractive. It suppresses lymphocyte function without damaging the phagocytic activity and migratory capacity of the reticulo-endothelial system. Cyclosporin A was first used clinically in 1978 and within a short period of time, the majority of the transplant centers in the world started using it for transplantation surgeries.[5,6]

In the mean time, much work has been put into the design of new therapeutic strategies that will present lower levels of side effects but will retain substantial efficacy. One efficient method to reach this goal was to increase the specificity of the therapeutic drugs. In 1975 Kohler and Milstein described a method by which antibodies could be made in vitro and the monoclonal antibody (mAb) era was born.[7] Then a major step was achieved toward the antigen-specific targeting of the immune system. Despite the generation of many mAbs against a series of surface or intracellular antigens, few of them underwent clinical evaluations due to a lack of efficacy or some adverse side effects that would have been unacceptable in humans. However, an antibody directed against the CD3 molecule was found to be particularly successful in delaying or treating several immune disorders.

PHARMACOLOGY OF ANTI-CD3 ANTIBODIES

The CD3 complex is a group of cell surface molecules found specifically on T lymphocytes (both on CD4+ and CD8+ T cells) and composed of three invariant subchains belonging to the immunoglobulin superfamily, γ, δ, and ε.[8] The CD3 molecule is associated with the T-cell antigen receptor (TCR) and functions in the cell surface expression of TCR and in the signaling transduction cascade that originates when a peptide/major histocompatibility complex (MHC) ligand, displayed by antigen-presenting cells (APCs), binds to the TCR (Figure 43.1). In 1979, Kung and colleagues generated the first murine mAb directed against the human CD3 molecule, called OKT3.[9] OKT3 is a mouse IgG2 mAb that shows potent mitogenic properties on T cells.[10] This property specific to all anti-CD3 antibodies promotes an extensive T-cell proliferation and cytokine production both *in vitro* and

in vivo.[11–13] This was considered to be one major side effect observed upon anti-CD3 administration *in vivo*. The antibody recipients commonly suffered from a 'flu-like' syndrome associated with fever, headache, nausea, vomiting, and gastrointestinal disturbance. These symptoms are transient, lasting from 2 to 3 days, and are due to the ability of the fragment crystallized (Fc) portion of the mAb to interact with the Fc receptor on monocytes/macrophages inducing a massive systemic release of both T-helper 1 (TNF-α, IFN-γ, IL-2) and T-helper 2 (IL-6 and IL-10) cytokines.[14–20] Other side effects, described in rodents or in humans, are inherent with strong immunosuppression and consist of partial lymphopenia (as long as the antibody is found in the body), virus infection or reactivation (mainly cytomegalovirus and Epstein–Barr virus), and tumors, but also production of human anti-mouse antibodies (HAMAs).[21–26] To circumvent such adverse effects, the OKT3 mAb was

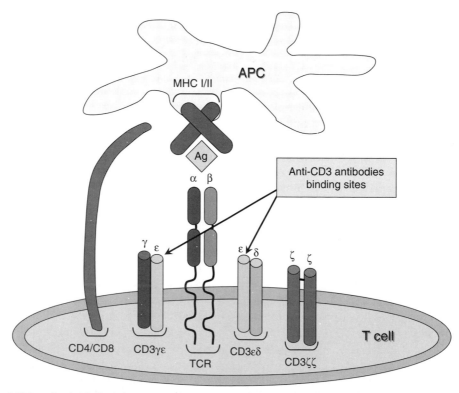

Figure 43.1 Anti-CD3 antibody binding sites shown in the context of the immune synapse. OKT3 as well as 145-2C11 anti-CD3 monoclonal antibodies recognize an epitope on the CD3e molecule. APC, antigen-presenting cells; MHC I/II, major histocompatibility complex class I or II; Ag, antigen; TCR, T-cell receptor.

engineered to avoid binding of the Fc portion to their receptors, namely CD16, CD32, and CD64 (Table 43.1). For preclinical evaluations a hamster anti-mouse CD3 mAb (145-2C11) was derived by immunizing Armenian hamsters with a murine cytolytic T-cell clone.[27] The anti-CD3 145-2C11 antibody is also specific for the ε chain of the CD3 complex and reacts with all mature T cells, with the ability to activate or inhibit certain T-cell functions similar to what was observed with OKT3.

Recently, the crystal structure of human CD3ε-γ in complex with a fragment antigen binding (Fab) of OKT3 has been solved.[28] Consequently, the Rossjohn's group described that the OKT3 antibody interacts exclusively with a conformational epitope of the CD3ε subunit and has a low affinity for the isolated CD3ε-γ heterodimer.

ANTI-CD3 ANTIBODY IN ORGAN TRANSPLANTATION

In 1985, the results from the first randomized clinical trial with the murine mAb OKT3 were published.[24] This trial aimed at exploring its effectiveness in treating T-cell-mediated rejection of renal allografts. Among the 63 patients, undergoing acute rejection of cadaveric renal transplants and treated with daily injections of OKT3 for 14 days, 93% showed rapid reversal of allograft rejection with a 1-year graft survival of 62%. In the mean time, 60 patients who received conventional high dose steroids as immunosuppressor demonstrated a reversal rate of 75%, which was significantly lower than the antibody therapy. Based on these very promising observations, in 1984 the US Food and Drug Agency (FDA) as well as other regulatory authorities worldwide approved the use of Orthoklone (OKT3), manufactured by Ortho-Biotech, for treating acute kidney transplant rejection. Importantly, this antibody was the first licensed for therapy in humans. Even though the efficacy of OKT3 in reversing and preventing acute allograft rejection was reported many times,[24,25,29–34] the cytokine release syndrome described above impaired its value as a therapeutic compound in humans. Therefore, development of engineered OKT3 antibodies was an essential milestone in their clinical application (Table 43.1). A series of non-Fc-binding anti-CD3 antibodies was developed and tested clinically in kidney, islet, and bone marrow transplantation. They all share the same ability to induce transient lymphodepletion lasting from a couple of days to a couple of weeks after treatment has ended.

So far, four phase I/II clinical trials have been conducted to prevent acute renal allograft rejection. First, a humanized IgG1 form of OKT3 (hOKT3γ1(Ala-Ala)) was mutated in the Fc portion (amino acids 234 and 235 were replaced by alanines) to avoid binding to Fc receptors.[35] Seven patients were treated daily with hOKT3γ1(Ala-Ala) (from 5 to 10 mg/day) for 10 consecutive days to achieve serum levels of 1 µg/ml. Among them five patients showed a rapid reversal of rejection which was prolonged over a year without strong side effects. Second, nine patients received an aglycosylated humanized

Table 43.1 Engineered anti-CD3 antibodies in clinical trials

Name	Antibody	Trial	Clinical indication	References
hOKT3γ1(Ala-Ala)	Mutated humanized IgG[1]	Phase I	Kidney transplant	35
		Phase I	Islet transplantation	40
		Phase II	Arthritis	69
		Phase II/III	Type 1 diabetes mellitus	61, 62
Visilizumab (HuM291)	Mutated humanized IgG[2]	Phase I	Bone marrow transplantation	38, 41
		Phase I	Kidney transplant	77
T3/4.A	Mouse IgA	Phase II	Kidney transplant	39
Campath 3 (YTH12.5 or ChAglyCD3)	Aglycosylated humanized IgG1	Phase I	Kidney transplant	36
		Phase II/III	Type 1 diabetes mellitus	68

IgG1 (campath 3 or ChAglyCD3) for 8 consecutive days at 8 mg/day.[36] None of the patients demonstrated any antiglobulin response or any significant cytokine release syndrome. Almost 78% showed proof of resolution of their rejection, although some patients experienced re-rejection. The third trial was a phase I dose escalation study performed by using a humanized IgG2 (HuM291 or visilizumab), engineered to have less mitogenic activity in humans.[37,38] A single dose of 0.015 mg/kg was well tolerated with only mild to moderate side effects and was sufficient to induce T-cell depletion for up to 1 week post treatment. Lastly, a non-mitogenic murine IgA antibody (T3/4.A) to human CD3 was tested in a phase II clinical trial.[39] Fifteen patients were enrolled and received an intravenous injection with 5 mg per day for 10 consecutive days. Most of the patients developed transient vomiting and/or diarrhea, which coincided with elevated serum levels of proinflammatory cytokines. These side effects disappeared after antibody clearance.

In the field of autoimmune diabetes, one of the most attractive approaches is transplantation of insulin-secreting β cells into diabetic patients. Although islet transplantation protocols have been improved, clinicians are still seeking immunomodulating agents that could prolong graft survival with low adverse events. To reach this goal, the hOKT3γ1(Ala-Ala) mAb was applied for 12 consecutive days (4 mg/day), beginning 2 days before their islet allograft transplants.[40] Four of six patients achieved and maintained insulin independence with normal metabolic control. The side effects were limited to a transient rash in one patient and temporary neutropenia in three of them.

Finally, the HuM291 mAb showed great promise for the treatment of acute graft-versus-host disease (GVHD), mediated by donor T cells and presenting a major barrier to successful hematopoietic cell transplant. The risk-benefit ratio was found to be acceptable, with a single-dose regimen of HuM291 of 3 mg/m² corresponding to a dosage ranging from 0.5 to 6.15 mg/patient. The drug was well tolerated and some signs of GVHD amelioration were observed in a majority of recipients.[41] Further trials need to be performed to determine the efficacy of visilizumab in GVDH.

To conclude, engineered anti-CD3 mAbs constitute promising tools to prevent acute allograft rejection. However, it is worth noting that all therapeutic protocols cited before were associated with conventional immunosuppression. Thus, future improvements in acute allograft rejection therapies should avoid conventional immunosuppressive agents. Importantly, anti-CD3 antibodies were not solely efficient in transplantation but showed the unique property of restoring self-tolerance in the autoimmune setting.

TOLEROGENIC CAPACITY OF ANTI-CD3 ANTIBODIES IN AUTOIMMUNE DISEASES

Alloimmunity and autoimmunity share a number of important afferent, effector, and regulatory immunological pathways. It is likely that they also share overlapping specificities that at least partially explain the ability of allograft rejection to trigger autoimmune responses, the increased susceptibility of patients with autoimmune diseases to allograft rejection, and a strikingly similar histopathologic appearance of acute and chronic rejection to some organ-specific autoimmune diseases. Therefore, with regard to the potent tolerogenic effect of anti-CD3 mAbs in alloimmunity, it was highly relevant to evaluate their effect in autoimmune settings. Consequently, in the early 1990s, the group of A.R. Hayward and M. Shreiber observed for the first time that a single neonatal injection with anti-CD3 145-2C11 modulates the T-cell repertoire and stops or delays autoimmunity in non-obese diabetic (NOD) mice, the genetically predisposed mouse model for type 1 diabetes mellitus (T1DM).[42] From this date, much work has been accomplished to unravel the mechanisms involved in such a therapeutic potency and to bring anti-CD3 mAbs closer to the clinic for autoimmune diseases.

Non-mitogenic anti-CD3 antibodies restore self-tolerance in autoimmune diabetes

T1DM is one of the most common autoimmune diseases, with an estimated yearly incidence that ranges from 3.7 to 20 per 100 000. During pathogenesis, autoreactive CD4+ and CD8+ T cells are generated and progressively destroy the insulin-producing pancreatic β cells. A destruction of approximately 80% of β cells occurs before type 1 patients become symptomatic both in animal models and in humans. In the past two decades, immunomodulatory approaches to prevent or cure T1DM have been developed and tested with some encouraging results. However, development of a cure for T1DM has been particularly difficult, because insulin injected into the body as a palliative therapy affords a reasonable life quality and expectancy. Moreover, the disease frequently affects young adults and children and therefore, the ethical window for any treatment is rather small and long-term side effects have to be avoided. Thus, the risk-benefit ratio for potential therapeutic drugs has to be carefully weighed. Conversely, insulin cannot prevent all of the late complications of T1DM, and the life expectancy can be reduced by 10–15 years due to serious complications including retinopathy, nephropathy, cardiovascular diseases or neuropathy.[43] Thus, production of non-mitogenic anti-CD3 mAbs that are deprived of strong side effects resurrected the interest of the scientists in these molecules.

First, the anti-CD3 mAb 145 2C11 was engineered as a non-Fc-binding F(ab')$_2$ for preclinical studies. Short-course treatment with this antibody was shown to reverse diabetes in hyperglycemic NOD mice.[44,45] Therapeutic efficacy was related to two striking features. First, the treatment was most efficient when administered into already diabetic animals and injection into prediabetic mice was not effective in delaying or preventing T1DM. This was highly unusual since more than 200 treatments were capable of preventing T1DM but very few can reverse it after hyperglycemia has occurred.[46] Second, in contrast to what was observed with strong immunosuppressive agents, long-term immune suppression was not needed to maintain permanent tolerance to β cell autoantigens. A 5-day course of therapy with low dose anti-CD3 F(ab')$_2$ was sufficient to cure diabetes after onset in a majority of mice and hyperglycemia did not recur over time. It is worth noting that efficacy of anti-CD3 was not mouse strain-dependent, since a similar protection after new-onset diabetes was reported in the transgenic rat

insulin promoter-lymphocytic choriomeningitis virus (RIP-LCMV) mice, a second model where T1DM is induced by infection with LCMV.[47] In subsequent studies, the group of J.F Bach and L. Chatenoud shed light on potential mechanisms involved in the anti-diabetogenic effect observed with anti-CD3 F(ab')$_2$. They demonstrated that it induced active tolerance mediated by regulatory T cells (Tregs) expressing the surface markers CD4 (coreceptor in the immunological synapse), CD25 (interleukin-2 receptor: IL-2), and CD62L (lymphocyte adhesion molecule 1: L-selectin). When co-transferred with diabetogenic effector T cells into immunocompromised NOD-SCID mice, these Tregs induced protection from diabetes.[44,45,48 56] Such a strong protective effect was not observed when CD4$^+$CD25$^+$ T cells from anti-CD3-protected mice were adoptively transferred into immunocompetent RIP-LCMV recipient mice.[47,57] These observations raise the paramount question whether a systemic immune modulator such as anti-CD3 acting on virtually all T cells, and not only on islet-specific T cells, may expand sufficient number of islet-specific Tregs *in vivo* to induce full protection when transferred into immunocompetent recipients. In the mean time, it emphasizes that the tolerogenic capacity of anti-CD3-specific mAb involves two phases to be fully functional when administered into newly diabetic animals.[49,50] The first induction phase, lasting approximately a week after antibody injection ended, is associated with a direct action on autoaggressive effector T cells. The insulitis in anti-CD3-treated mice is rapidly cleared within 2 or 3 days leading to normoglycemia. Then, a second phase involving an expansion of Tregs is mandatory to maintain permanent tolerance to β cell aAgs. Therefore, adoptive transfer of anti-CD3-induced Tregs into immunocompetent mice only mimics the second phase of the treatment and does not reflect the full protective capacity of anti-CD3 therapy. Mechanistically, the transforming growth factor (TGF)-β secreted by the anti-CD3 expanded Tregs, but not IL-4, plays a central role in the restoration of peripheral active tolerance.[58]

For clinical application, the full humanized IgG1 with a mutated (hOKT3γ1(Ala-Ala)) or aglycosylated (ChAglyCD3) Fc region that prevents them from binding to the Fc receptors has been developed (Table 43.1).[59,60] Based on the preclinical data from mouse models and the early pilot studies of hOKT3γ1(Ala-Ala) in kidney transplantation, the group of J. Bluestone and K.C Herold initiated a trial in patients suffering from recent-onset T1DM.[61] A total of 24 patients, between the ages of 7.5 and 30 years, were enrolled in an open-label control trial and randomized to each of the study groups: a 14-day course treatment with the hOKT3γ1(Ala-Ala) mAb or no mAb. All patients underwent a mixed meal tolerance test and other immunologic studies every 6 months. Thanks to the mutations in the Fc region of the mAb, the adverse events that occurred with drug administration were generally mild and included most commonly rash, fever, and other flu-like symptoms but of less severity than those following administration of OKT3. Therapeutically, over a 24-month period, a single course of treatment within the first 6 weeks after diagnosis significantly preserved the C-peptide response, a cleavage product from the processing of proinsulin to insulin measured to differentiate insulin produced by the body from insulin injected into the body as a palliative therapy.[62] Improvement in the C-peptide levels was also accompanied by amelioration in glucose control reflected by HbA1c level as well as lower exogenous insulin requirements. At a cellular level, hOKT3γ1 (Ala-Ala) therapy significantly augmented IL-10 and IL-5 cytokines in the peripheral blood of responsive patients while IFN-γ and IL-6 cytokine levels were decreased[63,64] Phenotypic studies of peripheral lymphocytes revealed a higher number of IL-10-expressing CD4+ T cells after anti-CD3 treatment. These cells were heterogeneous but generally CD45RO+ (a memory marker), CD25+, CD62L-, and expressed CCR4 (CC chemokine receptor 4). More surprisingly, suppressor CD8+CD25+ Tregs were identified in clinical responders and expanded after therapy.[65–67] These cells were CTLA-4+ (cytotoxic T-lymphocyte-associated antigen 4, encoding a receptor involved in the control of T-cell proliferation and apoptosis) and Foxp3+ (Forkhead box P3, a transcription-repressor protein), and required cell–cell contact for inhibition.

In light of the success obtained with the hOKT3γ1(Ala-Ala) mAb, a European multicenter trial was conducted with the aglycosylated ChyAglyCD3 mAb (Table 43.1). Two major conclusions can be drawn from the first report published 18 months after treatment.[68] First, short-term therapy with ChyAglyCD3 mAb preserved residual β-cell function in patients with new-onset type 1 diabetes and showing the highest β-cell mass at trial entry (C-peptide levels superior to the 50th percentile). Second, the adverse side effects observed in the European trial were more severe than those reported in the American trial. Administration with ChAglyCD3 was associated with moderate flu-like symptoms and transient but generalized Epstein–Barr viral reactivation. Such activation of latent virus particles was probably due to an increase in the anti-CD3 dose, from 28 to 48 mg/patient in the American and European trials, respectively, and should be considered in future clinical applications with any non-Fc-binding anti-CD3 mAbs.

ANTI-CD3 THERAPY IN RHEUMATOLOGY

Psoriatic arthritis (PsA) is a chronic disease characterized by inflammation of the skin (psoriasis) and joints (arthritis). PsA is a systemic rheumatic disease that can also cause inflammation in body tissues away from the joints other than the skin, such as in the eyes, heart, lungs, and kidneys. This pathology shares many features with several other arthritic conditions, such as ankylosing spondylitis, reactive arthritis (formerly Reiter's syndrome), and arthritis associated with Crohn's disease and ulcerative colitis. The efficacy of hOKT3γ1(Ala-Ala) antibody in PsA was evaluated in a phase I/II clinical trial.[69] Seven patients were treated with increasing daily doses of anti-CD3 mAb for 12–14 consecutive days. A short-term decrease of the symptoms (such as inflamed joints and pain scale) was described in six out of seven patients. Unfortunately, at day 90 after treatment only two out of six responders had sustained improvement. No patients developed strong side effects; however, at the highest hOKT3γ1(Ala-Ala) concentration, mild cytokine release symptoms associated with elevation of IL-10 were detected. Such an increase in IL-10 serum levels correlates with the T-helper 2 cytokine shift observed in type 1 diabetic patients treated with similar anti-CD3 mAb.[63] A forthcoming phase II clinical trial will establish the *bona fide* efficacy and safety of the drug in patients suffering from PsA.

Non-mitogenic anti-CD3 antibodies reverse established experimental autoimmune encephalomyelitis

Multiple sclerosis (MS) is a chronic, inflammatory disease that affects the central nervous system (CNS), mainly the brain and spinal cord. MS is believed to be an autoimmune disease and causes a variety of symptoms, including changes in sensation, visual problems, muscle weakness, depression, and difficulties with coordination. In the most severe cases, MS can cause impaired mobility and disability. The course of the disease is difficult to predict and varies from patient to patient. It often combines an acute phase with several relapsing-remitting phases. There is no known definitive cure for MS, but several types of therapy have proven to be helpful. However, the immunosuppressive drugs that are currently used for treatment of MS have shown many adverse side effects. Ideally, the treatment will aim at returning function after an attack within the CNS, preventing new attacks, and preventing disability.

In 2005, the group of S.D. Miller extended the therapeutic efficacy of non-mitogenic anti-CD3 by using an experimental autoimmune encephalomyelitis (EAE) animal model for human MS. Similar to what was described in autoimmune diabetes, when injected intravenously, the Fc-altered anti-CD3 mAbs reversed EAE after new onset.[70] However, two striking differences with the diabetes settings have been found. More explicitly, although the protection correlated with an increase in the frequency of CD4+CD25+ T cells, neither anti-CD25 nor anti-TGF-β antibody treatment abrogated the efficacy. As recently reported, when administered orally in different EAE mouse models, anti-CD3 145-2C11 suppressed autoimmune encephalomyelitis by inducing CD4+CD25-LAP+ T cells that contain latency-associated peptide (LAP) on their surface, confirming a minor role for CD4+CD25+ Tregs.[71] In sharp contrast with the data obtained with intravenous anti-CD3,[70] an *in vitro* as well as *in vivo* TGF-β-dependent mechanism was found to be crucial to mediate permanent self-tolerance.

CONCLUDING REMARKS

In a quarter of a century, anti-CD3 immunotherapies became unavoidable due to their inimitable efficiency to prevent or delay a variety of acute allograft rejections and autoimmune diseases. Their mode of action possesses two main features that distinguish them from conventional immunosuppressive agents. First, a short-course treatment with anti-CD3 antibodies often results in a long-term tolerance as opposed to other compounds that lose efficacy as soon as the drug is withdrawn from the body. Second, adverse side effects following anti-CD3 therapy have been drastically diminished by generating non-Fc-binding antibodies. Despite major advances in the prevention of acute rejection in transplantation and in the treatment of autoimmune diseases, a single course of anti-CD3 mAb does not induce permanent tolerance and the patients usually enter a relapsing phase 1–2 years after anti-CD3 administration ended. Therefore, future immuno-interventions using anti-CD3 mAb will aim prolong the efficacy without increasing the side effects. Accordingly, several combination therapies have been tested in rodents and are envisioned in humans. For instance, short-term therapy with anti-CD3 145-2C11 mAb in combination with a proinsulin vaccine reversed autoimmune diabetes more forcefully than the monotherapies alone in two animal models.[57,72] Mechanistically, anti-CD3 mAb creates a temporal window that allows proinsulin-induced Tregs to develop. These cells have the capacity to dampen site-specifically multiple autoaggressive responses by a phenomenon called bystander suppression.[73] In addition, anti-CD3 can be administered together with drugs, such as exendin-4, that will exacerbate β-cell regeneration after recent onset T1DM.[74,75] Lastly, based on the promising data published after the first clinical trial in PsA, the hOKT3γ1(Ala-Ala) might be a good candidate for the treatment of rheumatoid arthritis, an autoimmune disease that affects approximately 1% of the world's population when defined by either the presence of serum rheumatoid factor (RF) or erosive changes on radiographs in a patient with a compatible clinical presentation.[76] To conclude, the recent new developments in anti-CD3 therapy might greatly improve the management of several immunological disorders in the near future.

ACKNOWLEDGMENTS

The authors thank Eleanor Ling for critically reading the manuscript. This work is supported by NIH grants AI51973 and DK51091 to M.G.V.H. and D.B. is recipient of a European Marie-Curie Outgoing Fellowship (2005–2008).

REFERENCES

1. Monaco AP. Immunosuppression and tolerance for clinical organ allografts. Curr Opin Immunol 1989; 1(6): 1174–7.

2. Collier SJ. Immunosuppressive drugs. Curr Opin Immunol 1989; 2(6): 854-8.

3. Fritsche L, Einecke G, Fleiner F et al. Reports of large immunosuppression trials in kidney transplantation: room for improvement. Am J Transplant 2004; 4(5): 738–43.

4. Fritsche L, Dragun D, Neumayer HH et al. Impact of cyclosporine on the development of immunosuppressive therapy. Transplant Proc 2004; 36(2 Suppl): 130S–134S.

5. Powles RL, Barrett AJ, Clink H et al. Cyclosporin A for the treatment of graft-versus-host disease in man. Lancet 1978; 2(8104–5): 1327–31.

6. Calne RY, White DJ, Thiru S et al. Cyclosporin A in patients receiving renal allografts from cadaver donors. Lancet 1978; 2(8104–5): 1323–7.

7. Kohler G, Milstein C. Continuous cultures of fused cells secreting antibody of predefined specificity. Nature 1975; 256(5517): 495–7.

8. Sun ZY, Kim ST, Kim IC et al. Solution structure of the CD3epsilondelta ectodomain and comparison with CD3epsilongamma as a basis for modeling T cell receptor topology and signaling. Proc Natl Acad Sci U S A 2004; 101(48): 16867–72.

9. Kung P, Goldstein G, Reinherz EL et al. Monoclonal antibodies defining distinctive human T cell surface antigens. Science 1979; 206(4416): 347–9.

10. Van Wauwe JP, De Mey JR, Goossens JG. OKT3: a monoclonal anti-human T lymphocyte antibody with potent mitogenic properties. J Immunol 1980; 124(6): 2708–13.

11. Davis L, Vida R, Lipsky PE. Regulation of human T lymphocyte mitogenesis by antibodies to CD3. J Immunol 1986; 137(12): 3758–67.

12. Van Wauwe J, Goossens J. Mitogenic actions of Orthoclone OKT3 on human peripheral blood lymphocytes: effects of monocytes and serum components. Int J Immunopharmacol 1981; 3(3): 203–8.

13. Walls EV, Borghetti AF, Benzie CR et al. Early events during the activation of human lymphocytes by the mitogenic monoclonal antibody OKT3. Cell Immunol 1984; 89(1): 30–8.

14. Alegre M, Depierreux M, Florquin S et al. Acute toxicity of anti-CD3 monoclonal antibody in mice: a model for OKT3 first dose reactions. Transplant Proc 1990; 22(4): 1920–1.

15. Ferran C, Sheehan K, Dy M et al. Cytokine-related syndrome following injection of anti-CD3 monoclonal antibody: further evidence for transient in vivo T cell activation. Eur J Immunol 1990; 20(3): 509–15.

16. Hirsch R, Gress RE, Pluznik DH et al. Effects of in vivo administration of anti-CD3 monoclonal antibody on T cell function in mice. II. In vivo activation of T cells. J Immunol 1989; 142(3): 737–43.

17. Hirsch R, Gress RE, Bluestone JA. Anti-CD3 antibody for autoimmune disease, a cautionary note. Lancet 1989; 1(8651): 1390.

18. Abramowicz D, Schandene L, Goldman M et al. Release of tumor necrosis factor, interleukin-2, and gamma-interferon in serum after injection of OKT3 monoclonal antibody in kidney transplant recipients. Transplantation 1989; 47(4): 606–8.

19. Chatenoud L, Legendre C, Ferran C et al. Corticosteroid inhibition of the OKT3-induced cytokine-related syndrome–dosage and kinetics prerequisites. Transplantation 1991; 51(2): 334–8.

20. Chatenoud L, Ferran C, Bach JF. The anti-CD3-induced syndrome: a consequence of massive in vivo cell activation. Curr Top Microbiol Immunol 1991; 174: 121–34.

21. Waid TH, Lucas BA, Thompson JS et al. Treatment of acute cellular rejection with T10B9.1A-31 or OKT3 in renal allograft recipients. Transplantation 1992; 53(1): 80–6.

22. Weinshenker BG, Bass B, Karlik S et al. An open trial of OKT3 in patients with multiple sclerosis. Neurology 1991; 41(7): 1047–52.

23. Sgro C. Side-effects of a monoclonal antibody, muromonab CD3/orthoclone OKT3: bibliographic review. Toxicology 1995; 105(1): 23–9.

24. A randomized clinical trial of OKT3 monoclonal antibody for acute rejection of cadaveric renal transplants. Ortho Multicenter Transplant Study Group. N Engl J Med 1985; 313(6): 337–42.

25. Cosimi AB, Burton RC, Colvin RB et al. Treatment of acute renal allograft rejection with OKT3 monoclonal antibody. Transplantation 1981; 32(6): 535–9.

26. Prentice HG, Blacklock HA, Janossy G et al. Use of anti-T-cell monoclonal antibody OKT3 to prevent acute graft-versus-host disease in allogeneic bone-marrow transplantation for acute leukaemia. Lancet 1982; 1(8274): 700–3.

27. Leo O, Foo M, Sachs DH et al. Identification of a monoclonal antibody specific for a murine T3 polypeptide. Proc Natl Acad Sci U S A 1987; 84(5): 1374–8.

28. Kjer-Nielsen L, Dunstone MA, Kostenko L et al. Crystal structure of the human T cell receptor CD3 epsilon gamma heterodimer complexed to the therapeutic mAb OKT3. Proc Natl Acad Sci U S A 2004; 101(20): 7675–80.

29. Bowen A, Edwards LC, Gailiunas P et al. Lymphocyte function in patients treated with monoclonal anti-T3 antibody for acute cadaveric renal allograft rejection. Transplantation 1984; 38(5): 489–93.

30. Goldstein G, Norman DJ, Shield CF 3rd et al. OKT3 monoclonal antibody reversal of acute renal allograft rejection unresponsive to conventional immunosuppressive treatments. Prog Clin Biol Res 1986; 224: 239–49.

31. Norman DJ, Shield CF 3rd, Barry JM et al. Therapeutic use of OKT3 monoclonal antibody for acute renal allograft rejection. Nephron 1987; 46 (Suppl 1): 41–7.

32. Monaco A, Goldstein G, Barnes L. Use of Orthoclone OKT3 monoclonal antibody to reverse acute renal allograft rejection unresponsive to treatment with conventional immunosuppressive regimens. Transplant Proc 1987; 19 (2 Suppl 1): 28–31.

33. Canafax DM, Draxler CA. Monoclonal antilymphocyte antibody (OKT3) treatment of acute renal allograft rejection. Pharmacotherapy 1987; 7(4): 121–4.

34. Delmonico FL, Cosimi AB. Monoclonal antibody treatment of human allograft recipients. Surg Gynecol Obstet 1988; 166(1): 89–98.

35. Woodle ES, Xu D, Zivin RA et al. Phase I trial of a humanized, Fc receptor nonbinding OKT3 antibody, huOKT3gamma1(Ala-Ala) in the treatment of acute renal allograft rejection. Transplantation 1999; 68(5): 608–16.

36. Friend PJ, Hale G, Chatenoud L et al. Phase I study of an engineered aglycosylated humanized CD3 antibody in renal transplant rejection. Transplantation 1999; 68(11): 1632–7.

37. Cole MS, Stellrecht KE, Shi JD et al. HuM291, a humanized anti-CD3 antibody, is immunosuppressive to T cells while exhibiting reduced mitogenicity in vitro. Transplantation 1999; 68(4): 563–71.

38. Cole MS, Anasetti C, Tso JY. Human IgG2 variants of chimeric anti-CD3 are nonmitogenic to T cells. J Immunol 1997; 159(7): 3613–21.

39. Meijer RT, Surachno S, Yong SL et al. Treatment of acute kidney allograft rejection with a non-mitogenic CD3 antibody. Clin Exp Immunol 2003; 133(3): 485–92.

40. Hering BJ, Kandaswamy R, Harmon JV et al. Transplantation of cultured islets from two-layer preserved pancreases in type 1 diabetes with anti-CD3 antibody. Am J Transplant 2004; 4(3): 390–401.

41. Carpenter PA, Appelbaum FR, Corey L et al. A humanized non-FcR-binding anti-CD3 antibody, visilizumab, for treatment of steroid-refractory acute graft-versus-host disease. Blood 2002; 99(8): 2712–19.

42. Hayward AR, Shreiber M. Neonatal injection of CD3 antibody into nonobese diabetic mice reduces the incidence of insulitis and diabetes. J Immunol 1989; 143(5): 1555–9.

43. Liu E, Eisenbarth GS. Type 1A diabetes mellitus-associated autoimmunity. Endocrinol Metab Clin North Am 2002; 31(2): 391–410, vii–viii.

44. Chatenoud L, Primo J, Bach JF. CD3 antibody-induced dominant self tolerance in overtly diabetic NOD mice. J Immunol 1997; 158(6): 2947–54.

45. Chatenoud L, Thervet E, Primo J et al. Anti-CD3 antibody induces long-term remission of overt autoimmunity in nonobese diabetic mice. Proc Natl Acad Sci U S A 1994; 91(1): 123–7.

46. Shoda LK, Young DL, Ramanujan S et al. A comprehensive review of interventions in the NOD mouse and implications for translation. Immunity 2005; 23(2): 115–26.

47. von Herrath MG, Coon B, Wolfe T et al. Nonmitogenic CD3 antibody reverses virally induced (rat insulin promoter-lymphocytic choriomeningitis virus) autoimmune diabetes without impeding viral clearance. J Immunol 2002; 168(2): 933–41.

48. Chatenoud L. The use of monoclonal antibodies to restore self-tolerance in established autoimmunity. Endocrinol Metab Clin North Am 2002; 31(2): 457–75, ix.

49. Chatenoud L. CD3 antibody treatment stimulates the functional capability of regulatory T cells. Novartis Found Symp 2003; 252: 279–86; discussion 86–90.

50. Chatenoud L. CD3-specific antibody-induced active tolerance: from bench to bedside. Nat Rev Immunol 2003; 3(2): 123–32.

51. Chatenoud L. CD3-specific antibodies restore self-tolerance: mechanisms and clinical applications. Curr Opin Immunol 2005; 17(6): 632–7.

52. Chatenoud L, Bach JF. Resetting the functional capacity of regulatory T cells: a novel immunotherapeutic strategy to promote immune tolerance. Expert Opin Biol Ther 2005; 5 (Suppl 1): S73–S81.

53. Chatenoud L, Bach JF. Regulatory T cells in the control of autoimmune diabetes: the case of the NOD mouse. Int Rev Immunol 2005; 24(3-4): 247–67.

54. Chatenoud L. [Anti-CD3 monoclonal antibodies: a new step towards therapy in new-onset type 1 diabetes.] Med Sci (Paris) 2006; 22(1): 5–6.

55. Chatenoud L, Salomon B, Bluestone JA. Suppressor T cells – they're back and critical for regulation of autoimmunity! Immunol Rev 2001; 182: 149–63.

56. Chatenoud L, Thervet E, Primo J et al. [Remission of established disease in diabetic NOD mice induced by anti-CD3 monoclonal antibody.] C R Acad Sci III 1992; 315(6): 225–8.

57. Bresson D, Togher L, Rodrigo E et al. Anti-CD3 and nasal proinsulin combination therapy enhances remission from recent-onset autoimmune diabetes by inducing Tregs. J Clin Invest 2006; 116(5): 1371–81.

58. Belghith M, Bluestone JA, Barriot S et al. TGF-beta-dependent mechanisms mediate restoration of self-tolerance induced by antibodies to CD3 in overt autoimmune diabetes. Nat Med 2003; 9(9): 1202–8.

59. Bolt S, Routledge E, Lloyd I et al. The generation of a humanized, non-mitogenic CD3 monoclonal antibody which retains in vitro immunosuppressive properties. Eur J Immunol 1993; 23(2): 403–11.

60. Xu D, Alegre ML, Varga SS et al. In vitro characterization of five humanized OKT3 effector function variant antibodies. Cell Immunol 2000; 200(1): 16–26.

61. Herold KC, Hagopian W, Auger JA et al. Anti-CD3 monoclonal antibody in new-onset type 1 diabetes mellitus. N Engl J Med 2002; 346(22): 1692–8.

62. Herold KC, Gitelman SE, Masharani U et al. A single course of anti-CD3 monoclonal antibody hOKT3{gamma}1(Ala-Ala) results in improvement in C-peptide responses and clinical parameters for at least 2 years after onset of type 1 diabetes. Diabetes 2005; 54(6): 1763–9.

63. Herold KC, Burton JB, Francois F et al. Activation of human T cells by FcR nonbinding anti-CD3 mAb, hOKT3gamma1(Ala-Ala). J Clin Invest 2003; 111(3): 409–18.

64. Herold KC. Achieving antigen-specific immune regulation. J Clin Invest 2004; 113(3): 346–9.

65. Bisikirska BC, Herold KC. Use of anti-CD3 monoclonal antibody to induce immune regulation in type 1 diabetes. Ann N Y Acad Sci 2004; 1037: 1–9.

66. Bisikirska BC, Herold KC. Regulatory T cells and type 1 diabetes. Curr Diab Rep 2005; 5(2): 104–9.

67. Bisikirska B, Colgan J, Luban J et al. TCR stimulation with modified anti-CD3 mAb expands CD8+ T cell population and induces CD8+CD25+ Tregs. J Clin Invest 2005; 115(10): 2904–13.

68. Keymeulen B, Vandemeulebroucke E, Ziegler AG et al. Insulin needs after CD3-antibody therapy in new-onset type 1 diabetes. N Engl J Med 2005; 352(25): 2598–608.

69. Utset TO, Auger JA, Peace D et al. Modified anti-CD3 therapy in psoriatic arthritis: a phase I/II clinical trial. J Rheumatol 2002; 29(9): 1907–13.

70. Kohm AP, Williams JS, Bickford AL et al. Treatment with nonmitogenic anti-CD3 monoclonal antibody induces CD4+ T cell unresponsiveness and functional reversal of established experimental autoimmune encephalomyelitis. J Immunol 2005; 174(8): 4525–34.

71. Ochi H, Abraham M, Ishikawa H et al. Oral CD3-specific antibody suppresses autoimmune encephalomyelitis by inducing CD4(+)CD25(–)LAP(+) T cells. Nat Med 2006; 12(6): 627–35.

72. Bresson D, von Herrath M. Immunotherapy after recent-onset type 1 diabetes: combinatorial treatment for achieving long-term remission in humans? Rev Diabet Stud 2004; 1(3): 108–12.

73. Bresson D, von Herrath M. Moving towards efficient therapies in type 1 diabetes: to combine or not to combine? Autoimmunity Reviews 2007; 6(S): 315–22.

74. Suarez-Pinzon WL, Lakey JR, Brand SJ et al. Combination therapy with epidermal growth factor and gastrin induces neogenesis of human islet {beta}-cells from pancreatic duct cells and an increase in functional {beta}-cell mass. J Clin Endocrinol Metab 2005; 90(6): 3401–9.

75. Suarez-Pinzon WL, Yan Y, Power R et al. Combination therapy with epidermal growth factor and gastrin increases {beta}-cell mass and reverses hyperglycemia in diabetic NOD mice. Diabetes 2005; 54(9): 2596–601.

76. Hartzheim LA, Goss GL. Rheumatoid arthritis: a case study. Nurs Clin North Am 1998; 33(4): 595–602.

77. Norman DJ, Vincenti F, de Mattos AM et al. Phase I trial of HuM291, a humanized anti-CD3 antibody, in patients receiving renal allografts from living donors. Transplantation 2000; 70(12): 1707–12.

44

Alefacept

Thomas A Luger

Introduction • Mechanism of action • Efficacy in psoriasis • Psoriatic arthritis and rheumatoid arthritis • Other T-cell-mediated diseases • Safety • Conclusion • References

INTRODUCTION

The treatment of immune-mediated and chronic inflammatory diseases of the skin usually involves topical as well as systemic interventions. Although most of these strategies allow for effective disease control they are frequently associated with sometimes severe side effects. Therefore, there is continuous need for novel efficient therapies with a favorable safety profile. The recent progress in the understanding of the complex pathomechanisms underlying chronic inflammation and the major advances in biotechnology prompted the development of several novel compounds targeting autoantigen recognition and autoantibody production, cytokine function and production, tolerance induction, and gene transcription.[1,2] Among several novel therapeutic avenues, the development of biologic agents (biologics) in particular has expanded recently. Strategies for biologic therapy are multiple and may consist of mediators that promote immune deviation, agents that inhibit the effects of proinflammatory cytokines, compounds that target pathogenic T cells and agents that disrupt the antigen-presentation/ T-cell activation.[3–5] Although most of these developments aimed to the improve graft rejection and the treatment of autoimmune diseases, more recently several compounds have primarily been developed for the treatment of chronic

inflammatory skin diseases such as psoriasis, which like rheumatoid arthritis (RA), Crohn's disease, and uveitis, is regarded as an immune-mediated inflammatory disease (IMID). Accordingly, alefacept (LFA-3TIP) and efalizumab (anti-CD11a) have been developed for the treatment of psoriasis and now are approved in many countries. This chapter will briefly review the efficacy and safety of alefacept in the treatment of psoriasis and related inflammatory diseases.

MECHANISM OF ACTION

Alefacept is a recombinant fully human fusion protein where the extracellular CD2 binding domain of LFA-3 (CD58) has been linked to the Fc (hinge, CH2 and CH3 domains) portion of IgG1 leading to functional blockade of the LFA-3/ CD2 pathway.[6] LFA-3 is the ligand for human CD2 and is expressed on many cell types, including antigen-presenting cells (APCs).[7] CD2 primarily has been detected on T cells and natural killer (NK) cells[8] and its expression is up-regulated on activated or memory effector CD45RO+ T cells.[6,9] Binding of CD2 on responder T or NK cells to LFA-3 on APCs provides a costimulatory signal required for T-cell activation.[8] Thus blocking costimulation by anti-CD2 antibodies or by the fusion protein alefacept has been shown to inhibit T-cell activation *in vitro* as well as *in vivo*.[6] Moreover, upon co-engagement of CD2[+] and CD16[+] (FcγRIII) alefacept was found to stimulate CD16[+] accessory cells (NK cells, macrophages) ultimately resulting in selective granzyme-mediated apoptosis of memory effector T cells[10] (Figure 44.1).

Alefacept is approved in the USA, Canada, Australia, Argentina, Switzerland, Kuwait, and Israel for the treatment of psoriasis vulgaris. It is indicated as monotherapy to treat adult patients with moderate to severe chronic plaque psoriasis requiring phototherapy or systemic therapy. Currently ~15 000 patients with psoriasis have been treated with alefacept.

EFFICACY IN PSORIASIS

The efficacy of alefacept given as i.v. bolus was evaluated in a phase 2, multicenter, randomized, double-blind, placebo-controlled study of 229 patients with chronic plaque psoriasis. Patients received 0.025, 0.075, or 0.15 mg/kg alefacept or placebo weekly for 12 weeks, followed by a 12-week follow-up. Two weeks after the last injection, the mean decrease in the Psoriasis Area and Severity Index (PASI) score was 38% vs 53% vs 53% in patients receiving alefacept (0.025 vs 0.075 vs 0.15 mg/kg), compared with 21% reduction in the placebo group ($p < 0.001$). Twelve weeks after treatment with alefacept 28 patients were clear or almost clear of psoriasis,

indicating that in some patients alefacept treatment may result in a long-lasting remission after cessation of treatment. In these patients responses were found to be sustained for a median of 10 months and there was no evidence of disease rebound, indicating that alefacept may function as disease-remitting therapy.[11,12] Alefacept reduced peripheral blood CD4[+] and CD8[+] memory cells in a dose-dependent fashion without affecting naive T cells. The decrease in the number of memory effector T cells was directly correlated with the clinical response.[12] Repeated courses of i.v. alefacept in patients previously treated in phase 2 trials did not result in cumulative effects on memory T cells and were at least as effective as the initial course.[13] Moreover, in patients who achieved a major PASI improvement a significant decrease in the Dermatology Life Quality Index (DLQI) was noted.[14]

In a phase 3 study 553 patients with chronic plaque psoriasis were randomized to two 12-week courses of alefacept (7.5 mg i.v. weekly) or placebo, and a 12-week follow-up phase after each course. Patients received either two courses of alefacept (cohort 1) or alefacept for the first and placebo for the second course (cohort 2) or placebo for the first and alefacept for the second course (cohort 3). A PASI 75 (≤ 75% reduction in PASI score) was achieved in 28% of the patients who received one course of alefacept and in

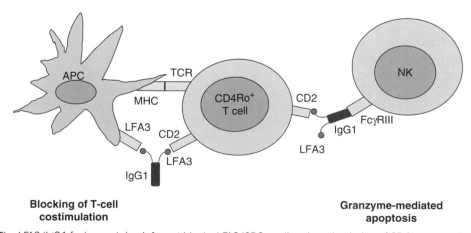

Blocking of T-cell costimulation

Granzyme-mediated apoptosis

Figure 44.1 The LFA3/IgG1 fusion protein alefacept blocks LFA3/CD2-mediated costimulation of CD4[+] memory T cells. However, upon co-engagement of CD2 and FcγRIII (CD16) on accessory cells (NK cells, macrophages) alefacept induces selective apoptosis of memory effector T cells.

8% of the placebo-treated patients ($p < 0.001$). Those patients who received a single course of alefacept and accomplished PASI 75 during or after the first course maintained PASI 50 for more than 7 months. Moreover, in these patients the second course of alefacept even augmented the efficacy. Accordingly, the overall response rate in patients who received two courses of alefacept demonstrated that 40% reached a PASI 75 and 71% a PASI 50.[15,16] Similar to the previous study,[12] a correlation of clinical improvement with reduction of memory effector T-cell counts was observed. In the majority of patients (~90%) CD4+ counts were at or greater than the lower limit (> 250 cells/µl).[17] Alefacept was well tolerated and did not result in antibody formation. However, the incidence of chills occurring within the 24 hours after the first few days was higher in the alefacept groups.[16] In patients who received alefacept and achieved PASI 75 or PASI 50 a significant decrease in the DLQI was observed.[18]

In an open-label parallel study in healthy volunteers comparing an i.m. and an i.v. formulation of alefacept, both preparations had a half-life of approximately 12 days and exhibited a comparable safety profile. In comparison to the i.v. formulation, the bioavailability of the i.m. preparation was around 50%.[19] Therefore in most of the subsequent clinical trials alefacept 15 mg i.m. weekly was used and this is the only formulation available today.

To examine the efficacy and safety of alefacept applied i.m., a randomized, double-blind, placebo-controlled phase 3 trial was performed in 507 patients with chronic plaque psoriasis. Patients were randomized to 10 mg of alefacept, 15 mg of alefacept or placebo administered i.m. once weekly. A dose-dependent significant improvement of the PASI score was observed in patients receiving alefacept. A PASI 75 was reached by 33% of patients in the 15 mg group, 28% of patients in the 10 mg group, and 13% of the placebo-treated patients.[20] In many patients the maximum PASI reduction was observed 6 weeks after finishing treatment.[21] Most of the patients who received a single course of 15 mg alefacept and achieved PASI 75 maintained at least PASI 50 for 7 months.[22] Moreover, a significant improvement in DLQI was observed in patients

responding to treatment, with the most significant amelioration occurring in those patients of the 15 mg group who achieved PASI 75.[23] As has been reported for i.v. application, alefacept given i.m. reduced the number of circulating effector memory T cells without affecting naïve T cells. A correlation between the reduction of CD4+ T-cell counts and clinical response was also observed. Irrespective of the dose, total lymphocyte as well as CD4+ T-cell counts returned to normal at 12 weeks after treatment in > 90% of the patients. No opportunistic infections and no cases of disease rebound have been reported.[24]

To improve the efficacy of alefacept the clinical outcome of multiple or extended courses was investigated. Accordingly, upon repeated courses of alefacept either 7.5 or 15 mg i.m. a continuous increase in the clinical improvement was observed even in patients who did not have a strong response with the first course of therapy.[25] In another study, one extended course of alefacept 15 mg i.m. administered weekly for 16 weeks appeared to have additional efficacy in some patients with a similar safety profile as observed in the 12-week dosing.[26] Recent studies have addressed the question whether high dose alefacept 30 mg weekly for 12 weeks would improve its efficacy. There appears to be no advantage for patients with psoriasis receiving a higher dose of alefacept.[27] The efficacy of alefacept was further evaluated in a subpopulation of patients with a history of systemic therapy such as methotrexate, retinoids, and cyclosporin A or phototherapy being ineffective or inappropriate. The results of this study indicate that alefacept is equally effective and safe in this difficult-to-treat group of patients as for the overall treated population in phase 3 clinical trials.[28] In a recent study the subcutaneous (s.c.) application of alefacept was compared to i.m. administration. Concerning pharmacodynamic profiles, efficacy, tolerability, and safety, no important difference between the two routes of administration has been observed. Thus because it is easier to use and less painful on injection s.c. application of alefacept may offer a certain advantage in certain patients.[29]

Recently alefacept 15 mg i.m. weekly for 12 weeks was investigated for its efficacy in the treatment of nail psoriasis in 15 and 6 patients, respectively, in two small open-label case studies. After a follow-up of 6 or 12 weeks an improvement of nail disease in several but not all patients was observed. Therefore, further controlled clinical trials are required to determine the value of alefacept for the treatment of psoriatic nails.[30,31] Alefacept also has been reported to achieve a significant improvement in patients with extensive and recalcitrant palmoplantar psoriasis.[32,33] In a recent open-label study 15 patients with palmoplantar psoriasis were treated with alefacept i.m. 15 mg weekly. The dose was increased if no noticeable response was observed after 8 weeks. These preliminary results indicate that alefacept may offer an effective alternative for the treatment of recalcitrant palmoplantar psoriasis.[33]

Alefacept monotherapy usually has a slow onset of action and the overall response rate of approximately 30% of patients reaching PASI 75 after one 12-week course may increase to approximately 40% with subsequent courses. Differences in the mechanism of action as well as the lack of carcinogenicity, hepatotoxicity, and nephrotoxicity suggest a potential additive advantage when alefacept is combined with topical, systemic or UV therapies currently used for the treatment of psoriasis. This promising possibility has been approached by several clinical trials and case studies.

Topical corticosteroids and vitamin D preparations are effective standard therapies for the treatment of psoriatic plaques. Therefore, in one randomized, double-blind, placebo-controlled study in patients with psoriasis the efficacy of combining alefacept with a topical corticosteroid was investigated. The additional use of betamethasone dipropionate cream for 4 weeks did not increase the overall clinical efficacy of alefacept i.m. 15 mg weekly for 12 weeks.[34] The effect of topical calcipotriol and alefacept was investigated in seven patients with psoriasis. The additive application of calcipotriol to alefacept (15 mg weekly) caused a more rapid clinical response but did not improve the overall clinical efficacy nor additionally stabilize the expression of markers of proliferation and differentiation on keratinocytes.[35]

The combination of alefacept and UVB phototherapy, a commonly used treatment for moderate and severe psoriasis, was evaluated in a two center open-label study in patients with chronic plaque psoriasis. In each center 30 patients were enrolled and either treated with alefacept (15 mg i.m. weekly for 12 weeks) or alefacept plus 6 weeks of UVB or alefacept plus 12 weeks of UVB. Patients were treated approximately three times per week with either broadband UVB (BB UVB) or narrowband UVB (311 nm, NB UVB). Both BB UVB and NB UVB provided a more rapid onset of clinical improvement compared with alefacept monotherapy. Twelve weeks of UVB did not result in an additional benefit over 6 weeks of UVB phototherapy. Alefacept alone and in combination with either of the UVB regimens was well tolerated and the mean CD4+ T-cell counts remained above the lower limit of normal. Therefore, alefacept in combination with UVB phototherapy is effective and safe, resulting in an accelerated clinical response without significantly ameliorating the overall outcome.[36,37] However, the efficacy of alefacept plus UVB was not compared to that of UVB monotherapy in any of these studies. Moreover, at present there are no data available on the combination of alefacept and photochemotherapy (PUVA).

There is recent evidence of an additive benefit when alefacept is combined with systemic retinoids. Accordingly, an improvement of the clinical response with no additional safety concerns has been reported.[38] Other possible combinations which are currently being evaluated include methotrexate and cyclosporine.[39] Because of the favorable safety profile of alefacept, transition of patients with moderate to severe from treatments such as methotrexate or cyclosporine frequently may be necessary. According to preliminary data, in most of these patients transition off either methotrexate or cyclosporine onto alefacept within 10–12 weeks was successful, with maintenance or improvement of the PASI score and no evidence of additional toxicity.[40]

The combination of alefacept with etanercept in patients with plaque psoriasis was evaluated in a series of three case reports. All patients experienced an improvement of their psoriatic arthritis upon monotherapy with etanercept (50 mg once or twice weekly) but skin involvement failed to respond even after several months of treatment. The addition of alefacept 15 mg i.m. weekly for 12 weeks resulted in a significant improvement of psoriatic skin disease, which was maintained for at least 8 weeks after completing alefacept. The combination was well tolerated, no adverse events or infections were observed and CD4[+] T-cell counts remained above normal limits. Although these results indicate that the combined use of biologics targeting different pathways may improve the efficacy this remains to be proven in larger controlled clinical trials.

PSORIATIC ARTHRITIS AND RHEUMATOID ARTHRITIS

A few clinical trials have addressed the question whether alefacept is an effective and safe treatment of psoriatic arthritis (PsA) or RA. In one first open-label explorative study 11 patients with active PsA received alefacept monotherapy (7.5 mg i.v.) weekly for 12 weeks with a 4-week follow-up period. A gradual decrease in disease activity with a sustained improvement during the follow-up phase was observed in most of the patients. Moreover, the clinical improvement was related to the reduction of circulating CD45RO[+] T cells and a decrease in infiltrating T cells and macrophages has been demonstrated in synovial tissue. Thus alefacept apparently is able to affect synovial tissue and to downregulate joint inflammation.[41] In a more recent randomized, double-blind, placebo-controlled study alefacept was evaluated in combination with methotrexate for the treatment of PsA. In this study 185 patients with three or more tender and swollen joints who had been on a stable dose of methotrexate (10–25 mg weekly) for at least 3 months were randomized to receive either alefacept 15 mg i.m. plus methotrexate ($n = 123$) or placebo plus methotrexate ($n = 62$). Alefacept or placebo was administered once weekly with a follow-up period of 12 weeks. Responders were regarded as those patients reaching a 20% improvement in disease activity according to the American College of Rheumatology criteria (ACR 20) at week 24. Using this as primary endpoint, 54% of patients in the alefacept group and 23% of patients in the

placebo group achieved ACR 20. The number of adverse events in both groups was comparable and no opportunistic infections or malignancies have been reported. Again this study strongly supports an additive efficacy and a favorable safety profile for alefacept in the treatment of PsA.[42] In a pilot study the efficacy of alefacept in combination with methotrexate was evaluated in 36 patients with RA. Patients received alefacept 7.5 mg i.v., alefacept 3.75 mg i.v. or placebo weekly for 12 weeks followed by a 12-week follow-up. At week 24, 58% of patients receiving alefacept 3.75 mg and 25% of patients receiving alefacept 7.5 mg versus 17% obtaining placebo achieved an ACR 20. Alefacept in combination with methotrexate was safe, well tolerated, and selectively reduced the number of circulating CD4[+] and CD8[+] T cells.[43] Alefacept therefore appears to be an effective alternative option for the treatment of RA with the optimal dose and regimen to be determined in future studies.

OTHER T-CELL-MEDIATED DISEASES

The efficacy of alefacept is currently being investigated in an increasing number of immune-mediated diseases characterized by T-cell infiltration in which conventional treatment was not successful. A significant clinical response to a single course of alefacept (15 mg i.m. weekly for 12 weeks) has been reported in two patients with recalcitrant lichen planus. The rapid onset of action was notable, with a remarkable improvement already after 4 weeks of treatment.[44] There is also some evidence indicating that alefacept may be useful to treat alopecia areata. In four patients with alopecia areata totalis a partial improvement with a 12-week course with alefacept 15 mg i.m. has been reported.[45] According to case reports alefacept may also be used successfully for the treatment of pyoderma gangrenosum and severe recalcitrant contact dermatitis.[46,47] Furthermore, alefacept appears to have beneficial effects in controlling steroid-resistant acute graft-versus-host disease (GVHD). In one trial seven patients received either 30 mg (adults) or 15 mg alefacept twice weekly. A rapid response to alefacept was observed within days even in grade 4 GVHD, especially in skin involvement, without evidence of alefacept-related adverse events.[48]

SAFETY

The safety profile of alefacept is very good even in patients who have received several courses. In general alefacept was well tolerated, with some mild adverse events that did not require discontinuation of treatment. The only adverse event which occurred more frequently in comparison to placebo after initiating the first course and tended to disappear during later courses was chills.[16,20] Even in individuals with a higher risk, such as elderly ($\geq$ 65 years), obese or diabetic patients, no increase in the incidence of adverse events was observed.[49] There was no evidence for an increased risk of opportunistic, mycobacterial or viral infections and no increased incidence of malignancies including skin cancer in patients receiving alefacept.[13,16,50] Moreover, no relation between low CD4+ T-cell counts and the overall risk of infections has been reported. Since a reduction of CD4+ and CD8+ T-cell counts usually occurs during alefacept treatment, peripheral CD4+ T-cell counts should be monitored before initiating therapy and weekly during the alefacept course. Treatment has to be stopped if CD4+ T-cell counts drop below 250 cells/μl and alefacept has to be discontinued in the case of CD4+ T-cell counts remaining low for 1 month. Usually T-cell counts return to normal limits with the termination of alefacept therapy.[16] The safety of less frequent monitoring of T-cell counts is currently being investigated. Because of the fully human composition of alefacept the incidence of antibodies to this biologic was observed only very rarely and there was no evidence for an association with the clinical response or hypersensitivity reactions.[16,20] In one study the effect of alefacept on T-cell-dependent humoral immune responses was investigated. Accordingly, alefacept did not impair the primary immune response to neoantigens nor the secondary immune response to recall antigens.[51] Thus it seems to be very unlikely that the immune response to microbial or tumor antigens is impaired during alefacept treatment.

According to the safety databases that have been established for alefacept, no currently unknown adverse events have been reported. Moreover, there is no evidence of rebound after discontinuation of alefacept. On the contrary, those patients achieving a significant clinical response continued to improve after the usual 12-week alefacept course.[16,20]

CONCLUSION

Alefacept was the first biologic to be developed and approved for the treatment of moderate to severe psoriasis. According to clinical studies alefacept has a favorable safety profile and monotherapy is effective, with approximately 50% of the patients achieving PASI 50 and 30% achieving PASI 75. Combination of alefacept with conventional antipsoriatic therapies such as phototherapy, retinoids, methotrexate or cyclosporin is safe and may increase the efficacy of either treatment. In addition, transition off immunosuppressive drugs such as methotrexate or cyclosporine onto alefacept maintained or improved the clinical response with no evidence of additional toxicity. Thus alefacept is a valuable and promising new addition which contributes substantially to treatment of psoriasis. Further trials are still required to improve dosing and combination strategies with alefacept and to perhaps identify a subgroup of patients which is most likely to respond to alefacept. The first promising results in patients with PsA and RA have to be evaluated in further clinical trials. Finally the efficacy of alefacept for the treatment of other T-cell-mediated diseases needs to be explored.

REFERENCES

1. Feldmann M, Steinman L. Design of effective immunotherapy for human autoimmunity. Nature 2005; 435(7042): 612–19.
2. Gottlieb AB. Psoriasis: emerging therapeutic strategies. Nat Rev Drug Discov 2005; 4(1): 19–34.
3. Saripalli YV, Gaspari AA. Focus on: biologics that affect therapeutic agents in dermatology. J Drugs Dermatol 2005; 4(2): 233–45.
4. Finucane KA, Archer CB. Recent advances in rheumatology: biological agents for the treatment of rheumatoid arthritis, the progression of psoriatic arthritis,

autoantibodies in systemic lupus erythematosus. Clin Exp Dermatol 2005; 30(2): 201–4.

5. Kourbeti IS, Boumpas DT. Biological therapies of autoimmune diseases. Curr Drug Targets Inflamm Allergy 2005; 4(1): 41–6.

6. Ormerod AD. Alefacept. Biogen. Curr Opin Investig Drugs 2003; 4(5): 608–13.

7. Springer TA, Dustin ML, Kishimoto TK, Marlin SD. The lymphocyte function-associated LFA-1, CD2, and LFA-3 molecules: cell adhesion receptors of the immune system. Annu Rev Immunol 1987; 5: 223–52.

8. Bierer BE, Sleckman BP, Ratnofsky SE, Burakoff SJ. The biologic roles of CD2, CD4, and CD8 in T-cell activation. Annu Rev Immunol 1989; 7: 579–99.

9. Davis SJ, van der Merwe PA. The structure and ligand interactions of CD2: implications for T-cell function. Immunol Today 1996; 17(4): 177–87.

10. da Silva AJ, Brickelmaier M, Majeau GR et al. Alefacept, an immunomodulatory recombinant LFA-3/IgG1 fusion protein, induces CD16 signaling and CD2/CD16-dependent apoptosis of CD2(+) cells. J Immunol 2002; 168(9): 4462–71.

11. Krueger GG, Ellis CN. Alefacept therapy produces remission for patients with chronic plaque psoriasis. Br J Dermatol 2003; 148(4): 784–8.

12. Ellis CN, Krueger GG. Treatment of chronic plaque psoriasis by selective targeting of memory effector T lymphocytes. N Engl J Med 2001; 345(4): 248–55.

13. Lowe NJ, Gonzalez J, Bagel J et al. Repeat courses of intravenous alefacept in patients with chronic plaque psoriasis provide consistent safety and efficacy. Int J Dermatol 2003; 42(3): 224–30.

14. Ellis CN, Mordin MM, Adler EY. Effects of alefacept on health-related quality of life in patients with psoriasis: results from a randomized, placebo-controlled phase II trial. Am J Clin Dermatol 2003; 4(2): 131–9.

15. Krueger GG. Clinical response to alefacept: results of a phase 3 study of intravenous administration of alefacept in patients with chronic plaque psoriasis. J Eur Acad Dermatol Venereol 2003; 17 (Suppl 2): 17–24.

16. Krueger GG, Papp KA, Stough DB et al. A randomized, double-blind, placebo-controlled phase III study evaluating efficacy and tolerability of 2 courses of alefacept in patients with chronic plaque psoriasis. J Am Acad Dermatol 2002; 47(6): 821–33.

17. McMichael AJ. The new biologics in psoriasis: possible treatments for alopecia areata. J Investig Dermatol Symp Proc 2003; 8(2): 217–18.

18. Feldman SR, Menter A, Koo JY. Improved health-related quality of life following a randomized controlled trial of alefacept treatment in patients with chronic plaque psoriasis. Br J Dermatol 2004; 150(2): 317–26.

19. Vaishnaw AK, TenHoor CN. Pharmacokinetics, biologic activity, and tolerability of alefacept by intravenous and intramuscular administration. J Pharmacokinet Pharmacodyn 2002; 29(5–6): 415–26.

20. Lebwohl M, Christophers E, Langley R et al. An international, randomized, double-blind, placebo-controlled phase 3 trial of intramuscular alefacept in patients with chronic plaque psoriasis. Arch Dermatol 2003; 139(6): 719–27.

21. Ortonne JP. Clinical response to alefacept: results of a phase 3 study of intramuscular administration of alefacept in patients with chronic plaque psoriasis. J Eur Acad Dermatol Venereol 2003; 17 (Suppl 2): 12–16.

22. Gordon KB, Langley RG. Remittive effects of intramuscular alefacept in psoriasis. J Drugs Dermatol 2003; 2(6): 624–8.

23. Finlay AY, Salek MS, Haney J. Intramuscular alefacept improves health-related quality of life in patients with chronic plaque psoriasis. Dermatology 2003; 206(4): 307–15.

24. Ortonne JP, Lebwohl M, Em GC. Alefacept-induced decreases in circulating blood lymphocyte counts correlate with clinical response in patients with chronic plaque psoriasis. Eur J Dermatol 2003; 13(2): 117–23.

25. Menter A, Cather JC, Baker D et al. The efficacy of multiple courses of alefacept in patients with moderate to severe chronic plaque psoriasis. J Am Acad Dermatol 2006; 54(1): 61–3.

26. Gribetz CH, Blum R, Brady C, Cohen S, Lebwohl M. An extended 16-week course of alefacept in the treatment of chronic plaque psoriasis. J Am Acad Dermatol 2005; 53(1): 73–5.

27. An open-label extended study evaluating an extended course of high-dose alefacept for the treatment of psoriasis. J Am Acad Dermatol 2006; 54: AB212 (abstract).

28. van de KP, Griffiths CE, Christophers E, Lebwohl M, Krueger GG. Alefacept in the treatment of psoriasis in patients for whom conventional therapies are inadequate. Dermatology 2005; 211(3): 256–63.

29. Sweetser MT, Woodworth J, Swan S, Ticho B. Results of a randomized open-label crossover study of the bioequivalence of subcutaneous versus intramuscular administration of alefacept. Dermatol Online J 2006; 12(3): 1.

30. Parrish CA, Sobera JO, Robbins CM et al. Alefacept in the treatment of psoriatic nail disease: a proof of concept study. J Drugs Dermatol 2006; 5(4): 339–40.

31. Cassetty CT, Alexis AF, Shupack JL, Strober BE. Alefacept in the treatment of psoriatic nail disease: a small case series. J Am Acad Dermatol 2005; 52(6): 1101–2.

32. Myers W, Christiansen L, Gottlieb AB. Treatment of palmoplantar psoriasis with intramuscular alefacept. J Am Acad Dermatol 2005; 53 (2 Suppl 1): S127–S129.

33. Pearce DJ, Feldman SR, Goffe B. Evaluation of alefacept for the treatment of palmoplantar psoriasis. J Am Acad Dermatol 2006; 54: AB218 (abstract).

34. Bovenschen HJ, Gerritsen WJ, de Jong EM, van de Kerkhof PC. Addition of a topical corticosteroid in the early phase of alefacept treatment for psoriasis. Acta Derm Venereol 2006; 86(3): 281–2.

35. van Duijnhoven MW, Korver JE, Vissers WH et al. Effect of calcipotriol on epidermal cell populations in alefacept-treated psoriatic lesions. J Eur Acad Dermatol Venereol 2006; 20(1): 27–33.

36. Koo JY, Bagel J, Sweetser MT, Ticho BS. Alefacept in combination with ultraviolet B phototherapy for the treatment of chronic plaque psoriasis: results from an open-label, multicenter study. J Drugs Dermatol 2006; 5(7): 623–8.

37. Ortonne JP, Khemis A, Koo JY, Choi J. An open-label study of alefacept plus ultraviolet B light as combination therapy for chronic plaque psoriasis. J Eur Acad Dermatol Venereol 2005; 19(5): 556–63.

38. Korman NJ, Koo JY, van de Kerkhof PC, Bagel J. The efficacy and safety of alefacept in combination with UVB light or systemic reinoids. J Am Acad Dermatol 2006; 54: AB226 (abstract).

39. van Duijnhoven MW, de Jong EM, Gerritsen WJ, Pasch MC, van de Kerkhof PC. Alefacept modifies long-term disease severity and improves the response to other treatments. Eur J Dermatol 2005; 15(5): 366–73.

40. Korman NJ, Moul DK. Alefacept for the treatment of psoriasis: a review of the current literature and practical suggestions for everyday clinical use. Semin Cutan Med Surg 2005; 24(1): 10–18.

41. Kraan MC, van Kuijk AW, Dinant HJ et al. Alefacept treatment in psoriatic arthritis: reduction of the effector T cell population in peripheral blood and synovial tissue is associated with improvement of clinical signs of arthritis. Arthritis Rheum 2002; 46(10): 2776–84.

42. Mease PJ, Gladman DD, Keystone EC. Alefacept in combination with methotrexate for the treatment of psoriatic arthritis: results of a randomized, double-blind, placebo-controlled study. Arthritis Rheum 2006; 54(5): 1638–45.

43. Schneider M, Stahl HD, Podrebarac T, Brown J. Tolerability and safety of combination and alefacept in rheumatoid arthritis: results of as pilot study. Arthritis Rheum 2006; 12: S654 (abstract).

44. Fivenson DP, Mathes B. Treatment of generalized lichen planus with alefacept. Arch Dermatol 2006; 142(2): 151–2.

45. Heffernan MP, Hurley MY, Martin KS, Smith DI, Anadkat MJ. Alefacept for alopecia areata. Arch Dermatol 2005; 141(12): 1513–16.

46. Feldman SR, McCarty A, Caroll C, Willard J. The use of alefacept for the treatment of pyoderma gangrenosum. J Am Acad Dermatol 2006; 54: AB226 (abstract).

47. Yeung-Yue K. Clinical improvement and apparent resolution of allergic contact dermatitis with alefacept. J Am Acad Dermatol 2006; 54: AB92 (abstract).

48. Shapira MY, Resnick IB, Bitan M et al. Rapid response to alefacept given to patients with steroid resistant or steroid dependent acute graft-versus-host disease: a preliminary report. Bone Marrow Transplant 2005; 36(12): 1097–101.

49. Gottlieb AB, Boehncke WH, Darif M. Safety and efficacy of alefacept in elderly patients and other special populations. J Drugs Dermatol 2005; 4(6): 718–24.

50. Goffe B, Papp K, Gratton D et al. An integrated analysis of thirteen trials summarizing the long-term safety of alefacept in psoriasis patients who have received up to nine courses of therapy. Clin Ther 2005; 27(12): 1912–21.

51. Gottlieb AB, Casale TB, Frankel E et al. CD4+ T-cell-directed antibody responses are maintained in patients with psoriasis receiving alefacept: results of a randomized study. J Am Acad Dermatol 2003; 49(5): 816–25.

45

Clinical targeting of interleukin-15

Iain B McInnes and Foo Y Liew

INTRODUCTION

There is considerable interest in understanding those mechanisms whereby innate and acquired immune responses interact in the context of chronic inflammation. In rheumatoid arthritis (RA) patients, the synovial membrane exhibits features suggesting that components of both compartments of the immune response are of functional importance.[1,2] A broad range of cells within inflamed synovium express relevant cytokine activities including macrophages, dendritic cells (DCs), synovial fibroblasts, mast cells, neutrophils, and T cells.[3,4] Interleukin-15 (IL-15) is a cytokine with quaternary structural similarities to IL-2,[5–7] that is produced primarily by macrophages and DCs. It exhibits inflammatory activities commensurate with the known pathogenesis of a number of chronic inflammatory disorders. In this chapter we will review evidence that indicates that IL-15 represents an intriguing therapeutic target. Clinical data are most advanced in inflammatory arthritis and will be given priority in this discussion.

IL-15 EXPRESSION IN INFLAMMATORY ARTHRITIS

The pleiotropic effects of IL-15 described in Chapter 14 clearly render it a candidate cytokine in the pathogenesis of inflammatory arthritis.

IL-15 mRNA and protein have been detected in RA synovial membrane by a number of investigators. IL-15 mRNA levels are present at higher levels in RA compared with reactive arthritis synovial biopsies.[8] Although cautious interpretation of mRNA data is required it is of interest that levels are higher in patients before commencement of immune suppressive therapy. Several ELISAs are now available, all of which detect IL-15 in around 60% of RA, but not osteoarthritis synovial fluids. Levels correlate directly with tumor necrosis factor (TNF)-α and remain after removal of rheumatoid factor, which likely interfered with earlier efforts to quantify IL-15, leading to overestimation of the concentrations present. Concentrations present are similar to levels of TNF-α or IL-12 detected in parallel assays,[9] but are lower than other monokines, e.g. IL-6, IL-18. These observations have recently been confirmed.[10–13] IL-15 has also been measured in RA synovial fluids using soluble IL-15Rα chain in a novel receptor capture assay,[9] in which IL-15 levels in RA synovial fluids correlate closely with those detected by ELISA. Moreover, recombinant soluble IL-15Rα interferes with the detection of IL-15 by ELISA (our unpublished observations). We have also detected IL-15 in synovial fluids derived from patients with psoriatic arthritis (H Wilson et al, unpublished observations), suggesting that IL-15 may be present in a broad range of inflammatory arthropathies.

Moreover, Raza and colleagues[14] examined very early arthritis patients using synovial lavage and observed high levels of IL-15 expression in those that subsequently met criteria for RA, suggesting that this cytokine may have an important early role commensurate with its activities in innate immune function.

Low levels of IL-15 are also present in sera of up to 40% of RA patients, although variable levels have been reported in distinct populations.[15–19] Serum IL-15 expression does not correlate with disease subsets thus far recognized. Whereas RA serum TNF-α levels correlate with the presence of germinal centers in parallel synovial biopsies, IL-15 levels were elevated in patents in whom either germinal centers or diffuse lymphocytic infiltrative patterns were observed.[16] IL-15 has also been detected in rheumatoid pleural effusions.[20] Circulating T cells in RA patients have also been reported to express IL-15, where its presence together with RANKL has been linked to osteoclast activation.[21]

IL-15 expression in inflamed synovium is found in lining layer macrophages, together with synovial fibroblasts and endothelial cells.[22–24] Synovial T cells have also been reported to express membrane IL-15.[21,23] The distribution of IL-15 is similar in psoriatic (PsA) and reactive arthritis (ReA) synovial membranes but expression is at reduced levels as compared with RA.[23,25] Of interest, both PsA and ReA synovium contain IL-2, with which IL-15 may exhibit counter-regulatory activities. IL-15 expression has also recently been detected in synovial membrane derived from juvenile RA patients,[26] associated with IL-18, IL-12, and interferon (IFN)-γ expression.

Spontaneous production of IL-15 by primary RA synovial membrane cultures and by isolated synovial fibroblasts is reported.[10,27] Such release is sensitive to cyclosporin (and FK-506) tractable pathway operating through cAMP.[27] In similar studies, we have observed up-regulation of IL-15 mRNA and intracellular IL-15 protein expression in purified synovial fibroblasts, although we have been unable to consistently detect IL-15 secretion thus far. In long-term cultures of mixed synovial tissues, outgrowth of tissues was found to be dependent upon the presence of T cells that in turn lead to local release of IL-15, IL-17, and fibroblast growth factor (FGF)-1.[28] Nevertheless, it has proven difficult to consistently achieve IL-15 secretion in *in vitro* systems and studies characterizing the regulation of intracellular processing events leading to long signal peptide (LSP)-IL-15 production in synovial membrane are urgently required, as is formal comparison of LSP and SSP (short signal peptide) isoform expression.[29]

Factors that in turn drive synovial IL-15 expression are unclear. We have recently identified that activated T cells can induce IL-15 expression in macrophages via cognate interactions. Exposure of synovial fibroblasts to TNF-α or IL-1β also induces high levels of IL-15 expression, although we have rarely detected this in secreted form. Recent studies in dermal fibroblasts similarly demonstrated that TNF-α but not IFN-γ induces membrane expression of IL-15 that in turn can sustain T-cell growth.[30] A further pathway promoting IL-15 production has been suggested in studies of synovial embryonic growth factor expression. Overexpression of the wingless (*Wnt*)5 and frizzled (*Fz*)5 ligand pair is associated with increased production and secretion of IL-15 by RA synovial fibroblasts, together with IL-6 and IL-8.[31] Furthermore, suppression of *Wnt5* or *Fz5* using antisense, dominant negative mutants or neutralizing antibodies led to reduction in IL-15 expression.[32] Thus a variety of stimuli including cellular feedback loops may promote IL-15 release in synovium (Figure 45.1). In contrast PGE$_2$ has been reported to inhibit IL-15 release in fibroblast cultures.[33]

Genetic evidence for IL-15 involvement in disease susceptibility or severity is thus far unconvincing. Polymorphisms in the IL-15 gene have been associated with juvenile idiopathic arthritis in small studies.[34] However, larger studies in RA are awaited and as such no firm conclusions can be reached yet. The role of promoter variation in regulating IL-15 expression and function is lacking thus far.

BIOACTIVITIES OF IL-15 RELEVANT TO INFLAMMATORY ARTHRITIS

The biologic effects of IL-15 in the context of tissue pathology have been discussed elsewhere (Chapter 14). These key properties are described

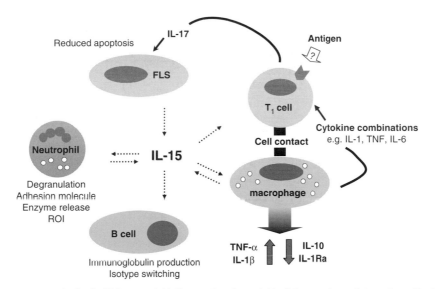

Figure 45.1 Data support a role for IL-15 in synovial inflammation through T-cell/macrophage interactions, T-cell cytokine release (IL-17), direct effects on neutrophil activation, and fibroblast activation. Synergy with other proinflammatory cytokines including IL-12 and IL-18 is necessary for optimal responses. Potential effects on dendritic cells and endothelial cell function remain to be explored.

in Table 45.1. IL-15 mediates proinflammatory activities potentially via a broad variety of effector pathways. Thus IL-15 activates synovial T cells and natural killer (NK) cells to directly secrete cytokines.[35,36] More importantly, it promotes and maintains a membrane phenotype, consisting of elevated CD69, LFA–1, CD40L, and perhaps cytokine (e.g. IFN-γ) expression, that promotes membrane–membrane interactions with adjacent macrophages and fibroblasts. This in turn provides a major route to macrophage cytokine release that is clearly central to RA pathogenesis, but also to release of matrix metalloproteinases that can promote cartilage degradation. Many chemokine activities have been detected in RA synovial membrane.[37,38] IL-15 represents part of this chemokinetic activity, in combination with at least IL-8, monocyte chemoattractant 1 (MCP-1), and macrophage inflammatory protein (MIP)-1α.[22,39] IL-15 also up-regulates chemokine receptors and induces redistribution of adhesion molecules, including intracellular adhesion molecule (ICAM)-1–3, CD43, and CD44, to uropods to further facilitate migration.[40,41] Finally, although numerous pathways provide for longevity of T cells in the synovial compartment including interactions with the extracellular matrix and adjacent

Table 45.1 Biologic effects of IL-15

Cell type	Key effects
T lymphocyte	• Activation/proliferation
	• Cytokine production Th/c1 and Th/c2
	• Cytotoxicity
	• Chemokinesis
	• Cytoskeletal rearrangement
	• Adhesion molecule expression
	• Reduced apoptosis
B lymphocyte	• Ig production
	• Proliferation
NK cell	• Cytotoxicity
	• Cytokine production
	• Reduced apoptosis
	• Lineage development
Macrophage	• Dose-dependent effect on activation
	• Membrane expression –costimulation
Osteoclast	• Maturation
	• Calcitonin receptor
Dendritic cell	• Maturation
	• Activation
Neutrophil	• Activation
	• Cytoskeletal rearrangement
	• Cytokine release
	• Reduced apoptosis
Fibroblast	• Reduced apoptosis
	• Cytokine release

inflammatory leukocyte populations, IL-15 may also contribute via amplification of anti-apoptotic intracellular signaling pathways. In this respect, however, IL-15 appears less important for T cells than IFNs present in low nanogram concentrations in synovium.[42]

IL-15 activity beyond lymphocyte subsets is also likely of importance. Neutrophils can be activated by IL-15,[43,44] and those derived from RA tissues may exhibit enhanced responsiveness compared with normal controls.[45] IL-15 enhances endothelial and fibroblast cell survival[46] and can enhance MMP release. This in turn promotes angiogenesis. It promotes osteoclastogenesis in synergy with RANKL via secretory and cell contact-mediated pathways.[21] A pathway of particular importance may be via activation of mast cells to release cytokines and serine protease enzymes capable in turn of promoting tissue damage and amplification of inflammation. Finally, IL-15 has been linked to hypernociception mediated via an IFN-γ-, endothelin (ET)-1-, PGE_2-dependent pathway.[47] In summary, these activities render IL-15 a candidate target in a variety of chronic inflammatory diseases and RA in particular (Figure 45.1).

STRATEGIES TO TARGET IL-15 *IN VIVO*

The complexities of IL-15 physiology pose considerable difficulties in determining what should be the optimal therapeutic strategy. Thus far three protein-based approaches have been considered, i.e. use of (i) neutralizing antibodies directed against either IL-15 or its receptor subcomponents, (ii) soluble IL-15Rα, and (iii) mutated IL-15 species, usually generated as fusion proteins. A further approach is to utilize small molecule signal pathway inhibitors aimed particularly at JAK/STAT pathways subserving IL-15-function. These are not yet specific to IL-15-mediated function but inhibit several common γ chain receptor-mediated events. Several studies utilizing these diverse approaches have been attempted, or are currently ongoing (Table 45.2).

INFLAMMATION MODEL STUDIES – IL-15 TARGETING *IN VIVO*

Several of the foregoing approaches have been tested in relevant disease models. We have used

Table 45.2 Strategies to target IL-15 in clinical studies

Modality	Comments
Anti-IL-15 antibody	• Specificity predictable • Requirement to block membrane and soluble cytokine • Human or humanized structure preferable
Soluble IL-15Rα	• High affinity and specificity • Pharmacokinetics unclear • Does not block IL-15Rβ and γ chain signaling • Human or humanized structure preferable
Mikβ1 anti-receptor	• High affinity • Blocks majority of IL-15-mediated signaling
Mutant IL-15 species	• Cytotoxic vs antagonistic benefits unclear • Specificity high • Pharmacokinetics unclear
Small molecule inhibitors	• Not IL-15-specific • Risk of idiosyncratic effects

full-length soluble IL-15Rα administration to manipulate IL-15 bioactivities *in vivo*. When sIL-15Rα is injected daily following antigen challenge the development of collagen-induced arthritis (CIA) is suppressed, associated with delayed development of anti-collagen-specific antibodies (IgG2a) and with reduced antigen-specific IFN-γ and TNF-α production *in vitro*.[48] On discontinuation of sIL-15Rα administration, CIA developed to levels comparable with controls, suggesting that anti-inflammatory effects are transient. In subsequent studies we have generated targeted mutants of IL-15Rα and identified the sushi domain as essential for functional cytokine neutralization.[49] Selected deletion of cysteine residues similarly disrupted folding to abrogate binding and function. Studies are ongoing to determine whether small molecule derivatives of sIL-15Rα are of therapeutic utility in the CIA model. This also provides opportunities to investigate the potential for dual targeting of synergistic cytokine activities, e.g. IL-15 and IL-18. An alternate approach has been to generate mutant IL-15 forms that can specifically modify IL-15 activities. An IL-15/Fcγ2a fusion protein that antagonizes the activities of IL-15 *in vitro* and lyses receptor-bearing cells, suppresses the onset of DTH responses *in vivo*, associated with reduction in CD4[+] T-cell infiltration.[50] This fusion protein has also proven effective *in vivo* in preventing rejection of murine islet cell allografts in combination with CTLA4/Fc.[51] Studies in CIA indicate that this fusion protein is effective in treating not only developing CIA but also established disease and that after treatment disease recurrence is suppressed. This effect is associated with suppression of expression of a broad range of inflammatory cytokines.[52] Finally anti-IL-15 antibody has been employed in informative studies *in vivo* using a psoriasis model in which human psoriatic biopsies engrafted to SCID mice have received human ati0IL-15 monoclonal antibody (mAb:AMG714) leading to rapid clearance of the psoriatic tissue pathogenesis.[53]

CLINICAL STUDIES TARGETING IL-15

Clinical studies in humans have been performed using a neutralizing antibody, AMG714, and a mAb targeting IL-2/15Rβ chain MIKβ2. The optimal approach in clinical trials has not yet been established.

The fully human IgG1 monoclonal anti-IL-15 antibody, AMG714, binds and neutralizes the activity of soluble and membrane-bound IL-15 *in vitro*. AMG714 has been tested in two clinical trials in RA. In a 12-week, dose-ascending, placebo-controlled study, RA patients (n = 30) that had failed several previous disease-modifying anti-rheumatic drugs (DMARDs) received a randomized, controlled, single dose of AMG714 (0.5–8 mg/kg) followed by open-label weekly doses for 4 weeks. IL-15 neutralization was well tolerated.[54] This study was not placebo-controlled throughout, however, encouraging signs of efficacy were obtained. Around 60% of patients achieved an ACR 20 response with some 25% achieving an ACR 70 improvement. In parallel studies, AMG714 was shown to inhibit endogenous RA synovial T-cell activation and to suppress IL-15-induced cytokine release.[54] A subsequent dose-finding study has now been performed[55] in which RA patients received increasing fixed doses (up to 280 mg per injection) of anti-IL-15 antibody every 2 weeks by s.c. injection for 3 months. An interim analysis indicated satisfactory tolerance compared with placebo and ACR 20 improvements were observed in approximately 60% of recipients receiving higher doses of AMG714. No significant alterations in the levels of circulating leukocyte subsets, including NK cells and CD8[+] memory T cells, were observed. Extension of this study was performed to compare the highest dose of AMG714 (*n* = 121) with placebo (*n* = 58). Significant improvements in ARC 20 responses occurred in AMG714 recipients compared with placebo at week 12 and week 16 of follow-up. Of note, however, ACR 20 responses were not significantly different from placebo at week 14 (reflecting a higher placebo response at this time point), the pre-designated primary outcome time for this study. Clear and significant improvements in acute phase reactants occurred in AMG714 recipients compared with placebo. Thus although there is clear evidence of biologic activity and biological proof of concept, larger confirmatory studies are now required to facilitate proper interpretation of these data and at this stage IL-15 should not as yet be considered a validated therapeutic target in RA.

Several outstanding issues remain in this clinical area. The relative role of IL-15 as a target compared with TNF and IL-6 is unclear. Its role in early T-cell/DC interactions suggests that it may have some role in tolerance induction and therefore manipulation of IL-15 may offer potential in early disease beyond its capability in later RA, the only subjects thus far treated. IL-15 mediates effects on epithelial cells of the gut, keratinocytes, myocytes, hepatocytes, and several central nervous system (CNS) subsets indicating broad tissue effector function in host defence.[56–64] Elevated levels are detected in a variety of inflammatory diseases and there is momentum currently to explore its therapeutic role across a range of disorders. In particular psoriasis offers attractive potential based on expression patterns in disease tissue, the beneficial effects of IL-15 blockade in relevant models, and the potential for interruption of IL-15 function in remitting relapsing inflammatory disease typical in some psoriatic disease patterns. Finally, it will now be necessary to extend the range of modalities of blockade. Preclinical studies are under way using IL-15 mutant proteins and additional anti-IL-15 mAbs are under consideration. A phase I trial has been performed in which IL-15 was blocked using Mikβ1 mAb in patients with large granular lymphocyte leukemia[65] – this reagent is now being tested in a variety of inflammatory conditions. In particular there is interest in utilizing either signal molecule inhibitors, e.g. JAK inhibitors. However, these do not yet facilitate specific cytokine targeting. This may not be a deficit in their strategic importance, as focusing on given pathologic signaling pathways may offer some advantages over pan cytokine inhibition.

CONCLUSIONS

IL-15 represents an intriguing cytokine activity with pleiotropic effects in RA synovial membrane. Recent studies suggest broader expression in a range of autoimmune diseases. Many data now support a proinflammatory role. The success of TNF-α blockade clearly illustrates the potential in effective targeting of regulatory cytokines. However, those patients in whom either a partial or absent response occurs demonstrate the need for further studies to determine factors that in turn regulate TNF-α production, operate in synergy with TNF-α or indeed operate independent of TNF-α. The data presented above provide compelling evidence to support such a role for IL-15 in synovial inflammation. Early clinical trials are encouraging but not yet conclusive in validating IL-15 as a target. Further preclinical and clinical studies will be required to determine what the optimal targeting mechanisms may be given the complex membrane and intracellular expression of IL-15 on a number of tissues. Nevertheless, it clearly represents a target worthy of exploration either alone or as a component of combination cytokine-targeting approaches.

ACKNOWLEDGMENTS

The support of the Nuffield Foundation (Oliver Bird Fund), the Wellcome Trust, and the Arthritis Research Campaign (UK) is acknowledged. Bernard P. Leung, J. Alastair Gracie, Ros Forsey, Morag Prach, Holger Ruchatz, Xiao Qing Wei, Max Field, Peter Wilkinson, and Roger D. Sturrock provided invaluable contributions. Clinical support from Hilary Capell, John Hunter, Duncan Porter, Andy Kininmonth, and Rajan Madhok is acknowledged.

REFERENCES

1. Fox DA. The role of T cells in the immunopathogenesis of rheumatoid arthritis: new perspectives. Arthritis Rheum 1997; 40: 598–609.

2. Panayi GS, Lanchbury JS, Kingsley GH. The importance of the T cell in initiating and maintaining the chronic synovitis of rheumatoid arthritis. Arthritis Rheum 1992; 35: 729–35.

3. Feldmann M, Brennan FM, Maini RN. Role of cytokines in rheumatoid arthritis. Annu Rev Immunol 1996; 14: 397–440.

4. Arend WP, Dayer JM. Inhibition of the production and effects of interleukin-1 and tumor necrosis factor alpha in rheumatoid arthritis. Arthritis Rheum 1995; 38: 151–60.

5. Grabstein KH, Eisenman J, Shanebeck K et al. Cloning of a T cell growth factor that interacts with the beta chain of the interleukin-2 receptor. Science 1994; 264: 965–8.

6. Bamford R, Grant A, Burton J et al. The interleukin (IL) 2 receptor β chain is shared by IL-2 and a cytokine, provisionally designated IL-T, that stimulates T-cell proliferation and the induction of lymphokine-activated killer cells. Proc Natl Acad Sci U S A 1994; 91: 4940–4.

7. Budagian V, Bulanova E, Paus R, Bulfone-Paus S. IL-15/IL-15 receptor biology: a guided tour through an expanding universe. Cytokine Growth Factor Rev 2006; 17: 259–80.

8. Kotake S, Schumacher HR Jr, Yarboro CH et al. In vivo gene expression of type 1 and type 2 cytokines in synovial tissues from patients in early stages of rheumatoid, reactive, and undifferentiated arthritis. Proc Assoc Am Physicians 1997; 109: 286–301.

9. McInnes IB, Leung BP, Feng GJ et al. A role for IL-15 in rheumatoid arthritis. Nat Med 1998; 4: 645.

10. Harada S, Yamamura M, Okamoto H et al. Production of interleukin-7 and interleukin-15 by fibroblast-like synoviocytes from patients with rheumatoid arthritis. Arthritis Rheum 1999; 42: 1508–16.

11. Shah MH, Hackshaw KV, Caligiuri MA. A role for IL-15 in rheumatoid arthritis? Nat Med 1998; 4: 643.

12. Ortiz AM, Garcia-Vicuna R, Sancho D et al. Cyclosporin A inhibits CD69 expression induced on synovial fluid

and peripheral blood lymphocytes by interleukin 15. J Rheumatol 2000; 27: 2329–38.

13. Ziolkowska M, Koc A, Luszczykiewicz G et al. High levels of IL-17 in rheumatoid arthritis patients: IL-15 triggers in vitro IL-17 production via cyclosporin A-sensitive mechanism. J Immunol 2000; 164: 2832–8.

14. Raza K, Falciani F, Curnow SJ et al. Early rheumatoid arthritis is characterized by a distinct and transient synovial fluid cytokine profile of T cell and stromal cell origin. Arthritis Res Ther 2005; 7(4): R784–95.

15. Aringer M, Stummvoll GH, Steiner G et al. Serum interleukin-15 is elevated in systemic lupus erythematosus. Rheumatology 2001; 40: 876–81.

16. Klimiuk PA, Sierakowski S, Latosiewicz R et al. Serum cytokines in different histological variants of rheumatoid arthritis. J Rheumatol 2001; 28: 1211–17.

17. Cordero OJ, Salgado FJ, Mera-Varela A, Nogueira M. Serum interleukin-12, interleukin-15, soluble CD26, and adenosine deaminase in patients with rheumatoid arthritis. Int Rheumatol 2001; 21: 69–74.

18. Hidaka T, Suzuki K, Kawakami M et al. Dynamic changes in cytokine levels in serum and synovial fluid following filtration leukocytapheresis therapy in patients with rheumatoid arthritis. J Clin Apheresis 2001; 16: 74–81.

19. Cho ML, Yoon CH, Hwang SY et al. Effector function of type II collagen-stimulated T cells from rheumatoid arthritis patients: cross-talk between T cells and synovial fibroblasts. Arthritis Rheum 2004; 50(3): 776–84.

20. Yanagawa H, Takeuchi E, Miyata J et al. Rheumatoid pleural effusion with detectable level of interleukin-15. J Intern Med 1998; 243: 331–2.

21. Miranda-Carus ME, Benito-Miguel M, Balsa A et al. Peripheral blood T lymphocytes from patients with early rheumatoid arthritis express RANKL and interleukin-15 on the cell surface and promote osteoclastogenesis in autologous monocytes. Arthritis Rheum 2006; 54(4): 1151 64.

22. McInnes IB, al-Mughales J, Field M et al. The role of interleukin-15 in T-cell migration and activation in rheumatoid arthritis. Nat Med 1996; 2: 175–82.

23. Thurkow EW, van der Heijden IM, Breedveld FC et al. Increased expression of IL-15 in the synovium of patients with rheumatoid arthritis compared with patients with Yersinia-induced arthritis and osteoarthritis. J Pathol 1997; 181: 444–50.

24. Oppenheimer-Marks N, Brezinschek RI, Mohamadzadeh M et al. Interleukin 15 is produced by endothelial cells and increases the transendothelial migration of T cells in vitro and in the SCID mouse-human rheumatoid arthritis model in vivo. J Clin Invest 1998; 101: 1261–72.

25. Danning CL, Illei GG, Hitchon C et al. Macrophage-derived cytokine and nuclear factor kappaB p65

26. expression in synovial membrane and skin of patients with psoriatic arthritis. Arthritis Rheum 2000; 43: 1244–56.

26. Scola MP, Thompson SD, Brunner HI et al. Interferon-gamma:interleukin 4 ratios and associated type 1 cytokine expression in juvenile rheumatoid arthritis synovial tissue. J Rheumatol 2002; 29: 369–78.

27. Cho ML, Kim WU, Min SY et al. Cyclosporine differentially regulates interleukin-10, interleukin-15, and tumor necrosis factor a production by rheumatoid synoviocytes. Arthritis Rheum 2002; 46: 42–51.

28. Wakisaka S, Suzuki N, Nagafuchi H et al. Characterization of tissue outgrowth developed in vitro in patients with rheumatoid arthritis: involvement of T cells in the development of tissue outgrowth. Int Arch Allergy Immunol 2000; 121: 68–79.

29. Waldmann TA, Tagaya Y. The multifaceted regulation of interleukin-15 expression and the role of this cytokine in NK cell differentiation and host response to intracellular pathogens. Annu Rev Immunol 1999; 17: 19–49.

30. Rappl G, Kapsokefalou A, Heuser C et al. Dermal fibroblasts sustain proliferation of activated T cells via membrane-bound interleukin-15 upon long-term stimulation with tumor necrosis factor-alpha. J Invest Dermatol 2001; 116: 102–9.

31. Sen M, Lauterbach K, El-Gabalawy H et al. Expression and function of wingless and frizzled homologs in rheumatoid arthritis. Proc Natl Acad Sci U S A 2000; 97: 2791–6.

32. Sen M, Chamorro M, Reifert J et al. Blockade of Wnt-5A/frizzled 5 signaling inhibits rheumatoid synoviocyte activation. Arthritis Rheum 2001; 44: 772–81.

33. Min SY, Kim WU, Cho Ml et al. Prostaglandin E2 suppresses nuclear factor-kappaB mediated interleukin 15 production in rheumatoid synoviocytes. J Rheumatol. 2002; 29(7): 1366–76.

34. Bierbaum S, Sengler C, Gerhold K, Berner R, Heinzmann A. Polymorphisms within interleukin 15 are associated with juvenile idiopathic arthritis. Clin Exp Rheumatol 2006; 24(2): 219.

35. McInnes IB, Leung BP, Sturrock RD et al. Interleukin-15 mediates T cell-dependent regulation of tumor necrosis factor-alpha production in rheumatoid arthritis. Nat Med 1997; 3: 189–95.

36. Dalbeth N, Callan MF. A subset of natural killer cells is greatly expanded within inflamed joints. Arthritis Rheum 2002; 46(7): 1763–72.

37. Szekanecz Z, Strieter RM, Kunkel SL, Koch AE. Chemokines in rheumatoid arthritis. Springer Semin Immunopathol 1998; 20: 115–32.

38. Szekanecz Z, Koch AE. Chemokines and angiogenesis. Curr Opin Rheumatol 2001; 13: 202–8.

39. Al-Mughales J, Blyth TH, Hunter JA, Wilkinson PC. The chemoattractant activity of rheumatoid synovial

fluid for human lymphocytes is due to multiple cytokines. Clin Exp Immunol 1996; 106: 230–6.

40. Nieto M, del Pozo MA, Sanchez-Madrid F. Interleukin-15 induces adhesion receptor redistribution in T lymphocytes. Eur J Immunol 1996; 26: 1302–7.

41. Nanki T, Shimaoka T, Hayashida K et al. Pathogenic role of the CXCL16-CXCR6 pathway in rheumatoid arthritis. Arthritis Rheum 2005; 52(10): 3004–14.

42. Pilling D, Akbar AN, Girdlestone J et al. Interferon-beta mediates stromal cell rescue of T cells from apoptosis. Eur J Immunol 1999; 29: 1041–50.

43. Girard D, Paquet ME, Paquin R, Beaulieu AD. Differential effects of interleukin-15 (IL-15) and IL-2 on human neutrophils: modulation of phagocytosis, cytoskeleton rearrangement, gene expression, and apoptosis by IL-15. Blood 1996; 88: 3176–84.

44. Girard D, Boiani N, Beaulieu AD. Human neutrophils express the interleukin-15 receptor alpha chain (IL-15Ralpha) but not the IL-9Ralpha component. Clin Immunol Immunopathol 1998; 88: 232–40.

45. Leung BP, Chaudhuri K, Forsey RJ et al. Interleukin-15 induces cytokine production by rheumatoid arthritis (RA) synovial neutrophils. Arthritis Rheum 1997; 40: s274 (1457).

46. Yang L, Thornton S, Grom AA. Interleukin-15 inhibits sodium nitroprusside-induced apoptosis of synovial fibroblasts and vascular endothelial cells. Arthritis Rheum 2002; 46(11): 3010–14.

47. Verri WA Jr, Cunha TM, Parada CA et al. IL-15 mediates immune inflammatory hypernociception by triggering a sequential release of IFN-gamma, endothelin, and prostaglandin. Proc Natl Acad Sci U S A 2006; 103(25): 9721–5.

48. Ruchatz H, Leung BP, Wei XQ et al. Soluble IL-15 receptor alpha-chain administration prevents murine collagen-induced arthritis: a role for IL-15 in development of antigen-induced immunopathology. J Immunol 1998; 160: 5654–60.

49. Wei X, Orchardson M, Gracie JA et al. The sushi domain of soluble IL-15 receptor alpha is essential for binding IL-15 and inhibiting inflammatory and allogenic responses in vitro and in vivo. J Immunol 2001; 167: 277–82.

50. Kim YS, Maslinski W, Zheng XX et al. Targeting the IL-15 receptor with an antagonist IL-15 mutant/Fc gamma2a protein blocks delayed-type hypersensitivity. J Immunol 1998; 160: 5742–8.

51. Ferrari-Lacraz S, Zheng XX, Kim YS et al. An antagonist IL-15/Fc protein prevents costimulation blockade-resistant rejection. J Immunol 2001; 167: 3478–85.

52. Ferrari-Lacraz S, Zanelli E, Neuberg M et al. Targeting IL-15 receptor-bearing cells with an antagonist mutant IL-15/Fc protein prevents disease development and progression in murine collagen-induced arthritis. J Immunol. 2004; 173(9): 5818–26.

53. Villadsen LS, Schuurman J, Beurskens F et al. Resolution of psoriasis upon blockade of IL-15 biological activity in a xenograft mouse model. J Clin Invest 2003; 112(10): 1571–80.

54. Baslund B, Tvede N, Danneskiold-Samsoe B et al. Targeting interleukin-15 in patients with rheumatoid arthritis: a proof-of-concept study. Arthritis Rheum 2005; 52(9): 2686–92.

55. Mcinnes IB, Martin R, I Zimmermann-gorska et al. Safety and efficacy of a human monoclonal antibody to IL-15 (AMG 714) in patients with rheumatoid arthritis: results of a multicenter, randomized, double-blind, placebo-controlled trial. Ann Rheum Dis 2006; OPOO22.

56. Kirman I, Nielsen OH. Increased numbers of interleukin-15-expressing cells in active ulcerative colitis. Am J Gastroenterol 1996; 91: 1789–94.

57. Sakai T, Kusugami K, Nishimura H et al. Interleukin 15 activity in the rectal mucosa of inflammatory bowel disease. Gastroenterology 1998; 114: 1237–43.

58. Kakumu S, Okumura A, Ishikawa T et al. Serum levels of IL-10, IL-15 and soluble tumour necrosis factor-alpha (TNF-alpha) receptors in type C chronic liver disease. Clin Exp Immunol 1997; 109: 458–63.

59. Kivisakk P, Matusevicius D, He B et al. IL-15 mRNA expression is up-regulated in blood and cerebrospinal fluid mononuclear cells in multiple sclerosis (MS). Clin Exp Immunol 1998; 111: 193–7.

60. Pashenkov M, Mustafa M, Kivisakk P, Link H. Levels of interleukin-15-expressing blood mononuclear cells are elevated in multiple sclerosis. Scand J Immunol 1999; 50: 302–8.

61. Stegall T, Krolick KA. Myocytes respond in vivo to an antibody reactive with the acetylcholine receptor by upregulating interleukin-15: an interferon-gamma activator with the potential to influence the severity and course of experimental myasthenia gravis. J Neuroimmunol 2001; 119: 377–86.

62. Agostini C, Trentin L, Facco M et al. Role of IL-15, IL-2, and their receptors in the development of T cell alveolitis in pulmonary sarcoidosis. J Immunol 1996; 157: 910–18.

63. Agostini C, Trentin L, Perin A et al. Regulation of alveolar macrophage-T cell interactions during Th1-type sarcoid inflammatory process. Am J Physiol 1999; 277: L240–250.

64. Muro S, Taha R, Tsicopoulos A et al. Expression of IL-15 in inflammatory pulmonary diseases. J Allergy Clin Immunol 2001; 108: 970–5.

65. Morris JC, Janik JE, White JD et al. Preclinical and phase I clinical trial of blockade of IL-15 using Mikbeta1 monoclonal antibody in T cell large granular lymphocyte leukemia. Proc Natl Acad Sci U S A 2006; 103(2): 401–6.

46

Clinical prospects of MAPK inhibitors

Susan E Sweeney and Gary S Firestein

Introduction • MAPK pathway • MAPK expression and regulation in rheumatoid arthritis synovium • Expression and regulation of MAPKs in cultured fibroblast-like synoviocytes • MAPKs in animal models of arthritis • MAPKs in other autoimmune diseases • MAPKs as therapeutic targets • Conclusion • References

INTRODUCTION

Intracellular signaling pathways, especially protein kinases, allow cells to respond to environmental stress. Diverse extracellular stimuli activate cascades of these kinases that ultimately result in nuclear localization of transcription factors and gene transcription. This process regulates expression of cytokines, chemokines, degradative enzymes, programmed cell death, and cell growth and proliferation. These pathways also initiate immune responses to protect the host from pathogens such as bacteria, viruses, and parasites. In genetically predisposed individuals with increased underlying immune reactivity, proinflammatory stimuli that engage this mechanism might not be self-limited and can direct a pathologic, destructive response that harms the host, as in rheumatoid arthritis (RA). Dissection of these cytokine and signal transduction pathways can potentially provide insight into the pathogenesis of chronic inflammatory diseases and lead to identification of potential therapeutic targets.

MAPK PATHWAY

Protein kinases are enzymes that phosphorylate serine, threonine, or tyrosine amino acid side chains on a variety of proteins, such as downstream kinases or transcription factors.

The resultant phosphorylation can alter the target protein kinase activity, initiate formation of intracellular complexes, or enhance enzymatic degradation of the phosphorylated proteins. One of these pathways, the mitogen-activated protein kinases (MAPKs), includes a family of kinase cascades that regulate many cellular activities including cell survival, proliferation, division, and metabolism, as well as cytokine and metalloproteinase gene expression.[1] MAPKs are divided into three subfamilies (Figure 46.1),

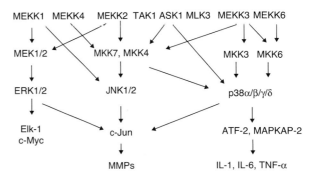

Figure 46.1 MAPK signaling pathways. Complex parallel and crossover signaling cascades link the three main MAPK families, ERK, JNK, and p38. The top level shows the MAP kinase kinase kinases (MAP3Ks), the second tier shows the MAP kinase kinases (MKKs), and the third tier consists of the MAPKs that regulate various genes through transcriptional and post-transcriptional mechanisms.

including extracellular signal-related kinases (ERK1 and 2), p38 MAPK (α, β, γ, δ), and c-Jun N-terminal kinase (JNK1, 2, 3).[2] The MAPK subfamilies differ in substrate specificity and response to extracellular stress, depending on the type of cell and stimulus. ERK1 and ERK2 are widely expressed and typically regulate cellular proliferation and differentiation. In contrast, p38 and JNK often increase inflammation and regulate apoptosis. However, the functions of individual MAPKs broadly overlap.

The MAPK pathways are parallel but interactive signal cascades that are composed of three sequentially activated kinases. MAPKs represent the terminal component of a three-tiered cascade and serve as phosphorylation substrates for MAPK kinases (MKKs). The MKKs are in turn regulated by upstream MKK kinases (MAP3Ks). MAP3Ks, MKKs, MAPKs, as well as the substrates of MAPKs, are regulated and activated via phosphorylation by upstream kinases and dephosphorylation by protein phosphatases.

Initiation of the MAPK cascade occurs when cells sense stress in the environment, such as cytokines, Toll-like receptor (TLR) ligands, growth factors, adhesion molecule ligation, ultraviolet irradiation, and oxidative stress. For instance, activation of certain cytokine receptors and growth factor receptors activates the ERKs. The p38 MAPKs are induced by lipopolysaccharide (LPS), proinflammatory cytokines, and osmotic shock. The JNK isoforms are also activated by a variety of stimuli, including ultraviolet light, protein synthesis inhibitors, and cytokines. While these general rules are useful, there is considerable cross-talk and promiscuity among the MAPKs. Engagement of cell surface receptors that initiate the MAPK cascade activates small intracellular GTPases (e.g. Ras, Rac), which in turn activate the MAP3Ks. MAP3Ks have distinct sequence motifs that provide selective activation capability in response to different extracellular stimuli. The many different MAP3Ks can then be matched with specific MKK-MAPK sets, allowing cells to respond to different circumstances with the activation of a specific MAPK pathway.

Although the four isoforms of p38 (p38α, β, γ, and δ) and two isoforms of ERK (ERK 1 and ERK2) are pivotal signaling pathways for inflammation and the cell cycle, respectively, JNK might be the primary MAPK involved in production of metalloproteinases (MMPs) and joint destruction in inflammatory arthritis. JNK was originally isolated and characterized as a stress-activated protein kinase on the basis of its activation in response to inhibition of protein synthesis by cycloheximide.[3] Three JNK genes exist, and each has multiple alternatively spliced subtypes, creating 10 JNK isoforms in total.[4] The pathway leading to JNK activation is complex, with both cell- and stimulus-specific responses controlled by phospho-relay systems among distinct intracellular complexes. A variety of receptor-associated signaling mechanisms then lead to activation of MAP3Ks, such as MEKK1–4, ASK1, TAK1, and MLK3, that subsequently activate downstream the two JNK kinases, MKK4 and MKK7. MKK4 can activate JNK or p38 MAPKs. MKK7, however, only activates JNK. MKK4 preferentially phosphorylates tyrosine 185 on JNK, whereas MKK7 prefers the threonine 183. Phosphorylation of both sites on JNK is required for full kinase function. JNK then phosphorylates two sites on the N-terminal activation domain of c-Jun, serine 63, and serine 73, which can then form hetero- and homo-dimers that bind the activator protein 1 (AP-1) site in promoter regions. AP-1 is widely distributed and regulates expression of MMP genes by binding to upstream regulatory regions. Similar cascades exist for the other two MAPK families: MEK1 and MEK2 are the MKKs that activate ERK, while MKK3 and MKK6 are the main kinases that regulate p38. In each case, the upstream kinases form stable complexes with the MAPK to provide an efficient method of signal transduction. Of the p38 proteins, the α isoform is thought to be most important for cytokine production by macrophages and is typically associated with MKK3.

MAPK EXPRESSION AND REGULATION IN RHEUMATOID ARTHRITIS SYNOVIUM

MAPKs are thought to participate in both the inflammatory and destructive components of RA. JNK, ERK, and p38 are expressed in synovial tissue and are present in their active phosphorylated forms in RA as demonstrated by immunohistochemistry and western blot analysis.[5,6] The relative distribution of each family is not random, but localized to specific regions of the synovium and independently contributes to disease pathogenesis. The MAPK p38 is widely distributed in the synovium, although the phosphorylated form is mainly found in the intimal lining where most of the cytokines and proteases are produced (Figure 46.2). Phospho-p38 is also expressed in synovial blood vessels. While p38δ is abundant in these locations, p38δ is overexpressed by synoviocytes at sites of invasion into the extracellular matrix.[7] The upstream regulators of p38, MKK3 and MKK6, are also more activated in RA than osteoarthritis (OA) and are located in the synovial intimal lining and, to a lesser extent, in perivascular lymphoid aggregates.[8] ERK activation

also appears to be localized primarily to blood vessels. In each case, the level of MAPK phosphorylation is significantly higher in RA than OA tissue.

p38 and ERK undoubtedly participate in the regulation of many of the genes known to contribute to rheumatoid synovitis, including tumor necrosis factor (TNF)-α, IL-1, and MMPs. p38, in particular, has complex mechanisms that modulate the expression of these genes, including regulation of transcription, mRNA stability, and translation. These proinflammatory genes are also regulated by JNK, albeit primarily at the transcriptional level. Activation of JNK in rheumatoid synovium was first demonstrated by western blot analysis, which confirmed that both 46 kD and 54 kD isoforms are phosphorylated to a greater extent in RA than OA[6] (Figure 46.3). Immunostaining has localized a significant percentage of the phospho-JNK to the sublining. However, its major substrate, c-Jun, and AP-1 are mainly activated in the synovial intimal lining. This is also the primary site for MMP gene expression and it is likely that JNK plays a prominent role in this process. The upstream activators of JNK, MKK4, and MKK7, are also expressed in rheumatoid synovium.[8] As with JNK, western blot shows that the JNK kinases (MKKs) are more highly phosphorylated in RA than OA synovium. Immunostaining confirms that MKK4 and MKK7 are mainly activated in

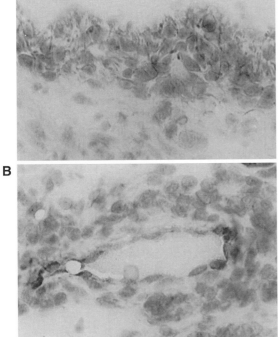

A

B

Figure 46.2 Immunostaining of activated p38 MAPK in synovial tissue from RA patients. Cryosections of synovial tissue from RA patients stained with P-p38 MAPK phosphospecific antibody (brown) demonstrate strong staining in RA, localized to the synovial lining (A) and endothelial cells of synovial blood vessels (B) Reproduced from Schett et al, Arthritis Rheum 2000; 43: 2501–12, with permission from John Wiley & Sons.[5]

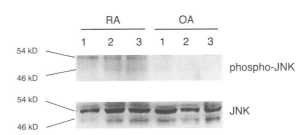

Figure 46.3 JNK phosphorylation in rheumatoid arthritis (RA) and osteoarthritis (OA) synovium. To evaluate the role of JNK *in vivo*, JNK phosphorylation was determined in extracts of intact RA and OA synovium by western blot analysis for JNK and phospho-JNK. Phospho-JNK was detected in the lysates of RA synovium tested but not in the OA tissue. Reproduced from Zuoning et al, J Pharmacol Exp Ther 1999; 291: 124–30, with permission from the American Society for Experimental Therapeutics.[6]

the intimal lining and also identifies this location as a key site for JNK function.

The top tier of the JNK cascade is also expressed in RA synovium. Multiple MAP3Ks have been identified using immunoassays to identify protein and polymerase chain reaction studies to quantify mRNA expression. Of these, MEKK1, MEKK2, TAK1, and ASK1 appear to be the most abundant in inflamed synovium.[9]

Immunohistochemistry to localize MEKK2 shows that it is primarily expressed in the intimal lining along with the other members of the JNK pathway.

EXPRESSION AND REGULATION OF MAPKs IN CULTURED FIBROBLAST-LIKE SYNOVIOCYTES

Of the three isoforms, JNK2 is the primary gene product in cultured fibroblast-like synoviocytes (FLS).[6] Approximately 90% of the JNK protein in synoviocytes is JNK2, with the remainder present as JNK1. JNK3 is mainly found in neural tissue and is not expressed in FLS or synovium. JNK, as well as p38 and ERK, are readily activated in synoviocytes as determined by phosphorylation and direct measures of kinase activity, by many proinflammatory factors known to be present in the rheumatoid joint, including IL-1 and TNF-α. *In vitro*, MAPK activation in FLS tends to be transient, often peaking after 15–30 minutes and declining to near baseline levels by 1 hour. Despite the decrease over time, the amount of phopshorylated MAPKs remains slightly above normal for up to 24 hours after stimulation. JNK activation and subsequent collagenase gene expression after IL-1 stimulation appear to be higher in RA than OA synoviocytes.[6]

The relative role of JNK, p38, and ERK in FLS function, especially related to AP-1 activation and MMP expression, was explored using small molecule inhibitors with relatively limited specificity.[6] Because a selective JNK inhibitor was not yet available, SB203580 was used to evaluate the mechanisms of increased collagenase expression in RA FLS. At low concentrations, this molecule is selective for p38. However, at 25–50 μM it also blocks some of the JNK isoforms. These studies suggested that blockade of p38 alone had less effect on collagenase gene expression than combination p38 and JNK blockade (i.e. by higher

SB203580 concentrations). However, in other cell lineages, such as chondrocytes, p38 played a prominent role in MMP13 expression. p38 blockade has a marked effect on IL-6 production, although the effects are mainly on protein production rather than mRNA levels. An ERK inhibitor, PD98059, has intermediate effects on MMP production in cultured synoviocytes.

More recent data using selective JNK inhibitors and genetic constructs have confirmed the pivotal role of JNK in the expression of MMPs by FLS. For instance, the JNK inhibitor SP600125 markedly decreased IL-1-induced c-Jun phosophorylation, AP-1 binding, and MMP gene expression in cultured synoviocytes.[10] Of interest, SP600125 did not suppress c-Jun phosphorylating activity below baseline levels, suggesting that other pathways (such as ERK or p38) can also contribute. This notion was confirmed by the observation that ERK inhibition also suppresses AP-1 activation and MMP expression.

Similar results were obtained by evaluating cultured synoviocytes isolated from JNK1$^{-/-}$ and JNK2$^{-/-}$ mice. Cells from both strains have a partial defect in IL-1-induced AP-1 activation and MMP3 and MMP13 gene expression. Of the two JNK isoforms, JNK2 appeared to be more important and is likely a reflection of the fact that this is the more abundant isoform in synoviocytes. The intermediate effect was probably due to the fact that only one of the two key JNK genes is deficient (double JNK knockout is embryonic lethal due to neural tube defects during development).

JNK also plays a role in the survival of synoviocytes and contributes to Fas-induced apoptosis. Nishioka and colleagues have shown that anti-Fas antibody induced cell death more readily in RA than OA synoviocytes.[11] This process was dependent on JNK phosphorylation and activation of AP-1. The authors speculated that overactivation of JNK signaling in RA FLS was due to prior exposure to cytokines *in situ*. To evaluate this possibility, OA FLS were pretreated with TNF-α, which increased their susceptibility to Fas-mediated apoptosis.[12] These data suggest that the cytokine environment in RA sensitizes to Fas-mediated cell death compared with non-inflammatory arthritis through a JNK-dependent mechanism.

Regulation of MAPKs in FLS by upstream kinases has also been evaluated. JNK is activated by the upstream MKKs, MKK4 and MKK7, that preferentially phosphorylate JNK on tyrosine 185 (MKK4) and threonine 183 (MKK7).[13] Both MKK4 and MKK7 are constitutively expressed by synoviocytes, and they are rapidly activated by exposure to cytokines like TNF-α and IL-1. Immunoprecipitation studies demonstrate that MKK4 and MKK7 form a complex with JNK, thereby providing a very efficient method for phosphorylating JNK and increasing expression of JNK-driven genes. This complex has been called the JNK signalsome and can also include scaffold proteins (e.g. JIP) or other upstream kinases (see below). The relative contribution of the two JNK kinases to FLS function has recently been examined using siRNA knockdown.[14] MKK4 appears to make little contribution to cytokine-stimulated JNK activation in FLS, while JNK phosphorylation and downstream transcriptional events were almost completely blocked by MKK7 knockdown. In contrast, non-receptor-mediated JNK activation, such as by anisomysin, is dependent on both MKK4 and MKK7. These data suggest that targeting an upstream kinase, especially MKK7, might interfere with pathogenic JNK activation in cytokine-driven diseases while allowing other stimuli to bypass this defect and engage JNK. While still highly speculative, this could potentially offer an improved risk-benefit profile compared with complete JNK blockade with a small molecule inhibitor.

Similarly, the upstream MKK3 and MKK6 are the primary activators of p38 in cultured FLS.[15] Both MKKs are rapidly activated by cytokines, but studies with dominant negative constructs suggest that MKK3 plays a more important role.[16] This was confirmed in MKK3$^{-/-}$ synoviocytes, where p38 phosphorylation and production of IL-1 and IL-6 after TNF-α stimulation was profoundly suppressed. Of interest, cytokine induction was normal in the MKK3$^{-/-}$ cells if they were treated with the TLR4 ligand LPS.[17] Upstream kinases MEK1 and MEK2 regulate the ERKs, although the relative contribution of each has not been elucidated.

The JNK signalsome, which includes JNK, MKK4, and MKK7, is regulated by the upstream MAP3Ks in synoviocytes. The upper tier of MAP3Ks is quite diverse and complex. Of the various members of the MAP3K family, TAK1, MEKK1, and MEKK2 are the most abundant in cultured FLS and are also expressed in intact synovium. Surprisingly, MEKK4, which is the most selective MAP3K for JNK, is only present at very low levels in FLS. MEKK2, in particular, can form a complex with the signalsome and is regulated by cytokines like IL-1. However, the relative hierarchy of these kinases in the activation of JNK and downstream genes is still uncertain. Preliminary data using siRNA knockdown methods suggest that TAK1, in particular, plays a key role in JNK phosphorylation and MMP expression in cytokine-stimulated FLS (unpublished data). Depending on the results of careful studies to dissect the pathway, new therapeutic targets might be identified that regulate JNK and other MAPKs in inflammation.

MAPKs IN ANIMAL MODELS OF ARTHRITIS

Given the key role that JNK plays in extracellular matrix degradation and cytokine production, the effect of JNK blockade in arthritis would be of considerable interest. Furthermore, data in JNK1$^{-/-}$ and JNK2$^{-/-}$ mice suggest that this pathway is also involved in the regulation of T-cell differentiation into the Th1 subset. Th1 cells, which produce cytokines like interferon (IFN)-γ, are thought to participate in the pathogenesis of animal models of arthritis as well as human RA. Hence, targeting JNK could alter the effector phase and the adaptive immune responses in inflammatory arthritis.

To evaluate the contribution of JNK to inflammatory joint disease, the JNK inhibitor SP600125 was evaluated in the rat adjuvant model. This anthrapyrazolone compound represented a major tool that advanced our understanding of JNK in inflammation.[18,19] It acts as a reversible ATP-competitive inhibitor with similar potency towards JNK1, JNK2, and JNK3. The adjuvant arthritis model is induced by immunization with complete Freund's adjuvant and results in T-cell-dependent, severe polyarticular, destructive arthritis. Rats were immunized with adjuvant on day 0 and treated daily with vehicle or SP600125 beginning on day 8. Administration of the JNK inhibitor modestly decreased paw swelling in treated rats (Figure 46.4).[10] More importantly, the SP600125-treated animals demonstrated a dramatic decrease in bone and cartilage damage as determined by radiographic analysis. Because the drug was administered over a week after immunization, its effect was more likely due to suppression of effector mechanisms than the initial immune response. This conclusion was substantiated by studies evaluating joint extracts from the SP600125-treated animals. *In vitro* kinase assays showed that JNK activity was suppressed and AP-1 binding was dramatically decreased. MMP13 gene expression was also much lower in the joints of the treated animals. These results were the first *in vivo* proof-of-concept that JNK inhibition could be effective in arthritis. The primary effect was on matrix destruction, although the modest anti-inflammatory effect

could have been due to the fact that the compound was not optimized for pharmacokinetics.

Because SP600125 inhibits all isoforms of JNK, and it is still possible that blocking only a single gene product would produce similar benefit. This has been explored using JNK1 and JNK2 knockout mice. Using the passive collagen arthritis model, Han and colleagues examined the course of disease in wild-type and JNK2$^{-/-}$ mice.[20] JNK2 was chosen first for evaluation because it is the major form expressed in FLS. The passive transfer model was used to determine the role of JNK2 in the effector phase of arthritis, which is independent of T cells. Although a modest degree of joint protection was noted, the benefit was much less than observed in the adjuvant arthritis model using a pan-JNK inhibitor. No effect was observed on the clinical severity of arthritis. Joint extract lysates also showed

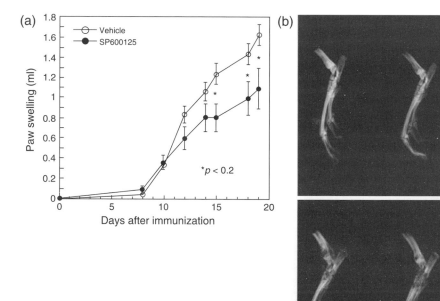

Figure 46.4 (a) Effect of the JNK inhibitor SP600125 on adjuvant arthritis in rats. Significantly less paw swelling was observed in the SP600125-treated animals. (b) Effect of SP600125 on radiographic damage in adjuvant arthritis. Ankle radiographs demonstrate decreased joint destruction in rats treated with SP600125 (upper panel) compared with vehicle (lower panel). Reproduced from Han et al, J Clin Invest 2001; 108: 73–81, with permission from the American Society for Clinical Investigation.[10]

similar amounts of AP-1 binding and MMP13 expression in the arthritic JNK2$^{-/-}$ and wild-type mice. These data suggest that an inhibitor might need to target both JNK1 and JNK2 to inhibit MMP expression.

More recently, the protective effect of JNK1 deficiency was examined in TNF-α transgenic mice. JNK1$^{-/-}$ mice were backcrossed with human TNF transgenic mice and the clinical course was evaluated. No differences in synovial inflammation, bone erosion, cartilage damage, or cellular infiltrate of the synovium were noted in the JNK1$^{-/-}$ hTNFtg compared with various controls.[21] Evaluation of JNK signaling in both genotypes demonstrated decreased phosphorylation of JNK in the JNK1$^{-/-}$ hTNFtg mice compared with hTNFtg mice. Expression of JNK2 and phospho-c-Jun in the synovial membrane was similar in both groups. The presence of intact JNK2 expression as well as JNK and c-Jun phosphorylation suggests that JNK2 can compensate for the deficiency of JNK1 in this model of TNF-α-mediated arthritis. These results agree with the concept that both JNK1 and JNK2 must be blocked to suppress joint destruction in arthritis.

Numerous studies have demonstrated that p38 inhibitors are effective in animal models of arthritis, including adjuvant arthritis and collagen-induced arthritis (CIA).[22,23] Treated animals have less synovial inflammation and cartilage destruction compared with vehicle-treated controls. p38 blockade also profoundly suppresses bone destruction. This appears to be due to a role of p38 in osteoclast differentiation and activation as well as suppression of RANKL expression[24] (Figure 46.5). The critical role of MKK3 as a key p38 regulator was recently confirmed *in vitro* using the passive K/BxN model in MKK3$^{-/-}$ mice. Deficiency of this MAPK kinase markedly decreased clinical arthritis as well as synovial phospho-p38, IL-1, and IL-6 levels.[17] The defect could be reversed by administration of exogenous IL-1 during the initial phases of the disease. As with cultured synoviocytes, LPS responses as measured by IL-6 production were normal in the MKK3$^{-/-}$ mice.

MAPKs IN OTHER AUTOIMMUNE DISEASES

JNK has been implicated in other rheumatic and inflammatory diseases including systemic lupus

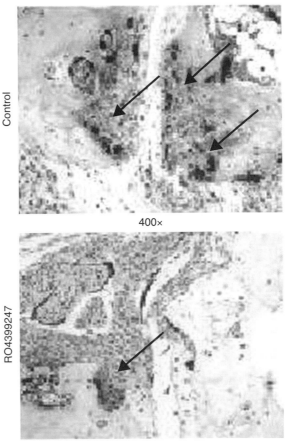

Figure 46.5 Effects of p38 MAPK blockade on bone erosion and synovial osteoclastogenesis. The numbers of synovial osteoclasts were determined in tartrate-resistant acid phosphatase (TRAP)-stained sections from TNF-transgenic mice ($n = 24$) that were treated with vehicle control (upper panel) or the p38 MAPK inhibitor RO4399247 (lower panel). Reductions in the number of synovial osteoclasts were statistically significant for the p38 MAPK inhibitor treated versus untreated control mice. Representative TRAP-stained sections of mice treated with vehicle (upper) or RO4399247 (lower) are shown. Reproduced from Zwerina et al, Arthritis Rheum 2006; 54: 463–72, with permission from John Wiley & Sons.[24]

erythematosus (SLE), psoriasis, asthma, and inflammatory bowel disease. Using intracellular flow cytometric assessment of SLE patients, B cells from the periphery of SLE patients contained higher levels of phosphorylated JNK, ERK, and p38 compared with normal individuals.[25] In psoriatic skin, JNK and ERK expression is increased in the nuclei of involved epidermis. In addition, western blot confirmed activation of JNK and ERK through detection of increased expression of phosphorylated forms of these kinases in the psoriatic epidermis.[26] Selective JNK and ERK activation might play a role in hyperproliferation and abnormal differentiation in psoriasis. Other studies, however, implicate ERK and p38 activation in psoriasis, rather than JNK.[27] It has also been proposed that blockade of JunB/AP-1 in epidermal keratinocytes triggers cytokine gene expression and cell recruitment that contributes to the epidermal alteration found in psoriasis. This alteration in gene expression could be sufficient to initiate both skin and joint manifestations in this disease.[28] p38 also is activated in many other inflammation models, including inflammatory bowel disease and allergic airway disease.[29,30]

Selective inhibition of JNK using SP600125 reduces inflammatory cell migration into the airway lumen after single allergen exposure in mice.[31] In addition, the JNK inhibitor SP600125 was used to evaluate the role of JNK in another murine model of airway inflammation and remodeling.[32] JNK inhibition results in fewer cells in the airways, suppressed eosinophilic inflammation in bronchial submucosa, and decreased allergen-induced bronchial responsiveness.

MAPKs AS THERAPEUTIC TARGETS

p38 inhibitors have been evaluated extensively in preclinical models of arthritis and have limited proof-of-concept in humans. Using the p38α/β selective inhibitor RWJ-67657, Fijen and colleagues evaluated the role of p38 in normal humans injected with low doses of LPS. The compound suppressed the fever response and the increase in serum cytokines like TNF-α.[33] A similar study with the Boehringer Ingelheim compound BIRB 796 showed that phosphorylation of the p38 substrate ATF-2 was inhibited after endotoxin injection.[34] This compound was also tested in a phase II study in RA, although the results have not been disclosed. VX-702 was examined in a short-term study of acute coronary syndrome and appeared to decrease the accompanying elevation in C-reactive protein.

This compound is also being evaluated in a phase II study as a single agent in RA. The VeRA study enrolled 315 patients and 278 completed 12 weeks of treatment. VX-702 led to a dose-dependent, statistically significant increase in ACR 20 response rates. The most common adverse events were rash, infection, and gastrointestinal intolerance, but no significant effects on lab measurements, including liver function tests, were noted. Overall the response was not robust, with a 44% ACR 20 response rate compared with 31% for placebo. However, the compound still needs to be evaluated in combination with methotrexate. Another Vertex compound, VX-745, was tested in a placebo-controlled study involving 44 patients; 43% of patients in the treatment arm achieved an ACR 20 response compared with 17% for placebo. Finally, the Scios compound SCI-469 has completed a phase I safety study in RA in patients. A larger phase II study comparing SCIO-469 to placebo has also recently been completed. This compound has also been studied in dental extraction pain and extended the time needed for ibuprofen rescue from 4.1 hours in the placebo group to 8.1 hours.

The major issues that have interfered with the development of these compounds relate to preclinical and clinical toxicity. For instance, several compounds have demonstrated an unusual inflammatory CNS condition in dogs, although this does not appear to occur in other species. As a result, new compounds with more limited CNS penetration have been proposed to solve this problem. In humans, hepatotoxicity has been a frequent dose-limiting concern. It is not clear whether this is compound-specific or mechanism-based. For instance, 16% of patients with RA treated with the lowest dose of VX-745 had elevated liver enzymes. The fact that structurally distinct compounds have similar profiles suggests the latter, although this is certainly not proven. Greater selectivity for p38 over other kinases, increased specificity for the α isoform of p38, or the development of allosteric inhibitors rather than ATP competitors might improve the toxicity profile. Alternatively, one could target downstream kinases, such as MAPKAPK-2, instead of p38 itself because MAPKAP-2 is likely responsible for the cytokine-regulating properties of the p38. The studies of MKKs also suggest that inhibiting MKK3 might provide the benefits of p38 inhibition for cytokine-mediated inflammation while sparing host defense and TLR responses.

JNK is a potential therapeutic target for a wide range of diseases, including cancer, diabetes, and inflammatory disorders. As with other kinases, the major issues for small molecules involve specificity and toxicity. These problems can be related, because lack of specificity for a particular kinase can potentially lead to unanticipated side effects. Specificity issues can be especially difficult when drugs are targeted at the ATP site of a kinase because there is considerable homology between different enzymes in the kinome. Alternatively, allosteric inhibitors that bind to other sites could potentially offer greater selectivity. Although the first JNK inhibitor, SP600125, from Celgene had a number of issues related to this problem, the elucidation of the crystal structure of JNK3 helped guide medicinal chemists to develop more suitable compounds.[35] For instance, Celgene has recently disclosed a second series of JNK inhibitors, such as CC-401, which successfully completed a phase I, double-blinded, placebo-controlled, ascending single intravenous dose study in healthy human volunteers.

A series of JNK compounds developed by Serono were disclosed as inhibitors of JNK2 and/or JNK3 for the treatment of autoimmune and neuronal disorders. These benzazoles are more potent inhibitors of JNK3 than JNK2. Serono also introduced a series of sulfonamide, sulfonyl amino acid, and sulfonyl hydrazides, as inhibitors of JNK2 and JNK3. One of the initial sulfonamides was further screened for its structure activity relationship and allowed identification of the areas that impart potency to the kinase-inhibiting motif. This work led to the identification of AS600292, the first selective JNK inhibitor in this class.[36] AS600292 protected against neuronal death by serum and growth factor starvation *in vitro*.

Structure activity studies led to increased potency via chemical modifications and improved biologic profile, resulting in synthesis of a new JNK inhibitor AS601245.[37] This compound was tested in the endotoxic shock model in mice, resulting in dose-dependent inhibition of plasma TNF-α levels when administered orally. The same compound was tested in a mouse model of CIA. Oral administration of AS601245 at 60 mg/kg reduced paw swelling and clinical arthritis scores in the JNK inhibitor-treated animals. Histological analysis revealed decreased cartilage erosion and synovial inflammation. Unlike SP600125, this optimized compound demonstrated potent anti-inflammatory and matrix-protecting effects. Selectivity tests against a large panel of kinases suggested that the compound has little or no effect on closely related kinases, hence the *in vivo* effects are likely due to inhibition of JNK. Cephalon has also revealed that the compound CEP-1347 will be tested in early Parkinson's disease.

Finally, in Crohn's disease, inhibition of the MAPKs JNK and p38 in humans using the combined inhibitor CNI-1493 demonstrated some evidence of clinical benefit with more rapid ulcer healing.[38] After these initial promising results, larger studies were discontinued because of lack of efficacy at doses that could be tolerated and infusion site reactions.

In addition to the competitive JNK inhibitors mentioned above, the development and therapeutic potential of ATP non-competitive peptide inhibitors has been another area of research in JNK inhibitor drug discovery.[39] While small molecule allosteric inhibitors have considerable potential, there is limited information on this topic. However, peptide-based approaches that can target or disrupt JNK signaling complexes have been reported. The JNK pathway is distinct from other MAPK pathways in the use of JIP family scaffold proteins.[40] Evidence that JIP1 serves to facilitate signaling through the JNK pathway *in vivo* was demonstrated by prevention of JNK activation in Jip1 knockout mice.[41] Overexpression of full-length JIP1 and studies using fragments of JIP, such as the JNK-binding domain (JBD), have also demonstrated inhibition of JNK activity in a variety of cell types. Purified JBD protein (JIP1 127-202) inhibits JNK activity in an *in vitro* kinase assay, and residues 144–163 of JIP1 JBD are essential for interaction with JNK. The sequence was resolved to an 11 amino acid peptide in the JBD region of JIP1 that binds JNK and inhibits its kinase activity.[42] The specificity of the short JIP1 JBD-derived peptides was tested and confirmed to inhibit only JNK and its upstream activators MKK4 and MKK7.[43] Finally, the JIP1-derived peptide was further characterized as a unique competitive inhibitor of the kinase interaction motif of c-Jun substrate.[44] JIP1 JBD peptides represent potential therapeutic targets through ATP non-competitive peptide inhibitors that bind to the kinase interaction motif on the substrate rather than the ATP binding site. In addition, the region on JNK that interacts with JIP1 could provide another location, other than the ATP binding site, to target as a JNK inhibitor.

Peptide inhibitors of JNK have been designed based on the protein scaffold JIP. *In vivo* studies are limited to gene transfer of the JIP1 JBD protecting neurons in a mouse model of Parkinson's disease.[45] The advantages of ATP non-competitive peptide inhibitors such as JIP1 JBD are primarily due to their highly specific interactions. Disadvantages of the non-competitive peptide inhibitors include limited cell permeability and potential proteolytic degradation *in vivo*.[39] Synthesis of peptidomimetics that can interact with JIP-1 binding sites could potentially overcome some of these problems.

ERK inhibitors for rheumatic disease have not progressed as far as the other two MAPK families. Most of the attention has been focused on cancer due to the prominent role that ERK plays in the regulation of cell growth. Rather than target ERK itself, current efforts appear related to inhibition of the upstream kinases MEK1 and MEK2. For instance, PD 0323901 has been evaluated in a phase I study in melanoma and several other types of cancer. This compound successfully inhibits ERK phosphorylation in the tumors and several partial remissions were observed. Toxicity related to skin rash and visual changes were observed with some frequency.

CONCLUSION

Improved understanding of MAPK regulation and function has resulted from extensive biochemical, cellular, and molecular studies in cultured synoviocytes. In addition, various animal models have been used to evaluate the role of the MAPKs and have confirmed that they have

considerable potential as a therapeutic target. MAPK inhibitors may be relevant for the treatment of numerous inflammatory diseases, including RA. The role of JNK in both effector mechanisms and some aspects of adaptive immunity support this concept. There are many inhibitors but additional work is still being directed towards the development of more selective compounds and novel inhibitors that target JNK-associated proteins, the JNK signalsome, protein–protein interactions, upstream kinases, and conformational changes required for signal transduction. Peptide or peptidomimetic inhibitors of the signaling complexes might allow disease-specific inhibition of pathogenic JNK or p38 signaling.[46] These approaches will hopefully lead to targeted therapies for a broad range of human diseases.

REFERENCES

1. Johnson GL, Lapadat R. Mitogen-activated protein kinase pathways mediated by ERK, JNK, and p38 protein kinases. Science 2002; 298: 1911–12.
2. Manning A, Davis R. Targeting JNK for therapeutic benefit: from junk to gold? Nat Rev Drug Discov 2003; 2: 554–65.
3. Kyriakis J, Avruch J. pp54 microtubule-associated protein 2 kinase. A novel serine/threonine protein kinase regulated by phosphorylation and stimulated by poly-L-lysine. J Biol Chem 1990; 265: 17355–63.
4. Gupta S, Barrett T, Whitmarsh A et al. Selective interaction of JNK protein kinase isoforms with transcription factors. EMBO J 1996; 15: 2760–70.
5. Schett G, Tohidast-Akrad M, Smolen JS et al. Activation, differentiatial localization, and regulation of the stress-activated protein kinases, extracellular signal-regulated kinase, c-JUN N-terminal kinase, and p38 mitogen-activated protein kinase, in synovial tissue and cells in rheumatoid arthritis. Arthritis Rheum 2000; 43: 2501–12.
6. Han Z, Boyle DL, Aupperle KR et al. Jun N-terminal kinase in rheumatoid arthritis. J Pharmacol Exp Ther 1999; 291: 124–30.
7. Kuchen S, Seemayer C, Rethage J et al. The L1 retroelement-related p40 protein induces p38delta MAP kinase. Autoimmunity 2004; 37: 57–65.
8. Sundarrajan M, Boyle DL, Chabaud-Riou M, Hammaker D, Firestein GS. Expression of the MAPK kinases MKK-4 and MKK-7 in rheumatoid arthritis and their role as key regulators of JNK. Arthritis Rheum 2003; 48: 2450–60.

9. Hammaker DR, Boyle DL, Chabaud-Riou M, Firestein GS. Regulation of JNK1 by MEKK2 and MAP kinase kinase kinases in rheumatoid arthritis. J Immunol 2004; 172: 1612–18.

10. Han Z, Boyle D, Chang L et al. c-Jun N-terminal kinase is required for metalloproteinase expression and joint destruction in inflammatory arthritis. J Clin Invest 2001; 108: 73–81.

11. Okamoto K, Fujisawa K, Hasunuma T et al. Selective activation of the JNK/AP-1 pathway in Fas-mediated apoptosis of rheumatoid arthritis synoviocytes. Arthritis Rheum 1997; 40: 919–26.

12. Ohshima S, Mima T, Sasai M et al. Tumour necrosis factor alpha (TNF-alpha) interferes with Fas-mediated apoptotic cell death on rheumatoid arthritis (RA) synovial cells: a possible mechanism of rheumatoid synovial hyperplasia and a clinical benefit of anti-TNF-alpha therapy for RA. Cytokine 2000; 12: 281–8.

13. Fleming Y, Armstrong C, Morrice N et al. Synergistic activation of stress-activated protein kinase 1/c-Jun N-terminal kinase (SAPK1/JNK) isoforms by mitogen-activated protein kinase kinase 4 (MKK4) and MKK7. Biochem J 2000; 352: 145–54.

14. Inoue T, Hammaker D, Boyle D, Firestein GS. Regulation of JNK by MKK7 in fibroblast-like synoviocytes. Arthritis Rheum 2006; 54: 2127–35.

15. Chabaud-Riou M, Firestein GS. Expression and activation of MKK3 and MKK6 in rheumatoid arthritis. Am J Pathol 2004; 164: 177–84.

16. Inoue T, Hammaker D, Boyle D, Firestein G. Regulation of p38 MAPK by MAPK kinases 3 and 6 in fibroblast-like synoviocytes. J Immunol 2005; 174: 4301–6.

17. Inoue T, Boyle DL, Corr M et al. Mirogen – activated protein kinase 3 is the pivotal pathway regulating p38 activation in inflammatory arthritis. Proc Natl Acid Sci U S A 2006 Apr 4; 103(14): 5484–9.

18. Bennett B, Sasaki D, Murray B et al. SP600125, an anthrapyrazolone inhibitor of Jun N-terminal kinase. Proc Natl Acad Sci U S A 2001; 98: 13681–6.

19. Bain J, McLauchlan H, Elliot M, Cohen P. The specificity of protein kinase inhibitors: an update. Biochem J 2003; 371(pt 1): 199–204.

20. Han Z, Chang L, Yamanishi Y, Karin M, Firestein G. Joint damage and inflammation in c-Jun N-terminal kinase 2 knockout mice with passive murine collagen-induced arthritis. Arthritis Rheum 2002; 46: 818–23.

21. Koller M, Hayer S, Redlich K et al. JNK1 is not essential for TNF-mediated joint disease. Arthritis Res Ther 2005; 7: R166–73.

22. Badger AM, Griswold DE, Kapadia R et al. Disease–modifying activity of SB242235, a selective inhibition of P38 mitogen–activated protein kinase, in rat adjuvant–induced arthritis. Arthritis Rheum 2000; 43(1): 175–83.

23. Nishikawa M, Myoui A, Tomita T et al. Prevention of the onset and progression of collagen–induced arthritis in rats by the protein P38 mitogen–activated protein kinase inhibitor FR167653. Arthritis Rheum 2003; 48(9): 2670–81.

24. Zwerina J, Hayer S, Redlich K et al. Activation of p38 MAPK is a key step in tumor necrosis factor-mediated inflammatory bone destruction. Arthritis Rheum 2006; 54: 463–72.

25. Grammer A, Fischer R, Lee O, Zhang X, Lipsky P. Flow cytometric assessment of the signaling status of human B lymphocytes from normal and autoimmune individuals. Arthritis Res Ther 2004; 6: 28–38.

26. Takahashi H, Ibe M, Nakamura S et al. Extracellular regulated kinase and c-Jun N-terminal kinase are activated in psoriatic involved epidermis. J Dermatol Sci 2002; 30: 94–9.

27. Johansen C, Kragballe K, Westergaard M et al. The mitogen-activated protein kinases p38 and ERK1/2 are increased in lesional psoriatic skin. Br J Dermatol 2005; 152: 37–42.

28. Zenz R, Eferl R, Kenner L et al. Psoriasis-like skin disease and arthritis caused by inducible epidermal deletion of Jun proteins. Nature 2005; 437: 369–75.

29. Hollenbach E, Vieth M, Roessner A et al. Inhibition of RICK/nuclear factor-kappaB and p38 signaling attenuates the inflammatory response in a murine model of Crohn disease. J Biol Chem 2005; 280: 14981–8.

30. Escott K, Belvisi M, Birrell M et al. Effect of the p38 kinase inhibitor, SB 203580, on allergic airway inflammation in the rat. Br J Pharmacol 2000; 131: 173–6.

31. Eynott P, Xu L, Bennett B et al. Effect of an inhibitor of Jun N-terminal protein kinase, SP600125, in single allergen challenge in sensitized rats. Immunology 2004; 112: 446–53.

32. Nath P, Eynott P, Leung S et al. Potential role of c-Jun NH2-terminal kinase in allergic airway inflammation and remodelling: effects of SP600125. Eur J Pharmacol 2005; 506: 273–83.

33. Fijen J, Zijlstra J, De Boer P et al. Suppression of the clinical and cytokine response to endotoxin by RWJ-67657, a p38 mitogen-activated protein-kinase inhibitor, in healthy human volunteers. Clin Exp Immunol 2001; 124: 16–20.

34. Branger J, van den Blink B, Weijer S et al. Anti-inflammatory effects of a p38 mitogen-activated protein kinase inhibitor during human endotoxemia. J Immunol 2002; 168: 4070–7.

35. Scapin G, Patel S, Lisnock J, Becker J, LoGrasso P. The structure of JNK3 in complex with small molecule inhibitors: structural basis for potency and selectivity. Chem Biol 2003; 10: 705–12.

36. Ruckle T, Biamonte M, Grippi-Vallotton T et al. Design, synthesis, and biological activity of novel, potent, and selective (benzoylaminomethyl)thiophene sulfonamide

inhibitors of c-Jun-N-terminal kinase. J Med Chem 2004; 47: 6921–34.

37. Gaillard P, Jeanclaude-Etter I, Ardissone V et al. Design and synthesis of the first generation of novel potent, selective, and in vivo active (benzothiazol-2-yl)acetonitrile inhibitors of the c-Jun N-terminal kinase. J Med Chem 2005; 48: 4596–607.

38. Hommes D, van den Blink B, Plasse T et al. Inhibition of stress-activated MAP kinases induces clinical improvement in moderate to severe Crohn's disease. Gastroenterology 2002; 122: 7–14.

39. Bogoyevitch M. Therapeutic promise of JNK ATP-noncompetitive inhibitors. Trends Mol Med 2005; 11: 232–9.

40. Yasuda J, Whitmarsh A, Cavanagh J, Sharma M, Davis R. The JIP group of mitogen-activated protein kinase scaffold proteins. Mol Cell Biol 1999; 19: 7245–54.

41. Jaeschke A, Czech M, Davis R. An essential role of the JIP1 scaffold protein for JNK activation in adipose tissue. Genes Dev 2004; 18: 1976–80.

42. Barr R, Kendrick T, Bogoyevitch M. Identification of the critical features of a small peptide inhibitor of JNK activity. J Biol Chem 2002; 277: 10987–97.

43. Borsello T, Clarke P, Hirt L et al. A peptide inhibitor of c-Jun N-terminal kinase protects against excitotoxicity and cerebral ischemia. Nat Med. 2003; 9: 1180–6.

44. Barr R, Boehm I, Attwood P, Watt P, Bogoyevitch M. The critical features and the mechanism of inhibition of a kinase interaction motif-based peptide inhibitor of JNK. J Biol Chem 2004; 279: 36327–38.

45. Xia X, Harding T, Weller M et al. Gene transfer of the JNK interacting protein-1 protects dopaminergic neurons in the MPTP model of Parkinson's disease. Proc Natl Acad Sci U S A 2001; 98: 10433–8.

46. Waetzig V, Herdegen T. Context-specific inhibition of JNKs: overcoming the dilemma of protection and damage. Trends Pharmacol Sci 2005; 26: 455–61.

47

Clinical prospects of NF-κB inhibitors to further targeted therapies in rheumatology

Stefan K Drexler, Jeremy JO Turner, and Brian M Foxwell

Introduction • The NF-κB transcription factor family • Involvement of NF-κB in rheumatological diseases • Non-specific NF-κB inhibitors • Targeted therapies • Potential future targets • Conclusion • References

INTRODUCTION

Many anti-inflammatory drugs currently used in clinical rheumatology are limited by lack of target specificity and a broad range of side effects consequent upon this. Thus, there is much interest in the possibility of developing improved targeted therapies that will have greater clinical efficacy combined with a narrower range of side effects.

The most significant recent advance in the clinical management of auto-inflammatory conditions including rheumatoid arthritis (RA) has been the advent of the biopharmaceuticals that target cytokines. Chief amongst these are the blockers of tumor necrosis factor (TNF)-α, infliximab (Centocor), a chimeric murine-human anti-TNF monoclonal antibody (mAb);[1] etanercept (Amgen), a TNF receptor-Fc fusion protein;[2] and adalimumab (Abbott Laboratories), a fully human anti-TNF mAb.[3] In addition, there has been success with blockade of interleukin (IL)-1 in RA using recombinant IL-1 receptor antagonist (IL-1Ra; anakinra, Amgen),[4,5] and with blockade of IL-6 by the humanized anti-IL-6 receptor mAb, tocilizumab (Hoffman-La-Roche).[6] However, the biopharmaceuticals have problems associated with their use including, cost, route of administration, and side effects.[7] They are also not universally efficacious in all patients. Thus, there is still a great unmet medical need for

the development of targeted anti-inflammatory drugs that will overcome some of these problems.

In order to build on the clinical success of the biopharmaceuticals while circumventing some of the associated problems, attention has focused on alternative strategies for inhibiting cytokine signaling. The transcription factor nuclear factor-κB (NF-κB) is activated by TNF-α, IL-6, and IL-1, and these genes are also under regulation by NF-κB.[8] Thus, inhibition of components of the NF-κB signaling pathway has come to be regarded as a promising alternative strategy for development of novel drugs to block the effects of excessive cytokines in auto-inflammatory diseases.

As the understanding of pathological cellular signaling in disease states improves, it is becoming feasible to apply this knowledge to identify novel drug targets and then seek compounds that act on these as a route to develop novel drugs. The efficacy of this approach has already been demonstrated by the development of the tyrosine kinase inhibitor imatinib (Novartis)[9] that targets constitutive tyrosine kinase signaling in chronic myeloid leukemia. In the future it is likely that an increasing number of drugs will be developed in this way.

This chapter discusses evidence that several anti-inflammatory agents currently in routine clinical use, in part, owe their anti-inflammatory effects to NF-κB inhibition. Current work to develop more targeted inhibitors will then be reviewed before discussing potential routes for the development of novel NF-κB inhibitors in the future.

THE NF-κB TRANSCRIPTION FACTOR FAMILY

The transcription factor NF-κB is involved in numerous cellular processes including development, inflammation, and immunity.[10] It consists of homo- or hetero-dimers of the subunits, c-Rel (also known as Rel); RelA (also known as p65 and NF-κB3); RelB, NF-κB1 (also known as p50), and NF-κB2 (also known as p52). All five subunits contain the characteristic Rel homology domain (RHD), which enables the subunits to dimerize and to bind to the promoter of target genes.[8]

NF-κB signaling is divided into two distinct signaling pathways, known as the canonical and the alternative (non-canonical) NF-κB pathways. Central to the canonical pathway is the formation of the NEMO (NF-κB essential modulator)/IKK (inhibitor κB kinase)1/IKK2 complex, the degradation of inhibitor-κB (IκB)α, following its phosphorylation, and the translocation of p50/RelA heterodimers to the nucleus (Figure 47.1). In contrast, the alternative pathway is activated by IKK1 phosphorylating NF-κB2 and marking it for processing by the proteasome. The processed p52, dimerized with RelB, subsequently translocates to the nucleus (Figure 47.1).

The most common dimer in the canonical NF-κB pathway, consisting of p50/RelA, is bound to the inhibitor, IκBα, in the cytosol in the quiescent state (Figure 47.1). IκBα is the archetypical NF-κB inhibitor in an evolutionary conserved inhibitor family consisting of IκBβ, IκBε, B cell CLL/lymphoma (Bcl)-3, IκBζ, and IκBNS as well as IκBγ, which is a degradation product of NF-κB1 and of NF-κB2.[8,11,12] With the exception of Bcl-3 and IκBζ, these proteins can inhibit the translocation of NF-κB dimers to the nucleus by interacting with the RHD and thereby inactivate the nuclear localization signal (NLS). IκBβ resembles IκBα in its primary as well as tertiary structure. However, while IκBα degradation leads to a rapid oscillatory NF-κB activation, IκBβ degradation results in prolonged NF-κB

activation.[8,13,14] This prolonged activation appears to be required for numerous pathological conditions including asthma and cystic fibrosis.[13,15–21] The oscillatory propensity in the NF-κB signaling system is counteracted by a negative feedback mechanism mediated by IκBε, which is delayed and functions in anti-phase to IκBα.[22] This indicates that cells have the capacity to modulate NF-κB activity depending on cell type and stimuli. Beside the canonical inhibitors IκBα, IκBβ, and IκBε, the two IκB family members Bcl-3 and IκBζ seem to have a more multifaceted role. Bcl-3 specifically interacts with the intrinsically inactive NF-κB1 and NF-κB2 homodimers in the nucleus and is not degraded after cellular stimulation.[23–26] Depending on its phosphorylation status it can either act as an inhibitor, dissociating p50 or p52 homodimers from DNA, or as a co-activator that is recruited to the gene promoter by p50 or p52 homodimers.[23–28] The recently described IκBζ is highly homologous to Bcl-3.[29–34] Its transcription is rapidly induced upon stimulation with Toll-like receptor (TLR) ligands and IL-1. Cells from IκBζ-deficient mice show a severe impairment of IL-6 production in response to a variety of TLR ligands and IL-1 but not in response to TNF-α.[35] Similar results were obtained using NF-κB1 knockout mice, which might indicate that IκBζ specifically interacts with the NF-κB1 subunit.[35] On the other hand, IκBNS seems to have the opposite role to IκBζ, as it was shown to selectively inhibit IL-6 production in response to lipopolysaccharide (LPS).[36] Furthermore, mice deficient in IκBNS are highly susceptible to LPS-induced endotoxic shock and intestinal inflammation, most likely due to prolonged activation of NF-κB.[37]

In order to allow the release of NF-κB dimers IκBs need to become phosphorylated by IKKs.[38] The IKK complex, inducing the canonical NF-κB pathway, consists of the regulatory subunit NEMO and the catalytic subunits IKK1 and IKK2.[39] While NEMO and IKK2 appear to be essential for NF-κB activation, cells lacking IKK1 still show normal levels of NF-κB DNA binding activity.[40–45] Subsequently, IKK1 kinase activity was found to be involved in the resolution of inflammation, induced by NF-κB activation, by accelerating the turnover of NF-κB and its

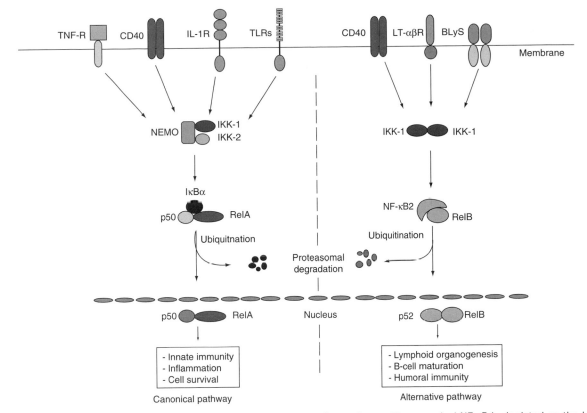

Figure 47.1 Illustration of the canonical and alternative NF-κB signaling pathways. The canonical NF-κB is depicted on the left side of the diagram. It is activated by proinflammatory mediators including TNF-α, IL-1, TLR ligands, and CD40L. Ligand binding ultimately leads to the activation of the IKK complex consisting of the regulatory subunit NEMO and the catalytic subunits IKK1 and IKK2. The endogenous inhibitor of NF-κB, IκBα, is phosphorylated by the IKK complex, which leads to its ubiquitination and as a result to its degradation by the proteasome. The released NF-κB dimer translocates to the nucleus where it induces transcription of genes involved in immunity, inflammation, and cell survival. The alternative NF-κB signaling pathway is depicted on the right. It is induced by lymphotoxin αβ, CD40L, and BLyS. Activation of these receptors leads to the activation of IKK1. IKK1 phosphorylates NF-κB2, which becomes degraded to p52 by the proteasome and as a result translocates to the nucleus as a dimer with RelB. The alternative pathway is involved in the organogenesis of lymphoid organs and in humoral immunity. NF-κB, nuclear factor-κB; TNF, tumor necrosis factor; IL, interleukin; TLR, Toll-like receptor; IKK, inhibitor of kappa kinase; NEMO, NF-κB essential modulator; IκBα, inhibitor-κBα; BLyS, B-lymphocyte stimulator.

release from the gene promoter.[46] In addition, IKK1 was shown to be an activator of the alternative NF-κB pathway[47–49] (Figure 47.1). IKK1 homo-dimer complexes induce the processing of NF-κB2 to p52 and consequently the nuclear translocation of p50/RelB hetero-dimers. While the NEMO/IKK1/IKK2 complex is required for NF-κB activation in response to most NF-κB stimuli, the role of the two non-canonical IKKs IKKε (also known as IKKi) and TBK-1 (TNF receptor associated factor family member-associated NF-κB activator binding kinase),

is unclear. Both were shown to be involved in the induction of interferon (IFN) regulatory factor (IRF)-3 in response to the TLR4 ligand LPS and the TLR3 ligand dsRNA.[50] Their role in the activation of NF-κB, however, is still not well understood.

Phosphorylation of IκBα by the IKKs and its subsequent proteasomal degradation releases NF-κB dimers to translocate to the nucleus and activate target genes.[47] However, NF-κB dimers need to undergo additional post-translational modifications, including site-specific phosphorylation and acetylation to produce a maximal transcriptional response.[51,52] The most well studied NF-κB subunit in terms of post-translational modifications is RelA. Several serine phosphorylation sites for RelA have been described including serines 276, 311, 529, and 536.[51] Kinases involved in the phosphorylation of these serine residues include protein kinase A (PKA), mitogen- and stress-activated kinase (MSK)-1, protein kinase C (PKC)ζ, ribosomal subunit kinase (RSK)-1, glycogen-synthase kinase (GSK)-3β, and phosphatidylinositol 3-kinase (PI3K), as well as the canonical IKKs and TBK1.[51] The kinases involved in serine phosphorylation appear to be stimuli-specific, e.g. PKA phosphorylates serine 276 in response to LPS while TNF-α triggers the phosphorylation of serine 276 by MSK1.[51] Ultimately serine phosphorylation leads to an enhancement in the overall transcriptional response. Similarly, acetylation is important for regulating NF-κB activity. Also, three main acetylation sites have been identified within RelA (lysines 218, 221, and 310).[53] The acetyltransferases p300 and cAMP response element binding protein (CBP) seem to be involved in RelA acetylation *in vivo*[53,54] and acetylation of RelA was reported to be regulated by phosphorylation of its serine residues 276 and 536, as phosphorylation increases the assembly of phosphoRelA-p300 complexes.[55] Acetylation of RelA results in different outcomes, as acetylation of lysine 221 enhances DNA binding and impairs assembly with IκBα, the acetylation of lysine 310 is required for full transcriptional activity of RelA.[51]

Inhibiting the amplification of NF-κB activity due to post-translational modification may provide a way to dampen the response generated by proinflammatory stimuli without affecting the basal activity of NF-κB, which is suggested to be beneficial by preventing undesired apoptosis.[56]

Nuclear translocation of NF-κB dimers allows their binding to κB sites in the promoter of the target gene. Several studies have attempted to identify DNA sequence specificity of different NF-κB dimers.[8,57–63] However, κB sites display a remarkably variable consensus sequence.[8] The classical κB nucleotide sequence is G-G-G-R-N-N-Y-Y-C-C[8] (where N = any base, R = purine, and Y = pyrimidine). This may suggest the possibility that the κB site, rather than

determining the ability of a particular dimer to bind effectively, affects which coactivator forms productive interactions with the bound NF-κB dimer. Unpublished results from our group suggest that even greater complexity of regulation of gene expression by κB sites exists. The κB sites of the TNF-α gene may be both inhibitory and stimulatory under specific conditions. One possible explanation is that the binding sites may affect the tertiary structure of the activation complex.

NF-κB activators and its outputs

The NF-κB pathway described above integrates signals from a wide range of stimuli and in turn activates numerous cellular responses.[64] This section will discuss NF-κB activation in the context of inflammation.

The canonical pathway is mainly stimulated by inflammatory signals including TNF-α, IL-1, IL-17, and CD40 ligand (CD40L), as well as pathogen-associated molecular patterns (PAMPs) recognized by TLRs and nucleotide oligomerization domain (NOD) receptors.[65–68] The activation of NF-κB by these stimuli leads to the expression of inflammatory mediators such as cytokines, chemokines, cell adhesion molecules, inducible nitric oxide synthase (iNOS), anti-apoptotic proteins, costimulatory molecules, matrix metalloproteinases (MMPs), and cyclooxygenase (COX).[69] The canonical NF-κB pathway leads to the maturation and activation of macrophages and dendritic cells (DCs) and consequently to the induction of the innate and adaptive immune response and inflammation. In the case of TNF-α-induced signaling, NF-κB has been shown to be an activator of anti-apoptotic gene expression.[70–73] This outcome of NF-κB signaling has been shown to depend on the termination of c-Jun N-terminal kinase (JNK) activation.[74,75] Therefore, TNF-α signaling may result in apoptosis, if JNK is activated, or proliferation, if NF-κB activation prevails.[76] This indicates that these signaling pathways are not strictly linear but that there is cross-talk between different signaling pathways taking place which influences the outcome of receptor stimulation. Therefore, inhibition of one signaling pathway may also affect the outcome of other signaling pathways.

In addition, NF-κB exhibits different activation dynamics depending on the stimulus. While showing an oscillatory dynamic when stimulated with TNF-α, this is not observed when stimulated with the TLR4 ligand LPS.[77] These differences are associated with distinct signaling pathways induced by those stimuli.

Strong inducers of the alternative NF-κB pathway are lymphotoxin (LT), CD40L, and B-lymphocyte stimulator (BLyS). Unlike the canonical pathway, activation of the alternative NF-κB pathway plays a major role in lymphoid organogenesis and humoral immunity through inducing B-cell maturation.[49]

The strong induction of immunity and inflammatory mediators requires a robust regulation of NF-κB activation. Evidence suggests that a defect or breakdown of regulatory mechanisms could lead to an exaggerated immune response and inflammatory diseases.[78] Therefore, NF-κB is a logical target for the treatment of inflammatory diseases.

INVOLVEMENT OF NF-κB IN RHEUMATOLOGICAL DISEASES

Initial evidence for an involvement of NF-κB in RA originated from the detection of NF-κB dimers in the nucleus of macrophages and fibroblast-like synoviocytes of patients with early and later stage RA.[79–81] This observation has also been made in other inflammatory diseases including sarcoidosis.[82] Overexpression of the endogenous NF-κB inhibitor IκBα in dissociated synovial membrane cultures from RA patients resulted in attenuation of proinflammatory mediators such as TNF-α, IL-1β, IL-6, and IL-8.[83,84] In contrast, expression of the anti-inflammatory IL-1Ra and IL-10 were unaffected, further confirming a specific functional role of NF-κB in driving inflammation in conditions such as RA[84] (Figure 47.2). Similarly, the overexpression of IκBα potently inhibited the expression of MMP-1, -3, and -13, while the expression of their endogenous inhibitor, tissue inhibitor of

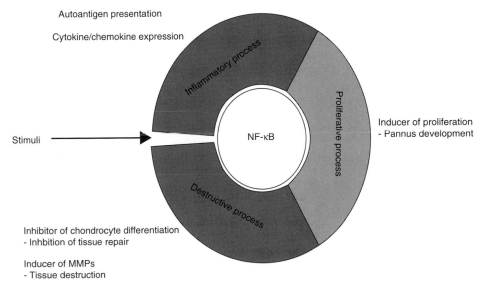

Figure 47.2 NF-κB activation affects numerous aspects of the disease process of RA. NF-κB activation leads to the expression of proinflammatory cytokines and chemokines as well as an enhancement of autoantigen presentation by DCs. This leads to inflammation through further recruitment of T cells and macrophages. The joint destruction observed in RA is also driven by NF-κB activation, which induces the expression of MMPs as well as inhibiting the differentiation of chondrocytes and therefore inhibiting repair of damaged cartilage. A third aspect of RA etiology is the formation of the pannus, which is driven by the induction of anti-apoptotic genes following NF-κB activation. NF-κB, nuclear factor-κB; RA, rheumatoid arthritis; DC, dendritic cell; MMP, matrix metalloproteinase.

metalloproteinase (TIMP)-1, was unaffected.[84] Comparable results were obtained in synovial cells obtained from osteoarthritis (OA) patients.[85] Further support for an involvement of NF-κB in the production of proinflammatory cytokines and destructive enzymes, such as MMPs, resulted from experiments using a dominant negative version of the upstream activator of NF-κB, IKK2 (IKK2dn). Overexpression of IKK2dn resulted in a significant inhibition of IL-6 and IL-8, as well as MMP-1, -2, -3, and -13. However, the expression of TNF-α was only marginally affected.[86] These results would suggest different mechanisms of NF-κB-dependent gene expression. Besides its function as an inducer of proinflammatory cytokine expression, NF-κB activation promotes another aspect of inflammation by up-regulating cell surface markers important for antigen presentation by DCs that lead to T-cell activation. This was shown to depend on the activation of the canonical NF-κB pathway, as the expression of IKK2dn inhibited this process.[87] Therefore, in the context of RA the activation of NF-κB could lead to enhanced autoantigen presentation by DCs (Figure 47.2).

Activation of NF-κB has an important role in the generation and maturation of osteoclasts, which are involved in bone resorption while at the same time inhibiting differentiation of chondrocytes that are essential for repair of damaged cartilage.[88–91] This contributes to the bone destruction observed in RA. Chondrogenesis requires activation of sex determining region Y-box (Sox) 9, which is down-regulated by TNF-α and IL-1 produced in response to NF-κB activation, thus inhibiting cartilage formation.[90] On the other hand, NF-κB drives synovial proliferation which leads to the formation of the pannus, characteristic of RA (Figure 47.2). Synovial tissue from patients with RA shows a significantly higher expression of NF-κB1 in cells at the cartilage–pannus junction compared with other areas.[92]

Animal models support this central role of NF-κB. Mice deficient in c-Rel or NF-κB1 are protected from the development of collagen-induced arthritis (CIA).[93] Similarly, transgenic expression of the constitutively active form of the inhibitor IκBα (N-terminally truncated from amino acids 37 to 317) in the T-cell lineage resulted in a decreased incidence and severity of CIA.[94] Furthermore, the use of decoy oligonucleotides, which obstruct the binding of NF-κB to the promoter of the target gene, prevented the recurrence of streptococcal cell wall (SCW)-induced arthritis as well as CIA, most probably due to inhibition of TNF-α and IL-1. Inhibition of IκBα degradation by the proteasome inhibitor PS-341 after the onset of polyarthritis in rats also showed beneficial effects as measured by the Total Arthritis Index.[95]

The evidence presented here indicates an involvement of NF-κB in numerous processes leading to inflammatory diseases and driving their progression, making NF-κB an attractive target for the treatment of rheumatological diseases.

NON-SPECIFIC NF-κB INHIBITORS

A number of anti-inflammatory drugs already in clinical use may produce some of their anti-inflammatory action by inhibiting components of the NF-κB signaling pathway. These include non-steroidal anti-inflammatory drugs (NSAIDs), sulfasalazine, glucocorticoids, thiazoledinediones (TZDs), triptolide, and thalidomide. However, in the case of all these drugs it must be emphasized that there is a multiplicity of targets in addition to NF-κB.

Non-steroidal anti-inflammatory drugs and derivatives

The prototypical NSAID is aspirin (aminosalicylic acid), the molecular target of which is COX, which leads to the formation of prostaglandins that cause inflammation, swelling, pain, and fever.[96] At high doses salicylic acid can also inhibit IKK2.[97] However, this effect is only seen at very high doses of salicylic acid, higher than would routinely be used in the treatment of RA.

Sulfasalazine

Sulfasalazine was originally developed in the 1940s as a combined antimicrobial/anti-inflammatory agent containing sulfapyridine and aminosalicylic acid. It is an established disease-modifying anti-rheumatoid drug (DMARD) and is also extensively used in the management of ankylosing spondylitis.[98] Its anti-inflammatory effects appear to be mediated through a number of mechanisms including induction of autocrine adenosine signaling,[99] COX inhibition, and inhibition of NF-κB signaling.[100] Although the endpoint of inhibited NF-κB signaling is reduced DNA binding (e.g. to the IL-12 subunit gene, p40-κB site),[100] it is not as yet clear at which exact point(s) along the NF-κB pathway sulfasalazine mediates its effects.

Glucocorticoids

Glucocorticoids remain among the most commonly used anti-inflammatory drugs. Their numerous anti-inflammatory actions are mediated by the glucocorticoid receptor (GR), a classical nuclear hormone receptor that dimerizes upon ligand binding and acts as a ligand-inducible transcription factor. The anti-inflammatory effects of glucocorticoids are mediated by numerous mechanisms including inhibition of the transcription factor activating protein-1 (AP-1), induction of lipocortin-1, and inhibition of NF-κB signaling.[101] Inhibition of NF-κB occurs by at least two distinct mechanisms. Firstly, the GR reportedly induces expression of the endogenous NF-κB inhibitor IκBα,[102,103] which forms a negative feedback loop inhibiting nuclear translocation of NF-κB. Secondly, the GR inhibits expression of NF-κB target genes,[104–106] which is probably mediated by direct protein–protein interaction between the GR and NF-κB.[107] However, glucocorticoids can have significant side effects including osteoporosis, type 2 diabetes, hypertension, upper gastrointestinal tract ulceration, and increased susceptibility to infection.[108] Therefore, the challenge is to design compounds that show comparable anti-inflammatory efficacy to glucocorticoids without major side effects. Other glucocorticoid derivatives with potent NF-κB-inhibiting effects but fewer side effects than traditional glucocorticoids are under development, such as the inhaled glucocorticoid derivative ciclesonide, for the treatment of asthma.[109]

Thiazoledinediones

The TZDs are synthetic agonists at the peroxisome proliferator-activated receptor (PPAR)γ, a nuclear receptor involved in the regulation of metabolic function in tissues including liver, muscle, and adipose.[110] This class of drugs was developed for the treatment of type 2 diabetes mellitus and includes troglitazone (now withdrawn due to several cases of liver failure),[111] pioglitazone (Takeda),[112] and rosiglitazone (Glaxo Smith Kline).[113] In addition to their anti-diabetic actions, several lines of evidence also suggest that these drugs have clinically useful anti-inflammatory properties and these have now been ascribed, at least in part, to inhibition of NF-κB signaling. In animal models including the carrageenin paw edema model of inflammation, the CIA model of arthritis,[114] and the dextran sodium sulfate (DSS) model of colitis, rosiglitazone reduces inflammation. While there are as yet no clinical trials of TZDs in arthritis, in an open-label trial of rosiglitazone in patients with ulcerative colitis, 4 mg twice daily led to a reduction of severity of the colitis.[115] Although congestive cardiac failure may be exacerbated in patients taking TZDs[116] and a small number also develop abnormal liver function tests,[117] these drugs are generally well tolerated and safe for the majority of patients. Several mechanisms of inhibition of NF-κB by TZDs have been hypothesized,[118–120] including reduction in RelA expression.[118,119]

Thalidomide

Thalidomide was originally developed in the 1950s as a treatment for hyperemesis gravidarum but was withdrawn in 1961 as its teratogenic effects became apparent. However, it has become recognized as an immunomodulatory agent and has been successfully used in the treatment of inflammatory conditions including human immunodeficiency virus (HIV)-associated aphthous ulceration and inflammatory bowel disease.[121] NF-κB inhibition has been suggested as a mechanism of action of thalidomide in inflammation.[122,123] In particular, it appears that thalidomide may inhibit the phosphorylation of IκBα.[124] There are as yet no reported trials of thalidomide in RA; however, clinical trials of thalidomide in inflammatory bowel disease indicate that not only is it a clinically efficacious anti-inflammatory agent but it also has an acceptable safety and side effect profile.[125]

Triptolide

The anti-rheumatic properties of extracts of the Chinese herbal remedy *Tripterygium wilfordii* Hook F (thunder god vine, lei gong teng)[126] have been recognized for many years. The active ingredient has been identified as a diterpene triepoxide, triptolide (Table 47.1).[127] *In vitro* triptolide inhibits TNF-α- and IL-1β-induced transcription of inflammatory cytokines. Inhibition occurs after NF-κB DNA-binding, by either interfering with post-transcriptional modifications of RelA or interfering with the recruitment of transcription cofactors.[128] Beside the inhibition of NF-κB, triptolide was also shown to inhibit the transcription factors, nuclear factor activating T cells (NF-AT) and AP-1 at the level of nuclear translocation.[128–130] A recent double-blind placebo-controlled trial of an ethanol/ethyl acetate extract of *Tripterygium wilfordii* Hook F in patients with long-standing RA that was resistant to conventional therapy showed that most patients achieved an American College of Rheumatalogists score (ACR) 20% response and significant improvements in objective markers of inflammation. No serious side effects were observed.[131]

TARGETED THERAPIES

Although a number of anti-inflammatory agents currently in clinical use may act in part by inhibition of NF-κB, they also have other targets and are all limited by significant side effects. It is therefore desirable that drugs with more specific mechanisms of action are developed providing a decreased risk of undesirable side effects. In this section we will therefore review some of the compounds currently under development that are designed to inhibit specific components of the NF-κB signaling pathways.

IKK2 inhibitors

Numerous elements in the activation pathway of NF-κB are currently under investigation for their feasibility as therapeutic targets. Inhibitors for the kinases IKK1 and IKK2 would provide a specific inhibition of NF-κB activation while leaving other signaling pathways intact. Therefore, intensive

effort has been made in the development of these inhibitors (reviewed by Karin et al.).[132] Although IKK1 would be an attractive target for the treatment of autoimmune diseases, no potent and specific inhibitor has been described so far. However, several IKK2 inhibitors are in their preclinical developmental stages and showed an effect in models of arthritis.

SPC-839 is a quinazoline analog and an ATP-competitive inhibitor of IKK2.[132] It inhibits IKK2 with an IC_{50} of 62 nM compared with inhibition of IKK1 with an IC_{50} of 13 μM.[132] Treatment of rat adjuvant arthritis with SPC-839 led to a reduction in paw swelling and radiographic damage.[133] An inhibition of NF-κB activation in LPS-challenged rats was already detectable at a dose of 10 mg/kg.[132] Another well-studied IKK2 inhibitor is BMS-345541. Tested in the human monocytic cell line THP-1, this compound blocked the release of LPS-induced TNF-α, IL-1β, IL-8, and IL-6 with an IC_{50} in a range between 1 and 5 μM.[134] More recently, it was shown that BMS-345541 successfully blocks the release of MMP-9 in RAW 264.7 cells in response to the TLR9 ligand CpG DNA.[135] Furthermore, CIA mice treated with BMS-345541 showed significantly reduced joint inflammation and destruction.[136] However, this effect was only observed if BMS-345541 was administered prophylactically before the induction of disease.

A more recently described IKK2 inhibitor is ML120B, with an IC_{50} of 60 nM, as evaluated in an *in vitro* kinase assay.[137] ML120B inhibited the induction of RANTES (regulated on activation, normal T-cell expressed and secreted) in TNF-α- or IL-1β-stimulated human fibroblast-like synoviocytes.[137] Moreover, the expression of TNF-α, IL-1β, and IL-6 was also inhibited in LPS- or peptidoglycan (PGN)-stimulated human mast cells as well as the expression of MMP-1 and MMP-13 in human chondrocytes stimulated with IL-1.[137] These results suggest that ML120B is a potent inhibitor of NF-κB in RA-relevant cell systems. Furthermore, ML120B was shown to block the differentiation and maturation of T cells and B cells and to inhibit the expression of numerous proinflammatory mediators such as IL-6, IL-8, and RANTES in human airway smooth muscle cells.[138] The inhibition of these cytokines and chemokines using ML120B was

Table 47.1 NF-κB targeted anti-inflammatory drugs in current clinical use and undergoing development

Drug	Structure	Target/mode of action	Trials	Refs
Triptolide		p65 post-transcriptional modifications NF-κB co-activator recruitment	RA, phase II	127–130,163
Sulfasalazine		NF-κB DNA binding	RA, RCTs	100,164
NFkappaB decoy oligo	5′-CCTTGAAGGGATTT CCCTCC-3′ (phosphorothioate)	NF-κB DNA binding	Phase I in HIV skin disease, phase II in atopic dermatitis	143,165, 166,167
Steroids, e.g. prednisolone		Trans-repression of NF-κB	RA, RCTs	106,107,168
PPARγ agonists, e.g. rosiglitazone		Trans-repression of NF-κB	DM, RCTs	114
SPC-839		IKK2 inhibitor	No clinical trial data available	132,133

Continued

Table 47.1 NF-κB targeted anti-inflammatory drugs in current clinical use and undergoing development—cont'd

Drug	Structure	Target/mode of action	Trials	Refs
BMS-345541		IKK2 inhibitor	No clinical trial data available	134–136,140
ML120B		IKK2 inhibitor	No clinical trial data available	138,137
Bortezomib		Proteasome inhibitor	Approved by FDA for multiple myeloma	142,141
NBD	C-terminus of IKK1 and IKK2	NF-κB dimerization	No clinical trial data available	89,152–154
SN50	NLD of NF-kappaB1	Nuclear localization of NF-kappaB	No clinical trial data available	144–149
PTP-p65-P1	Amino acids 271–282 of RelA	Transactivation of RelA	No clinical trial data available	150
Thalidomide		IKK	IBD, juvenile RA, and ankylosing spondylitis	124,169–171

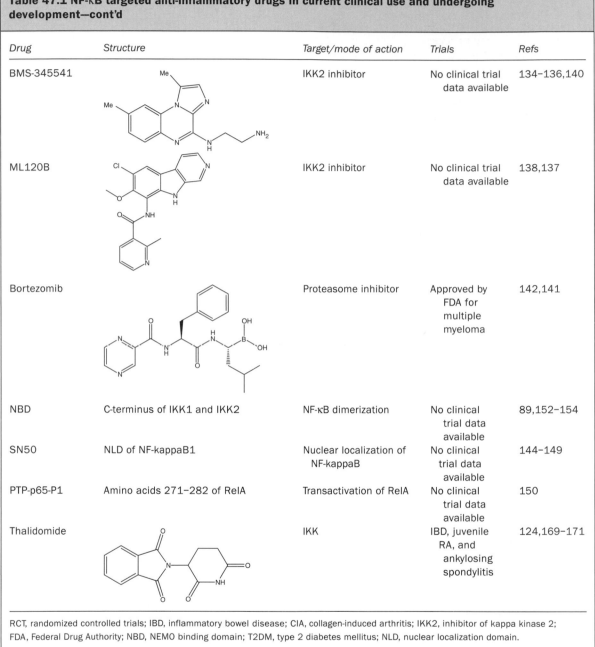

RCT, randomized controlled trials; IBD, inflammatory bowel disease; CIA, collagen-induced arthritis; IKK2, inhibitor of kappa kinase 2; FDA, Federal Drug Authority; NBD, NEMO binding domain; T2DM, type 2 diabetes mellitus; NLD, nuclear localization domain.

either as effective as or more effective than dexamethasone.[138]

Proteasome inhibitors

Following the phosphorylation and ubiquitination of IκBα, it is degraded by the proteasome and releases the NF-κB dimer to translocate to the nucleus.[139] Therefore, targeting the proteasome could prevent the nuclear translocation of NF-κB. A proteasome inhibitor already approved by the US Food and Drug Administration (FDA) for the treatment of multiple myeloma is bortezomib (Millenium).[140] Another proteasome inhibitor currently in clinical trials for multiple myeloma is PR171 (Proteolix). However, because the proteasome is involved in a great variety of regulatory processes, the effects generated are non-specific. Adverse effects observed after bortezomib treatment include infections of the upper respiratory tract, lymphopenia, and thrombocytopenia.[141,142] Because the treatment of chronic inflammatory diseases such as RA makes it necessary to administer therapies over a long period of time, such side effects are likely to be unacceptable.

NF-κB decoy oligos

Since NF-κB functions by binding specific DNA sequences in the promoters of target genes, novel NF-κB targeted anti-inflammatory drugs utilizing the DNA-binding properties of the NF-κB heterodimers may provide future therapies. One approach to achieve this is the therapeutic use of phosphothiorate deoxyribonucleic acid oligomers. Several *in vitro* experimental models of this approach have been reported, such as the use of folate-linked lipid-based nanoparticles to transfect macrophages with NF-κB decoy oligos.[143] In the RAW264.7 murine macrophage cell line, these were found to potently inhibit the translocation of NF-κB from cytoplasm to the nucleus, following LPS stimulation.[143] Such agents are already in clinical trials for atopic dermatitis (NIH Clinical Trials Identifier NCT 00125333). These trials are ongoing and no results are available yet. If it were possible to safely and effectively deliver such decoy oligos to the inflamed joint then these would also form attractive treatments for RA.

NF-κB inhibitory peptides

An alternative approach to inhibit NF-κB activation is to block the interaction of molecules involved in NF-κB signaling using short peptide sequences. The first member of this class of inhibitors described was SN50, which contained the nuclear localization domain sequence of NF-κB1.[144] SN50 was shown to block NF-κB in numerous cell lines in response to the HIV envelope protein glycoprotein (gp) 120 and staphylococcal enterotoxin B.[145,146] Furthermore, SN50

was reported to protect rats from acute pancreatitis as well as showing efficacy in the treatment of corneal alkali burns in mice.[147,148] However, SN50 also affects the nuclear translocation of STATs (signal transducer and activator of transcription), AP-1, and NF-AT.[149] This proof of principle of inhibiting NF-κB through blocking specific interaction of signaling components led to the development of several other inhibitory peptides. In contrast to SN50, the PTD-p65-P1 peptide was reported to specifically inhibit TNF α induced NF κB activation without affecting other transcription factors.[150] PTD-p65-P1 corresponds to the amino acid residues 271–282 of RelA. It was reported to block the phosphorylation of serines 276, 529, and 536 of RelA, thereby inhibiting transactivation of RelA without affecting IκBα degradation.[150] However, no *in vivo* studies confirming the inhibitory effect of PTD-p65-P1 are available so far. The cell-permeable peptide NBD consists of six amino acids (Leu, Asp, Trp, Ser, Trp, Leu), which correspond to the C-terminus of IKK1 as well as IKK2 that is responsible for the association with NEMO.[151] Numerous studies have investigated the effect of NBD administration on NF-κB activation in models of inflammatory arthritis. The administration of NBD to mice before the onset of inflammatory arthritis inhibited cytokine-induced osteoclasts formation and thereby inhibited bone erosion in the joints of those mice.[152] Similarly, the administration of NBD into mice at the onset of CIA reduced the severity of the inflammatory arthritis by impairing the production of TNF-α and IL-1 and thereby reducing joint swelling and the destruction of bone and cartilage.[89] Also, NBD given at the onset of carrageenin-induced paw edema led to a reduction in edema formation and cellular infiltration into the paws of the mice.[153] In all of the animal studies described above NBD was administered before or at the onset of inflammation, therefore, it is unclear if NBD exhibits an effect on an already established inflammatory disease. However, initial results obtained from *in vitro* studies using fibroblast-like synoviocytes and macrophages from RA patients also suggest a positive effect of NBD on RA treatment in humans.[154] When given to *ex vivo* cultured RA synovial tissue or RA fibroblast-like synoviocytes, it inhibited the spontaneous release of IL-1β, TNF-α, and IL-6.[154] Moreover, NBD inhibited IL-1β-induced expression of TNF-α in human macrophages.[154] These results indicate that NBD might be a promising future therapeutic in rheumatological diseases, which is able to inhibit NF-κB specifically. However, the use of peptide drugs is limited by the requirement for a parenteral route of administration. The ultimate goal would therefore be to identify peptidometic, orally bioavailable, small molecular weight compounds to replace such peptides.

POTENTIAL FUTURE TARGETS

In addition to the targets describe above, there remain a number of targets in the NF-κB signaling pathway that have so far not been exploited for development of targeted anti-inflammatory drugs. In this section, the potential for developing targeted therapies to inhibit some of these will be discussed.

Ubiquitin ligase inhibition

Following IκBα phosphorylation by IKKs, E3 ubiquitin ligase targets IκBα for proteasomal degradation by addition of poly-ubiquitin side chains. Inhibition of the E3 ligase is therefore a potential mechanism for modulating NF-κB signaling. Such an approach is already being utilized in the oncology field[155] by means of high throughput screening to identify inhibitors of anaphase promoting complex (APC) E3 ligase. However, E3 ubiquitin ligases are involved in numerous cellular processes, therefore, their inhibition might lead to a broad range of adverse effects as is observed with proteasome inhibitors.

Phosphorylation of RelA

Post-translational covalent modification of Rel family members appears to be a key regulatory step in NF-κB signaling.[46,156] Thus phosphorylation of serine residues in RelA represents potential targets. Since kinase inhibition is a well established route of drug development, such an approach should be readily amenable to a high throughput small molecule screening approach similar to that used in the identification of IKK inhibitors.[157] Kinases reported to be involved in serine phosphorylation of RelA include PKA, MSK-1, PKCζ, RSK-1, GSK-3β, PI3K, IKK1, IKK2, TBK1,[51] and Bruton's tyrosine kinase (Btk).[156,158] As some of these kinases appear to be restricted to particular stimuli, their inhibition raises the prospect of highly specific future therapies. Moreover, this approach would potentially have the advantage of inhibiting the amplification of the stimulated NF-κB signal while leaving its basal activity unaffected.

Inhibition of translocation

One of the key steps in NF-κB activation is nuclear translocation. Thus, nuclear–cytoplasmic shuttling presents an attractive potential target for inhibition of NF-κB-induced inflammation and it can be envisaged that drugs to inhibit transport through the nuclear pore complex (NPC)[159] could be developed. Some interest has already been shown in this target for drug development by researchers in other areas such as HIV.[160,161]

Gene therapy

An approach to circumvent potential systemic toxicity of NF-κB targeted therapies for arthritis is to administer therapy selectively to the affected joints by means of gene therapy. A study of the use of recombinant adeno-associated virus (rAAV) in the rat adjuvant arthritis model[162] showed that a single intra-articular injection of rAAV encoding IKK2dn produced significant reductions in paw swelling and production of IL-6 and TNF-α in the treated joint. Such work raises the possibility of NF-κB targeted gene therapy becoming a viable option for the treatment of arthritis in humans. Indeed, a phase II gene therapy trial sponsored by the Targeted Genetics Coporation, USA is already recruiting (clinical trials identifier, NCT00126724) in which patients with inflammatory arthritis (including patients who are already on anti-TNF therapy or on classical DMARDS) receive repeat intra-articular injections of an adeno-associated vector designed to express human TNF receptor (TNFR)-immunoglobulin (IgG1) Fc fusion protein.

CONCLUSION

The central role of NF-κB in inflammation and immunity makes it a legitimate target for the treatment of inflammatory diseases. *In vitro* as well as *in vivo* studies confirm the central involvement of NF-κB in rheumatological diseases including RA and OA. NF-κB inhibition causes significant reduction in the disease activity of CIA and SCW models of RA and the improvement observed in these models of RA appears to be due to inhibition of NF-κB-dependent expression of proinflammatory mediators as well as enzymes including MMPs that are responsible for joint destruction.

Considerable effort has been made to develop therapeutically useful inhibitors of NF-κB. However, the treatment of chronic inflammation requires a therapy to be administered over a long period of time, making significant side effects – as is observed, for example, with proteasome inhibitors – unacceptable.

The NF-κB pathway shows a high degree of convergence, whereby signals from a wide range of receptors are processed through a central signalling pathway comprising the IKK/IκB/NF-κB cascade (Figure 47.3). Subsequently, NF-κB signaling diverges and results in numerous cellular responses due to the induction of a great variety of genes (Figure 47.3). However, more recent work is beginning to unveil the complexity of the NF-κB system and its regulation. For example, the discovery of the role of NF-κB transactivation in 'fine tuning' gene induction adds another layer of complexity to this signaling system.[51]

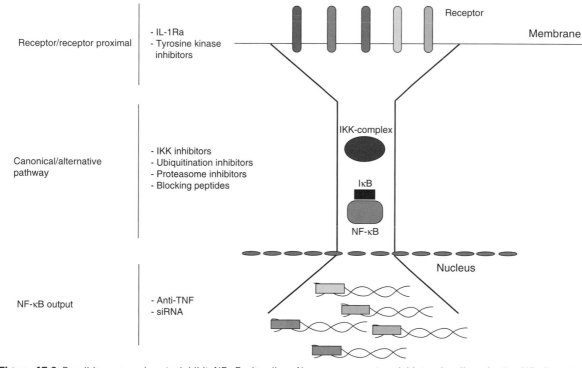

Figure 47.3 Possible approaches to inhibit NF-κB signaling. Numerous receptors initiate signaling via the NF-κB pathway. Signaling then converges through either the canonical or non-canonical pathway before diverging through induction of a wide range of genes. Examples of classes of compounds that inhibit signaling upstream of the convergence of this pathway (Receptor/receptor proximal in the diagram) include receptor antagonists (e.g. IL1-Ra). Examples of inhibitors that act on the canonical and alternative pathways include IKK inhibitors, ubiquitination inhibitors, proteasome inhibitors, and blocking peptides. Examples of inhibitors acting after divergence of the pathway (NF-κB output in the diagram) include anti-TNF agents and siRNA-based therapies. NF-κB, nuclear factor-κB; IL-1Ra, interleukin-1 receptor antagonist; TNF, tumor necrosis factor; siRNA, small interfering RNA.

Future therapies based on inhibiting NF-κB signaling could be divided into three possible categories (Figure 47.3). Inhibition of the receptor or receptor proximal signal transducers would be specific for one stimulus; however, it might affect, several signaling pathways induced by this receptor. This would be a promising therapy if the stimulus, responsible for the condition which is treated, is already identified. On the other hand, while inhibiting central components of the NF-κB pathway (e.g. IKK complex, IκBα degradation) would exert only limited effects on other signaling pathways, it may be expected to produce a more global inhibition of NF-κB and therefore result in significant adverse effects. A third possibility would be the targeting of specific NF-κB outputs. Anti-TNF therapy is one such example; in the future siRNA-based therapies may provide another approach.

However, in addition to mediating pathological inflammation, NF-κB is also necessary for host defense and thus global inhibition of NF-κB would lead to an unacceptable range of side effects including serious infections. In order to utilize the therapeutic potential of NF-κB inhibition, it will be necessary to further study the regulation of NF-κB and its involvement in specific conditions including RA and OA. This knowledge will facilitate future development of compounds that are more precisely targeted, thereby giving greater therapeutic efficacy with fewer side effects.

REFERENCES

1. Feldmann M, Maini RN. Lasker Clinical Medical Research Award. TNF defined as a therapeutic target for rheumatoid arthritis and other autoimmune diseases. Nat Med 2003; 9: 1245–50.
2. Weinblatt ME, Kremer JM, Bankhurst AD et al. A trial of etanercept, a recombinant tumor necrosis factor receptor: Fc fusion protein, in patients with rheumatoid arthritis receiving methotrexate. N Engl J Med 1999; 340: 253–9.
3. Feldmann M, Brennan FM, Foxwell BM et al. Anti-TNF therapy: where have we got to in 2005? J Autoimmun 2005; 25 (Suppl): 26–8.
4. Bresnihan B, Alvaro-Gracia JM, Cobby M et al. Treatment of rheumatoid arthritis with recombinant human interleukin-1 receptor antagonist. Arthritis Rheum 1998; 41: 2196–204.
5. Campion GV, Lebsack ME, Lookabaugh J et al. Dose-range and dose-frequency study of recombinant human interleukin-1 receptor antagonist in patients with rheumatoid arthritis. The IL-1Ra Arthritis Study Group. Arthritis Rheum 1996; 39: 1092–101.
6. Nishimoto N, Yoshizaki K, Miyasaka N et al. Treatment of rheumatoid arthritis with humanized anti-interleukin-6 receptor antibody: a multicenter, double-blind, placebo-controlled trial. Arthritis Rheum 2004; 50: 1761–9.
7. Feldmann M, Brennan FM, Williams RO et al. The transfer of a laboratory based hypothesis to a clinically useful therapy: the development of anti-TNF therapy of rheumatoid arthritis. Best Pract Res Clin Rheumatol 2004; 18: 59–80.
8. Ghosh S, May MJ, Kopp EB. NF-kappa B and Rel proteins: evolutionarily conserved mediators of immune responses. Annu Rev Immunol 1998; 16: 225–60.
9. Kovacsovics T, Maziarz RT. Philadelphia chromosome-positive acute lymphoblastic leukemia: impact of imatinib treatmenton remission induction and allogeneic stem cell transplantation. Curr Oncol Rep 2006; 8: 343–51.
10. Karin M, Lin A. NF-kappaB at the crossroads of life and death. Nat Immunol 2002; 3: 221–7.
11. Baldwin AS Jr. The NF-kappa B and I kappa B proteins: new discoveries and insights. Annu Rev Immunol 1996; 14: 649–83.
12. Verma IM, Stevenson JK, Schwarz EM et al. Rel/NF-kappa B/I kappa B family: intimate tales of association and dissociation. Genes Dev 1995; 9: 2723–35.
13. Thompson JE, Phillips RJ, Erdjument-Bromage H et al. I kappa B-beta regulates the persistent response in a biphasic activation of NF-kappa B. Cell 1995; 80: 573–82.
14. Tran K, Merika M, Thanos D. Distinct functional properties of IkappaB alpha and IkappaB beta. Mol Cell Biol 1997; 17: 5386–99.
15. Bitko V, Barik S. Persistent activation of RelA by respiratory syncytial virus involves protein kinase C, underphosphorylated IkappaBbeta, and sequestration of protein phosphatase 2A by the viral phosphoprotein. J Virol 1998; 72: 5610–18.
16. Blackwell TS, Stecenko AA, Christman JW. Dysregulated NF-kappaB activation in cystic fibrosis: evidence for a primary inflammatory disorder. Am J Physiol Lung Cell Mol Physiol 2001; 281: L69–70.
17. DeLuca C, Petropoulos L, Zmeureanu D et al. Nuclear IkappaBbeta maintains persistent NF-kappaB activation in HIV-1-infected myeloid cells. J Biol Chem 1999; 274: 13010–16.
18. Hiscott J, Kwon H, Genin P. Hostile takeovers: viral appropriation of the NF-kappaB pathway. J Clin Invest 2001; 107: 143–51.
19. Johnson DR, Douglas I, Jahnke A et al. A sustained reduction in IkappaB-beta may contribute to persistent NF-kappaB activation in human endothelial cells. J Biol Chem 1996; 271: 16317–22.
20. Palmer GH, Machado J Jr, Fernandez P et al. Parasite-mediated nuclear factor kappaB regulation in

lymphoproliferation caused by *Theileria parva* infection. Proc Natl Acad Sci U S A 1997; 94: 12527–32.

21. Stecenko AA, King G, Torii K et al. Dysregulated cytokine production in human cystic fibrosis bronchial epithelial cells. Inflammation 2001; 25: 145–55.

22. Kearns JD, Basak S, Werner SL et al. IkappaBepsilon provides negative feedback to control NF-kappaB oscillations, signaling dynamics, and inflammatory gene expression. J Cell Biol 2006; 173: 659–64.

23. Bours V, Franzoso G, Azarenko V et al. The oncoprotein Bcl-3 directly transactivates through kappa B motifs via association with DNA-binding p50B homodimers. Cell 1993; 72: 729–39.

24. Nolan GP, Fujita T, Bhatia K et al. The bcl-3 proto-oncogene encodes a nuclear I kappa B-like molecule that preferentially interacts with NF-kappa B p50 and p52 in a phosphorylation-dependent manner. Mol Cell Biol 1993; 13: 3557–66.

25. Fujita T, Nolan GP, Liou IIC et al. The candidate proto-oncogene bcl-3 encodes a transcriptional coactivator that activates through NF-kappa B p50 homodimers. Genes Dev 1993; 7: 1354–63.

26. Heissmeyer V, Krappmann D, Wulczyn FG et al. NF-kappaB p105 is a target of IkappaB kinases and controls signal induction of Bcl-3-p50 complexes. EMBO J 1999; 18: 4766–78.

27. Franzoso G, Bours V, Park S et al. The candidate oncoprotein Bcl-3 is an antagonist of p50/NF-kappa B-mediated inhibition. Nature 1992; 359: 339–42.

28. Dechend R, Hirano F, Lehmann K et al. The Bcl-3 onco-protein acts as a bridging factor between NF-kappaB/Rel and nuclear co-regulators. Oncogene 1999; 18: 3316–23.

29. Takeda K, Kaisho T, Akira S. Toll-like receptors. Annu Rev Immunol 2003; 21: 335–76.

30. Janeway CA Jr, Medzhitov R. Innate immune recognition. Annu Rev Immunol 2002; 20: 197–216.

31. O'Neill LA. Therapeutic targeting of Toll-like receptors for inflammatory and infectious diseases. Curr Opin Pharmacol 2003; 3: 396–403.

32. Yamazaki S, Muta T, Takeshige K. A novel IkappaB protein, IkappaB-zeta, induced by proinflammatory stimuli, negatively regulates nuclear factor-kappaB in the nuclei. J Biol Chem 2001; 276: 27657–62.

33. Kitamura H, Kanehira K, Okita K et al. MAIL, a novel nuclear I kappa B protein that potentiates LPS-induced IL-6 production. FEBS Lett 2000; 485: 53–6.

34. Haruta H, Kato A, Todokoro K. Isolation of a novel interleukin-1-inducible nuclear protein bearing ankyrin-repeat motifs. J Biol Chem 2001; 276: 12485–8.

35. Yamamoto M, Yamazaki S, Uematsu S et al. Regulation of Toll/IL-1-receptor-mediated gene expression by the inducible nuclear protein IkappaBzeta. Nature 2004; 430: 218–22.

36. Hirotani T, Lee PY, Kuwata H et al. The nuclear IkappaB protein IkappaBNS selectively inhibits lipopolysaccharide-induced IL-6 production in macrophages of the colonic lamina propria. J Immunol 2005; 174: 3650–7.

37. Kuwata H, Matsumoto M, Atarashi K et al. IkappaBNS inhibits induction of a subset of Toll-like receptor-dependent genes and limits inflammation. Immunity 2006; 24: 41–51.

38. Karin M, Ben-Neriah Y. Phosphorylation meets ubiquitination: the control of NF-[kappa]B activity. Annu Rev Immunol 2000; 18: 621–63.

39. Rothwarf DM, Zandi E, Natoli G et al. IKK-gamma is an essential regulatory subunit of the IkappaB kinase complex. Nature 1998; 395: 297–300.

40. Makris C, Godfrey VL, Krahn-Senftleben G et al. Female mice heterozygous for IKK gamma/NEMO deficiencies develop a dermatopathy similar to the human X-linked disorder incontinentia pigmenti. Mol Cell 2000; 5: 969–79.

41. Li Q, Van Antwerp D, Mercurio F et al. Severe liver degeneration in mice lacking the IkappaB kinase 2 gene. Science 1999; 284: 321–5.

42. Li ZW, Chu W, Hu Y et al. The IKKbeta subunit of IkappaB kinase (IKK) is essential for nuclear factor kappaB activation and prevention of apoptosis. J Exp Med 1999; 189: 1839–45.

43. Chen LW, Egan L, Li ZW et al. The two faces of IKK and NF-kappaB inhibition: prevention of systemic inflammation but increased local injury following intestinal ischemia-reperfusion. Nat Med 2003; 9: 575–81.

44. Hu Y, Baud V, Delhase M et al. Abnormal morphogenesis but intact IKK activation in mice lacking the IKKalpha subunit of IkappaB kinase. Science 1999; 284: 316–20.

45. Hu Y, Baud V, Oga T et al. IKKalpha controls formation of the epidermis independently of NF-kappaB. Nature 2001; 410: 710–14.

46. Lawrence T, Bebien M, Liu GY et al. IKKalpha limits macrophage NF-kappaB activation and contributes to the resolution of inflammation. Nature 2005; 434: 1138–43.

47. Ghosh S, Karin M. Missing pieces in the NF-kappaB puzzle. Cell 2002; 109 (Suppl): S81–S96.

48. Dejardin E, Droin NM, Delhase M et al. The lympho-toxin-beta receptor induces different patterns of gene expression via two NF-kappaB pathways. Immunity 2002; 17: 525–35.

49. Senftleben U, Cao Y, Xiao G et al. Activation by IKKalpha of a second, evolutionary conserved, NF-kappa B signaling pathway. Science 2001; 293: 1495–9.

50. Takeda K, Akira S. TLR signaling pathways. Semin Immunol 2004; 16: 3–9.

51. Chen LF, Greene WC. Shaping the nuclear action of NF-kappaB. Nat Rev Mol Cell Biol 2004; 5: 392–401.

52. Schmitz ML, Mattioli I, Buss H et al. NF-kappaB: a multifaceted transcription factor regulated at several levels. Chembiochem 2004; 5: 1348–58.

53. Chen LF, Mu Y, Greene WC. Acetylation of RelA at discrete sites regulates distinct nuclear functions of NF-kappaB. EMBO J 2002; 21: 6539–48.

54. Kiernan R, Bres V, Ng RW et al. Post-activation turn-off of NF-kappa B-dependent transcription is regulated by acetylation of p65. J Biol Chem 2003; 278: 2758–66.

55. Chen LF, Williams SA, Mu Y et al. NF-kappaB RelA phosphorylation regulates RelA acetylation. Mol Cell Biol 2005; 25: 7966–75.

56. Kucharczak J, Simmons MJ, Fan Y et al. To be, or not to be: NF-kappaB is the answer – role of Rel/NF-kappaB in the regulation of apoptosis. Oncogene 2003; 22: 8961–82.

57. Fujita T, Nolan GP, Ghosh S et al. Independent modes of transcriptional activation by the p50 and p65 subunits of NF-kappa B. Genes Dev 1992; 6: 775–87.

58. Kunsch C, Ruben SM, Rosen CA. Selection of optimal kappa B/Rel DNA-binding motifs: interaction of both subunits of NF-kappa B with DNA is required for transcriptional activation. Mol Cell Biol 1992; 12: 4412–21.

59. Hoffmann A, Leung TH, Baltimore D. Genetic analysis of NF-kappaB/Rel transcription factors defines functional specificities. EMBO J 2003; 22: 5530–9.

60. Berkowitz B, Huang DB, Chen-Park FE et al. The x-ray crystal structure of the NF-kappa B p50.p65 heterodimer bound to the interferon beta -kappa B site. J Biol Chem 2002; 277: 24694–700.

61. Chen FE, Ghosh G. Regulation of DNA binding by Rel/NF-kappaB transcription factors: structural views. Oncogene 1999; 18: 6845–52.

62. Chen-Park FE, Huang DB, Noro B et al. The kappa B DNA sequence from the HIV long terminal repeat functions as an allosteric regulator of HIV transcription. J Biol Chem 2002; 277: 24701–8.

63. Escalante CR, Shen L, Thanos D et al. Structure of NF-kappaB p50/p65 heterodimer bound to the PRDII DNA element from the interferon-beta promoter. Structure 2002; 10: 383–91.

64. Hayden MS, Ghosh S. Signaling to NF-kappaB. Genes Dev 2004; 18: 2195–224.

65. Osborn L, Kunkel S, Nabel GJ. Tumor necrosis factor alpha and interleukin 1 stimulate the human immunodeficiency virus enhancer by activation of the nuclear factor kappa B. Proc Natl Acad Sci U S A 1989; 86: 2336–40.

66. O'Neill LA. How Toll-like receptors signal: what we know and what we don't know. Curr Opin Immunol 2006; 18: 3–9.

67. Martinon F, Tschopp J. NLRs join TLRs as innate sensors of pathogens. Trends Immunol 2005; 26: 447–54.

68. Kolls JK, Linden A. Interleukin-17 family members and inflammation. Immunity 2004; 21: 467–76.

69. Kopp E, Medzhitov R, Carothers J et al. ECSIT is an evolutionarily conserved intermediate in the Toll/IL-1 signal transduction pathway. Genes Dev 1999; 13: 2059–71.

70. Liu ZG, Hsu H, Goeddel DV et al. Dissection of TNF receptor 1 effector functions: JNK activation is not linked to apoptosis while NF-kappaB activation prevents cell death. Cell 1996; 87: 565–76.

71. Beg AA, Baltimore D. An essential role for NF-kappaB in preventing TNF-alpha-induced cell death. Science 1996; 274: 782–4.

72. Van Antwerp DJ, Martin SJ, Kafri T et al. Suppression of TNF-alpha-induced apoptosis by NF-kappaB. Science 1996; 274: 787–9.

73. Wang CY, Mayo MW, Baldwin AS Jr. TNF- and cancer therapy-induced apoptosis: potentiation by inhibition of NF-kappaB. Science 1996; 274: 784–7.

74. Kamata H, Honda S, Maeda S et al. Reactive oxygen species promote TNFalpha-induced death and sustained JNK activation by inhibiting MAP kinase phosphatases. Cell 2005; 120: 649–61.

75. Pham CG, Bubici C, Zazzeroni F et al. Ferritin heavy chain upregulation by NF-kappaB inhibits TNFalpha-induced apoptosis by suppressing reactive oxygen species. Cell 2004; 119: 529–42.

76. Karin M. Nuclear factor-kappaB in cancer development and progression. Nature 2006; 441: 431–6.

77. Covert MW, Leung TH, Gaston JE et al. Achieving stability of lipopolysaccharide-induced NF-kappaB activation. Science 2005; 309: 1854–7.

78. Andreakos E, Sacre S, Foxwell BM et al. The toll-like receptor-nuclear factor kappaB pathway in rheumatoid arthritis. Front Biosci 2005; 10: 2478–88.

79. Asahara H, Asanuma M, Ogawa N et al. High DNA-binding activity of transcription factor NF-kappa B in synovial membranes of patients with rheumatoid arthritis. Biochem Mol Biol Int 1995; 37: 827–32.

80. Handel ML, McMorrow LB, Gravallese EM. Nuclear factor-kappa B in rheumatoid synovium. Localization of p50 and p65. Arthritis Rheum 1995; 38: 1762–70.

81. Marok R, Winyard PG, Coumbe A et al. Activation of the transcription factor nuclear factor-kappaB in human inflamed synovial tissue. Arthritis Rheum 1996; 39: 583–91.

82. Drent M, van den Berg R, Haenen GR et al. NF-kappaB activation in sarcoidosis. Sarcoidosis Vasc Diffuse Lung Dis 2001; 18: 50–6.

83. Foxwell B, Browne K, Bondeson J et al. Efficient adenoviral infection with IkappaB alpha reveals that macrophage tumor necrosis factor alpha production in rheumatoid arthritis is NF-kappaB dependent. Proc Natl Acad Sci U S A 1998; 95: 8211–15.

84. Bondeson J, Foxwell B, Brennan F et al. Defining therapeutic targets by using adenovirus: blocking NF-kappaB inhibits both inflammatory and destructive mechanisms in rheumatoid synovium but spares anti-inflammatory mediators. Proc Natl Acad Sci U S A 1999; 96: 5668–73.

85. Amos N, Lauder S, Evans A et al. Adenoviral gene transfer into osteoarthritis synovial cells using the endogenous inhibitor IkappaBalpha reveals that most,

but not all, inflammatory and destructive mediators are NFkappaB dependent. Rheumatology (Oxford) 2006; 45: 1201–9.

86. Andreakos E, Smith C, Kiriakidis S et al. Heterogeneous requirement of IkappaB kinase 2 for inflammatory cytokine and matrix metalloproteinase production in rheumatoid arthritis: implications for therapy. Arthritis Rheum 2003; 48: 1901–12.

87. Andreakos E, Smith C, Monaco C et al. Ikappa B kinase 2 but not NF-kappa B-inducing kinase is essential for effective DC antigen presentation in the allogeneic mixed lymphocyte reaction. Blood 2003; 101: 983–91.

88. Iotsova V, Caamano J, Loy J et al. Osteopetrosis in mice lacking NF-kappaB1 and NF-kappaB2. Nat Med 1997; 3: 1285–9.

89. Jimi E, Aoki K, Saito H et al. Selective inhibition of NF-kappa B blocks osteoclastogenesis and prevents inflammatory bone destruction in vivo. Nat Med 2004; 10: 617–24.

90. Murakami S, Lefebvre V, de Crombrugghe B. Potent inhibition of the master chondrogenic factor Sox9 gene by interleukin-1 and tumor necrosis factor-alpha. J Biol Chem 2000; 275: 3687–92.

91. de Crombrugghe B, Lefebvre V, Behringer RR et al. Transcriptional mechanisms of chondrocyte differentiation. Matrix Biol 2000; 19: 389–94.

92. Benito MJ, Murphy E, Murphy EP et al. Increased synovial tissue NF-kappa B1 expression at sites adjacent to the cartilage-pannus junction in rheumatoid arthritis. Arthritis Rheum 2004; 50: 1781–7.

93. Campbell IK, Gerondakis S, O'Donnell K et al. Distinct roles for the NF-kappaB1 (p50) and c-Rel transcription factors in inflammatory arthritis. J Clin Invest 2000; 105: 1799–806.

94. Seetharaman R, Mora AL, Nabozny G et al. Essential role of T cell NF-kappa B activation in collagen-induced arthritis. J Immunol 1999; 163: 1577–83.

95. Palombella VJ, Conner EM, Fuseler JW et al. Role of the proteasome and NF-kappaB in streptococcal cell wall-induced polyarthritis. Proc Natl Acad Sci U S A 1998; 95: 15671–6.

96. Vane JR, Botting RM. The mechanism of action of aspirin. Thromb Res 2003; 110: 255–8.

97. Yuan M, Konstantopoulos N, Lee J et al. Reversal of obesity- and diet-induced insulin resistance with salicylates or targeted disruption of Ikkbeta. Science 2001; 293: 1673–7.

98. Chen J, Liu C. Is sulfasalazine effective in ankylosing spondylitis? A systematic review of randomized controlled trials. J Rheumatol 2006; 33: 722–31.

99. Cronstein BN, Montesinos MC, Weissmann G. Salicylates and sulfasalazine, but not glucocorticoids, inhibit leukocyte accumulation by an adenosine-dependent mechanism that is independent of inhibition of prostaglandin synthesis and p105 of NFkappaB. Proc Natl Acad Sci U S A 1999; 96: 6377–81.

100. Kang BY, Chung SW, Im SY et al. Sulfasalazine prevents T-helper 1 immune response by suppressing interleukin-12 production in macrophages. Immunology 1999; 98: 98–103.

101. Hayashi R, Wada H, Ito K et al. Effects of glucocorticoids on gene transcription. Eur J Pharmacol 2004; 500: 51–62.

102. Auphan N, DiDonato JA, Rosette C et al. Immunosuppression by glucocorticoids: inhibition of NF-kappa B activity through induction of I kappa B synthesis. Science 1995; 270: 286–90.

103. Scheinman RI, Cogswell PC, Lofquist AK et al. Role of transcriptional activation of I kappa B alpha in mediation of immunosuppression by glucocorticoids. Science 1995; 270: 283–6.

104. Drouin J, Sun YL, Chamberland M et al. Novel glucocorticoid receptor complex with DNA element of the hormone-repressed POMC gene. EMBO J 1993; 12: 145–56.

105. Sakai DD, Helms S, Carlstedt-Duke J et al. Hormone-mediated repression: a negative glucocorticoid response element from the bovine prolactin gene. Genes Dev 1988; 2: 1144–54.

106. Webster JC, Cidlowski JA. Mechanisms of glucocorticoid-receptor-mediated repression of gene expression. Trends Endocrinol Metab 1999; 10: 396–402.

107. Hermoso MA, Cidlowski JA. Putting the brake on inflammatory responses: the role of glucocorticoids. IUBMB Life 2003; 55: 497–504.

108. D'Acquisto F, Ianaro A. From willow bark to peptides: the ever widening spectrum of NF-kappaB inhibitors. Curr Opin Pharmacol 2006; 6: 387–92.

109. Bateman E, Karpel J, Casale T et al. Ciclesonide reduces the need for oral steroid use in adult patients with severe, persistent asthma. Chest 2006; 129: 1176–87.

110. Peraldi P, Xu M, Spiegelman BM. Thiazolidinediones block tumor necrosis factor-alpha-induced inhibition of insulin signaling. J Clin Invest 1997; 100: 1863–9.

111. Tolman KG, Chandramouli J. Hepatotoxicity of the thiazolidinediones. Clin Liver Dis 2003; 7: 369–79, vi.

112. Hofmann CA, Edwards CW 3rd, Hillman RM et al. Treatment of insulin-resistant mice with the oral antidiabetic agent pioglitazone: evaluation of liver GLUT2 and phosphoenolpyruvate carboxykinase expression. Endocrinology 1992; 130: 735–40.

113. Oakes ND, Kennedy CJ, Jenkins AB et al. A new antidiabetic agent, BRL 49653, reduces lipid availability and improves insulin action and glucoregulation in the rat. Diabetes 1994; 43: 1203–10.

114. Cuzzocrea S, Mazzon E, Dugo L et al. Reduction in the evolution of murine type II collagen-induced arthritis by treatment with rosiglitazone, a ligand of the peroxisome proliferator-activated receptor gamma. Arthritis Rheum 2003; 48: 3544–56.

115. Lewis JD, Lichtenstein GR, Stein RB et al. An open-label trial of the PPAR-gamma ligand rosiglitazone for active ulcerative colitis. Am J Gastroenterol 2001; 96: 3323–8.

116. Hartung DM, Touchette DR, Bultemeier NC et al. Risk of hospitalization for heart failure associated with thiazolidinedione therapy: a Medicaid claims-based case-control study. Pharmacotherapy 2005; 25: 1329–36.

117. Belcher G, Schernthaner G. Changes in liver tests during 1-year treatment of patients with Type 2 diabetes with pioglitazone, metformin or gliclazide. Diabetic Med 2005; 22: 973–9.

118. Ghanim H, Garg R, Aljada A et al. Suppression of nuclear factor-kappaB and stimulation of inhibitor kappaB by troglitazone: evidence for an anti-inflammatory effect and a potential antiatherosclerotic effect in the obese. J Clin Endocrinol Metab 2001; 86: 1306–12.

119. Aljada A, Garg R, Ghanim H et al. Nuclear factor-kappaB suppressive and inhibitor-kappaB stimulatory effects of troglitazone in obese patients with type 2 diabetes: evidence of an antiinflammatory action? J Clin Endocrinol Metab 2001; 86: 3250–6.

120. Mohanty P, Aljada A, Ghanim H et al. Evidence for a potent antiinflammatory effect of rosiglitazone. J Clin Endocrinol Metab 2004; 89: 2728–35.

121. Hershfield NB. Disappearance of Crohn's ulcers in the terminal ileum after thalidomide therapy. Can J Gastroenterol 2004; 18: 101–4.

122. Yasui K, Kobayashi N, Yamazaki T et al. Thalidomide as an immunotherapeutic agent: the effects on neutrophil-mediated inflammation. Curr Pharm Des 2005; 11: 395–401.

123. Kim YS, Kim JS, Jung HC et al. The effects of thalidomide on the stimulation of NF-kappaB activity and TNF-alpha production by lipopolysaccharide in a human colonic epithelial cell line. Mol Cells 2004; 17: 210–16.

124. Jin SH, Kim TI, Han DS et al. Thalidomide suppresses the interleukin 1beta-induced NFkappaB signaling pathway in colon cancer cells. Ann N Y Acad Sci 2002; 973: 414–18.

125. Bariol C, Meagher AP, Vickers CR et al. Early studies on the safety and efficacy of thalidomide for symptomatic inflammatory bowel disease. J Gastroenterol Hepatol 2002; 17: 135–9.

126. Lipsky PE, Tao XL. A potential new treatment for rheumatoid arthritis: thunder god vine. Semin Arthritis Rheum 1997; 26: 713–23.

127. Tao X, Cai JJ, Lipsky PE. The identity of immunosuppressive components of the ethyl acetate extract and chloroform methanol extract (T2) of Tripterygium wilfordii Hook. F. J Pharmacol Exp Ther 1995; 272: 1305–12.

128. Qiu D, Zhao G, Aoki Y et al. Immunosuppressant PG490 (triptolide) inhibits T-cell interleukin-2 expression at the level of purine-box/nuclear factor of activated T-cells and NF-kappaB transcriptional activation. J Biol Chem 1999; 274: 13443–50.

129. Qiu D, Kao PN. Immunosuppressive and anti-inflammatory mechanisms of triptolide, the principal active diterpenoid from the Chinese medicinal herb Tripterygium wilfordii Hook. f. Drugs R D 2003; 4: 1–18.

130. Jiang XH, Wong BC, Lin MC et al. Functional p53 is required for triptolide-induced apoptosis and AP-1 and nuclear factor-kappaB activation in gastric cancer cells. Oncogene 2001; 20: 8009–18.

131. Tao X, Younger J, Fan FZ et al. Benefit of an extract of Tripterygium Wilfordii Hook F in patients with rheumatoid arthritis: a double-blind, placebo-controlled study. Arthritis Rheum 2002; 46: 1735–43.

132. Karin M, Yamamoto Y, Wang QM. The IKK NF-kappa B system: a treasure trove for drug development. Nat Rev Drug Discov 2004; 3: 17–26.

133. Hammaker D, Sweeney S, Firestein GS. Signal transduction networks in rheumatoid arthritis. Ann Rheum Dis 2003; 62 (Suppl 2): ii86–9.

134. Burke JR, Pattoli MA, Gregor KR et al. BMS-345541 is a highly selective inhibitor of I kappa B kinase that binds at an allosteric site of the enzyme and blocks NF-kappa B-dependent transcription in mice. J Biol Chem 2003; 278: 1450–6.

135. Rhee JW, Lee KW, Sohn WJ et al. Regulation of matrix metalloproteinase-9 gene expression and cell migration by NF-kappaB in response to CpG-oligodeoxynucleotides in RAW 264.7 cells. Mol Immunol 2007; 44: 1393–400.

136. McIntyre KW, Shuster DJ, Gillooly KM et al. A highly selective inhibitor of I kappa B kinase, BMS-345541, blocks both joint inflammation and destruction in collagen-induced arthritis in mice. Arthritis Rheum 2003; 48: 2652–9.

137. Wen D, Nong Y, Morgan JG et al. A selective small molecule IkappaB Kinase beta inhibitor blocks nuclear factor kappaB-mediated inflammatory responses in human fibroblast-like synoviocytes, chondrocytes, and mast cells. J Pharmacol Exp Ther 2006; 317: 989–1001.

138. Catley MC, Sukkar MB, Chung KF et al. Validation of the anti-inflammatory properties of small-molecule IκB kinase (IKK)-2 inhibitors by comparison with adenoviral-mediated delivery of dominant-negative IKK1 and IKK2 in human airways smooth muscle. Mol Pharmacol 2006; 70: 697–705.

139. Alkalay I, Yaron A, Hatzubai A et al. Stimulation-dependent I kappa B alpha phosphorylation marks the NF-kappa B inhibitor for degradation via the ubiquitin-proteasome pathway. Proc Natl Acad Sci U S A 1995; 92: 10599–603.

140. Spano JP, Bay JO, Blay JY et al. Proteasome inhibition: a new approach for the treatment of malignancies. Bull Cancer 2005; 92: E61–6, 945–52.

141. Jagannath S, Barlogie B, Berenson J et al. A phase 2 study of two doses of bortezomib in relapsed or refractory myeloma. Br J Haematol 2004; 127: 165–72.

142. O'Connor OA, Wright J, Moskowitz C et al. Phase II clinical experience with the novel proteasome inhibitor bortezomib in patients with indolent non-Hodgkin's lymphoma and mantle cell lymphoma. J Clin Oncol 2005; 23: 676–84.

143. Hattori Y, Sakaguchi M, Maitani Y. Folate-linked lipid-based nanoparticles deliver a NFkappaB decoy into activated murine macrophage-like RAW264.7 cells. Biol Pharm Bull 2006; 29: 1516–20.

144. Lin YZ, Yao SY, Veach RA et al. Inhibition of nuclear translocation of transcription factor NF-kappa B by a synthetic peptide containing a cell membrane-permeable motif and nuclear localization sequence. J Biol Chem 1995; 270: 14255–8.

145. Ledeboer A, Gamanos M, Lai W et al. Involvement of spinal cord nuclear factor kappaB activation in rat models of proinflammatory cytokine-mediated pain facilitation. Eur J Neurosci 2005; 22: 1977–86.

146. Liu D, Liu XY, Robinson D et al. Suppression of staphylococcal enterotoxin B-induced toxicity by a nuclear import inhibitor. J Biol Chem 2004; 279: 19239–46.

147. Letoha T, Somlai C, Takacs T et al. A nuclear import inhibitory peptide ameliorates the severity of cholecystokinin-induced acute pancreatitis. World J Gastroenterol 2005; 11: 990–9.

148. Saika S, Miyamoto T, Yamanaka O et al. Therapeutic effect of topical administration of SN50, an inhibitor of nuclear factor-kappaB, in treatment of corneal alkali burns in mice. Am J Pathol 2005; 166: 1393–403.

149. Torgerson TR, Colosia AD, Donahue JP et al. Regulation of NF-kappa B, AP-1, NFAT, and STAT1 nuclear import in T lymphocytes by noninvasive delivery of peptide carrying the nuclear localization sequence of NF-kappa B p50. J Immunol 1998; 161: 6084–92.

150. Takada Y, Singh S, Aggarwal BB. Identification of a p65 peptide that selectively inhibits NF-kappa B activation induced by various inflammatory stimuli and its role in down-regulation of NF-kappaB-mediated gene expression and up-regulation of apoptosis. J Biol Chem 2004; 279: 15096–104.

151. May MJ, D'Acquisto F, Madge LA et al. Selective inhibition of NF-kappaB activation by a peptide that blocks the interaction of NEMO with the IkappaB kinase complex. Science 2000; 289: 1550–4.

152. Dai S, Hirayama T, Abbas S et al. The IkappaB kinase (IKK) inhibitor, NEMO-binding domain peptide, blocks osteoclastogenesis and bone erosion in inflammatory arthritis. J Biol Chem 2004; 279: 37219–22.

153. di Meglio P, Ianaro A, Ghosh S. Amelioration of acute inflammation by systemic administration of a cell-permeable peptide inhibitor of NF-kappaB activation. Arthritis Rheum 2005; 52: 951–8.

154. Tas SW, Vervoordeldonk MJ, Hajji N et al. Local treatment with the selective IkappaB kinase beta inhibitor NEMO-binding domain peptide ameliorates synovial inflammation. Arthritis Res Ther 2006; 8: R86.

155. Huang J, Sheung J, Dong G et al. High-throughput screening for inhibitors of the E3 ubiquitin ligase APC. Methods Enzymol 2005; 399: 740–54.

156. Doyle SL, Jefferies CA, O'Neill LA. Bruton's tyrosine kinase is involved in p65-mediated transactivation and phosphorylation of p65 on serine 536 during NFkappaB activation by lipopolysaccharide. J Biol Chem 2005; 280: 23496–501.

157. McInnes C. Improved lead-finding for kinase targets using high-throughput docking. Curr Opin Drug Discov Devel 2006; 9: 339–47.

158. Mansell A, Smith R, Doyle SL et al. Suppressor of cytokine signaling 1 negatively regulates Toll-like receptor signaling by mediating Mal degradation. Nat Immunol 2006; 7: 148–55.

159. Tran EJ, Wente SR. Dynamic nuclear pore complexes: life on the edge. Cell 2006; 125: 1041–53.

160. Zhao LJ, Zhu H. Structure and function of HIV-1 auxiliary regulatory protein Vpr: novel clues to drug design. Curr Drug Targets Immune Endocr Metabol Disord 2004; 4: 265–75.

161. Wakamatsu K, Nanki T, Miyasaka N et al. Effect of a small molecule inhibitor of nuclear factor-kappaB nuclear translocation in a murine model of arthritis and cultured human synovial cells. Arthritis Res Ther 2005; 7: R1348–59.

162. Tas SW, Adriaansen J, Hajji N et al. Amelioration of arthritis by intraarticular dominant negative Ikkbeta gene therapy using adeno-associated virus type 5. Hum Gene Ther 2006; 17: 821–32.

163. Lu H, Hachida M, Enosawa S et al. Immunosuppressive effect of triptolide in vitro. Transplant Proc 1999; 31: 2056–7.

164. Suarez-Almazor ME, Belseck E, Shea B et al. Sulfasalazine for rheumatoid arthritis. Cochrane Database Syst Rev 2000: CD000958.

165. Breuer-McHam J, Simpson E, Dougherty I et al. Activation of HIV in human skin by ultraviolet B radiation and its inhibition by NFkappaB blocking agents. Photochem Photobiol 2001; 74: 805–10.

166. A phase 1/2 multicenter, randomized, double-blind, placebo-controlled, parallel-group, dose-ranging study to evaluate the safety of repeated topical application of three concentrations of NF-kappaB decoy in adults with mild-to-moderate atopic dermatitis/

http://clinicaltrials.gov/ct/show/NCT00153337?
order=1 accessed 12, April 2007.

167. Tomita T, Takeuchi E, Tomita N et al. Suppressed severity of collagen-induced arthritis by in vivo transfection of nuclear factor kappaB decoy oligodeoxynucleotides as a gene therapy. Arthritis Rheum 1999; 42: 2532–42.

168. Gotzsche PC, Johansen HK. Short-term low-dose corticosteroids vs placebo and nonsteroidal antiinflammatory drugs in rheumatoid arthritis. Cochrane Database Syst Rev 2004: CD000189.

169. Akkoc N, van der Linden S, Khan MA. Ankylosing spondylitis and symptom-modifying vs disease-modifying therapy. Best Pract Res Clin Rheumatol 2006; 20: 539–57.

170. Moutsopoulos NM, Angelov N, Sankar V et al. Immunological consequences of thalidomide treatment in Sjogren's syndrome. Ann Rheum Dis 2006; 65: 112–14.

171. Adams A, Lehman TJ. Update on the pathogenesis and treatment of systemic onset juvenile rheumatoid arthritis. Curr Opin Rheumatol 2005; 17: 612–16.

48

Outcomes assessment in rheumatic disease

Daniel Aletaha and Josef Smolen

Introduction • Domains – The 'core set' measures and more • Combination of domains • Summary • References

INTRODUCTION

Outcomes assessment is a crucial element in the optimal care of patients with rheumatic diseases. The term 'outcome', however, relates to different aspects of the disease depending on which surrogate of the pathophysiology one is looking at and whose perspective one is taking. From a pathophysiological aspect, disease activity, accumulating damage, and the ultimate consequences of the underlying events, functional impairment: are three essential features. From a more individual perspective, the trialist will use the term outcome(s) in relation to those attributes of the disease that constitute the primary endpoints to be influenced by short- or intermediate-term therapeutic interventions in clinical trials. The clinician will primarily be interested in improvement of disease activity and those elements that reflect patient's satisfaction; the patient's perspective will be best mirrored by patient-reported 'outcomes', such as pain and physical and social functioning. Finally, epidemiologists and health service researchers will often consider 'outcome' as something more remote, some characteristic future disease states that need to be prevented, or focus on long-term economic aspects.

In general, outcome measures can consist of measures that reflect individual disease characteristics or composite indices. Moreover, they can be disease-specific, organ-specific (if defining an organ as a group of tissues that fulfill particular functions, such as in the current context the joints or the spine), or generic (referring to an instrument's applicability to various diseases as opposed to 'disease-specificity' or 'organ-specificity'). The purpose of this chapter is to give an overview of the most common measures that are used to follow the clinical course of inflammatory joint diseases, which are the entities that have the worst disease outcomes (in the meaning of the epidemiologist),[1–3] while at the same time, they are clearly the ones that are most amenable to improvement by current therapies. They comprise rheumatoid arthritis (RA), psoriatic arthritis (PsA), and ankylosing spondylitis (AS).

Since, as discussed above, the term 'outcomes' is very wide, the focus of this chapter is to present the various *disease activity* measures that are commonly used. In this sense, we will rather take the perspective of the patient, the physician, or the trialist, and we do not focus on long-term consequences (the epidemiologist's perspective). Therefore radiographic damage, which is a chapter on its own for these three diseases, will also not be discussed here. However, in some instances, the trade-off between the disease process and disease outcome is not always separable, as in the instance of measures of function, which can be used as surrogates of disease activity to follow patients in clinical practice,[4] while they also partly represent a component that is related to the destructive consequences of the disease.[5]

DOMAINS – THE 'CORE SET' MEASURES AND MORE

One term that is closely linked to the assessment of disease activity is 'core set'. Partly independently, the American College of Rheumatology (ACR), the European League Against Rheumatism (EULAR), and the World Health Organization (WHO), have developed sets of disease activity attributes in an effort to create consistency in applied measures and trial reports.[6–8]

For RA, these measures included swollen and tender joint counts (SJC, TJC), patient assessment of pain, patient and evaluator global assessment of disease activity (PGA, EGA), and a measure of the acute phase response (APR). It seems reasonable that these measures, at least partly, should be used for actual disease activity evaluation and response to therapy also in clinical practice. The ACR and WHO disease activity core sets also include measures of physical function, which are regarded as outcome measures in the EULAR core set. Structural damage is yet another outcome measure; as explained in the introduction, the respective measures will not be covered within the scope of this chapter. Table 48.1 provides a synopsis of domains and measures.

The RA core set measures are usually evaluated also in PsA. PGA and EGA as well as the assessment of pain are most commonly measured on visual analog scales (VAS). APR are also evaluated, although their elevation, even in active PsA, is less reliably associated with the active arthritic process. Joint counts and functional measures have been partly adapted for PsA.

In 1999, a core set to assess outcome in AS was proposed by the Assessment in Ankylosing Spondylitis (ASAS) International Working Group.[9] This AS outcome core set consists of the following domains: physical function, spinal mobility, patient global, pain, morning stiffness, fatigue, number of swollen joints, erythrocyte sedimentation rate, radiographs of the spine and the hips, and enthesitis. The ASAS also outlined the specific instruments for each domain; they will be discussed in the appropriate sections below.

Pain levels

Pain is the most prominent symptom of rheumatic diseases. There are numerous reliable methods of pain assessment,[10–12] but most commonly, pain is measured on a 100 mm horizontal VAS.[13–15]

Usually, the past week is evaluated. Horizontal and vertical VAS are well correlated, but vertical scales tend to produce higher values.[15] There is evidence suggesting that patients might differ considerably in their ability to use the VAS,[13] but the VAS remains the most prominent instrument for the evaluation of pain in rheumatic diseases.

Patient and evaluator assessment of global disease activity (PGA, EGA)

The global level of disease activity can also be directly rated by a patient or physician/evaluator. Like pain scores, these two further core set variables for RA are also typically assessed on 100 mm VAS and, at least in RA, one of them is rarely assessed without the other. While PGA is a patient-derived measure (a 'subjective' measure), and EGA is observer-derived (i.e. a more 'objective' measure), they still correlate relatively well, although PGA is frequently rated higher than EGA.[16] This systematic difference is seen in most clinical trial and observational databases and is a good argument for evaluating both[6,8] ('averaging' effect), which in fact is a requirement of several composite indices of disease activity.[16,17]

In AS, a single VAS to assess global well-being has also been proposed, the *Bath Ankylosing Spondylitis Global Score (BAS-G)*,[18] which has been shown to be reliable and to correlate well with the BASDAI (see section on composite indices). However, the BAS-G assesses the impact of AS on a patient's well-being, and can therefore be regarded as a measure of disease activity, a measure of functional limitation, or both.

Acute phase reactants

Acute phase reactants (APRs) are most important in peripheral joint disease, that is, especially RA and (less so) PsA, but not in isolated spinal disease, as commonly seen in AS. The most frequently used APRs are C-reactive protein (CRP) and erythrocyte sedimentation rate (ESR). These markers are universally employed in studies and clinical practice; the APR correlates well with clinical disease activity, and the time integrated APR also correlates well with disease

Table 48.1 Synopsis of domains and measures

Variable	Rheumatoid arthritis	Psoriatic arthritis	Ankylosing spondylitis
Individual domains			
Pain levels	VAS (horizontal; patients differ in their ability of to complete scales)		
Patient global assessment (PGA)	VAS for both (rarely one without the other, 'averaging effect'; EGA systematically lower than PGA		BAS-G (evaluates global health rather than mere disease activity)
Evaluator global assessment (EGA)			Less frequently assessed than in RA/PsA
Acute phase reactants (APRs)	C-reactive protein ESR	Less important than in RA	Not relevant if no peripheral joint disease
Swollen and tender joint counts (SJC/TJC)	ACR joint count (66/68) used in clinical trials; 28-joint count in both trials and practice (most feasible, high validity)	Joint counts adapted from RA (ACR joint + DIP joints of the feet and CMCs on both sides as one joint; 76/78)	Not applicable
Dactylitis	Not applicable	Simple count of digits has been used in trials (poor sensitivity to change)	Not applicable
Tendonitis	Not applicable	No measure available	Not applicable
Enthesitis	Not applicable	Mander index (66 tendon sites) MASES (13 sites)	Mander index MASES
Spine	Not applicable	No specific measures available	
Skin assessment	Not applicable	PASI score (most relevant) Lattice index	Not applicable
Physical function	HAQ (and modifications) SF-36 AIMS (AIMS2, AIMS2-SF) Metrologic functional measures (e.g. grip strength)	HAQ HAQ-SK HAQ-S	HAQ-S BASMI BASFI
Combined measures			
Composite indices	DAS DAS28 SDAI CDAI	No measure available	No measure available
Self-report instruments	RADAR RADAI	No measure available	BASDAI
Response criteria	ACR response EULAR response SDAI/CDAI response ACR-N ACR-hybrid	PsARC ACR response EULAR response	ASAS response

outcomes, such as radiographic progression.[19–22] In most cases, APRs do not add information if clinical information from joint counts, PGA, and EGA are available.[16] In cases where APR is clearly higher than the respective clinical measures, this is usually due to infection or other causes of inflammation not related to the rheumatic disease. On the other hand, if APR is low and as such discrepant to high clinical disease activity, it is likely to be neglected in the assessment of a patient with a rheumatic disease and in the respective therapeutic considerations. In addition, APR measures are normal in many patients with RA at their first presentation[23] and, therefore, some clinical trials of early RA allowed inclusion of patients with normal CRP and ESR.[24] Many other APRs are known, such as serum amyloid A (SAA), IL-6, or hepcidin, and likewise many other immunoinflammatory biomarkers, such as tumor necrosis factor (TNF)-α, RANKL, matrix metalloproteinases, are well known. However, for many of them, the clinical usefulness of determination has not yet been clearly established, partly because they are currently too expensive or too tedious to perform.

Swollen and tender joint counts

Joint assessment is a very obvious element of disease activity evaluation in polyarticular diseases. Therefore, counting the number of affected joints seems to be most reasonable in RA and PsA, while in AS, due to its infrequent involvement of peripheral joints, is seems to be less informative. Joint involvement is typically evaluated for soft tissue swelling and effusion (swollen joint count, SJC) and tenderness on pressure or motion (tender joint count, TJC). There is evidence of some usefulness of counting deformed joints,[25,26] but this is not commonly done. Several joint indices and counts have been developed over the past 50 years,[27,28] which mostly differ simply by the number of joints assessed. There are some exceptions, including the 'weighted' joint counts, which weight joints by their surface area, and 'graded' joint counts, which weight joints by severity of swelling or tenderness.[29–38]

The chronology of their development dates back to the *Lansbury Index*,[29] in which swelling and tenderness in 86 joints were graded as minimal, slight, moderate, or maximal, and also weighted for joint surface area. Another early index, the *Ritchie Articular Index*, which is also used in the original Disease Activity Score (DAS; see below) assesses graded tenderness in 26 joint areas[32] and was later simplified by Hart to exclude the grading by severity, which is a major cause of inter-rater disagreement.[33] Today, the most commonly employed indices are the comprehensive *66/68-joint count*, as suggested by the American Rheumatism Association (ARA; now American College of Rheumatology, ACR) in 1965,[30] and its simplification to the *28-joint count*.[36] They have been shown to have similar validity and reliability.[39,40] Among other regions, the 28-joint counts also spare the assessment of the foot and ankle joints, since both swelling and tenderness in these joints are frequently confounded by disorders other than RA.[36,40] The feet can be included using a 32-joint count, although it is not more reliable than the 28-joint count, even for the assessment of remission.[35] At the present time, it seems most sensible to use the 28-joint count as a simple and validated measure, unless the more comprehensive joint counts are easily obtainable from a logistic and a cost perspective in trials and practice. The 28-joint count has been adopted by the EULAR, and is widely accepted.[41] Importantly, the 28-joint count has also been reliably employed in clinical trials,[42,43] especially as the joint count contained in several composite indices (see below) employed as primary and secondary endpoints for disease activity assessment.

In patients with PsA, the 66/68 (ACR) joint count[30] has also been shown to be a reliable instrument.[44,45] A modification of the ACR joint count that includes assessment of the distal interphalangeal (DIP) joints of the feet and the carpometacarpal joints of the hands (counted as 1 unit on each side) was also derived, resulting in 76/78 joints. Also, a graded (0–3) version of the ACR joint count is used;[46] however, this index was shown to be less reliable compared with the ungraded ACR joint count.[47] Although not validated, the 28-joint count[36] has also been used in PsA, especially for the purpose of calculation of composite indices, such as the DAS28 (see below). However, the high prevalence of

DIP joint involvement makes it a potentially less sensible instrument in PsA.

Dactylitis

Dactylitis is a feature that is typical for PsA. It is defined as the swelling of a whole digit, which is often referred to as a 'sausage' digit. Approximately 40% of patients with PsA develop dactylitis.[48] It is most likely related to inflammation of the tendons and the joints in the affected digit and it can have an acute (swelling, redness, pain) or chronic (swelling without signs of acute inflammation) presentation. Dactylitis carries an increased risk of radiographic progression of joint damage.[49] The simple number of digits with dactylitis has been used in several clinical trials,[50,51] but more quantitative methods may be needed to enhance sensitivity to change.

Tendonitis and Enthesitis

Tendonitis frequently occurs in patients with PsA, but no measure of tendon inflammation has yet been used in clinical trials, let alone been validated. Enthesitis, relates to inflammation of tendon insertion sites and is a common feature in spondylarthropathies including AS and PsA. These sites most frequently include the insertions of the Achilles tendon and the plantar fascia to the calcaneus, and tendon insertions to the pelvis and thorax. Two measures have been proposed for use in spondylarthropathies, but have been derived in patients with ankylosing spondylitis. The *Mander Index*[52] requires assessment of 66 sites, which limits its feasibility in clinical trials or practice. Also, it is often difficult to discern true enthesitis from trigger points in (secondary) fibromyalgia. The *Maastricht Ankylosing Spondylitis Enthesitis Score (MASES)*[53] evaluates only 13 sites. However, the reliability of the assessment of enthesitis is moderate at best, and is different depending on the site of enthesitis.[45] A simple count of enthesitic sites has been used in clinical trials.[51,54]

Spine

The most characteristic clinical symptoms of spondylitis are back pain and stiffness, which tend to worsen after prolonged periods of inactivity. Unlike in ankylosing spondylitis, axial involvement in PsA is less consistent, less severe, and more heterogeneous. Spondylitis is found in up to half,[55] and sacroiliitis in up to one of four patients with PsA.[48,56] The clinical measures used to evaluate spondylitis and sacroiliitis do not differ between PsA and AS, and have mostly been developed for AS. However, aside from the BASDAI (discussed in the section on composite indices below), the BAS-G (discussed in the section on global scores above), and the ASAS response criteria (discussed in the section on response criteria), there are no other specific instruments that measure or at least include the assessment of spondylitis.

Skin

Skin involvement is only an issue in PsA, and psoriatic skin involvement is highly reflected in the quality of life measures and patient global assessments. Various physician global assessment scales are available to quantify the severity of psoriasis. These scales are widely used,[57] and have been primary outcomes in trials of psoriasis.[58] However, the most common instrument is the *Psoriasis Area and Severity Index (PASI)*.[59] In the PASI, the body is divided into four areas (head, upper and lower extremity, and trunk). Each area is rated from 0 to 4 for average redness, induration, and scaling of lesions and the numbers are summed and weighted by surface area. The total PASI is the sum of all four areas. It has been a reliable tool in clinical trials of biologics in psoriasis and PsA,[51,58,60] and 50% and 75% improvement in PASI is a clinically meaningful endpoint.[61]

There are a number of alternatives in patients with less severe psoriasis,[57] of which the *Lattice Index*[62] appears to be better understood by patients and physicians than the PASI due to its static step score. In contrast to the PASI, it evaluates patients globally rather than by areas, and rates the different qualities on an eight-step scale. It has been shown to be well correlated with both the PASI and the physician global score, and may have even better reliability than the PASI.[62]

Physical function

Instruments that allow measurement of physical function can be divided into self-report questionnaires and quantitative objective instruments.

Likely the most important generic self-reported measure of physical function is the *Medical Outcomes Study Short Form-36 (SF-36)*.[63] Two main summary scores can be calculated from the 36 items and 8 scales of the SF-36, the physical component and the mental component. By virtue of its validity, reliability, and good psychometric properties,[64,65] the SF-36 allows evaluation of healthy individuals as well as patients with different diseases[65] and likewise assessment of response to therapy.

The most prominent disease-specific instrument for the assessment of physical function is the *Health Assessment Questionnaire (HAQ)*.[66] In particular, the HAQ Disability Index (HAQ-DI) is widely used to evaluate the ability to perform activities of daily living. The HAQ-DI consists of 20 questions related to the upper and/or lower extremity; these questions are organized in 8 categories: dressing, rising, eating, walking, hygiene, reach, grip, and usual activities. For each question there is a four-level difficulty scale ranging from 0 to 3, representing no difficulty (0), some difficulty (1), much difficulty (2), and inability to do (3). The mean of the highest individual scores across the eight categories is the final HAQ score; it ranges from 0 to 3: higher levels indicate more disability and levels < 0.3 are close to normal. The HAQ-DI is now used in virtually every RA trial. It increases with duration of RA, reflecting the accumulated joint damage;[67] and over the long term the correlation between HAQ-DI and radiographic changes increases.[67,68]

Pincus and colleagues have modified the HAQ *(modified HAQ, MHAQ)*,[69] simplifying the scoring for daily clinical care. To this end, the questions of the original HAQ were reduced to one or two per category; the total score is derived by calculating the average of the eight categories. Pincus also introduced the *multidimensional HAQ (MDHAQ)*,[4] expanding the 8-item MHAQ to 14 items and reducing the floor effect that had been noticed with the use of the MHAQ.

On the original HAQ scale, the intervals between scores at different points do not translate into similar changes in functional impairment. Therefore, Wolfe et al. recently developed the *HAQ-II*, in which this psychometric problem has been addressed.[70]

While the minimal clinically important difference of the HAQ has been suggested to be 0.22,[71] in many clinical trials this cut-off point has been modified to 0.25 to better reflect the true increments of the HAQ-DI. Recent studies showed that the potential for HAQ score improvement differs depending on average RA duration.[72] The degree of the underlying damage may reduce the reversibility of HAQ scores in individual patients.[73] The HAQ as a measure of functional limitation is determined by both activity (reversible component) and accrued damage (irreversible component).[73,74] In terms of therapeutic strategies, the irreversible proportion of functional impairment constitutes an 'unavoidable' component in patients with accrued damage after long-standing disease, but likewise a 'preventable' long-term component of disability in patients with early disease that needs to be targeted intensively.

The *Arthritis Impact Measurement Scale (AIMS)*[11] encompasses nine domains, two of which are depression and anxiety. The domains are composed of 4–7 questions totalling 49 questions. The *AIMS2* is a longer version comprising 12 domains and 78 questions[75] and there is a shorter versions (*AIMS2-short form*: 5 domains and 26 questions).[76] The AIMS2-SF can be filled out in about 5 minutes.[77] Wolfe et al. developed *the clinical HAQ (CLINHAQ)*,[78] which, in addition to the eight categories of the original HAQ, borrowed the depression and anxiety scales from the AIMS, and included five additional VAS and a pain diagram.

This group of quantitative instruments includes measures of hand function, and timed measures of locomotor function.[79] *Grip strength* is usually measured using a vigorimeter or a dynamometer;[80] the readout is the pressure attained by squeezing a compressible rubber bulb. The *Moberg picking-up* test has been standardized as a timed measurement of the ability to pick up small metallic items randomly placed in three lines on the table, and to put them into a box.[81] In the *Button test* patients are timed while undoing and rebuttoning five buttons on a board with one hand.[82] The *Walking time* is a timed measurement of the patient's ability to walk a particular distance. It has been shown that, using standardized protocols, all these instruments have excellent reliability[82] and predict long-term morbidity and mortality in patients with RA.[79]

Several instruments to assess function and quality of life have been developed for patients with PsA. The *SF-36 (see above)*[63] has been validated for the assessment of patients with PsA[83,84] and showed significant changes in PsA clinical trials.[50,60] The *HAQ-DI*, originally developed for RA[66] has meanwhile been modified for patients with spondylarthropathies *(HAQ-S)*[85] and psoriasis *(HAQ-SK)*.[86] Both scores show similar results to the original HAQ-DI in patients with PsA.[85,86] This indicates that inclusion of the spinal and the skin domains does not systematically impact the overall assessment of physical function in patients with PsA systematically. Consequently, the original HAQ can be employed in PsA clinical trials.[87] The *AIMS*[11] and *AIMS2*,[75] have also been validated for PsA.[88,89]

In AS, functional impairment can be evaluated by the *Bath Ankylosing Spondylitis Metrology Index (BASMI)*,[90] which combines assessments of the ability to perform cervical rotation, lumbar flexion (modified Schober test), lumbar side flexion, tragus-to-wall distance, and intermalleolar distance and serves as a clinical index of spine mobility. It ranges from 0 to 10, correlates with radiographic damage, and has shown excellent inter-rater and intra-rater reliability.[91]

Other functional measures in AS apply self-reporting. The *Bath Ankylosing Spondylitis Functional Index (BASFI)*[92] is a 10-item questionnaire, each of which is rated on a 10-cm VAS (0 indicating no limitation and 10 indicating inability to do). The BASFI is the mean of all 10 VAS. The other self-report instruments are based on categorical ratings of the ability to perform daily life activities. The *Dougados Functional Index (DFI)* comprises 20 items[93] related to daily life activities and scored as 0 (no difficulty), 1 (some difficulty), or 2 (impossible to do). While there are specifically

designed instruments for AS based on the *Health Assessment Questionnaire (HAQ for Spondylarthropathies; HAQ-S)*,[85] the addition of the AS subscales did not improve sensitivity to detect functional problems in patients with AS.[94] As mentioned above, the HAQ-S is also used in PsA.[95,96] The *Revised Leeds Disability Questionnaire (RLDQ)*[97] comprises four questions for each of four scales (mobility, bending down, neck movements, and posture). It is calculated as the mean of the highest scores in each section like the HAQ-S, giving a final range of 0–3, offers four categorical responses, and appears to be sensitive to change.[97]

All these scores were shown to have various degrees of reliability and validity, although different sensitivities to change have been reported in studies. The DFI has a narrow grading (scale of 0–2), which may not allow many patients to accurately assign their responses accordingly. This limits sensitivity to change in comparison with HAQ, HAQ-S, BASFI,[98] pain, and stiffness.[94] On the other hand, BASFI scores are skewed and have been shown to exhibit a ceiling effect,[98] although sensitivity to change of the BASFI was reported to be higher than for the HAQ-S.[99]

COMBINATION OF DOMAINS

Composite indices

RA varies in its presentation and course. Consequently, disease activity expresses itself variably. This is reflected by the many surrogates that have been employed (see sections above). They all put emphasis on just a single or a limited aspect of disease activity. Given this heterogeneity of RA, none of these measures allows the clinician to quantify disease activity or response to therapy sufficiently reliably – neither in an individual nor in groups of patients. Therefore, an independent evaluation of all variables in clinical trials leads to methodological issues.[100] To overcome these limitations, composite endpoints have been employed[100–102] and combined ('composite') indices developed.

Composite scores have been mainly built to evaluate disease activity of RA patients in clinical trials, where differential response to drugs is of major interest and the use of such indices allows reduction of sample sizes. However, composite indices should also be used to follow patients in clinical practice.[103] On the one hand, absolute changes in these scores can be compared, but on the other hand criteria exist that allow classification of the extent of the response (see below).

Older scores, such as those propagated by Steinbrocker[104] and Lansbury[105] included items characteristic of disease activity beyond the core set variables (e.g. anemia or fever). The Mallya index encompassed hemoglobin, morning stiffness, and grip strength aside from tender joints, ESR, and pain.[106] Pain and grip strength were later excluded by van Riel et al. in a trial.[107] The newer indices, in current use, are based on the core set variables[6–8] and their detailed characteristics are shown in Table 48.2. These are the *Disease Activity Score (DAS)* and its modification employing 28-joint counts, the DAS 28, as well as the *Simplified Disease Activity Index (SDAI)* and its modification sparing CRP, the *Clinical Disease Activity Index (CDAI)*.

The gold standard for the derivation of the DAS[108] was the start or stop of disease-modifying anti-rheumatic therapy by a physician, reflecting high and low disease activity, respectively. The statistical procedures used for this purpose led to a complex formula, which involves different weighting of each variable, square root and logarithmic transformation of some variables. The original DAS employs an extended 44 swollen joint count[109] as well as the Ritchie Articular Index,[32] a graded joint tenderness score. Both these types of joint assessments are rarely employed in clinical practice and trials. Therefore, the DAS was modified towards the use of condensed, ungraded, and unweighted 28-joint counts,[110] the DAS28.[111] Meanwhile, there are various modifications of the DAS and the DAS28: these scores may comprise CRP instead of ESR (DAS-CRP and DAS28-CRP) or may exclude the assessment of global health, i.e. are composed of only three variables (DAS-3 and DAS28-3). However, none of these modifications has been fully validated. Therefore, the values of these various modifications are not mutually interchangeable, and care must be taken to ascertain which of the many varying DAS instruments has been employed when interpreting respective clinical data. For example, extrapolating DAS-4-CRP results to DAS-4-ESR data may be misleading. Finally, the complexity of the DAS and the DAS28 formulae necessitates the use of a pocket calculator or computer program, and does not make the score transparent for patients.

Therefore, simpler indices have been developed. Interestingly, calculating a linear sum of values of variables that were untransformed and unweighted, as done for the first time in the *Simplified Disease Activity Index (SDAI)*, resulted in a very high correlation with the DAS28.[17] The variables had been selected based on the ACR and the EULAR core sets,[6,7] as well as on previous studies on reactive arthritis.[112] Meanwhile, the SDAI has been widely validated using clinical trial data, in daily settings and across different cultures,[17,113–117] and recently cut-off points for remission and activity states have been derived.[118] The SDAI, DAS, and DAS28 all require laboratory measures (CRP or ESR), which might limit their usefulness in clinical practice, when lab results are missing or not yet available. While no modification of the DAS or DAS28 exists that spares an APR, the Clinical Disease Activity Index (CDAI) has been validated as a modification of the SDAI;[114,119] this index does well without CRP and has been validated using several different cohorts of patients. It correlates highly with the DAS28 and the ACR response, but also with the HAQ and radiographic changes.[114] It makes prompt assessment of disease activity possible and consequently facilitates immediate decision making regarding treatment. Moreover, it can be easily understood by the patients.[103]

No validated composite disease activity indices have yet been developed for PsA and AS.

Self-report instruments of disease activity

RA disease activity can also be assessed using patient-reported questionnaires. The *Rapid Assessment of Disease Activity in Rheumatology (RADAR)*,[120] is a two-page self-administered questionnaire that comprises six items which are scored. While the individual RADAR items can be interpreted using expert opinion or other

Table 48.2 Commonly used composite indices in rheumatoid arthritis

Indices	Formulae (CRP in mg/L for DAS and LAS28, and in mg/dl for SDAI; GH: VAS in mm; PGA and EGA: VAS in cm)	Cut-off points	Possible range[a]
DAS, 4 var, ESR	$= 0.54 \times \sqrt{(Ritchie)} + 0.065 \times SJC44 + 0.33 \times \log_{nat}(ESR) + 0.0072 \times GH$	REM < 1.6	0.23–9.87
DAS, 4 var, CRP	$= 0.54 \times \sqrt{(Ritchie)} + 0.065 \times SJC44 + 0.17 \times \log_{nat}(CRP+1) + 0.0072 \times GH + 0.45$	LDA < 2.4; MDA < 3.7; HDA ≥ 3.7	0.57–9.58
DAS, 3 var, ESR	$= 0.54 \times \sqrt{(Ritchie)} + 0.065 \times SJC44 + 0.33 \times \log_{nat}(ESR) + 0.22$		0.45–9.37
DAS, 3 var, CRP	$= 0.54 \times \sqrt{(Ritchie)} + 0.065 \times SJC44 + 0.17 \times \log_{nat}(CRP+1) + 0.65$		0.77–9.06
DAS28, 4 var, ESR	$= 0.56 \times \sqrt{(TJC28)} + 0.28 \times \sqrt{(SJC28)} + 0.70 \times \log_{nat}(ESR) + 0.014 \times GH$	REM < 2.6	0.49–9.07
DAS28, 4 var, CRP	$= 0.56 \times \sqrt{(TJC28)} + 0.28 \times \sqrt{(SJC28)} + 0.36 \times \log_{nat}(CRP+1) + 0.014 \times GH + 0.96$	LDA < 3.2	1.21–8.47
DAS28, 3 var, ESR	$= [0.56 \times \sqrt{(TJC28)} + 0.28 \times \sqrt{(SJC28)} + 0.70^* \times \log_{nat}(ESR)] \times 1.08 + 0.16$	MDA ≤ 5.1	0.68–8.44
DAS28, 3 var, CRP	$= [0.56 \times \sqrt{(TJC28)} + 0.28^* \sqrt{(SJC28)} + 0.36^* \log_{nat}(CRP+1)] \times 1.10 + 1.15$	HDA > 5.1	1.42–7.87
SDAI	SJC28 + TJC28 + PGA + EGA + CRP	[b]REM ≤ 3.3; LDA ≤ 11; MDA ≤26; HDA > 26	0.1–86
CDAI	SJC28 + TJC28 + PGA + EGA	[b]REM ≤2.8; LDA ≤ 10; MDA ≤22; HDA > 22	0–76

[a]Range of ESR assumed as 2–100, and range of CRP assumed as 1–100 mg/L.

[b]Cut-off points have recently been revised for SDAI,[118] and p esented for the CDAI (*Clin Exp Rheum*); traditional cut-off points for the SDAI were: REM ≤ 5, LDA ≤ 20, MDA ≤ 40, and HDA > 40.

DAS, Disease Activity Score; DAS28, DAS based on 28 joint counts; Ritchie, Ritchie Articular Index; SJC28, SJC44, swollen joint counts based on the evaluation of 28 or 44 joints, respectively; TJC28, tender joint count based on 28 joints; ESR, erythrocyte sedimentation rate; CRP C-reactive protein; GH, global health; PGA, EGA, patient and evaluator global; REM, remission; LDA, low disease activity; MDA, moderate disease activity; HAD, high disease activity Adapted from Aletaha and smolen.[28]

studies as references, there is no total score for this instrument. The application of the *Rheumatoid Arthritis Disease Activity Index (RADAI)*,[121] a questionnaire that includes five items, has also been proposed for clinical practice. Completion and scoring of both the RADAR and RADAI questionnaires takes less than 10 minutes; however, evaluation of the RADAI requires a calculator.[122] Both scores are reliable and valid when compared to functional or other disease activity measures.[123,124] However, it is important to distinguish between symptom questionnaires, such as those just mentioned, and health status questionnaires (see below), since they provide complementary information.[123] Moreover, it is also important to appreciate that the composite clinical indices described above incorporate 'objective' evaluation based on clinical examination and/or laboratory variables, while symptom questionnaires are restricted to subjective judgment. This may be one reason why both the RADAR and the RADAI are rarely used in clinical practice or in clinical trials.

A self-report instrument has also been developed to measure disease activity in AS, namely the *Bath Ankylosing Spondylitis Disease Activity Index (BASDAI)*.[125] This instrument assesses severity of fatigue, spinal joint pain, peripheral joint pain, localized tenderness, and morning stiffness by employing 10 cm VAS. Morning stiffness is evaluated separately qualitatively and quantitatively. The final BASDAI is an average of these six scales, ranges from 0 to 10, and is reliable and sensitive to change; active disease is usually regarded a BASDAI ≥ 4.[126]

Response criteria

Response criteria express improvement relative to a baseline and are therefore useful to assess drug effects in clinical trials. The Paulus RA response criteria[127] required at least 20% improvement in four of six measures, namely joint pain/tenderness score, joint swelling score, morning stiffness, and ESR, and two or more grades on a five-grade scale (or from grade 2 to grade 1) for PGA and EGA. This index allowed discrimination between placebo and DMARD-treated patients.

Also, the ACR response criteria,[128] which are based on the ACR core set variables,[6] require 20% improvement (ACR 20) in several variables: swollen and tender joint counts on the one hand as well as three of the five remaining core set variables on the other hand. Like the Paulus criteria, the ACR criteria aimed to discriminate active drug from placebo in clinical trials. With better therapies, the criteria were broadened toward 50% (ACR 50) and 70% (ACR 70) improvement. This allowed judgment of frequencies of more substantial responses, but discrimination of active drug from placebo was not better than using the ACR 20 criteria.[129]

The ACR-N response[130,131] grades a 0–100% improvement by evaluating the smallest relative improvement seen for following three measures: swollen joint count, tender joint count, and median of the five remaining core set variables. This transposition of the ACR criteria from a dichotomous to a continuous scale allows for a more quantitative (rather than categorical) readout. However, deterioration from baseline may be calculated as a negative value or as zero, and its time-integrated use as ACR-N area under the curve does not provide valid discrimination between regimens.[132,133]

Finally, a new measure, the 'hybrid' measure of ACR response has recently been presented,[134] aiming to provide a continuous scale using a complex formula. Since it has not yet been used in clinical trials nor validated outside the original study, it will not be detailed herein.

The EULAR response criteria are based on the DAS and the DAS28 and classify three categories: good response, moderate response, and no response.[135] EULAR response (good + moderate) is often more frequent than ACR 20 response, and good EULAR responses are usually higher than ACR 70 responses.

In clinical practice, regular (3-monthly) evaluation of disease activity by composite scores (CDAI, SDAI or DAS28) should be performed, aiming to reach remission or at least the low disease activity range by switching therapies according to the respective disease activity.[103,136,137]

Interestingly, the *ACR response criteria for RA*[128] have also been employed for PsA trials,[50,51,60,138] usually using the 78/76-joint counts to account for the DIP of the feet.

Despite the fact that they had not been developed nor originally validated for PsA, they showed good discrimination between active drug and placebo.

In contrast, the *Psoriatic Arthritis Response Criteria (PsARC)* have been developed specifically for PsA.[54] Mostly they showed good discrimination between active drug and placebo.[50,51,60,138]

The *EULAR response criteria* for RA (using the DAS28) have also recently been applied in a clinical trial of PsA.[51] Like the ACR criteria, they showed good discrimination between active drug and placebo. However, most patients in most recent trials had symmetric polyarthritis.

Clearly, more methodological work is needed. This should not only be devoted to validate currently available composite scores, such as the DAS28, the SDAI or the CDAI, but also to develop new ones specifically for PsA. In this context it is worthwhile mentioning that an index that has already been validated in an oligoarticular disease involving DIP joints, namely reactive arthritis, the DAREA,[112] may also be of interest for further evaluation in PsA.

Response criteria have also been developed for AS. The response criteria of the Assessment in Ankylosing Spondylitis (ASAS) International Working Group are defined as a 20% improvement (*and* at least 10 unit change on a 0–100 scale) in at least three of the following four measures: PGA (VAS), pain (VAS), function (BASFI), and inflammation (mean of duration and intensity of morning stiffness on 100 mm VAS, such as in the BASDAI); these constitute the *ASAS20* criteria.[139] The fourth measure must not deteriorate by the same margins. Analogous definitions lead to achievement of ASAS50 and ASAS70 responses.[139] ASAS partial remission is defined as a score of < 20 mm in each of these four domains.[139]

SUMMARY

Outcome assessment in clinical trials comprises disease activity evaluation of RA core set variables and respective sets of variables in PsA and AS, assessments of quality of life and physical function. However, such assessments are also needed in daily clinical practice, especially given today's costly biological therapies. To this end,

reliable and – of note – simple tools are available, allowing clinicians to define therapeutic goals in collaboration with the patient. The value of these instruments lies in the follow-up of changes in the patient's state and consequent dynamic therapeutic adaptations to achieve low disease activity or remission, optimal physical functioning, and prevention of damage.

REFERENCES

1. Wolfe F, Hawley DJ. The longterm outcomes of rheumatoid arthritis: work disability: a prospective 18 year study of 823 patients. J Rheumatol 1998; 25(11): 2108–17.
2. Wong K, Gladman DD, Husted J, Long JA, Farewell VT. Mortality studies in psoriatic arthritis: results from a single outpatient clinic. I. Causes and risk of death. Arthritis Rheum 1997; 40(10): 1868–72.
3. Gran JT, Skomsvoll JF. The outcome of ankylosing spondylitis: a study of 100 patients. Br J Rheumatol 1997; 36(7): 766–71.
4. Pincus T, Swearingen C, Wolfe F. Toward a multidimensional Health Assessment Questionnaire (MDHAQ): assessment of advanced activities of daily living and psychological status in the patient-friendly health assessment questionnaire format. Arthritis Rheum 1999; 42(10): 2220–30.
5. Aletaha D, Smolen J, Ward MM. Measuring function in rheumatoid arthritis: identifying reversible and irreversible components. Arthritis Rheum 2006; 54(9): 2784–92.
6. Felson DT, Anderson JJ, Boers M et al. The American College of Rheumatology preliminary core set of disease activity measures for rheumatoid arthritis clinical trials. The Committee on Outcome Measures in Rheumatoid Arthritis Clinical Trials. Arthritis Rheum 1993; 36(6): 729–40.
7. Smolen JS. The work of the EULAR Standing Committee on International Clinical Studies Including Therapeutic Trials (ESCISIT). Br J Rheumatol 1992; 31(4): 219–20.
8. Boers M, Tugwell P, Felson DT et al. World Health Organization and International League of Associations for Rheumatology core endpoints for symptom modifying antirheumatic drugs in rheumatoid arthritis clinical trials. J Rheumatol Suppl 1994; 41: 86–9.
9. van der Heijde DM, Calin A, Dougados M et al. Selection of instruments in the core set for DC-ART, SMARD, physical therapy, and clinical record keeping in ankylosing spondylitis. Progress report of the ASAS Working Group. Assessments in Ankylosing Spondylitis. J Rheumatol 1999; 26(4): 951–4.
10. Williamson A, Hoggart B. Pain: a review of three commonly used pain rating scales. J Clin Nurs 2005; 14(7): 798–804.

11. Meenan RF, Gertman PM, Mason JH. Measuring health status in arthritis. The arthritis impact measurement scales. Arthritis Rheum 1980; 23(2): 146–52.

12. Melzack R. The short-form McGill Pain Questionnaire. Pain 1987; 30(2): 191–7.

13. Carlsson AM. Assessment of chronic pain. I. Aspects of the reliability and validity of the visual analogue scale. Pain 1983; 16(1): 87–101.

14. Huskisson EC. Measurement of pain. Lancet 1974; 2(7889): 1127–31.

15. Scott J, Huskisson EC. Vertical or horizontal visual analogue scales. Ann Rheum Dis 1979; 38(6): 560.

16. Aletaha D, Nell VP, Stamm T et al. Acute phase reactants add little to composite disease activity indices for rheumatoid arthritis: validation of a clinical activity score. Arthritis Res Ther 2005; 7(4): R796-R806.

17. Smolen JS, Breedveld FC, Schiff MH et al. A simplified disease activity index for rheumatoid arthritis for use in clinical practice. Rheumatology (Oxford) 2003; 42(2): 244–57.

18. Jones SD, Steiner A, Garrett SL, Calin A. The Bath Ankylosing Spondylitis Patient Global Score (BAS-G). Br J Rheumatol 1996; 35(1): 66–71.

19. Dawes PT, Fowler PD, Clarke S et al. Rheumatoid arthritis: treatment which controls the C-reactive protein and erythrocyte sedimentation rate reduces radiological progression. Br J Rheumatol 1986; 25(1): 44–9.

20. van Leeuwen MA, van Rijswijk MH, van der Heijde DM et al. The acute-phase response in relation to radiographic progression in early rheumatoid arthritis: a prospective study during the first three years of the disease. Br J Rheumatol 1993; 32 (Suppl 3): 9–13.

21. Plant MJ, Williams AL, O'Sullivan MM et al. Relationship between time-integrated C-reactive protein levels and radiologic progression in patients with rheumatoid arthritis. Arthritis Rheum 2000; 43(7): 1473–7.

22. Combe B, Dougados M, Goupille P et al. Prognostic factors for radiographic damage in early rheumatoid arthritis: a multiparameter prospective study. Arthritis Rheum 2001; 44(8): 1736–43.

23. Wolfe F, Michaud K. The clinical and research significance of the erythrocyte sedimentation rate. J Rheumatol 1994; 21(7): 1227–37.

24. St Clair EW, van der Heijde DM, Smolen JS et al. Combination of infliximab and methotrexate therapy for early rheumatoid arthritis: a randomized, controlled trial. Arthritis Rheum 2004; 50(11): 3432–43.

25. Pincus T, Brooks RH, Callahan LF. A proposed 30–45 minute 4 page standard protocol to evaluate rheumatoid arthritis (SPERA) that includes measures of inflammatory activity, joint damage, and longterm outcomes. J Rheumatol 1999; 26(2): 473–80.

26. Escalante A, del Rincon I. The disablement process in rheumatoid arthritis. Arthritis Rheum 2002; 47(3): 333–42.

27. Ward MM. Clinical and laboratory measures. In: St Clair EW, Pisetsky DS, Haynes BF, eds. Rheumatoid Arthritis. Philadelphia: Lippincott Williams & Wilkins 2004: 51–63.

28. Aletaha D, Smolen JS. The definition and measurement of disease modification in inflammatory rheumatic diseases. Rheum Dis Clin North Am 2006; 32(1): 9–44.

29. Lansbury J. Quantitation of the manifestations of rheumatoid arthritis. 4. Area of joint surfaces as an index to total joint inflammation and deformity. Am J Med Sci 1956; 232(2): 150–5.

30. deAndrade JR, Casagrgande PA. A seven-day variability study of 499 patients with peripheral rheumatoid arthritis. Arthritis Rheum 1965; 19: 302–34.

31. Williams HJ, Ward JR, Reading JC et al. Low-dose D-penicillamine therapy in rheumatoid arthritis. A controlled, double-blind clinical trial. Arthritis Rheum 1983; 26(5): 581–92.

32. Ritchie DM, Boyle JA, McInnes JM et al. Clinical studies with an articular index for the assessment of joint tenderness in patients with rheumatoid arthritis. Q J Med 1968; 37(147): 393–406.

33. Hart LE, Tugwell P, Buchanan WW et al. Grading of tenderness as a source of interrater error in the Ritchie articular index. J Rheumatol 1985; 12(4): 716–17.

34. Egger MJ, Huth DA, Ward JR, Reading JC, Williams HJ. Reduced joint count indices in the evaluation of rheumatoid arthritis. Arthritis Rheum 1985; 28(6): 613–19.

35. Kapral T, Dernoschnig F, Machold KP et al. Condensed joint counts in rheumatoid arthritis: are ankles and feet decisive? Ann Rheum Dis 2005; 64 (Suppl III): 220.

36. Fuchs HA, Brooks RH, Callahan LF, Pincus T. A simplified twenty-eight-joint quantitative articular index in rheumatoid arthritis. Arthritis Rheum 1989; 32(5): 531–7.

37. Stucki G, Sangha O, Bruhlmann P, Stucki S, Michel BA. Weighting for joint surface area improves the information provided by a reduced 28-joint articular index of swollen joints. Scand J Rheumatol 1998; 27(2): 125–9.

38. Wolfe F, O'Dell JR, Kavanaugh A, Wilske K, Pincus T. Evaluating severity and status in rheumatoid arthritis. J Rheumatol 2001; 28(6): 1453–62.

39. Prevoo ML, van Riel PL, 't Hof MA et al. Validity and reliability of joint indices. A longitudinal study in patients with recent onset rheumatoid arthritis. Br J Rheumatol 1993; 32(7): 589–94.

40. Smolen JS, Breedveld FC, Eberl G et al. Validity and reliability of the twenty-eight-joint count for the assessment of rheumatoid arthritis activity. Arthritis Rheum 1995; 38(1): 38–43.

41. Felson DT, Anderson JJ, Boers M et al. For the ACR Committee on Outcome Measures. Reduced joint count in rheumatoid arthritis clinical trials. Arthritis Rheum 1994; 37: 463–4.

42. Smolen JS, Kalden JR, Scott DL et al. Efficacy and safety of leflunomide compared with placebo and sulphasalazine in active rheumatoid arthritis: a double-blind, randomised, multicentre trial. European Leflunomide Study Group. Lancet 1999; 353(9149): 259–66.

43. Emery P, Breedveld FC, Lemmel EM et al. A comparison of the efficacy and safety of leflunomide and methotrexate for the treatment of rheumatoid arthritis. Rheumatology (Oxford) 2000; 39(6): 655–65.

44. Gladman DD, Farewell V, Buskila D et al. Reliability of measurements of active and damaged joints in psoriatic arthritis. J Rheumatol 1990; 17(1): 62–4.

45. Gladman DD, Cook RJ, Schentag C et al. The clinical assessment of patients with psoriatic arthritis: results of a reliability study of the spondyloarthritis research consortium of Canada. J Rheumatol 2004; 31(6): 1126–31.

46. Daunt AO, Cox NL, Robertson JC, Cawley MI. Indices of disease activity in psoriatic arthritis. J R Soc Med 1987; 80(9): 556–8.

47. Thompson PW, Hart LE, Goldsmith CH et al. Comparison of four articular indices for use in clinical trials in rheumatoid arthritis: patient, order and observer variation. J Rheumatol 1991; 18(5): 661–5.

48. Veale D, Rogers S, Fitzgerald O. Classification of clinical subsets in psoriatic arthritis. Br J Rheumatol 1994; 33(2): 133–8.

49. Brockbank JE, Stein M, Schentag CT, Gladman DD. Dactylitis in psoriatic arthritis: a marker for disease severity? Ann Rheum Dis 2005; 64(2): 188–90.

50. Mease PJ, Kivitz AJ, Burch FX et al. Etanercept treatment of psoriatic arthritis: safety, efficacy, and effect on disease progression. Arthritis Rheum 2004; 50(7): 2264–72.

51. Antoni CE, Kavanaugh A, Kirkham B et al. Sustained benefits of infliximab therapy for dermatologic and articular manifestations of psoriatic arthritis: results from the infliximab multinational psoriatic arthritis controlled trial (IMPACT). Arthritis Rheum 2005; 52(4): 1227–36.

52. Mander M, Simpson JM, McLellan A et al. Studies with an enthesis index as a method of clinical assessment in ankylosing spondylitis. Ann Rheum Dis 1987; 46(3): 197–202.

53. Heuft-Dorenbosch L, Spoorenberg A, van Tubergen A et al. Assessment of enthesitis in ankylosing spondylitis. Ann Rheum Dis 2003; 62(2): 127–32.

54. Clegg DO, Reda DJ, Mejias E et al. Comparison of sulfasalazine and placebo in the treatment of psoriatic arthritis. A Department of Veterans Affairs Cooperative Study. Arthritis Rheum 1996; 39(12): 2013–20.

55. Gladman DD, Brubacher B, Buskila D, Langevitz P, Farewell VT. Psoriatic spondyloarthropathy in men and women: a clinical, radiographic, and HLA study. Clin Invest Med 1992; 15(4): 371–5.

56. Gladman DD, Shuckett R, Russell ML, Thorne JC, Schachter RK. Psoriatic arthritis (PSA) – an analysis of 220 patients. Q J Med 1987; 62(238): 127–41.

57. Feldman SR, Krueger GG. Psoriasis assessment tools in clinical trials. Ann Rheum Dis 2005; 64 (Suppl 2): ii65-ii68.

58. Chaudhari U, Romano P, Mulcahy LD et al. Efficacy and safety of infliximab monotherapy for plaque-type psoriasis: a randomised trial. Lancet 2001; 357(9271): 1842–7.

59. Fredriksson T, Pettersson U. Severe psoriasis – oral therapy with a new retinoid. Dermatologica 1978; 157(4): 238–44.

60. Mease PJ, Goffe BS, Metz J et al. Etanercept in the treatment of psoriatic arthritis and psoriasis: a randomised trial. Lancet 2000; 356(9227): 385–90.

61. Carlin CS, Feldman SR, Krueger JG, Menter A, Krueger GG. A 50% reduction in the Psoriasis Area and Severity Index (PASI 50) is a clinically significant endpoint in the assessment of psoriasis. J Am Acad Dermatol 2004; 50(6): 859–66.

62. Langley RG, Ellis CN. Evaluating psoriasis with Psoriasis Area and Severity Index, Psoriasis Global Assessment, and Lattice System Physician's Global Assessment. J Am Acad Dermatol 2004; 51(4): 563–9.

63. Ware JE Jr, Sherbourne CD. The MOS 36-item short-form health survey (SF-36). I. Conceptual framework and item selection. Med Care 1992; 30(6): 473–83.

64. McHorney CA, Ware JE Jr, Raczek AE. The MOS 36-Item Short-Form Health Survey (SF-36): II. Psychometric and clinical tests of validity in measuring physical and mental health constructs. Med Care 1993; 31(3): 247–63.

65. McHorney CA, Ware JE Jr., Lu JF, Sherbourne CD. The MOS 36-item Short-Form Health Survey (SF-36): III. Tests of data quality, scaling assumptions, and reliability across diverse patient groups. Med Care 1994; 32(1): 40–66.

66. Fries JF, Spitz P, Kraines RG, Holman HR. Measurement of patient outcome in arthritis. Arthritis Rheum 1980; 23(2): 137–45.

67. Scott DL, Pugner K, Kaarela K et al. The links between joint damage and disability in rheumatoid arthritis. Rheumatology (Oxford) 2000; 39(2): 122–32.

68. Drossaers-Bakker KW, de Buck M, Van Zeben D et al. Long-term course and outcome of functional capacity in rheumatoid arthritis: the effect of disease activity and radiologic damage over time. Arthritis Rheum 1999; 42(9): 1854–60.

69. Pincus T, Summey JA, Soraci SA Jr, Wallston KA, Hummon NP. Assessment of patient satisfaction in activities of daily living using a modified Stanford

Health Assessment Questionnaire. Arthritis Rheum 1983; 26(11): 1346–53.

70. Wolfe F, Michaud K, Pincus T. Development and validation of the health assessment questionnaire II: a revised version of the health assessment questionnaire. Arthritis Rheum 2004; 50(10): 3296–305.

71. Kosinski M, Zhao SZ, Dedhiya S, Osterhaus JT, Ware JE Jr. Determining minimally important changes in generic and disease-specific health-related quality of life questionnaires in clinical trials of rheumatoid arthritis. Arthritis Rheum 2000; 43(7): 1478–87.

72. Aletaha D, Ward M. Duration of rheumatoid arthritis influences the degree of functional improvement in clinical trials. Ann Rheum Dis 2006; 65: 227–33.

73. Aletaha D, Smolen JS, Ward MM.Measuring function in rheumatoid arthritis: identifying reversible and irreversible components. Arthritis Rheum. 2006 sep; 54(9): 2784–92.

74. Smolen JS, Aletaha D. Patients with rheumatoid arthritis in clinical care. Ann Rheum Dis 2004; 63(3): 221–5.

75. Meenan RF, Mason JH, Anderson JJ, Guccione AA, Kazis LE. AIMS2. The content and properties of a revised and expanded Arthritis Impact Measurement Scales Health Status Questionnaire. Arthritis Rheum 1992; 35(1): 1–10.

76. Guillemin F, Coste J, Pouchot J et al. The AIMS2-SF: a short form of the Arthritis Impact Measurement Scales 2. French Quality of Life in Rheumatology Group. Arthritis Rheum 1997; 40(7): 1267–74.

77. Taal E, Rasker JJ, Riemsma RP. Sensitivity to change of AIMS2 and AIMS2-SF components in comparison to M-HAQ and VAS-pain. Ann Rheum Dis 2004; 63(12): 1655–8.

78. Wolfe F. Data collection and utilization: a methodology for clinical practice and clinical research. In: Wolfe F, Pincus T, eds. Rheumatoid Arthritis: Pathogenesis, Assessment, Outcome, and Treatment, 32 edn. New York: Marcel Dekker, 1994: 463–514.

79. Pincus T, Callahan LF. Rheumatology function tests: grip strength, walking time, button test and questionnaires document and predict longterm morbidity and mortality in rheumatoid arthritis. J Rheumatol 1992; 19(7): 1051–7.

80. Jones E, Hanly JG, Mooney R et al. Strength and function in the normal and rheumatoid hand. J Rheumatol 1991; 18(9): 1313–18.

81. Ng CL, Ho DD, Chow SP. The Moberg pickup test: results of testing with a standard protocol. J Hand Ther 1999; 12(4): 309–12.

82. Pincus T, Brooks RH, Callahan LF. Reliability of grip strength, walking time and button test performed according to a standard protocol. J Rheumatol 1991; 18(7): 997–1000.

83. Husted JA, Gladman DD, Farewell VT, Long JA, Cook RJ. Validating the SF-36 health survey questionnaire in patients with psoriatic arthritis. J Rheumatol 1997; 24(3): 511–17.

84. Husted JA, Gladman DD, Cook RJ, Farewell VT. Responsiveness of health status instruments to changes in articular status and perceived health in patients with psoriatic arthritis. J Rheumatol 1998; 25(11): 2146–55.

85. Daltroy LH, Larson MG, Roberts NW, Liang MH. A modification of the Health Assessment Questionnaire for the spondyloarthropathies. J Rheumatol 1990; 17(7): 946–50.

86. Husted JA, Gladman DD, Long JA, Farewell VT. A modified version of the Health Assessment Questionnaire (HAQ) for psoriatic arthritis. Clin Exp Rheumatol 1995; 13(4): 439–43.

87. Gladman DD, Helliwell P, Mease PJ et al. Assessment of patients with psoriatic arthritis: a review of currently available measures. Arthritis Rheum 2004; 50(1): 24–35.

88. Husted J, Gladman DD, Farewell VT, Long JA. Validation of the revised and expanded version of the Arthritis Impact Measurement Scales for patients with psoriatic Arthritis. J Rheumatol 1996; 23(6): 1015–19.

89. Husted J, Gladman DD, Long JA, Farewell VT. Relationship of the arthritis impact measurement scales to changes in articular status and functional performance in patients with psoriatic arthritis. J Rheumatol 1996; 23(11): 1932–7.

90. Jenkinson TR, Mallorie PA, Whitelock HC et al. Defining spinal mobility in ankylosing spondylitis (AS). The Bath AS Metrology Index. J Rheumatol 1994; 21(9): 1694–8.

91. Kennedy LG, Jenkinson TR, Mallorie PA et al. Ankylosing spondylitis: the correlation between a new metrology score and radiology. Br J Rheumatol 1995; 34(8): 767–70.

92. Calin A, Garrett S, Whitelock H et al. A new approach to defining functional ability in ankylosing spondylitis: the development of the Bath Ankylosing Spondylitis Functional Index. J Rheumatol 1994; 21(12): 2281–5.

93. Dougados M, Gueguen A, Nakache JP et al. Evaluation of a functional index and an articular index in ankylosing spondylitis. J Rheumatol 1988; 15(2): 302–7.

94. Ward MM, Kuzis S. Validity and sensitivity to change of spondylitis-specific measures of functional disability. J Rheumatol 1999; 26(1): 121–7.

95. Blackmore MG, Gladman DD, Husted J, Long JA, Farewell VT. Measuring health status in psoriatic arthritis: the Health Assessment Questionnaire and its modification. J Rheumatol 1995; 22(5): 886–93.

96. Queiro R, Sarasqueta C, Belzunegui J et al. Psoriatic spondyloarthropathy: a comparative study between HLA-B27 positive and HLA-B27 negative disease. Semin Arthritis Rheum 2002; 31(6): 413–18.

97. Abbott CA, Helliwell PS, Chamberlain MA. Functional assessment in ankylosing spondylitis: evaluation of a new self-administered questionnaire and correlation with anthropometric variables. Br J Rheumatol 1994; 33(11): 1060–6.

98. Eyres S, Tennant A, Kay L, Waxman R, Helliwell PS. Measuring disability in ankylosing spondylitis: comparison of bath ankylosing spondylitis functional index with revised Leeds Disability Questionnaire. J Rheumatol 2002; 29(5): 979–86.

99. Heikkila S, Viitanen JV, Kautiainen H, Kauppi M. Functional long-term changes in patients with spondylarthropathy. Clin Rheumatol 2002; 21(2): 119–22.

100. Tugwell P, Bombardier C. A methodologic framework for developing and selecting endpoints in clinical trials. J Rheumatol 1982; 9(5): 758–62.

101. Goldsmith CH, Smythe HA, Helewa A. Interpretation and power of a pooled index. J Rheumatol 1993; 20(3): 575–8.

102. Schulz KF, Grimes DA. Multiplicity in randomised trials I: endpoints and treatments. Lancet 2005; 365(9470): 1591–5.

103. Grigor C, Capell H, Stirling A et al. Effect of a treatment strategy of tight control for rheumatoid arthritis (the TICORA study): a single-blind randomised controlled trial. Lancet 2004; 364(9430): 263–9.

104. Steinbrocker O, Bloch DA. A therapeutic score card for rheumatoid arthritis. N Engl J Med 1946; 14. 501–6.

105. Lansbury J. Quantitation of the activity of rheumatoid arthritis. 5. A method for summation of the systemic indices of rheumatoid activity. Am J Med Sci 1956; 232(3): 300–10.

106. Mallya RK, Mace BE. The assessment of disease activity in rheumatoid arthritis using a multivariate analysis. Rheumatol Rehabil 1981; 20(1): 14–17.

107. van Riel PL, Reekers P, van de Putte LB, Gribnau FW. Association of HLA antigens, toxic reactions and therapeutic response to auranofin and aurothioglucose in patients with rheumatoid arthritis. Tissue Antigens 1983; 22(3): 194–9.

108. van der Heijde DM, 't Hof MA, van Riel PL et al. Judging disease activity in clinical practice in rheumatoid arthritis: first step in the development of a disease activity score. Ann Rheum Dis 1990; 49(11): 916–20.

109. van der Heijde DM, van't Hof MA, van Riel PL et al. Validity of single variables and composite indices for measuring disease activity in rheumatoid arthritis. Ann Rheum Dis 1992; 51(2): 177–81.

110. Smolen JS, Breedveld FC, Eberl G et al. Validity and reliability of the twenty-eight-joint count for the assessment of rheumatoid arthritis activity. Arthritis Rheum 1995; 38(1): 38–43.

111. Prevoo ML, 't Hof MA, Kuper HH et al. Modified disease activity scores that include twenty-eight-joint counts. Development and validation in a prospective longitudinal study of patients with rheumatoid arthritis. Arthritis Rheum 1995; 38(1): 44–8.

112. Eberl G, Studnicka-Benke A, Hitzelhammer H, Gschnait F, Smolen JS. Development of a disease activity index for the assessment of reactive arthritis (DAREA). Rheumatology (Oxford) 2000; 39(2): 148–55.

113. Aletaha D, Stamm T, Smolen JS. Validation of the Simplified Disease Activity Index (SDAI) in an observational cohort of patients with rheumatoid arthritis. Ann Rheum Dis 2004; 63 (Suppl 1): 111.

114. Aletaha D, Nell VK, Stamm T et al. Acute phase reactants add little to composite disease activity indices for rheumatoid arthritis:validation of a clinical activity score. Arthritis Res Ther 2005; 7: R796–806.

115. Wong AL, Harker JO, Park GS, Paulus HE. Longitudinal measurement of RA disease activity in a clinical practice setting: usefulness of the SDAI. Arthritis Rheum 2004; 50 (Suppl): S 386–7.

116. Soubrier M, Zerkak D, Dougados M. Should we revisit the definition of higher disease activity state in rheumatoid arthritis (RA)? Arthritis Rheum 2004; 50 (Suppl): S387.

117. Leeb BF, Andel I, Sautner J et al. Disease activity measurement of rheumatoid arthritis: comparison of the simplified disease activity index (SDAI) and the disease activity score including 28 joints (DAS28) in daily routine. Arthritis Rheum 2005; 53(1): 56–60.

118. Aletaha D, Ward MM, Machold KP et al. Remission and active disease in rheumatoid arthritis: defining criteria for disease activity states. Arthritis Rheum 2005; 52: 2625–36.

119. Lissiane K, Guedes N, Kowalski SC, Ieda M, Laurindo M. The new indices Sdai and Cdai in early arthritis: similar performance to the Das28 index. Arthritis Rheum 2006; 54 (Suppl): S206-S207.

120. Mason JH, Anderson JJ, Meenan RF et al. The rapid assessment of disease activity in rheumatology (RADAR) questionnaire. Validity and sensitivity to change of a patient self-report measure of joint count and clinical status. Arthritis Rheum 1992; 35(2): 156–62.

121. Stucki G, Liang MH, Stucki S, Bruhlmann P, Michel BA. A self-administered rheumatoid arthritis disease activity index (RADAI) for epidemiologic research. Psychometric properties and correlation with parameters of disease activity. Arthritis Rheum 1995; 38(6): 795–8.

122. Fransen J, Stucki G, Van Riel PC. Rheumatoid arthritis measures. Arthritis Care Res 2001; 49 (Suppl 5): S214-S224.

123. Mason JH, Meenan RF, Anderson JJ. Do self-reported arthritis symptom (RADAR) and health status (AIMS2) data provide duplicative or complementary information? Arthritis Care Res 1992; 5(3): 163–72.

124. Fransen J, Hauselmann H, Michel BA, Caravatti M, Stucki G. Responsiveness of the self-assessed rheumatoid arthritis disease activity index to a flare of disease activity. Arthritis Rheum 2001; 44(1): 53–60.

125. Garrett S, Jenkinson T, Kennedy LG et al. A new approach to defining disease status in ankylosing spondylitis: the Bath Ankylosing Spondylitis Disease Activity Index. J Rheumatol 1994; 21(12): 2286–91.

126. Braun J, Pham T, Sieper J et al. International ASAS consensus statement for the use of anti-tumour necrosis factor agents in patients with ankylosing spondylitis. Ann Rheum Dis 2003; 62(9): 817–24.

127. Paulus HE, Egger MJ, Ward JR, Williams HJ. Analysis of improvement in individual rheumatoid arthritis patients treated with disease-modifying antirheumatic drugs, based on the findings in patients treated with placebo. The Cooperative Systematic Studies of Rheumatic Diseases Group. Arthritis Rheum 1990; 33(4): 477–84.

128. Felson DT, Anderson JJ, Boers M et al. American College of Rheumatology. Preliminary definition of improvement in rheumatoid arthritis. Arthritis Rheum 1995; 38(6): 727–35.

129. Felson DT, Anderson JJ, Lange ML, Wells G, LaValley MP. Should improvement in rheumatoid arthritis clinical trials be defined as fifty percent or seventy percent improvement in core set measures, rather than twenty percent? Arthritis Rheum 1998; 41(9): 1564–70.

130. Schiff M, Waever A, Keystone E, Moreland L, Spencer-Gree G. Comparison of ACR response, numeric ACR, ACR AUC as measures of clinical improvement in RA clinical trials. Arthritis Rheum 1999; 42 (Suppl 9): S81.

131. Siegel JN, Zhen BG. Use of the American College of Rheumatology N (ACR-N) index of improvement in rheumatoid arthritis: argument in favor. Arthritis Rheum 2005; 52(6): 1637–41.

132. Boers M. Use of the American College of Rheumatology N (ACR-N) index of improvement in rheumatoid arthritis: argument in opposition. Arthritis Rheum 2005; 52(6): 1642–5.

133. Aletaha D, Smolen JS. The American College of Rheumatology N (ACR-N) debate: going back into the middle of the tunnel? Comment on the articles by Siegel and Zhen and by Boers. Arthritis Rheum 2006; 54(1): 377–8.

134. American College of Rheumatology Committee to Reevaluate Improvment Criteria. A proposed revision to the ACRLO: the hybrid measure of American College of Reumatology response ARTHRITIS RHEUM 2007; 57: 193–2002.

135. van Gestel AM, Prevoo ML, 't Hof MA et al. Development and validation of the European League Against Rheumatism response criteria for rheumatoid arthritis. Comparison with the preliminary American College of Rheumatology and the World Health Organization/International League Against Rheumatism Criteria. Arthritis Rheum 1996; 39(1): 34–40.

136. Smolen JS, Sokka T, Pincus T, Breedveld FC. A proposed treatment algorithm for rheumatoid arthritis: aggressive therapy, methotrexate, and quantitative measures. Clin Exp Rheumatol 2003; 21 (5 Suppl 31): S209–S210.

137. Goekoop-Ruiterman YP, Vries-Bouwstra JK, Allaart CF et al. Clinical and radiographic outcomes of four different treatment strategies in patients with early rheumatoid arthritis (the BeSt study): a randomized, controlled trial. Arthritis Rheum 2005; 52(11): 3381–90.

138. Kaltwasser JP, Nash P, Gladman D et al. Efficacy and safety of leflunomide in the treatment of psoriatic arthritis and psoriasis: a multinational, double-blind, randomized, placebo-controlled clinical trial. Arthritis Rheum 2004; 50(6): 1939–50.

139. Anderson JJ, Baron G, van der HD, Felson DT, Dougados M. Ankylosing spondylitis assessment group preliminary definition of short-term improvement in ankylosing spondylitis. Arthritis Rheum 2001; 44(8): 1876–86.

Index

Note: Page references in *italics* refer to Figures and Tables